Health, United States, 2007

With Chartbook on Trends in the Health of Americans

U.S. DEPARTMENT OF HEALTH AND HUMAN SERVICES
Centers for Disease Control and Prevention
National Center for Health Statistics

November 2007
DHHS Publication No. 2007-1232

Preface

Health, United States, 2007 is the 31st report on the health status of the Nation and is submitted by the Secretary of the Department of Health and Human Services to the President and the Congress of the United States in compliance with Section 308 of the Public Health Service Act. This report was compiled by the National Center for Health Statistics (NCHS), Centers for Disease Control and Prevention (CDC). The National Committee on Vital and Health Statistics served in a review capacity.

The *Health, United States* series presents national trends in health statistics. Each report includes an executive summary, highlights, a chartbook, trend tables, extensive appendixes, and an index.

Chartbook

The *Chartbook on Trends in the Health of Americans* updates and expands information from previous chartbooks and introduces this year's special feature on access to care. The chartbook assesses the Nation's health by presenting trends and current information on selected determinants and measures of health status and utilization of health care. Many measures are shown separately for persons of different ages because of the strong effect of age on health. Selected figures also highlight differences in determinants and measures of health status and utilization of health care by such characteristics as sex, race, Hispanic origin, education, and poverty level.

Trend Tables

The chartbook section is followed by 151 trend tables organized around four major subject areas: health status and determinants, health care utilization, health care resources, and health care expenditures. A major criterion used in selecting the trend tables is availability of comparable national data over a period of several years. The tables present data for selected years to highlight major trends in health statistics. Earlier editions of *Health, United States* may present data for additional years that are not included in the current printed report. Where possible, these additional years of data are available in Excel spreadsheet files on the *Health, United States* website. Tables with additional data years are listed in Appendix III.

Racial and Ethnic Data

Many tables in *Health, United States* present data according to race and Hispanic origin consistent with Department-wide emphasis on expanding racial and ethnic detail when presenting health data. Trend data on race and ethnicity are presented in the greatest detail possible after taking into account the quality of data, the amount of missing data, and the number of observations. Standards for classification of federal data on race and ethnicity are described in Appendix II, Race.

Education and Income Data

Many tables in *Health, United States* present data according to socioeconomic status, using education and family income as proxy measures. Education and income data are generally obtained directly from survey respondents and are not generally available from records-based data collection systems. State vital statistics systems currently report mother's education on the birth certificate and, based on an informant, decedent's education on the death certificate. See Appendix II, Education; Family income; and Poverty.

Disability Data

Disability is a complex concept and can include presence of physical or mental impairments that limit a person's ability to perform an important activity and affect the use of or need for accommodations or interventions required to improve functioning. Information on disability in the U.S. population is critical to health planning and policy. Although some information is currently available from federal data collection systems, the information is limited by lack of standard definitions and survey questions on disability. Several current initiatives are underway to coordinate and standardize measurement of disability across federal data systems. Until such standardized information is available, *Health, United States* includes the following disability-related information for the civilian noninstitutionalized population: prevalence of limitations of activity due to chronic conditions (Table 58), vision and hearing limitations for adults (Table 59), and limitations in Activities of Daily Living (ADL) and Instrumental Activities of Daily Living (IADL) for the population age 65 and over (Table 58). In addition, disability-related information is provided for Medicare enrollees (Table 143), Medicaid recipients (Table 144), and veterans with service-connected disabilities (Table 146).

Changes in This Edition

Each volume of *Health, United States* is prepared to maximize its usefulness as a standard reference source while maintaining its continuing relevance. Comparability is fostered by including similar trend tables in each volume. Timeliness is maintained by (1) adding new tables each year to reflect emerging topics in public health and (2) improving the content of ongoing tables. *Health, United States, 2007* includes five new trend tables on the following: estimates of the prevalence of selected health conditions (Table 69), based on data from the National Health and Nutrition Examination Survey; reduced access to medical care due to cost in selected states (Table 80), based on data from the National Health Interview Survey; international comparisons of magnetic resonance imaging (MRI) and computed tomography (CT) scanners (Table 119), based on data from the Organisation for Economic Co-operation and Development and the CT and MRI Census; and mental health and substance abuse treatment expenditures (Tables 126 and 127), based on data from the Substance Abuse and Mental Health Services Administration.

The *Health, United States, 2007* Chartbook section includes new charts on the foreign-born population (Figure 2), expenditures for mental health services and substance abuse treatment (Figures 7 and 8), blood cotinine levels among children (Figure 10), emergency department visits among adolescents for alcohol-related reasons (Figure 11), and restaurant meal consumption (Figure 12). The Special Feature includes 16 charts on access to care (Figures 21–36).

Appendixes

Appendix I describes each data source used in the report and provides references for further information about the sources. Data sources are listed alphabetically within two broad categories: (1) Government Sources and (2) Private and Global Sources.

Appendix II is an alphabetical listing of terms used in the report. It also presents standard populations used for age-adjustment (Tables I, II, and III); ICD codes for causes of death shown in *Health, United States* from the Sixth through Tenth Revisions and the years when the Revisions were in effect (Tables IV and V); comparability ratios between ICD–9 and ICD–10 for selected causes (Table VI); ICD–9–CM codes for external cause-of-injury, diagnostic, and procedure categories (Tables VII, X, and XI); effects on health insurance rates of adding probe questions for Medicare and Medicaid coverage in the National Health Interview Survey (Table VIII); industry codes according to the 2002 North American Industry Classification System (Table IX); National Drug Code (NDC) Therapeutic Class recodes of generic analgesic drugs (Table XII); and sample tabulations of NHIS data comparing the 1977 and 1997 Standards for the Classification of Federal Data on Race and Ethnicity (Tables XIII and XIV).

Appendix III lists tables for which additional years of trend data are available electronically in Excel spreadsheet files on the *Health, United States* website and CD-ROM, described below under Electronic Access.

Index

The Index to Trend Tables and Chartbook Figures is a useful tool for locating data by topic. Tables are cross-referenced by such topics as Child and adolescent health; Older population age 65 years and over; Women's health; Men's health; state data; American Indian, Asian, Black, and Hispanic origin populations; Education; Injury; Disability; and Metropolitan and nonmetropolitan data.

Electronic Access

Health, United States may be accessed in its entirety on the World Wide Web at www.cdc.gov/nchs/hus.htm. From the *Health, United States* website, one may also register for the *Health, United States* electronic mailing list to receive announcements about release dates and notices of updates to tables.

Health, United States, 2007, the chartbook, and each of the trend tables are available as Acrobat PDF files on the website. Chartbook figures are available as downloadable PowerPoint® slides. Trend tables and chartbook data tables are available as downloadable Excel spreadsheet files. Trend tables listed in Appendix III include additional years of data not shown in the printed report or PDF files. Both PDF and spreadsheet files for selected tables will be updated on the website if more current data become available near the time when the printed report is released. Readers who register with the electronic mailing list will be notified of these table updates. Previous editions of *Health, United States* and chartbooks, starting with the 1993 edition, also may be accessed from the *Health, United States* website.

Health, United States is also available on CD-ROM, where it can be viewed, searched, printed, and saved using Adobe Acrobat software on the CD-ROM.

Copies of the Report

Copies of *Health, United States, 2007*, and the CD-ROM can be purchased from the Government Printing Office (GPO) through links to GPO on the National Center for Health Statistics website, Publications and Information Products page.

Questions?

For answers to questions about this report, contact:

Office of Information Services
Information Dissemination Staff
National Center for Health Statistics
Centers for Disease Control and Prevention
3311 Toledo Road, Fifth Floor
Hyattsville, MD 20782
Phone: 1-800-232-4636
E-mail: nchsquery@cdc.gov
Internet: www.cdc.gov/nchs

Acknowledgments

Overall responsibility for planning and coordinating the content of this volume rested with the Office of Analysis and Epidemiology, National Center for Health Statistics (NCHS), under the direction of Amy B. Bernstein, Diane M. Makuc, and Linda T. Bilheimer.

Production of ***Health, United States, 2007***, highlights, trend tables, and appendixes was managed by Amy B. Bernstein, Sheila Franco, and Virginia M. Freid. Trend tables were prepared by Amy B. Bernstein, Mary Ann Bush, Alan J. Cohen, Margaret A. Cooke, La-Tonya D. Curl, Catherine R. Duran, Sheila Franco, Virginia M. Freid, Ji-Eun Lee, Andrea P. MacKay, Livia Navon, Patricia N. Pastor, Mitchell B. Pierre, Rebecca A. Placek, Cynthia A. Reuben, and Henry Xia, with assistance from Anita L. Powell and Ilene B. Rosen. Appendix II tables and the index were assembled by Anita L. Powell. Production planning and coordination of trend tables were managed by Rebecca A. Placek. Review and clearance books were assembled by Ilene B. Rosen. Administrative and word processing assistance were provided by Lillie C. Featherstone and Rhonda Williams-Robinson.

Production of the ***Chartbook on Trends in the Health of Americans*** was managed by Virginia M. Freid. Data and analysis for specific charts were provided by Amy B. Bernstein, Margaret A. Cooke, Sheila Franco, Virginia M. Freid, Deborah D. Ingram, Ji-Eun Lee, Livia Navon, Patricia N. Pastor, and Cynthia A. Reuben. Graphs were drafted by La-Tonya D. Curl, and data tables were prepared by Rebecca A. Placek. Technical assistance and programming were provided by Alan J. Cohen, Catherine R. Duran, Mitchell B. Pierre, and Henry Xia.

Publications management and editorial review were provided by Demarius V. Miller, CDC/CCHIS/NCHM/Division of Creative Services, Writer-Editor Services Branch. Oversight review for publications and electronic products was provided by Margot A. Palmer, Acting Director, Office of Information Services. The designer was Sarah Hinkle, CDC/CCHIS/NCHM/Division of Creative Services; production was done by Jacqueline M. Davis and Zung T. Le, CDC/CCHIS/NCHM/Division of Creative Services; and printing was managed by Patricia L. Wilson, CDC/OCOO/MASO.

Electronic access through the NCHS Internet site and CD-ROM was provided by Christine J. Brown, Jacqueline M. Davis, Zung T. Le, Demarius V. Miller, Sharon L. Ramirez, Ilene B. Rosen, and Patricia L. Wilson.

Data and technical assistance were provided by staff of the following NCHS organizations: *Division of Health Care Statistics*: Catharine W. Burt, Frederic Decker, Carol J. DeFrances, Marni J. Hall, Lauren Harris-Kojetin, Esther Hing, Adrienne Jones, Lola Jean Kozak, Karen L. Lipkind, Maria F. Owings, Robert Pokras, Robin E. Remsburg, Susan M. Schappert, and Ingrid Vassanelli; *Division of Health Examination Statistics*: Margaret D. Carroll, Lester R. Curtin, Bruce Dye, Susan E. Schober, and Jacqueline D. Wright; *Division of Health Interview Statistics*: Patricia F. Adams, Veronica E. Benson, Barbara Bloom, Robin A. Cohen, Achintya Dey, Margaret Lethbridge-Cejku, Eve Powell-Griner, Jeannine Schiller, and Charlotte A. Schoenborn; *Division of Vital Statistics*: Robert N. Anderson, Elizabeth Arias, Thomas D. Dunn, Donna L. Hoyert, Joyce A. Martin, Kenneth D. Kochanek, T.J. Mathews, Arialdi M. Miniño, Sherry L. Murphy, and Stephanie J. Ventura; *Office of Analysis and Epidemiology*: Liming Cai, Lois Fingerhut, Yelena Gorina, Margie Goulding, Deborah D. Ingram, Patricia A. Knapp, Thomas Socey, and Rashmi Tandon; *Office of the Center Director*: Juan Rafael Albertorio-Diaz and Francis C. Notzon; and *Office of Research and Methodology*: Meena Khare.

Additional data and technical assistance were also provided by the following organizations of the Centers for Disease Control and Prevention: *Epidemiology Program Office*: Samuel L. Groseclose and Patsy A. Hall; *National Center for Chronic Disease Prevention and Health Promotion*: Laura Kann, Steve Kinchen, Shari L. Shanklin, and Lilo Strauss; *National Center for HIV, STD, and TB Prevention*: Michael Campsmith, Rachel S. Wynn, and Jill Wasserman; by the following organizations within the Department of Health and Human Services: *Agency for Healthcare Research and Quality*: Jessica S. Banthin, David Kashihara, Steven R. Machlin, and Marc W. Zodet; *Centers for Medicare & Medicaid Services*: Cathy A. Cowan, Frank Eppig, David A. Gibson, Deborah W. Kidd, Olivia Nuccio, and Joseph S. Regan; *Health Resources and Services Administration*: Virginia McBride; *National Institutes of Health*: Moira O'Brien and Lynn A. G. Ries; *Substance Abuse and Mental Health Services Administration*: Jeff Buck, Daniel Foley, and Rita Vandivort-Warren; and by the following governmental and nongovernmental organizations: *U.S. Census Bureau*: Bernadette D. Proctor; *Bureau of Justice Statistics*: Allen Beck and William Sabol; *Bureau of Labor Statistics*: Stella Cromartie, Kay Ford, Daniel Ginsburg, Diane Herz, Sara Kline, and Stephen Pegula; *Department of Veterans Affairs*: William Kloiber, Dat Tran, and Henry Caplan; *American Association of Colleges of Pharmacy*: Jennifer M. Patton; *American Association of Colleges of Podiatric Medicine*: Moraith G. North; *American Dental Education Association*: Richard Weaver; *Association of Schools of Public Health*: Mah-Sere K. Sow; *Cowles Research Group*: C. McKeen Cowles; *HealthLeaders-InterStudy*: Tracy Coats; *Thomson Medstat*: Rosanna Coffey, Katharine Levit, Tami Mark, and Katheryn Ryan; and *United Network for Organ Sharing*: Sarah Taranto and Denise Tripp.

Contents

Contents

Preface iii
Acknowledgments vi
List of Chartbook Figures xiii
List of Trend Tables xv

Executive Summary and Highlights

Executive Summary 3
- Overall Health of the Nation 3
- Health Status by Sociodemographic Characteristics 3
- Health Care Resources 4
- Expenditures and Payors 4
- Access to Health Care and Utilization of Health Services 5

Highlights 8
- Life Expectancy and Mortality 8
- Health Behaviors and Risk Factors 9
- Health Status and Health Conditions 10
- Health Care Expenditures and Payors 11
- Health Care System Influences, Personnel, and Resources 11
- Special Feature: Access to Health Care 12

Chartbook on Trends in the Health of Americans

Population 16
- Age 16
- Foreign-Born Population 18
- Race and Ethnicity 20
- Poverty 22

Health Care Expenditures 26
- Personal Health Care Expenditures 26
- Expenditures for Mental Health Services and Substance Abuse Treatment 28

Health Risk Factors 32
- Cigarette Smoking 32
- Blood Cotinine Levels in Children 34
- Alcohol-Related Emergency Department Visits: Adolescents and Young Adults 36
- Frequency of Restaurant Meals 38
- Overweight and Obesity 40

Morbidity and Limitation of Activity 42
- Limitation of Activity Due to Chronic Conditions: Children 42
- Limitation of Activity Due to Chronic Conditions: Working-Age and Older Adults 44
- Three or More Chronic Conditions 48

Mortality 50
- Life Expectancy 50
- Infant Mortality 52
- Leading Causes of Death for All Ages 54

Special Feature: Access to Health Care 56
- Introduction 56
- Physician Supply 60
- Kidney Transplants 64
- No Usual Source of Medical Care 68
- Delayed Medical Care Due to Lack of Transportation 70
- Health Insurance at the Time of Interview 72
- Length of Time Without Health Insurance 74
- Profile of the Uninsured Population 76
- Burden of Out-of-Pocket Expenditures 78
- Undiagnosed Medical Conditions 80
- Foregone Medical Care Due to Cost by Length of Time Without Health Insurance 82
- Dental Care Utilization 84
- Colorectal Scope Procedures 86
- Antidepressant Drugs: Adults 88

Technical Notes 90
- Data Sources and Comparability 90
- Data Presentation 90
- Survey Questions and Coding 90

Data Tables for Figures 1–36 93

Trend Tables

Health Status and Determinants 125
- Population 125
- Fertility and Natality 132
- Mortality 159
- Determinants and Measures of Health 239

Utilization of Health Resources 295
Ambulatory Care 295
Inpatient Care 338

Health Care Resources 355
Personnel 355
Facilities 365

Health Care Expenditures and Payors 375
National Health Expenditures 375
Health Care Coverage and Major Federal Programs 399
State Health Expenditures and Health Insurance 418

Appendixes

Contents 429
I. Sources of Data 433
Government Sources 434
Private and Global Sources 478
II. Definitions and Methods 484
III. Additional Data Years Available 538

Index to Trend Tables 541

List of Chartbook Figures

Population

1. Total population and older population: United States, 1950–2050 17
2. Foreign-born population, by citizenship: United States, 1970–2004 19
3. Population in selected race and Hispanic origin groups, by age: United States, 1980–2006 21
4. Poverty by age: United States, 1966–2005 23
5. Low income by age, race, and Hispanic origin: United States, 2005 25

Health Care Expenditures

6. Personal health care expenditures, by source of funds and type of expenditures: United States, 2005 27
7. National expenditures for mental health services, by source of funds: United States, 1986–2003 29
8. National expenditures for substance abuse treatment, by source of funds: United States, 1986–2003 31

Health Risk Factors

9. Cigarette smoking among men, women, high school students, and mothers during pregnancy: United States, 1965–2005 33
10. Blood cotinine levels among children 4–17 years of age, by percent of poverty level: United States, 1988–1994 and 2001–2004 35
11. Alcohol-related emergency department (ED) visit rates among persons 14–28 years of age, by age and sex: United States, 2002–2004 37
12. Weekly restaurant meal consumption among people 1 year of age and over, by age: United States, 1999–2004 39
13. Overweight and obesity, by age: United States, 1960–2004 41

Morbidity and Limitation of Activity

14. Limitation of activity caused by selected chronic health conditions among children, by age: United States, 2004–2005 43
15. Limitation of activity caused by selected chronic health conditions among working-age adults, by age: United States, 2004–2005 45
16. Limitation of activity caused by selected chronic health conditions among older adults, by age: United States, 2004–2005 47
17. Three or more chronic conditions among adults 45 years of age and over, by age and percent of poverty level: United States, 2005 49

Mortality

18. Life expectancy at birth and at 65 years of age, by race and sex: United States, 1970–2004 51
19. Infant, neonatal, and postneonatal mortality rates: United States, 1950–2004 53
20. Death rates for leading causes of dealth for all ages: United States, 1950–2004 55

Special Feature: Access to Health Care

21. Adults 18 years of age and over reporting they did not receive needed health-related services in the past 12 months because they could not afford them, by age and type of service: United States, 2005 57
22. Patient care physicians per 10,000 population, by county: United States, 2004 61
23. Obstetricians or gynecologists per 10,000 females age 15 years and over, by county: United States, 2004 63
24. Active kidney transplant waiting list patients at end of year, by race and Hispanic origin: United States, 1988, 1996, and 2006 65
25. Active waiting list patients who received a kidney transplant within 2 years, by race and Hispanic origin: United States, 1988, 1996, and 2004 67
26. No usual source of care among adults 45–64 years of age, by selected diagnosed chronic conditions and race and Hispanic origin: United States, 2004–2005 69
27. Delayed medical care in the past 12 months due to lack of transportation among adults 18 years of age and over, by sex, percent of poverty level, and age: United States, 2004–2005 71
28. Health insurance coverage at the time of interview among persons under 65 years of age: United States, 1984–2005 73
29. Uninsured for at least part of the 12 months prior to interview among persons under 65 years of age, by length of time uninsured and selected characteristics: United States, 2005 75

30. The uninsured population under 65 years of age, by selected characteristics: United States, 2005 77
31. Persons under 65 years of age who spent more than 10% of after-tax family income on out-of-pocket medical expenditures, by percent of poverty level: United States, 1996 and 2004 79
32. Adults 20–64 years of age with undiagnosed high cholesterol or elevated blood pressure, by health insurance status and age: United States, 1999–2004 81
33. Persons under 65 years of age who did not get needed medical care in the past year due to cost, by duration of health insurance coverage and percent of poverty level: United States, 2005 83
34. No dental visit in the past year among persons with natural teeth, by age and percent of poverty level: United States, 2005 85
35. Adults 50 years of age and over ever having a colorectal scope procedure, by selected characteristics: United States, annual average 2000, 2003, and 2005 87
36. Adults 18 years of age and over reporting antidepressant drug use in the past month by sex and race and Hispanic origin: United States, 1988–1994 and 1999–2002 89

Summary List of Trend Tables by Topic

All Topics (Tables 1–151)

Population (Tables 1–3)

Resident population
Persons in poverty
and more . . .

Fertility and Natality (Tables 4–18)

Births
Low birthweight
Breastfeeding
and more . . .

Mortality (Tables 19–49)

Infant mortality
Life expectancy
Death rates, by cause
and more . . .

Determinants and Measures of Health (Tables 50–76)

Health status
Cigarette smoking
Alcohol consumption
High blood pressure
Overweight and obese
and more . . .

Ambulatory Care (Tables 77–97)

Visits: health care, dentists, emergency departments, and more . . .

Prevention: mammograms, pap smears, vaccinations

Inpatient Care (Tables 98–104)

Hospital stays and procedures
Nursing homes
and more . . .

Personnel (Tables 105–112)

Physicians
Dentists
Nurses
Health professions school enrollment
and more . . .

Facilities (Tables 113–119)

Hospitals
Nursing homes
and more . . .

National Health Expenditures (Tables 120–135)

Personal health expenditures
Out-of-pocket costs
Prescription drugs
Nursing home costs
and more . . .

Health Care Coverage and Major Federal Programs (Tables 136–146)

Insurance coverage:
Medicare
Medicaid
Private coverage
Uninsured
HMOs
and more . . .

State Health Expenditures and Health Insurance (Tables 147–151)

Medicare, Medicaid, HMO expenditures/enrollees
Uninsured persons
and more . . .

List of Trend Tables

Health Status and Determinants

Population

1. **Resident population,** by age, sex, race, and Hispanic origin: United States, selected years 1950–2005 125

2. **Inmates in state or federal prisons and local jails,** by sex, race, Hispanic origin, and age: United States, selected years 1999–2005 128

3. Persons and families below **poverty** level, by selected characteristics, race, and Hispanic origin: United States, selected years 1973–2005 130

Fertility and Natality

4. Crude birth rates, **fertility rates, and birth rates** by age, race, and Hispanic origin of mother: United States, selected years 1950–2004 132

5. **Live births**, by plurality, and detailed race and Hispanic origin of mother: United States, selected years 1970–2004 . . . 135

6. **Twin and higher order multiple births,** by race, Hispanic origin, and age of mother: United States, selected years 1971–2004 137

7. **Prenatal care** for live births, by detailed race and Hispanic origin of mother: United States, selected years 1970–2004 . . . 138

8. **Early prenatal care** by race and Hispanic origin of mother, geographic division, and state: United States, average annual 1996–1998, 1999–2001, and 2002–2004 139

9. **Teenage childbearing,** by detailed race and Hispanic origin of mother: United States, selected years 1970–2004 . . . 142

10. **Nonmarital childbearing** by detailed race and Hispanic origin of mother, and maternal age: United States, selected years 1970–2004 143

11. **Maternal education** for live births, by detailed race and Hispanic origin of mother: United States, selected years 1970–2004 144

12. **Mothers who smoked cigarettes** during pregnancy, by detailed race, Hispanic origin, age, and education of mother: United States, selected years, 1989–2004 145

13. **Low-birthweight** live births, by detailed race, Hispanic origin, and smoking status of mother: United States, selected years 1970–2004 146

14. **Low-birthweight** live births among mothers 20 years of age and over, by detailed race, Hispanic origin, and education of mother: United States, selected years 1989–2004 147

15. **Low-birthweight** live births, by race and Hispanic origin of mother, geographic division, and state: United States, average annual 1996–1998, 1999–2001, and 2002–2004 . . . 149

16. Legal **abortions** and legal **abortion ratios,** by selected patient characteristics: United States, selected years 1973–2003 152

17. **Contraceptive** use in the past month among women 15–44 years of age, by age, race, Hispanic origin, and method of contraception: United States, selected years 1982–2002 154

18. **Breastfeeding** among mothers 15–44 years of age, by year of baby's birth, and selected characteristics of mother: United States, average annual 1986–1988 through 1999–2001 158

Mortality

19. **Infant, neonatal, and postneonatal mortality rates,** by detailed race and Hispanic origin of mother: United States, selected years 1983–2004 159

20. **Infant mortality rates** among mothers 20 years of age and over, by education, detailed race, and Hispanic origin of mother: United States, selected years 1983–2004 162

21. **Infant mortality rates** by birthweight: United States, selected years 1983–2004 164

22. **Infant mortality rates,** fetal mortality rates, and perinatal mortality rates, by race: United States, selected years 1950–2004 165

23. **Infant mortality rates,** by race and Hispanic origin of mother, geographic division, and state: United States, average annual 1989–1991, 1999–2001, and 2002–2004 166

24. **Neonatal mortality rates,** by race and Hispanic origin of mother, geographic division, and state: United States, average annual 1989–1991, 1999–2001, and 2002–2004 169

25. **Infant mortality rates** and international rankings: Selected countries and territories, selected years 1960–2004 172

26. **Life expectancy** at birth and at 65 years of age, by sex: Selected countries and territories, selected years 1980–2003 173

27. **Life expectancy** at birth, at 65 years of age, and at 75 years of age, by race and sex: United States, selected years 1900–2004 175

28. **Age-adjusted death rates,** by race, Hispanic origin, geographic division, and state: United States, average annual 1979–1981, 1989–1991, and 2002–2004 176

29. **Age-adjusted death rates** for selected causes of death, by sex, race, and Hispanic origin: United States, selected years 1950–2004 178

30. **Years of potential life lost** before age 75 for selected causes of death, by sex, race, and Hispanic origin: United States, selected years 1980–2004 182

31. **Leading causes of death** and numbers of deaths, by sex, race, and Hispanic origin: United States, 1980 and 2004 186

32. **Leading causes of death** and numbers of deaths, by age: United States, 1980 and 2004 190

33. Age-adjusted death rates, by race, sex, region, and **urbanization** level: United States, average annual 1996–1998, 1999–2001, and 2002–2004 192

34. Age-adjusted death rates among persons 25–64 years of age for selected causes of death, by sex and **educational attainment:** Selected states, 1994–2004 195

35. **Death rates** for all causes, by sex, race, Hispanic origin, and age: United States, selected years 1950–2004 197

36. Death rates for **diseases of heart,** by sex, race, Hispanic origin, and age: United States, selected years 1950–2004 201

37. Death rates for **cerebrovascular diseases,** by sex, race, Hispanic origin, and age: United States, selected years 1950–2004 204

38. Death rates for **malignant neoplasms,** by sex, race, Hispanic origin, and age: United States, selected years 1950–2004 207

39. Death rates for **malignant neoplasms of trachea, bronchus, and lung,** by sex, race, Hispanic origin, and age: United States, selected years 1950–2004 211

40. Death rates for **malignant neoplasm of breast** among females, by race, Hispanic origin, and age: United States, selected years 1950–2004 214

41. Death rates for **chronic lower respiratory diseases,** by sex, race, Hispanic origin, and age: United States, selected years 1980–2004 216

42. Death rates for **human immunodeficiency virus (HIV) disease,** by sex, race, Hispanic origin, and age: United States, selected years 1987–2004 219

43. **Maternal mortality** for complications of pregnancy, childbirth, and the puerperium, by race, Hispanic origin, and age: United States, selected years 1950–2004 221

44. Death rates for **motor vehicle-related injuries,** by sex, race, Hispanic origin, and age: United States, selected years 1950–2004 222

45. Death rates for **homicide,** by sex, race, Hispanic origin, and age: United States, selected years 1950–2004 226

46. Death rates for **suicide,** by sex, race, Hispanic origin, and age: United States, selected years 1950–2004 230

47. Death rates for **firearm-related injuries,** by sex, race, Hispanic origin, and age: United States, selected years 1970–2004 233

48. Deaths from selected **occupational diseases** among persons 15 years of age and over: United States, selected years 1980–2004 236

49. **Occupational injury deaths** and rates, by industry, sex, age, race, and Hispanic origin: United States, selected years 1992–2005 237

Determinants and Measures of Health

50. **Occupational injuries** and illnesses with days away from work, job transfer, or restriction, by industry: United States, 2003–2005 239

51. Selected **notifiable disease rates** and number of cases: United States, selected years 1950–2005 240

52. Acquired immunodeficiency syndrome **(AIDS)** cases, by year of diagnosis and selected characteristics: United States, 2001–2005 242

53. Age-adjusted **cancer incidence rates** for selected cancer sites, by sex, race, and Hispanic origin: United States, selected geographic areas, selected years 1990–2004 244

54. Five-year relative **cancer survival rates** for selected cancer sites, by race and sex: United States, selected geographic areas, selected years 1975–1977 through 1996–2003 247

55. **Diabetes** among adults 20 years of age and over, by sex, age, and race and Hispanic origin: United States, 1988–1994 and 2001–2004 248

56. **Severe headache or migraine, low back pain, and neck pain** among adults 18 years of age and over, by selected characteristics: United States, 1997, 2004, and 2005 249

57. **Joint pain** among adults 18 years of age and over, by selected characteristics: United States, 2002, 2004, and 2005 251

58. **Limitation of activity** caused by chronic conditions, by selected characteristics: United States, selected years 1997–2005 255

59. **Vision and hearing limitations** among adults 18 years of age and over, by selected characteristics: United States, selected years 1997–2005 258

60. **Respondent-assessed health status,** by selected characteristics: United States, selected years 1991–2005 ... 260

61. **Serious psychological distress** among adults 18 years of age and over, by selected characteristics: United States, average annual selected years, 1997–1998 through 2004–2005 262

62. **Suicidal ideation, suicide attempts, and injurious suicide attempts** among students in grades 9–12, by sex, grade level, race, and Hispanic origin: United States, selected years 1991–2005 264

63. Current **cigarette smoking** among adults 18 years of age and over, by sex, race, and age: United States, selected years 1965–2005 266

64. Age-adjusted prevalence of current **cigarette smoking** among adults 25 years of age and over, by sex, race, and education level: United States, selected years 1974–2005 268

65. Current **cigarette smoking** among adults, by sex, race, Hispanic origin, age, and education level: United States, average annual 1990–1992, 1995–1998, and 2003–2005 ... 269

66. **Use of selected substances** in the past month among persons 12 years of age and over, by age, sex, race, and Hispanic origin: United States, 2002, 2004, and 2005 271

67. **Use of selected substances** among high school seniors, tenth-, and eighth-graders, by sex and race: United States, selected years 1980–2006 273

68. **Alcohol consumption** among adults 18 years of age and over, by selected characteristics: United States, 1997, 2004, and 2005 276

69. **Selected health conditions and risk factors:** United States, 1988–1994 through 2003–2004 279

70. **Hypertension** and elevated blood pressure among persons 20 years of age and over, by sex, age, race and Hispanic origin, and poverty level: United States, 1988–1994 and 2001–2004 280

71. **Serum total cholesterol levels** among persons 20 years of age and over, by sex, age, race and Hispanic origin, and poverty level: United States, selected years 1960–1962 through 2001–2004 282

72. **Mean energy and macronutrient intake** among persons 20–74 years of age, by sex and age: United States, 1971–1974 through 2001–2004 285

73. **Leisure-time physical activity** among adults 18 years of age and over, by selected characteristics: United States, 1998, 2004, and 2005 286

74. **Overweight, obesity, and healthy weight** among persons 20 years of age and over, by sex, age, race and Hispanic origin, and poverty level: United States, 1960–1962 through 2001–2004 288

75. **Overweight among children and adolescents** 6–19 years of age, by age, sex, race and Hispanic origin, and poverty level: United States, 1963–1965 through 2001–2004 292

76. **Untreated dental caries,** by age, sex, race and Hispanic origin, and poverty level: United States, 1971–1974, 1988–1994, and 2001–2004 293

Utilization of Health Resources

Ambulatory Care

77. **No usual source of health care** among children under 18 years of age, by selected characteristics: United States, average annual 1993–1994, 2001–2002, and 2004–2005 ... 295

78. **No usual source of health care** among adults 18–64 years of age, by selected characteristics: United States, average annual selected years 1993–1994 through 2004–2005 297

79. **Reduced access to medical care** during the past 12 months due to cost, by selected characteristics: United States, 1997, 2004, and 2005 299

80. **Reduced access to medical care** during the past 12 months due to cost, by state: 25 largest states and United States, 1997–1998, 2000–2001, and 2004–2005 301

81. **No health care visits** to an office or clinic within the past 12 months among children under 18 years of age, by selected characteristics: United States, average annual 1997–1998, 2001–2002, and 2004–2005 302

82.**Health care visits** to doctor offices, emergency departments, and home visits within the past 12 months, by selected characteristics: United States, 1997, 2004, and 2005 304

83. **Vaccinations** of children 19–35 months of age for selected diseases, by race, Hispanic origin, poverty level, and residence in metropolitan statistical area (MSA): United States, selected years 1995–2006 307

84. **Vaccination** coverage among children 19–35 months of age, by geographic division, state, and selected urban area: United States, selected years 1995–2006 309

85. **Influenza vaccination** among adults 18 years of age and over, by selected characteristics: United States, selected years 1989–2005 311

86. **Pneumococcal vaccination** among adults 18 years of age and over, by selected characteristics: United States, selected years 1989–2005 313

87. Use of **mammography** among women 40 years of age and over, by selected characteristics: United States, selected years 1987–2005 315

88. Use of **Pap smears** among women 18 years of age and over, by selected characteristics: United States, selected years 1987–2005 317

89. **Emergency department visits** within the past 12 months among children under 18 years of age, by selected characteristics: United States, 1997, 2004, and 2005 319

90. **Emergency department visits** within the past 12 months among adults 18 years of age and over, by selected characteristics: United States, selected years 1997–2005 ... 322

91. **Injury-related visits** to hospital emergency departments, by sex, age, and intent and mechanism of injury: United States, average annual 1995–1996, 1999–2000, and 2004–2005 324

92. **Visits to physician offices, hospital outpatient departments, and hospital emergency departments,** by selected characteristics: United States, selected years 1995–2005 326

93. **Visits to primary care generalist and specialist physicians,** by selected characteristics and type of physician: United States, selected years 1980–2005 329

94. **Dental visits** in the past year, by selected characteristics: United States, 1997, 2004, and 2005 331

95. **Selected prescription and nonprescription drugs** recorded during physician office visits and hospital outpatient department visits, by sex and age: United States, 1995–1996 and 2004–2005 333

96. **Prescription drug** use in the past month by sex, age, race and Hispanic origin: United States, 1988–1994 and 1999–2002 336

97. **Admissions to mental health organizations,** by type of service and organization: United States, selected years 1986–2004 337

Inpatient Care

98. **Persons with hospital stays** in the past year, by selected characteristics: United States, selected years 1997, 2004, and 2005 338

99. **Discharges,** days of care, and average length of stay in nonfederal short-stay hospitals, by selected characteristics: United States, selected years 1980–2005 341

100. **Discharges** and days of care in nonfederal short-stay hospitals, by sex, age, and selected first-listed diagnoses: United States, 1990, 2000, and 2005 343

101. **Discharges** and average length of stay in nonfederal short-stay hospitals, by sex, age, and selected first-listed diagnoses: United States, 1990, 2000, and 2005 346

102. **Discharges** with at least one procedure in nonfederal short-stay hospitals, by sex, age, and selected procedures: United States, average annual 1994–1995 and 2004–2005 . . . 349

103. **Hospital admissions,** average length of stay, outpatient visits, and outpatient surgery, by type of ownership and size of hospital: United States, selected years 1975–2005 352

104. **Nursing home residents** 65 years of age and over, by age, sex, and race: United States, selected years 1973–2004 353

Health Care Resources

Personnel

105. **Persons employed** in health service sites, by site and sex: United States, 2000–2006 355

106. Active **physicians** and doctors of medicine in patient care, by geographic division and state: United States, selected years 1975–2005 356

107. **Doctors of medicine,** by activity and place of medical education: United States and outlying U.S. areas, selected years 1975–2005 358

108. **Doctors of medicine** in primary care, by specialty: United States and outlying U.S. areas, selected years 1949–2005 359

109. **Employees and wages,** by selected healthcare occupations: United States, selected years 1999–2005 360

110. First-year enrollment and **graduates of health professions schools,** and number of schools, by selected profession: United States, selected years 1980–2005 361

111. **Total enrollment of minorities** in schools for selected health occupations, by race and Hispanic origin: United States, selected academic years 1980–1981 through 2004–2005 362

112. First-year and total **enrollment of women** in schools for selected health occupations: United States, selected academic years 1980–1981 through 2004–2005 364

Facilities

113. **Hospitals,** beds, and occupancy rates, by type of ownership and size of hospital: United States, selected years 1975–2005 365

114. **Mental health organizations** and beds for 24-hour hospital and residential treatment, by type of organization: United States, selected years 1986–2004 366

115. **Community hospital beds** and average annual percentage change, by geographic division and state: United States, selected years 1960–2005 367

116. **Occupancy rates** in community hospitals and average annual percent change, by geographic division and state: United States, selected years 1960–2005 369

117. **Nursing homes,** beds, occupancy, and residents, by geographic division and state: United States, selected years 1995–2006 371

118. **Medicare-certified providers and suppliers:** United States, selected years 1980–2005 373

119. Number of Magnetic Resonance Imaging **(MRI) units** and Computed Tomography **(CT) scanners:** Selected countries, selected years 1990–2004 374

Health Care Expenditures and Payors

National Health Expenditures

120. **Total health expenditures** as a percent of gross domestic product and per capita health expenditures in dollars, by selected countries: Selected years 1960–2004 375

121. Gross domestic product, federal, and state and local government expenditures, **national health expenditures,** and average annual percent change: United States, selected years 1960–2005 376

122. **Consumer Price Index** and average annual percent change for all items, selected items, and medical care components: United States, selected years 1960–2006 377

123. **Growth in personal health care expenditures** and percent distribution of factors affecting growth: United States, 1960–2005 378

124. **National health expenditures,** average annual percent change, and percent distribution, by type of expenditure: United States, selected years 1960–2005 379

125. **Personal health care expenditures,** by source of funds and type of expenditure: United States, selected years 1960–2005 381

126. **National health expenditures for mental health services,** average annual percent change and percent distribution, by type of expenditure: United States, selected years 1986–2003 383

127. **National health expenditures for substance abuse treatment,** average annual percent change and percent distribution, by type of expenditure: United States, selected years 1986–2003 384

128. **Expenses for health care and prescribed medicine,** by selected population characteristics: United States, selected years 1987–2004 385

129. **Sources of payment for health care,** by selected population characteristics: United States, selected years 1987–2004 388

130. **Out-of-pocket health care expenses** among persons with medical expenses, by age: United States, selected years 1987–2004 391

131. **Expenditures for health services** and supplies and percent distribution, by type of payer: United States, selected years 1987–2005 392

132. **Employers'** costs per employee-hour worked for total compensation, wages and salaries, and **health insurance,** by selected characteristics: United States, selected years 1991–2006 394

133. **Hospital expenses,** by type of ownership and size of hospital: United States, selected years 1980–2005 396

134. **Nursing home average monthly charges** per resident, by selected facility characteristics: United States, 1985–2004 397

135. **Mental health expenditures,** percent distribution, and per capita expenditures, by type of mental health organization: United States, selected years 1975–2002 398

Health Care Coverage and Major Federal Programs

136. **Private health insurance** coverage among persons under 65 years of age, by selected characteristics: United States, selected years 1984–2005 399

137. **Private health insurance** coverage obtained through the workplace among persons under 65 years of age, by selected characteristics: United States, selected years 1984–2005 401

138. **Medicaid coverage** among persons under 65 years of age, by selected characteristics: United States, selected years 1984–2005 403

139. **No health insurance coverage** among persons under 65 years of age, by selected characteristics: United States, selected years 1984–2005 405

140. **Health insurance coverage** for persons 65 years of age and over, by type of coverage and selected characteristics: United States, selected years 1992–2005 . . . 407

141. **Medicare** enrollees and expenditures and percent distribution, by Medicare program and type of service: United States and other areas, selected years 1970–2006 409

142. **Medicare** enrollees and program payments among fee-for-service Medicare beneficiaries, by sex and age: United States and other areas, selected years 1994–2004 411

143. **Medicare** beneficiaries by race, ethnicity, and selected characteristics: United States, 1992, 2003, and 2004 412

144. **Medicaid** recipients and medical vendor payments, by basis of eligibility, and race and ethnicity: United States, selected fiscal years 1972–2004 414

145. **Medicaid** recipients and medical vendor payments, by type of service: United States, selected fiscal years 1972–2004 415

146. **Department of Veterans Affairs** health care expenditures and use, and persons treated, by selected characteristics: United States, selected fiscal years 1970–2005 417

State Health Expenditures and Health Insurance

147. State mental health agency per capita **expenditures for mental health services** and average annual percent change, by geographic region and state: United States, selected fiscal years 1981–2004 418

148. **Medicare** enrollees, enrollees in managed care, payment per enrollee, and short-stay hospital utilization by geographic region and state: United States, 1994 and 2004 420

149. **Medicaid** recipients, recipients in managed care, payments per recipient, and recipients per 100 persons below the poverty level, by geographic region and state: United States, selected fiscal years 1989–2004 422

150. Persons enrolled in **health maintenance organizations** (HMOs) by geographic region and state: United States, selected years 1980–2006 424

151. **Persons without health insurance coverage by state:** United States, average annual 1995–1997 through 2003–2005 426

Executive Summary and Highlights

Executive Summary

Health, United States, 2007, is the 31st annual report on the health status of the Nation prepared by the Secretary of the Department of Health and Human Services for the President and Congress. In a chartbook and 151 detailed tables, it provides an annual picture of the health of the entire Nation. Trends are presented on health status and health care utilization, resources, and expenditures. This year's report includes a focus on access to needed or recommended health care services.

For those entrusted with safeguarding the Nation's health, monitoring the health of the American people is an essential step in making sound health policy and setting research and program priorities. Health measures provide essential information for assessing how the Nation's resources should be directed to improve the population's health. Examination of emerging trends identifies diseases, conditions, and risk factors that warrant study and intervention. *Health, United States* presents trends and current information on measures and determinants of the Nation's health. It also identifies variation in health and health care among people by race and ethnicity, gender, education and income level, and geographic location. Given the increasing diversity of the Nation and the continuing changes in the health care infrastructure, this is a challenging and critically important task.

Overall Health of the Nation

Life expectancy in the United States continues to increase. In 2004, American men could expect to live more than 3 years longer, and women more than 1 year longer, than they did in 1990 (Figure 18 and Table 27). Mortality from heart disease, stroke, and cancer has continued to decline in recent years (Figure 20 and Table 29). Infant mortality, one major determinant of overall life expectancy, declined (Figure 19 and Table 22) through 2001 and has changed little since then.

Yet, even as progress is made in improving life expectancy, increased longevity is accompanied by increased prevalence of chronic conditions and their associated pain and disability. In recent years, progress in some areas has not been as rapid as in earlier years, or trends have been moving in the wrong direction. Moreover, improvements have not been equally distributed by income, race, ethnicity, education, and geography.

Of concern for all Americans is the high prevalence of people with unhealthy lifestyles and behaviors, such as insufficient exercise and overweight, which are risk factors for many chronic diseases and disabilities including heart disease, diabetes, hypertension, and back pain. The rising number of overweight children and adults and the large percentage of those who are physically inactive (Figures 12–13 and Tables 72–75) raise additional concerns about Americans' future health (1).

Prevalence of risky behaviors among children and young adults remains at unacceptable levels. About 20% of adolescents age 16–17 years, and more than 40% of young adults age 18–25 years, reported binge alcohol use in 2005, and 20% of young adults age 18–25 years reported using illicit drugs in the past month (Table 66). The percentage of high school students who seriously considered suicide has declined since 1991, but the percentage who attempted suicide has remained stable (7%–9%) (Table 62).

Health Status by Sociodemographic Characteristics

Efforts to improve Americans' health in the 21st century will be influenced by important changes in demographics. Ours is a nation growing older and becoming more racially and ethnically diverse. The percentage of the population 75 years of age and over was 6% in 2005 and is projected to increase to 12% by 2050 (Figure 1). With an aging population and longer life expectancy comes increasing total prevalence of chronic diseases and conditions associated with aging, such as disability and limitation of activity. In 2005, 44% of those age 75 years and over living in the community reported having a limitation in their usual activity due to a chronic condition, compared with 12% of people 45–54 years of age (Table 58). Many of the diseases associated with aging, including diabetes and hypertension, produce cumulative damage if not properly treated. Others, such as emphysema and some cancers, develop slowly or after long periods of environmental exposure. Almost 70% of men and more than 80% of women age 75 years and over had either high blood pressure or were taking antihypertension medication in 2001–2004, compared with about 35% of adults age 45–54 years (Table 70). The proportion of the population with high serum cholesterol rates has been dropping, in large part due to increased use of cholesterol-lowering drugs (Table 71). In 2001–2004, 17% of adults had either diagnosed or undiagnosed high serum cholesterol, and older women (age 55 and over) were substantially more likely to have high cholesterol than older men (Table 71). Vision and hearing also decline with age (Table 59) and many types of pain, particularly those associated with the musculoskeletal system such as joint pain, are more common at older ages (Table 57).

Socioeconomic and cultural differences among racial and ethnic groups in the United States will likely also influence future patterns of disease, disability, and health care use. *Health, United States, 2007,* identifies major disparities in health and health care by socioeconomic status, race, ethnicity, and insurance status. In 2006, 15% of Americans were of Hispanic origin, 12% were African American, 4% were Asian, and about 1% were American Indian or Alaska Native or were of more than one race (Figure 3). Significant racial and ethnic disparities exist across a wide range of health measures. The gap in life expectancy between the black and white populations has narrowed, but persists (Figure 18 and Table 27). Disparities in risk factors and morbidity also exist. Obesity, a major risk factor for many chronic diseases, varies by race and ethnicity—51% of non-Hispanic black women age 20 years and over were obese in 2001–2004, compared with 39% of women of Mexican origin and 31% of non-Hispanic white women (Table 74, age-adjusted). The differences in health status by race and Hispanic origin documented in this report may be explained by several factors including socioeconomic status, health practices, psychosocial stress and limited resources, environmental exposures, discrimination, and access to health care, the focus of this year's Special Feature (2,3).

In 2004, the number of noncitizen foreign-born persons reached 21.1 million, representing 7.3% of the U.S. civilian noninstitutionalized population (Figure 2). Noncitizen foreign-born persons may be either legal or illegal U.S. residents. They are disproportionately low-income and uninsured (4,5). They are also more likely to face other barriers to accessing health care including ineligibility for many government-sponsored programs and difficulty in finding providers who speak their language and provide culturally-sensitive care (5).

Health Care Resources

Health care technologies, facilities, equipment, and provider specialties have changed over recent decades. Sophisticated imaging equipment is more available in the United States, compared with almost all other countries (Table 119). Until the mid-20th century, hospitals and primary care physicians were the major providers of health care, with few specialized facilities. There are now more physician subspecialties and specialized health care facilities including imaging centers, outpatient surgical centers, and dialysis centers (Tables 107, 118). More procedures are being furnished on an outpatient basis and the length of inpatient hospital stays has shortened (Tables 99, 103). The supply of assisted living facilities is increasing rapidly, whereas the number of nursing home beds has declined (Table 117) (6). The number of physicians per capita has been increasing, but they are not distributed equally across the Nation (Figures 22, 23, and Table 106). The supply of allied health professionals is shifting. The numbers of dental hygienists and dental assistants, pharmacy technicians, diagnostic medical sonographers, massage therapists, medical assistants, and medical equipment preparers have increased by 5% or more per year since 1999, whereas the numbers of respiratory therapy technicians and occupational therapist aides have declined by 5% or more per year (Table 109). Projections indicate that there may be an increasing shortage of nurses and pharmacists as well as other health professionals needed to care for our aging population (7,8).

Expenditures and Payors

The United States spends more on health per capita than any other country, and health spending continues to increase (Table 120). In 2005, national health care expenditures in the United States totaled $2 trillion, a 7% increase from 2004 (Table 121). Hospital spending, which accounts for 31% of national health expenditures (Table 124), increased by 8% in 2005 (Table 125). Spending for prescription drugs accounted for 10% of national health expenditures in 2005. This spending increased 6% in 2005, down from an average annual growth of 12% from 2000 to 2004 (Table 124).

Overall, private health insurance paid 36% of total personal health care expenditures in 2005, the federal government 34%, state and local governments 11%, and out-of-pocket payments 15% (Figure 6). Expenditures on mental health services and substance abuse treatment constituted 7.5% of national health expenditures in 2003 and have grown at a slower rate than that of overall health expenditures since 1993 despite an increase in the number of people treated (Figures 7, 8 and Tables 126, 127) (9). The distribution of funding sources for mental health services differs from that for substance abuse treatment, with Medicaid and private health insurance paying the largest shares of mental health expenditures, whereas other state and local government funds account for the largest share of substance abuse expenditures.

Access to Health Care and Utilization of Health Services

The health care delivery system is evolving, and with its evolution, the types of services that are available are changing. New technological advances can prevent, treat, or ameliorate conditions and diseases that were once thought untreatable. Yet, some Americans have difficulty accessing these services because they may be unavailable, difficult to obtain, or too expensive to purchase. In its 1993 report, Access to Health Care in America, the Institute of Medicine defined access as "the timely use of personal health services to achieve the best possible health outcomes" (3). Tracking which Americans do not receive the increasing number of potentially beneficial services or who do not receive them in a timely manner, and the reasons underlying suboptimal use of services, is essential to identifying solutions that can improve access to health care and improve the health of our population.

In 2005, more than 40 million adults (about 19%) did not receive "needed services" because they could not afford them (Figure 21). Nearly 15 million adults did not obtain eyeglasses, 25 million did not get dental care, 19 million did not get needed prescribed medicine, and 15 million did not get needed medical care due to cost. In 2004–2005, reported access problems varied among the 25 most populous states: 3%–9% of people in these states did not get needed medical care, 5%–11% delayed medical care, and 4%–14% did not get prescription drugs because they could not afford them (Table 80).

Health care resources are not distributed equally throughout the country (Figures 22, 23). Many rural areas experience a shortage of physicians and other providers (10). People living in rural areas, or areas without specific services, may have to travel long distances to obtain some health care services. They may experience long waiting times for appointments or be unable to obtain timely urgent or emergency care. Supply shortages of some health care services may affect all population groups, regardless of geography. For example, the supply of donated kidneys falls far short of the demand from people with end-stage renal disease (Figures 24, 25).

In addition to geographic distribution and supply of health care services, there are other obstacles to receiving needed health care. Lack of health insurance coverage has been well documented as a major barrier to receiving health care and has often been used as a proxy for overall access to health care (3). The percentage of the population under 65 years of age with no health insurance coverage fluctuated around 16%–17% between 1999 and 2005 (Figure 28 and Table 139). Uninsured people are substantially less likely to receive health care than their insured counterparts (Figures 33, 35, and Tables 81, 82, 87, 88, 98). Hispanic and American Indian or Alaska Native persons under 65 years are more likely to be uninsured than those in other racial and ethnic groups, and lower insurance rates in these populations is reflected in large part by lower utilization of most health care services (Tables 81, 82, 139). More than 60% of the uninsured population is age 18–44 years and almost one-half are non-Hispanic white persons. More than 40% of the uninsured population had a family income of at least 200% of the poverty level (Figure 30).

Poverty can also be a barrier to receiving health care, particularly for people without health insurance or for certain types of services where insurance coverage is less generous or less common, such as dental and mental health care. In 2005, about one-half of adults with any natural teeth in families with income below 200% of the poverty level did not have a recent dental visit, compared with less than one-quarter of adults with family income more than 400% of poverty (Figure 34).

The burden of out-of-pocket medical-related expenses is greatest for poor and uninsured people. In 2004, more than one-quarter of persons under 65 years of age living below the poverty level reported spending more than 10% of their disposable income on out-of-pocket medical care costs and health insurance premiums (Figure 31). For families with income between 100%–400% of poverty, the out-of-pocket cost of health insurance premiums may impose a substantial burden relative to their income, even with employer subsidies for their workers' health insurance. Higher-income families with health insurance who have catastrophic illnesses also may devote a substantial portion of their income to medical care, health insurance premiums, or both (11). Those lacking insurance through the workplace face individual insurance policy premiums that can cost substantially more than employer-sponsored plans—particularly for people with pre-existing conditions (12).

For both uninsured and insured populations, there may be nonfinancial barriers to health care. These barriers include, but are not limited to, transportation problems, lack of knowledge of where to obtain care or when to seek care, communication difficulties with the provider due to language or cultural barriers, and covert or overt discrimination. In 2004–2005, about 6% of adults living in poverty reported delaying needed medical care because they did not have transportation (Figure 27). Data from 2004–2005 also show that about 11% of adults 45–64 years of age—a time in life when chronic illnesses become more common—did not have a usual source of health care, and about 5%–6% of adults 45–64 years of age with hypertension, serious heart disease, or diabetes did not report a usual source of care (Figure 26 and Table 78).

The relationship between insurance coverage, low-income, and other barriers to access is complex because people who cannot pay for uncovered services may try to limit their health care utilization (13). It is possible that because access to needed health care is in part a function of the perception of need, people with less contact with physicians and other health care providers may not be aware of their undiagnosed conditions or recommended screening and preventive services. However, uninsured people are not significantly less likely than insured people to have undiagnosed elevated blood pressure and high cholesterol (Figure 32).

Differences in utilization among socioeconomic groups also may indicate access issues. Educational or cultural barriers to care may prevent people from knowing when to seek care, or prevent them from seeking or receiving care. If one racial, ethnic, or other population has a lower use rate even among insured members of the group, it could be that other barriers to access including availability, overt or covert discrimination, care-seeking behaviors, or barriers that are difficult to measure, may be obstacles to care. For example, colorectal screening is recommended for all adults age 50 and over, yet rates of scope procedures remain lower for insured black and Hispanic adults than for insured non-Hispanic white adults (Figure 35). Recent use of mammography remains lower for Asian women than for non-Hispanic black or white women, although differences in recent use of these tests between non-Hispanic black and white women have disappeared over time (Table 87). These screening differences may be explained by the propensity to seek care or comply with treatment recommendations. They also may be due in part to barriers in accessing these services, such as the inability to communicate with the provider due to language or cultural barriers or the lack of effective education of these populations about the importance of the procedures. Although differences in use of mammography and colorectal scope procedures may not necessarily indicate a barrier to health care access, highlighting these differences may spur more in-depth investigations that determine the source of these differences. If barriers to receiving these services are uncovered, programs or solutions to eliminate these barriers may be developed.

To improve the health of all Americans and enable policymakers to chart future trends, target resources most effectively, and set program priorities, it is critical that the Nation keep collecting and disseminating reliable and accurate information about all components of health, including current health status, the determinants of health, resources, and outcomes. Equally important is documenting trends in access to and utilization of health care services that improve the health of our population. The trends may identify barriers in access to needed or recommended services. The following highlights from *Health, United States, 2007 With Chartbook on Trends in the Health of Americans* summarize the latest findings gathered from the public and private health care sectors to help the Department of Health and Human Services, the President, and the Congress in carrying out their mission of monitoring and improving the health of the Nation.

References

1. Ogden CL, Carroll MD, Curtin LR, McDowell MA, Tabak CJ, Flegal KM. Prevalence of overweight and obesity in the United States, 1999–2004. JAMA 2006;295(13):1549–55.
2. Williams DR, Rucker TD. Understanding and addressing racial disparities in health care. Health Care Finan Rev 2000;21(4):75–90.
3. Institute of Medicine (U.S.). Committee on Monitoring Access to Personal Health Care Services. Access to health care in America. Washington, DC: National Academy Press. 1993.
4. Kaiser Commission on Medicaid and the Uninsured. Immigrants' health care coverage and access. Washington, DC: Kaiser Family Foundation. 2003.
5. Ku L, Matani S. Left out: Immigrants' access to health care and insurance. Health Aff 2001; 20(1):247–56.
6. Harrington C, Chapman S, Miller E, Miler N, Newcomer R. Trends in the supply of long-term-care facilities and beds in the United States. Journal of Applied Gerontology 2005;24(4):265–82.
7. Kenreigh CA, Wagner LT. The pharmacist shortage: Where do we stand? Medscape Pharmacists 2006;7(1). Medscape posted 01/13/2006.
8. Buerhaus PI, Staiger DO, Auerbach DI. New signs of a strengthening U.S. nurse labor market? Health Aff 2004;23(6):w526–33.
9. Mark TL, Levit KL, Coffey RM, McKusick DR, Harwood H, King E, et al. National expenditures for mental health services and substance abuse treatment, 1993–2003. SAMHSA pub. no. SMA 07–4227. Rockville, MD: Substance Abuse and Mental Health Services Administration. 2007.
10. Ricketts TC. The changing nature of rural health care. Annu Rev Public Health 2000;21:639–57.
11. Banthin JS, Bernard DM. Changes in financial burdens for health care: National estimates for the population younger than 65 years, 1996 to 2003. JAMA 2006;296(22):2712–9.
12. Pauly MV, Nichols LM. The nongroup health insurance market: Short on facts, long on opinions and policy disputes. Health Aff 2002;Suppl web exclusives:w325–44.
13. Ross JS, Bradley EH, Busch SH. Use of health care services by lower-income and higher-income uninsured adults. JAMA 2006;295(17):2027–36.

Highlights

Health, United States, 2007, is the 31st report on the health status of the Nation. In a chartbook and 151 trend tables, it presents current and historic information on the health of the U.S. population. The trend tables are organized around four major subject areas: health status and determinants, health care utilization, health care resources, and health care expenditures and payors. The 2007 Chartbook on Trends in the Health of Americans focuses on selected determinants and measures of health and includes a special feature on access to health care .

Life Expectancy and Mortality

Life expectancy and infant mortality rates are often used to gauge the overall health of a population. Life expectancy shows a long-term upward trend and infant mortality shows a long-term downward trend. As overall death rates have declined, racial and ethnic disparities in mortality have persisted, but the gap in life expectancy between the black and white populations has narrowed.

In 2004, **life expectancy** at birth for the total population reached a record high of 77.8 years, up from 75.4 years in 1990 (Table 27).

Between 1990 and 2004, **life expectancy at birth** increased 3.4 years for **males** and 1.6 years for **females**. The gap in life expectancy between males and females narrowed from 7.0 years in 1990 to 5.2 years in 2004 (Table 27).

Between 1990 and 2004, **life expectancy at birth** increased more for the **black** than for the **white population**, thereby narrowing the gap in life expectancy between these two racial groups. In 1990, life expectancy at birth for the white population was 7.0 years longer than for the black population. By 2004, the difference had narrowed to 5.2 years (Figure 18 and Table 27).

Overall mortality was 31% higher for **black Americans** than for white Americans in 2004 compared with 37% higher in 1990. In 2004, age-adjusted death rates for the black population exceeded those for the white population by 46% for **stroke** (cerebrovascular disease), 32% for **heart disease**, 23% for **cancer** (malignant neoplasms), and 787% for **HIV disease** (Table 29).

In 2004, the **infant mortality** rate decreased to 6.8 infant deaths per 1,000 live births (Figure 19 and Table 22).

Large disparities in **infant mortality** rates among **racial and ethnic groups** continue to exist. In 2004, infant mortality rates were highest for infants of non-Hispanic black mothers (13.6 deaths per 1,000 live births), American Indian mothers (8.4 per 1,000), and Puerto Rican mothers (7.8 per 1,000); and lowest for infants of Cuban mothers (4.6 per 1,000 live births) and Asian or Pacific Islander mothers (4.7 per 1,000) (Table 19).

The **leading cause of death** differs by age group. In 2004, the leading cause of death was congenital malformations for infants, unintentional injuries for people age 1–44 years, cancer for middle-age adults age 45–64 years, and heart disease for adults age 65 years and over (Table 32).

Age-adjusted mortality from **heart disease**, the leading cause of death overall, declined 33% between 1990 and 2004, continuing a long-term downward trend (Figure 20 and Table 36).

Age-adjusted mortality from **cancer** (malignant neoplasms), the second leading cause of death overall, decreased 14% between 1990 and 2004 (Figure 20 and Table 38).

The age-adjusted death rate for **motor vehicle-related injuries** has remained stable since the early 1990s following a period of decline. Death rates for motor vehicle-related injuries are higher at age 15–24 years and 75 years and over than at other ages (Table 44).

The age-adjusted death rate for **HIV disease** has declined slowly since 1998, after a sharp decrease between 1995 and 1998. The death rate for HIV disease is higher at age 35–54 years than at other ages (Table 42).

The **homicide** rate for **black males 15–24 years of age** decreased sharply from the early to the late 1990s and has remained relatively stable since then (Table 45). Homicide continues to be the leading cause of death for young black males 15–24 years of age.

In 2004, young **American Indian males 15–24 years of age** continued to have substantially higher death rates for motor vehicle-related injuries and for suicide than young males in other race or ethnicity groups. Death rates for the American Indian population are known to be underestimated (Tables 44 and 46).

The **suicide rate for non-Hispanic white men 65 years of age and over** is higher than in other groups. In 2004, the suicide rate for older non-Hispanic white men was about two to three times the rate for older men in other race or ethnicity groups and nearly 8 times the rate for older non-Hispanic white women (Table 46).

Health Behaviors and Risk Factors

Health behaviors have a significant effect on health status. Pregnant teenagers are less likely to receive early prenatal care and more likely to drop out of school and to live in poverty, than are other parents. Heavy and chronic use of alcohol and use of illicit drugs increase the risk of disease and injuries. Cigarette smoking increases the risk of lung cancer, heart disease, emphysema, and other diseases. Obesity increases the risk of heart disease, diabetes, and stroke. Regular physical activity reduces the risk of disease and enhances mental and physical functioning.

The **birth rate for teenagers** declined in 2005 (preliminary data) for the 14th consecutive year, to 40.4 births per 1,000 women age 15–19 years, 2% lower than in 2004. Rates declined 3% for teenagers age 15–17 years and remained unchanged for teenagers age 10–14 years and 18–19 years (Table 4).

In 2005 (preliminary data), the **birth rate for unmarried women** reached a record high of 47.6 births per 1,000 unmarried women age 15–44 years, up 3% from 2004. In 2005, 37% of all births were to unmarried women and the percentages generally increased for all age, race, and Hispanic origin subgroups (Table 10).

Low birthweight is associated with elevated risk of death and disability in infants. In 2005 (preliminary data), the low birthweight rate (less than 2,500 grams, or 5.5 pounds, at birth) increased to 8.2%, up from 7.0% in 1990 (Table 13).

Between 1988–1994 and 2003–2004, the prevalence of **overweight among preschool-age children** 2–5 years of age almost doubled, from about 7% to 14% (Figure 13 and Table 69).

The prevalence of **overweight among school-age children** increased more than 60% between 1988–1994 and 2003–2004. Among children 6–11 years of age, overweight increased from 11% to 19%. The prevalence of overweight among adolescents 12–19 years of age grew from 11% to 17% (Figure 13 and Tables 69 and 75).

Between 1993 and 2005, the percentage of **high school students** who reported attempting suicide (8%–9%) and whose **suicide attempts** required medical attention (2%–3%) remained fairly constant. Girls were more likely than boys to consider or attempt suicide. However, in 2004, adolescent boys (15–19 years of age) were almost 4 times as likely to die from suicide as were adolescent girls, in part reflecting their choice of more lethal methods, such as firearms (Tables 46 and 62).

In 2005, among current drinkers 18 years of age and over, about one-third reported consuming **five or more alcoholic drinks in one day** during the past year, with the highest proportion among young adults 18–24 years of age (55%). In 2005, among current drinkers 18–24 years of age, 67% of men and 41% of women reported consuming five or more alcoholic drinks on at least one day in the past year (Table 68).

Between 2003 and 2005, the percentage of **high school students who reported smoking cigarettes** in the past month remained stable at 22%–23% after declining from 36% in 1997 (Figure 9).

In 2005, 21% of U.S. adults were current **cigarette smokers,** the same percentage as in 2004, suggesting that the decline in cigarette smoking prevalence might be stalling (Figure 9 and Table 63).

Children with low family income are more likely to have high **blood cotinine** levels (a marker for exposure to secondhand smoke) than children living in higher income families. In 2001–2004, children living in families with income below 200% of the poverty level were at least twice as likely to have had a high blood cotinine level as children living in higher income families (22%–28% compared with 10%) (Figure 10).

Among **adults** 20–74 years of age, **overweight and obesity** rates have increased since 1960–1962. These increases were driven largely by increases in the percentage of adults who were obese. From 1960–1962 through 2003–2004, the percentage of adults who were overweight but not obese remained steady at 32%–34% (age-adjusted). During that time period, the percentage of adults who were obese increased from 13% to 34% (age-adjusted) (Figure 13 and Table 74).

In 1999–2004, **weekly restaurant meal** consumption varied by age. Eating four or more weekly restaurant meals ranged from 9% among children 1–12 years to 32% among adults 18–44 years of age. Adults 65 years and over had the lowest likelihood of eating at least one weekly restaurant meal (Figure 12).

In 2005, almost one-third of **adults** 18 years of age and over engaged in **regular leisure-time physical activity**. Adults in families with income above twice the poverty level were more likely to engage in regular leisure-time physical activity (34%) than adults in lower income families (20%–22%) (age-adjusted) (Table 73).

Health Status and Health Conditions

Measures of health status include respondent-assessed health status, limitation in activity caused by chronic conditions, and serious psychological distress. Measures of morbidity presented in this report include the incidence and prevalence of selected specific diseases and conditions.

In 2005, the percentage of noninstitutionalized **adults** reporting their **health as fair or poor** ranged from 6% of those age 18–44 years to 30% of those age 75 years and over. The proportion of adults with fair or poor health was higher among non-Hispanic black and Hispanic persons compared with non-Hispanic white persons (Table 60).

In 2005, **activity limitation** caused by chronic health conditions was reported for 7% of **children** under the age of 18 years. Among school-age children (5–17 years of age), learning disabilities and Attention Deficit/Hyperactivity Disorder (ADHD or ADD) were frequently reported as a cause of activity limitation (Figure 14 and Table 58).

Arthritis and other musculoskeletal conditions were the **leading causes of activity limitation** among working-age **adults 18–64 years** of age in 2004–2005. Mental illness was the second most frequently mentioned condition causing activity limitation among adults 18–44 years of age and the third most frequently mentioned among adults 45–54 years of age (Figure 15).

In 2004–2005, 3% of the noninstitutionalized population reported having **serious psychological distress**. Adults living below the poverty level were more than five times as likely to report serious psychological distress as adults in families with income of at least twice the poverty level (8.6% compared with 1.7%) (Table 61).

The prevalence of **hypertension**, defined as elevated blood pressure or taking antihypertensive medication, increases with age. In 2001–2004, 36% of men and 35% of women age 45–54 years had hypertension, compared with 67% of men and 82% of women age 75 years and over (Table 70).

Between 1988–1994 and 2001–2004, the percentage of both men and women 55 years and over with **high total serum cholesterol levels** (greater than 240 mg/dL) declined substantially. However, older women were more likely to have high serum cholesterol than older men. In 2001–2004, 26% of women age 65–74 years had high serum cholesterol, compared with 11% of men age 65–74 years (Table 71).

In 2001–2004, the prevalence of **diabetes** (including both diagnosed and undiagnosed) increased with age from 11% among adults 40–59 years of age to 23% among adults 60 years of age and over. The percentage of adults with undiagnosed diabetes was 3% among those 40–59 years of age and 6% among those 60 years of age and over (Table 55).

Between 1988–1994 and 2001–2004, approximately one-quarter of **adults 20–64** years of age had **untreated dental caries**, down from nearly one-half in 1971–1974 (Table 76).

In 2005, 28% of adults 18 years of age and over had any **low back pain** in the past 3 months and 15% reported having a **severe headache or migraine** in the past 3 months (age-adjusted) (Table 56).

In 2005, approximately 2.2 million **workplace injuries and illnesses** in the private sector involved days away from work, job transfer, or restricted duties at work for a rate of 2.4 cases per 100 full-time workers (FTW). The transportation and warehousing industry reported the highest injury and illness rate, with 4.6 cases per 100 FTW. The next highest rates were reported by the manufacturing industry (3.5 per 100 FTW) and the construction industry (3.4 per 100 FTW) (Table 50).

Health Care Expenditures and Payors

The United States spends more on health per capita than any other country, and U.S. health spending continues to increase, though the rate of increase has slowed for the third consecutive year. Spending increases are due to increased intensity and cost of services and a higher volume of services needed to treat an aging population. Major payors for health care include private health insurers and public programs such as Medicare and Medicaid. Medicaid is jointly funded by the federal and state governments to provide health care for certain groups of low-income persons. Medicare is funded by the federal government and covers the health care of most persons 65 years of age and over and disabled persons.

The United States spends a larger **share of its gross domestic product (GDP) on health** than does any other major industrialized country. In 2004, the United States devoted 15% of its GDP to health compared with 12% in Switzerland and more than 10% in France, Germany, Iceland, and Portugal, the countries with the next highest shares (Table 120).

In 2005, **national health care expenditures** in the United States totaled $2 trillion, a 6.9% increase from 2004. The rate of increase slowed for the third consecutive year, though it was still higher than the growth in the gross domestic product (GDP) (Tables 121).

Prescription drug expenditures increased almost 6% in 2005, a much slower rate than in previous years. The price of prescription drugs and medical supplies increased 4% in the Consumer Price Index in 2005 and 2006 (Tables 122 and 124).

Expenditures for hospital care accounted for 31% of all national health expenditures in 2005. Physician and clinical services accounted for 21% of the total in 2005, prescription drugs for 10%, and nursing home care for 6% (Table 124).

In 2005, 34% of **personal health care expenditures** were paid by the federal government and 11% by state and local government; private health insurance paid 36% and consumers paid 15% out-of-pocket (Figure 6 and Table 125).

In 2003, Medicaid (26%) and private health insurance (24%) funded the largest shares of mental health services expenditures (Figure 7). In contrast, other state and local government expenditures (excluding Medicaid) funded the largest share (40%) of **substance abuse treatment expenditures** (Figures 7 and 8).

In 2003, national health **expenditures for mental health services** were about $100 billion. Almost one-quarter of these expenditures were for retail prescription drugs ($23 billion) (Table 126).

National health **expenditures for substance abuse treatment** increased by about 50% from 1986 to 2003 (inflation-adjusted). In 2003, national health expenditures for substance abuse treatment exceeded $20 billion (unadjusted dollars) (Table 127).

In 2004, 97% of persons 65 years of age and over in the civilian noninstitutionalized population had **medical expenses** that averaged about $8,900 per person with expenses. Almost one-fifth of expenses was paid out-of-pocket, 16% by private insurance, and 64% by public programs (primarily Medicare) (Tables 128 and 129).

In 2006, the **Medicare** program had about 43 million **enrollees and expenditures** of $408 billion, up from $336 billion the previous year. Expenditures for the first year of the new Medicare drug program (Part D), introduced in 2006, were $47 billion (Table 141).

Of the 33 million **Medicare enrollees in the fee-for-service program** in 2004, 12% were 85 years of age and over and 16% were under 65 years of age (Table 142).

In 2004, children under 21 years of age accounted for 48% of **Medicaid recipients** but only 17% of expenditures. Aged, blind, and disabled persons accounted for 22% of recipients and 66% of expenditures (Table 144).

Health Care System Influences, Personnel, and Resources

Major changes continue to occur in the delivery of health care in the United States, driven in part by changes in payment policies intended to rein in rising costs and by advances in technology that have allowed more complex treatments to be performed on an outpatient basis. Hospital inpatient utilization has been stable in recent years. The ratio of physicians per population continues to increase slowly, but supply is not equally distributed across the country. The supply of other practitioners, including pharmacists and nurses, may not be increasing as rapidly as needed to keep pace with our aging population.

In 2005, 41% of doctor visits were to **specialty care physicians**, up from 34% in 1980. During this period, the proportion of office-based doctor visits to **general and family practice physicians** decreased from 34% to 22% (Table 93).

Physician supply varied greatly by geographic area in 2004 with only 11% of **counties having a patient care physician to population ratio** above the overall national ratio of 24 physicians per 10,000 population. Similarly, 14% of counties had a ratio of obstetricians or gynecologists greater than the national ratio of 3 obstetricians or gynecologists per 10,000 females 15 years of age and over. In 2004, almost 50% of counties had no practicing obstetricians or gynecologists (Figures 22 and 23).

Between 1999 and 2005, the **number** of dental hygienists and assistants, massage therapists, diagnostic medical sonographers, medical equipment preparers, medical assistants, and pharmacy technicians increased by 5%–10% annually. During this period, the **hourly wages** of radiation therapists, nuclear medicine technologists, massage therapists, pharmacists, and physician assistants rose the most, at 6%–7% annually (Table 109).

In 2004, the United States had among the highest number of **Magnetic Resonance Imaging (MRI) units and Computed Tomography (CT) scanners** per population among OECD countries reporting 2004 data. The U.S. had 27 MRI units and 32 CT scanners per one million population. Other countries with high numbers of MRI units included Austria (15 MRI units per one million population), Iceland (17), and Switzerland (14). Countries with high numbers of CT scanners included Austria (29 CT scanners per one million population), Italy (21), and South Korea (32) (Table 119).

In 2005, 63% of **surgeries** were performed on an **outpatient** basis compared with 51% in 1990 and 16% in 1980 (Table 103).

Between 1990 and 2005, the number of **community hospital beds** declined 13%, from about 927,000 to 802,000. Since 1990, the community hospital occupancy rate has remained steady at 62%–67% (Table 113).

Between 1990 and 2004, the overall rate of **inpatient mental health beds** per 100,000 civilian population in the United States declined by 45%. In state and county mental hospitals, the number of mental health beds per population declined by 53%, in private psychiatric hospitals the decline was 48%, and in nonfederal general hospital psychiatric services the decline was 34% (Table 114).

In 2006, there were about 1.7 million **nursing home beds** in about 16,000 nursing homes certified for use by Medicare and Medicaid beneficiaries. Between 1995 and 2006, nursing home bed occupancy was relatively stable, estimated at 84% in 2006. **Occupancy rates** were 90% or higher in 14 states and the District of Columbia in 2006 (Table 117).

Special Feature: Access to Health Care

Identifying which Americans do not receive potentially beneficial health care services, and the reasons underlying suboptimal use of services, is essential to identifying solutions that can improve access to needed health care.

Foregone or delayed health care due to cost

The percentage of Americans who reported not receiving needed health care services (as determined by the respondents) varies by age, family income, insurance coverage, and state of residence.

In 2005, 19% of adults 18 years of age and over—more than 40 million people—reported that they needed and **did not receive one or more of the following services in the past year because they could not afford them:** medical care, prescription medicines, mental health care, dental care, or eyeglasses (Figure 21).

In 2005, about 12% of adults 18 years of age and over reported that they **did not receive needed dental care;** 7% did **not purchase needed eyeglasses,** and about 9% **did not purchase needed prescription drugs due to cost** (Figure 21).

Adults 18–64 years of age were more likely than older adults or children to report not receiving needed medical care or delaying their medical care due to cost. In 2005, 7% of adults 18–64 years of age reported that they did **not get needed medical care** during the past 12 months, 9%–10%

delayed medical care, and 9%–10% **did not get needed prescription drugs** due to the cost. Compared with 1997, in 2005, more adults 18–64 years of age reported not getting needed medical care and needed prescription drugs due to cost (Table 79).

Almost all **adults 65 years of age** and over have Medicare coverage. Despite this health insurance coverage, in 2005, 4%–6% of those with income below or near the poverty level **did not get needed medical care** during the past 12 months, 6%–9% **delayed their medical care**, and 9%–12% **did not get the prescription drugs** they needed due to the cost. Medicare coverage for prescription drugs began in 2006 (Table 79).

In 2004–2005, **reduced access to medical care due to cost** varied across the 25 most populous **states**. The percentage of residents who reported not getting needed care due to cost ranged from 3%–9%. The range of those reporting delaying medical care due to cost was 5%–11%. The percentage reporting not getting needed prescription drugs due to cost varied among the 25 states from 4%–14% (Table 80).

In 2005, 19% of people under age 65 years of age who were uninsured for all or part of the preceding year **did not receive needed medical care** in the past 12 months **due to cost**, compared with 2% of people covered by health insurance for the full year (Table 79 and Figure 33).

In 2004, 27% of people with family income below the poverty line paid more than 10% of their **after-tax family income on out-of-pocket health care expenditures** (including health insurance premiums) (Figure 31).

The burden of **out-of-pocket expenses** for health care varies considerably by age. In 2004, more than one-half of people 75 years of age and over with health care expenses paid $1,000 or more out-of-pocket, compared with 28% of those 45–64 years of age, and 13% of adults 18–44 years of age (Table 130).

Barriers to health care use

Often-cited barriers to accessing needed health care include a lack of transportation and not having a usual source of medical care. Supply shortages or maldistribution of services can also create obstacles to the timely receipt of health care services.

In 2004–2005, about 5%–6% of **adults 45–64 years** of age with hypertension, a serious heart condition, or diabetes did not report a **usual source of care** (Figure 26).

In 2004–2005, 6% of adults living below the poverty level reported **delaying health care** in the past 12 months due to a **lack of transportation** compared with less than 1% of adults living at 200% or more of the poverty level. On average, women were more likely to report delaying care due to a lack of transportation than men (data table for Figure 27).

From 1988 to 2004 the percentage of patients receiving **kidney transplants** within two years of being added to the waiting list declined 56% for white patients and about 65% for black patients, in large part because the increase in the number of patients on the waiting list has not been met by a concurrent increase in the number of donated kidneys (Figure 25).

Lack of health insurance

Access to health care is often equated with lack of health insurance coverage, which has been established as a major barrier to receiving most health care services.

In 2005, the percentage of the **population under 65 years of age with no health insurance coverage** (public or private) **at a point in time** was 16.4%. Between 1995 and 2005, this percentage fluctuated between 16.1% and 17.5% (Figure 28 and Table 139).

Among the under 65 years of age population, the **poor and near poor** (those with family income less than 200% of poverty) were much more likely to be **uninsured at a point in time** than persons in higher income families (Table 139).

In 2005, 9% of **children** under 18 years of age were **uninsured at a point in time**. Between 2000 and 2005, among children in families with income just above the poverty level (100%–150% of poverty), the percentage uninsured dropped from 25% to 15% (Table 139) , while the percentage with Medicaid or State Children's Health Insurance Program (SCHIP) coverage increased from 35% to 49% (Table 138).

In 2005, 29% of **young adults** 18–24 years of age were **uninsured at a point in time.** This age group was more than twice as likely to be uninsured as those 45–64 years of age (Table 139).

In 2005, among persons under 65 years of age, those of **Hispanic origin and American Indians and Alaska Natives** were more likely to be **uninsured at a point in time** than were those in other racial and ethnic groups (Table 139).

Many people under 65 years of age, particularly those with a low family income, do not have health insurance coverage consistently throughout the year. In 2005, one-fifth of people under 65 years of age **were uninsured for at least part of the 12 months prior to interview.** Two-fifths of people of Mexican origin were uninsured for at least part of the 12 months prior to interview (Figure 29).

The likelihood of being **uninsured** varied among the **states.** In 2003–2005, the average percentage of the population with no health insurance coverage ranged from less than 10% in Minnesota, Hawaii, and Iowa, to 25% in Texas (Table 151).

About one-half of the **uninsured population** were non-Hispanic white persons with the other half being people of other **races and ethnicities** (Figure 30).

Differential utilization of services by population group

Access is often studied by examining whether rates of service use are at recommended or expected levels, or whether population groups differ in use of services. Lower rates of service use among a population group may reflect an access barrier in the lower-use group.

The percentage of mothers receiving **prenatal care** in the first trimester of pregnancy remained unchanged from 2003 to 2004 at 84% for the 43 reporting areas for which comparable trend data were available. In 2004, the percentage of mothers with early prenatal care varied substantially by **race and ethnicity,** from 70% for American Indian or Alaska Native mothers to 89% for non-Hispanic white mothers (Table 7).

In 2006, 77% of children 19–35 months of age received the **combined vaccination** series of four doses of DTaP (diphtheria-tetanus-acellular pertussis) vaccine, three doses of polio vaccine, one dose of MMR (measles-mumps-rubella vaccine), three doses of Hib (Haemophilus influenzae type b) vaccine, three doses of hepatitis B vaccine, and one dose of varicella vaccine. Children living below the poverty threshold were less likely than were children living at or above poverty to have received the combined vaccination series (74% compared with 78%) (Table 83).

Between 1987 and 1999, **mammography usage** in the past 2 years among women 40 years of age and over rose from 29% to 70% and has been between 67%–70% through 2005. Mammography levels are lower among Hispanic and Asian women compared with non-Hispanic black and white women (Table 87).

In 2004–2005, 6% of **children** under 6 years of age and 14% of children 6–17 years of age had **no health care visit** to a doctor or clinic within the past 12 months. Uninsured children under age 18 were almost three times as likely as those with insurance to have no recent health care visits (Table 81).

In 2005, about one-fourth of **children** 2–17 years of age did not have a **dental visit** in the past year. Children with family income below 200% of poverty were more likely to lack a recent dental visit than those with higher family income (Table 94).

In 2005, about one-half of adults with family income below 200% of the **poverty** level **did not have a dental visit** in the past year (Figure 34).

In 1999–2002, nearly 13% of non-Hispanic white women reported **antidepressant drug use** in the past month, more than twice the percentage of non-Hispanic black women and women of Mexican origin (age-adjusted; Figure 36).

In 2000–2005, about 44% of adults 50 years of age and over reported ever having had a procedure for detecting colorectal cancer using **colonoscopy, proctoscopy, or sigmoidoscopy.** Among insured adults 50–64 years of age, the proportion who ever had a scope procedure was lower among Hispanic and non-Hispanic black adults than non-Hispanic white adults (Figure 35).

In 1973–1974, the **nursing home resident** rate for the white population 65 years of age and over was more than twice that for the black population (61.2 compared with 28.2 per 1,000 population; age-adjusted). By 2004, the resident rate for the black population (49.9) exceeded that for the white population (34.0) (Table 104).

Population

Age

The population age 65 and over is increasing at a faster rate than the total population.

From 1950 to 2005, the total resident population of the United States increased from 151 million to 296 million, representing an average annual growth rate of 1.2% (Figure 1). During the same period, the population 65 years of age and over grew, on average, 2.0% per year, increasing from 12 to 37 million persons. The population 75 years of age and over grew the fastest (on average, 2.8% per year), increasing from 4 to 18 million persons.

Projections indicate that the rate of growth for the total population from now until 2050 will be slower, but older age groups will continue to grow more rapidly than the total population (1). By 2029, all of the baby boomers (those born in the post World War II period 1946–1964) will be age 65 years and over. As a result, the population age 65–74 years will increase from 6% to 10% of the total population between 2005 and 2030 (data table for Figure 1). As the baby boomers age, the population 75 years of age and over will rise from 6% to 9% of the population by 2030 and continue to grow to 12% in 2050. By 2040, the population age 75 years and over will exceed the population 65–74 years of age.

Reference

1. Day JC. National population projections. 2001. U.S. Census Bureau. Available from: www.census.gov/population/www/pop-profile/natproj.html.

Figure 1. Total population and older population: United States, 1950-2050

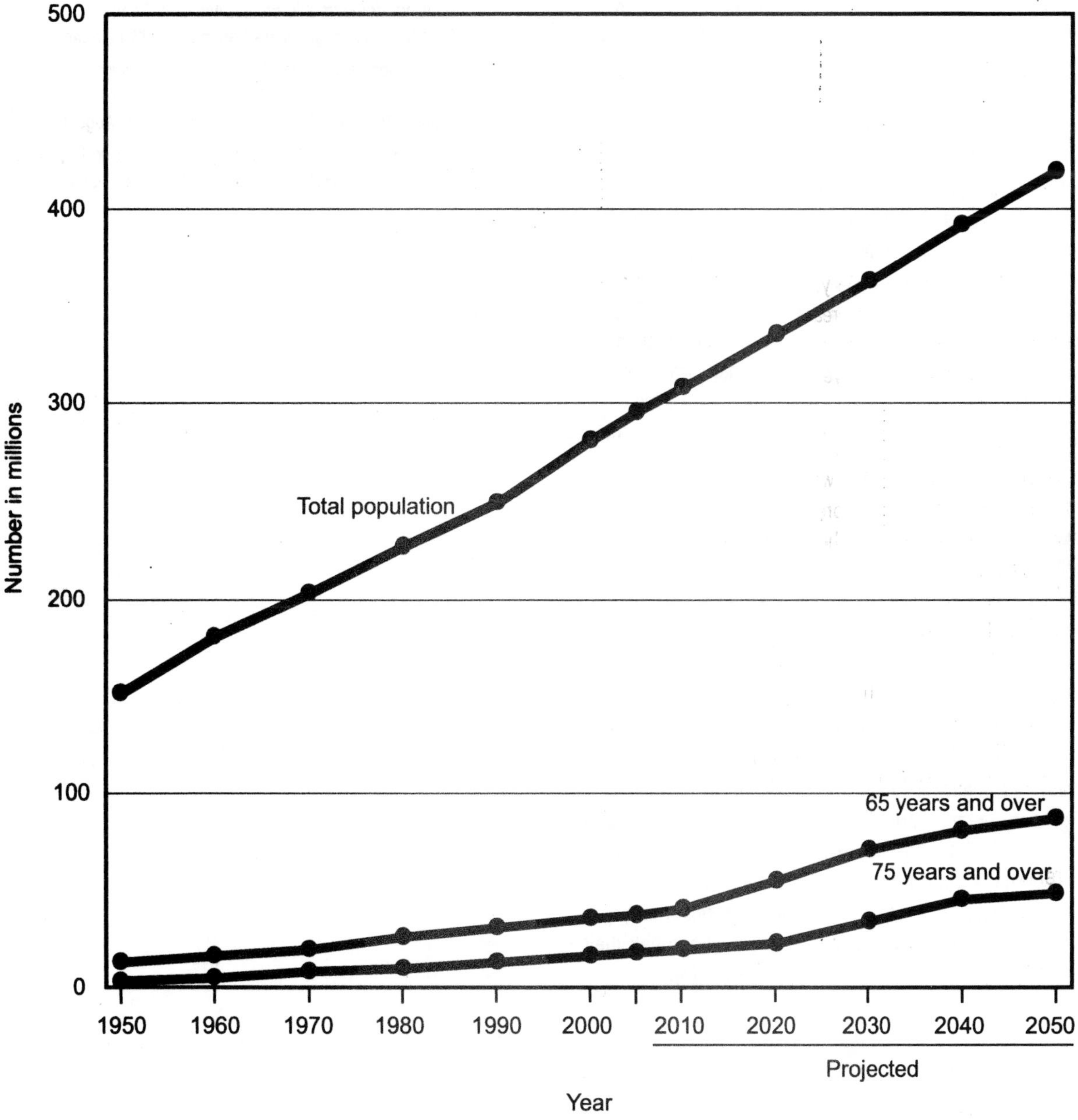

NOTE: See data table for Figure 1 for data points graphed and additional notes.

SOURCE: U.S. Census Bureau.

Foreign-Born Population

The proportion of the United States' population that is foreign-born more than doubled between 1970 and 2004.

According to the U.S. Census Bureau, foreign-born persons are defined as those who were not U.S. citizens at birth and include immigrants (legal permanent residents), temporary migrants (e.g., students, visiting scientists), humanitarian migrants (refugees), and unauthorized migrants (people illegally residing in the United States). Persons born abroad of U.S. citizen parents or born in Puerto Rico or other U.S. island areas are not considered foreign-born. Foreign-born persons may be United States citizens by naturalization or they may be noncitizens of the United States (1). Foreign-born noncitizens may be either legal or illegal U.S. residents.

In 2004, there were 34.2 million foreign-born people, representing nearly 12% of the civilian noninstitutionalized population of the United States (data table for Figure 2). Between 1970 and 2004, the percentage of the U.S. population that was foreign-born more than doubled (Figure 2).

The proportion of foreign-born noncitizens living in the United States is growing more rapidly than that of naturalized citizens. In 2004, the number of foreign-born noncitizens reached 21.1 million, representing 7.3% of the U.S. civilian noninstitutionalized population. Noncitizen foreign-born persons are disproportionately low-income and uninsured (2). They are also more likely than naturalized citizens to face other barriers to accessing health care including ineligibility for many government-sponsored programs and difficulty in finding providers who speak their language and provide culturally-sensitive care (3).

References

1. U.S. Census Bureau. 2000 census of population and housing, demographic profile. Available from: factfinder.census.gov/home/saff/main.html?_lang=en.
2. Kaiser Commission on Medicaid and the Uninsured. Immigrants' health care: Coverage and access. Washington, DC: Kaiser Family Foundation, August, 2003.
3. Ku L, Matani S. Left out: Immigrants' access to health care and insurance. Health Affairs 2001;20 (1):247–56.

Figure 2. Foreign-born population, by citizenship: United States, 1970–2004

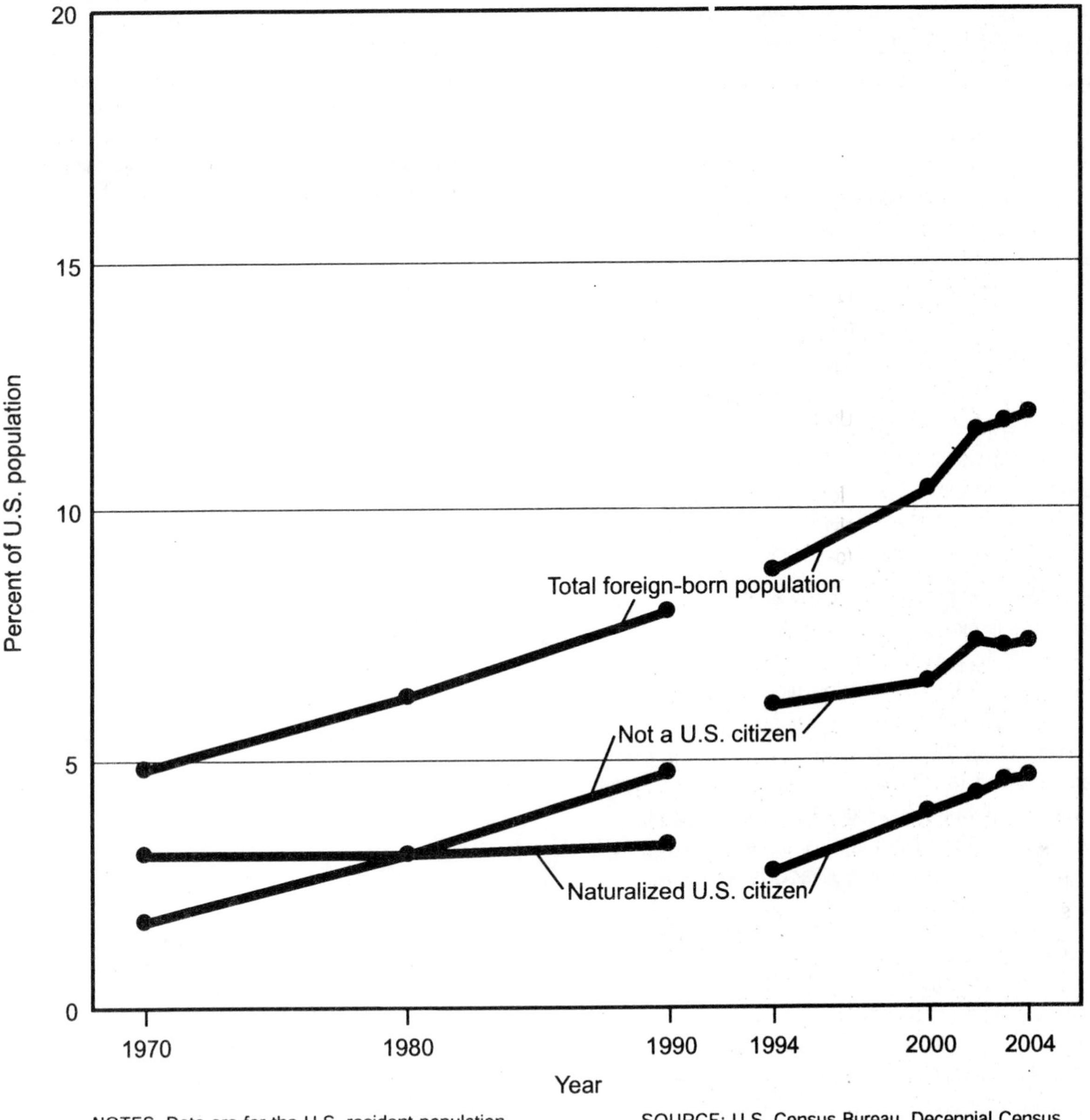

NOTES: Data are for the U.S. resident population (1970, 1980, and 1990). Starting in 1994, data are for the U.S. civilian noninstitutionalized population. See data table for Figure 2 for data points graphed and additional notes.

SOURCE: U.S. Census Bureau. Decennial Census (1970, 1980, and 1990) and Current Population Survey (1994–2004).

Race and Ethnicity

The percentage of Americans who identify themselves as Hispanic or Asian continues to increase.

Changes in the racial and ethnic composition of the population have important consequences for the Nation's health because many measures of disease and disability differ significantly by race and ethnicity. One of the overarching goals of U.S. public health policy is elimination of racial and ethnic disparities in health.

Diversity has long been a characteristic of the U.S. population, but the racial and ethnic composition of the Nation has changed over time. In 2006, about 30% of adults and over 40% of children were members of racial or ethnic minority populations (data table for Figure 3). Moreover, the percentage of the population that is of Hispanic origin or Asian has more than doubled in recent decades (data table for Figure 3).

In the 1980 and 1990 decennial censuses, Americans could choose only one racial category to describe their race (1). Beginning with the 2000 census, the question on race was modified to allow the choice of more than one racial category. Although, overall, a small percentage of persons of non-Hispanic origin selected two or more races in 2006, the percentage of children described as being of more than one race was more than twice as high as the percentage of adults (Figure 3). The number of American adults identifying themselves or their children as multiracial is expected to increase in the future (2).

The percentage of persons reporting two or more races varies considerably among racial groups. For example, the percentage of persons reporting a specified race in combination with one or more additional racial groups was 1.7% for white persons and 35.5% for American Indian or Alaska Native persons in 2006 (3).

References

1. Grieco EM, Cassidy RC. Overview of race and Hispanic origin. Census 2000 brief. U.S. Census Bureau. March 2001.
2. Waters MC. Immigration, intermarriage, and the challenges of measuring racial/ethnic identities. Am J Public Health 2000;90(11):1735–7.
3. U.S. Census Bureau. Monthly postcensal resident population, by single year of age, sex, race, and Hispanic origin. Available from: www.census.gov/popest/national/asrh/2005_nat_res.html. (Data for July 1, 2006.)

Figure 3. Population in selected race and Hispanic origin groups, by age: United States, 1980–2006

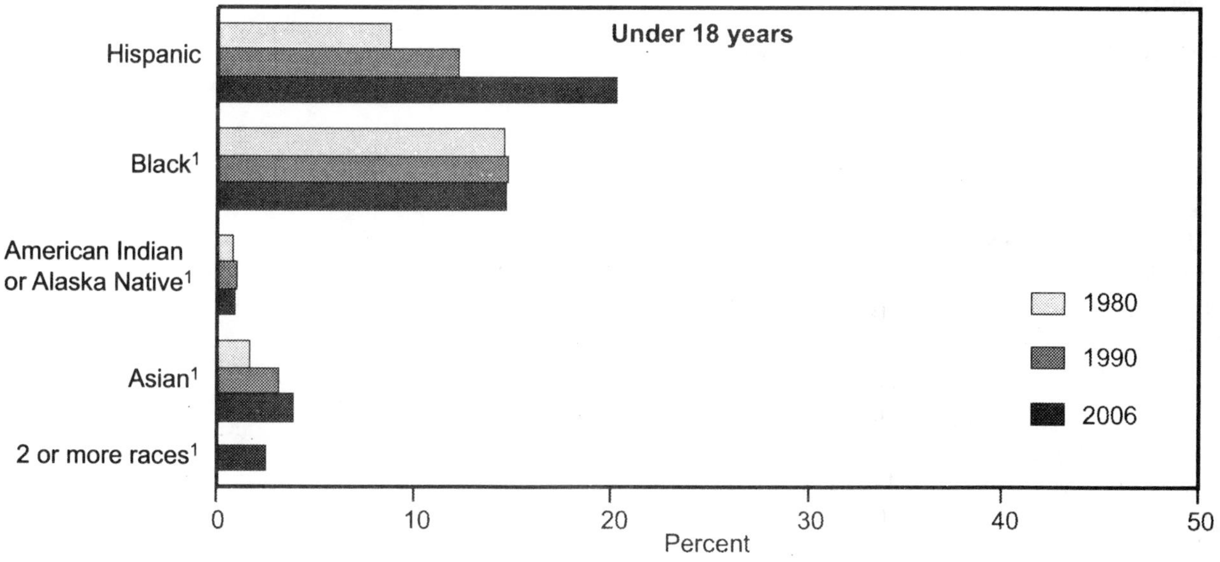

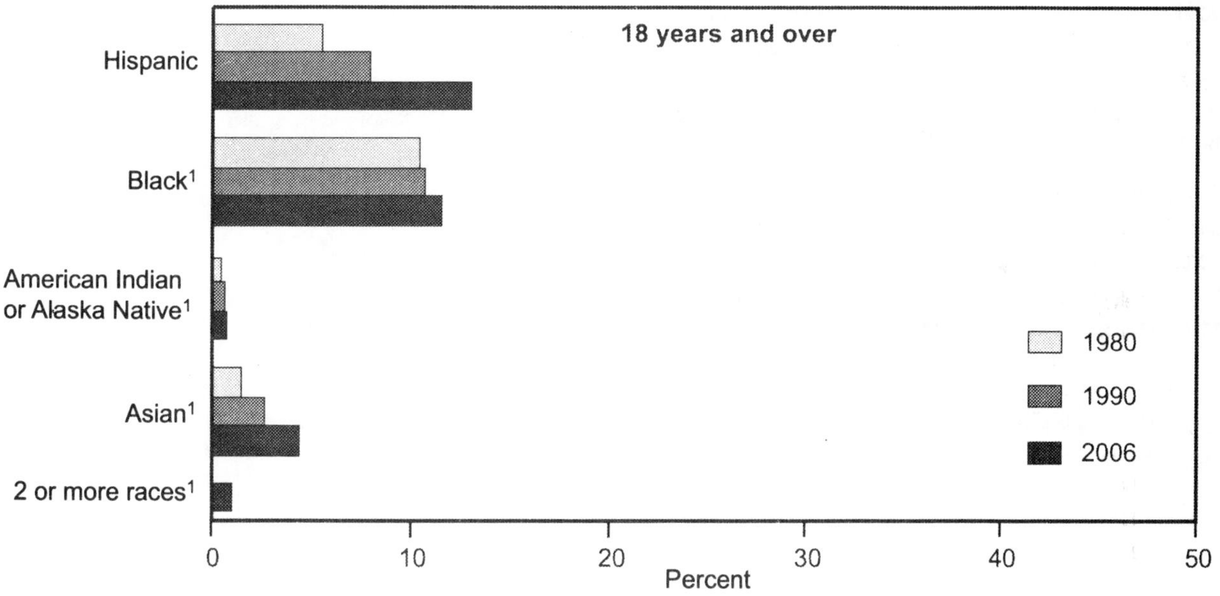

[1]Not Hispanic.

NOTES: Persons of Hispanic origin may be of any race. Race data for 2006 are not directly comparable with data for 1980 and 1990. Individuals could report only one race in 1980 and 1990, and more than one race in 2006. Persons who selected only one race in 2006 are included in single-race categories; persons who selected more than one race in 2006 are shown as having 2 or more races and are not included in single-race categories. In 1980 and 1990, the Asian category included Asian and Native Hawaiian or Other Pacific Islander; in 2006, this category includes only Asian. See data table for Figure 3 for data points graphed and data for Native Hawaiian or Other Pacific Islander.

SOURCE: U.S. Census Bureau.

Poverty

The poverty rate continues to be highest among children under 18 years of age.

Children and adults in families with income below or near the federal poverty level have worse health than those with higher income (see Appendix II, Poverty, for a definition of the federal poverty level). Although in some cases illness can lead to poverty, more often poverty causes poor health by its connection with inadequate nutrition, substandard housing, exposure to environmental hazards, unhealthy lifestyles, and decreased access to and use of health care services (1).

In 2005, the overall percentage of the U.S. population living in poverty was 12.6%, up from 11.3% in 2000 (2). The poverty rate increased for people 65 years of age and over from 2004 to 2005, but declined slightly for other ages (data table for Figure 4).

Starting in 1974, children have been more likely than either working-age or older adults to be living in poverty (Figure 4). In 2005, 13 million children (17.6%) lived in poverty and another 15.6 million children (21.3%) were classified as near-poor with family income of 100% to less than 200% of the poverty level (data table for Figure 5).

Prior to 1974, persons 65 years of age and over were more likely to live in poverty than people of other ages. With the increased benefits provided by government social insurance programs such as Social Security, the poverty rate of older adults declined rapidly until 1974 and continued a gradual decline to a low of 9.7% in 1999 (3). In 2005, 3.6 million persons age 65 years and over or 10.1% of older adults lived in poverty. An additional 9.5 million (26.7%) were near-poor (data table for Figure 5).

Figure 4. Poverty by age: United States, 1966-2005

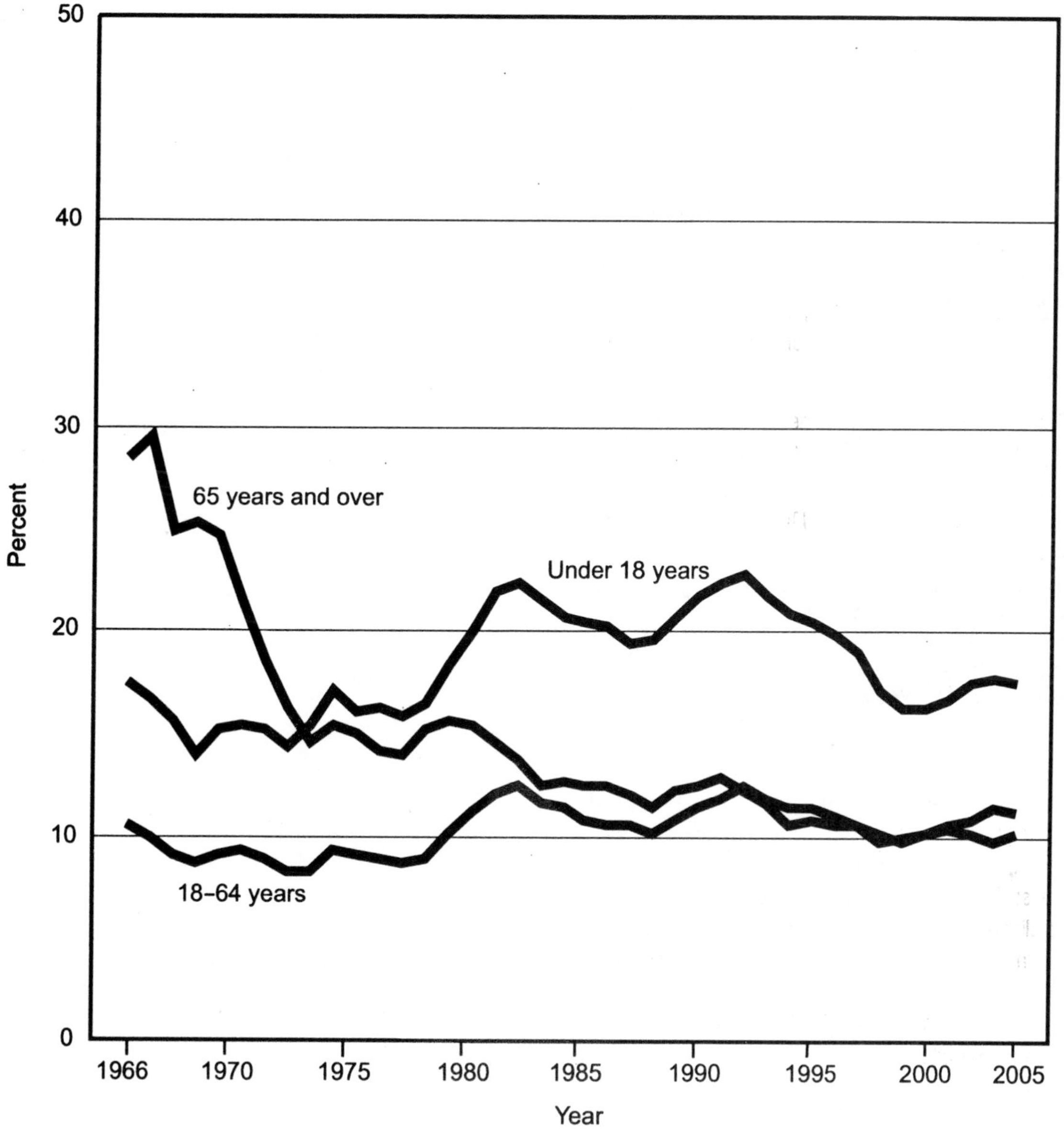

NOTES: Data shown are the percentage of persons with family income below the poverty level. See data table for Figure 4 for data points graphed and additional notes.

SOURCE: U.S. Census Bureau, Current Population Survey.

Poverty *(Continued)*

At all ages, a higher percentage of Hispanic and black persons than non-Hispanic white persons were poor (Figure 5). In 2005, 28%–35% of Hispanic and black children were poor compared with 10%–11% of non-Hispanic white and Asian children. Similarly, among persons 65 years of age and over, almost one-fifth of Hispanic and one-quarter of black persons were poor, compared with 8% of non-Hispanic white persons and 13% of Asians. In 2003–2005, one-quarter of American Indian or Alaska Native persons lived in poverty (estimate based on 3 years of data) (2).

References

1. Pamuk E, Makuc D, Heck K, Reuben C, Lochner K. Socioeconomic Status and Health Chartbook. Health, United States, 1998. Hyattsville, MD: National Center for Health Statistics. 1998.
2. DeNavas-Walt C, Proctor B, Hill LC. Income, poverty, and health insurance coverage in the United States: 2005. Current population reports, series P-60 no 231. Washington, DC: U.S. Government Printing Office. 2006. Available from: www.census.gov/prod/2006pubs/p60–231.pdf.
3. Clark RL, Quinn JF. The economic status of the elderly. Medicare Brief 1999;4:1–12.

Figure 5. Low income by age, race, and Hispanic origin: United States, 2005

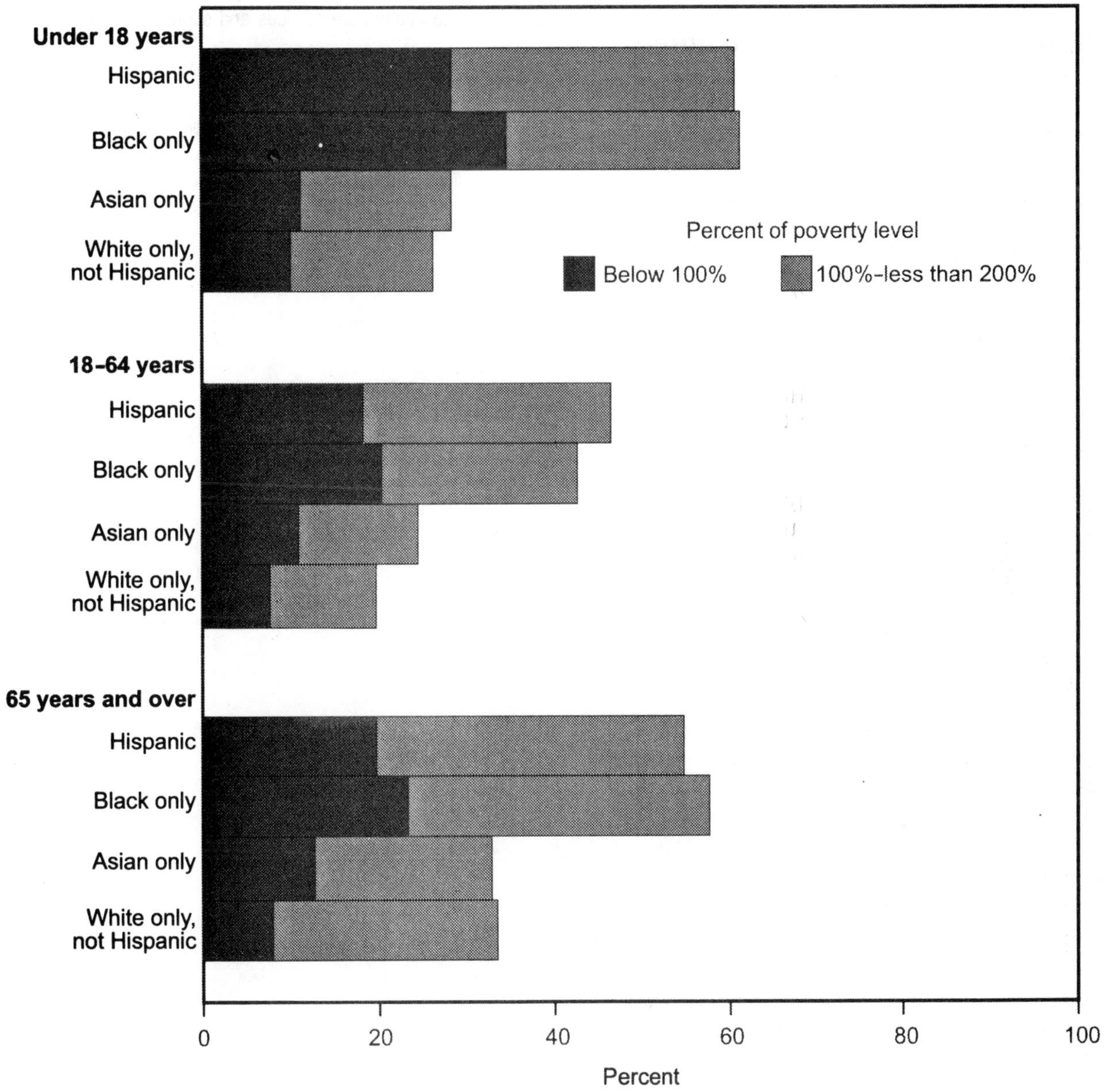

NOTES: Percent of poverty level is based on family income and family size and composition using U.S. Census Bureau poverty thresholds. Persons of Hispanic origin may be of any race. Black and Asian races include persons of Hispanic and non-Hispanic origin. See data table for Figure 5 for data points graphed and additional notes.

SOURCE: U.S. Census Bureau, Current Population Survey.

Health Care Expenditures

Personal Health Care Expenditures

In 2005, the largest shares of personal health care expenditures were paid by private health insurance and the federal government.

In 2005, the United States spent 16% (up from 14% in 2000) of its Gross Domestic Product (GDP) on health care, a greater share than any other developed country for which data are collected by the Organisation of Economic Co-operation and Development (Tables 120 and 121).

In 2005, the United States spent $2 trillion on health care, an average of $6,700 per person (Table 121). Personal health care expenditures, a component of national health expenditures that includes spending for hospital care, physician services, prescription drugs, nursing home care, dental care, and other types of medical care accounted for 84% of national health expenditures in 2005. The remaining 16% was spent on administration, government public health activities, research, and structures and equipment (Table 124) (1).

Overall, private health insurance paid for 36% of total personal health expenditures in 2005, the federal government 34%, state and local government 11%, and out-of-pocket payments accounted for 15% (Figure 6). The share of total expenditures paid out-of-pocket has declined from 27% in 1980 to 15% in 2005 (Table 125). This decline resulted from an expansion of benefits in both private health insurance plans and in government programs. Despite the decline in the share of health care expenditures paid out-of-pocket, the growth in health care costs over recent years means that consumers may still have significant out-of-pocket expenditures for their health care.

In 2005, 37% of personal health care expenditures were for hospital care, 25% for physician care, 12% for prescription drugs, 7% for nursing home care, and the remaining 18% for other personal health care, including visits to nonphysician medical providers, medical supplies, and other health services (Figure 6). The share of total personal health care expenditures devoted to hospital care has declined from 40% in 1980 to 31% in 2005 and the prescription drug expenditure share has doubled from 5% to 10% over the same period, reflecting the shift in health care from inpatient to ambulatory care settings and the increasing contribution of prescription drugs to health care services and spending (Table 124).

Reference

1. Smith C, Cowan C, Heffler S, Catlin A. National health spending in 2005: the slowdown continues. Health Aff (Millwood) 2007;26(1):142–153.

Figure 6. Personal health care expenditures, by source of funds and type of expenditures: United States, 2005

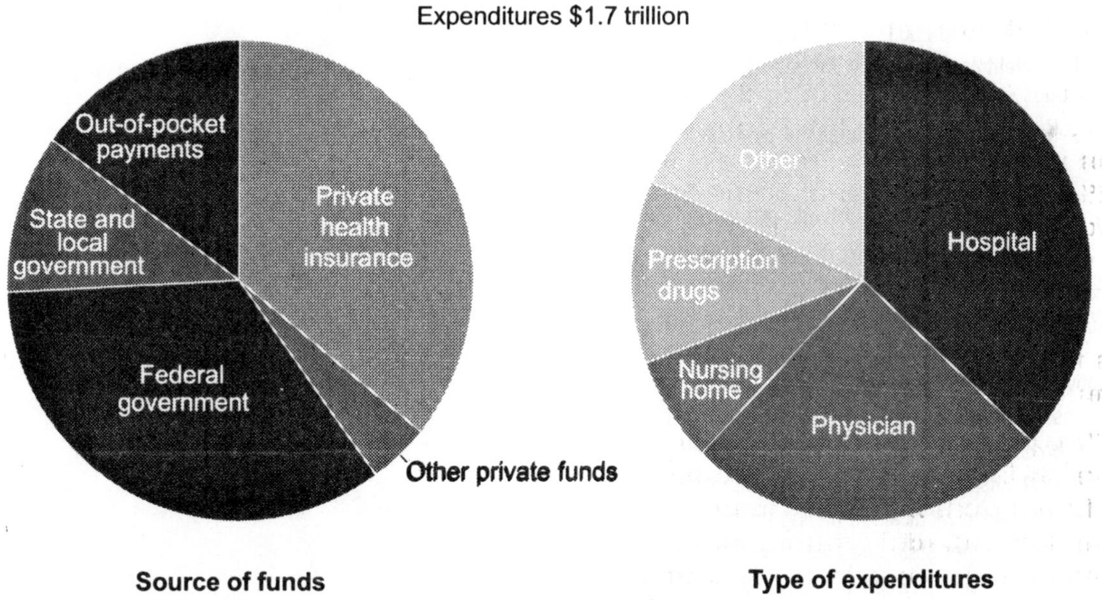

NOTE: See data table for Figure 6 for data points graphed and additional notes.

SOURCE: Centers for Medicare & Medicaid Services, Office of the Actuary, National Health Statistics Group, National Health Expenditure Accounts.

Expenditures for Mental Health Services and Substance Abuse Treatment

Medicaid and private insurance pay the largest shares of mental health expenditures, whereas the largest share of substance abuse expenditures come from other state and local government funds (excluding Medicaid expenditures).

Mental health treatment has often been considered the stepchild of the medical care system with patients reluctant to use these services and insurers reluctant to pay for them. Estimates from a survey covering the years 2001 to 2003 found that about 30% of people 18–54 years of age suffered from a mental disorder during the year, yet only one-third of them received treatment (1).

A recent report estimated mental health services and substance abuse treatment (MHSA) expenditures from 1986 to 2003 (2). Combined expenditures for these services accounted for 7.5% of national health expenditures ($121 billion) in 2003. The MHSA expenditures have grown at a slower rate than overall health expenditures since 1986 (2), despite an increase in the number of people treated (1). Inflation-adjusted expenditures on mental health services doubled between 1986 and 2003, while expenditures on substance abuse treatment increased by one-half during this same period (data tables for Figures 7 and 8). From 1986 to 2003 national health expenditures increased by nearly two and one-half times (3).

The relative importance of sources of funds differed between mental health services and substance abuse treatment. By 2003, Medicaid accounted for the largest share of mental health services expenditures (26%), up from 16% in 1986 (Figure 7). Starting in 1998, Medicaid surpassed other state and local government funding as the largest payer for mental health services. Other state and local government payments cover mental health programs run by state, county, and municipal governments. Since 2001, private health insurance has been second behind Medicaid in paying for mental health services, followed by other state and local government expenditures, out-of-pocket payments, and Medicare.

Figure 7. National expenditures for mental health services, by source of funds: United States, 1986–2003

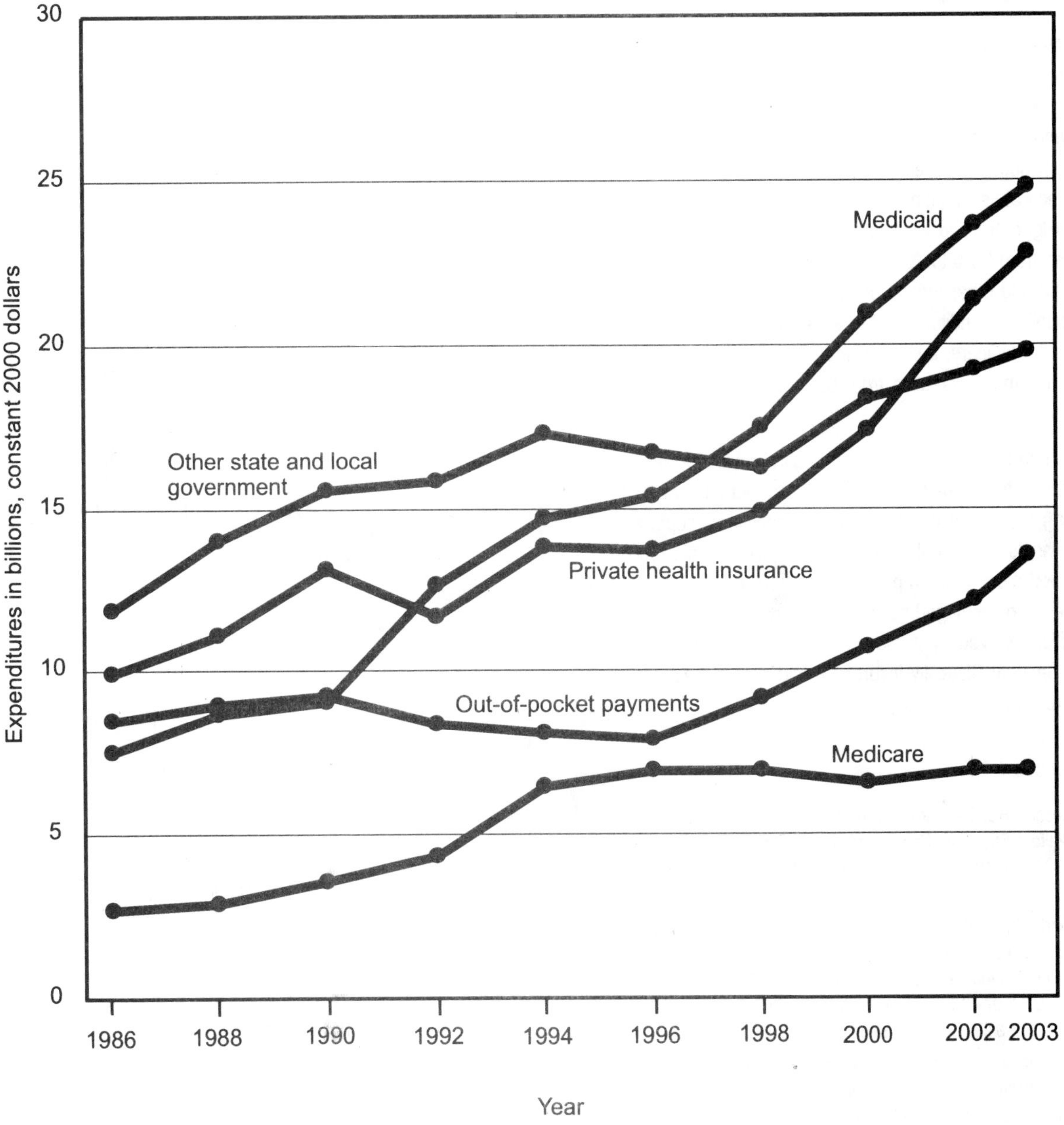

NOTES: Estimates have been inflation-adjusted to 2000 U.S. dollars using the Gross Domestic Product implicit price deflator developed by the U.S. Department of Commerce, Bureau of Economic Analysis. Excludes other private funding and other federal government expenditures, which combined are 7% of total mental health expenditures in 2003. See data table for Figure 7 for data points graphed and additional notes.

SOURCE: Substance Abuse and Mental Health Services Administration.

Expenditures for Mental Health Services and Substance Abuse Treatment *(Continued)*

In contrast, other state and local government funds have paid the largest share of substance abuse treatment expenditures since 1987, and that share has grown steadily. In 2003, other state and local government payments (not including the state share of Medicaid expenditures) accounted for 40% of substance abuse treatment expenditures, up from 29% in 1986 (Figure 8). The share of private health insurance declined from 30% to 10% during this time while the share of Medicaid and other federal government funding increased. Total public expenditures (other state and local government, Medicaid, Medicare, and other federal sources) for substance abuse treatment increased from 50% of total expenditures in 1986 to 77% in 2003.

Changes in the funding of mental health services and substance abuse treatment resulted from many factors including population growth; increased societal acceptance of mental health treatment; more effective psychotropic drugs prescribed more often in primary care settings; the emergence of managed health care; expansions in populations served by public programs such as Medicaid and Social Security Disability Insurance; and cost containment measures (2).

References

1 Kessler RC, Demler O, Frank RG, Olfson M, Pincus HA, Walters EE, et al. Prevalence and treatment of mental disorders, 1990 to 2003. N Engl J Med 2005;352(24):3095–105.

2. Mark TL, Levit KL, Coffey RM, McKusick DR, Harwood H, King E, et al. National expenditures for mental health services and substance abuse treatment, 1993–2003. SAMHSA pub. no. SMA 07–4227. Rockville, MD: Substance Abuse and Mental Health Services Administration, 2007.

3. Calculated using the gross domestic product implicit price deflator from Table 126 and national health expenditure estimates from the Centers for Medicare & Medicaid Services. Available from: www.cms.gov/NationalHealthExpendData/downloads/nhegdp05.zip.

Figure 8. National expenditures for substance abuse treatment, by source of funds: United States, 1986–2003

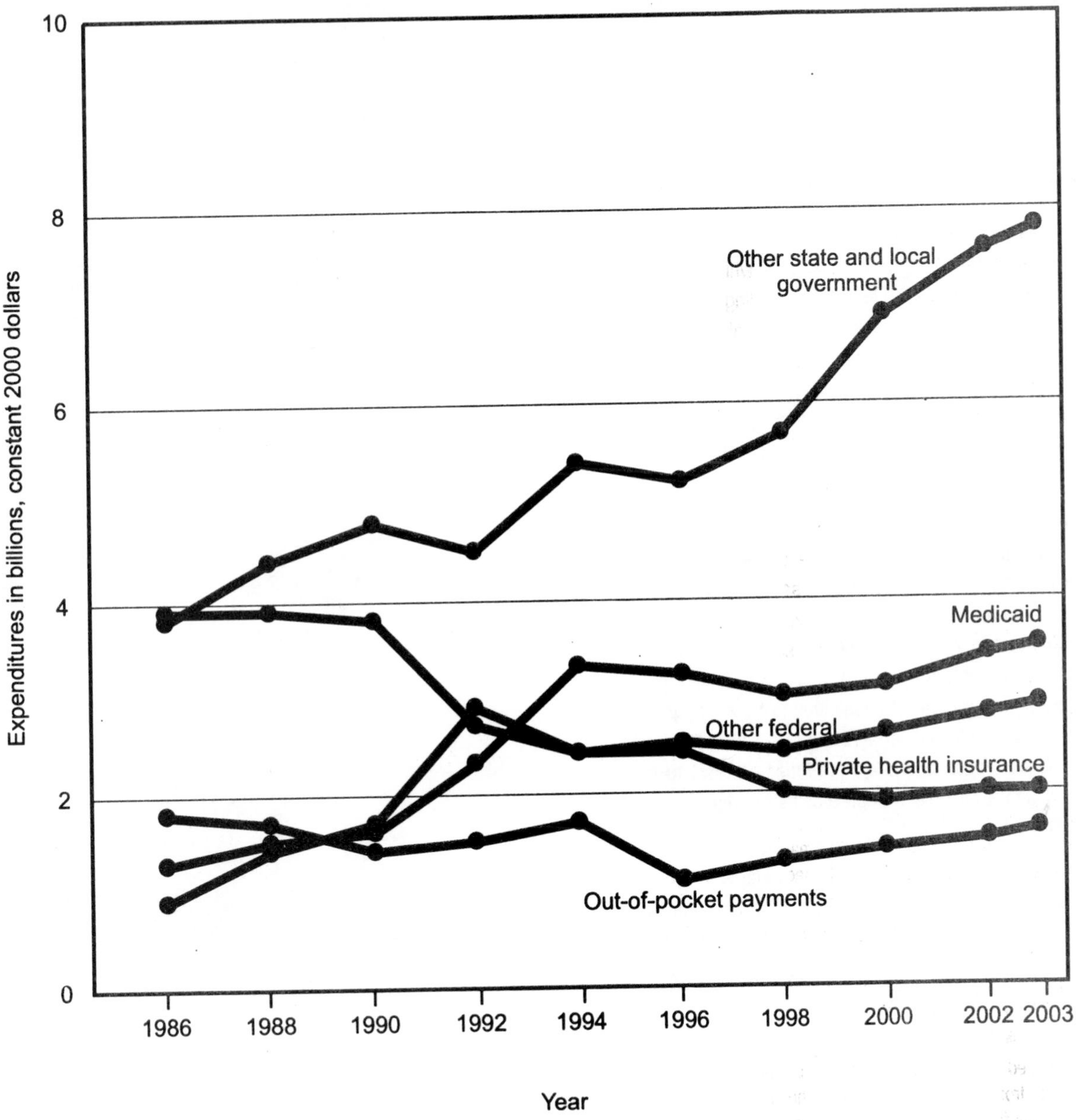

NOTES: Estimates have been inflation-adjusted to 2000 U.S. dollars using the Gross Domestic Product implicit price deflator developed by the U.S. Department of Commerce, Bureau of Economic Analysis. Not shown are other private funding and Medicare expenditures, which combined are 9% of total substance abuse treatment expenditures in 2003. See data table for Figure 8 for data points graphed and additional notes.

SOURCE: Substance Abuse and Mental Health Services Administration.

Health Risk Factors

Cigarette Smoking

Fewer Americans are smoking cigarettes, but nearly one-fifth of women and one-quarter of men and high school students still are current cigarette smokers, as are 10% of pregnant women.

Smoking is associated with a significantly increased risk of heart disease, stroke, lung and other types of cancer, and chronic lung diseases (1). Decreasing cigarette smoking among adolescents and adults is a major public health objective for the Nation. Preventing smoking among teenagers and young adults is critical because smoking usually begins in adolescence (2). Smoking during pregnancy contributes to elevated risk of miscarriage, premature delivery, and having a low birthweight infant (3).

Following the first Surgeon General's Report on smoking in 1964, cigarette smoking declined sharply for men and at a slower pace for women (Figure 9). The percentage of men and women who smoke declined more slowly between 1990 and 2004, and in 2005 the proportion did not change (4). In 2005, 23% of men and 18% of women were smokers. Cigarette smoking by adults continues to be strongly associated with educational attainment. Adults with less than a high school education were three times as likely to smoke as those with a bachelor's degree or more education (Table 64).

Cigarette smoking among high school students in grades 9–12 decreased between 1997 and 2003 after increasing in the early 1990s. In 2005, 23% of high school students had smoked cigarettes in the past month, 14% had smoked cigars, and 8% had used smokeless tobacco (5).

Among mothers with a live birth, the percentage reporting on the birth certificate that they smoked cigarettes during pregnancy declined between 1989 and 2004 from 20% to 10%. Maternal smoking has declined for all racial and ethnic groups, but differences among these groups persist (Table 12).

References:

1. U.S. Department of Health and Human Services. The health consequences of smoking: A report of the Surgeon General. Atlanta, GA: Centers for Disease Control and Prevention; 2004. Available from: www.cdc.gov/tobacco/sgr/sgr_2004/index.htm.
2. U.S. Department of Health and Human Services. Preventing tobacco use among young people: A report of the Surgeon General. Atlanta, GA: Centers for Disease Control and Prevention; 1994. Available from: www.cdc.gov/tobacco/sgr/sgr_1994/.
3. Mathews TJ. Smoking during pregnancy in the 1990s. National vital statistics reports 2001; vol 49 no 7. Hyattsville, MD: National Center for Health Statistics. 2001. Available from: www.cdc.gov/nchs/data/nvsr/nvsr49/nvsr49_07.pdf.
4. CDC. Tobacco use among adults—United States, 2005. MMWR 2006;55(42):1145–48. Available from: www.cdc.gov/mmwr/preview/mmwrhtml/mm5542a1.htm.
5. CDC. Youth Risk Behavior Surveillance—United States, 2005. MMWR 2006;55(SS-5):1–33. Available from: www.cdc.gov/mmwr/PDF/ss/ss5505.pdf.

Figure 9. Cigarette smoking among men, women, high school students, and mothers during pregnancy: United States, 1965–2005

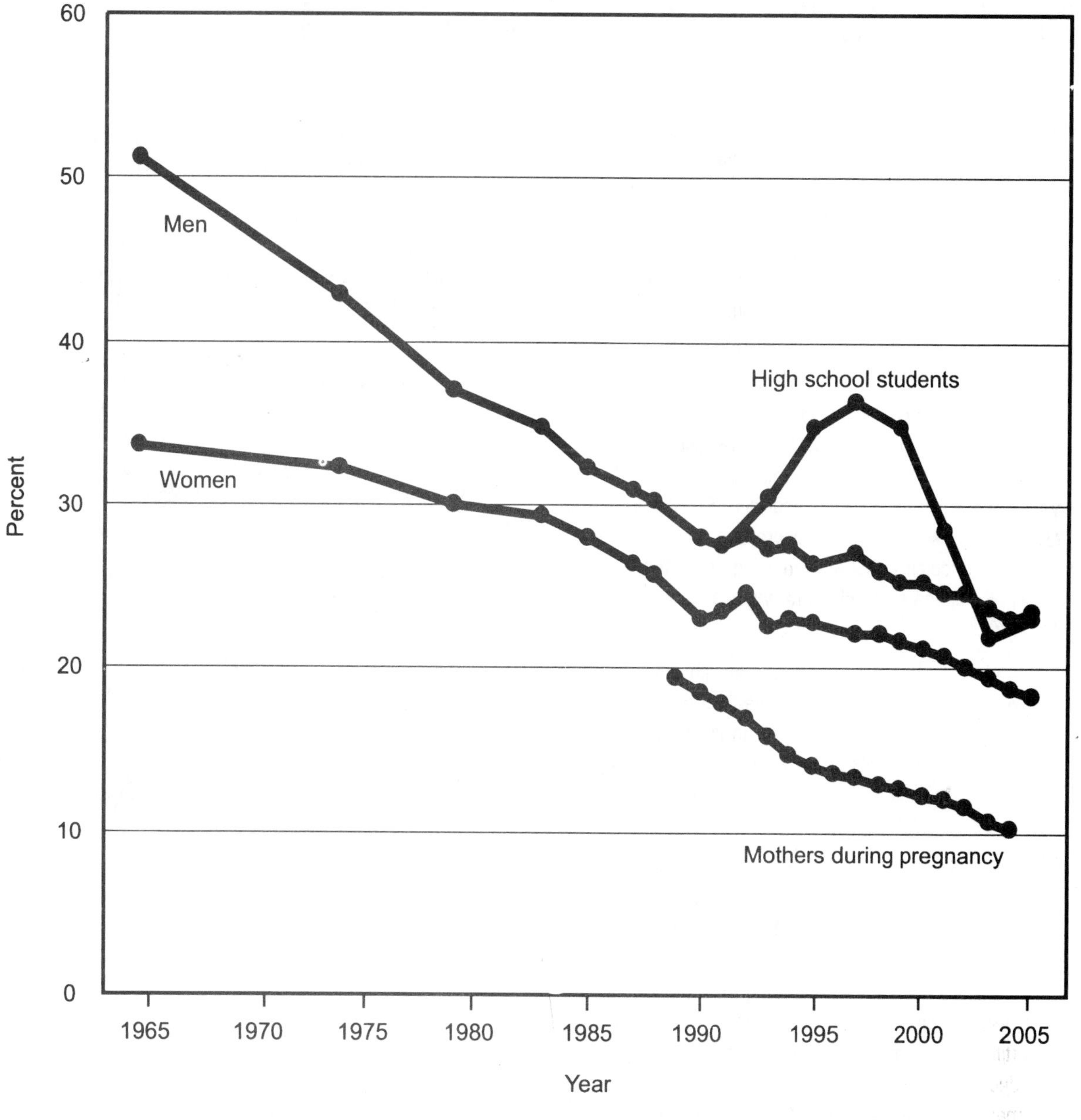

NOTES: Estimates for men and women are age-adjusted. Cigarette smoking is defined as: (for men and women 18 years and over) at least 100 cigarettes in lifetime and now smoke every day or some days; (for students in grades 9-12) 1 or more cigarettes in the 30 days preceding the survey; and (for mothers with a live birth) during pregnancy. See data table for Figure 9 for data points graphed, standard errors, and additional notes.

SOURCES: Centers for Disease Control and Prevention, National Center for Health Statistics, National Health Interview Survey (data for men and women); National Vital Statistics System (data for mothers during pregnancy); National Center for Chronic Disease Prevention and Health Promotion, Youth Risk Behavior Survey (data for high school students).

Blood Cotinine Levels in Children

Children living below or near the poverty level are more likely to have high blood cotinine levels than children living in higher income families.

Secondhand tobacco smoke exposure or environmental tobacco smoke (ETS) is an important and preventable cause of morbidity among children. Children exposed to ETS are at an increased risk for acute lower respiratory tract infections, asthma induction and exacerbation, and middle-ear infections (1). The primary source of children's exposure to ETS is in the home (2). In 1992, the Environmental Protection Agency classified ETS as a Group A carcinogen known to cause cancer in humans (1).

Cotinine, a breakdown product of nicotine, is a marker for exposure to secondhand smoke (3,4). Heavy exposure to ETS usually produces blood cotinine levels above 1.0 ng/ml (defined as high cotinine level in this analysis) (5). Higher cotinine levels are associated with an increased prevalence of respiratory health problems such as wheezing apart from colds among all children and asthma for younger children 4–6 years of age (6).

The percentage of children 4–17 years of age with any detectable blood cotinine levels (at or above 0.05 ng/ml) decreased from 84% in 1988–1994 to 57% in 2001–2004 (Figure 10). High cotinine levels (more than 1.0 ng/ml) among children 4–17 years of age decreased from 23% in 1988–1994 to 17% in 2001–2004.

Children living below or near the poverty level are more likely to have high blood cotinine levels than children living in higher income families. In 2001–2004, children living below 200% of poverty were more than twice as likely to have had a high blood cotinine level as children living in higher income families (22%–28% compared with 10%) (Figure 10). Some studies indicate that factors such as less spacious housing, including fewer rooms in the home, and low parental education are among the many predictors of high cotinine levels in children (6,7). Such factors are more common in lower-income households.

High blood cotinine level varies by race and ethnicity. In 2001–2004, children of Mexican origin had the lowest rate of high blood cotinine levels at 5%, compared with non-Hispanic black children (22%) and non-Hispanic white children (19%) (data table for Figure 10).

References

1. U.S. Environmental Protection Agency. Respiratory health effects of passive smoking: Lung cancer and other disorders. Washington, DC: U.S. Environmental Protection Agency, 1992; pub. no. EPA/600/6–90/006F.
2. CDC. State-specific prevalence of cigarette smoking among adults, and children's and adolescents' exposure to environmental tobacco smoke—United States, 1996. MMWR 1997;46(44):1038–43.
3. U.S. Department of Health and Human Services. The health consequences of involuntary exposure to tobacco smoke: A report of the surgeon general. Atlanta, GA. 2006.
4. Federal Interagency Forum on Child and Family Statistics. America's children: Key national indicators of well-being, 2005. Washington, DC: U.S. Government Printing Office. 2005.
5. Centers for Disease Control and Prevention. Third national report on human exposure to environmental chemicals. 2005. Available from: www.cdc.gov.exposurereport/report.htm.
6. Mannino DM, Moorman JE, Kingsley B, et al. Health effects related to environmental tobacco smoke exposure in children in the United States: Data from the Third National Health and Nutrition Examination Survey. Arch Pediatr Adolesc Med 2001;155:36–41.
7. Wilson SE, Kahn RS, Khoury J, et al. Racial differences in exposure to environmental tobacco smoke among children. Environmental Health Perspectives 2005;113(3):362–7.

Figure 10. Blood cotinine levels among children 4–17 years of age, by percent of poverty level: United States, 1988–1994 and 2001–2004

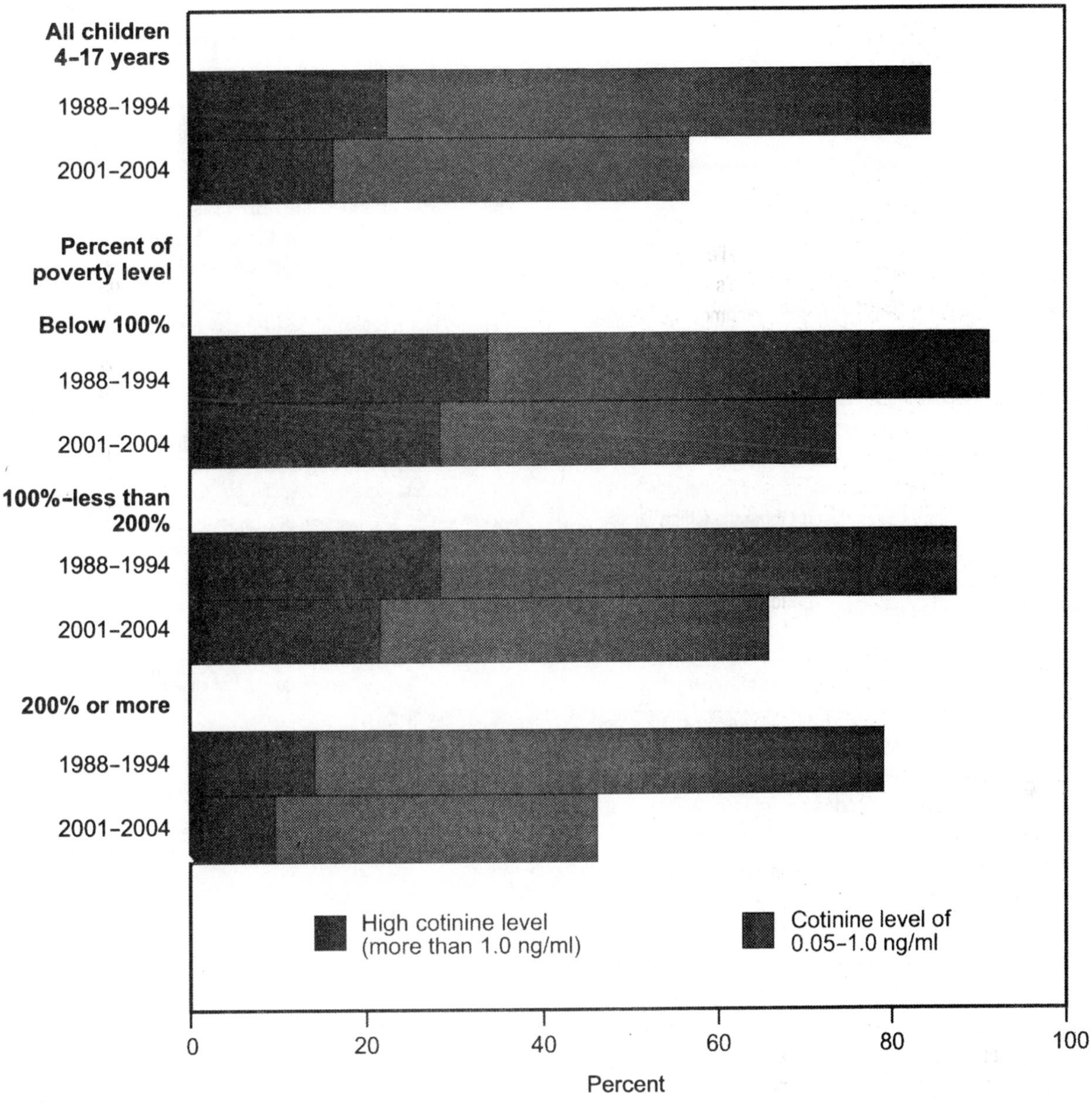

NOTES: Cotinine levels are for nonsmoking children only. Percent of poverty level is based on family income and family size and composition using U.S. Census Bureau poverty thresholds. See data table for Figure 10 for data points graphed, standard errors, and additional notes.

SOURCE: Centers for Disease Control and Prevention, National Centers for Health Statistics, National Health and Nutrition Examination Survey.

Alcohol-Related Emergency Department Visits: Adolescents and Young Adults

During 2002–2004, there were on average each year, more than 230,000 alcohol-related emergency department visits among underage adolescents 14–20 years of age.

Alcohol is the most widely used drug among youth (1). Alcohol use causes serious and potentially life-threatening problems for adolescents and young adults. Research indicates that drinking is associated with risk-taking and sensation-seeking behavior, and alcohol has disinhibiting effects that may increase the likelihood of unsafe activities. In 1984, the Uniform Drinking Age Act was enacted that mandated reduced federal transportation funds to those states that did not raise the minimum legal drinking age to 21, and by 1988 all states had increased the legal drinking age to 21 years (2). In 2007, the U.S. Surgeon General's Office issued a *Call to Action* against underage drinking, which has remained at consistently high levels (3). Currently, there are approximately 11 million underage drinkers in the U.S.

The National Hospital Ambulatory Medical Care Survey (NHAMCS) collects data on visits to hospital emergency departments (ED). In this analysis, an emergency department visit was considered alcohol-related based on a review of the ED record including the patient's reasons for the ED visit, and the diagnoses and the injury codes recorded (see Technical Notes for detailed information related to the definition of an alcohol-related visit). Because alcohol can be a contributing or underlying cause of ED visits, different algorithms for identifying alcohol-related ED visits exist (4). Our analysis uses a conservative approach to identify alcohol-related ED visits.

During 2002–2004, there were, on average each year, more than 230,000 alcohol-related ED visits among underage adolescents 14–20 years of age (data table for Figure 11). Alcohol-related ED visits among underage adolescents accounted for 2% of all ED visits for this age group (5).

Alcohol-related ED visit rates differed by sex and age, for both underage and legal drinkers (Figure 11). Visit rates among males were higher than among their female counterparts in every age group except for adolescents 18–20 years of age. Alcohol-related ED visit rates increased with age from early to late adolescence and then remained at that level through young adulthood (data table for Figure 11). In 2002–2004, rates for older male adolescents 18–20 years of age were more than twice those of male adolescents 14–17 years of age and rates for older female adolescents were more than three times those of younger female adolescents. Alcohol-related ED visit rates did not differ significantly between young adults who had reached legal drinking age and late adolescent drinkers 18–20 years of age.

Most (89%) alcohol-related ED visits resulted in patients being treated and released from the ED, 5% were admitted to inpatient units, and a small number of patients were transferred to other health facilities, left before being seen, or left against medical advice (5).

References

1. Substance Abuse and Mental Health Services Administration. Consequences of underage alcohol use. Available from: ncadi.samhsa.gov/govpubs/rpo992/.
2. French MT, Maclean JC. Underage alcohol use, delinquency, and criminal activity. Health Economics 2006;15:1261–81.
3. U.S. Department of Health and Human Services. The Surgeon General's call to prevent and reduce underage drinking. U.S. Department of Health and Human Services, Office of the Surgeon General, 2007. Available from: www.surgeongeneral.gov/topics/underagedrinking/calltoaction.pdf.
4. McDonald AJ, Wang N, Camargo CA. U.S. emergency department visits for alcohol-related diseases and injuries between 1992 and 2000. Arch Int Med 2004;164:531–7.
5. National Center for Health Statistics, National Hospital Ambulatory Medical Care Survey, unpublished analysis.

Figure 11. Alcohol-related emergency department (ED) visit rates among persons 14–28 years of age, by age and sex: United States, 2002–2004

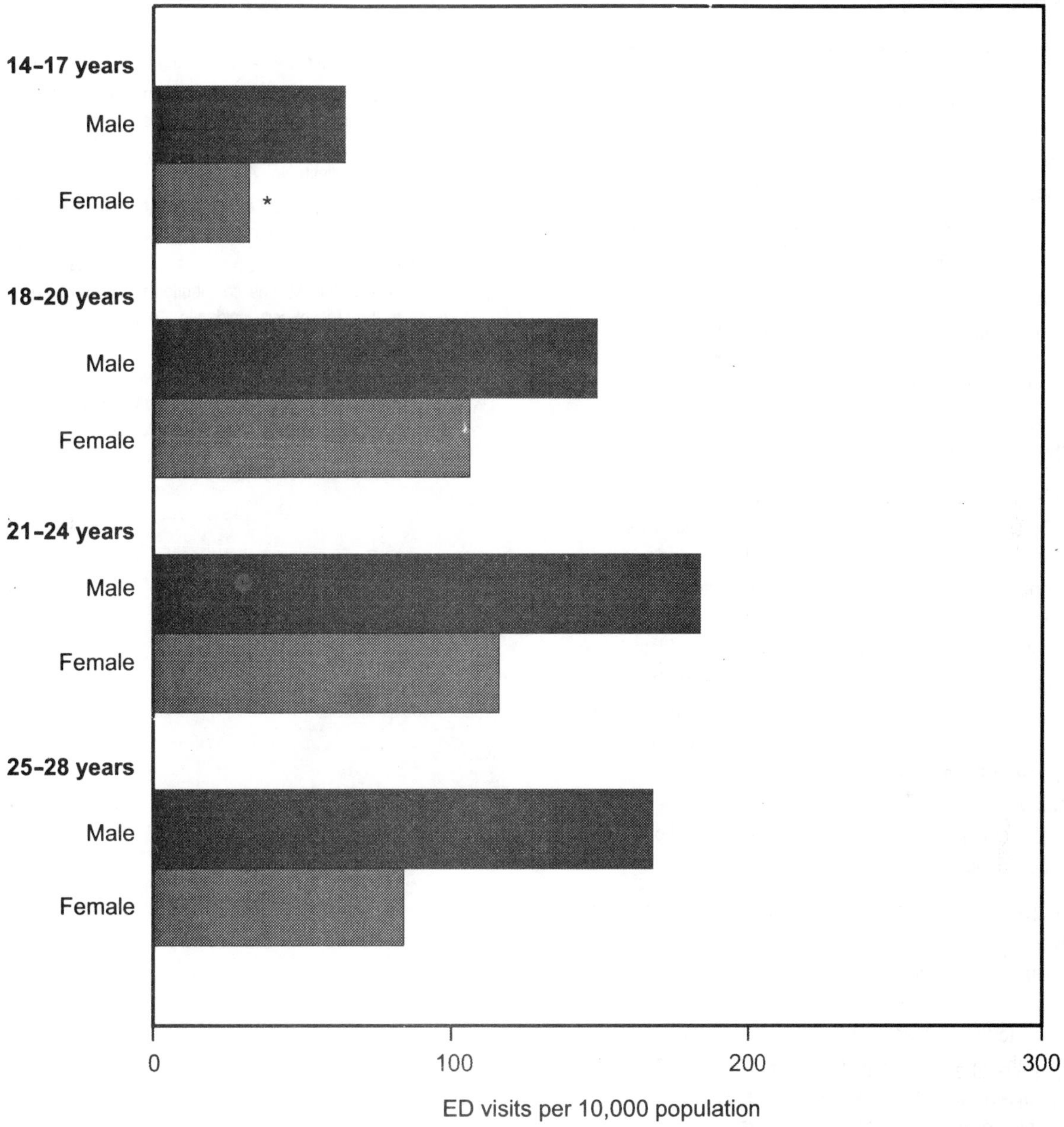

* Estimates are considered unreliable. Data shown with an asterisk have a relative standard error of 20%–30%.

NOTES: An emergency department visit was considered alcohol-related if the checkbox for alcohol was indicated, the physician's diagnoses (any-listed) were alcohol-related, alcohol-related external cause-of-injury codes were present, or the patient's reasons for visit were alcohol-related. See data table for Figure 11 for data points graphed, standard errors, and additional notes.

SOURCE: Centers for Disease Control and Prevention, National Center for Health Statistics, National Hospital Ambulatory Medical Care Survey.

Frequency of Restaurant Meals

Over one-half of Americans reported eating an average of one to three restaurant meals weekly.

Between 1972 and 2004, the number of food service establishments in the United States nearly doubled from 491,000 to 878,000 (1). In 2004, spending on food away from home, including restaurant meals, catered affairs, and food on out-of-town trips accounted for 42% of average annual food expenditures compared with 26% in 1970 (2,3).

Although away-from-home meals can be healthy, research has shown that, on average, they are higher in overall calories, fat, saturated fat, and sodium content than foods eaten at home (3,4). Restaurant meal portion sizes tend to be larger than at home portion sizes and have been increasing over the past 30 years (5).

In 1999–2004, frequency of restaurant meal consumption varied by age (Figure 12). Restaurant meals included meals eaten at eat-in restaurants, carryout restaurants, and restaurants that deliver food (see Technical Notes). Adults 65 years and older were least likely to consume restaurant meals, whereas 18–24 year olds were most likely (data table for Figure 12). Although children 1–12 years of age had the lowest percentage of eating four or more restaurant meals a week (9%), this group had one of the highest percentages of eating one to three restaurant meals a week (63%). Restaurant meal consumption was consistently higher among males and among individuals with family income above 200% of the poverty level (6).

The frequent consumption of restaurant meals, coupled with the overall poor nutritional profile of these foods, has coincided with the significant increase in the percentage of Americans who are obese (Figure 13). Several factors contribute to the frequent consumption of restaurant meals including the high percentage of women employed outside the home, smaller households, and the increased supply of restaurants, including the proliferation of relatively inexpensive fast-food restaurants (3,4).

References

1. The Keystone Center. The Keystone Forum on away-from-home foods: Opportunities for preventing weight gain and obesity. Final Report. May, 2006.
2. U.S. Department of Labor, U.S. Bureau of Labor Statistics. Consumer expenditures in 2004. Report 992, April 2006.
3. Lin BH, Guthrie J, Frazao E. Away-from-home foods increasingly important to quality of American diet. Economic Research Service, U.S. Department of Agriculture, Agriculture Information Bulletin No. 749; 1999.
4. Kant AK, Graubard BI. Eating out in America, 1987–2000: Trends and nutritional correlates. Preventive Medicine 2004;38:243–9.
5. Young LR, Nestle M. The contribution of expanding portion sizes to the U.S. obesity epidemic. Am J Public Health 2002;92:246–9.
6. Centers for Disease Control and Prevention, National Center for Health Statistics, National Health and Nutrition Examination Survey, unpublished analysis.

Figure 12. Weekly restaurant meal consumption among people 1 year of age and over, by age: United States, 1999-2004

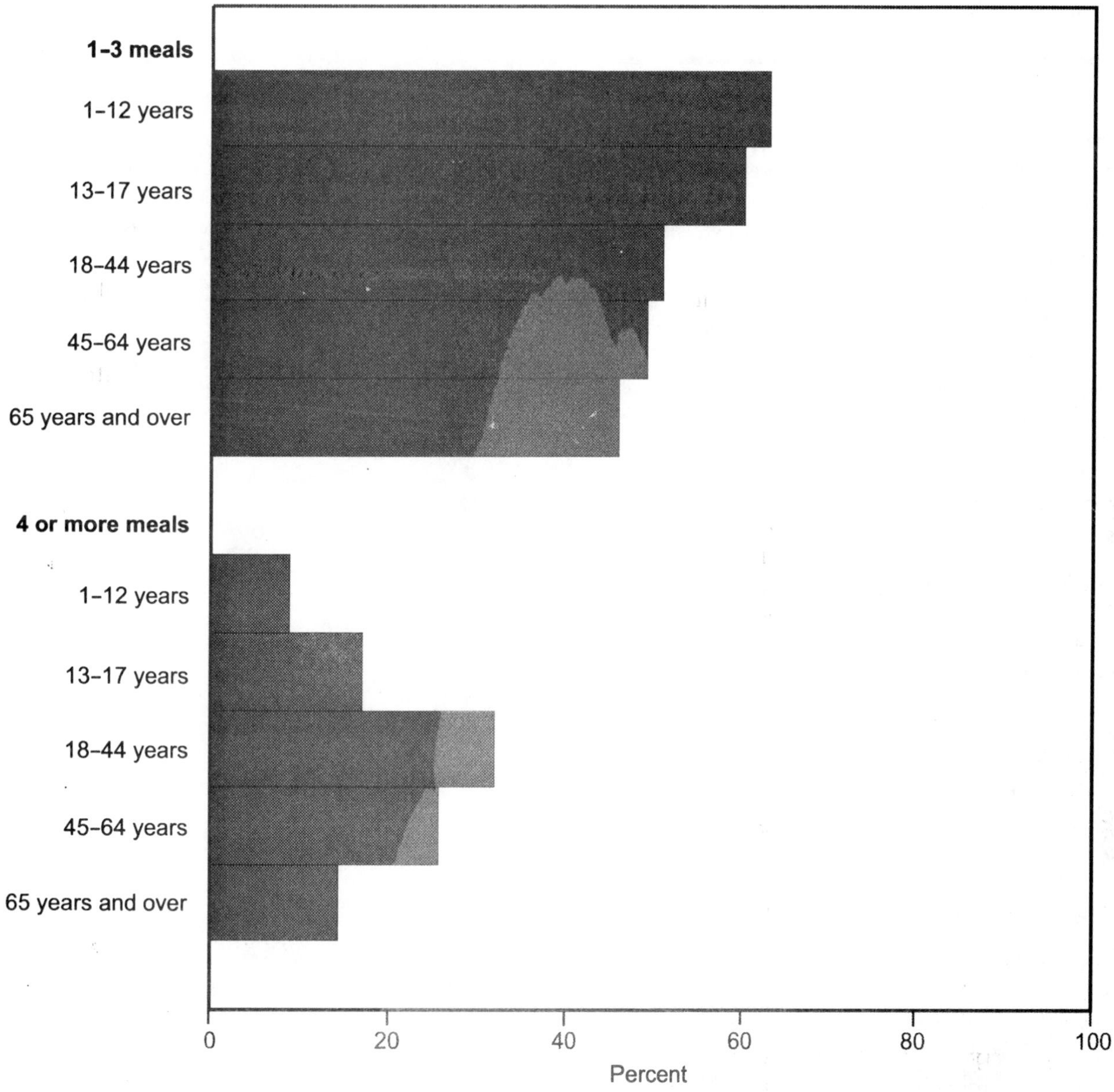

NOTES: Data for children 1–15 years of age are collected from proxy respondents. Data for persons 16 years of age and over are self-reported. Restaurant meals include meals eaten at eat-in restaurants, carry-out restaurants, and restaurants that deliver food. See data table for Figure 12 for data points graphed, standard errors, and additional notes.

SOURCE: Centers for Disease Control and Prevention, National Center for Health Statistics, National Health and Nutrition Examination Survey.

Overweight and Obesity

Two-thirds of American adults are overweight and one-third are obese.

Surplus body weight is associated with excess morbidity and mortality (1). Among adults, overweight and obesity are associated with an elevated risk of heart disease, diabetes, and some types of cancer. Overweight and obesity also increase the severity of disease associated with hypertension, arthritis, and other musculoskeletal problems (2). Additionally, overweight has serious health consequences among younger persons. Among children and adolescents, overweight is associated with an increased risk of high cholesterol, liver abnormalities, diabetes, and becoming an overweight adult (3). Diet, physical inactivity, genetic factors, environment, and health conditions all contribute to overweight in children and adults. The potential health benefits from reduction in the prevalence of overweight and obesity are of significant public health importance.

The prevalence of overweight and obesity changed little between the early 1960s and 1976–1980 (Figure 13). Findings from the 1988–1994 and 1999–2004 National Health and Nutrition Examination Surveys, however, showed substantial increases in overweight among adults. The upward trend in overweight since 1980 reflects primarily an increase in the percentage of adults 20–74 years of age who are obese. In 2003–2004, 67% of adults in that age group were overweight (includes obese); 34% of adults 20–74 years of age were obese (age-adjusted). Since 1960–1962, the percentage of adults who were overweight but not obese has remained steady at 32%–34% (age-adjusted).

The percentage of children (6–11 years of age) and adolescents (12–19 years of age) who are overweight has risen since 1976–1980. In 2003–2004, 17%–19% of children and adolescents were overweight. The percentage of preschool-age children (2–5 years of age) who are overweight almost doubled from 1988–1994 (7%) to 2003–2004 (14%).

The prevalence of obesity varies among adults by sex, race, and ethnicity (Table 74). In 2001–2004, 30% of men and 34% of women 20–74 years of age were obese (age-adjusted). The prevalence of obesity among women differed significantly by racial and ethnic group (among the groups presented). In 2001–2004, one-half of non-Hispanic black women were obese compared with nearly one-third of non-Hispanic white women. In contrast, the prevalence of obesity among men was similar by race and ethnicity.

References

1. National Institutes of Health. Clinical guidelines on the identification, evaluation, and treatment of overweight and obesity in adults: The evidence report. NIH pub. no. 98–4083. 1998. Available from: www.nhlbi.nih.gov/guidelines/obesity/ob_gdlns.htm.
2. U.S. Department of Health and Human Services. The Surgeon General's call to action to prevent and decrease overweight and obesity. Rockville, MD: U.S. Department of Health and Human Services; 2001. Available from: www.surgeongeneral.gov/topics/obesity/.
3. Dietz WH. Health consequences of obesity in youth: Childhood predictors of adult disease. Pediatrics 1998;101(3 Pt 2):518–25.

Figure 13. Overweight and obesity, by age: United States, 1960–2004

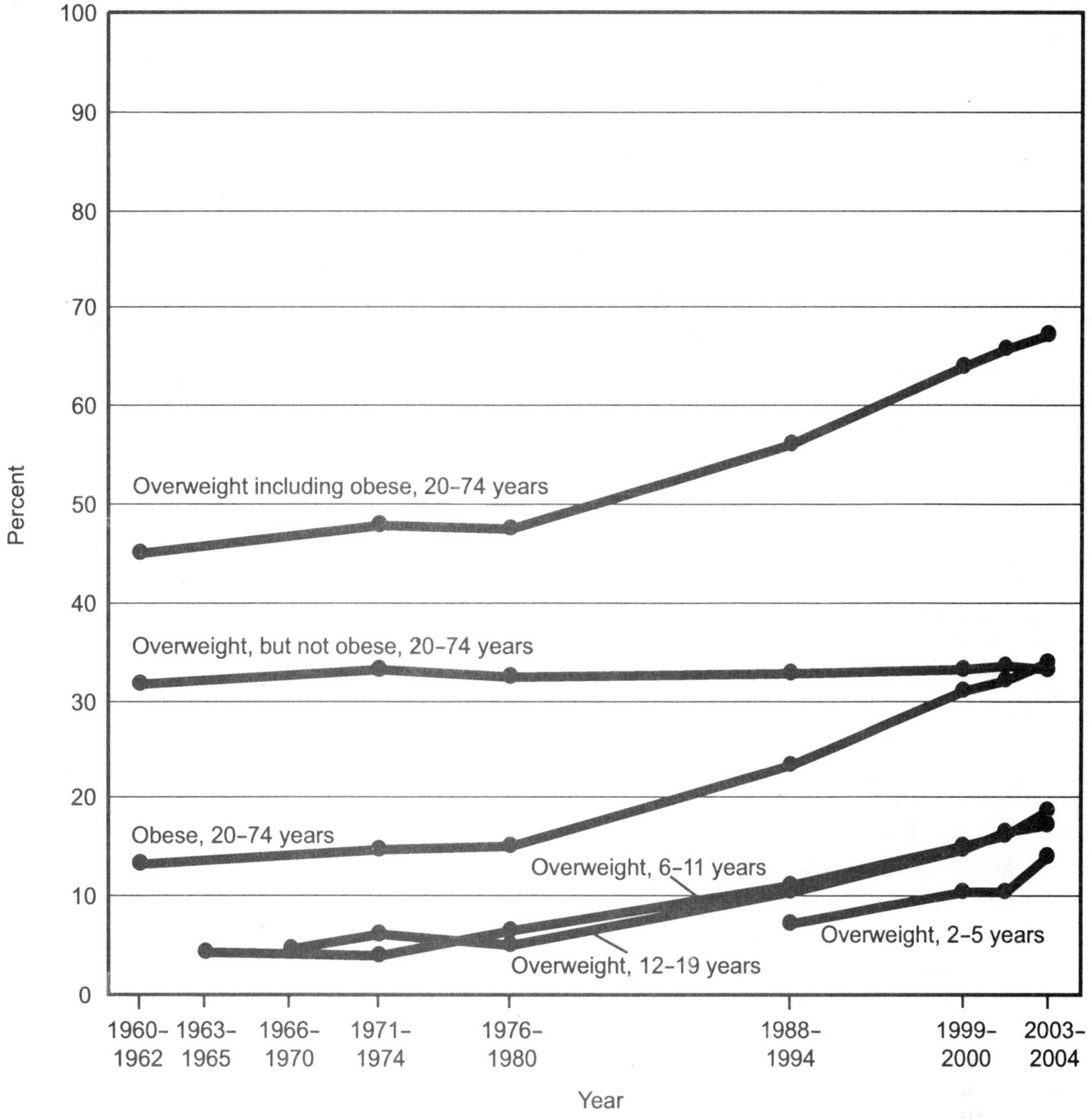

NOTES: Estimates for adults are age-adjusted. For adults: overweight including obese is defined as a body mass index (BMI) greater than or equal to 25, overweight but not obese as a BMI greater than or equal to 25 but less than 30, and obese as a BMI greater than or equal to 30. For children: overweight is defined as a BMI at or above the sex- and age-specific 95th percentile BMI cut points from the 2000 CDC Growth Charts: United States. Obese is not defined for children. See data table for Figure 13 for data points graphed, standard errors, and additional notes.

SOURCES: Centers for Disease Control and Prevention, National Center for Health Statistics, National Health Examination Survey and National Health and Nutrition Examination Survey.

Morbidity and Limitation of Activity

Limitation of Activity Due to Chronic Conditions: Children

Conditions associated with learning, emotional, and behavioral problems are leading causes of activity limitation among children.

Limitation of activity due to chronic physical, mental, or emotional conditions is a broad measure of health and functioning that gauges a child's ability to engage in major age-appropriate activities and is related to a child's need for special educational and medical services. The National Health Interview Survey identifies children with activity limitation through questions about specific limitations in activities such as play, self-care, walking, memory, and other activities, and the current use of special education or early intervention services. Estimates of the number of children with an activity limitation may differ depending on the type of limitations included and the methods used to identify them (1).

Between 1997 and 2005, the percentage of children with activity limitation was 7% (Table 58). In 2004–2005, the percentage of school-age children with activity limitation (8%) was double the percentage of preschoolers with activity limitation (4%) primarily due to the large number of school-age children who were identified as limited solely by their participation in special education (2).

In 2004–2005, chronic health conditions causing activity limitation in children varied by age (Figure 14). Speech problems, mental retardation, and asthma were the leading causes of activity limitation among preschool children. Learning disability and Attention Deficit/Hyperactivity Disorder (ADHD or ADD) were reported as leading causes of activity limitation among all school-age children. Among younger school-age children, speech problems were also a leading cause of activity limitation, and among older school-age children, other mental, emotional, and behavioral problems were an additional important cause.

References

1. Newacheck PW, Strickland B, Shonkoff JP, et al. An epidemiologic profile of children with special health care needs. Pediatrics 1998;102(1):117–23.
2. Federal Interagency Forum on Child and Family Statistics. America's children: Key national indicators of well-being, 2007. Washington, DC: U.S. Government Printing Office; 2007. Available from: www.childstats.gov/.

Figure 14. Limitation of activity caused by selected chronic health conditions among children, by age: United States, 2004–2005

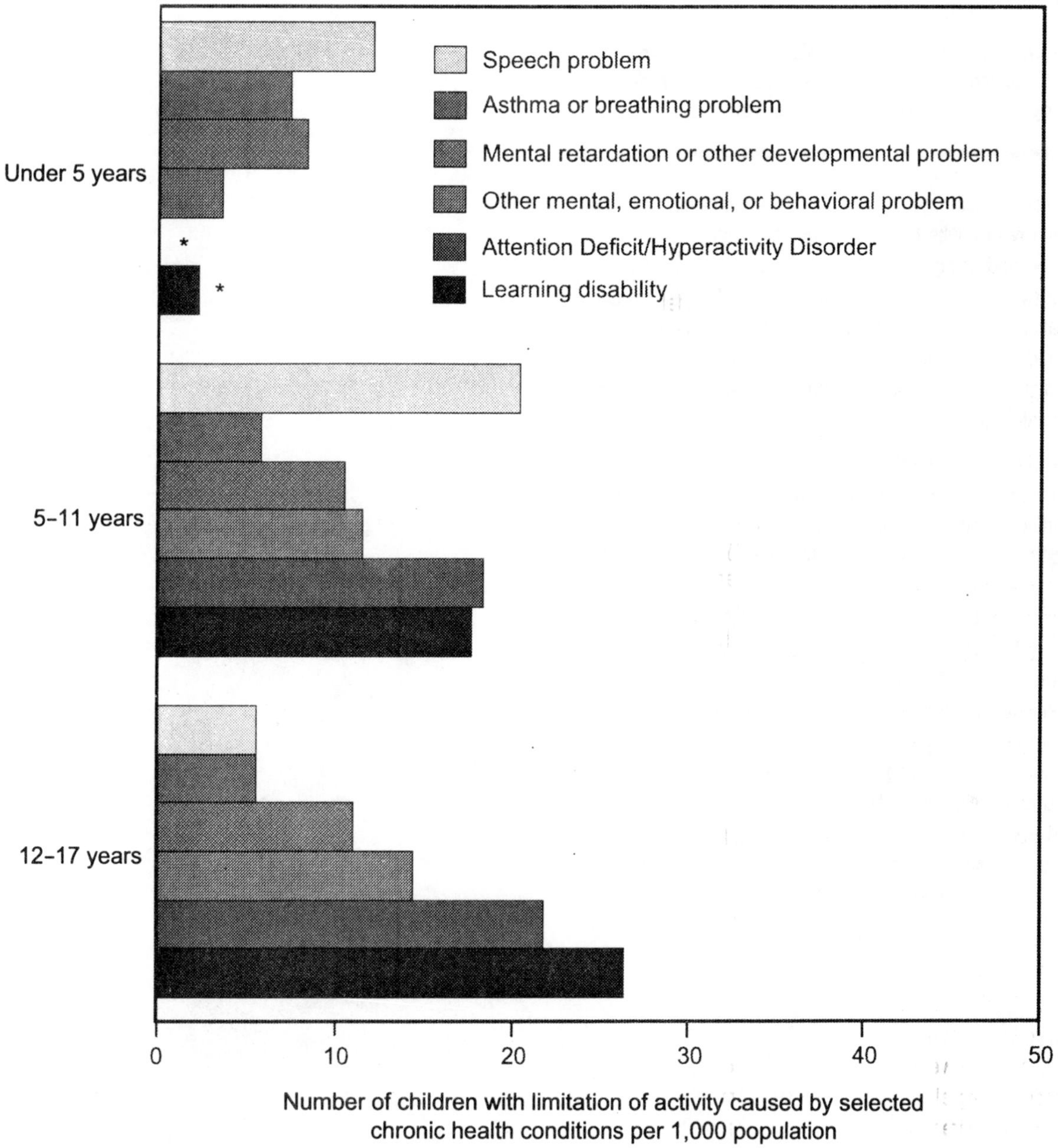

* Estimates are considered unreliable. Data shown with an asterisk have a relative standard error (RSE) of 20%–30%. Data not shown have an RSE of greater than 30%.

NOTES: Children with more than one chronic health condition causing activity limitation are counted in each category. See data table for Figure 14 for data points graphed, standard errors, and additional notes.

SOURCE: Centers for Disease Control and Prevention, National Center for Health Statistics, National Health Interview Survey.

Limitation of Activity Due to Chronic Conditions: Working-Age and Older Adults

Arthritis and other musculoskeletal conditions are the most frequently reported cause of activity limitation among both working-age and older adults.

Chronic physical, mental, and emotional conditions can limit the ability of adults to perform important activities such as working and doing everyday household chores. With advancing age, an increasing percentage of adults experience limitation of activity. Estimates of the number of working-age and older adults with limitation of activity are important for determining current and future types of health care needs and associated costs (1).

Between 1997 and 2005, the percentage of noninstitutionalized working-age adults 18–64 years of age reporting an activity limitation caused by a chronic health condition remained relatively stable (Table 58). In 2004–2005, the percentage of working-age adults who reported limitations ranged from 6% at age 18–44 years to 20% at age 55–64 years (2). Arthritis and other musculoskeletal conditions were the most frequently mentioned conditions causing limitation among working-age adults of all ages in 2004–2005 (Figure 15). Among adults 18–44 years of age, mental illness was the second leading cause of activity limitation followed by fractures or joint injury. Among adults 45–64 years of age, heart and circulatory conditions were the second leading cause of limitation. Other frequently mentioned conditions included mental illness and diabetes.

Figure 15. Limitation of activity caused by selected chronic health conditions among working-age adults, by age: United States, 2004–2005

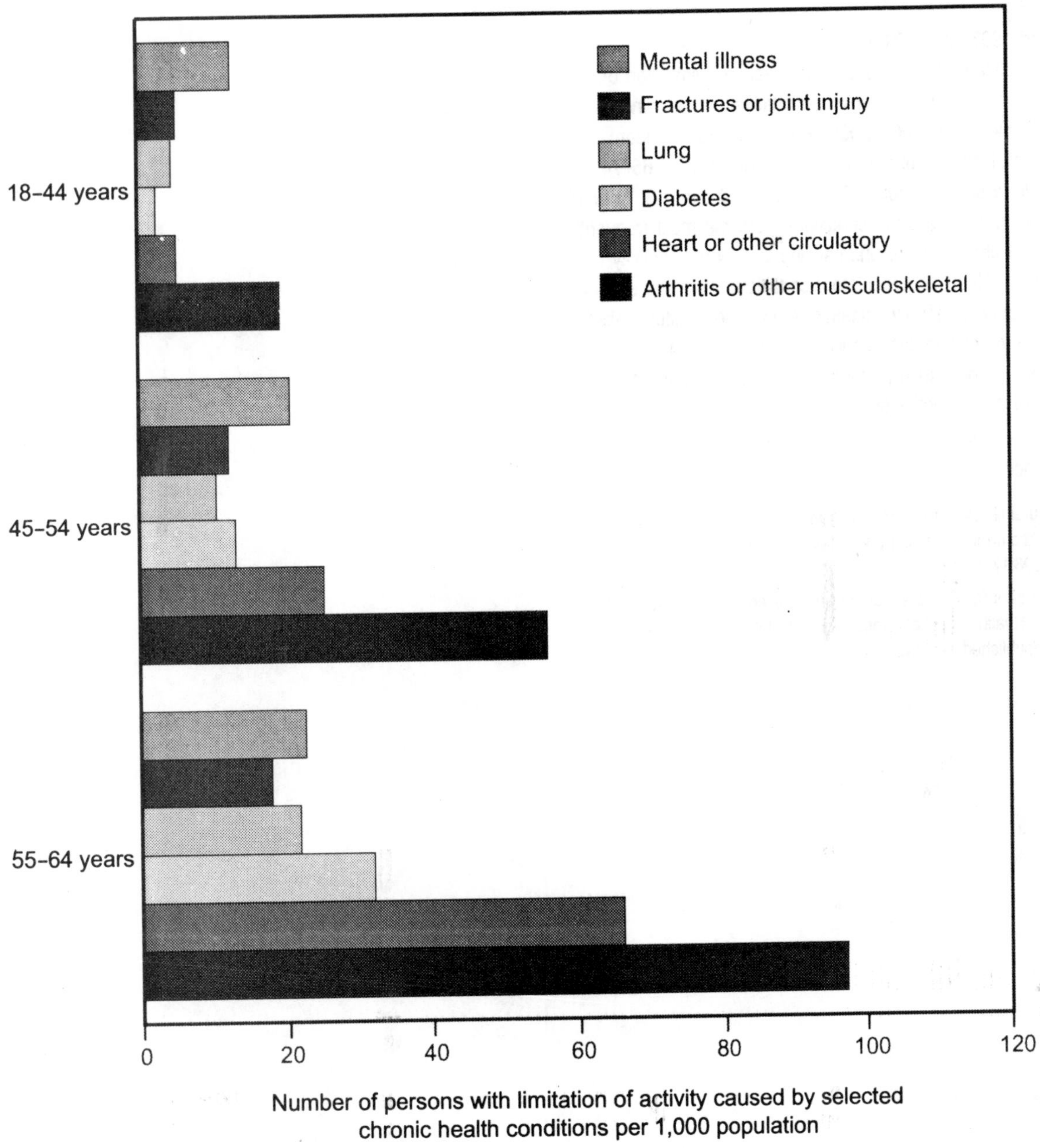

NOTES: Data are for the civilian noninstitutionalized population. Adults with more than one chronic condition causing activity limitation are counted in each category. See data table for Figure 15 for data points graphed, standard errors, and additional notes.

SOURCE: Centers for Disease Control and Prevention, National Center for Health Statistics, National Health Interview Survey.

Limitation of Activity Due to Chronic Conditions: Working-Age and Older Adults *(Continued)*

Between 1997 and 1999, the percentage of non-institutionalized adults 65 years and over with limitation of activity declined and has remained relatively stable since 1999. (Table 58). In 2004–2005, the percentage of older adults with limitation of activity ranged from 25% of 65–74 year olds to 60% of adults 85 years old and over (2). Arthritis and other musculoskeletal conditions were the most frequently mentioned chronic conditions causing limitation of activity (Figure 16). Heart and circulatory conditions were the second leading cause of activity limitation. Among noninstitutionalized adults 85 years and over, senility or dementia, vision conditions, and hearing problems were frequently mentioned causes of activity limitation.

References

1. Guralnik JM, Fried LP, Salive ME. Disability as a public health outcome in the aging population. Annu Rev Public Health 1996;17:25–46.
2. Centers for Disease Control and Prevention, National Center for Health Statistics, National Health Interview Survey, unpublished analysis.

Figure 16. Limitation of activity caused by selected chronic health conditions among older adults, by age: United States, 2004-2005

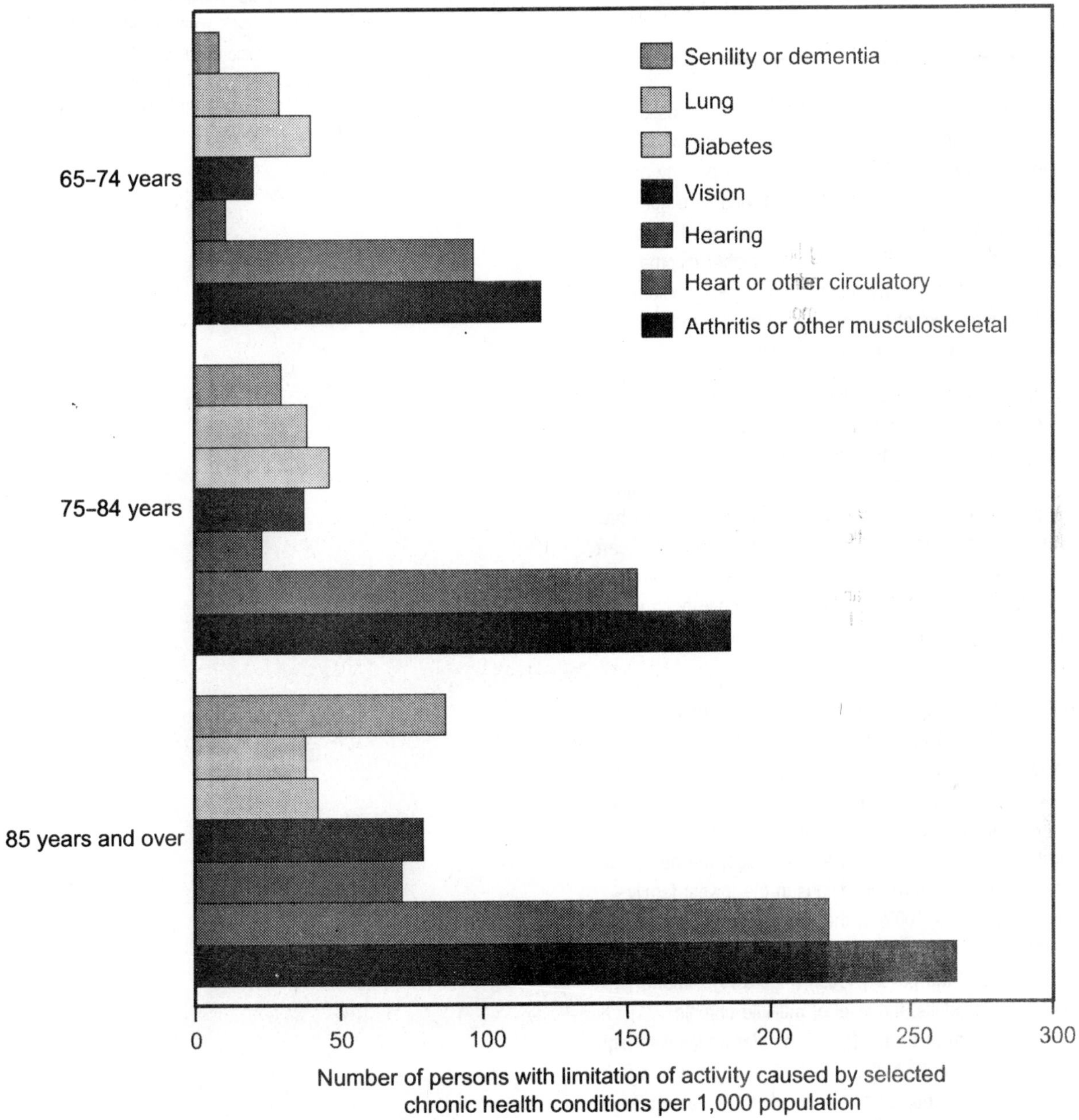

NOTES: Data are for the civilian noninstitutionalized population. Adults with more than one chronic health condition causing activity limitation are counted in each category. See data table for Figure 16 for data points graphed, standard errors, and additional notes.

SOURCE: Centers for Disease Control and Prevention, National Center for Health Statistics, National Health Interview Survey.

Three or More Chronic Conditions

Poverty is strongly associated with having three or more chronic conditions, especially among adults 45–64 years of age.

Many studies of adult health have shown a strong association between poverty and a wide array of chronic health conditions (1). Given the association between poverty and the risk factors for many chronic health conditions, it is not surprising that low-income adults more often report multiple serious health conditions than those with higher income. The relationship between poverty and serious health problems reflects both the effect of low income on health and the effect of poor health on the ability to earn a living (1,2).

Data from the National Health Interview Survey were used to assess chronic health conditions of adults age 45 years and over living in the community. Adults were identified as having three or more chronic conditions if they reported ever being told by a physician or other health professional that they had three or more of the following conditions: hypertension, heart disease, stroke, emphysema, diabetes, cancer, or arthritis. Among adults ever diagnosed with asthma, only those who reported currently having asthma were considered to have a chronic condition.

In 2005, the percentage of adults with three or more chronic conditions increased with age from 7% of adults 45–54 years of age to 37% of adults 75 years of age and over. Among adults 45–64 years of age, the prevalence of three or more chronic conditions was strongly related to family income. Among adults 45–54 and 55–64 years of age, the percentage with three or more chronic conditions in the lowest family income group (below 100% of the poverty level) was two to three times the level in the highest family income category (400% or more of the poverty level) (Figure 17). Among middle-age poor adults, the level of multiple chronic conditions was similar to that for much older adults with high family income. In 2005, 30% of adults 55–64 years of age in the lowest income group and 31% of adults 75 years of age and over in the highest income group had three or more chronic conditions.

References

1. Pamuk E, Makuc D, Heck K, Reuben C, Lochner K. Socioeconomic Status and Health Chartbook. Health, United States, 1998. Hyattsville, MD: National Center for Health Statistics. 1998. Available from: www.cdc.gov/nchs/hus.htm.
2. Freidland RB. Multiple chronic conditions. Data Profiles, Challenges for the 21st Century: Chronic and Disabling Conditions: Number 12. Georgetown University Center on an Aging Society. November 2003.

Figure 17. Three or more chronic conditions among adults 45 years of age and over, by age and percent of poverty level: United States, 2005

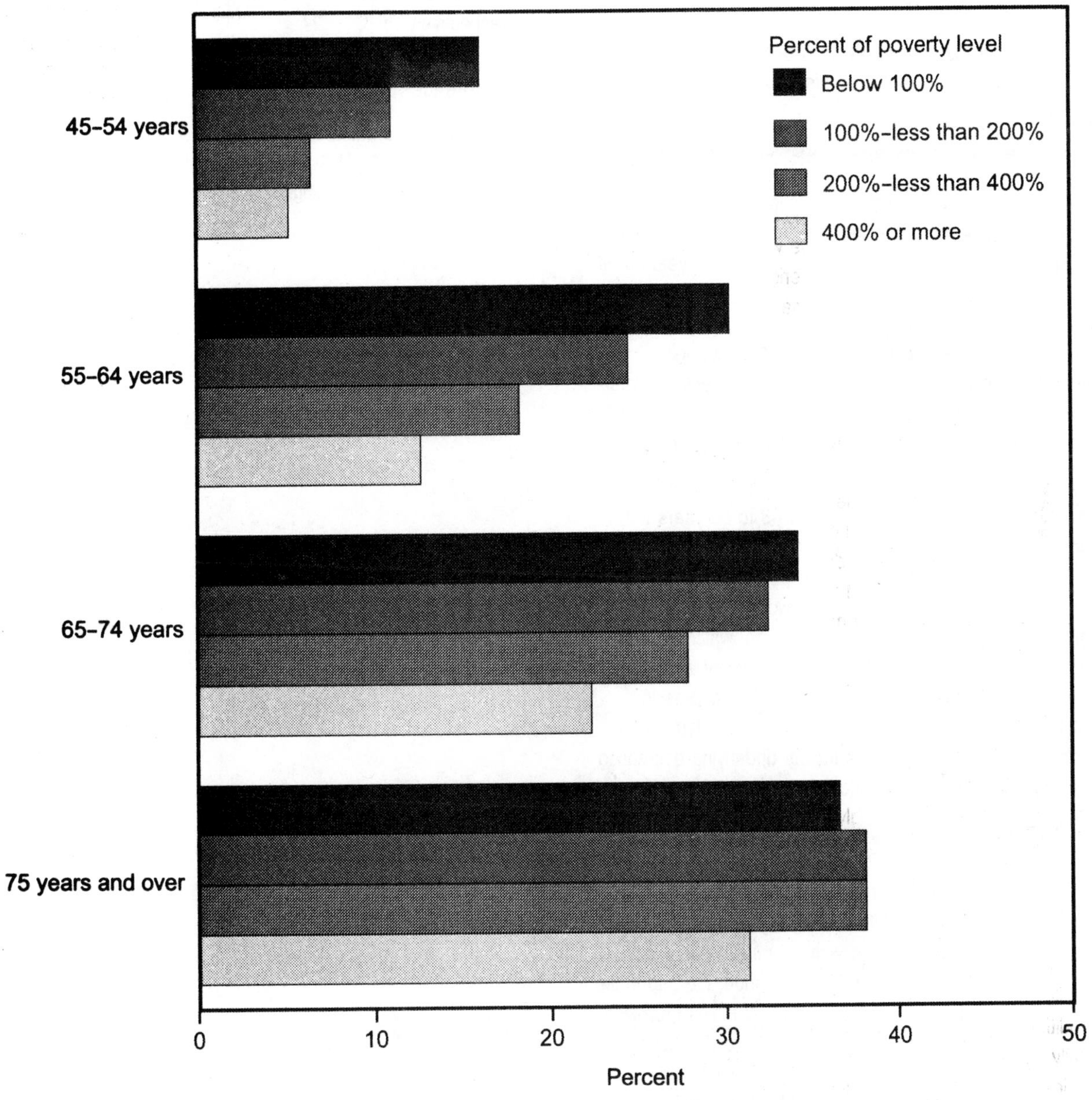

NOTES: Adults who had ever been told by a physician they had three or more of the following conditions: hypertension, heart disease, stroke, emphysema, diabetes, cancer, arthritis and related diseases, or current asthma. Percent of poverty level is based on family income and family size and composition using U.S. Census Bureau poverty thresholds. See data table for Figure 17 for data points graphed, standard errors, and additional notes.

SOURCE: Centers for Disease Control and Prevention, National Center for Health Statistics, National Health Interview Survey.

Mortality

Life Expectancy

The gap in life expectancy at birth between white persons and black persons persists, but has narrowed since 1990.

Life expectancy is a measure often used to gauge the overall health of a population. As a summary measure of mortality, life expectancy represents the average number of years of life that could be expected if current death rates were to remain constant. Shifts in life expectancy are often used to describe trends in mortality. Life expectancy at birth is strongly influenced by infant and child mortality. Life expectancy later in life reflects death rates at or above a given age and is independent of the effect of mortality at younger ages (1).

From 1900 through 2004, life expectancy at birth increased from 46 to 75 years for men and from 48 to 80 years for women (Table 27). Life expectancy at age 65 also increased during this period. Among men, life expectancy at age 65 rose from 12 to 17 years and among women from 12 to 20 years. In contrast to life expectancy at birth, which increased sharply early in the 20th century, life expectancy at age 65 improved primarily after midcentury. Improved access to health care, advances in medicine, healthier lifestyles, and better health before age 65 are factors underlying decreased death rates among older Americans (2).

In 2004, life expectancy at birth was 76 years for white males compared with 70 years for black males and 81 years for white females compared with 76 years for black females (data table for Figure 18). Life expectancy at birth increased more for the black than for the white population between 1990 and 2004 (Figure 18). During this period, the gap in life expectancy between white males and black males narrowed from 8 years to 6 years (data table for Figure 18). During the same period, the gap in life expectancy between white females and black females decreased from 6 years to 5 years.

The gap in life expectancy between white and black people at age 65 is narrower than at birth. Between 1990 and 2004, the difference in life expectancy at age 65 between white males and black males remained stable at 2 years. In 2004, life expectancy at age 65 was 17 years for white males and 15 years for black males. The difference in life expectancy between white and black females has also been stable in recent years; in 2004, at age 65, white females and black females could expect to live an additional 20 and 19 years, respectively.

References

1. Arriaga EE. Measuring and explaining the change in life expectancies. Demography 1984;21(1):83–96.
2. Fried LP. Epidemiology of aging. Epidemiol Rev 2000;22(1): 95–106.

Figure 18. Life expectancy at birth and at 65 years of age, by race and sex: United States, 1970–2004

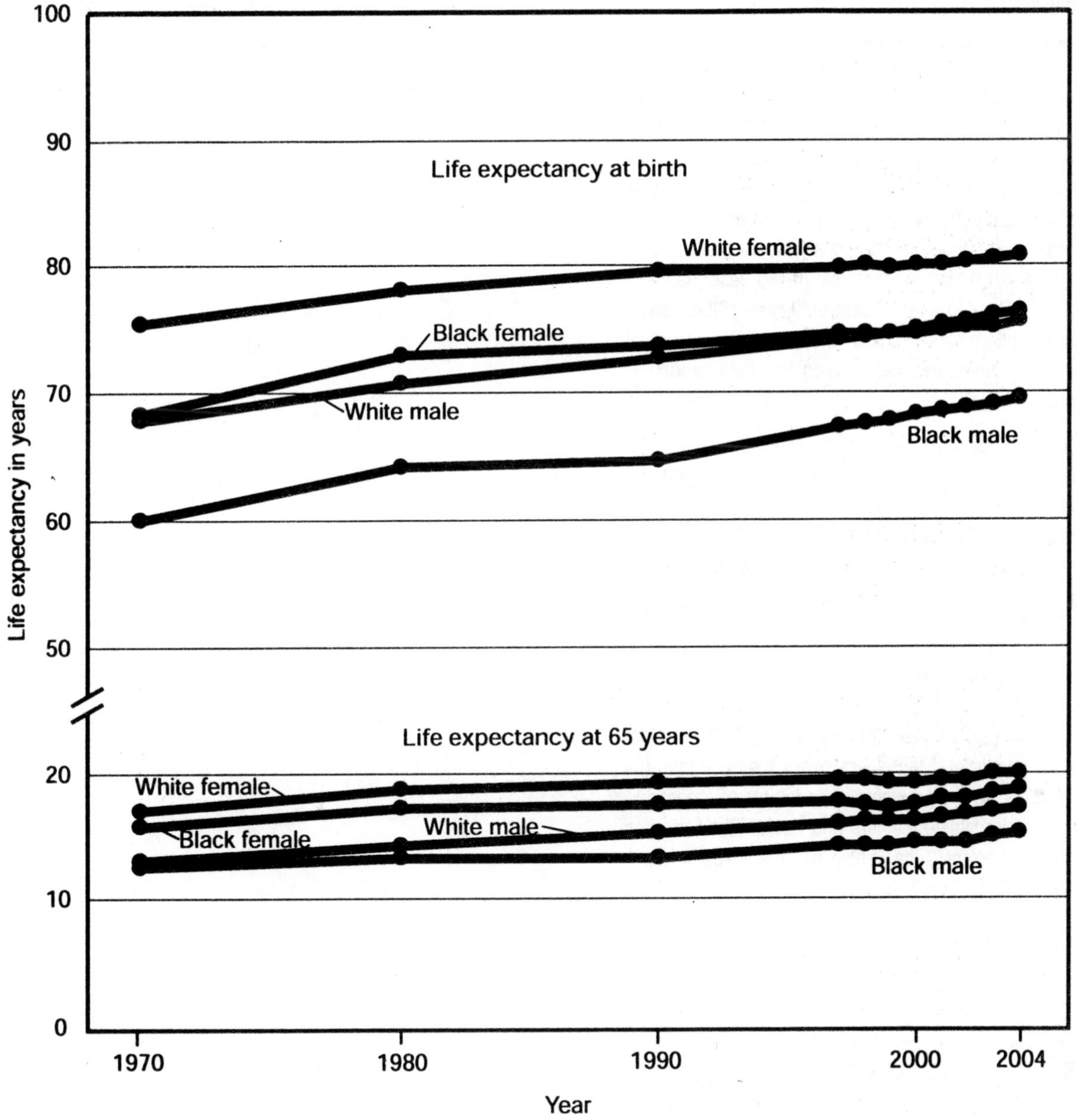

NOTES: Life expectancies prior to 1997 are from decennial life tables based on census data and deaths for a 3-year period around the census year. Therefore, the middle year in each 3-year period is plotted in this figure. Beginning in 1997, the annual life tables are complete life tables based on a methodology similar to that used for decennial life tables. See data table for Figure 18 for data points graphed and additional notes.

SOURCE: Centers for Disease Control and Prevention, National Center for Health Statistics, National Vital Statistics System.

Infant Mortality

Both neonatal and postneonatal mortality rates have declined substantially since 1950.

The infant mortality rate, the risk of death during the first year of life, is related to the underlying health of the mother, public health practices, socioeconomic conditions, and availability and use of appropriate health care for infants and pregnant women. Disorders related to short gestation and low birthweight, and congenital malformations are the leading causes of death during the neonatal period (less than 28 days of life). Sudden Infant Death Syndrome (SIDS) and congenital malformations rank as the leading causes of infant deaths during the postneonatal period (28 days through 11 months of life) (1).

After decades of decline, there has been little progress in lowering the U.S. infant mortality rate from 2000–2004. In 2004, the infant mortality rate was 6.8 infant deaths per 1,000 live births, compared with 6.9 in 2000. The 2004 infant mortality rate was 77% lower than in 1950, due primarily to annual declines in the infant mortality rate from 1960–2000 (Figure 19).

Infant mortality rates have declined for most racial and ethnic groups, but large disparities among the groups remain (Table 19). During 2001–2003, the infant mortality rate was highest for infants of non-Hispanic black mothers. Infant mortality rates were also high among infants of American Indian or Alaska Native mothers and Puerto Rican mothers. Infants of mothers of Cuban origin had the lowest infant mortality rates.

Reference

1. Heron MP, Smith BL. Deaths: Leading causes for 2003. National vital statistics reports; vol 55 no 10. Hyattsville, MD: National Center for Health Statistics. 2007. Available from: www.cdc.gov/nchs/data/nvsr/nvsr55/nvsr55_10.pdf.

Figure 19. Infant, neonatal, and postneonatal mortality rates: United States, 1950–2004

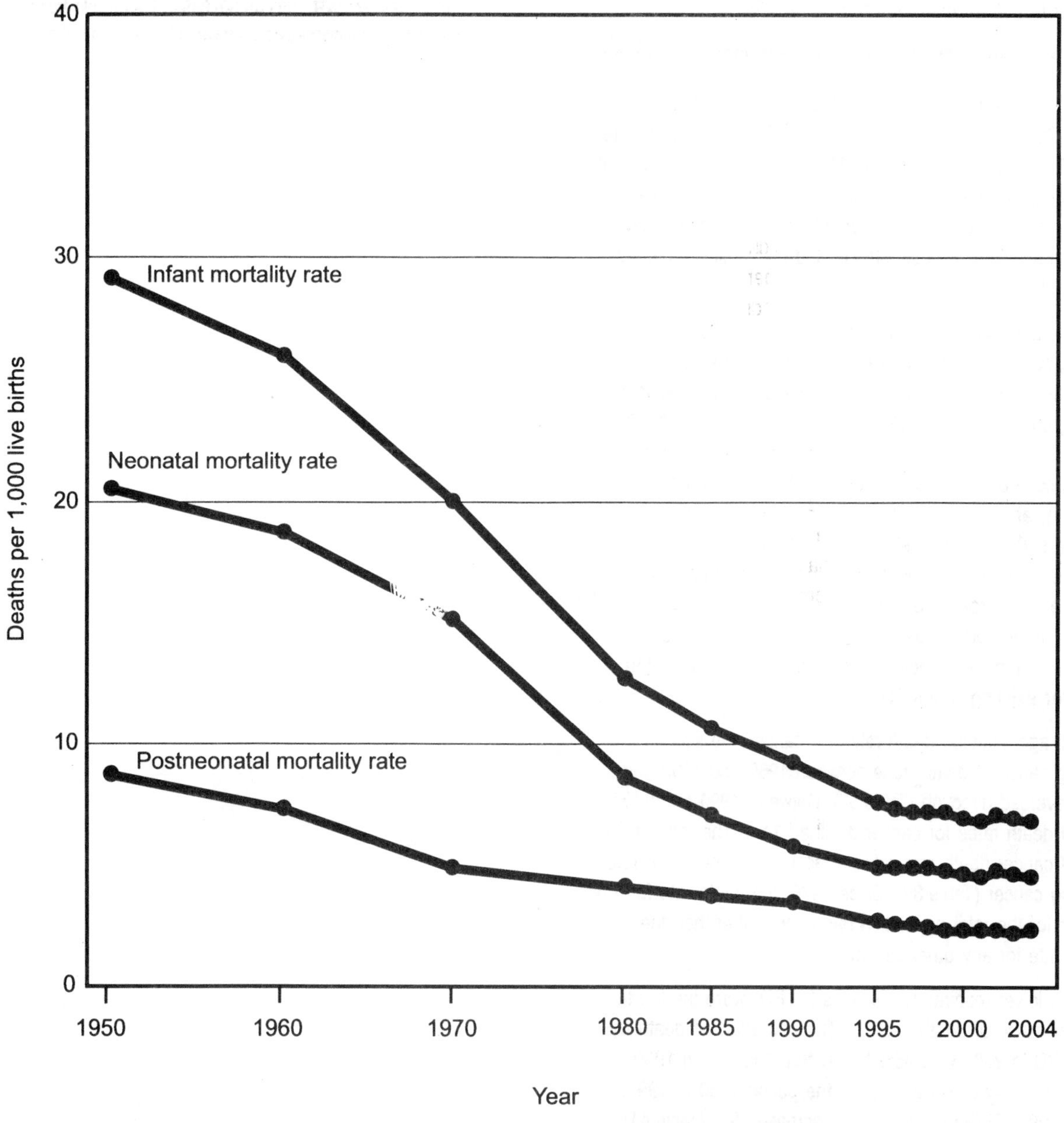

NOTES: Infant is defined as under 1 year of age, neonatal as under 28 days of age, and postneonatal as between 28 days and 1 year of age. See data table for Figure 19 for data points graphed and additional notes.

SOURCE: Centers for Disease Control and Prevention, National Center for Health Statistics, National Vital Statistics System.

Leading Causes of Death for All Ages

Mortality from heart disease, stroke, and unintentional injuries is substantially lower than in 1950.

In 2004, a total of 2.4 million deaths were reported in the United States (Table 31). The overall age-adjusted death rate was 45% lower in 2004 than in 1950. The reduction in overall mortality during the last half of the twentieth century was driven mostly by declines in mortality for such leading causes of death as heart disease, stroke, and unintentional injuries (Figure 20).

In 2004, the age-adjusted death rate for heart disease, the leading cause of death, was 63% lower than the rate in 1950 (Table 36). The age-adjusted death rate for stroke, the third leading cause of death, declined 72% since 1950 (Table 37). Heart disease and stroke mortality are associated with risk factors such as high cholesterol, high blood pressure, smoking, and dietary factors. Other important factors include socioeconomic status, obesity, and physical inactivity. Factors contributing to the decline in heart disease and stroke mortality include better control of risk factors, improved access to early detection, and better treatment and care, including new drugs and expanded uses for existing drugs (1).

Overall age-adjusted death rates for cancer, the second leading cause of death, rose between 1960 and 1990 and then reversed direction (Table 38). Between 1990 and 2004 overall death rates for cancer declined 14%. The trend in the overall cancer death rate reflects the trend in the death rate for lung cancer (Table 39). Since 1970, the death rate for lung cancer for the total population has been higher than the death rate for any other cancer site.

Chronic lower respiratory diseases (CLRD) were the fourth leading cause of death in 2004. The age-adjusted death rate for CLRD in 2004 was 45% higher than the rate in 1980. CLRD mortality increased during the period 1980 to 1999. Since 1999, CLRD mortality has decreased 9% (Table 41).

The fifth leading cause of death in 2004 was unintentional injuries. Age-adjusted death rates for unintentional injuries declined during the period 1950–1992 (Table 29). Since 1992, the unintentional injury mortality rate has gradually increased. Despite recent increases, the death rate for unintentional injuries in 2004 was still 52% lower than the rate in 1950.

Reference

1. CDC. Achievements in public health, 1990–1999: Decline in deaths from heart disease and stroke—United States, 1990–1999. MMWR 1999;48(30):649–56. Available from: www.cdc.gov/mmwr/preview/mmwrhtml/mm4830a1.htm.

Figure 20. Death rates for leading causes of death for all ages: United States, 1950–2004

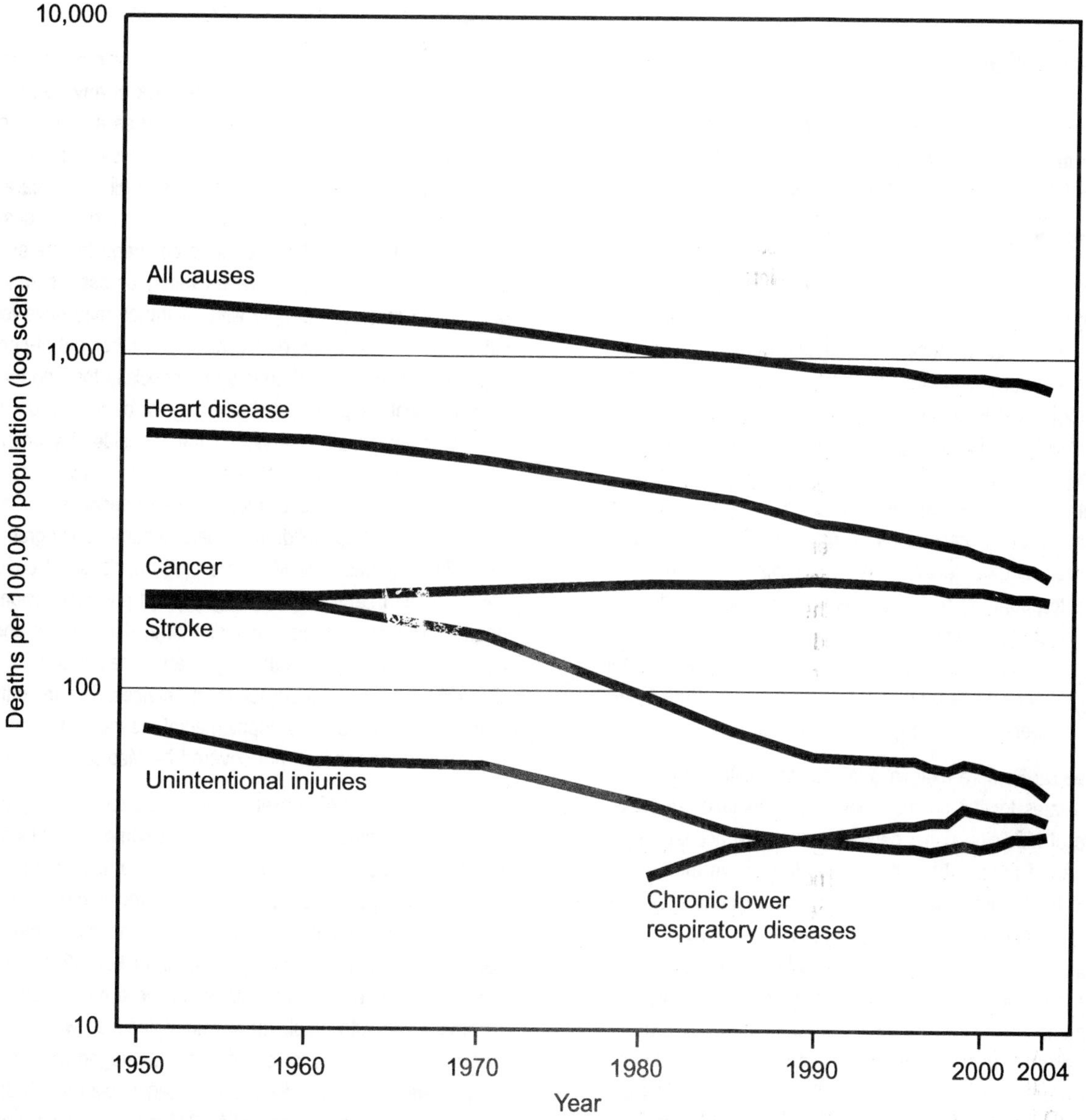

NOTES: Estimates are age-adjusted. Causes of death shown are the five leading causes of death for all ages in 2004. Starting with 1999 data, causes of death were coded according to ICD–10. See data table for Figure 20 for data points graphed and additional notes.

SOURCE: Centers for Disease Control and Prevention, National Center for Health Statistics, National Vital Statistics System.

Special Feature: Access to Health Care

Introduction

In 2005, almost 20% of adults reported they did not receive needed health-related services in the past 12 months because they could not afford them.

The American health care delivery system is evolving, and as it changes, so do the types of services that are available. New technological advances can prevent, treat, or ameliorate conditions and diseases that were once thought untreatable. Yet many people who could benefit from these services do not receive them. Identifying which Americans do not receive potentially beneficial services, and the reasons underlying suboptimal use of services, is essential to identifying solutions that can improve access to health care. Providing needed preventive, curative, rehabilitative, and palliative health care services to people in need benefits not only the individuals but also their communities, in terms of having a healthier population, increasing productivity, and reducing spending for expensive types of care such as emergency department care or care for persons who are needlessly ill or disabled (1).

This Special Feature examines access to health care in the United States for the noninstitutionalized population. A 1993 Institute of Medicine panel defined health care access as "the timely use of personal health services to achieve the best possible health outcomes" (2). Due to the difficulty of directly measuring need for services, appropriate timeliness of services, and health outcomes, access is usually studied indirectly by examining whether rates of service use are at recommended or expected levels, or whether population groups differ in use of services. Lower rates of service use among a group may reflect a barrier to access but must be further studied to determine if there is differing need for services among the groups, and whether services are underutilized in the lower-use group or overutilized in the higher-use group. However, having equal access to health care services does not guarantee that needed services are received or that outcomes are optimal. Not everyone who has access to services receives them when needed, and people who live in areas with few services may still obtain them (2). Additionally, the relationship between health care and outcomes is influenced by a myriad of factors other than access, including propensity to seek care, health status, compliance with medical advice, and quality of services provided.

Health insurance coverage is also used as a proxy measure of access to health care because the lack of any health insurance coverage has been established as a major barrier to receiving most health care services. However, insurance alone is not sufficient to ensure access to all health care services. Few insurance policies cover all needed or desired services, and many policies exclude coverage for pre-existing conditions (2). Cost-sharing varies widely across insurance policies, so that even people with insurance may have to pay substantial copayments, deductibles, and other out-of-pocket expenses. Generosity of coverage, especially for long-term care, medical supplies, psychotherapy, or dental, vision, home health, or rehabilitative services varies considerably among private health insurance policies. States also vary in the extent to which they cover these types of services in their Medicaid and State Children's Health Insurance Program (SCHIP) programs. The Medicare program does not cover several health services, including general physical, vision, or hearing exams; long-term custodial care; dental care; and the cost of eyeglasses or hearing aids, and it requires a deductible and copayment for most services. The majority of Medicare enrollees have supplemental insurance to cover some costs for services not covered by Medicare (Table 140).

The burden of out-of-pocket health care expenses is greatest for poor and uninsured people (3). But some higher-income families with health insurance who have catastrophic illnesses or high out-of-pocket expenditures for noncovered services may devote a substantial portion of their income to medical care, or to health insurance premiums, or both (2, Figure 31). Health insurance premiums alone can be a burden on family income. Even with employer subsidies for their workers' health insurance, worker contributions averaged $627 for a single-person plan and $2,973 for a family plan in 2006; employers paid an average of $3,615 per worker for single plans and $8,508 for family coverage (4). Individual insurance policies paid entirely by the beneficiary can cost substantially more—particularly for people with pre-existing conditions—and can account for a large share of disposable income in poorer families (5).

Figure 21. Adults 18 years of age and over reporting they did not receive needed health-related services in the past 12 months because they could not afford them, by age and type of service: United States, 2005

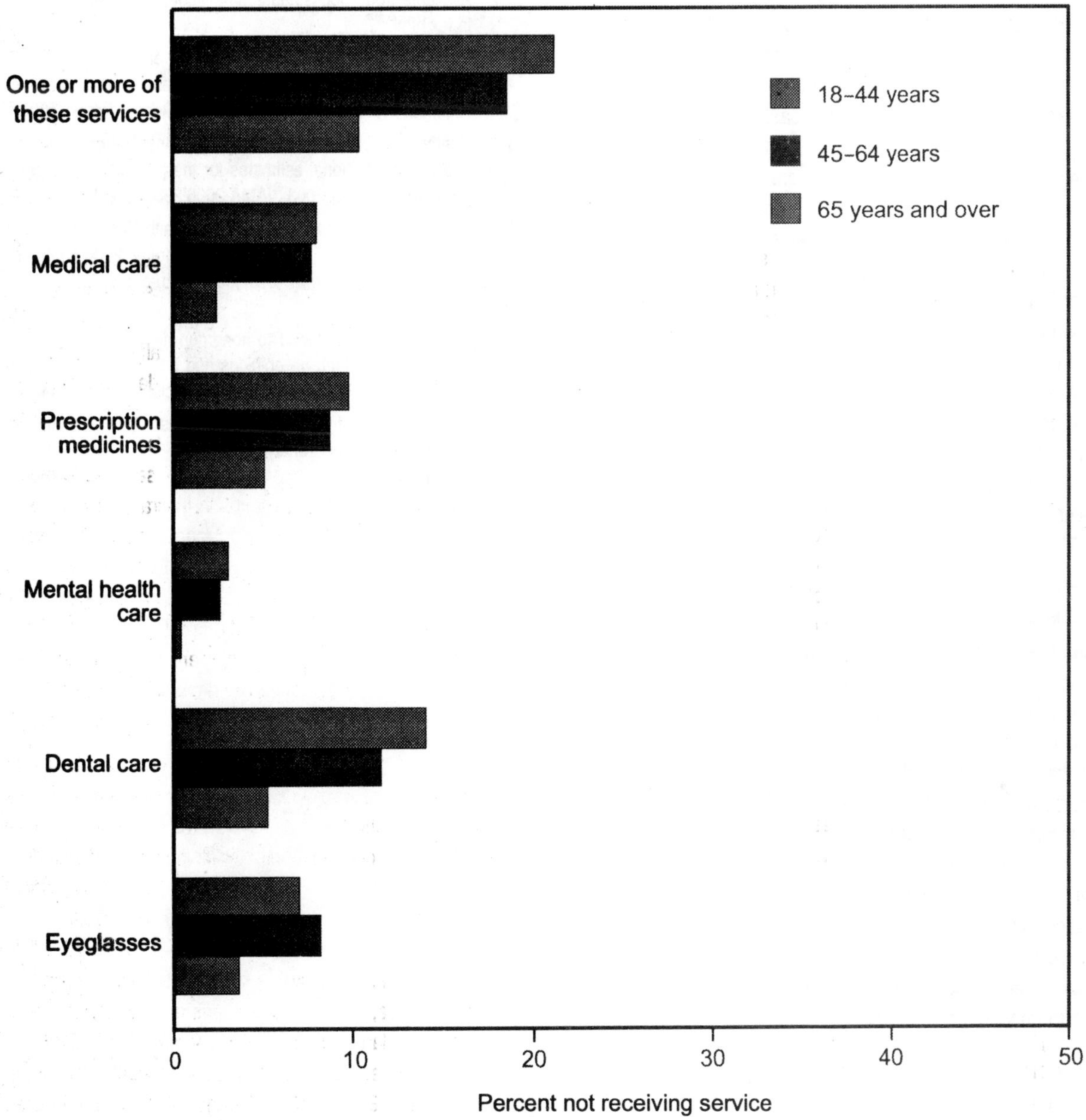

NOTE: See data table for Figure 21 for data points graphed, standard errors, and additional notes.

SOURCE: Centers for Disease Control and Prevention, National Center for Health Statistics, National Health Interview Survey.

Access to Health Care: Introduction

(Continued)

The majority of Americans do not report having problems accessing health care services due to cost. In 2005, 19% of adults 18 years of age and over—more than 40 million people—reported they did not receive one or more of the following health-related services in the past year because they could not afford them: medical care, prescription medicines, mental health care, dental care, or eyeglasses (see Technical Notes for the survey questions). About 12% of adults reported they did not receive needed dental care and 7% did not purchase needed eyeglasses due to cost (data table for Figure 21). About 7% of adults (representing about 15 million people) reported they did not receive needed medical care in 2005 because they could not afford it. The percentage of adults who did not receive prescription drugs because they could not afford them increased from 6% in 1997 to 9% in 2005 (6). Fewer problems in obtaining needed services were reported for children and adults age 65 years and over than working-age adults 18–64 years of age (Table 79, Figure 21).

This Special Feature explores several dimensions of access to care, including supply of medical care providers and services (distribution of primary care physicians and obstetricians or gynecologists by county, and supply relative to demand for transplantable kidneys), nonfinancial barriers to care (lack of usual source of care and delayed care due to lack of transportation), and financial barriers to care (insurance and the burden of health care expenditures by family income). It also presents data on utilization of selected services—dental care, colorectal scope procedures, and antidepressant drugs—to highlight differences in use rates by population groups. Population groups with lower use rates may have some barriers to accessing these services. Taken together, these charts present some major issues related to access to health care in our Nation.

References

1. Institute of Medicine (U.S.). Coverage matters: Insurance and health care. Washington, DC: National Academy Press; 2001. Available from: books.nap.edu/html/coverage_matters/index.html.
2. Institute of Medicine (U.S.). Committee on Monitoring Access to Personal Health Care Services. Access to health care in America. Washington, DC: National Academy Press; 1993.
3. Banthin JS, Bernard DM. Changes in financial burdens for health care: National estimates for the population younger than 65 years, 1996 to 2003. JAMA 2006;296(22):2712–9.
4. The Kaiser Family Foundation and Health Research and Educational Trust. Employer health benefits: 2006 summary of findings. Available from: www.kff.org/insurance/7527/upload/7528.pdf.
5. Pauly MV, Nichols LM. The nongroup health insurance market: Short on facts, long on opinions and policy disputes. Health Aff (Millwood) 2002;Jul–Dec;suppl web exclusives:w325–44.
6. National Center for Health Statistics, National Health Interview Survey, unpublished analysis.

Physician Supply

The supply of physicians varies by metropolitan status and geography, and nearly one-half of U.S. counties had no obstetricians or gynecologists in 2004.

A shortage of physicians in a geographic area can increase travel time to see a physician and serve as a deterrent to timely and appropriate health care. Scarcity of physicians can also lead to higher caseloads for physicians and consequently, increased time to getting an appointment, as well as increased waiting time for receiving care.

The supply of patient care physicians in the United States has increased by 50% since 1980 (1). In 2004, there were 24 active, nonfederal, patient care physicians per 10,000 population in the United States (data table for Figure 22) compared to 16 per 10,000 population in 1980 (1). However, the supply of physicians varied substantially across the country (Figure 22, see Technical Notes). Only 11% of counties had a ratio of physicians to population above the national ratio, while 4% of counties had no physicians and an additional 7% met the criteria to be designated as health professional shortage areas (HPSA). HPSAs are defined by the Health Resources and Services Administration as a geographic area with less than 2.86 primary care physicians per 10,000 population (2).

In 2004, about 50 million people or 17% of the U.S. population lived in nonmetropolitan counties (see Appendix II, Metropolitan statistical area). Of the 707,380 active, nonfederal, patient care physicians, only 9% were located in nonmetropolitan counties. More than 90% of the 134 U.S. counties with no physicians were nonmetropolitan. Most of the counties with no physicians are located in the Plains states and parts of the Southwest (Figure 22).

Figure 22. Patient care physicians per 10,000 population, by county: United States, 2004

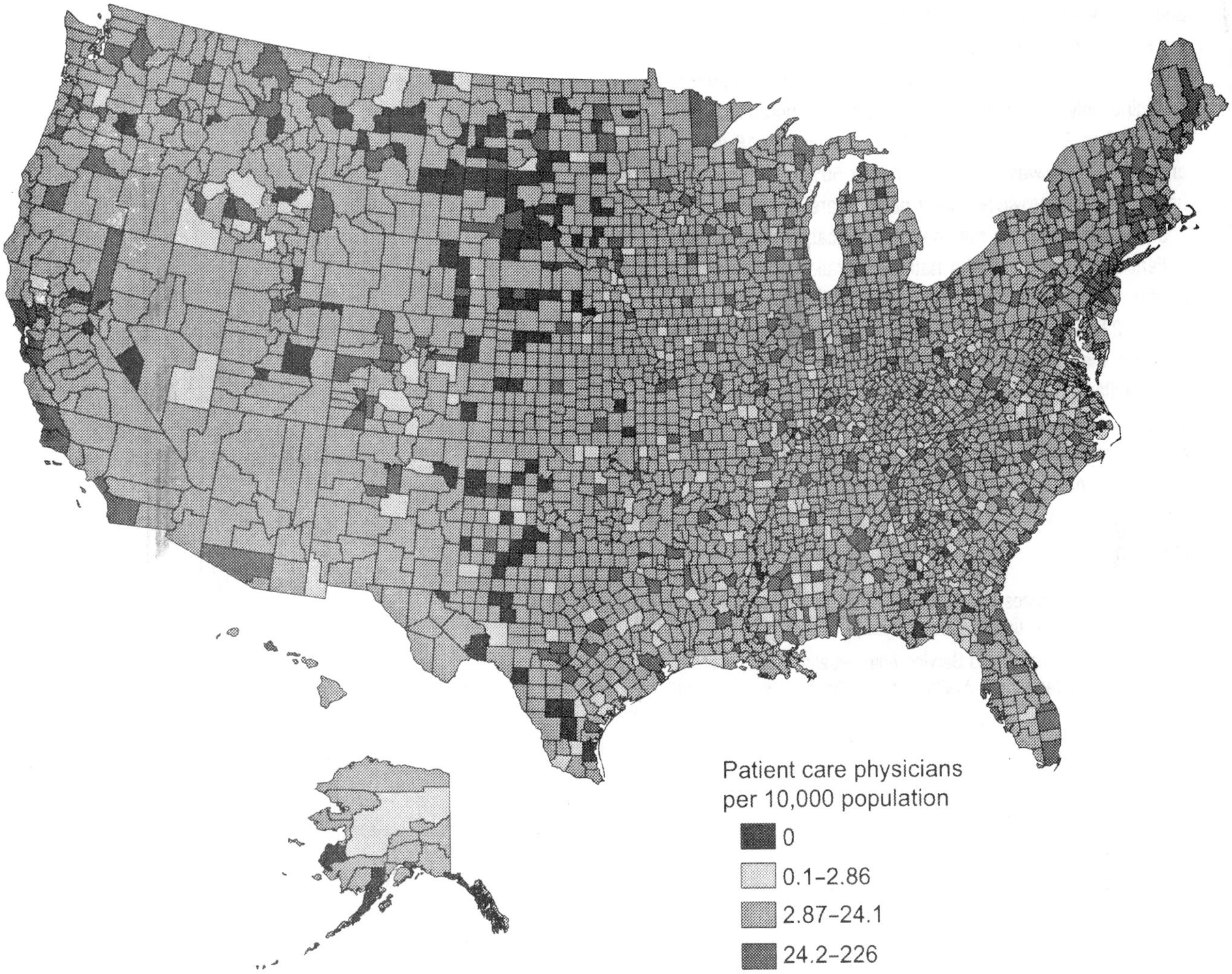

NOTES: Data are for active, nonfederal, patient care physicians. Doctors of medicine and doctors of osteopathy are included. See data table for Figure 22 for additional notes.

SOURCE: Health Resources and Services Administration, 2005 Area Resource File.

Physician Supply *(Continued)*

Obstetricians or gynecologists (obgyns) are physician specialists who provide medical and surgical care to women and have expertise in pregnancy, childbirth, and disorders of the female reproductive system. Between 1980 and 2004, the national supply of nonfederal, patient care, obgyns (doctors of medicine only, see data table for Figure 23) increased from about 2.5 to 3.0 obgyns per 10,000 females age 15 years and over (1). However, in 2004, nearly 50% of U.S. counties had no obgyns providing direct patient care, and 85% of counties fell below the national ratio indicating that, as with patient care physicians, the nationwide ratio is being driven by the counties that have high concentrations of obgyns (Figure 23). Relative to population, nonmetropolitan counties had less than one-half the number of obgyns compared with metropolitan counties (1.4 obgyns versus 3.3 per 10,000 females 15 years of age and over) (data table for Figure 23). Ninety-three percent of counties that had no obgyns also had no certified nurse midwives in 2003 (1).

References

1. Health Resources and Services Administration, 2005 Area Resource File, unpublished analysis.
2. Health Resources and Service Administration, Bureau of Health Professionals. Available from: bhpr.hrsa.gov/shortage/.

Figure 23. Obstetricians or gynecologists per 10,000 females age 15 years and over, by county: United States, 2004

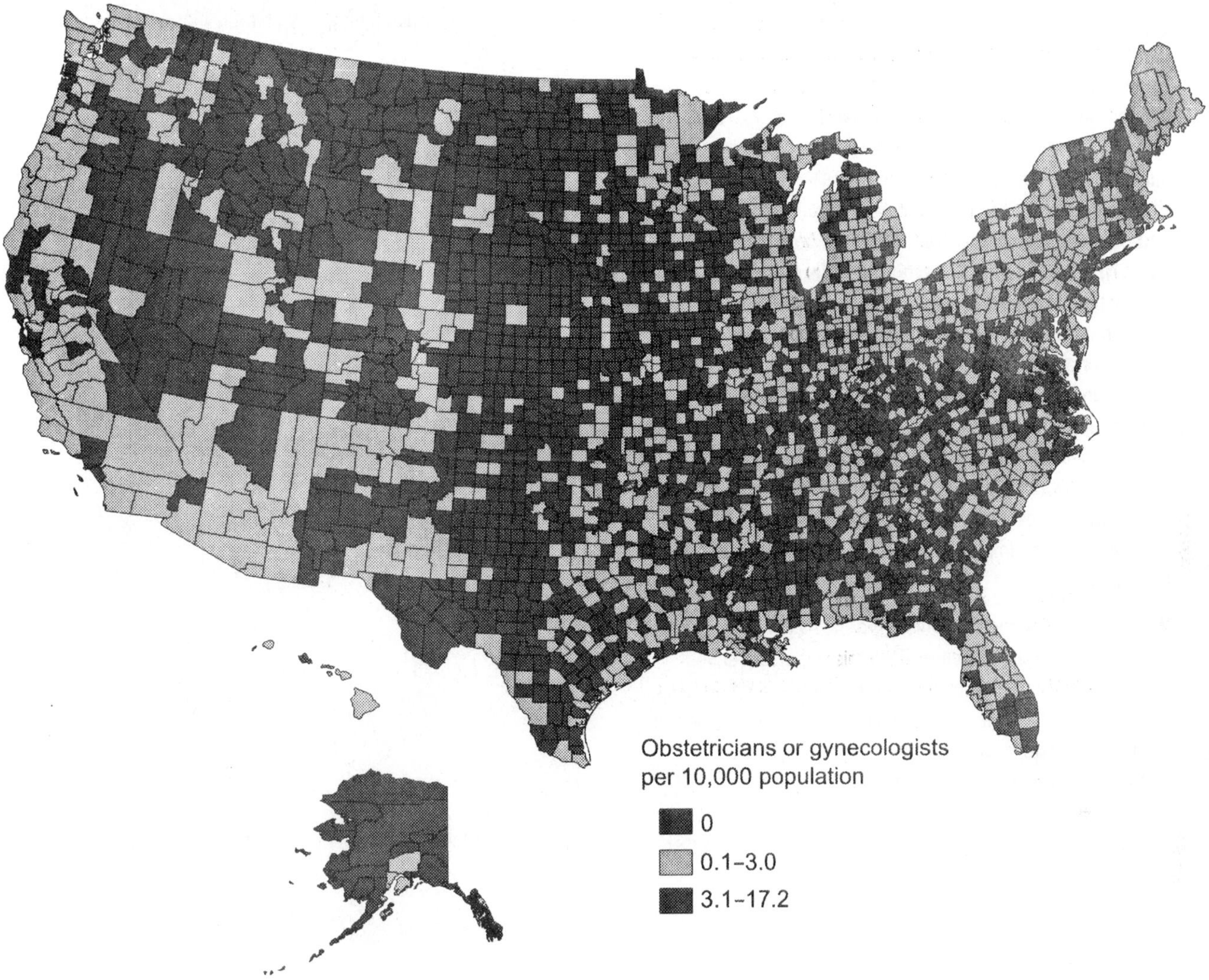

NOTES: Data are for active, nonfederal, patient care obgyn doctors of medicine and exclude doctors of osteopathy. See data table for Figure 23 for additional notes.

SOURCE: Health Resources and Services Administration, 2005 Area Resource File.

Kidney Transplants

The supply of donated kidneys available for people with end-stage renal disease is not keeping up with demand.

End-stage renal disease (ESRD) is defined as a permanent loss of the kidneys' ability to filter wastes from the circulatory system. Its prevalence and treatment costs have increased substantially over the past few decades. In 2004, Medicare's End-Stage Renal Disease program paid almost $19 billion, and other sources paid more than $10 billion, for ESRD care (1). ESRD can result from a number of medical conditions, but the most common causes are diabetic nephropathy, systemic arterial hypertension, glomerulonephritis, and polycystic kidney disease. Once kidney function declines to less than 12%–15%, patient survival is dependent on renal replacement therapy—either ongoing dialysis treatments or kidney transplant. For eligible candidates, transplant and subsequent anti-rejection therapy is preferable because it eliminates the need for dialysis, reduces mortality, improves quality of life, and is less costly than dialysis (2).

With the aging of the population and increases in diabetes prevalence, the prevalence of ESRD and the subsequent need for kidney transplantation is expected to continue to increase. Black people are significantly more likely to develop ESRD than white people. Diabetes and hypertension prevalence rates are higher in black than in white populations. The progression of these diseases differs between the black and white populations, producing earlier onset of ESRD in black people. However, the causes of higher rates of ESRD in black people have not yet been fully explained (3).

The U.S. Organ Procurement and Transplantation Network and the Scientific Registry of Transplant Recipients contain data regarding every organ donation and transplant event occurring in the United States since 1987. This database shows that the number of new registrations on the kidney transplant waiting list increased more than 300% between 1988 and 2006, and 67% between 1996 and 2006 (data table for Figure 24). Non-Hispanic black people made up 33% of the active waiting list (patients eligible for an immediate transplantation) in 2006, more than three times their proportion of the United States population (13%, Table 1). The percentage of non-Hispanic black people on the waiting list remained relatively stable over the past decade, whereas the percentage of non-Hispanic white people declined, and the percentages of Hispanic and non-Hispanic Asian people increased. In 2006, there were 19,247 non-Hispanic white and 16,452 non-Hispanic black patients on the active kidney transplant waiting list (Figure 24).

Although the majority of the costs of kidney transplantation are paid by Medicare's End-Stage Renal Disease program or by private insurance, the ability to pay for transplantation does not ensure access to a kidney. The supply of available and donor-recipient compatible kidneys has not kept pace with demand, and the percentage of patients who remain on the active waiting list for multiple years is increasing in large part because of lack of availability of organs. At the end of 2006, 23% of all active waiting list patients had been waiting for three years or more for their transplant (4).

Figure 24. Active kidney transplant waiting list patients at end of year, by race and Hispanic origin: United States, 1988, 1996, and 2006

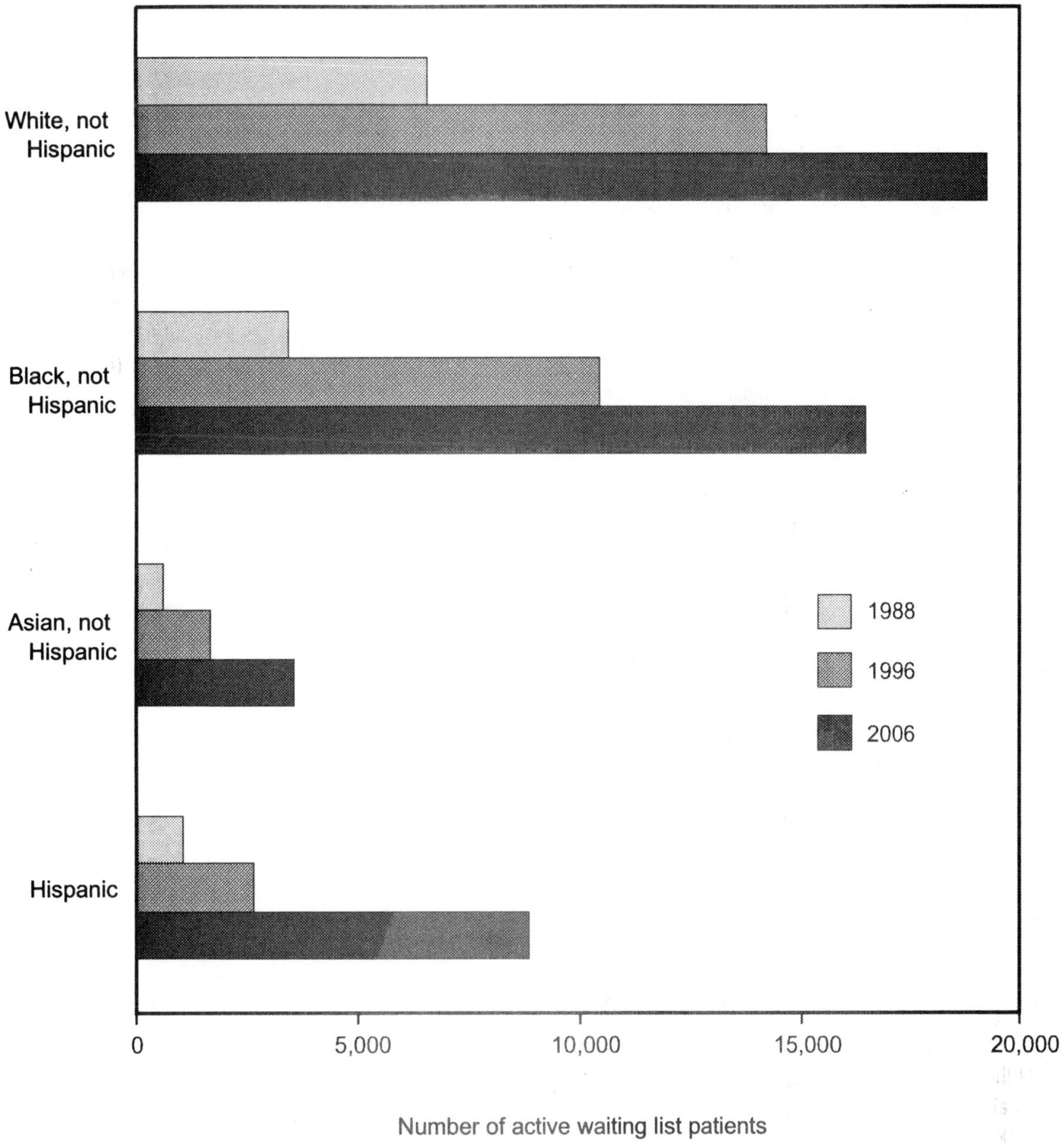

NOTES: Race and ethnicity are reported together as a single data element—either race or ethnicity, but not both. Persons listed as Hispanic are considered Hispanic and all others are classified by their recorded race. See data table for Figure 24 for data points graphed and additional notes.

SOURCE: Organ Procurement and Transplantation Network (OPTN) data as of March 9, 2007, supported in part by Health Resources and Services Administration contract 234–2005–370011C.

Kidney Transplants *(Continued)*

Between 1988 and 2004, the percentage of patients transplanted within two years of being added to the active waiting list declined 56% for non-Hispanic white patients, about 65% for non-Hispanic black or non-Hispanic Asian patients, and 69% for Hispanic patients (data table for Figure 25). In 2004, non-Hispanic white patients were more likely to receive a transplant within two years than non-Hispanic black, non-Hispanic Asian or Hispanic patients (30% compared to 20%–21%) (Figure 25). Racial disparities in rates of organ donation and renal transplantation may be influenced by genetic and biological factors, the request and consent procedures of organ procurement organizations, patient registration practices for a center or region, organ acceptance practices at each transplant center, geographic location, socioeconomic status, cultural attitudes and beliefs about organ donation, rates of organ donation within each local area, and the donor pool (5,6).

References

1. U.S. Renal Data System, USRDS 2006 annual data report: Atlas of end-stage renal disease in the United States. 2006. National Institutes of Health, National Institute of Diabetes and Digestive and Kidney Diseases, Bethesda, MD. Available from: www.usrds.org/.
2. Wolfe RA, Ashby VB, Milford EL, et al. Comparison of mortality in patients on dialysis, patients on dialysis awaiting transplantation, and recipients of a first cadaveric transplant. N Engl J Med 1999; 341:1725–30.
3. Young CJ, Kew C. Health disparities in transplantation: Focus on complexity and challenge of renal transplantation in African Americans. Med Clin N Am 2005;89:1003–31.
4. U.S. Department of Health and Human Services, Health Resources and Services Administration, Healthcare Systems Bureau, Division of Transplantation, Rockville, MD; United Network for Organ Sharing, Richmond, VA. Unpublished data from the Organ Procurement and Transplantation Network as of March 9, 2007.
5. Sanfilippo FP, Vaughn WK, Peters TG, et al. Factors affecting the waiting time of cadaveric kidney transplant candidates in the United States. JAMA 1992;267:247–52.
6. Healthy People 2010: Objectives for improving health. Volume 1 (Part A, chapter 4). 2000. Available from: www.healthypeople.gov/Document/RTF/Volume1/04CKD.rtf.

Figure 25. Active waiting list patients who received a kidney transplant within 2 years, by race and Hispanic origin: United States, 1988, 1996, and 2004

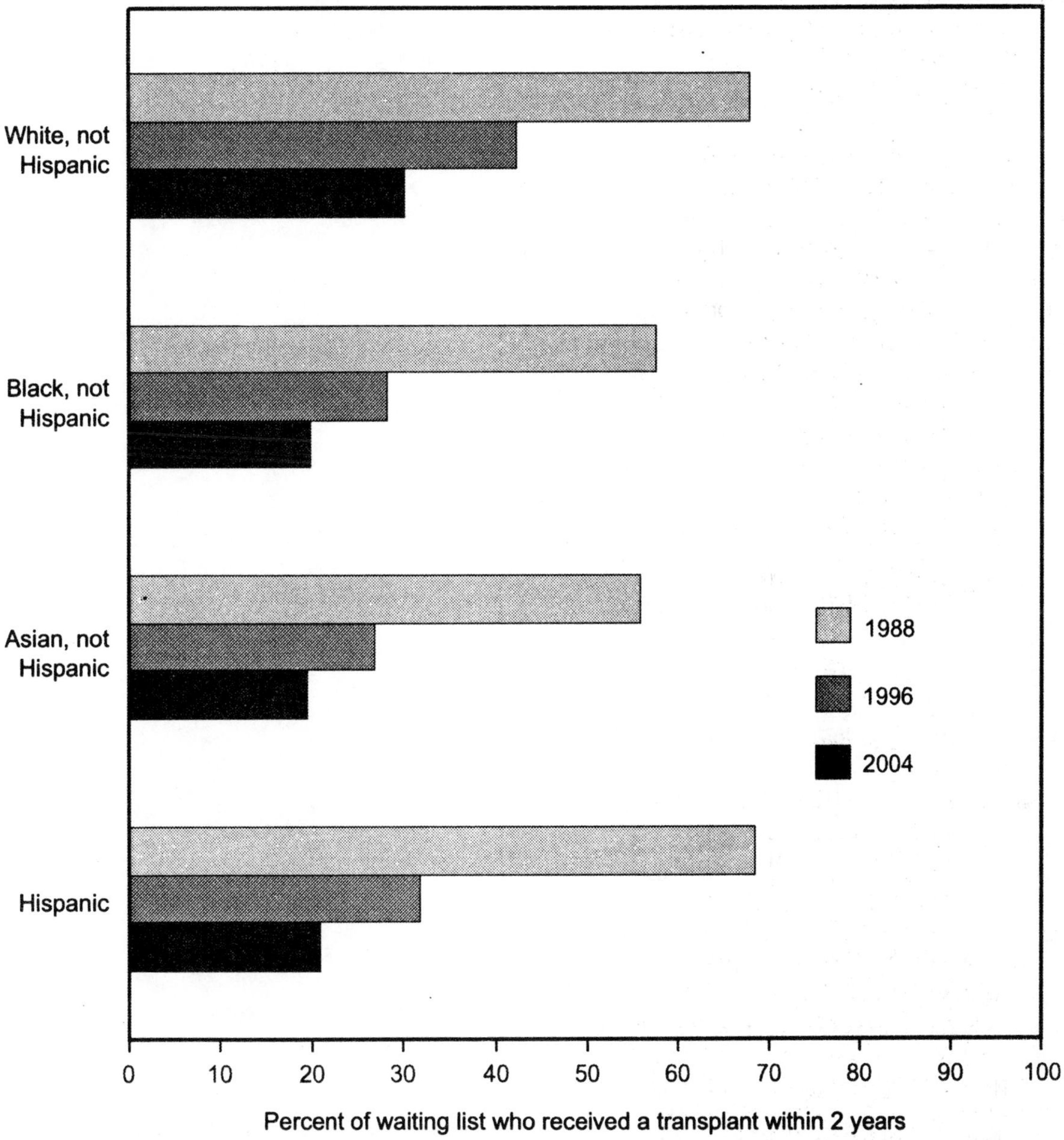

NOTES: Race and ethnicity are reported together as a single data element—either race or ethnicity, but not both. Persons listed as Hispanic are considered Hispanic and all others are classified by their recorded race. See data table for Figure 25 for data points graphed and additional notes.

SOURCE: Organ Procurement and Transplantation Network (OPTN) data as of March 9, 2007, supported in part by Health Resources and Services Administration contract 234-2005-370011C.

No Usual Source of Medical Care

Between 5% and 6% of adults 45–64 years of age with diagnosed hypertension, serious heart conditions, or diabetes report not having a usual source of medical care.

Not having a medical home or usual source of health care may be a barrier to accessing health care. Lacking a usual source of care is associated with poorer control of chronic conditions such as hypertension and lower receipt of preventive services (1,2). Lack of a usual source of care is most common among young adults 18–44 years of age (Table 78). However, about 10% of adults 45–64 years of age—a time in life when chronic illnesses become more common—did not have a usual source of health care in 2004–2005. The proportion of adults 45–64 years of age without a usual source of care has been stable over the past decade.

In 2004–2005, adults 45–64 years of age who did not report diagnosed chronic conditions were nearly three times as likely to lack a usual source of care as adults who reported hypertension, a serious heart condition, or diabetes (Figure 26, see Technical Notes for definitions of categories). Among those not reporting chronic conditions, Hispanic adults were considerably more likely than others to lack a usual source of care.

About 5%–6% of adults 45–64 years of age with diagnosed hypertension, serious heart disease, and diabetes reported not having a usual source of care. Among midlife adults with diagnosed hypertension, Hispanic and non-Hispanic black adults were more likely than non-Hispanic white adults to lack a usual source of care. For midlife adults with diagnosed diabetes, Hispanic adults were at least twice as likely to lack a usual source of care as other racial or ethnic groups.

References

1. Jiang H, Muntner P, Chen J, Roccella EJ, Streiffer RH, Whelton PK. Factors associated with hypertension control in the general population of the United States. Arch Intern Med 2002;162:1051–8. Available from: archinte.ama-assn.org/cgi/content/abstract/162/9/1051.
2. Corbie-Smith G, Flagg EW, Doyle JP, O'Brien MA. Influence of usual source of care on differences by race/ethnicity in receipt of preventive services. J Gen Intern Med 2002;17(6):458–64.

Figure 26. No usual source of care among adults 45–64 years of age, by selected diagnosed chronic conditions and race and Hispanic origin: United States, 2004–2005

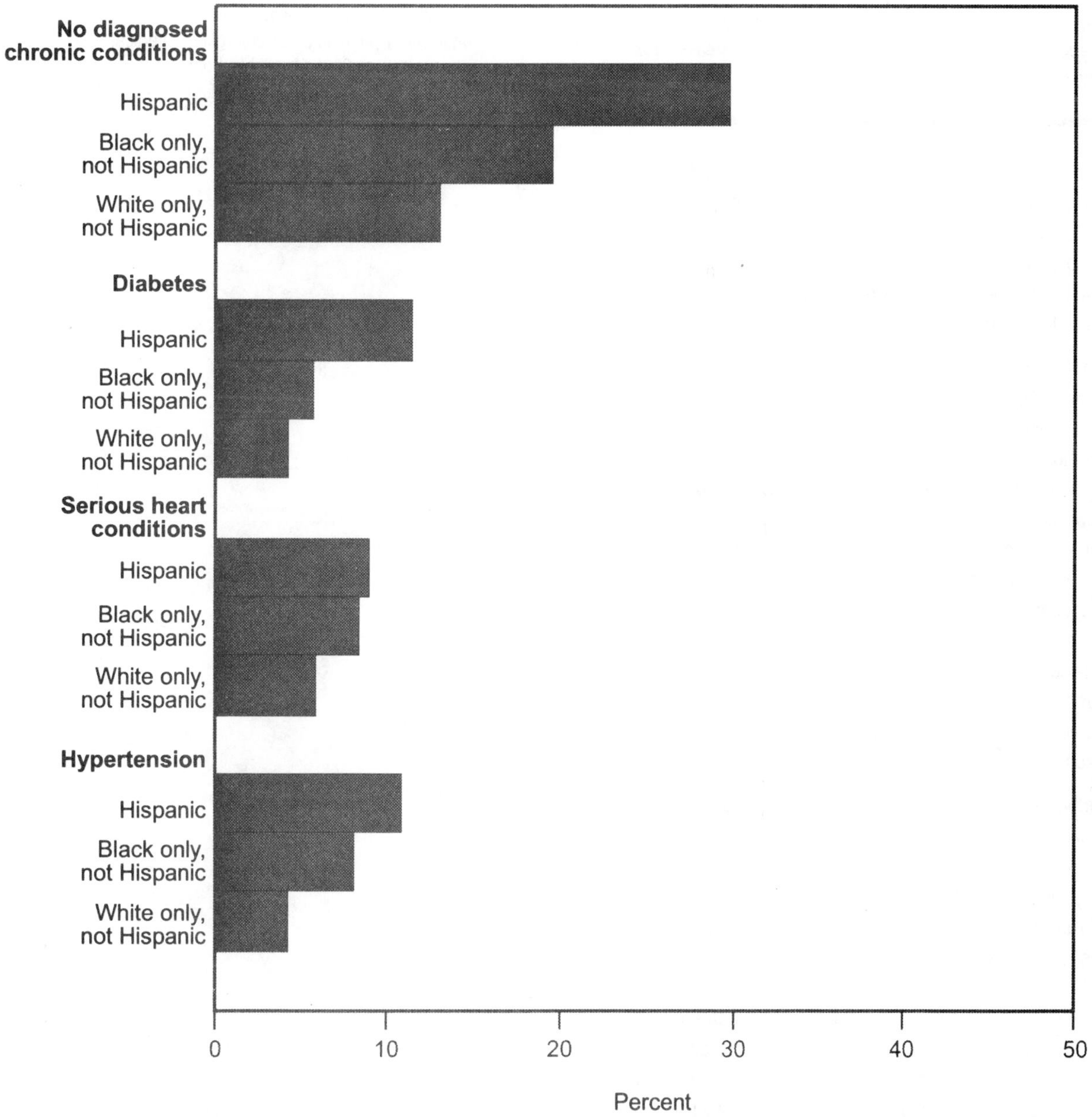

NOTES: Diagnosed chronic conditions were identified by asking if a physician or other health provider ever told the respondent they had the condition. Respondents who reported more than one chronic condition were counted in each reported category. See data table for Figure 26 for data points graphed, standard errors, definition of conditions, and additional notes.

SOURCE: Centers for Disease Control and Prevention, National Center for Health Statistics, National Health Interview Survey.

Delayed Medical Care Due to Lack of Transportation

Poor adults are more likely than those with higher incomes to delay medical care due to lack of transportation, with poor women age 45–64 years most likely to report this problem.

Missing routine or preventive medical care can lead to the need for emergency care or even to preventable hospitalizations. Lack of access to transportation due to not owning a vehicle, not having a vehicle available via a friend or family member, or not having access to public transportation can lead to difficulty in seeking medical care.

According to the 2001 National Household Transportation Survey, 27% of households with income below $20,000 did not own a vehicle, compared with 5% among households earning $20,000 to $39,999 and 8% of all U.S. households (1). Although public transit is an option, cost can be prohibitive and routes may not correspond with the location of medical facilities. In many communities, various forms of paratransit, alternative modes of flexible passenger transportation that do not follow fixed routes or schedules such as van services and demand-responsive buses, are available for medically-related trips (2). However, publicly funded transportation programs are usually targeted to specific vulnerable groups, such as Medicaid enrollees, persons with disabilities, or older persons.

In 2004–2005, adults living in families with income below 100% of the poverty level reported delaying care due to lack of transportation at 10 times the rate of adults with family incomes of 200% or more of the poverty level (data table for Figure 27; see Technical Notes for exact question wording). Among those with family income below 100% of the poverty level, adults 45–64 years of age reported the highest rates of delaying medical care due to lack of transportation (Figure 27). The problem was most commonly reported among poor women age 45–64 years, with almost 10% reporting that they delayed obtaining medical care due to lack of transportation.

References

1. Pucher J, Renne JL. Socioeconomics of urban travel: Evidence from the 2001 NHTS. Transportation Quarterly 2003;75:49–77.
2. Transit Cooperative Research Board. Cost-benefit analysis of providing non-emergency medical transportation. 2005. Available from: onlinepubs.trb.org/onlinepubs/tcrp/tcrp_webdoc_29.pdf.

Figure 27. Delayed medical care in the past 12 months due to lack of transportation among adults 18 years of age and over, by sex, percent of poverty level, and age: United States, 2004-2005

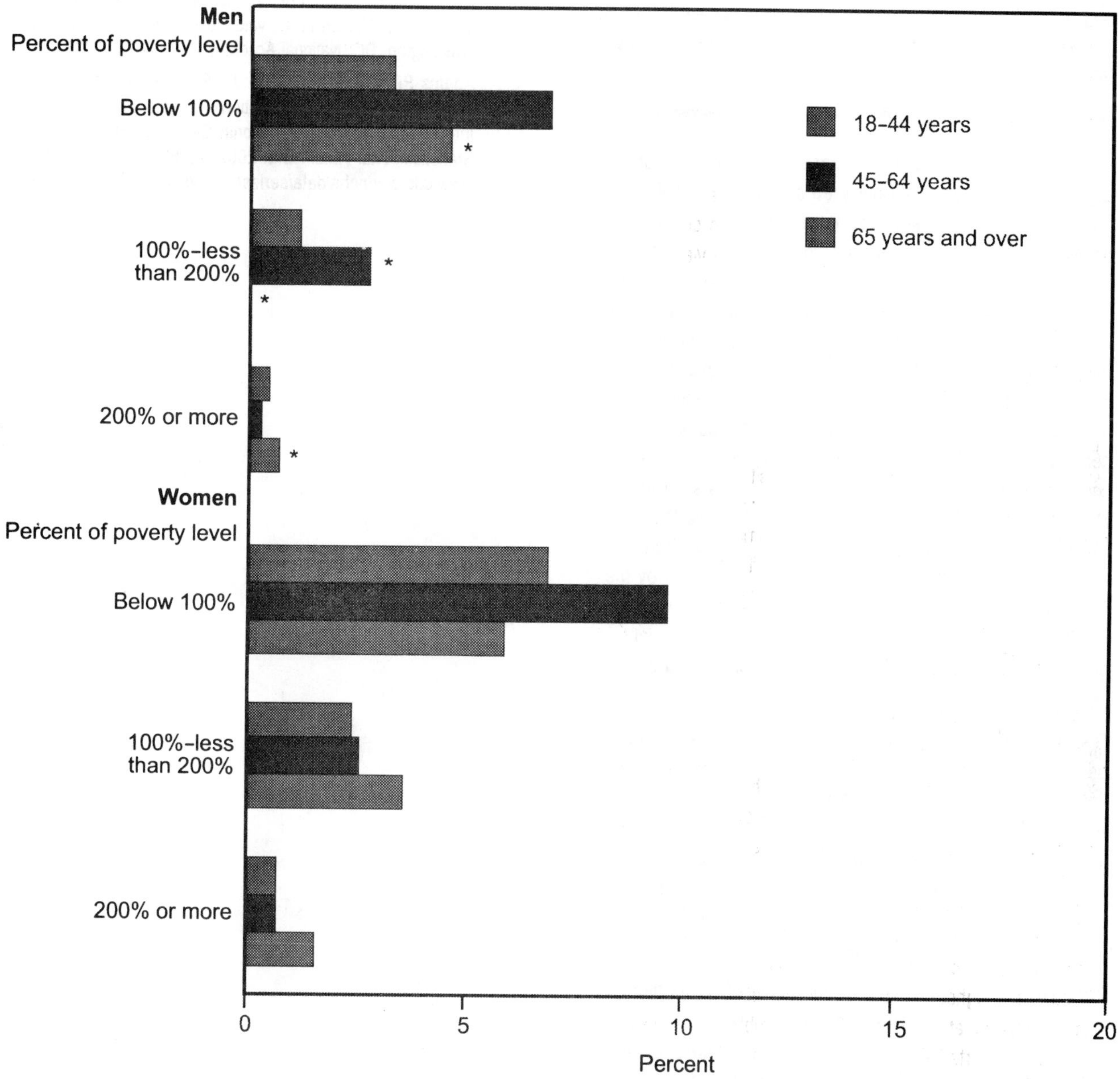

* Estimates are considered unreliable. Data shown with an asterisk have a relative standard error (RSE) of 20%–30%. Data not shown have an RSE of greater than 30%.

NOTES: Percent of poverty level is based on family income and family size and composition using U.S. Census Bureau poverty thresholds. See data table for Figure 27 for data points graphed, standard errors, and additional notes.

SOURCE: Centers for Disease Control and Prevention, National Center for Health Statistics, National Health Interview Survey.

Health Insurance at the Time of Interview

Between 1999 and 2005, the percentage of people under age 65 with private health insurance declined while public coverage programs expanded leaving the uninsured rate unchanged.

Health insurance coverage is an important determinant of access to health care (1). Uninsured children and adults under 65 years of age are substantially less likely to have a usual source of health care or a recent health care visit than their insured counterparts (Tables 77, 78, 79, 81). Uninsured people are more likely to forego needed health care because they cannot afford it (Table 79). The major source of coverage for persons under 65 years of age is private employer-sponsored group health insurance. Private health insurance may also be purchased on an individual basis, but is generally more costly and tends to provide less adequate coverage than group insurance. Public programs such as Medicaid and the State Children's Health Insurance Program (SCHIP) provide coverage for many low-income children and adults. Almost all adults age 65 and over are covered by the Medicare program, resulting in very few older adults without health insurance. Medicare enrollees may have additional private or public coverage to supplement their Medicare benefit package.

Between 1984 and 1994, private coverage declined among people under 65 years of age while Medicaid coverage and the percentage with no health insurance increased (Figure 28, Appendix II, Health insurance coverage). After rising to 73% in 1999, the percentage with private health insurance has declined each year, reaching 68% in 2005. This decrease has been offset by an increase in the percentage with Medicaid or SCHIP, resulting in little change in the percentage uninsured.

In recent years, 16%–17% of people under 65 years had no health insurance at the time of their interview. In 2005, cost was cited by more than one-half of these uninsured as the reason for their lack of coverage (2). Other reasons given were having lost a job or a change in employment (24%), Medicaid benefits stopped (10%), and ineligibility for family insurance coverage due to age or leaving school (8%).

References

1. Institute of Medicine. Committee on the consequences of uninsurance. Series of reports: Coverage matters: Insurance and health care; Care without coverage; Health insurance is a family matter; A shared destiny: Community effects of uninsurance; Hidden costs, value lost: Uninsurance in America. Washington, DC: National Academy Press. 2001–2003.
2. Adams PF, Dey AN, Vickerie JL. Summary health statistics for the U.S. population: National Health Interview Survey, 2005. National Center for Health Statistics. Vital Health Stat 2007;10(233). Available from: www.cdc.gov/nchs/data/series/sr_10/sr10_233.pdf.

Figure 28. Health insurance coverage at the time of interview among persons under 65 years of age: United States, 1984-2005

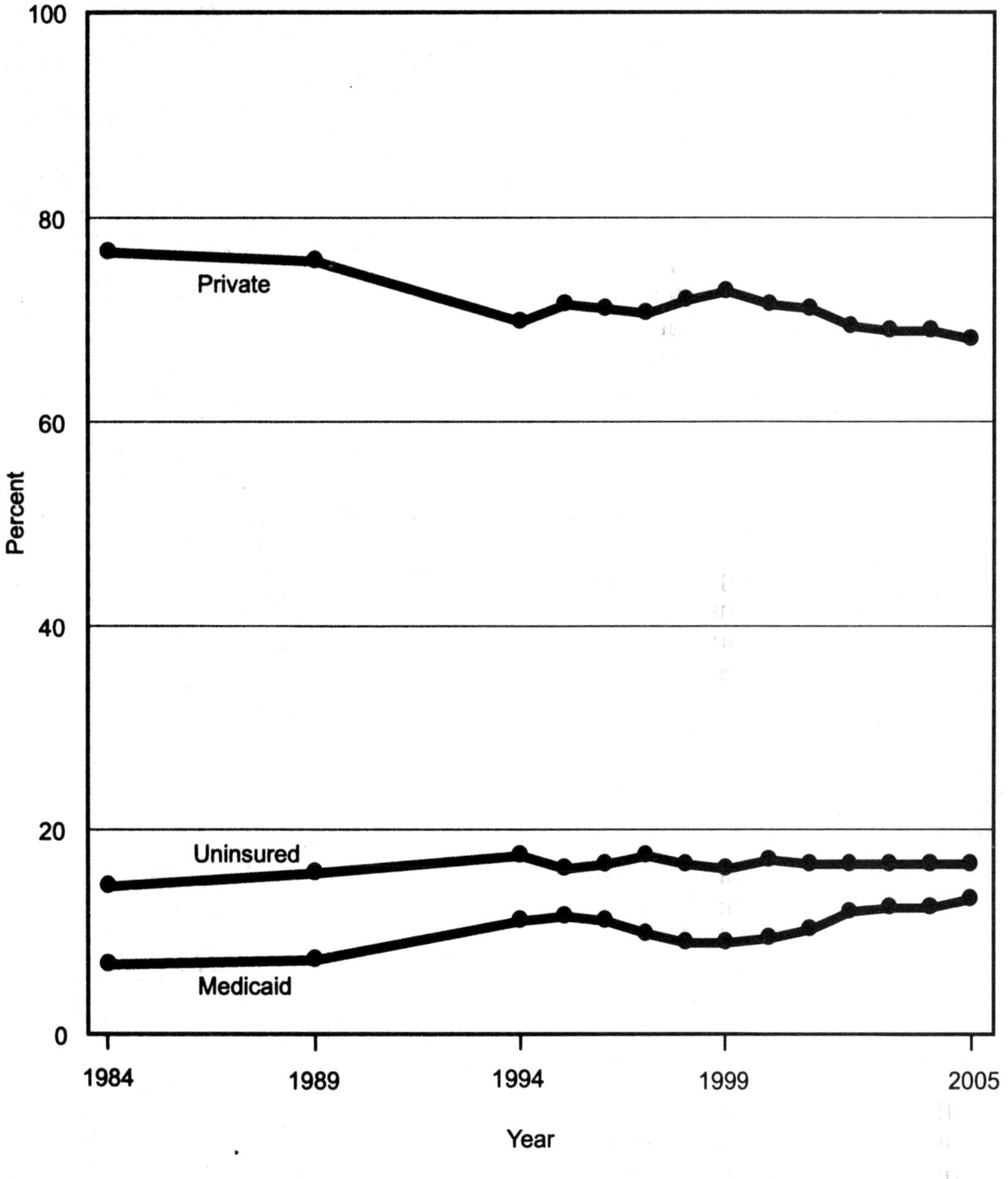

NOTE: See data table for Figure 28 for data points graphed, standard errors, and additional notes.

SOURCE: Centers for Disease Control and Prevention, National Center for Health Statistics, National Health Interview Survey.

Length of Time Without Health Insurance

Persons of Mexican origin are more likely than those in other race or ethnic groups to be uninsured for more than 12 months.

Many people under age 65, particularly those with low incomes, do not have health insurance coverage consistently throughout the year. Reasons for discontinuities in coverage may include loss or change of employment and financial reversals, divorce, births and other changes in life circumstances, and migration between states. Respondents to the National Health Interview Survey (NHIS) were asked whether they had health insurance at the time of their interview and the type of coverage (see Appendix II, Health insurance coverage). Those covered by health insurance at the time of interview were asked whether there was any time during the 12 months prior to the interview when they did not have health insurance. People who were uninsured at the time of interview were asked how long it had been since they last had health coverage. These questions provide estimates of the percentage of persons without coverage at a point-in-time (Figure 28), as well as estimates of the percentage without coverage for different lengths of time (Figure 29).

In 2005, 20% of people under 65 years of age reported being uninsured for at least part of the 12 months prior to interview. Among those who reported any time without insurance coverage during the 12 months prior to interview, the majority reported being uninsured for more than 12 months. About 11% of persons under 65 years reported being uninsured for more than 12 months, 8% reported being uninsured for any period up to 12 months, and 1% reported being uninsured and had missing data for the length of time they were uninsured (data table for Figure 29).

Children under 18 years of age were less likely to be uninsured than adults were because low income children are eligible for public programs such as SCHIP designed specifically for them. The percentage of adults under 65 years of age without health insurance coverage decreased with age (Figure 29). In 2005, adults 18–24 years of age were more likely than adults age 55–64 years to lack coverage for at least part of the 12 months prior to interview (35% compared with 13%). About 20% of persons 18–24 years of age lacked coverage for more than 12 months.

More than one-third of people with low family income (less than twice the poverty level) had no health insurance coverage for at least part of the 12 months prior to interview compared with 13 percent of those with higher family income. More than one-fifth of people in these lower income families were uninsured for more than 12 months, compared with only 6% of people in higher income families. Persons of Mexican origin were more likely than those in any other race or ethnic group to be uninsured for at least part of the 12 months prior to interview. In 2005, 40% of Mexican-origin persons lacked coverage for at least part of the 12 months prior to interview with 29% lacking coverage for more than 12 months.

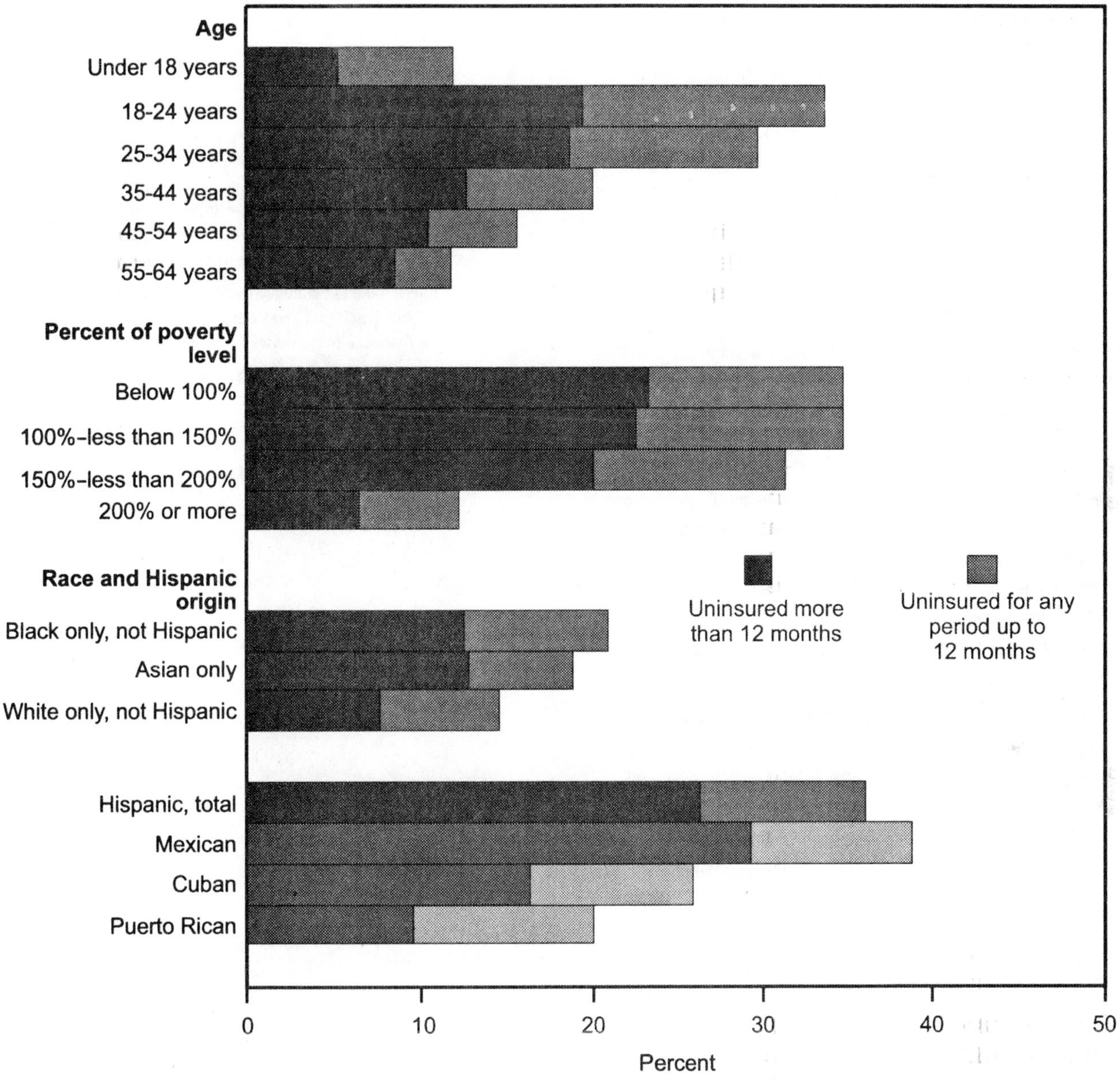

NOTES: Persons of Hispanic origin may be of any race. Asian only race includes persons of Hispanic and non-Hispanic origin. Percent of poverty level is based on family income and family size and composition using U.S. Census Bureau poverty thresholds. See data table for Figure 29 for data points graphed, standard errors, and additional notes.

SOURCE: Centers for Disease Control and Prevention, National Center for Health Statistics, National Health Interview Survey.

Profile of the Uninsured Population

Two-thirds of uninsured adults are currently working for pay.

People without health insurance coverage are more likely than their insured counterparts to forego needed medical care or prescription drugs (Table 79) and not to have a usual source of health care (Tables 77 and 78). They are also three times as likely to have not had a doctor's visit in the past year (Table 82). In 2005, 42.1 million persons under 65 years of age were uninsured on the day of their interview accounting for 16% of the nonelderly population (Table 139, see Appendix II, Health insurance coverage).

About two-thirds of uninsured adults were working for pay in the week prior to their interview in 2005 (data table for Figure 30). Employment is the major source of private health insurance coverage (Table 137). However, many uninsured people work for firms that do not offer coverage, are not eligible for coverage, or decline offers of health insurance for financial or other reasons (1). Since 2000, the percentage of private firms offering private health insurance benefits has declined. Small firms, those with a large percentage of low-income earners, and those with a high percentage of part-time workers were less likely to offer their employees health insurance coverage (2).

In 2005, the majority of the uninsured population was comprised of young adults 18–44 years of age who accounted for more than 60% of the uninsured population (Figure 30). More than one-fifth of the uninsured were 45–64 years of age, a time in life when chronic illness becomes more prevalent (Tables 55, 70, 71). Children comprised 16% of the uninsured.

The uninsured population was about equally divided between non-Hispanic white people and people of other races and ethnicities. People of Hispanic origin accounted for nearly one-third of the uninsured population, and 14% of the uninsured population were non-Hispanic black (data table for Figure 30).

Although Medicaid and the State Children's Health Insurance Program cover some poor and near poor people, private health insurance can be expensive, particularly when it is not subsidized by employers (1,3). Low-income families may have difficulty affording health insurance, but not all uninsured people have low family income. In 2005, more than 40% of uninsured people had a family income of at least 200% of the poverty level (data table for Figure 30).

About 60% of the uninsured population was unmarried (data table for Figure 30). Married people have the advantage of two potential sources of health insurance coverage.

References

1. Department of Health and Human Services. Office of the Assistant Secretary for Planning and Evaluation. Overview of the uninsured in the United States: An analysis of the 2005 Current Population Survey. 2005. Available from: aspe.hhs.gov/health/reports/05/uninsured-cps/index.htm#work.
2. The Kaiser Family Foundation and Health Research and Educational Trust. Employer Health Benefits: 2006 Annual Survey. Available from: www.kff.org/insurance/7527/index.cfm.
3. Banthin JS, Bernard DM. Changes in financial burdens for health care: National estimates for the population younger than 65 years, 1996 to 2003. JAMA 2006;296:2712–9.

Figure 30. The uninsured population under 65 years of age, by selected characteristics: United States, 2005

42.1 million persons uninsured at the time of interview

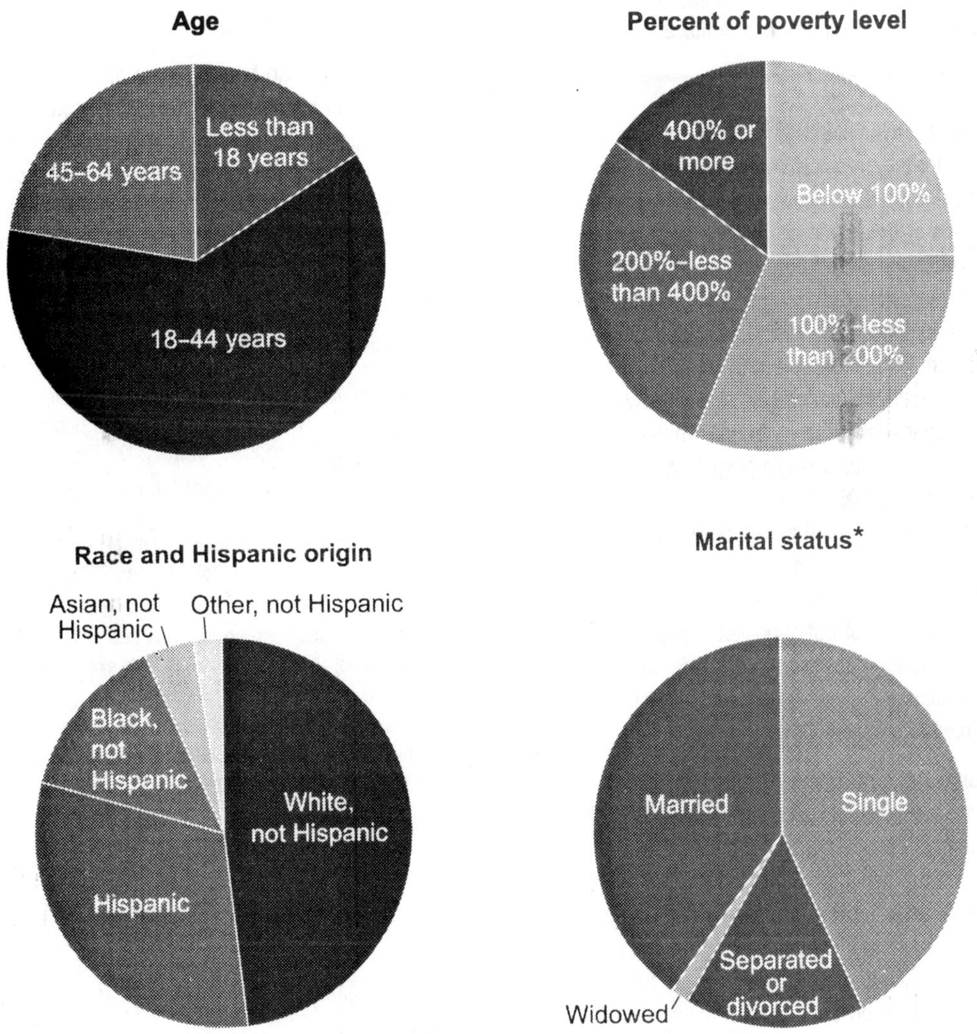

*Marital status is for adults 18–64 years of age (35.3 million uninsured persons).

NOTES: Percent of poverty level is based on family income and family size and composition using U.S. Census Bureau poverty thresholds. Persons of Hispanic origin may be of any race. See data table for Figure 30 for data points graphed and additional notes.

SOURCE: Centers for Disease Control and Prevention, National Center for Health Statistics, National Health Interview Survey.

Burden of Out-of-Pocket Expenditures

More than one-quarter of people under 65 years of age living in poverty are paying more than 10% of their after-tax family income on out-of-pocket medical expenses, including health insurance premiums.

Although health insurance substantially reduces the amount enrolled people pay for their medical care, out-of-pocket expenditures for non-covered services, copayments, deductibles, and caps on total amounts paid by insurance may impose a considerable financial burden even for insured people (1). In 2004, an estimated 15% of all aggregate personal health care expenditures—more than $236 billion dollars—were paid out-of-pocket (Table 125). Annual premiums for private health insurance can be expensive, and for people with employer-sponsored coverage, worker contributions averaged $627 for a single-person plan and $2,973 for a family plan in 2006 (2). Individual policies (nonemployer-sponsored, nongroup) paid entirely by the beneficiary often cost substantially more than group policies (3). Low-income and uninsured people are at a greater risk of a high burden of out-of-pocket expenditures, but insured wealthier people can also pay considerable amounts for their health care if they experience catastrophic illness or chronic disabling conditions (4).

The Medical Expenditure Panel Survey (MEPS) collects information on costs for health insurance premiums, utilization of medical care services, and expenses and source of payment for medical care services (See Technical Notes). It also collects detailed family income data. Figure 31 presents the percentage of people under 65 years of age who lived in families that spent more than 10% of their after-tax family income (disposable income) on out-of-pocket medical costs, including any costs for health insurance premiums, by family poverty level.

The financial burden of out-of-pocket health care costs is greatest for the poor. More than one-quarter of people under age 65 with family income below the poverty line paid more than 10% of their after-tax family income on out-of-pocket health care expenditures in both 1996 and 2004 (Figure 31). Almost one-quarter of people living in families with income of 100%–less than 200% of the poverty level paid more than 10% of their disposable income for health care costs in both these years (24% in 1996 and 22% in 2004), as did 16%–17% of people with family income of 200%–less than 400% of the poverty level. Among people in the highest income group (more than 400% of the poverty level), 10% paid more than 10% of their after-tax family income on out-of-pocket health care and premiums in 2004, an increase from 7% of this income group in 1996.

Health insurance can be expensive and financially burdensome to families, particularly nongroup, individually purchased policies. In 2003, persons with nongroup plans were nearly three times as likely to spend more than 10% of their disposable income on health care, including health insurance premiums as individuals in any other insurance category, including the uninsured (1).

References

1. Banthin JS, Bernard DM. Changes in financial burdens for health care: National estimates for the population younger than 65 years, 1996 to 2003. JAMA 2006;296:2712–9.
2. The Kaiser Family Foundation and Health Research and Educational Trust. Employer health benefits: 2006 summary of findings. Available from: www.kff.org/insurance/7527/upload/7528.pdf.
3. Pauly MV, Nichols LM. The nongroup health insurance market: Short on facts, long on opinions and policy disputes. Health Aff (Millwood) 2002 Jul-Dec;suppl web exclusives:w325–44.
4. Hoffman C, Rowland D, Hamel E. Medical debt and access to health care. Kaiser Commission on Medicaid and the Uninsured, September 2005. Available from: kff.org/uninsured/7403.cfm.

Figure 31. Persons under 65 years of age who spent more than 10% of after-tax family income on out-of-pocket medical expenditures, by percent of poverty level: United States, 1996 and 2004

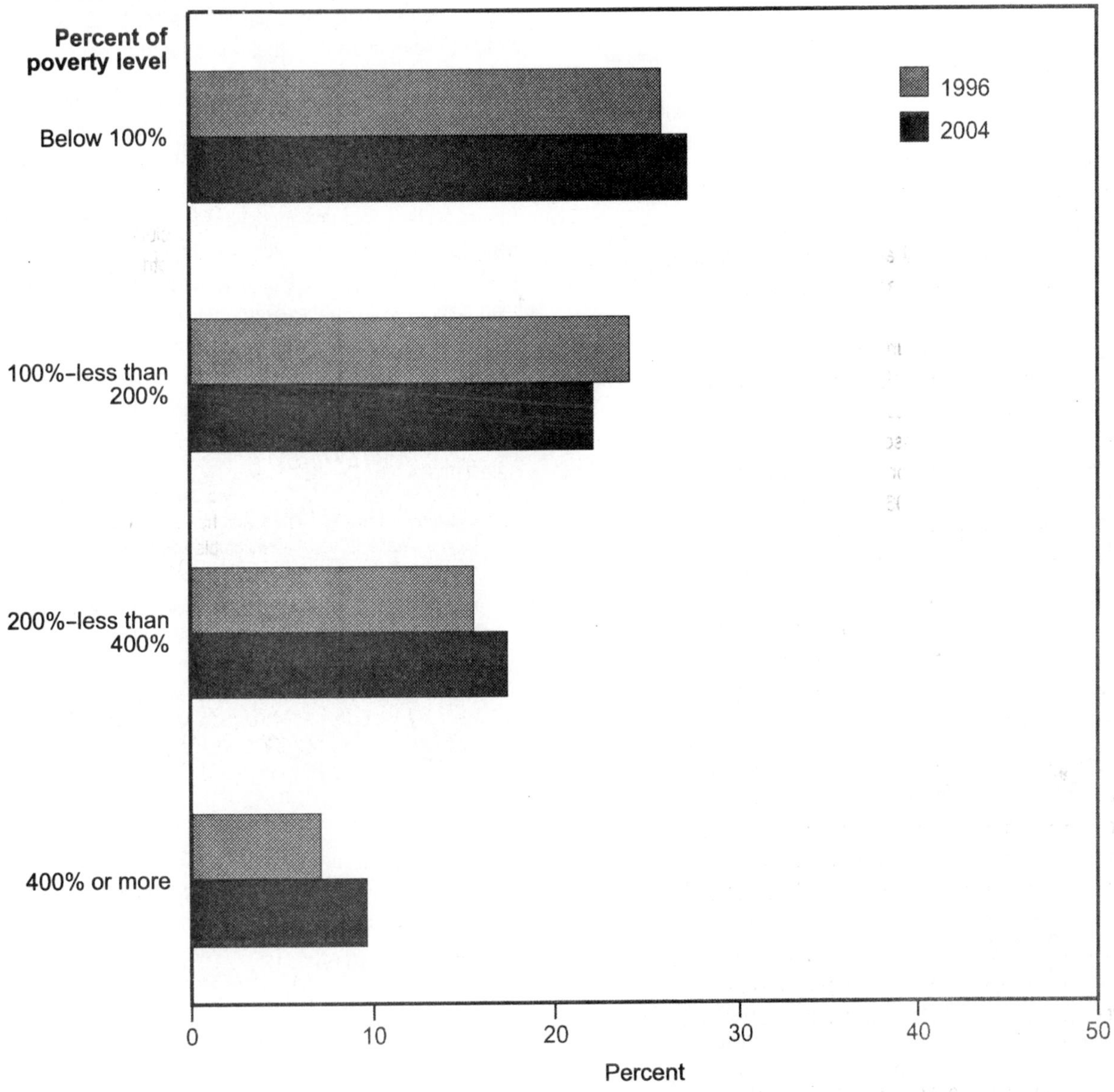

NOTES: Out-of-pocket medical expenditures include health insurance premiums. See data table for Figure 31 for data points graphed and additional notes.

SOURCE: Agency for Healthcare Research and Quality, Medical Expenditure Panel Survey.

Undiagnosed Medical Conditions

The percentage of adults 20–64 years of age who have undiagnosed high cholesterol or elevated blood pressure does not differ significantly by health insurance coverage.

Appropriate ongoing health care is necessary to prevent, reduce, or delay morbidity and disability, and to delay premature death from chronic conditions. In order to obtain appropriate health care and make any needed lifestyle adjustments, people must first be diagnosed with the medical condition. Uninsured people are less likely to have a usual source of care, have fewer ambulatory care visits per year, but are as likely to use emergency departments as insured persons (Tables 78, 82, and 90). This differential pattern of health care use may increase the likelihood that uninsured persons have undiagnosed medical conditions.

High cholesterol and elevated blood pressure are common, serious, treatable medical conditions. Both conditions are risk factors for heart disease, the leading cause of death (Table 31; 1). Elevated blood pressure is also a risk factor for stroke, the third leading cause of death (2).

In the National Health and Nutrition Examination Survey, respondents were asked about the presence of chronic health conditions, including whether a physician or other health professional had ever told them they had high cholesterol or high blood pressure. They were also asked about health insurance coverage at the time of their interview. Following their interview, respondents were examined at the mobile examination center (MEC); the examination included laboratory and other tests. The presence of high cholesterol was defined as a total cholesterol reading of 240 mg/dL or higher (6.20 mmol/L) and elevated blood pressure as an average systolic blood pressure of 140 mm Hg or higher, or an average diastolic reading of 90 mm Hg or higher. Persons were considered undiagnosed if they failed to report in the interview that the medical condition had been previously diagnosed but the condition was detected as a result of the examination at the MEC. Because nearly all persons 65 years of age and over are insured, this analysis was limited to adults 20–64 years of age. For more information, see the Technical Notes.

Overall, 10% of adults 20–64 years of age had undiagnosed high cholesterol and 8% had undiagnosed elevated blood pressure in 1999–2004 (data table for Figure 32). Adults 45–64 years of age were more likely to have undiagnosed conditions than those 20–44 years of age. In particular, they were more than three times as likely as adults 20–44 years of age to have undiagnosed elevated blood pressure.

Although it appears from Figure 32 that uninsured adults were more likely than insured adults to have undiagnosed high cholesterol or elevated blood pressure based on data from 1999–2004, these differences were not statistically significant. The percentage with undiagnosed conditions did not differ by insurance status for adults 20–44 years of age or those 45–64 years of age. These chronic conditions could have been diagnosed when they were previously insured or during the use of free or subsidized care, or care paid for out-of-pocket or during the use of emergency health care services.

References

1. Centers for Disease Control and Prevention. Heart disease risk factors. Available from: www.cdc.gov/heartdisease/risk_factors.htm.
2. American Heart Association. Stroke risk factors. Available from: www.americanheart.org/presenter.jhtml?identifier=4716.

Figure 32. Adults 20–64 years of age with undiagnosed high cholesterol or elevated blood pressure, by health insurance status and age: United States, 1999–2004

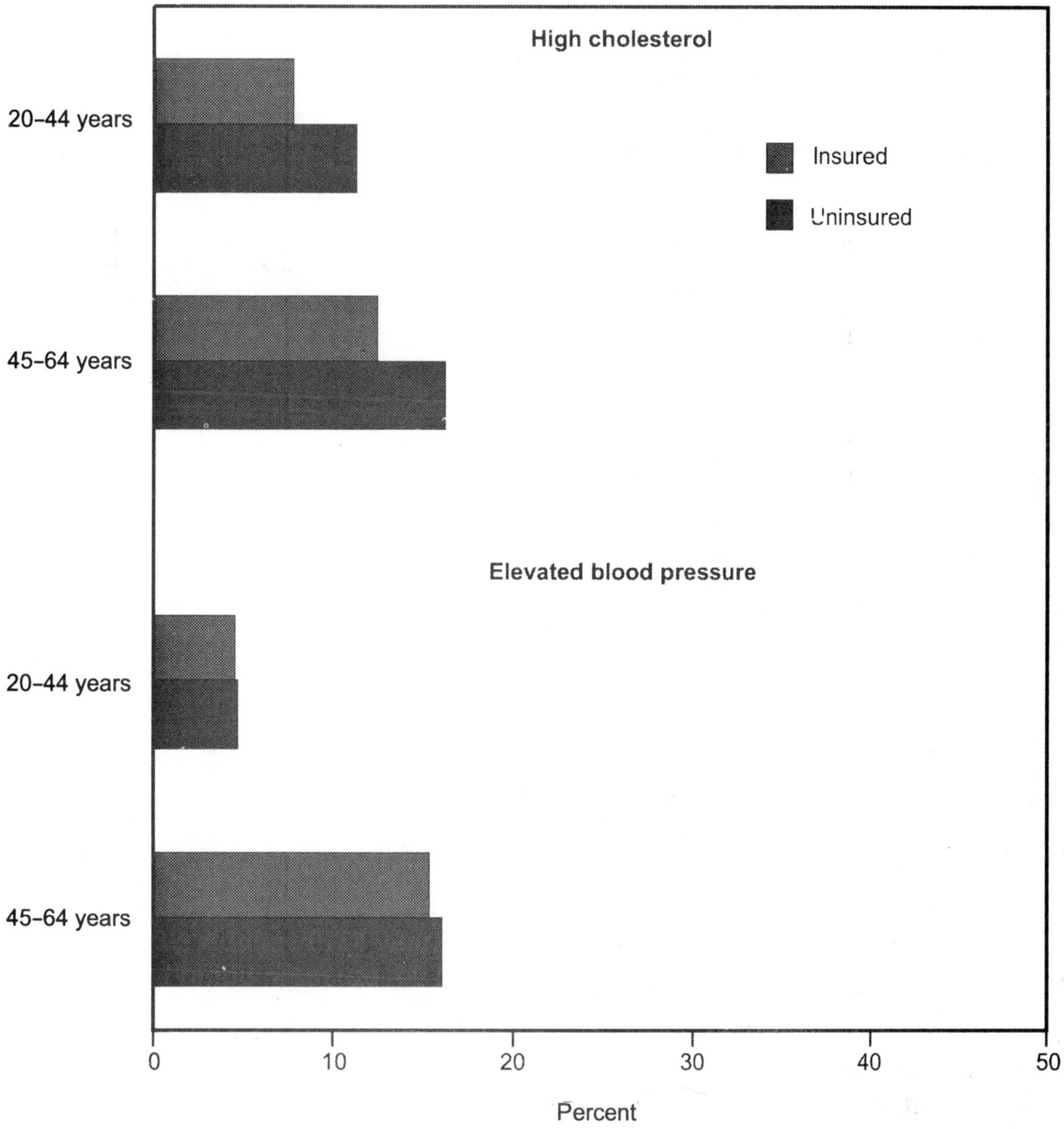

NOTES: Insurance coverage is as of the day of interview. Undiagnosed refers to the condition not being reported during the interview, but detected upon examination. See data table for Figure 32 for data points graphed, standard errors, and additional notes.

SOURCE: Centers for Disease Control and Prevention, National Center for Health Statistics, National Health and Nutrition Examination Survey.

Foregone Medical Care Due to Cost by Length of Time Without Health Insurance

Persons with some period during the previous 12 months without health insurance are more likely to forego needed medical care due to cost than those who had coverage the whole 12 months.

Because health care can be expensive, people without health insurance may not receive needed medical care because of the cost. Even people with health insurance may find that deductibles, copayments, and coinsurance place some medical care out of their financial reach. As shown in Figure 29, many people under age 65, particularly those with low incomes, do not have health insurance coverage consistently throughout the year. Nearly all persons 65 years of age and older are covered continuously by Medicare, the federal health program for the elderly, and are therefore excluded from Figure 33.

In 2005, health insurance was a major determinant of whether people were likely to forego needed health care because of the cost (see Technical Notes). People under 65 years who had been uninsured for more than 12 months or who had been uninsured for any time up to 12 months prior to their survey interview were much more likely to have foregone needed medical care because of the cost than were those who had been insured continuously the whole 12 months (Figure 33). There was little difference between people uninsured for any part of the year and those who were continuously uninsured for more than a year in their likelihood of foregoing medical care.

Children under 18 years of age were less likely to have foregone needed medical care because of cost than were adults 18–64 years of age (Figure 33). Children are less likely than adults to have chronic conditions, which often require higher-cost medical care. In 2004, annual expenses for health care for children averaged $1144 compared with $3053 for adults 18–64 years of age (calculated from Table 128). In addition, because decisions concerning children's medical care are usually made by their parents, these data suggest that adults may be more likely to forego needed medical care for themselves than for their children.

The likelihood of foregoing needed medical care because of cost also differed according to family income. In 2005, people living in families with income less than twice the poverty level were more likely to forego such care than people with higher income, irrespective of age or health insurance.

Figure 33. Persons under 65 years of age who did not get needed medical care in the past year due to cost, by duration of health insurance coverage and percent of poverty level: United States, 2005

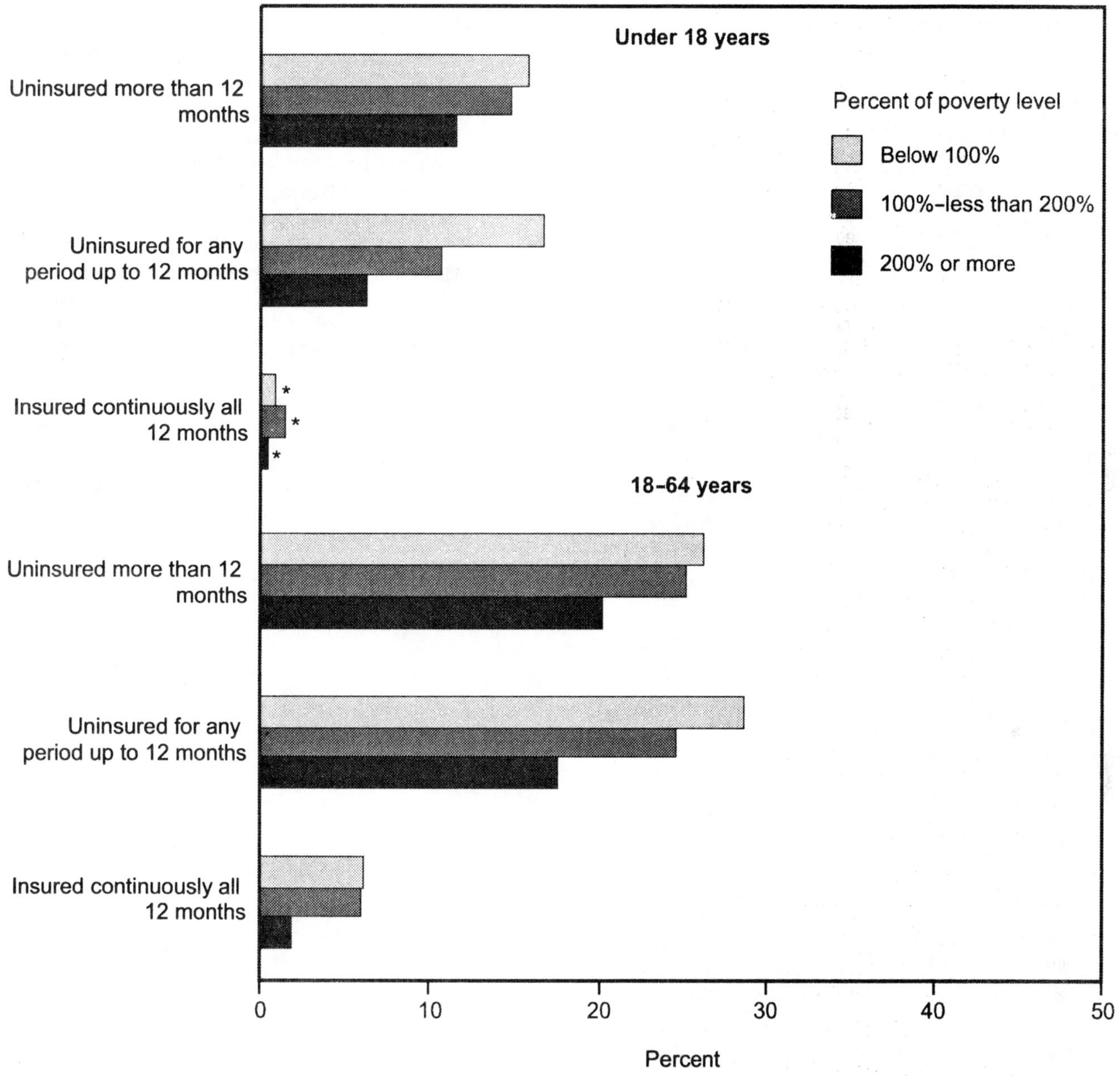

* Estimates are considered unreliable. Data shown with an asterisk have a relative standard error of 20%–30%.

NOTES: See data table for Figure 33 for data points graphed, standard errors, and additional notes.

SOURCE: Centers for Disease Control and Prevention, National Center for Health Statistics, National Health Interview Survey.

Dental Care Utilization

Poor or near-poor persons are more likely to lack a recent dental visit than higher income persons.

Lack of regular dental care can result in pain, infection, and delayed diagnosis of oral diseases including periodontal or gingival diseases and oral cancers (1). Barriers to accessing dental care include paying for care, navigating government assistance programs, finding a dentist who will accept Medicaid, locating a dentist close to home (especially true for inner-city and rural residents), getting to a dental office, and cultural or language barriers (2). For some people, lack of knowledge concerning the need for periodic oral health care is also a barrier to seeking care. Certain subpopulation groups—the poor, black persons, and persons of Mexican origin—were more likely to have untreated dental caries (Table 76). Untreated dental caries indicates that needed dental care was not received.

Accessing dental care may be more difficult than accessing medical care because a smaller percentage of Americans have dental insurance than medical coverage. In 2001, 61% of adults had any dental insurance compared with 86% of adults with any medical insurance (3). On average, Americans paid about one-half of the cost of dental care out-of-pocket in 2003 (4). More adults reported they did not get needed dental care due to the cost (12%) than did not receive needed medical care due to cost (7%) (Figure 21).

An additional factor affecting use of dental care is the absence or presence of natural teeth (5). Edentulous persons (without any natural teeth) should see a dentist periodically for maintenance of any dental prostheses and oral cancer screening. About one-quarter of persons 65 years of age and over were edentulous in 2005 (6). Edentulous persons 65 years of age and over were almost three times as likely to lack a recent dental visit as their dentate counterparts (with at least one natural tooth) (data table for Figure 34).

Use of dental care varied by family income and age (Figure 34, see Technical Notes). Within each age group, persons living below 200% of the poverty level were substantially more likely to lack a dental visit within the past year than those living in families with higher income. About one-third of all children (dentate status is not assessed for children) living below 200% of the poverty level did not have a recent dental visit. About one-half of dentate adults with family income below 200% of the poverty level did not have a recent dental visit (data table for Figure 34).

References

1. Oral Health in America: A Report of the Surgeon General. May 2000. Available from: www.surgeongeneral.gov/library/oralhealth.
2. Guay AH. Access to dental care: Solving the problem for underserved populations. JADA 2004; 135:1599–605.
3. Dental, Oral and Craniofacial Data Research Center. Oral health U.S., 2002. Bethesda, MD. Available from: drc.hhs.gov/report/inside_cover.htm.
4. Agency for Healthcare Research and Quality. Medical Expenditure Panel Survey. Center for Financing, Access, and Cost Trends. Dental services expenditures table 2. 2003. Available from: www.meps.ahrq.gov/mepsweb/data_stats/summ_tables/hc/state_expend/2003/table2.htm.
5. Macek MD, Cohen LA, Reid BC, Manski RJ. Dental visits among older U.S. adults, 1999: The roles of dentition status and cost. JADA 2004;135:1154–62.
6. Centers for Disease Control and Prevention, National Health Interview Survey, unpublished analysis.

Figure 34. No dental visit in the past year among persons with natural teeth, by age and percent of poverty level: United States, 2005

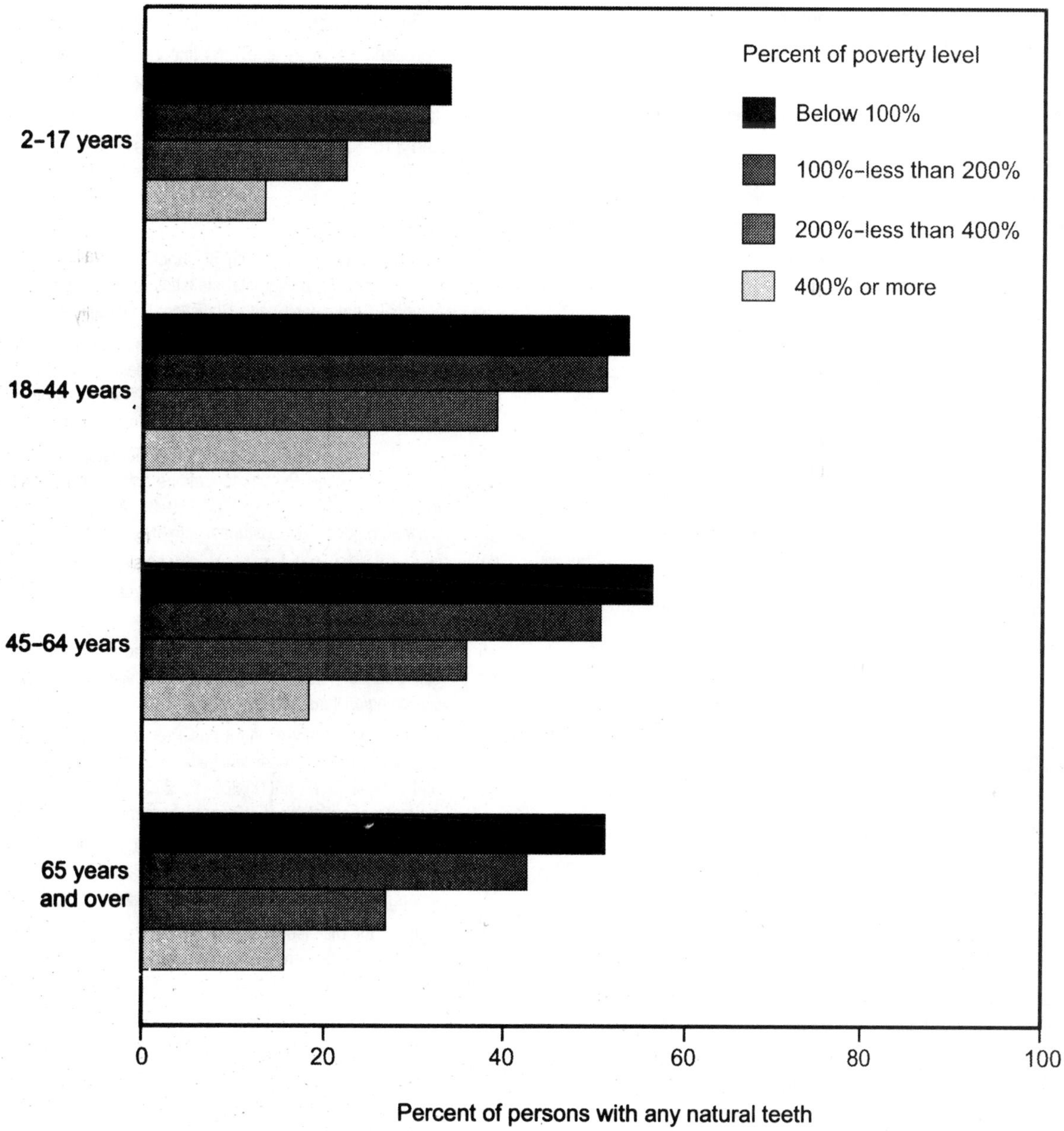

NOTES: Data are for all children 2–17 years. Dentate status is not assessed for children. Data are for the civilian noninstitutionalized population. See data table for Figure 34 for data points graphed, standard errors, and additional notes.

SOURCE: Centers for Disease Control and Prevention, National Center for Health Statistics, National Health Interview Survey.

Colorectal Scope Procedures

The percentage of adults ever having a colorectal scope procedure remains low; racial and ethnic disparities persist even among adults with health insurance coverage.

Colorectal cancer, or cancer of the colon or rectum, is the second leading cause of cancer-related death in the United States. In 2004, about 54,000 people in the United States died from colorectal cancer (1). Reducing the number of deaths from colorectal cancer depends on detecting and removing precancerous polyps or growths as well as detecting and treating the cancer in its early stages (2). The U.S. Preventive Services Task Force (UPSTF) recommends regular screening for colorectal cancer for all adults 50 years of age and over. Recommendations call for one or more of the following tests: fecal occult blood test (FOBT) every year, flexible sigmoidoscopy every 5 years, double-contrast barium enema every 5 years, or colonoscopy every 10 years (3).

About 44% of adults 50 years of age and over reported ever having had a colonoscopy, sigmoidoscopy, or proctoscopy (scope procedure) (data table for Figure 35, Technical Notes). Uninsured adults were less than half as likely as their insured counterparts to have been screened. The average procedure cost was estimated at $800–$2,000 for colonoscopy and $150–$300 for sigmoidoscopy (4,5). The Medicare program covers much of the cost of scope procedures among adults 65 years and over, and scope procedure rates among older insured persons are higher than for younger insured adults. More than one-half (52%) of older insured adults reported ever having a scope procedure compared with about 40% of insured adults 50–64 years of age (data table for Figure 35).

Although use of scope procedures has been increasing in recent years (6), racial and ethnic disparities persist even among adults who have health insurance coverage. Among insured adults 50–64 years of age, the percentage ever having a scope procedure was lower among Hispanic and non-Hispanic black adults than non-Hispanic white adults (Figure 35). Access barriers such as language, health literacy, and cultural perceptions of risk may contribute to the racial and ethnic disparities in scope procedure rates (7). The percentage ever having a scope procedure also varied by educational attainment. About 30% of insured adults age 50–64 years with less than a high school education, compared to 45% of adults with more than a high school education, reported ever having a scope procedure (Figure 35).

Population groups that were less likely to have ever had scope procedures were also less likely to have fecal occult blood tests in the past year, so it is unlikely that they are substituting more affordable annual fecal occult tests (between $10–$25) for scope procedures (5,8).

References

1. Miniño AM, Heron M, Smith BL, Kochanek KD. Deaths: Final data for 2004. National vital statistics reports. Hyattsville, MD: National Center for Health Statistics. Forthcoming.
2. Centers for Disease Control and Prevention. National Center for Chronic Disease Prevention and Health Promotion. Cancer—Colorectal cancer screening. 2006. Available from: www.cdc.gov/cancer/colorectal/basic_info/screening/.
3. U.S. Preventive Services Task Force. Screening for colorectal cancer: Recommendations and rationale. Ann Intern Med 2002. Jul 16;137(2):129–31. Available from: www.ahrq.gov/clinic/uspstf/uspscolo.htm.
4. Sonnenberg A, Delcò F, Inadomi JM. Cost-effectiveness of colonoscopy in screening for colorectal cancer. Ann Intern Med 2000;133:573–84.
5. Myers D. Colon cancer screening for the uninsured. About colon cancer. Available from: coloncancer.about.com/od/screening/a/Uninsured.htm.
6. Centers for Disease Control and Prevention. Increased use of colorectal cancer tests—United States, 2002 and 2004. MMWR 55(11);308–11. 2006. Available from: www.cdc.gov/mmwr/preview/mmwrhtml/mm5511a4.htm.
7. Shih YT, Zhao L, Elting LS. Does Medicare coverage of colonoscopy reduce racial/ethnic disparities in cancer screening among the elderly? Health Affairs 2006;25(4):1153–62.
8. Centers for Disease Control and Prevention, National Health Interview Survey, unpublished analysis.

Figure 35. Adults 50 years of age and over ever having a colorectal scope procedure, by selected characteristics: United States, annual average 2000, 2003, and 2005

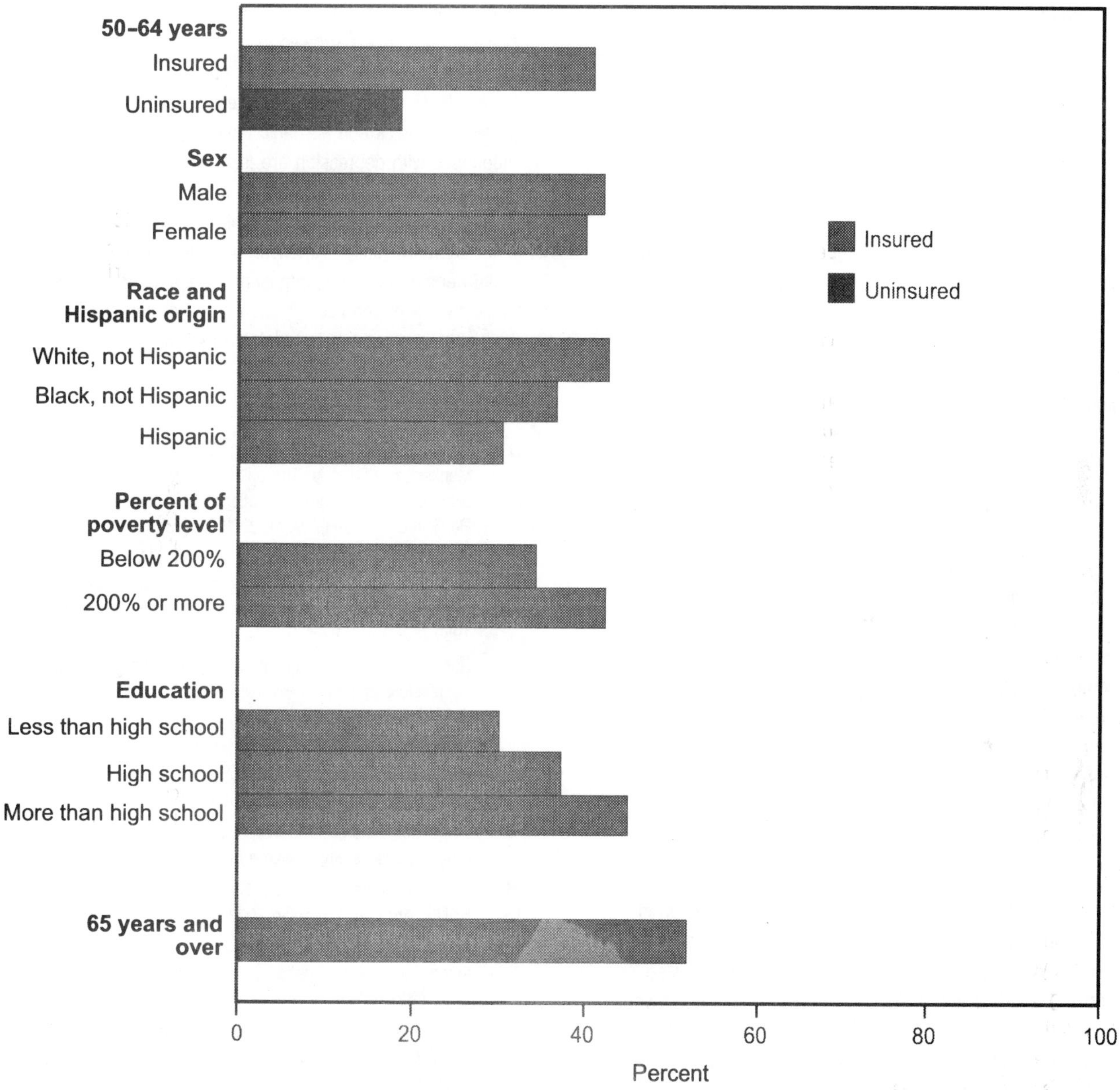

NOTES: Colorectal scope procedures include colonoscopy, sigmoidoscopy, or proctoscopy. See data table for Figure 35 for data points graphed, standard errors, and additional notes.

SOURCE: Centers for Disease Control and Prevention, National Center for Health Statistics, National Health Interview Survey.

Antidepressant Drugs: Adults

Non-Hispanic white women are more likely to have used antidepressant drugs in the past month than non-Hispanic black women or women of Mexican origin.

Depression and other forms of mental illness are critical public health issues in America today. In 2001–2002, an estimated 16% of noninstitutionalized adults had a major depressive disorder at some point in their lifetime, with 7% having had a major depressive episode during the 12 months prior to interview (1). The detrimental effects of depressive symptoms on quality of life and daily functioning have been estimated to equal or exceed those of heart disease and exceed those of diabetes, arthritis, and gastrointestinal disorders (2,3). Access to both accurate diagnosis and appropriate treatment of depression is necessary to combat this prevalent and debilitating disease.

Prescriptions for antidepressants have been rising, associated with the introduction in 1988 of a new class of drugs known as selective serotonin reuptake inhibitors (SSRIs) (4). Current SSRIs include the brand names Celexa®, Lexapro®, Luvox®, Paxil®, Prozac®, and Zoloft®. In addition to their use as antidepressants, SSRIs are approved and marketed for the treatment of other mental disorders including obsessive compulsive disorder, panic disorder, anxiety disorders, and premenstrual dysphoric disorder. The substantial increase in prescriptions for antidepressants also suggests widespread "off-label" (other than FDA-approved uses) use for subsyndromal mental health conditions and a variety of physical disorders (5,6).

Between 1988–1994 and 1999–2002 the percentage of adults in the civilian noninstitutionalized population who reported using an antidepressant drug during the past month more than tripled, increasing from 2.5% to 8.0% (age-adjusted; data table for Figure 36, Technical Notes). Use among women rose from 3.3% to 10.6% and use among men from 1.6% to 5.2%. In both time periods, antidepressant use by women was about twice that of men.

In 1999–2002, the percentage of non-Hispanic white adults who reported the use of antidepressants was more than double that reported by non-Hispanic black and Mexican adults. Nearly 13% of non-Hispanic white women reported use of antidepressants in the past month, compared with about 5% of non-Hispanic black and Mexican women. In the same time period, 6% of non-Hispanic white men reported antidepressant drug use in the past month, compared with about 3% of non-Hispanic black men and less than 2% of men of Mexican origin. Disparities in the diagnosis of depression of black and Hispanic patients compared to white patients may have narrowed in recent years. However, racial or ethnic disparities in the treatment—including prescriptions for antidepressant drugs—of depression once diagnosed persist (7). Black and Hispanic patients who have been diagnosed with depression are less likely to obtain counseling and drug therapy to treat their depression than are white patients. Factors contributing to this disparity may include a belief by more African American and Hispanic persons than white persons that antidepressant therapy is unacceptable or ineffective, a preference for other types of therapy, or financial and insurance barriers to obtaining treatment (7,8).

References

1. Kessler RC, Berglund P, Demler O, Jin R, Koretz D, Merikangas KR, et al. The epidemiology of major depressive disorder: Results from the National Comorbidity Survey Replication (NCS-R). JAMA 2003;289(23):3095–105.
2. Wells KB, Stewart A, Hays RD, Burnam MA, Rogers W, Daniels M, et al. The functioning and well-being of depressed patients: Results from the Medical Outcomes Study. JAMA 1989;262(7):914–9.
3. Burvill PW. Recent progress in the epidemiology of major depression. Epidemiol Rev 1995;17(1):21–31.
4. Pincus HA, Tanielian TL, Marcus SC, Olfson M, Zarin DA, Thompson J, et al. Prescribing trends in psychotropic medications: Primary care, psychiatry, and other medical specialties. JAMA 1998;279(7):526–31.
5. Foote SM, Etheredge L. Increasing use of new prescription drugs: A case study. Health Aff 2000;19(4):165–70.
6. Stone KJ, Viera AJ, Parman CL. Off-label applications for SSRIs. Am Fam Physician 2003;68(3):498–504.
7. Miranda J, Cooper LA. Disparities in care for depression among primary care patients. J Gen Intern Med 2004;19(2):120–6.
8. Schraufnagel TJ, Wagner AW, Miranda J, Roy-Byrne PP. Treating minority patients with depression and anxiety: What does the evidence tell us? Gen Hosp Psychiatry 2006 Jan-Feb;28(1):27–36.

Figure 36. Adults 18 years of age and over reporting antidepressant drug use in the past month, by sex and race and Hispanic origin: United States, 1988–1994 and 1999–2002

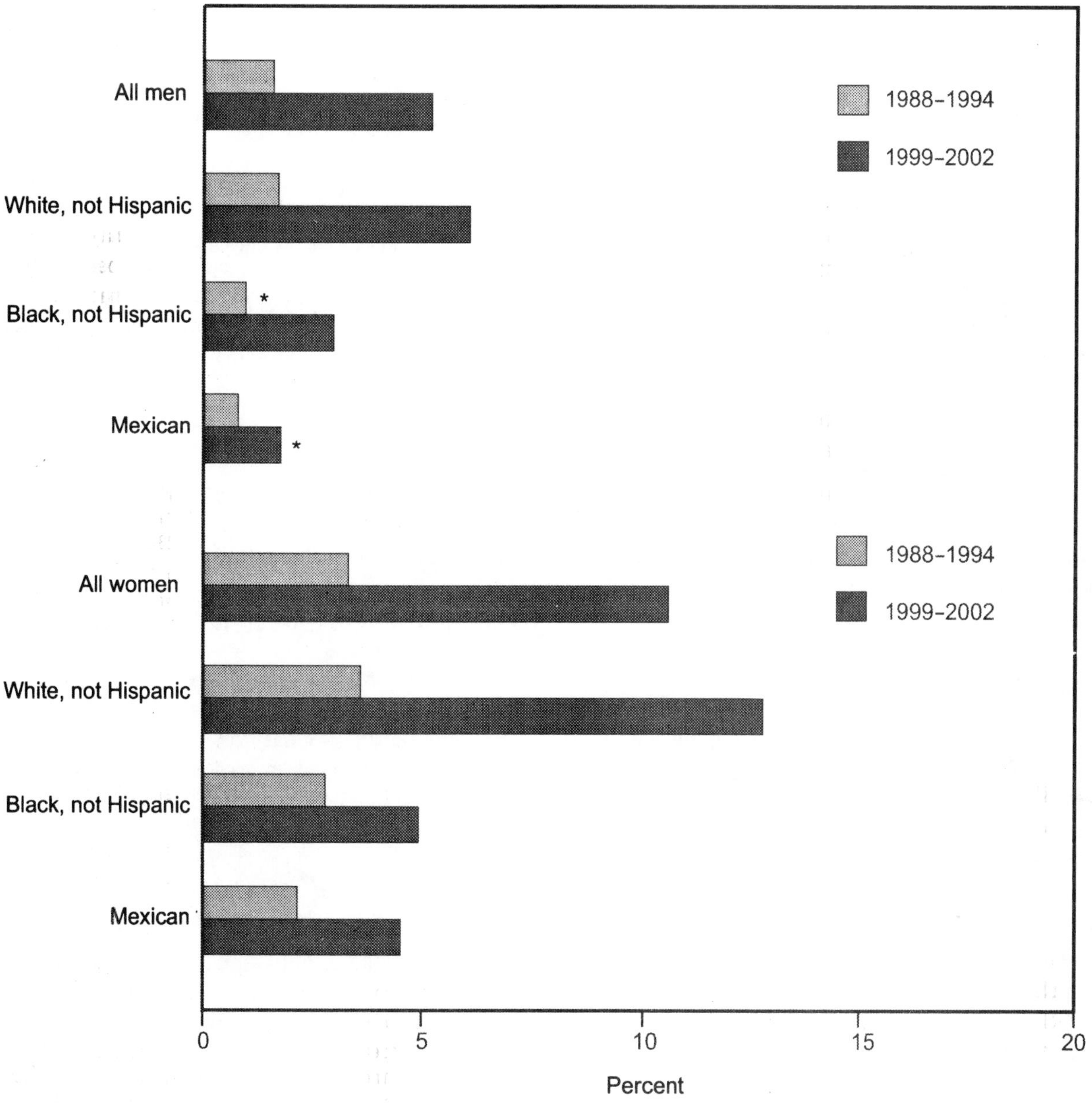

NOTES: * Estimates are considered unreliable. Data shown with an asterisk have a relative standard error of 20%–30%. Data are age-adjusted. Data are for the civilian non-institutionalized population. See data table for Figure 36 for data points graphed, specific drugs included, standard errors, and additional notes.

SOURCE: Centers for Disease Control and Prevention, National Center for Health Statistics, National Health and Nutrition Examination Survey.

Technical Notes

Data Sources and Comparability

Data for *The Chartbook on Trends in the Health of Americans* come from many different surveys and data systems and cover a broad range of years. Detailed descriptions of data sources are contained in Appendix I.

Data Presentation

Many measures in *The Chartbook on Trends in the Health of Americans* are shown for people in specific age groups because of the strong effect age has on most health outcomes. Some estimates are age-adjusted using the age distribution of the 2000 standard population, and this is noted in the data tables that accompany each Figure (see Appendix II, Age adjustment). Age-adjusted rates are computed to eliminate differences in observed rates that result from age differences in population composition. For some Figures, data years are combined to increase sample size and reliability of the estimates. Some charts present time trends and others focus on differences in estimates among population subgroups for the most recent time point available.

Graphic Presentation

Most line charts, for which only selected years of data are displayed, have dot markers on the data years. Line charts for which data are displayed for every year in the trend are shown without the use of dot markers. Figure 20 does not show dot markers, although selected years of data are graphed for years prior to 1995. Most trends are shown on a linear scale to emphasize absolute differences over time. The linear scale is the scale most frequently used and recognized, and it emphasizes the absolute changes between data points over time (1). The time trend for overall mortality measures is shown on a logarithmic (or log) scale to emphasize the rate of change and to enable measures with large differences in magnitude to be shown on the same chart. Log scales emphasize the relative or percentage change between data points. Readers are cautioned that one potential disadvantage to log scale is that the absolute magnitude of changes may appear smaller than the untransformed statistics would indicate (2). When interpreting data on a log scale, the following points should be kept in mind:

1. A sloping straight line indicates a constant rate (not amount) of increase or decrease in the values,
2. A horizontal line indicates no change,
3. The slope of the line indicates the rate of increase or decrease,
4. Parallel lines, regardless of their magnitude, depict similar rates of change (1).

Tabular Presentation

Following the Technical Notes are data tables that present the data points graphed in each Figure. Some data tables contain additional data that were not graphed because of space considerations. Standard errors for data points are provided for many measures. Additional information clarifying and qualifying the data are included in table notes and Appendix I and II references.

Survey Questions and Coding:

Additional information on data used in the Chartbook and Special Feature, including exact wording of questions and coding schemes, is detailed below.

National Health Interview Survey (NHIS)

Figures 21 and 33: The following questions were about the use of health care. Do not include dental care. "DURING THE PAST 12 MONTHS, was there any time when [you/someone in the family] needed medical care, but did not get it because [you/the family] couldn't afford it?" (In Figure 21, results are presented only for sample adults to be consistent with the rest of the chart. Therefore, estimates in this Figure for not receiving needed medical care due to cost may differ slightly from those presented in Table 79.)

Figure 21: "DURING THE PAST 12 MONTHS, was there any time when you needed any of the following, but didn't get it because you couldn't afford it?" (asked of sample adults)

___ prescription medicines

___ mental health care or counseling

___ dental care (including checkups)

___ eyeglasses

Figure 26: Respondents were asked whether they have a place they usually go to when they are sick or need advice about their health. Persons who reported the emergency department as their usual source of care were considered to lack a usual source in this analysis. Diagnosed chronic health conditions were identified by asking if a doctor or other health professional ever told the respondent they had hypertension (told at least two times), a serious heart condition (told they had coronary heart disease, heart attack, or angina), or diabetes (excluding during pregnancy). Adults classified in this analysis as without chronic conditions did not report being diagnosed with serious heart conditions, hypertension, cancer (excluding non-melanoma skin cancer), diabetes, arthritis, emphysema, asthma, stroke, ulcer, and not told in the past year had: chronic bronchitis, liver or kidney disease. See Appendix II, Usual source of care.

Figure 27: "There are many reasons people delay getting medical care. Have you delayed getting care for any of the following reasons in the PAST 12 MONTHS?"

___ you didn't have transportation (asked of sample adults).

Figures 28–30: See Appendix II, Health insurance coverage.

Figure 34: See Appendix II, Dental visit.

Figure 35: "Have you EVER HAD a sigmoidoscopy, colonoscopy, or proctoscopy? These are exams in which a health care professional inserts a tube into the rectum to look for signs of cancer or other problems." Data from 2000, 2003, and 2005 were combined to produce estimates.

National Health and Nutrition Examination Survey (NHANES)

Figure 12: "On average, how many times per week do you/does sample person eat meals that were prepared in a restaurant? Please include eat-in restaurants, carry-out restaurants and restaurants that deliver food to your house." ['Meals' mean more than a beverage or snack food like candy bars or bag of chips].

Figure 32: To determine if a respondent had undiagnosed high cholesterol or high blood pressure, information from the interview, examination, and laboratory sections of the NHANES was used. The questionnaire administered to all participants included questions about whether the respondent had been told by a health professional that he or she had certain medical conditions. The questions for high blood cholesterol and high blood pressure were: "Have you **ever** been told by a doctor or other health professional that your blood cholesterol level was high?" and "Have you **ever** been told by a doctor or other health professional that you had hypertension, also called high blood pressure?"

Respondents answering yes were classified as diagnosed with the condition. Respondents answering no were classified as not diagnosed with the condition. Respondents without a yes or no response were excluded from the relevant analysis. For more information on the questionnaire, see www.cdc.gov/nchs/data/nhanes/nhanes_03_04/sp_bpq_c.pdf. Most respondents, regardless of their responses to the questionnaire, were examined at the mobile examination center (MEC); the examination included laboratory and other tests. The presence of high cholesterol was defined as a total cholesterol reading of 240 mg/dL or higher (6.20 mmol/L). Most participants have at least three blood pressure readings taken. High blood pressure is defined as an average systolic blood pressure of 140 mm Hg or higher, or an average diastolic reading of 90 mm Hg or higher. Blood pressure readings of zero were assumed to be in error and were not included in our calculations. Respondents who did not have their cholesterol or blood pressure measured were excluded from the corresponding analysis. For more information on cholesterol testing, see www.cdc.gov/nchs/data/nhanes/nhanes_03_04/l13_c.pdf. For more information on blood pressure readings, see www.cdc.gov/nchs/data/nhanes/nhanes_03_04/bpx_c.pdf. Persons were considered undiagnosed if during the interview they reported that they did not have the medical condition but the condition was detected as a result of the examination at the MEC. To determine insurance coverage, respondents were asked: "Are you covered by health insurance or some other kind of health care plan?" [Include health insurance obtained through employment or purchased directly as well as government programs like Medicare and Medicaid that provide medical care or help pay medical bills.]

Respondents answering yes were classified as insured; respondents answering no were classified as uninsured. For more information on the health insurance questions, see www.cdc.gov/nchs/data/nhanes/nhanes_03_04/sp_hiq_c.pdf.

Figure 36: The questionnaire administered to all participants also included a question on whether they had taken a prescription drug in the past month. Those who answered "yes" were asked to show the interviewer the medication containers for all the prescriptions. For each drug reported, the interviewer entered the product's complete name from the container. If no container was available, the interviewer asked the participant to verbally report the name of the drug. Additionally, participants were asked how long they had been taking the drug and the main reason for use. All reported medication names were converted to their standard generic ingredient name. For multi-ingredient products, the ingredients were listed in alphabetical order (i.e., Tylenol #3 would be listed as Acetaminophen; Codeine). No trade or proprietary names were provided on the data file. Antidepressant drugs include: amitriptyline, amoxapine, bupropion, citalopram, clomipramine, desipramine, doxepin, escitalopram, fluoxetine, fluvoxamine, imipramine, isocarboxazid, maprotiline, mirtazapine, nefazodone, nortriptyline, paroxetine, phenelzine, protriptyline, sertraline, tranylcypromine, trazodone, trimipramine, and venlafaxine. More information on prescription drug data collection and coding in the NHANES is available from: www.cdc.gov/nchs/data/nhanes/frequency/rxq_rxdoc.pdf. More information on NHANES III prescription drug data collection and coding is available from: www.cdc.gov/nchs/data/nhanes/nhanes3/PUPREMED-acc.pdf. Also see Appendix I, National Health and Nutrition Examination Survey.

Medical Expenditure Panel Survey (MEPS)

Figure 31: The Medical Expenditure Panel Survey produces nationally representative estimates of health care use, expenditures, source of payment, and insurance coverage for the civilian noninstitutionalized population. For each medical care visit or prescription drug during a 1-year period, the respondent reports the condition for which the visit was made. Expenses associated with each visit or prescription drug are recorded. For information on family income measurement, see Banthin JS, Selden TM. Income measurement in the Medical Expenditure Panel Survey. Agency for Healthcare Research and Quality working paper No. 06005, July 2006. Available from: //207.188.212.220/mepsweb/data_files/publications/workingpapers/wp_06005.pd. Also see Appendix I: Medical Expenditure Panel Survey.

Area Resource File

Figures 22 and 23: Data are for active, nonfederal, patient care physicians. Patient care physicians include office-based physicians, full-time hospital staff, and residents or fellows. Estimates for Figure 22 include doctors of medicine and doctors of osteopathic medicine, whereas estimates for Figure 23 only includes data for doctors of medicine (35,799 and excludes 1,502 obgyn doctors of osteopathy (D.O.) in 2004. Obgyn D.O. data were not available at the county level.) County metropolitan status was determined using the Office of Management and Budget definition. See Appendix II, Metropolitan statistical area. The highest category of physician to population on each map represents counties that have physician to population ratios greater than the national ratio. For Figure 22, the category with less than 2.86 patient care physicians per 10,000 population indicates counties that meet the Health Resources and Services Administration definition of a health professional shortage area. Available from: bhpr.hrsa.gov/shortage/.

National Hospital Ambulatory Medical Care Survey

Figure 11: An emergency department (ED) visit was considered alcohol-related if the checkbox for alcohol was indicated, the physician's diagnoses (any-listed) were alcohol-related (ICD–9–CM 291, 303, 305.0, 425.5, 535.30, 571.1–.3, 760.71, 790.3, 980, or V–113), alcohol-related external cause-of-injury codes were present (ICD–9–CM E860 or 710, an alcohol use or abuse cause-of-injury code developed by the National Center for Health Statistics), or the patient's reasons for the visit codes were alcohol-related (alcohol-related problem, including alcohol abuse, drinking problem (1145.0), alcoholism, including alcohol dependence (2320.0), or adverse effects of alcoholism, including acute intoxication, drunk, intoxication (5915.0). The checkbox for alcohol can indicate use among the patient or some other person. Among adolescents and young adults, 0.2% of ED visits were related to use among someone other than the patient.

References

1. Page RM, Cole GE, Timmreck TC. Basic epidemiological methods and biostatistics: A practical guidebook. Sudbury, MA: Jones and Bartlett Publishers, 1995.
2. Jekel JF, Elmore JG, Katz DL. Epidemiology biostatistics and preventive medicine. Philadelphia, PA: W.B. Saunders Company, 1996.

Data Tables for Figures 1–36

Data table for Figure 1. Total population and older population: United States, 1950–2050

Year	All ages	65 years and over	65–74 years	75 years and over
		Number		
1950	150,697,361	12,194,612	8,339,960	3,854,652
1960	179,323,175	16,559,580	10,996,842	5,562,738
1970	203,211,926	20,065,502	12,435,456	7,630,046
1980	226,545,805	25,549,427	15,580,605	9,968,822
1990	248,709,873	31,078,895	18,045,495	13,033,400
2000	281,421,906	34,991,753	18,390,986	16,600,767
2005	296,410,404	36,790,113	18,639,813	18,150,300
2010	308,935,581	40,243,713	21,269,509	18,974,204
2020	335,804,546	54,631,891	31,779,159	22,852,732
2030	363,584,435	71,453,471	37,947,933	33,505,538
2040	391,945,658	80,049,634	35,469,908	44,579,726
2050	419,853,587	86,705,637	37,942,437	48,763,200
		Percent		
1950	100.0	8.1	5.5	2.6
1960	100.0	9.2	6.1	3.1
1970	100.0	9.9	6.1	3.8
1980	100.0	11.3	6.9	4.4
1990	100.0	12.5	7.3	5.2
2000	100.0	12.4	6.5	5.9
2005	100.0	12.4	6.3	6.1
2010	100.0	13.0	6.9	6.1
2020	100.0	16.3	9.5	6.8
2030	100.0	19.7	10.4	9.2
2040	100.0	20.4	9.0	11.4
2050	100.0	20.7	9.0	11.6

NOTES: Data are for the resident population. Data for 1950 exclude Alaska and Hawaii. Data for 2010–2050 are projected. See Appendix II, Population.

SOURCES: U.S. Bureau of the Census: 1950 Nonwhite population by race. Special Report P-E, No.3B. Washington: U.S. Government Printing Office, 1951 [data for 1950]; U.S. Census of Population: 1960, Number of inhabitants, PC(1)-A1, United States Summary, 1964 [data for 1960]; Number of inhabitants, final report PC(1)-A1, United States Summary, 1971 [data for 1970]; U.S. Census Bureau, 1980 Census of Population, General population characteristics, United States Summary (PC80-1-B1) [data for 1980]; 1990 Census of Population, General population characteristics, United States Summary (CP-1-1) [data for 1990]; Table 1. Annual estimates of the population by sex and five-year age groups for the United States: April 1, 2000 to July 1, 2004 (NC-EST2004-01) available from: www.census.gov/popest/national/asrh/NC-EST2004/NC-EST2004-01.xls [data for Census 2000]; U.S. Census Bureau: Annual estimates of the population by sex and five-year age groups for the United States: April 1, 2000, to July 1, 2005 (NC-EST2005-01), available from: www.census.gov/popest/national/asrh/NC-EST2005-sa.html [data for 2005]; U.S. interim projections by age, sex, race, and Hispanic origin, 2004. Detail File available from: www.census.gov/ipc/www/usinterimproj/ [data for projections].

Data table for Figure 2. Foreign-born population, by citizenship: United States, 1970–2004

Year	*Total foreign-born population*	*Naturalized U.S. citizen*	*Not a U.S. citizen*
		Numbers in thousands	
1970	9,740	6,198	3,542
1980	14,080	7,110	6,969
1990	19,767	7,997	11,770
1994	22,568	6,975	15,593
1995	24,493	7,601	16,892
1996	24,557	7,904	16,653
1997	25,779	9,043	16,736
1998	26,281	9,739	16,542
1999	26,447	9,868	16,579
2000	28,380	10,622	17,758
2002	32,453	11,962	20,491
2003	33,471	12,837	20,634
2004	34,244	13,128	21,116
		Percent of U.S. population	
1970	4.8	3.1	1.7
1980	6.2	3.1	3.1
1990	7.9	3.2	4.7
1994	8.7	2.7	6.0
1995	9.3	2.9	6.4
1996	9.3	3.0	6.3
1997	9.7	3.4	6.3
1998	9.8	3.6	6.1
1999	9.7	3.6	6.1
2000	10.4	3.9	6.5
2002	11.5	4.2	7.3
2003	11.7	4.5	7.2
2004	11.9	4.6	7.3

NOTES: Data for 1970, 1980, and 1990 are based on the U.S. resident population, enumerated from the decennial censuses. Prior to 1994, the decennial census was the sole source for the foreign-born population. Starting in 1994, data are for the U.S. civilian noninstitutionalized population from the Current Population Survey, March Supplements, which began collecting data on nativity, citizenship, year-of-entry, and parental nativity of respondents. Because of theses changes, the data in this table slightly understate the growth in the foreign-born population in the years after 1994. See Appendix II, Foreign-born persons. Estimates for foreign-born persons include immigrants (legal permanent residents), temporary migrants (e.g., students, visiting scientists), humanitarian migrants (e.g., refugees), and unauthorized migrants (people illegally residing in the United States).

SOURCE: U.S. Census Bureau. 1970 census, Vol. I, Characteristics of the Population, Ch. D, Part 1, PC(1)-D1, Table 191, p.596 [data for 1970]; 1980 census, Vol. 1, Characteristics of the Population, Ch. D, Part 1, Sect. A, PC80-D1-A, Table 253, p.7 [data for 1980]; 1990 census, Social and Economic Characteristics, 1990 CP-2-1, Table 18, p.18 [data for 1990]; Current Population Survey, March Supplements [data for 1994–2004].

Data table for Figure 3. Population in selected race and Hispanic origin groups, by age: United States, 1980–2006

Race and Hispanic origin	*All ages* 1980	1990	2000	2006	*Under 18 years* 1980	1990	2000	2006	*18 years and over* 1980	1990	2000	2006
						Percent distribution						
Total	100.0	100.0	100.0	100.0	100.0	100.0	100.0	100.0	100.0	100.0	100.0	100.0
Hispanic or Latino	6.4	9.0	12.5	14.7	8.8	12.2	17.1	20.2	5.5	7.9	11.0	13.0
Not Hispanic or Latino:												
White	79.9	75.7	69.5	66.5	74.2	68.9	61.3	57.7	82.1	78.1	72.3	69.3
Black or African American	11.5	11.8	12.2	12.3	14.5	14.7	14.9	14.6	10.4	10.7	11.3	11.5
American Indian or Alaska Native	0.6	0.7	0.7	0.8	0.8	1.0	1.0	0.9	0.5	0.6	0.7	0.7
Asian	1.6	2.8	3.7	4.3	1.7	3.1	3.5	3.9	1.5	2.7	3.8	4.4
Native Hawaiian or Other Pacific Islander	...	...	0.1	0.1	...	...	0.2	0.2	...	...	0.1	0.1
2 or more races	...	...	1.2	1.4	...	...	2.2	2.5	...	...	0.9	1.0

...Category not applicable.

NOTES: Data are for the resident population. Persons of Hispanic origin may be of any race. Race data for 2000 and beyond are not directly comparable with data for 1980 and 1990. Individuals could report only one race in 1980 and 1990, and more than one race beginning in 2000. Persons who selected only one race in 2000 and beyond are shown in single-race categories; persons who selected more than one race in 2000 and beyond are shown as having 2 or more races and are not included in the single-race categories. In 1980 and 1990, the Asian category included Asian and Native Hawaiian or Other Pacific Islander; in 2000 and beyond this category includes only Asian. See Appendix II, Hispanic origin; Race.

SOURCES: U.S. Census Bureau: U.S. population estimates, by age, sex, race, and Hispanic origin: 1980 to 1991. Current population reports, series P-25, no 1095. Washington, DC. U.S. Government Printing Office, February 1993 [data for April 1, 1980 and April 1, 1990]; U.S. Census Bureau: Monthly postcensal resident populations, from July 1, 2000 to July 1, 2006 by age, sex, race, and Hispanic origin. Available from: www.census.gov/popest/national/asrh/2005_nat_res.html [data for April 1, 2000 and July 1, 2006].

Data table for Figure 4. Poverty by age: United States, 1966–2005

Year	*All ages*	*Under 18 years*	*18–64 years*	*65 years and over*
	Percent of persons with family income below the poverty level			
1966	14.7	17.6	10.5	28.5
1967	14.2	16.6	10.0	29.5
1968	12.8	15.6	9.0	25.0
1969	12.1	14.0	8.7	25.3
1970	12.6	15.1	9.0	24.6
1971	12.5	15.3	9.3	21.6
1972	11.9	15.1	8.8	18.6
1973	11.1	14.4	8.3	16.3
1974	11.2	15.4	8.3	14.6
1975	12.3	17.1	9.2	15.3
1976	11.8	16.0	9.0	15.0
1977	11.6	16.2	8.8	14.1
1978	11.4	15.9	8.7	14.0
1979	11.7	16.4	8.9	15.2
1980	13.0	18.3	10.1	15.7
1981	14.0	20.0	11.1	15.3
1982	15.0	21.9	12.0	14.6
1983	15.2	22.3	12.4	13.8
1984	14.4	21.5	11.7	12.4
1985	14.0	20.7	11.3	12.6
1986	13.6	20.5	10.8	12.4
1987	13.4	20.3	10.6	12.5
1988	13.0	19.5	10.5	12.0
1989	12.8	19.6	10.2	11.4
1990	13.5	20.6	10.7	12.2
1991	14.2	21.8	11.4	12.4
1992	14.8	22.3	11.9	12.9
1993	15.1	22.7	12.4	12.2
1994	14.5	21.8	11.9	11.7
1995	13.8	20.8	11.4	10.5
1996	13.7	20.5	11.4	10.8
1997	13.3	19.9	10.9	10.5
1998	12.7	18.9	10.5	10.5
1999	11.9	17.1	10.1	9.7
2000	11.3	16.2	9.6	9.9
2001	11.7	16.3	10.1	10.1
2002	12.1	16.7	10.6	10.4
2003	12.5	17.6	10.8	10.2
2004	12.7	17.8	11.3	9.8
2005	12.6	17.6	11.1	10.1

NOTES: Data are for the civilian noninstitutionalized population. Poverty level is based on family income and family size and composition using U.S. Census Bureau poverty thresholds. See Appendix II, Poverty. See related Table 3.

SOURCES: U.S. Census Bureau, Current Population Survey, March 1967–2006. DeNavas-Walt C, Proctor BD, Hill LC. Income, poverty, and health insurance coverage in the United States: 2005. Current population reports, series P-60, no 231. Washington, DC: U.S. Government Printing Office. 2006.

Data table for Figure 5. Low income by age, race, and Hispanic origin: United States, 2005

Characteristic	Percent of poverty level: Below 100% (Percent)	Percent of poverty level: 100%–less than 200% (Percent)	Percent of poverty level: Below 100% (Number in millions)	Percent of poverty level: 100%–less than 200% (Number in millions)
All ages				
All races and origins	12.6	18.4	37.0	53.9
Hispanic or Latino	21.8	30.0	9.4	12.9
Black or African American only	24.9	24.5	9.2	9.0
Asian only	11.1	15.1	1.4	1.9
White only, not Hispanic or Latino	8.3	14.8	16.2	29.1
Under 18 years				
All races and origins	17.6	21.3	12.9	15.6
Hispanic or Latino	28.3	32.4	4.1	4.8
Black or African American only	34.5	26.8	3.8	3.0
Asian only	11.1	17.3	0.3	0.5
White only, not Hispanic or Latino	10.0	16.2	4.3	6.9
18–64 years				
All races and origins	11.1	15.6	20.5	28.8
Hispanic or Latino	18.3	28.1	4.8	7.3
Black or African American only	20.4	22.1	4.6	5.0
Asian only	11.0	13.5	0.9	1.2
White only, not Hispanic or Latino	7.8	11.9	9.7	14.8
65 years and over				
All races and origins	10.1	26.7	3.6	9.5
Hispanic or Latino	19.9	34.7	0.5	0.8
Black or African American only	23.3	34.5	0.7	1.0
Asian only	12.8	20.1	0.1	0.3
White only, not Hispanic or Latino	7.9	25.4	2.3	7.3

NOTES: Data are for the civilian noninstitutionalized population. Persons of Hispanic origin may be of any race. Black and Asian races include persons of both Hispanic and non-Hispanic origin. Percent of poverty level is based on family income and family size and composition using U.S. Census Bureau poverty thresholds. See related Table 3. See Appendix II, Hispanic origin; Poverty; Race.

SOURCES: U.S. Census Bureau, Current Population Survey, March 1967–2006. DeNavas-Walt C, Proctor BD, Hill LC. Income, poverty, and health insurance coverage in the United States: 2005. Current population reports, series P-60, no 231. Washington, DC: U.S. Government Printing Office. 2006. Age and sex of all people, family members, and unrelated individuals iterated by income-to-poverty ratio and race: 2005. Available from: pubdb3.census.gov/macro/032006/pov/new01_000.htm.

Data table for Figure 6. Personal health care expenditures, by source of funds and type of expenditures: United States, 2005

Personal health care expenditures and source of funds	*Type of expenditures*					
	Total	*Hospital care*	*Physician services*	*Nursing home*	*Prescription drugs*	*Other*
			Amount in billions			
All personal health care expenditures	$1,661.4	$611.6	$421.2	$121.9	$200.7	$306.1
			Percent distribution			
All personal health care expenditures	100.0	36.8	25.4	7.3	12.1	18.4
Source of funds			Percent distribution			
All sources of funds	100.0	100.0	100.0	100.0	100.0	100.0
Out-of-pocket payments	15.0	3.3	10.1	26.5	25.4	33.9
Private health insurance	35.9	35.5	48.3	7.5	47.4	23.5
Other private funds	4.1	4.5	6.4	3.7	0.0	3.2
Government	45.0	56.8	35.3	62.3	27.2	39.5
Medicaid	17.5	17.3	7.1	43.9	18.6	21.2
Medicare	19.9	29.5	21.2	15.7	2.0	12.6
Other government	7.5	10.0	7.0	2.7	6.6	5.6
Federal	34.2	45.7	28.9	42.7	16.4	26.9
State and local	10.7	11.1	6.3	19.6	10.8	12.5

0.0 Quantity more than zero but less than 0.05.

NOTES: Other expenditures include dental services, other professional services, home health care, nonprescription drugs and other medical nondurables, vision products and other medical durables, and other personal health care, not shown separately. See related Tables 124–125. See Appendix I, National Health Expenditure Accounts.

SOURCE: Centers for Medicare & Medicaid Services, Office of the Actuary, National Health Statistics Group, National Health Expenditure Accounts.

Data table for Figure 7. National expenditures for mental health services, by source of funds: United States, 1986–2003

		Private				*Public*				
Year	*All*	*Total private*	*Out-of-pocket*	*Private health insurance*	*Other private*	*Total public*	*Medicare*	*Medicaid*	*Other federal*	*Other state and local*
					Expenditures in billions inflation-ad usted 2000 U.S. dollars					
1986	$46.5	$21.6	$8.5	$9.9	$3.2	$24.9	$2.7	$7.5	$2.9	$11.9
1987	49.0	22.0	8.4	10.1	3.5	27.0	2.6	8.2	3.1	13.1
1988	52.7	23.7	9.0	11.1	3.7	29.0	2.9	8.7	3.3	14.0
1989	54.8	24.9	9.0	12.2	3.7	29.9	3.4	8.7	3.0	14.7
1990	56.9	25.9	9.3	13.1	3.5	31.1	3.6	9.1	2.9	15.5
1991	57.8	24.7	8.8	12.5	3.4	33.1	3.8	11.0	2.8	15.4
1992	59.0	23.4	8.4	11.7	3.3	35.5	4.3	12.6	2.9	15.8
1993	62.4	24.2	8.1	12.6	3.4	38.3	5.4	13.3	3.1	16.6
1994	67.0	25.1	8.1	13.8	3.3	41.9	6.5	14.7	3.3	17.3
1995	67.1	25.2	7.9	14.0	3.3	41.9	6.5	15.2	3.2	17.0
1996	66.4	24.4	7.9	13.7	2.8	42.0	6.9	15.3	3.0	16.7
1997	67.4	24.9	8.3	14.3	2.4	42.5	7.1	16.1	2.9	16.5
1998	69.8	26.4	9.2	14.9	2.3	43.5	6.9	17.5	2.8	16.2
1999	73.5	28.1	9.6	16.0	2.6	45.3	6.6	18.8	2.8	17.1
2000	79.2	30.7	10.7	17.4	2.5	48.5	6.6	20.9	2.8	18.3
2001	84.6	33.3	11.5	19.3	2.5	51.3	6.9	22.6	3.0	18.8
2002	89.4	36.4	12.2	21.3	2.9	53.0	6.9	23.6	3.2	19.2
2003	94.3	39.5	13.5	22.8	3.2	54.8	6.9	24.8	3.3	19.8
					Percent distribution					
1986	100.0	46.5	18.2	21.3	6.9	53.5	5.8	16.1	6.2	25.5
1987	100.0	44.9	17.2	20.6	7.0	55.1	5.4	16.7	6.4	26.6
1988	100.0	45.0	17.0	21.0	6.9	55.0	5.6	16.5	6.3	26.6
1989	100.0	45.4	16.4	22.3	6.8	54.6	6.3	15.9	5.5	26.9
1990	100.0	45.5	16.3	22.9	6.2	54.5	6.3	16.1	5.0	27.2
1991	100.0	42.7	15.2	21.7	5.9	57.3	6.6	19.1	4.9	26.7
1992	100.0	39.7	14.2	19.9	5.6	60.3	7.3	21.3	4.8	26.8
1993	100.0	38.7	13.0	20.3	5.5	61.3	8.6	21.3	5.0	26.5
1994	100.0	37.5	12.1	20.5	4.9	62.5	9.7	21.9	5.0	25.9
1995	100.0	37.5	11.8	20.8	4.9	62.5	9.7	22.7	4.8	25.3
1996	100.0	36.8	12.0	20.7	4.2	63.2	10.5	23.1	4.5	25.1
1997	100.0	37.0	12.3	21.2	3.5	63.0	10.6	23.8	4.3	24.4
1998	100.0	37.8	13.1	21.4	3.3	62.2	9.9	25.1	4.1	23.2
1999	100.0	38.3	13.1	21.7	3.5	61.7	9.0	25.6	3.8	23.3
2000	100.0	38.7	13.6	21.9	3.2	61.3	8.3	26.4	3.5	23.1
2001	100.0	39.4	13.6	22.8	2.9	60.6	8.2	26.7	3.6	22.2
2002	100.0	40.7	13.7	23.8	3.3	59.3	7.7	26.4	3.6	21.5
2003	100.0	41.9	14.3	24.2	3.4	58.1	7.3	26.3	3.5	21.0

NOTES: Estimates have been inflation-ad usted to 2000 U.S. dollars using the Gross omestic Product implicit price deflator developed by the U.S. epartment of Commerce, ureau of Economic Analysis. Other private funds include philanthropy and other nonpatient revenues received by providers. Other federal funds include mental health block grants to the states and epartments of eterans Affairs and efense programs. Other state and local funding includes dollars from state and local government budgets allocated to community health centers, psychiatric hospitals and other types of mental health services. See related Table 126.

SOURCE: Mark T , evit , Coffey RM, Mc usick R, Harwood H, ing E, et al. National Expenditures for Mental Health Services and Substance Abuse Treatment, 1993–2003. SAMHSA pub. no. SMA 07-4227. Rockville, M : Substance Abuse and Mental Health Services Administration, 2007 and unpublished data.

Data table for Figure 8. National expenditures for substance abuse treatment, by source of funds: United States, 1986–2003

		Private				*Public*				
Year	*All*	*Total private*	*Out-of-pocket*	*Private health insurance*	*Other private*	*Total public*	*Medicare*	*Medicaid*	*Other federal*	*Other state and local*
	Expenditures in billions inflation-ad usted 2000 U.S. dollars									
1986	$13.1	$6.5	$1.8	$3.9	$0.8	$6.6	$0.6	$1.3	$0.9	$3.8
1987	13.7	6.5	1.8	3.8	0.9	7.2	0.6	1.4	1.0	4.2
1988	14.6	6.6	1.7	3.9	1.0	7.9	0.5	1.5	1.4	4.4
1989	14.8	6.6	1.6	4.0	1.0	8.3	0.6	1.5	1.5	4.7
1990	14.8	6.2	1.4	3.8	0.9	8.6	0.6	1.6	1.7	4.8
1991	14.4	5.3	1.3	3.2	0.8	9.1	0.5	1.9	2.8	3.9
1992	15.4	5.0	1.5	2.7	0.8	10.3	0.6	2.3	2.9	4.5
1993	17.0	5.4	2.2	2.3	0.9	11.6	0.8	2.7	2.9	5.2
1994	16.9	4.9	1.7	2.4	0.8	11.9	0.9	3.3	2.4	5.4
1995	16.9	4.5	1.2	2.6	0.7	12.4	0.9	3.7	2.3	5.6
1996	15.9	4.1	1.1	2.4	0.6	11.8	1.0	3.2	2.5	5.2
1997	15.9	3.9	1.2	2.1	0.6	11.9	1.0	3.0	2.4	5.6
1998	16.1	3.9	1.3	2.0	0.6	12.2	1.0	3.0	2.4	5.7
1999	16.7	3.9	1.3	1.9	0.7	12.8	1.0	3.0	2.5	6.4
2000	17.5	4.0	1.4	1.9	0.8	13.5	0.9	3.1	2.6	6.9
2001	18.2	4.1	1.4	1.9	0.8	14.1	0.9	3.2	2.7	7.3
2002	19.1	4.4	1.5	2.0	0.8	14.7	0.9	3.4	2.8	7.6
2003	19.5	4.4	1.6	2.0	0.9	15.1	0.9	3.5	2.9	7.8
	Percent distribution									
1986	100.0	49.6	13.8	29.6	6.2	50.4	4.3	10.0	7.1	29.0
1987	100.0	47.4	13.1	27.6	6.8	52.6	4.2	10.4	7.5	30.5
1988	100.0	45.6	11.8	26.9	6.9	54.4	3.8	10.4	9.8	30.5
1989	100.0	44.2	10.9	26.7	6.6	55.8	3.7	10.3	10.0	31.8
1990	100.0	41.7	9.8	25.5	6.4	58.3	3.8	10.8	11.3	32.4
1991	100.0	36.8	9.1	22.2	5.5	63.2	3.4	13.3	19.1	27.3
1992	100.0	32.6	9.7	17.6	5.3	67.4	4.1	15.1	18.9	29.3
1993	100.0	31.6	12.9	13.7	5.0	68.4	4.4	16.1	17.2	30.6
1994	100.0	29.3	10.2	14.5	4.6	70.7	5.2	19.3	14.4	31.9
1995	100.0	26.5	7.1	15.2	4.3	73.5	5.2	21.9	13.4	33.0
1996	100.0	25.8	7.1	14.8	3.8	74.2	6.0	20.2	15.5	32.6
1997	100.0	24.7	7.3	13.4	4.0	75.3	6.1	18.9	15.1	35.2
1998	100.0	24.2	8.1	12.4	3.7	75.8	6.5	18.4	15.2	35.8
1999	100.0	23.4	8.0	11.3	4.1	76.6	5.7	18.0	14.8	38.1
2000	100.0	22.8	7.8	10.6	4.4	77.2	5.1	17.5	15.1	39.5
2001	100.0	22.6	7.7	10.4	4.5	77.4	4.8	17.8	14.9	39.9
2002	100.0	22.9	8.0	10.5	4.4	77.1	4.6	18.0	14.9	39.7
2003	100.0	22.6	8.0	10.1	4.5	77.4	4.5	17.9	14.8	40.3

NOTES: Estimates have been inflation-ad usted to 2000 U.S. dollars using the Gross omestic Product implicit price deflator developed by the U.S. epartment of Commerce, ureau of Economic Analysis. Other private funds include philanthropy and other nonpatient revenues received by providers. Other federal funds include block grants to the states and epartments of eterans Affairs and efense programs. Other state and local funding includes dollars from state and local government budgets allocated to substance abuse treatment. See related Table 127.

SOURCE: Mark T , evit , Coffey RM, Mc usick R, Harwood H, ing E, et al. National Expenditures for Mental Health Services and Substance Abuse Treatment, 1993–2003. SAMHSA pub. no. SMA 07-4227. Rockville, M : Substance Abuse and Mental Health Services Administration, 2007 and unpublished data.

Data table for Figure 9. Cigarette smoking among men, women, high school students, and mothers during pregnancy: United States, 1965–2005

Year	*Men*		*Women*		*High school students*		*Mothers during pregnancy*
	Percent	*SE*	*Percent*	*SE*	*Percent*	*SE*	*Percent*
1965	51.2	0.3	33.7	0.3	---	---	---
1974	42.8	0.5	32.2	0.4	---	---	---
1979	37.0	0.5	30.1	0.5	---	---	---
1983	34.8	0.6	29.4	0.4	---	---	---
1985	32.2	0.5	27.9	0.4	---	---	---
1987	30.9	0.4	26.5	0.4	---	---	---
1988	30.3	0.4	25.7	0.3	---	---	---
1989	---	---	---	---	---	---	19.5
1990	28.0	0.4	22.9	0.3	---	---	18.4
1991	27.6	0.4	23.5	0.3	27.5	1.4	17.8
1992	28.1	0.5	24.6	0.5	---	---	16.9
1993	27.3	0.6	22.6	0.4	30.5	1.0	15.8
1994	27.6	0.5	23.1	0.5	---	---	14.6
1995	26.5	0.6	22.7	0.5	34.8	1.2	13.9
1996	---	---	---	---	---	---	13.6
1997	27.1	0.4	22.2	0.4	36.4	1.1	13.2
1998	25.9	0.4	22.1	0.4	---	---	12.9
1999	25.2	0.5	21.6	0.4	34.8	1.3	12.6
2000	25.2	0.4	21.1	0.4	---	---	12.2
2001	24.6	0.4	20.7	0.4	28.5	1.0	12.0
2002	24.6	0.4	20.0	0.4	---	---	11.4
2003	23.7	0.4	19.4	0.4	21.9	1.1	10.7
2004	23.0	0.4	18.7	0.4	---	---	10.2
2005	23.4	0.5	18.3	0.4	23.0	1.2	---

SE is standard error.

--- ata not available.

NOTES: ata for men and women are for the civilian noninstitutionalized population. Estimates for men and women are age-ad usted to the 2000 standard population using five age groups: 18–24 years, 25–34 years, 35–44 years, 45–64 years, and 65 years and over. Age-ad usted estimates in this table may differ from other age-ad usted estimates based on the same data and presented elsewhere if different age groups are used in the ad ustment procedure. Cigarette smoking is defined as follows: among men and women 18 years and over, those who ever smoked 100 cigarettes in their lifetime and now smoke every day or some days among high school students in grades 9–12, those who smoked cigarettes on 1 or more of the 30 days preceding the survey and among mothers with a live birth, those who smoked during pregnancy. ata for mothers who smoked during pregnancy are based on the 1989 Revision of the U.S. Certificate of ive irth. Some states did not re uire the reporting of mother s tobacco use during pregnancy on the birth certificate and are not included in this analysis. Reporting of tobacco use during pregnancy increased from 43 states and the istrict of Columbia C in 1989 to 49 states and C in 2000–2002. Starting with 2003 data, some reporting areas adopted the 2003 Revision of the U.S. Standard Certificate of ive irth and one state continued to not report data. Tobacco use during pregnancy data based on the 2003 Revision are not comparable with data based on the 1989 Revision of the U.S. Standard Certificate of ive irth and are excluded from this analysis. See Appendix II, Age ad ustment Cigarette smoking Tobacco use. See related Tables 12 and 63.

SOURCES: Centers for isease Control and Prevention, National Center for Health Statistics, National Health Interview Survey data for men and women National ital Statistics System data for mothers during pregnancy National Center for Chronic isease Prevention and Health Promotion, outh Risk ehavior Survey data for high school students .

Data table for Figure 10. Blood cotinine levels among children 4–17 years of age, by age, race and Hispanic origin, and percent of poverty level: United States, 1988–1994 and 2001–2004

	Any detectable cotinine level (at or above 0.05 ng/ml)			
	1988–1994		*2001–2004*	
Characteristic	*Percent*	*SE*	*Percent*	*SE*
Age				
4–17 years	84.4	1.5	56.8	2.8
4–11 years	84.5	1.7	59.4	2.9
12–17 years	84.3	2.0	53.7	3.0
Race and Hispanic origin				
Not Hispanic or atino:				
hite only	83.7	1.9	56.0	3.8
lack only	94.7	1.0	79.3	2.2
Mexican	76.5	2.2	41.1	3.1
Percent of poverty level				
elow 100	91.3	1.6	73.7	3.5
100 –less than 200	87.5	2.2	65.8	4.2
200 or more	78.9	2.5	46.0	2.7
	High cotinine level (more than 1.0 ng/ml)			
	Percent	*SE*	*Percent*	*SE*
Age				
4–17 years	22.5	1.2	16.6	1.5
4–11 years	24.3	1.4	18.4	1.9
12–17 years	20.1	1.6	14.3	1.3
Race and Hispanic origin				
Not Hispanic or atino:				
hite only	23.1	1.7	18.8	2.1
lack only	33.7	2.1	22.1	1.6
Mexican	8.3	1.1	4.8	1.1
Percent of poverty level				
elow 100	33.8	2.7	28.4	2.5
100 –less than 200	28.5	2.8	21.5	3.0
200 or more	14.2	1.2	9.7	1.3

NOTES: Cotinine levels are for nonsmoking children only. The cotinine value of 0.05 ng ml was the limit of detection in 1988–1994. Persons of Mexican origin may be of any race. Percent of poverty level is based on family income and family size and composition using U.S. Census ureau poverty thresholds. Family income data were missing for 4 –5 of children 4–17 years of age. See Appendix II, Poverty Race.

SOURCE: Centers for isease Control and Prevention, National Center for Health Statisics, National Health and Nutrition Examination Survey.

Data table for Figure 11. Alcohol-related emergency department (ED) visits among persons 14–28 years of age, by age and sex: United States, 2002–2004

Age	*Average annual number of alcohol-related ED visits*					
	Total		*Male*		*Female*	
14–20 years	233,000		144,100		89,000	
14–17 years	80,600		54,300		26,200	
18–20 years	152,500		89,700		62,800	
21–24 years	238,400		146,100		92,300	
25–28 years	187,100		124,700		62,500	
	Alcohol-related ED visits per 10,000 population					
	Rate	*SE*	*Rate*	*SE*	*Rate*	*SE*
14–20 years	82.1	6.7	99.9	9.6	63.7	8.4
14–17 years	49.0	6.5	64.7	10.7	32.5	7.3
18–20 years	127.7	13.4	148.8	20.1	106.1	17.4
21–24 years	149.8	12.5	184.0	18.5	115.8	15.7
25–28 years	125.5	12.6	167.8	17.6	83.5	16.6

SE is standard error.

Estimates are considered unreliable. ata preceded by an asterisk have a relative standard error RSE of 20 –30

NOTES: Rates are computed using the civilian noninstitutionalized population as the denominator. An emergency department visit was considered alcohol-related if the checkbox for alcohol was indicated, the physician s diagnoses any-listed were alcohol-related IC –9–CM 291, 303, 305.0, 425.5, 535.30, 571.1–.3, 760.71, 790.3, 980, or -113 , alcohol-related external cause-of-in ury codes were present IC –9–CM E860 or 710, an alcohol use abuse cause-of-in ury code developed by the National Center for Health Statistics , or the patient s reasons for the visit codes were alcohol-related alcohol-related problem, including alcohol abuse, drinking problem 1145.0 , alcoholism, including alcohol dependence 2320.0 , or adverse effects of alcoholism, including acute intoxication, drunk, intoxication 5915.0 . The checkbox for alcohol can indicate use among the patient or some other person. Among adolescents and young adults, 0.2 of visits were related to use among someone other than the patient.

SOURCE: Centers for isease Control and Prevention, National Center for Health Statistics, National Hospital Ambulatory Medical Care Survey.

Data table for Figure 12. Weekly restaurant meal consumption among people 1 year of age and over, by age: United States, 1999–2004

Age	*Average restaurant meals per week*					
	Less than 1 meal		*1–3 meals*		*4 or more meals*	
	Percent	*SE*	*Percent*	*SE*	*Percent*	*SE*
Total	24.1	0.6	52.7	0.6	23.2	0.6
1–12 years	28.2	0.9	63.0	1.1	8.8	0.7
13–17 years	22.6	1.1	60.1	1.1	17.3	0.8
18–44 years	17.1	0.7	50.9	0.8	32.0	0.8
18–24 years	15.3	0.9	49.4	1.3	35.3	1.3
25–34 years	17.2	0.9	50.1	1.5	32.7	1.3
35–44 years	18.3	1.1	52.4	1.4	29.3	1.2
45–64 years	25.2	1.0	49.2	1.3	25.6	1.1
45–54 years	23.8	1.2	48.4	1.5	27.8	1.3
55–64 years	27.5	1.6	50.5	1.8	22.0	1.7
65 years and over	39.7	1.6	45.9	1.3	14.4	1.3

SE is standard error.

NOTES: ata are for the civilian noninstitutionalized population. ata for children 1–15 years of age are collected from proxy respondents ata for persons 16 years of age and over are self-reported. Restaurant meals include meals eaten at eat-in restaurants, carry-out restaurants, and restaurants that deliver food. The less than one meal a week category includes respondents who seldom or never consumed restaurant meals.

SOURCE: Centers for isease Control and Prevention, National Center for Health Statistics, National Health and Nutrition Examination Survey.

Data table for Figure 13. Overweight and obesity, by age: United States, 1960–2004

Year	*Preschool-age children 2–5 years*		*School-age children 6–11 years*		*Adolescents 12–19 years*		*Adults 20–74 years*					
	Overweight						*Overweight including obese*		*Overweight but not obese*		*Obese*	
	Percent	*SE*	*Percent*	*SE*	*Percent*	*SE*	*Percent*	*SE*	*Percent*	*SE*	*Percent*	*SE*
1960–1962	- - -	- - -	- - -	- - -	- - -	- - -	44.8	1.0	31.5	0.5	13.3	0.6
1963–1965	- - -	- - -	4.2	0.4	- - -	- - -	- - -	- - -	- - -	- - -	- - -	- - -
1966–1970	- - -	- - -	- - -	- - -	4.6	0.3	- - -	- - -	- - -	- - -	- - -	- - -
1971–1974	- - -	- - -	4.0	0.5	6.1	0.6	47.7	0.7	33.1	0.6	14.6	0.5
1976–1980	- - -	- - -	6.5	0.6	5.0	0.5	47.4	0.8	32.3	0.6	15.1	0.5
1988–1994	7.2	0.7	11.3	1.0	10.5	0.9	56.0	0.9	32.7	0.6	23.3	0.7
1999–2000	10.3	1.7	15.1	1.4	14.8	0.9	64.1	1.9	33.1	1.1	31.0	1.5
2001–2002	10.6	1.8	16.3	1.6	16.7	1.1	65.7	0.9	33.6	1.1	32.1	1.2
2003–2004	13.9	1.6	18.8	1.3	17.4	1.7	67.1	1.3	33.2	1.1	33.9	1.3

SE is standard error.

- - - ata not available.

NOTES: ata are for the civilian noninstitutionalized population. Estimates for adults are age-ad usted to the 2000 standard population using five age groups: 20–34 years, 35–44 years, 45–54 years, 55–64 years, and 65–74 years. Age-ad usted estimates in this table may differ from other age-ad usted estimates based on the same data and presented elsewhere if different age groups are used in the ad ustment procedure. For children and adolescents: overweight is defined as a body mass index MI at or above the sex- and age-specific 95th percentile MI cut points from the 2000 C C Growth Charts: United States See: www.cdc.gov growthcharts obese is not defined for children. For adults: overweight including obese is defined as a MI greater than or e ual to 25 overweight but not obese as a MI greater than or e ual to 25 but less than 30 and obese as a MI greater than or e ual to 30. ata for 1966–1970 are for adolescents 12–17 years, not 12–19 years. Pregnant adolescents were excluded beginning in 1971–1974. Pregnant women 20 years of age and over were excluded in all years. See Appendix II, Age ad ustment ody mass index MI . See related Tables 69, 74, and 75.

SOURCES: Centers for isease Control and Prevention, National Center for Health Statistics. National Health Examination Survey and National Health and Nutrition Examination Survey.

Data table for Figure 14. Limitation of activity caused by selected chronic health conditions among children, by age: United States, 2004–2005

Type of chronic health condition	*Under 5 years*		*5–11 years*		*12–17 years*	
	Rate	*SE*	*Rate*	*SE*	*Rate*	*SE*
	Number of children with limitation of activity caused by selected chronic health conditions per 1,000 population					
Speech problem	12.1	1.1	20.4	1.2	5.6	0.6
Asthma or breathing problem	7.5	0.8	5.8	0.6	5.6	0.7
Mental retardation or other developmental problem	8.4	1.0	10.5	0.9	11.0	0.9
Other mental, emotional, or behavioral problem	3.6	0.7	11.5	0.9	14.4	1.0
Attention eficit Hyperactivity isorder.			18.3	1.2	21.8	1.3
earning disability	2.3	0.6	17.7	1.2	26.3	1.4

SE is standard error.

Estimates are considered unreliable. ata preceded by an asterisk have a relative standard error RSE of 20 –30 . ata not shown have an RSE of greater than 30 .

NOTES: ata are for noninstitutionalized children. Children with limitation of activity caused by chronic health conditions were either identified by enrollment in special programs special education or early intervention services or by a limitation in their ability to perform activities usual for their age group because of a physical, mental, or emotional problem. Conditions refer to response categories in the National Health Interview Survey. Children who were reported to have more than one chronic health condition as the cause of their activity limitation were counted in each reported category. Starting in 2001, the condition list for children was expanded to include categories for Attention eficit Hyperactivity isorder A H or A and learning disability. Thus, comparable data for this figure are not available prior to 2001. See Appendix II, Condition imitation of activity. See related Table 58.

SOURCE: Centers for isease Control and Prevention, National Center for Health Statistics, National Health Interview Survey.

Data table for Figure 15. Limitation of activity caused by selected chronic health conditions among working-age adults, by age: United States, 2004–2005

Type of chronic health condition	*18–44 years*		*45–54 years*		*55–64 years*	
	Rate	*SE*	*Rate*	*SE*	*Rate*	*SE*
	Number of persons with limitation of activity caused by selected chronic health conditions per 1,000 population					
Mental illness	13.0	0.5	20.7	1.1	22.6	1.2
Fractures or oint in ury	5.5	0.3	12.4	0.7	17.9	1.0
ung	4.8	0.3	10.6	0.7	21.8	1.4
iabetes	2.5	0.2	13.2	0.7	31.9	1.5
Heart or other circulatory	5.3	0.3	25.3	1.0	66.0	2.1
Arthritis or other musculoskeletal	19.5	0.7	55.8	1.7	97.1	2.6

SE is standard error.

NOTES: ata are for the civilian noninstitutionalized population. Conditions refer to response categories in the Nationai Health Interview Survey some conditions include several response categories. Mental illness includes depression, anxiety or emotional problem, and other mental conditions. Heart or other circulatory includes heart problem, stroke problem, hypertension or high blood pressure, and other circulatory system conditions. Arthritis or other musculoskeletal includes arthritis or rheumatism, back or neck problem, and other musculoskeletal system conditions. Persons may report more than one chronic health condition as the cause of their activity limitation. See Appendix II, Condition imitation of activity. See related Table 58.

SOURCE: Centers for isease Control and Prevention, National Center for Health Statistics, National Health Interview Survey.

Data table for Figure 16. Limitation of activity caused by selected chronic health conditions among older adults, by age: United States, 2004–2005

Type of chronic health condition	*65–74 years*		*75–84 years*		*85 years and over*	
	Rate	*SE*	*Rate*	*SE*	*Rate*	*SE*
	Number of persons with limitation of activity caused by selected chronic health conditions per 1,000 population					
Senility or dementia	8.8	0.9	30.2	2.2	86.9	6.3
ung	29.9	1.8	39.0	2.3	38.5	4.1
iabetes	40.6	1.9	47.2	2.6	42.6	4.5
ision	20.8	1.5	38.4	2.5	78.7	6.1
Hearing	11.1	1.0	23.3	2.0	71.8	5.8
Heart or other circulatory	96.7	3.2	153.5	5.0	220.7	9.8
Arthritis or other musculoskeletal	120.4	3.4	186.3	5.2	266.2	10.1

SE is standard error.

NOTES: ata are for the civilian noninstitutionalized population. Conditions refer to response categories in the National Health Interview Survey some conditions include several response categories. ision includes vision conditions or problems seeing, and hearing includes hearing problems. Heart or other circulatory includes heart problem, stroke problem, hypertension or high blood pressure, and other circulatory system conditions. Arthritis or other musculoskeletal includes arthritis or rheumatism, back or neck problem, and other musculoskeletal system conditions. Senility is the term offered to respondents on a flashcard, but this category may include Alzheimer s disease or other types of dementia reported by the respondent. Persons may report more than one chronic health condition as the cause of their activity limitation. See Appendix II, Condition imitation of activity. See related Table 58.

SOURCE: Centers for isease Control and Prevention, National Center for Health Statistics, National Health Interview Survey.

Data table for Figure 17. Three or more chronic conditions among adults 45 years of age and over, by age and percent of poverty level: United States, 2005

	45–54 years		*55–64 years*		*65–74 years*		*75 years and over*	
Percent of poverty level	*Percent*	*SE*	*Percent*	*SE*	*Percent*	*SE*	*Percent*	*SE*
Total	7.3	0.4	17.6	0.6	27.8	0.9	36.6	1.0
elow 100	16.2	1.9	30.4	2.4	34.2	3.1	36.6	2.8
100 –less than 200	11.1	1.4	24.6	1.9	32.5	2.0	38.1	2.1
200 –less than 400	6.6	0.8	18.3	1.3	27.9	1.7	38.1	2.1
400 or more	5.3	0.5	12.7	0.9	22.4	1.5	31.4	2.5

SE is standard error.

NOTES: ata are for the civilian noninstitutionalized population. Chronic health conditions, except for asthma, were determined by asking if a doctor or health professional ever told the respondent that he or she had a specified condition. The health measure, three or more chronic conditions, includes three or more of the following conditions: hypertension, heart disease, stroke, emphysema, diabetes, cancer, arthritis and related diseases, or current asthma. Current asthma was determined by asking if a doctor or health professional ever told the respondent he or she had asthma and whether the respondent still had asthma. Heart disease includes coronary heart disease, angina or angina pectoris, heart attack or myocardial infarction, and any other kind of heart condition or heart disease. iabetes includes all types with the exception of diabetic conditions related to pregnancy. Cancer includes all types with the exception of non-melanoma skin cancer. Arthritis includes arthritis, rheumatoid arthritis, gout, lupus, or fibromyalgia. Percent of poverty level is based on family income and family size and composition using U.S. Census ureau poverty thresholds. Missing family income data were imputed for 38 of adults 45 years of age and over in 2005. See Appendix II, Condition Family income Poverty.

SOURCE: Centers for isease Control and Prevention, National Center for Health Statistics, National Health Interview Survey.

Data table for Figure 18. Life expectancy at birth and at 65 years of age, by race and sex: United States, 1970–2004

Year	*Male*	*Female*	*White male*	*Black male*	*White female*	*Black female*
			ife expectancy at birth in years			
1969–1971	67.0	74.6	67.9	60.0	75.5	68.3
1979–1981	70.1	77.6	70.8	64.1	78.2	72.9
1989–1991	71.8	78.8	72.7	64.5	79.5	73.7
1997	73.6	79.4	74.3	67.2	79.9	74.7
1998	73.8	79.5	74.5	67.6	80.0	74.8
1999	73.9	79.4	74.6	67.8	79.9	74.7
2000	74.3	79.7	74.8	68.2	80.0	74.9
2001	74.4	79.8	75.0	68.6	80.2	75.5
2002	74.5	79.9	75.1	68.8	80.3	75.6
2003	74.8	80.1	75.3	69.0	80.5	76.1
2004	75.2	80.4	75.7	69.5	80.8	76.3
			ife expectancy at age 65 in years			
1969–1971	13.0	16.8	13.0	12.5	16.9	15.7
1979–1981	14.2	18.4	14.3	13.3	18.6	17.1
1989–1991	15.1	19.0	15.2	13.3	19.1	17.4
1997	15.9	19.2	16.0	14.2	19.3	17.6
1998	16.0	19.2	16.1	14.3	19.3	17.4
1999	16.1	19.1	16.1	14.3	19.2	17.3
2000	16.2	19.3	16.3	14.5	19.2	17.4
2001	16.4	19.4	16.5	14.4	19.5	17.9
2002	16.6	19.5	16.6	14.6	19.5	18.0
2003	16.8	19.8	16.9	14.9	19.8	18.5
2004	17.1	20.0	17.2	15.2	20.0	18.6

NOTES: eath rates used to calculate life expectancies for 1997–1999 are based on postcensal 1990-based population estimates life expectancies for 2000 and beyond are calculated with death rates based on census 2000. See Appendix I, Population Census and Population Estimates. ife expectancies prior to 1997 are from decennial life tables based on census data and deaths for a 3-year period around the census year. The middle year in each 3-year period is plotted in Figure 18. eginning in 1997, the annual life tables are complete life tables based on a methodology similar to that used for decennial life tables. eaths to nonresidents were excluded beginning in 1970. See Appendix II, ife expectancy. See related Table 27.

SOURCE: Arias, E. United States life tables, 2004. National vital statistics reports. Hyattsville, M : National Center for Health Statistics. 2006, forthcoming.

Data table for Figure 19. Infant, neonatal, and postneonatal mortality rates: United States, 1950–2004

Year	*Infant*	*Neonatal*	*Postneonatal*
		eaths per 1,000 live births	
1950	29.2	20.5	8.7
1960	26.0	18.7	7.3
1970	20.0	15.1	4.9
1980	12.6	8.5	4.1
1985	10.6	7.0	3.7
1990	9.2	5.8	3.4
1995	7.6	4.9	2.7
1996	7.3	4.8	2.5
1997	7.2	4.8	2.5
1998	7.2	4.8	2.4
1999	7.1	4.7	2.3
2000	6.9	4.6	2.3
2001	6.8	4.5	2.3
2002	7.0	4.7	2.3
2003	6.9	4.6	2.2
2004	6.8	4.5	2.3

NOTES: Infant is defined as under 1 year of age, neonatal as under 28 days of age, and postneonatal as between 28 days and 1 year of age. See related Table 22.

SOURCE: Centers for isease Control and Prevention, National Center for Health Statistics, National ital Statistics System.

Data table for Figure 20. Death rates for leading causes of death for all ages: United States, 1950–2004

Year	All causes	Heart disease	Cancer	Stroke	Chronic lower respiratory diseases	Unintentional injuries
			eaths per 100,000 population			
1950	1,446.0	586.8	193.9	180.7	---	78.0
1960	1,339.2	559.0	193.9	177.9	---	62.3
1970	1,222.6	492.7	198.6	147.7	---	60.1
1980	1,039.1	412.1	207.9	96.2	28.3	46.4
1985	988.1	375.0	211.3	76.4	34.5	38.5
1990	938.7	321.8	216.0	65.3	37.2	36.3
1995	909.8	293.4	209.9	63.1	40.1	34.4
1996	894.1	285.7	206.7	62.5	40.6	34.5
1997	878.1	277.7	203.4	61.1	41.1	34.2
1998	870.6	271.3	200.7	59.3	41.8	34.5
1998 Comparability-modified	870.6	267.4	202.1	62.8	43.8	35.6
1999	875.6	266.5	200.8	61.6	45.4	35.3
2000	869.0	257.6	199.6	60.9	44.2	34.9
2001	854.5	247.8	196.0	57.9	43.7	35.7
2002	845.3	240.8	193.5	56.2	43.5	36.9
2003	832.7	232.3	190.1	53.5	43.3	37.3
2004	800.8	217.0	185.8	50.0	41.1	37.7

--- ata not available.

NOTES: Estimates are age-ad usted to the year 2000 standard population using the following age groups: under 1 year, 1–4 years, 10-year age groups from 5–14 through 75–84 years, and 85 years and over. Causes of death shown are the five leading causes of death for all ages in 2004. The 1950 death rates are based on the 6th revision of the International Classification of isease IC -6 , 1960 death rates on the IC -7, 1970 death rates on the IC -8, and 1980–1998 death rates on the IC -9. The 1998 comparability-modified death rates use comparability ratios to ad ust the rate to be comparable to records classified according to IC -10. Starting with 1999 data, death rates are based on IC -10. Comparability ratios across revisions for selected causes are available from: www.cdc.gov nchs data statab comp2.pdf. eath rates for chronic lower respiratory diseases are available from 1980 when a category that included bronchitis, emphysema, asthma, and other chronic lung diseases was introduced in IC -9. Cancer refers to malignant neoplasms stroke to cerebrovascular diseases and unintentional in uries is preferred to accidents in the public health community. Rates for 1991–1999 were computed using intercensal population estimates based on the 2000 census. Rates for 2000 were computed using 2000 census counts. Rates for 2001 and beyond were computed using postcensal estimates based on the 2000 census. See Appendix I, Population Census and Population Estimates. See Appendix II, Age ad ustment Cause of death Comparability ratio. See related Tables 29, 31, 32, 35, 36, 37, 38, 39, and 41.

SOURCE: Centers for isease Control and Prevention, National Center for Health Statistics, National ital Statistics System.

Data table for Figure 21. Adults 18 years of age and over reporting they did not receive needed health-related services in the past 12 months because they could not afford them, by age and type of service: United States, 2005

	18 years and over		*18–44 years*		*45–64 years*		*65 years and over*	
Needed service but could not afford it	*Percent*	*SE*	*Percent*	*SE*	*Percent*	*SE*	*Percent*	*SE*
			Percent not receiving needed service					
One or more of these services:	18.6	0.3	21.2	0.4	18.6	0.4	10.4	0.5
Medical care	7.1	0.2	8.1	0.3	7.7	0.3	2.5	0.2
Prescription medicines	8.7	0.2	9.8	0.3	8.7	0.3	5.1	0.3
Mental health care	2.6	0.1	3.1	0.2	2.6	0.2	0.5	0.1
ental care	11.8	0.2	14.1	0.4	11.5	0.4	5.2	0.3
Eyeglasses	6.9	0.2	7.0	0.3	8.2	0.3	3.7	0.3
			Number not receiving needed services in thousands					
One or more of these services:	40,438		23,373		13,417		3,648	
Medical care	15,385		8,933		5,574		878	
Prescription medicines	18,682		10,707		6,217		1,758	
Mental health care	5,502		3,438		1,880		183	
ental care	25,377		15,359		8,234		1,784	
Eyeglasses	14,805		7,635		5,884		1,286	

NOTES: ata are for the civilian noninstitutionalized population. ased on persons responding yes to the uestion, uring the past 12 months was there any time when person needed service but did not get it because person couldn t afford it Estimates were calculated using the sample adult weight, see Technical Notes.

SOURCE: Centers for isease Control and Prevention, National Center for Health Statistics, National Health Interview Survey.

Data table for Figure 22. Patient care physician supply and distribution among United States counties, by county metropolitan status: United States, 2004

Characteristic	*Total*	*Metropolitan counties*[1]	*Nonmetropolitan counties*
All counties:			
Number of patient care physicians	707,380	646,571	60,809
Patient care physicians per 10,000 population	24.1	26.5	12.2
istribution among counties:			
Patient care physicians per 10,000 population		Number of counties	
0	134	11	123
0.1–2.86	205	74	131
2.87–24.1	2,454	731	1,723
24.2–226	348	274	74
Patient care physicians per 10,000 population		Percent of counties	
0	4.3	1.0	6.0
0.1–2.86	6.5	6.8	6.4
2.87–24.1	78.1	67.1	84.0
24.2–226	11.1	25.1	3.6
Patient care physicians per 10,000 population		Population in counties	
0	419,773	72,270	347,503
0.1–2.86	3,199,705	1,634,433	1,565,272
2.87–24.1	164,762,304	119,992,662	44,769,642
24.2–226	125,273,622	122,257,377	3,016,245

[1]Metropolitan counties are defined using the Office of Management and udget definition. See Appendix II, Metropolitan statistical area.

NOTES: ata are for active, nonfederal, patient care physicians. octors of medicine and doctors of osteopathy are included. Patient care physicians include office-based physicians, full-time hospital staff, and residents or fellows. See Appendix II, Physician.

SOURCE: Health Resources and Services Administration, 2005 Area Resource File.

Data table for Figure 23. Obstetrician or gynecologist supply and distribution among United States counties, by county metropolitan status: United States, 2004

Characteristic	*Total*	*Metropolitan counties[1]*	*Nonmetropolitan counties*
All counties:			
Number of obstetricians or gynecologists	35,799	32,853	2,946
Obstetricians or gynecologists per 10,000 population[2]	3.0	3.3	1.4
istribution among counties:			
Obstetricians or gynecologists per 10,000 population[2]		Number of counties	
0	1,481	272	1,209
0.1–3.0	1,208	531	677
3.1–17.2	452	287	165
Obstetricians or gynecologists per 10,000 population[2]		Percent of counties	
0	47.2	25.0	59.0
0.1–3.0	38.5	48.7	33.0
3.1–17.2	14.4	26.3	8.0
Obstetricians or gynecologists per 10,000 population[2]		Population in counties	
0	8,339,693	2,494,091	5,845,602
0.1–3.0	56,094,638	44,029,217	12,065,421
3.1–17.2	54,996,721	52,561,665	2,435,056

[1]Metropolitan counties are defined using the Office of Management and udget definition. See Appendix II, Metropolitan statistical area.
[2]Ratio for female population 15 years of age and over.

NOTES: ata are for active, nonfederal, patient care obgyn doctors of medicine and exclude 1,502 obgyn doctors of osteopathy .O. in 2004. Obgyn .O. data were not available at the county level. Patient care doctors of medicine include office-based physicians, full-time hospital staff, and residents or fellows. See Appendix II, Physician.

SOURCES: Health Resources and Services Administration, 2005 Area Resource File. Female population 15 years of age and over from the National Center for Health Statistics NCHS estimates of uly 1, 2005 United States resident population by county, age, sex, race, and Hispanic origin, prepared under a collaborative arrangement with the U.S. Census ureau, Population Estimates Program. Available from: www.cdc.gov nchs about ma or dvs popbridge datadoc.htm vintage2005. American Osteopathic Association: Fact Sheet 2004, updated August 2004.

Data table for Figure 24. Active kidney transplant waiting list patients at end of year, by race and Hispanic origin: United States, 1988, 1996, and 2006

Race and Hispanic origin	*1988*	*1996*	*2006*
		Number	
Total	11,706	29,443	49,268
Not Hispanic:			
hite	6,594	14,248	19,247
lack or African American	3,447	10,472	16,452
Asian	603	1,685	3,576
American Indian or Alaska Native	0	372	517
Native Hawaiian or Other Pacific Islander	0	0	349
Multiracial	- - -	- - -	271
Hispanic or atino	1,062	2,666	8,856
		Percent	
Total	100.0	100.0	100.0
Not Hispanic:			
hite	56.3	48.4	39.1
lack or African American	29.4	35.6	33.4
Asian	5.2	5.7	7.3
American Indian or Alaska Native	0.0	1.3	1.0
Native Hawaiian or Other Pacific Islander	0.0	0.0	0.7
Multiracial	- - -	- - -	0.6
Hispanic or atino	9.1	9.1	18.0

- - - ata not available.

NOTES: Race and ethnicity are reported together as a single data element either race or ethnicity, but not both. Patients indicated to be Hispanic have been grouped together, with the remaining patients grouped into non-Hispanic categories. Starting in 1999, the category non-Hispanic multiracial was added.

SOURCE: Organ Procurement and Transplantation Network OPTN data as of March 9, 2007, supported in part by Health Resources and Services Administration contract 234–2005–370011C.

Data table for Figure 25. Active waiting list patients who received a kidney transplant within 2 years, by race and Hispanic origin: United States, 1988, 1996, and 2004

Race and Hispanic origin	*1988*	*1996*	*2004*
Total		Percent	
Not Hispanic:			
hite	67.8	42.3	30.1
lack or African American	57.5	28.2	19.9
Asian	55.9	26.8	19.5
American Indian or Alaska Native	57.8	26.6	23.7
Multiracial	- - -	24.9	22.7
Hispanic or atino	68.5	31.8	20.9

- - - ata not available.

NOTES: Race and ethnicity are reported together as a single data element either race or ethnicity, but not both. Patients indicated to be Hispanic have been grouped together, with the remaining patients grouped into non-Hispanic categories. Starting in 1999, the category non-Hispanic multiracial was added.

SOURCE: Unpublished data based on Organ Procurement and Transplantation Network OPTN data as of March 9, 2007, supported in part by Health Resources and Services Administration contract 234–2005–370011C.

Data table for Figure 26. No usual source of care among adults 45–64 years of age, by selected diagnosed chronic conditions and race and Hispanic origin: United States, 2004–2005

	No diagnosed chronic conditions		*Diabetes*		*Serious heart conditions*		*Hypertension*	
Race and Hispanic origin	*Percent*	*SE*	*Percent*	*SE*	*Percent*	*SE*	*Percent*	*SE*
Total	15.8	0.5	5.4	0.6	6.4	0.7	5.3	0.3
Hispanic or atino	29.8	1.5	11.4	2.1	9.0	2.5	10.9	1.4
Not Hispanic or atino:								
lack or African American only	19.5	1.4	5.7	1.3	8.3	1.9	8.0	1.0
hite only	13.1	0.6	4.2	0.7	5.8	0.8	4.3	0.4
Asian only	20.2	2.6						

SE is standard error.

Estimates are considered unreliable. ata not shown have a relative standard error greater than 30

NOTES: ata are for the civilian noninstitutionalized population. Respondents who reported more than one chronic condition were counted in each reported category. Persons of Hispanic origin may be of any race. iagnosed chronic conditions were identified by asking if a physician or other health provider ever told the respondent they had the condition. Serious heart conditions include coronary heart disease, heart attack, or angina. Hypertension is told on two or more occasions. iabetes excludes during pregnancy only. Respondents who reported borderline diabetes were recoded to no. No chronic conditions is never told had: serious heart condition, hypertension on two or more occasions, cancer excluding non-melanoma skin cancer , diabetes, arthritis, emphysema, asthma, stroke, ulcer and not told in the past year had: chronic bronchitis, liver disease, or kidney disease. See Appendix II, Hispanic origin Race Usual source of care.

SOURCE: Centers for isease Control and Prevention, National Center for Health Statistics, National Health Interview Survey.

Data table for Figure 27. Delayed medical care in the past 12 months due to lack of transportation among adults 18 years of age and over, by sex, percent of poverty level, and age: United States, 2004–2005

			Percent of poverty level					
	All income levels		*Below 100%*		*100%–less than 200%*		*200% or more*	
Sex and age	*Percent*	*SE*	*Percent*	*SE*	*Percent*	*SE*	*Percent*	*SE*
Total								
18 years and over	1.6	0.1	6.1	0.3	2.3	0.1	0.6	0.0
18–44 years	1.5	0.1	5.3	0.4	1.9	0.2	0.6	0.1
45–64 years	1.5	0.1	8.5	0.7	2.7	0.3	0.5	0.1
65 years and over	2.1	0.2	5.5	0.7	2.9	0.4	1.2	0.2
Men								
18 years and over	1.0	0.1	4.3	0.4	1.7	0.2	0.4	0.1
18–44 years	1.0	0.1	3.3	0.5	1.2	0.2	0.5	0.1
45–64 years	1.1	0.1	6.9	0.9	2.8	0.6	0.3	0.1
65 years and over	1.2	0.2	4.6	1.0			0.7	0.2
omen								
18 years and over	2.1	0.1	7.4	0.4	2.8	0.2	0.8	0.1
18–44 years	2.0	0.1	6.9	0.6	2.4	0.3	0.7	0.1
45–64 years	1.9	0.1	9.7	0.9	2.6	0.4	0.7	0.1
65 years and over	2.7	0.2	5.9	0.9	3.6	0.5	1.6	0.3

0.0 Quantity more than zero but less than 0.05.

SE is standard error.

Estimates are considered unreliable. ata preceded by an asterisk have a relative standard error RSE of 20 –30 . ata not shown have an RSE of greater than 30

NOTES: ata are for the civilian noninstitutionalized population. Percent of poverty level is based on family income and family size and composition using U.S. Census ureau poverty thresholds. Missing family income data were imputed for 35 of adults in 2004–2005. See Appendix II, Family income Poverty.

SOURCE: Centers for isease Control and Prevention, National Center for Health Statistics, National Health Interview Survey.

Data table for Figure 28. Health insurance coverage at the time of interview among persons under 65 years of age: United States, 1984–2005

	Health insurance coverage at the time of interview					
	Private		*Medicaid*		*Uninsured*	
Year	*Percent*	*SE*	*Percent*	*SE*	*Percent*	*SE*
1984	76.8	0.6	6.8	0.3	14.5	0.4
1989	75.9	0.4	7.2	0.2	15.6	0.3
1994	69.9	0.4	11.2	0.3	17.5	0.3
1995	71.3	0.4	11.5	0.2	16.1	0.2
1996	71.2	0.5	11.1	0.3	16.6	0.3
1997	70.7	0.4	9.7	0.2	17.5	0.2
1998	72.1	0.4	8.9	0.2	16.6	0.2
1999	72.8	0.3	9.1	0.2	16.1	0.2
2000	71.5	0.4	9.5	0.2	17.0	0.3
2001	71.2	0.4	10.4	0.2	16.4	0.3
2002	69.4	0.4	11.8	0.2	16.8	0.2
2003	68.9	0.4	12.3	0.2	16.5	0.3
2004	68.8	0.4	12.5	0.2	16.4	0.2
2005	68.2	0.4	13.0	0.2	16.4	0.2

SE is standard error.

NOTES: ata are for the civilian noninstitutionalized population. Medicaid includes other public assistance through 1996 includes state-sponsored health plans starting in 1997 and includes State Children s Health Insurance Program SCHIP starting in 1999. Uninsured persons are not covered by private insurance, Medicaid, SCHIP, public assistance through 1996 , state-sponsored or other government-sponsored health plans starting in 1997 , Medicare, or military plans. Persons with Indian Health Service only are considered to have no coverage. Percents do not add to 100 because the percentage of persons with Medicare, military plans, and other government-sponsored plans is not shown and because persons with both private insurance and Medicaid appear in both categories. Starting with data from the third uarter of 2004, persons under 65 years of age with no reported coverage were asked explicitly about Medicaid coverage. Estimates for Medicaid coverage shown in this table include the additional information. See Appendix II, Health insurance coverage. See related Tables 136, 138, and 139.

SOURCE: Centers for isease Control and Prevention, National Center for Health Statistics, National Health Interview Survey.

Data table for Figure 29. Uninsured for at least part of the 12 months prior to interview among persons under 65 years of age, by length of time uninsured and selected characteristics: United States, 2005

			Length of time uninsured prior to interview			
	Total uninsured prior to interview		*More than 12 months*		*Any period up to 12 months*	
Characteristic	*Percent*	*SE*	*Percent*	*SE*	*Percent*	*SE*
Age						
Under 65 years	20.3	0.3	11.4	0.2	7.6	0.1
Under 18 years	13.0	0.3	5.3	0.2	6.6	0.2
18–24 years	35.4	0.7	19.5	0.6	14.2	0.4
25–34 years	31.1	0.5	18.8	0.5	10.9	0.3
35–44 years	21.6	0.4	12.7	0.3	7.3	0.3
45–54 years	16.8	0.4	10.5	0.3	5.2	0.2
55–64 years	13.0	0.4	8.5	0.3	3.3	0.2
Percent of poverty level						
Below 100%	36.1	0.8	23.3	0.7	11.4	0.4
100%–less than 150%	35.6	0.9	22.5	0.8	12.1	0.6
150%–less than 200%	32.6	0.9	20.0	0.8	11.2	0.6
200% or more	13.5	0.2	6.5	0.2	5.7	0.2
Race and Hispanic origin						
Black or African American only, not Hispanic or Latino	22.2	0.6	12.6	0.5	8.3	0.5
Asian only	20.0	1.2	12.9	1.0	6.0	0.7
White only, not Hispanic or Latino	15.8	0.3	7.6	0.2	7.0	0.2
Hispanic or Latino (total)	37.1	0.6	26.3	0.6	9.7	0.4
Mexican	39.9	0.8	29.2	0.7	9.6	0.5
Cuban	26.4	2.6	16.3	1.9	9.5	1.6
Puerto Rican	21.2	1.6	9.6	1.0	10.4	1.3
Marital status (18–64 years)						
Single	33.8	0.5	20.4	0.4	11.7	0.3
Married	16.7	0.3	9.8	0.3	5.7	0.2
Separated or divorced	30.5	0.6	18.4	0.5	10.7	0.4
Widowed	25.1	1.5	16.2	1.2	7.4	1.0
Working status (18–64 years)						
Employed	21.6	0.3	12.9	0.2	7.3	0.2

SE is standard error.

NOTES: Data are for the civilian noninstitutionalized population. Total uninsured prior to interview includes people uninsured more than 12 months, people uninsured any period up to 12 months, and people uninsured for an unknown length of time (1.3% for persons under 65 years). Persons of Hispanic origin may be of any race. Total for Hispanic includes groups not shown separately. Asian only race includes persons of Hispanic and non-Hispanic origin. Uninsured persons are not covered by private insurance, Medicaid, State Children's Health Insurance Program (SCHIP), state-sponsored or other government-sponsored health plans, Medicare, or military plans. Persons with Indian Health Service only are considered uninsured. Percent of poverty level is based on family income and family size and composition using U.S. Census Bureau poverty thresholds. Missing family income data were imputed for 32% of persons under 65 years of age in 2005. See Appendix II, Family income; Health insurance coverage; Hispanic origin; Poverty; Race.

SOURCE: Centers for Disease Control and Prevention, National Center for Health Statistics, National Health Interview Survey.

Data table for Figure 30. Uninsured and insured populations under 65 years of age by selected characteristics: United States, 2005

Characteristic	*Insurance status at time of interview*			
	Uninsured		*Insured*	
	Percent distribution	*SE*	*Percent distribution*	*SE*
Under 65 years of age				
Total	100.0		100.0	
Under 18 years	16.2	0.4	31.2	0.2
18–44 years	61.6	0.5	39.4	0.2
45–64 years	22.2	0.4	29.4	0.3
Percent of poverty level				
Total	100.0		100.0	
Below 100%	25.1	0.6	11.2	0.3
100%–less than 200%	31.6	0.7	15.5	0.3
200%–less than 400%	28.7	0.8	30.3	0.5
400% or more	14.6	0.6	43.0	0.6
Race and Hispanic origin				
Total	100.0		100.0	
Hispanic or Latino	31.3	0.7	12.5	0.3
Not Hispanic or Latino:				
White only	48.0	0.9	69.2	0.4
Black or African American only	13.9	0.6	12.2	0.3
Asian only	4.3	0.3	4.1	0.2
All other not Hispanic persons	2.4	0.3	2.0	0.2
Marital status (18–64 years)				
Total	100.0		100.0	
Single	40.2	0.6	24.0	0.3
Married	41.8	0.6	62.8	0.3
Separated or divorced	16.3	0.4	11.6	0.2
Widowed	1.7	0.1	1.5	0.1
Working status				
Total 18–64 years	100.0		100.0	
Employed	68.7	0.5	76.5	0.3
Not employed	31.3	0.5	23.5	0.3
Total 18–44 years	100.0		100.0	
Employed	70.7	0.5	78.7	0.3
Not employed	29.3	0.5	21.3	0.3
Total 45–64 years	100.0		100.0	
Employed	62.8	0.9	73.5	0.4
Not employed	37.2	0.9	26.5	0.4

SE is standard error.

NOTES: Data are for the civilian noninstitutionalized population. Percentages exclude persons unknown on health insurance status. These persons are included in the estimate of the total uninsured population (see Figure 30, Table 139). Persons of Hispanic origin may be of any race. Uninsured persons are not covered by private insurance, Medicaid, State Children's Health Insurance Program (SCHIP), state-sponsored or other government-sponsored health plans, Medicare, or military plans. Persons with Indian Health Service only are considered uninsured. Percent of poverty level is based on family income and family size and composition using U.S. Census Bureau poverty thresholds. Missing family income data were imputed for 32% of persons under 65 years of age in 2005. Employment status is in the previous week. Not employed includes all reasons not employed such as not working, looking for work, retired, disabled, taking care of house or family, or going to school. See Appendix II, Family income; Health insurance coverage; Hispanic origin; Poverty; Race.

SOURCE: Centers for Disease Control and Prevention, National Center for Health Statistics, National Health Interview Survey.

Data table for Figure 31. Persons under 65 years of age who spent more than 10% of after-tax family income on out-of-pocket medical expenditures, by percent of poverty level: United States, 1996 and 2004

Characteristic	1996		2004	
	Percent	SE	Percent	SE
Under 65 years	15.8	0.5	16.6	0.4
Percent of poverty level				
Less than 100%	25.9	1.5	27.3	1.3
100%–less than 200%	24.1	1.5	22.2	1.1
200%–less than 400%	15.6	0.9	17.4	0.8
400% or more	7.1	0.6	9.6	0.5

NOTES: Data are for the civilian noninstitutionalized population. Percent of poverty level is based on family income and family size and composition using U.S. Census Bureau poverty thresholds. Dollar values for 1996 were inflated to 2003 values using the Consumer Price Index for urban areas. Out-of-pocket medical expenditures include health insurance premiums. For information on family income measurement see Banthin JS, Selden TM, Income measurement in the Medical Expenditure Panel Survey. Agency for Healthcare Research and Quality working paper No. 06005, July 2006. Available from: www.meps.ahrq.gov/mepsweb/data_files/publications/workingpapers/wp_06005.pdf#xml=http://207.188.212.220/cgi-bin/texis/webinator/search/pdfhi.txt?query=working+paper+06005&pr=MEPSFULLSITE&prox=page&rorder=500&rprox=500&rdfreq=500&rwfreq=500&rlead=500&sufs=0&order=r&cq=&id=465e84c92a.

SOURCE: Agency for Healthcare Research and Quality, Medical Expenditure Panel Survey.

Data table for Figure 32. Adults 20–64 years of age with undiagnosed high cholesterol or elevated blood pressure, by health insurance status and age: United States, 1999–2004

Medical condition and age	Total		Insured		Uninsured	
	Percent	SE	Percent	SE	Percent	SE
High cholesterol						
20–64 years	10.3	0.6	9.9	0.6	12.7	1.7
20–44 years	8.4	0.7	7.8	0.7	11.2	2.0
45–64 years	12.7	1.0	12.4	1.0	16.2	3.2
Elevated blood pressure						
20–64 years	8.2	0.5	8.5	0.6	7.1	0.8
20–44 years	4.5	0.5	4.5	0.5	4.7	0.6
45–64 years	15.5	1.2	15.4	1.2	16.1	2.3

SE is standard error.

NOTES: Insurance coverage is as of the day of interview. Undiagnosed is defined as during the interview, the respondent reporting never being told by a physician or other health professional that they had high cholesterol or elevated blood pressure, but on examination, in the mobile examination center, having a total cholesterol reading of 240 mg/dL or higher or an average of readings for systolic blood pressure of 140 mm Hg or higher or for diastolic blood pressure of 90 mm Hg or higher. Elevated blood pressure estimates exclude pregnant women.

SOURCE: Centers for Disease Control and Prevention, National Center for Health Statistics, National Health and Nutrition Examination Survey.

Data table for Figure 33. Persons under 65 years of age who did not get needed medical care in the past year due to cost, by duration of health insurance coverage and percent of poverty level: United States, 2005

	Health insurance status during 12 months prior to interview					
	Uninsured more than 12 months		*Uninsured for any period up to 12 months*		*Insured continuously all 12 months*	
Age and percent of poverty level	*Percent*	*SE*	*Percent*	*SE*	*Percent*	*SE*
Under 18 years						
All incomes	14.1	1.3	10.5	1.0	0.7	0.1
Below 100%	15.8	2.4	16.7	2.9	*0.9	0.2
100%–less than 200%	14.8	2.4	10.6	1.7	*1.4	0.3
200% or more	11.5	2.2	6.3	1.1	*0.4	0.1
18–64 years						
All incomes	23.4	0.6	21.4	0.7	2.8	0.1
Below 100%	26.1	1.2	28.7	1.8	6.1	0.5
100%–less than 200%	25.2	1.1	24.6	1.5	6.0	0.4
200% or more	20.2	0.9	17.5	0.9	1.9	0.1

SE is standard error.

* Estimates are considered unreliable. Data preceded by an asterisk have a relative standard error of 20%–30%.

NOTES: Data are for the civilian noninstitutionalized population. Uninsured persons are not covered by private insurance, Medicaid, State Children's Health Insurance Program (SCHIP), state-sponsored or other government-sponsored health plans, Medicare, or military plans. Persons with Indian Health Service only are considered uninsured. Percent of poverty level is based on family income and family size and composition using U.S. Census Bureau poverty thresholds. Missing family income data were imputed for 32% of persons under 65 years of age in 2005. See Appendix II, Family income; Health insurance coverage; Hispanic origin; Poverty; Race.

SOURCE: Centers for Disease Control and Prevention, National Center for Health Statistics, National Health Interview Survey.

Data table for Figure 34. No dental visit in the past year by dentition status (presence of natural teeth), age, and percent of poverty level: United States, 2005

Dentate persons (with any natural teeth)	*2 years and over*		*2–17 years*		*18 years and over*		*18–44 years*		*45–64 years*		*65 years and over*	
	Percent	*SE*	*Percent*	*SE*	*Percent*	*SE*	*Percent*	*SE*	*Percent*	*SE*	*Percent*	*SE*
Percent of poverty level												
All persons	31.8	0.3	23.8	0.5	34.5	0.4	38.4	0.5	30.2	0.6	28.8	0.8
Below 100%	47.2	0.9	33.8	1.4	54.0	1.2	53.6	1.5	56.2	2.0	51.2	3.7
100%–less than 200%	44.3	0.7	31.4	1.2	49.7	0.8	51.3	1.2	50.6	1.7	42.6	2.0
200%–less than 400%	32.7	0.6	22.2	0.9	36.2	0.6	39.0	1.0	35.9	1.1	26.8	1.4
400% or more	19.7	0.5	13.4	0.7	21.1	0.5	24.8	0.8	18.4	0.7	15.6	1.3

Edentate persons (without any natural teeth)	*65 years and over*	
	Percent	*SE*
Percent of poverty level		
All persons	79.7	1.2
Below 100%	83.6	2.8
100%–less than 200%	83.8	1.9
200%–less than 400%	77.9	2.3
400% or more	68.2	4.3

NOTES: Data are for all children 2–17 years because dentate status is not assessed for children. Data are for the civilian noninstitutionalized population. Percent of poverty level is based on family income and family size and composition using U.S. Census Bureau poverty thresholds. Missing family income data were imputed for 34% of persons 2 years of age and over in 2005. See Appendix II, Dental visit; Family income; Poverty.

SOURCE: Centers for Disease Control and Prevention, National Center for Health Statistics, National Health Interview Survey.

Data table for Figure 35. Adults 50 years of age and over ever having a colorectal scope procedure, by selected characteristics: United States, annual average 2000, 2003, and 2005

	Total		*Insured*		*Uninsured*	
Characteristic	*Percent*	*SE*	*Percent*	*SE*	*Percent*	*SE*
50 years and over	43.8	0.4	45.7	0.4	18.6	0.9
65 years and over	51.4	0.5	51.7	0.5	*	*
50–64 years						
Total, 50–64 years	38.2	0.4	40.8	0.5	18.5	0.9
Male	39.3	0.6	41.9	0.7	18.4	1.4
Female	37.2	0.6	39.9	0.6	18.5	1.2
Race and Hispanic origin						
White, not Hispanic	40.6	0.5	42.6	0.5	21.1	1.3
Black, not Hispanic	33.8	1.1	36.7	1.2	18.1	2.1
Hispanic	25.3	1.1	30.5	1.4	12.9	1.5
Percent of poverty level						
Below 200%	29.2	0.8	34.3	1.1	16.9	1.2
200% or more	40.7	0.5	42.2	0.5	20.4	1.5
Education						
Less than high school	25.8	0.9	30.2	1.2	13.2	1.3
High school	34.8	0.7	37.4	0.8	17.5	1.6
More than high school	43.6	0.6	45.1	0.6	24.5	1.7

* Estimates are considered unreliable. Data not shown have a relative standard error of greater than 30%.

NOTES: Data are for the civilian noninstitutionalized population. Persons of Hispanic origin may be of any race. Respondents from the National Interview Survey were asked: "Have you ever had a sigmoidoscopy, colonoscopy, or proctoscopy?" These are exams in which a health care professional inserts a tube into the rectum to look for signs of cancer or other problems. Percent of poverty level is based on family income and family size and composition using U.S. Census Bureau poverty thresholds. See Appendix II, Education; Hispanic origin; Poverty; Race.

SOURCE: Centers for Disease Control and Prevention, National Center for Health Statistics, National Health Interview Survey.

Data table for Figure 36. Adults 18 years of age and over reporting antidepressant drug use in the past month, by sex and race and Hispanic origin: United States, 1988–1994 and 1999–2002

Sex, race and ethnicity	1988–1994		1999–2002	
	Percent	SE	Percent	SE
Total, age-adjusted	2.5	0.2	8.0	0.4
White only, not Hispanic	2.7	0.3	9.5	0.5
Black only, not Hispanic	2.0	0.3	4.1	0.5
Mexican	1.5	0.2	3.1	0.5
Total, crude	2.4	0.2	8.1	0.4
White only, not Hispanic	2.7	0.2	9.6	0.5
Black only, not Hispanic	1.7	0.2	3.8	0.5
Mexican	1.3	0.1	2.3	0.4
Men, age-adjusted	1.6	0.2	5.2	0.4
White only, not Hispanic	1.7	0.2	6.1	0.5
Black only, not Hispanic	*1.0	0.2	3.0	0.6
Mexican	0.8	0.1	*1.8	0.5
Men, crude	1.5	0.2	5.2	0.3
White only, not Hispanic	1.7	0.2	6.2	0.4
Black only, not Hispanic	*0.9	0.2	2.7	0.5
Mexican	*0.7	0.2	*	*
Women, age-adjusted	3.3	0.3	10.6	0.6
White only, not Hispanic	3.6	0.4	12.8	0.8
Black only, not Hispanic	2.8	0.4	4.9	0.6
Mexican	2.2	0.3	4.5	0.7
Women, crude	3.2	0.3	10.7	0.6
White only, not Hispanic	3.5	0.4	12.9	0.8
Black only, not Hispanic	2.4	0.3	4.7	0.6
Mexican	1.8	0.3	*3.6	0.7

SE is standard error.

* Estimates are considered unreliable. Data preceded by an asterisk have a relative standard error (RSE) of 20%–30%. Data not shown have a RSE of greater than 30%.

NOTES: Data are for the civilian noninstitutionalized population. Totals include persons of all races and Hispanic origins, not just those shown separately. Age-adjusted estimates were adjusted to the 2000 standard population using three age groups: 18–44 years, 45–64 years, and 65 years and over. See Appendix II, Age adjustment. Antidepressant drugs include: amitriptyline, amoxapine, bupropion, citalopram, clomipramine, desipramine, doxepin, escitalopram, fluoxetine, fluvoxamine, imipramine, isocarboxazid, maprotiline, mirtazapine, nefazodone, nortriptyline, paroxetine, phenelzine, protriptyline, sertraline, tranylcypromine, trazodone, trimipramine, venlafaxine.

SOURCE: Centers for Disease Control and Prevention, National Center for Health Statistics, National Health and Nutrition Examination Survey.

Trend Tables

Table 1 (page 1 of 3). Resident population, by age, sex, race, and Hispanic origin: United States, selected years 1950–2005

[Data are based on decennial census updated with data from multiple sources]

Sex, race, Hispanic origin, and year	Total resident population	Under 1 year	1–4 years	5–14 years	15–24 years	25–34 years	35–44 years	45–54 years	55–64 years	65–74 years	75–84 years	85 years and over
	Number in thousands											
All persons												
1950	150,697	3,147	13,017	24,319	22,098	23,759	21,450	17,343	13,370	8,340	3,278	577
1960	179,323	4,112	16,209	35,465	24,020	22,818	24,081	20,485	15,572	10,997	4,633	929
1970	203,212	3,485	13,669	40,746	35,441	24,907	23,088	23,220	18,590	12,435	6,119	1,511
1980	226,546	3,534	12,815	34,942	42,487	37,082	25,635	22,800	21,703	15,581	7,729	2,240
1990	248,710	3,946	14,812	35,095	37,013	43,161	37,435	25,057	21,113	18,045	10,012	3,021
2000	281,422	3,806	15,370	41,078	39,184	39,892	45,149	37,678	24,275	18,391	12,361	4,240
2003	290,811	4,004	15,766	40,969	41,206	39,873	44,371	40,805	27,900	18,337	12,869	4,713
2004	293,655	4,077	15,994	40,751	41,701	40,032	44,109	41,619	29,079	18,463	12,971	4,860
2005	296,410	4,107	16,197	40,397	42,077	40,143	43,862	42,482	30,356	18,640	13,054	5,096
Male												
1950	74,833	1,602	6,634	12,375	10,918	11,597	10,588	8,655	6,697	4,024	1,507	237
1960	88,331	2,090	8,240	18,029	11,906	11,179	11,755	10,093	7,537	5,116	2,025	362
1970	98,912	1,778	6,968	20,759	17,551	12,217	11,231	11,199	8,793	5,437	2,436	542
1980	110,053	1,806	6,556	17,855	21,419	18,382	12,570	11,009	10,152	6,757	2,867	682
1990	121,239	2,018	7,581	17,971	18,915	21,564	18,510	12,232	9,955	7,907	3,745	841
2000	138,054	1,949	7,862	21,043	20,079	20,121	22,448	18,497	11,645	8,303	4,879	1,227
2003	143,037	2,046	8,060	20,977	21,183	20,222	22,134	20,044	13,424	8,349	5,154	1,445
2004	144,537	2,085	8,178	20,860	21,438	20,336	22,034	20,453	13,999	8,428	5,218	1,508
2005	146,000	2,101	8,280	20,675	21,647	20,421	21,940	20,895	14,627	8,529	5,279	1,604
Female												
1950	75,864	1,545	6,383	11,944	11,181	12,162	10,863	8,688	6,672	4,316	1,771	340
1960	90,992	2,022	7,969	17,437	12,114	11,639	12,326	10,393	8,036	5,881	2,609	567
1970	104,300	1,707	6,701	19,986	17,890	12,690	11,857	12,021	9,797	6,998	3,683	969
1980	116,493	1,727	6,259	17,087	21,068	18,700	13,065	11,791	11,551	8,824	4,862	1,559
1990	127,471	1,928	7,231	17,124	18,098	21,596	18,925	12,824	11,158	10,139	6,267	2,180
2000	143,368	1,857	7,508	20,034	19,105	19,771	22,701	19,181	12,629	10,088	7,482	3,013
2003	147,773	1,958	7,706	19,992	20,024	19,650	22,237	20,761	14,475	9,988	7,714	3,269
2004	149,118	1,992	7,817	19,890	20,263	19,696	22,075	21,166	15,079	10,036	7,753	3,352
2005	150,411	2,005	7,917	19,721	20,430	19,722	21,922	21,587	15,729	10,110	7,775	3,492
White male												
1950	67,129	1,400	5,845	10,860	9,689	10,430	9,529	7,836	6,180	3,736	1,406	218
1960	78,367	1,784	7,065	15,659	10,483	9,940	10,564	9,114	6,850	4,702	1,875	331
1970	86,721	1,501	5,873	17,667	15,232	10,775	9,979	10,090	7,958	4,916	2,243	487
1980	94,976	1,487	5,402	14,773	18,123	15,940	11,010	9,774	9,151	6,096	2,600	621
1990	102,143	1,604	6,071	14,467	15,389	18,071	15,819	10,624	8,813	7,127	3,397	760
2000	113,445	1,524	6,143	16,428	15,942	16,232	18,568	15,670	10,067	7,343	4,419	1,109
2003	116,875	1,594	6,296	16,322	16,726	16,159	18,129	16,807	11,590	7,308	4,638	1,307
2004	117,916	1,625	6,381	16,229	16,896	16,205	17,994	17,116	12,062	7,358	4,688	1,361
2005	118,932	1,636	6,456	16,090	17,027	16,230	17,866	17,453	12,571	7,425	4,733	1,445
White female												
1950	67,813	1,341	5,599	10,431	9,821	10,851	9,719	7,868	6,168	4,031	1,669	314
1960	80,465	1,714	6,795	15,068	10,596	10,204	11,000	9,364	7,327	5,428	2,441	527
1970	91,028	1,434	5,615	16,912	15,420	11,004	10,349	10,756	8,853	6,366	3,429	890
1980	99,835	1,412	5,127	14,057	17,653	15,896	11,232	10,285	10,325	7,951	4,457	1,440
1990	106,561	1,524	5,762	13,706	14,599	17,757	15,834	10,946	9,698	9,048	5,687	2,001
2000	116,641	1,447	5,839	15,576	14,966	15,574	18,386	15,921	10,731	8,757	6,715	2,729
2003	119,474	1,525	5,999	15,488	15,658	15,310	17,813	17,034	12,263	8,576	6,859	2,950
2004	120,353	1,551	6,081	15,405	15,831	15,302	17,625	17,329	12,741	8,595	6,874	3,020
2005	121,203	1,561	6,158	15,278	15,942	15,288	17,447	17,637	13,248	8,634	6,872	3,138
Black or African American male												
1950	7,300	- - -	[1]944	1,442	1,162	1,105	1,003	772	459	299	[2]113	- - -
1960	9,114	281	1,082	2,185	1,305	1,120	1,086	891	617	382	137	29
1970	10,748	245	975	2,784	2,041	1,226	1,084	979	739	461	169	46
1980	12,585	269	967	2,614	2,807	1,967	1,235	1,024	854	567	228	53
1990	14,420	322	1,164	2,700	2,669	2,592	1,962	1,175	878	614	277	66
2000	17,407	313	1,271	3,454	2,932	2,586	2,705	1,957	1,090	683	330	87
2003	18,190	336	1,301	3,444	3,180	2,613	2,705	2,218	1,232	711	355	96
2004	18,417	337	1,320	3,414	3,248	2,650	2,695	2,278	1,293	722	359	101
2005	18,658	339	1,334	3,367	3,318	2,691	2,687	2,345	1,367	737	366	108

See footnotes at end of table.

Table 1 (page 2 of 3). Resident population, by age, sex, race, and Hispanic origin: United States, selected years 1950–2005

[Data are based on decennial census updated with data from multiple sources]

Sex, race, Hispanic origin, and year	Total resident population	Under 1 year	1–4 years	5–14 years	15–24 years	25–34 years	35–44 years	45–54 years	55–64 years	65–74 years	75–84 years	85 years and over
	Number in thousands											
Black or African American female												
1950	7,745	- - -	[1]941	1,446	1,300	1,260	1,112	796	443	322	[2]125	- - -
1960	9,758	283	1,085	2,191	1,404	1,300	1,229	974	663	430	160	38
1970	11,832	243	970	2,773	2,196	1,456	1,309	1,134	868	582	230	71
1980	14,046	266	951	2,578	2,937	2,267	1,488	1,258	1,059	776	360	106
1990	16,063	316	1,137	2,641	2,700	2,905	2,279	1,416	1,135	884	495	156
2000	19,187	302	1,228	3,348	2,971	2,866	3,055	2,274	1,353	971	587	233
2003	19,958	323	1,260	3,337	3,140	2,862	3,052	2,579	1,531	999	627	247
2004	20,184	324	1,279	3,306	3,193	2,886	3,037	2,651	1,607	1,011	636	254
2005	20,416	324	1,292	3,260	3,244	2,909	3,024	2,727	1,695	1,029	645	267
American Indian or Alaska Native male												
1980	702	17	59	153	161	114	75	53	37	22	9	2
1990	1,024	24	88	206	192	183	140	86	55	32	13	3
2000	1,488	28	109	301	271	229	229	165	88	45	18	5
2003	1,553	21	96	293	294	240	232	187	107	53	24	6
2004	1,572	22	90	290	300	244	233	192	114	56	25	7
2005	1,579	22	86	282	303	248	231	197	119	58	26	7
American Indian or Alaska Native female												
1980	718	16	57	149	158	118	79	57	41	27	12	4
1990	1,041	24	85	200	178	186	148	92	61	41	21	6
2000	1,496	26	106	293	254	219	236	174	95	54	28	10
2003	1,558	21	93	286	278	224	235	198	115	62	33	13
2004	1,576	21	88	282	285	227	233	204	122	65	35	14
2005	1,582	21	83	274	289	229	230	209	129	67	36	15
Asian or Pacific Islander male												
1980	1,814	35	130	321	334	366	252	159	110	72	30	6
1990	3,652	68	258	598	665	718	588	347	208	133	57	12
2000	5,713	84	339	861	934	1,073	947	705	399	231	112	27
2003	6,419	94	367	917	983	1,211	1,068	832	496	277	138	36
2004	6,633	101	387	927	994	1,238	1,112	866	531	292	146	39
2005	6,831	104	404	937	1,000	1,252	1,156	900	569	309	154	44
Asian or Pacific Islander female												
1980	1,915	34	127	307	325	423	269	192	126	71	33	9
1990	3,805	65	247	578	621	749	664	371	264	166	65	17
2000	6,044	81	336	817	914	1,112	1,024	812	451	305	152	41
2003	6,783	89	354	882	947	1,254	1,137	950	565	351	196	59
2004	7,005	96	368	898	954	1,281	1,179	983	609	365	208	64
2005	7,209	99	384	909	955	1,295	1,221	1,014	657	380	222	73

See footnotes at end of table.

Table 1 (page 3 of 3). Resident population, by age, sex, race, and Hispanic origin: United States, selected years 1950–2005

[Data are based on decennial census updated with data from multiple sources]

Sex, race, Hispanic origin, and year	Total resident population	Under 1 year	1–4 years	5–14 years	15–24 years	25–34 years	35–44 years	45–54 years	55–64 years	65–74 years	75–84 years	85 years and over
	Number in thousands											
Hispanic or Latino male												
1980	7,280	187	661	1,530	1,646	1,256	761	570	364	200	86	19
1990	11,388	279	980	2,128	2,376	2,310	1,471	818	551	312	131	32
2000	18,162	395	1,506	3,469	3,564	3,494	2,653	1,551	804	474	203	50
2003	20,599	442	1,682	3,832	3,759	4,016	3,101	1,910	991	542	261	65
2004	21,347	463	1,769	3,919	3,794	4,163	3,242	2,023	1,058	566	280	71
2005	22,065	476	1,837	3,996	3,823	4,295	3,376	2,155	1,137	591	299	80
Hispanic or Latino female												
1980	7,329	181	634	1,482	1,546	1,249	805	615	411	257	117	30
1990	10,966	268	939	2,039	2,028	2,073	1,448	868	632	403	209	59
2000	17,144	376	1,441	3,318	3,017	3,016	2,476	1,585	907	603	303	101
2003	19,300	424	1,611	3,659	3,235	3,363	2,815	1,908	1,097	680	380	128
2004	19,975	443	1,694	3,744	3,303	3,454	2,919	2,006	1,164	705	405	139
2005	20,622	456	1,763	3,815	3,370	3,532	3,015	2,115	1,242	731	430	153
White, not Hispanic or Latino male												
1980	88,035	1,308	4,772	13,317	16,554	14,739	10,284	9,229	8,803	5,906	2,519	603
1990	91,743	1,351	5,181	12,525	13,219	15,967	14,481	9,875	8,303	6,837	3,275	729
2000	96,551	1,163	4,761	13,238	12,628	12,958	16,088	14,223	9,312	6,894	4,225	1,062
2003	97,660	1,173	4,718	12,797	13,237	12,393	15,225	15,025	10,660	6,796	4,390	1,245
2004	97,986	1,184	4,706	12,623	13,376	12,301	14,957	15,228	11,071	6,824	4,422	1,294
2005	98,327	1,186	4,710	12,409	13,482	12,203	14,703	15,441	11,507	6,868	4,448	1,369
White, not Hispanic or Latino female												
1980	92,872	1,240	4,522	12,647	16,185	14,711	10,468	9,700	9,935	7,707	4,345	1,411
1990	96,557	1,280	4,909	11,846	12,749	15,872	14,520	10,153	9,116	8,674	5,491	1,945
2000	100,774	1,102	4,517	12,529	12,183	12,778	16,089	14,446	9,879	8,188	6,429	2,633
2003	101,555	1,121	4,488	12,125	12,673	12,188	15,201	15,261	11,236	7,935	6,499	2,829
2004	101,789	1,128	4,477	11,964	12,783	12,095	14,916	15,466	11,652	7,932	6,491	2,888
2005	102,031	1,130	4,483	11,767	12,833	12,008	14,647	15,673	12,087	7,946	6,466	2,992

- - - Data not available.
[1]Population for age group under 5 years.
[2]Population for age group 75 years and over.

NOTES: The race groups, white, black, American Indian or Alaska Native, and Asian or Pacific Islander, include persons of Hispanic and non-Hispanic origin. Persons of Hispanic origin may be of any race. Starting with *Health, United States, 2003*, intercensal population estimates for the 1990s and 2000 are based on the 2000 census. Population estimates for 2001 and later years are 2000-based postcensal estimates. Population figures are census counts as of April 1 for 1950, 1960, 1970, 1980, 1990, and 2000; estimates as of July 1 for other years. See Appendix I, Population Census and Population Estimates. Populations for age groups may not sum to the total due to rounding. Although population figures are shown rounded to the nearest 1,000, calculations of birth rates and death rates shown in this volume are based on unrounded population figures for decennial years and for all years starting with 1991. See Appendix II, Rate. Unrounded population figures are available in the spreadsheet version of this table. Available from: www.cdc.gov/nchs/hus.htm. Data for additional years are available. See Appendix III.

SOURCES: U.S. Census Bureau: 1950 Nonwhite Population by Race. Special Report P-E, No. 3B. Washington, DC: U.S. Government Printing Office, 1951; U.S. Census of Population: 1960, Number of Inhabitants, PC(1)-A1, United States Summary, 1964; 1970, Number of Inhabitants, Final Report PC(1)-A1, United States Summary, 1971; U.S. population estimates, by age, sex, race, and Hispanic origin: 1980 to 1991. Current population reports, series P–25, no 1095. Washington, DC: U.S. Government Printing Office, Feb. 1993; National Center for Health Statistics. Estimates of the July 1, 1991–July 1, 1999, April 1, 2000, and July 1, 2001–July 1, 2005 United States resident population by age, sex, race, and Hispanic origin, prepared under a collaborative arrangement with the U.S. Census Bureau, Population Estimates Program. Available from: www.cdc.gov/nchs/about/major/dvs/popbridge/popbridge.htm.

Table 2 (page 1 of 2). Inmates in state or federal prisons and local jails, by sex, race, Hispanic origin, and age: United States, selected years 1999–2005

[Data are based on reporting by a census of departments of correction and the Federal Bureau of Prisons and a sample of jails]

Sex, race, Hispanic origin, and age	*1999*	*2000*	*2003*	*2004*	*2005*	*1999*	*2000*	*2003*	*2004*	*2005*
	Number of inmates in thousands [1]					Inmates per 100,000 population [2]				
Total [3,4]	1,861	1,932	2,079	2,131	2,186	- - -	686	716	726	738
Male [3,4]	1,711	1,776	1,902	1,948	1,993	1,261	1,297	1,331	1,348	1,371
Female [3,4]	149	156	176	183	194	106	110	119	123	129
White, not Hispanic: [4]										
Male	610	664	665	696	689	630	683	681	717	709
Female	54	64	76	82	89	53	63	75	81	88
Black, not Hispanic: [4]										
Male	757	792	832	843	806	4,617	4,777	4,834	4,919	4,682
Female	68	70	67	68	66	375	380	352	359	347
Hispanic: [4]										
Male	296	291	364	367	403	1,802	1,715	1,778	1,717	1,856
Female	23	20	28	29	29	142	117	148	143	144
Male										
18–19	79	81	72	73	74	1,868	1,917	1,709	1,727	1,739
20–24	299	310	346	352	357	3,130	3,177	3,316	3,255	3,291
25–29	317	330	332	340	351	3,363	3,580	3,417	3,390	3,462
30–34	321	334	314	316	320	3,193	3,362	2,944	3,060	3,122
35–39	282	294	292	292	291	2,474	2,613	2,641	2,755	2,765
40–44	190	198	241	250	256	1,699	1,747	2,096	2,187	2,240
45–54	157	165	224	238	251	896	903	1,129	1,162	1,214
55 and over	49	51	66	72	77	193	199	238	247	260
Female										
18–19	4	4	4	5	5	92	96	109	112	116
20–24	19	20	25	27	28	205	210	255	264	277
25–29	29	30	26	27	29	303	324	277	283	299
30–34	37	39	33	34	34	370	391	316	330	342
35–39	29	31	36	36	38	257	272	322	346	364
40–44	16	17	27	29	31	144	149	232	247	264
45–54	12	12	20	22	23	63	64	97	101	110
55 and over	3	3	4	4	4	8	8	11	11	12
White, not Hispanic male										
18–19	24	26	24	24	24	885	942	882	911	905
20–24	91	100	103	107	107	1,462	1,560	1,610	1,641	1,627
25–29	96	105	93	98	99	1,535	1,732	1,607	1,666	1,682
30–34	114	125	104	107	105	1,674	1,861	1,545	1,691	1,693
35–39	106	116	109	111	106	1,302	1,460	1,467	1,607	1,562
40–44	74	81	99	105	103	897	972	1,206	1,314	1,299
45–54	71	78	94	101	100	522	553	626	664	658
55 and over	27	30	37	40	40	129	139	162	170	167
Black, not Hispanic male										
18–19	35	37	33	33	32	5,787	6,027	5,365	5,473	5,306
20–24	136	143	161	162	154	10,407	10,593	11,329	11,054	10,486
25–29	152	160	154	156	150	12,334	13,118	12,809	12,603	11,955
30–34	142	150	135	135	127	11,225	11,892	10,627	10,979	10,472
35–39	130	136	127	125	116	9,548	10,054	9,570	10,036	9,425
40–44	79	83	102	105	99	6,224	6,399	7,639	7,993	7,575
45–54	59	62	93	99	97	3,399	3,409	4,425	4,546	4,401
55 and over	13	13	19	21	21	611	635	842	898	879

See footnotes at end of table.

Table 2 (page 2 of 2). Inmates in state or federal prisons and local jails, by sex, race, Hispanic origin, and age: United States, selected years 1999–2005

[Data are based on reporting by a census of departments of correction and the Federal Bureau of Prisons and a sample of jails]

Sex, race, Hispanic origin, and age	*1999*	*2000*	*2003*	*2004*	*2005*	*1999*	*2000*	*2003*	*2004*	***2005***
Hispanic male	Number of inmates in thousands[1]					Inmates per 100,000 population[2]				
18–19	16	16	13	14	14	2,524	2,419	1,888	1,957	**2,072**
20–24	62	60	74	75	80	4,141	3,885	3,620	3,577	**3,878**
25–29	60	58	78	79	86	4,220	4,084	3,719	3,606	**3,884**
30–34	56	55	68	69	74	3,844	3,756	3,451	3,438	**3,640**
35–39	40	40	51	50	55	2,898	2,781	2,975	2,866	**3,111**
40–44	31	31	36	36	41	2,746	2,621	2,537	2,403	**2,649**
45–54	22	22	33	34	39	1,521	1,426	1,761	1,652	**1,873**
55 and over	7	8	9	9	11	460	468	501	473	**562**
White, not Hispanic female										
18–19	2	2	2	2	2	63	71	68	71	**76**
20–24	7	8	11	12	13	121	137	178	191	**206**
25–29	10	11	11	12	13	154	187	191	203	**220**
30–34	13	15	14	15	16	185	224	211	237	**255**
35–39	10	13	16	16	18	128	159	211	238	**260**
40–44	6	7	12	13	14	73	87	143	162	**177**
45–54	5	6	9	10	11	33	39	58	63	**70**
55 and over	1	2	2	2	3	5	7	8	8	**9**
Black, not Hispanic female										
18–19	1	1	2	2	2	224	231	254	262	**257**
20–24	7	7	9	9	9	524	525	607	625	**611**
25–29	13	14	10	10	10	956	993	744	746	**720**
30–34	19	19	13	12	12	1,362	1,409	891	905	**855**
35–39	14	14	14	14	13	940	962	926	993	**957**
40–44	7	8	11	11	11	512	513	732	764	**751**
45–54	4	5	8	8	8	214	209	318	327	**323**
55 and over	1	1	1	1	1	27	28	28	29	**26**
Hispanic female										
18–19	1	1	1	1	1	94	87	166	162	**168**
20–24	4	4	5	5	5	284	246	295	304	**317**
25–29	5	4	5	5	5	357	296	268	268	**287**
30–34	5	4	5	5	5	372	301	319	313	**312**
35–39	4	3	5	5	5	308	247	333	331	**322**
40–44	2	2	4	4	4	203	168	276	271	**264**
45–54	2	2	3	3	3	133	106	149	136	**138**
55 and over	0	0	1	1	1	11	9	29	25	**26**

- - - Data not available.
0 is greater than 0 but less than 500.
[1]Estimates as of June 30 of year shown.
[2]Inmate estimates as of June 30 of year shown. For data prior to 2005, population is U.S. resident population for July 1 of year shown. For 2005 data, population is U.S. resident population for January 1, 2005.
[3]Includes all other races not shown separately. See Appendix II, Hispanic origin; Race.
[4]Includes all other ages not shown separately. A small number of inmates are under age 18.

NOTES: Data are for inmates in custody. See Appendix I, The Annual Survey and Census of Jails; National Prisoner Statistics. Starting with 2004 data, inmates reporting more than one race are excluded. Some estimates of the total number of inmates have been revised and differ from previous editions of *Health, United States*. Because of revisions, some categories may not sum to the total. Data for additional years are available. See Appendix III.

SOURCES: Harrison PM, Beck AJ. Prison and jail inmates at midyear 2005. Bureau of Justice Statistics Bulletin. Washington, DC: U.S. Department of Justice, 2006. Reports for earlier years are available from: www.ojp.usdoj.gov/bjs/prisons.htm.

Table 3 (page 1 of 2). Persons and families below poverty level, by selected characteristics, race, and Hispanic origin: United States, selected years 1973–2005

[Data are based on household interviews of the civilian noninstitutionalized population]

Selected characteristics, race, and Hispanic origin[1]	1973	1980	1985	1990	1995	2000[2]	2003	2004[3]	2005
All persons					Percent below poverty				
All races	11.1	13.0	14.0	13.5	13.8	11.3	12.5	12.7	12.6
White only	8.4	10.2	11.4	10.7	11.2	9.5	10.5	10.8	10.6
Black or African American only	31.4	32.5	31.3	31.9	29.3	22.5	24.4	24.7	24.9
Asian only	- - -	- - -	- - -	12.2	14.6	9.9	11.8	9.8	11.1
Hispanic or Latino	21.9	25.7	29.0	28.1	30.3	21.5	22.5	21.9	21.8
Mexican	- - -	- - -	28.8	28.1	31.2	22.9	- - -	- - -	- - -
Puerto Rican	- - -	- - -	43.3	40.6	38.1	25.6	- - -	- - -	- - -
White only, not Hispanic or Latino	7.5	9.1	9.7	8.8	8.5	7.4	8.2	8.7	8.3
Related children under 18 years of age in families									
All races	14.2	17.9	20.1	19.9	20.2	15.6	17.2	17.3	17.1
White only	9.7	13.4	15.6	15.1	15.5	12.4	13.9	14.3	13.9
Black or African American only	40.6	42.1	43.1	44.2	41.5	30.9	33.6	33.4	34.2
Asian only	- - -	- - -	- - -	17.0	18.6	12.5	12.1	9.4	11.0
Hispanic or Latino	27.8	33.0	39.6	37.7	39.3	27.6	29.5	28.6	27.7
Mexican	- - -	- - -	37.4	35.5	39.3	29.5	- - -	- - -	- - -
Puerto Rican	- - -	- - -	58.6	56.7	53.2	32.1	- - -	- - -	- - -
White only, not Hispanic or Latino	- - -	11.3	12.3	11.6	10.6	8.5	9.3	9.9	9.5
Related children under 18 years of age in families with female householder and no spouse present									
All races	- - -	50.8	53.6	53.4	50.3	40.1	41.8	41.9	42.8
White only	- - -	41.6	45.2	45.9	42.5	33.9	37.0	38.2	38.8
Black or African American only	- - -	64.8	66.9	64.7	61.6	49.3	49.8	49.2	50.2
Asian only	- - -	- - -	- - -	32.2	42.4	38.0	37.4	18.7	25.6
Hispanic or Latino	- - -	65.0	72.4	68.4	65.7	49.8	50.6	51.9	50.2
Mexican	- - -	- - -	64.4	62.4	65.9	51.4	- - -	- - -	- - -
Puerto Rican	- - -	- - -	85.4	82.7	79.6	55.3	- - -	- - -	- - -
White only, not Hispanic or Latino	- - -	- - -	- - -	39.6	33.5	28.0	30.7	31.5	33.1
All persons					Number below poverty in thousands				
All races	22,973	29,272	33,064	33,585	36,425	31,581	35,861	37,040	36,950
White only	15,142	19,699	22,860	22,326	24,423	21,645	24,272	25,327	24,872
Black or African American only	7,388	8,579	8,926	9,837	9,872	7,982	8,781	9,014	9,168
Asian only	- - -	- - -	- - -	858	1,411	1,258	1,401	1,201	1,402
Hispanic or Latino	2,366	3,491	5,236	6,006	8,574	7,747	9,051	9,122	9,368
Mexican	- - -	- - -	3,220	3,764	5,608	5,460	- - -	- - -	- - -
Puerto Rican	- - -	- - -	1,011	966	1,183	814	- - -	- - -	- - -
White only, not Hispanic or Latino	12,864	16,365	17,839	16,622	16,267	14,366	15,902	16,908	16,227
Related children under 18 years of age in families									
All races	9,453	11,114	12,483	12,715	13,999	11,005	12,340	12,473	12,335
White only	5,462	6,817	7,838	7,696	8,474	6,834	7,624	7,876	7,652
Black or African American only	3,822	3,906	4,057	4,412	4,644	3,495	3,750	3,702	3,743
Asian only	- - -	- - -	- - -	356	532	407	331	265	312
Hispanic or Latino	1,364	1,718	2,512	2,750	3,938	3,342	3,982	3,985	3,977
Mexican	- - -	- - -	1,589	1,733	2,655	2,537	- - -	- - -	- - -
Puerto Rican	- - -	- - -	535	490	610	329	- - -	- - -	- - -
White only, not Hispanic or Latino	- - -	5,174	5,421	5,106	4,745	3,715	3,957	4,190	3,973

See footnotes at end of table.

Table 3 (page 2 of 2). Persons and families below poverty level, by selected characteristics, race, and Hispanic origin: United States, selected years 1973–2005

[Data are based on household interviews of the civilian noninstitutionalized population]

Selected characteristics, race, and Hispanic origin[1]	*1973*	*1980*	*1985*	*1990*	*1995*	*2000*[2]	*2003*	*2004*[3]	*2005*
Related children under 18 years of age in families with female householder and no spouse present				Number below poverty in thousands					
All races	- - -	5,866	6,716	7,363	8,364	6,300	7,085	7,152	7,210
White only	- - -	2,813	3,372	3,597	4,051	3,090	3,580	3,782	3,747
Black or African American only	- - -	2,944	3,181	3,543	3,954	2,908	3,026	2,963	2,993
Asian only	- - -	- - -	- - -	80	145	162	119	55	68
Hispanic or Latino	- - -	809	1,247	1,314	1,872	1,407	1,727	1,840	1,774
Mexican	- - -	- - -	553	615	1,056	938	- - -	- - -	- - -
Puerto Rican	- - -	- - -	449	382	459	242	- - -	- - -	- - -
White only, not Hispanic or Latino	- - -	- - -	- - -	2,411	2,299	1,832	2,033	2,114	2,158

- - - Data not available.

[1]The race groups, white, black, and Asian, include persons of Hispanic and non-Hispanic origin. Persons of Hispanic origin may be of any race. Starting with 2002 data, race-specific estimates are tabulated according to the 1997 Revisions to the Standards for the Classification of Federal Data on Race and Ethnicity and are not strictly comparable with estimates for earlier years. The three single-race categories shown in the table conform to the 1997 Standards. For 2002 and later years, race-specific estimates are for persons who reported only one racial group. Prior to data year 2002, data were tabulated according to the 1977 Standards in which the Asian only category included Native Hawaiian and Other Pacific Islander. Estimates for single-race categories prior to 2002 are based on answers to the Current Population Survey questionnaire which asked respondents to choose only a single race. See Appendix II, Hispanic origin; Race.

[2]Estimates are consistent with 2001 data through implementation of the 2000 census-based population controls and a 28,000 household sample expansion.

[3]The 2004 data have been revised to reflect a correction to the weights in the 2005 Annual Social and Economic Supplements (ASEC).

NOTES: Estimates of poverty for 1991–1998 are based on 1990 postcensal population estimates. Estimates for 1999 and later years are based on 2000 census population controls. Poverty level is based on family income and family size using U.S. Census Bureau poverty thresholds. See Appendix II, Poverty. The Current Population Survey is not large enough to produce reliable annual estimates for American Indian or Alaska Native persons, or for Native Hawaiians. The 2003–2005 average poverty rate for American Indian or Alaska Natives only was 25.3%, representing 573,000 persons. Data for additional years are available. See Appendix III.

SOURCES: U.S. Census Bureau, Current Population Survey 2000–2006 Annual Social and Economic Supplements; DeNavas-Walt C, Proctor BD, Lee CH. Income, poverty, and health insurance coverage in the United States: 2005. Current population reports, series P–60, no 231. Washington, DC: U.S. Government Printing Office. 2006.

Table 4 (page 1 of 3). Crude birth rates, fertility rates, and birth rates by age, race, and Hispanic origin of mother: United States, selected years 1950–2004

[Data are based on birth certificates]

			Age of mother									
				15–19 years								
Race, Hispanic origin, and year	*Crude birth rate* [1]	*Fertility rate* [2]	*10–14 years*	*Total*	*15–17 years*	*18–19 years*	*20–24 years*	*25–29 years*	*30–34 years*	*35–39 years*	*40–44 years*	*45–54 years* [3]
All races			Live births per 1,000 women									
1950	24.1	106.2	1.0	81.6	40.7	132.7	196.6	166.1	103.7	52.9	15.1	1.2
1960	23.7	118.0	0.8	89.1	43.9	166.7	258.1	197.4	112.7	56.2	15.5	0.9
1970	18.4	87.9	1.2	68.3	38.8	114.7	167.8	145.1	73.3	31.7	8.1	0.5
1980	15.9	68.4	1.1	53.0	32.5	82.1	115.1	112.9	61.9	19.8	3.9	0.2
1985	15.8	66.3	1.2	51.0	31.0	79.6	108.3	111.0	69.1	24.0	4.0	0.2
1990	16.7	70.9	1.4	59.9	37.5	88.6	116.5	120.2	80.8	31.7	5.5	0.2
1995	14.6	64.6	1.3	56.0	35.5	87.7	107.5	108.8	81.1	34.0	6.6	0.3
2000	14.4	65.9	0.9	47.7	26.9	78.1	109.7	113.5	91.2	39.7	8.0	0.5
2002	13.9	64.8	0.7	43.0	23.2	72.8	103.6	113.6	91.5	41.4	8.3	0.5
2003	14.1	66.1	0.6	41.6	22.4	70.7	102.6	115.6	95.1	43.8	8.7	0.5
2004	14.0	66.3	0.7	41.1	22.1	70.0	101.7	115.5	95.3	45.4	8.9	0.5
Race of child: [4] White												
1950	23.0	102.3	0.4	70.0	31.3	120.5	190.4	165.1	102.6	51.4	14.5	1.0
1960	22.7	113.2	0.4	79.4	35.5	154.6	252.8	194.9	109.6	54.0	14.7	0.8
1970	17.4	84.1	0.5	57.4	29.2	101.5	163.4	145.9	71.9	30.0	7.5	0.4
1980	14.9	64.7	0.6	44.7	25.2	72.1	109.5	112.4	60.4	18.5	3.4	0.2
Race of mother: [5] White												
1980	15.1	65.6	0.6	45.4	25.5	73.2	111.1	113.8	61.2	18.8	3.5	0.2
1985	15.0	64.1	0.6	43.3	24.4	70.4	104.1	112.3	69.9	23.3	3.7	0.2
1990	15.8	68.3	0.7	50.8	29.5	78.0	109.8	120.7	81.7	31.5	5.2	0.2
1995	14.1	63.6	0.8	49.5	29.6	80.2	104.7	111.7	83.3	34.2	6.4	0.3
2000	13.9	65.3	0.6	43.2	23.3	72.3	106.6	116.7	94.6	40.2	7.9	0.4
2002	13.5	64.8	0.5	39.4	20.5	68.0	101.6	117.4	95.5	42.4	8.2	0.5
2003	13.6	66.1	0.5	38.3	19.8	66.2	100.6	119.5	99.3	44.8	8.7	0.5
2004	13.5	66.1	0.5	37.7	19.5	65.0	99.2	118.6	99.1	46.4	8.9	0.5
Race of child: [4] Black or African American												
1960	31.9	153.5	4.3	156.1	---	---	295.4	218.6	137.1	73.9	21.9	1.1
1970	25.3	115.4	5.2	140.7	101.4	204.9	202.7	136.3	79.6	41.9	12.5	1.0
1980	22.1	88.1	4.3	100.0	73.6	138.8	146.3	109.1	62.9	24.5	5.8	0.3
Race of mother: [5] Black or African American												
1980	21.3	84.9	4.3	97.8	72.5	135.1	140.0	103.9	59.9	23.5	5.6	0.3
1985	20.4	78.8	4.5	95.4	69.3	132.4	135.0	100.2	57.9	23.9	4.6	0.3
1990	22.4	86.8	4.9	112.8	82.3	152.9	160.2	115.5	68.7	28.1	5.5	0.3
1995	17.8	71.0	4.1	94.4	68.5	135.0	133.7	95.6	63.0	28.4	6.0	0.3
2000	17.0	70.0	2.3	77.4	49.0	118.8	141.3	100.3	65.4	31.5	7.2	0.4
2002	15.7	65.8	1.8	66.6	40.0	107.6	127.1	99.0	64.4	31.5	7.4	0.4
2003	15.7	66.3	1.6	63.8	38.2	103.7	126.1	100.4	66.5	33.2	7.7	0.5
2004	16.0	67.6	1.6	63.3	37.2	104.4	127.7	103.6	67.9	34.0	7.9	0.5
American Indian or Alaska Native mothers [5]												
1980	20.7	82.7	1.9	82.2	51.5	129.5	143.7	106.6	61.8	28.1	8.2	*
1985	19.8	78.6	1.7	79.2	47.7	124.1	139.1	109.6	62.6	27.4	6.0	*
1990	18.9	76.2	1.6	81.1	48.5	129.3	148.7	110.3	61.5	27.5	5.9	*
1995	15.3	63.0	1.6	72.9	44.6	122.2	123.1	91.6	56.5	24.3	5.5	*
2000	14.0	58.7	1.1	58.3	34.1	97.1	117.2	91.8	55.5	24.6	5.7	0.3
2002	13.8	58.0	0.9	53.8	30.7	89.2	112.6	91.8	56.4	25.4	5.8	0.3
2003	13.8	58.4	1.0	53.1	30.6	87.3	110.0	93.5	57.4	25.4	5.5	0.4
2004	14.0	58.9	0.9	52.5	30.0	87.0	109.7	92.8	58.0	26.8	6.0	0.2

See footnotes at end of table.

This table will be updated on the Web. Go to www.cdc.gov/nchs/hus.htm.

Table 4 (page 2 of 3). Crude birth rates, fertility rates, and birth rates by age, race, and Hispanic origin of mother: United States, selected years 1950–2004

[Data are based on birth certificates]

Race, Hispanic origin, and year	Crude birth rate[1]	Fertility rate[2]	Age of mother: 10–14 years	15–19 years: Total	15–19 years: 15–17 years	15–19 years: 18–19 years	20–24 years	25–29 years	30–34 years	35–39 years	40–44 years	45–54 years[3]
			Live births per 1,000 women									
Asian or Pacific Islander mothers[5]												
1980	19.9	73.2	0.3	26.2	12.0	46.2	93.3	127.4	96.0	38.3	8.5	0.7
1985	18.7	68.4	0.4	23.8	12.5	40.8	83.6	123.0	93.6	42.7	8.7	1.2
1990	19.0	69.6	0.7	26.4	16.0	40.2	79.2	126.3	106.5	49.6	10.7	1.1
1995	16.7	62.6	0.7	25.5	15.6	40.1	64.2	103.7	102.3	50.1	11.8	0.8
2000	17.1	65.8	0.3	20.5	11.6	32.6	60.3	108.4	116.5	59.0	12.6	0.8
2002	16.5	64.1	0.3	18.3	9.0	31.5	60.4	105.4	109.6	56.5	12.5	0.9
2003	16.8	66.3	0.2	17.4	8.8	29.8	59.6	108.5	114.6	59.9	13.5	0.9
2004	16.8	67.1	0.2	17.3	8.9	29.6	59.8	108.6	116.9	62.1	13.6	1.0
Hispanic or Latino mothers[5,6]												
1980	23.5	95.4	1.7	82.2	52.1	126.9	156.4	132.1	83.2	39.9	10.6	0.7
1990	26.7	107.7	2.4	100.3	65.9	147.7	181.0	153.0	98.3	45.3	10.9	0.7
1995	24.1	98.8	2.6	99.3	68.3	145.4	171.9	140.4	90.5	43.7	10.7	0.6
2000	23.1	95.9	1.7	87.3	55.5	132.6	161.3	139.9	97.1	46.6	11.5	0.6
2002	22.6	94.4	1.4	83.4	50.7	133.0	164.3	139.4	95.1	47.8	11.5	0.7
2003	22.9	96.9	1.3	82.3	49.7	132.0	163.4	144.4	102.0	50.8	12.2	0.7
2004	22.9	97.8	1.3	82.6	49.7	133.5	165.3	145.6	104.1	52.9	12.4	0.7
White, not Hispanic or Latino mothers[5,6]												
1980	14.2	62.4	0.4	41.2	22.4	67.7	105.5	110.6	59.9	17.7	3.0	0.1
1990	14.4	62.8	0.5	42.5	23.2	66.6	97.5	115.3	79.4	30.0	4.7	0.2
1995	12.5	57.5	0.4	39.3	22.0	66.2	90.2	105.1	81.5	32.8	5.9	0.3
2000	12.2	58.5	0.3	32.6	15.8	57.5	91.2	109.4	93.2	38.8	7.3	0.4
2002	11.7	57.4	0.2	28.5	13.1	51.9	84.3	109.3	94.4	40.9	7.6	0.5
2003	11.8	58.5	0.2	27.4	12.4	50.0	83.5	110.8	97.6	43.2	8.1	0.5
2004	11.6	58.4	0.2	26.7	12.0	48.7	81.9	110.0	97.1	44.8	8.2	0.5
Black or African American, not Hispanic or Latino mothers[5,6]												
1980	22.9	90.7	4.6	105.1	77.2	146.5	152.2	111.7	65.2	25.8	5.8	0.3
1990	23.0	89.0	5.0	116.2	84.9	157.5	165.1	118.4	70.2	28.7	5.6	0.3
1995	18.2	72.8	4.2	97.2	70.4	139.2	137.8	98.5	64.4	28.8	6.1	0.3
2000	17.3	71.4	2.4	79.2	50.1	121.9	145.4	102.8	66.5	31.8	7.2	0.4
2002	16.1	67.4	1.9	68.3	41.0	110.3	131.0	102.1	66.1	32.1	7.5	0.4
2003	15.9	67.1	1.6	64.7	38.7	105.3	128.1	102.1	67.4	33.4	7.7	0.5
2004	15.8	67.0	1.6	63.1	37.1	103.9	126.9	103.0	67.4	33.7	7.8	0.5

See footnotes at end of table.

This table will be updated on the Web. Go to www.cdc.gov/nchs/hus.htm.

Table 4 (page 3 of 3). Crude birth rates, fertility rates, and birth rates by age, race, and Hispanic origin of mother: United States, selected years 1950–2004

[Data are based on birth certificates]

- - - Data not available.
* Rates based on fewer than 20 births are considered unreliable and are not shown.
[1]Live births per 1,000 population.
[2]Total number of live births regardless of age of mother per 1,000 women 15–44 years of age.
[3]Prior to 1997, data are for live births to mothers 45–49 years of age per 1,000 women 45–49 years of age. Starting with 1997 data, rates are for live births to mothers 45–54 years of age per 1,000 women 45–49 years of age. See Appendix II, Age.
[4]Live births are tabulated by race of child. See Appendix II, Race, Birth File.
[5]Live births are tabulated by race and/or Hispanic origin of mother. See Appendix II, Race, Birth File.
[6]Prior to 1993, data from states lacking an Hispanic-origin item on the birth certificate were excluded. See Appendix II, Hispanic origin. Rates in 1985 were not calculated because estimates for the Hispanic and non-Hispanic populations were not available.

NOTES: Data are based on births adjusted for underregistration for 1950 and on registered births for all other years. Starting with 1970 data, births to persons who were not residents of the 50 states and the District of Columbia are excluded. Starting with *Health, United States, 2003,* rates for 1991–1999 were revised using intercensal population estimates based on the 2000 census. Rates for 2000 were computed using the 2000 census counts and starting in 2001 rates were computed using 2000-based postcensal estimates. See Appendix I, Population Census and Population Estimates. The race groups, white, black, American Indian or Alaska Native, and Asian or Pacific Islander, include persons of Hispanic and non-Hispanic origin. Persons of Hispanic origin may be of any race. Starting with 2003 data, some states reported multiple-race data. The multiple-race data for these states were bridged to the single-race categories of the 1977 Office of Management and Budget standards for comparability with other states. See Appendix II, Race. Interpretation of trend data should take into consideration expansion of reporting areas and immigration. Data for additional years are available. See Appendix III.

SOURCES: Centers for Disease Control and Prevention, National Center for Health Statistics, National Vital Statistics System, Birth File. Martin JA, Hamilton BE, Sutton PD, Ventura SJ, Menacker F, Kirmeyer S. Births: Final Data for 2004. National vital statistics reports. vol 55 no 1. Hyattsville, MD: National Center for Health Statistics. 2006; Hamilton BE, Sutton PD, Ventura SJ. Revised birth and fertility rates for the 1990s and new rates for Hispanic populations, 2000 and 2001: United States. National vital statistics reports. vol 51 no 12. Hyattsville, MD: National Center for Health Statistics. 2003; Ventura SJ. Births of Hispanic parentage, 1980 and 1985. Monthly vital statistics report. vol 32 no 6 and vol 36 no 11, suppl. Public Health Service. Hyattsville, MD. 1983 and 1988; Internet release of *Vital statistics of the United States, 2000, vol 1, natality*, tables 1–1 and 1–7 available from: www.cdc.gov/nchs/datawh/statab/unpubd/natality/natab2000.htm.

This table will be updated on the Web. Go to www.cdc.gov/nchs/hus.htm.

Table 5 (page 1 of 2). Live births, by plurality, and detailed race and Hispanic origin of mother: United States, selected years 1970–2004

[Data are based on birth certificates]

Plurality of birth and race and Hispanic origin of mother	*1970*	*1971*	*1975*	*1980*	*1985*	*1990*	*1995*	*2000*	*2003*	*2004*
All births					Number of live births					
All races	3,731,386	3,555,970	3,144,198	3,612,258	3,760,561	4,158,212	3,899,589	4,058,814	4,089,950	4,112,052
White	3,109,956	2,939,568	2,576,818	2,936,351	3,037,913	3,290,273	3,098,885	3,194,005	3,225,848	3,222,928
Black or African American	561,992	553,750	496,829	568,080	581,824	684,336	603,139	622,598	599,847	616,074
American Indian or Alaska Native	22,264	23,254	22,690	29,389	34,037	39,051	37,278	41,668	43,052	43,927
Asian or Pacific Islander[1]	- - -	27,004	28,884	74,355	104,606	141,635	160,287	200,543	221,203	229,123
Chinese	7,044	7,222	7,778	11,671	16,405	22,737	27,380	34,271	- - -	- - -
Japanese	7,744	7,846	6,725	7,482	8,035	8,674	8,901	8,969	- - -	- - -
Filipino	8,066	7,946	10,359	13,968	20,058	25,770	30,551	32,107	- - -	- - -
Hawaiian	- - -	3,718	3,711	4,669	4,938	6,099	5,787	6,608	- - -	- - -
Other Asian or Pacific Islander	- - -	272	311	36,565	55,170	78,355	87,668	118,588	- - -	- - -
Hispanic or Latino[2]	- - -	- - -	- - -	307,163	372,814	595,073	679,768	815,868	912,329	946,349
Mexican	- - -	- - -	- - -	215,439	242,976	385,640	469,615	581,915	654,504	677,621
Puerto Rican	- - -	- - -	- - -	33,671	35,147	58,807	54,824	58,124	58,400	61,221
Cuban	- - -	- - -	- - -	7,163	10,024	11,311	12,473	13,429	14,867	14,943
Central and South American	- - -	- - -	- - -	21,268	40,985	83,008	94,996	113,344	135,586	143,520
Other and unknown Hispanic or Latino	- - -	- - -	- - -	29,622	43,682	56,307	47,860	49,056	48,972	49,044
Not Hispanic or Latino:[2]										
White	- - -	- - -	- - -	1,256,777	1,407,460	2,626,500	2,382,638	2,362,968	2,321,904	2,296,683
Black or African American	- - -	- - -	- - -	300,480	337,448	661,701	587,781	604,346	576,033	578,772
Twin births										
All races	- - -	63,298	59,192	68,339	77,102	93,865	96,736	118,916	128,665	132,219
White	- - -	49,972	46,715	53,104	60,351	72,617	76,196	93,235	101,297	103,438
Black or African American	- - -	12,452	11,375	13,638	14,646	18,164	17,000	20,626	20,633	21,618
American Indian or Alaska Native	- - -	362	348	491	537	699	769	900	1,047	1,086
Asian or Pacific Islander[1]	- - -	320	505	1,045	1,536	2,320	2,771	4,155	5,688	6,077
Chinese	- - -	80	120	135	232	368	507	748	- - -	- - -
Japanese	- - -	98	115	103	131	161	217	218	- - -	- - -
Filipino	- - -	92	176	173	247	388	542	612	- - -	- - -
Hawaiian	- - -	46	92	69	74	101	98	109	- - -	- - -
Other Asian or Pacific Islander	- - -	4	2	565	852	1,302	1,407	2,468	- - -	- - -
Hispanic or Latino[2]	- - -	- - -	- - -	5,154	6,550	10,713	12,685	16,470	19,472	20,351
Mexican	- - -	- - -	- - -	3,599	4,292	6,701	8,341	11,130	12,954	13,485
Puerto Rican	- - -	- - -	- - -	631	705	1,226	1,248	1,461	1,666	1,759
Cuban	- - -	- - -	- - -	102	201	228	312	371	465	562
Central and South American	- - -	- - -	- - -	371	665	1,463	1,769	2,361	3,141	3,393
Other and unknown Hispanic or Latino	- - -	- - -	- - -	451	687	1,095	1,015	1,147	1,246	1,152
Not Hispanic or Latino:[2]										
White	- - -	- - -	- - -	23,004	28,402	60,210	62,370	76,018	81,691	83,346
Black or African American	- - -	- - -	- - -	7,278	8,400	17,646	16,622	20,173	20,010	20,605
Triplet and higher order multiple births										
All races	- - -	1,034	1,066	1,337	1,925	3,028	4,973	7,325	7,663	7,275
White	- - -	834	909	1,104	1,648	2,639	4,505	6,551	6,733	6,326
Black or African American	- - -	196	151	211	240	321	352	521	650	605
American Indian or Alaska Native	- - -	0	2	9	13	4	20	18	33	22
Asian or Pacific Islander[1]	- - -	0	4	9	23	61	96	235	247	322
Chinese	- - -	0	0	3	2	13	21	29	- - -	- - -
Japanese	- - -	0	4	6	0	0	3	8	- - -	- - -
Filipino	- - -	0	0	0	4	15	15	57	- - -	- - -
Hawaiian	- - -	0	0	0	0	3	3	6	- - -	- - -
Other Asian or Pacific Islander	- - -	0	0	0	17	30	54	135	- - -	- - -
Hispanic or Latino[2]	- - -	- - -	- - -	78	106	235	355	659	784	723
Mexican	- - -	- - -	- - -	43	82	121	202	391	480	483
Puerto Rican	- - -	- - -	- - -	12	14	28	35	73	88	103
Cuban	- - -	- - -	- - -	0	3	9	24	15	28	*
Central and South American	- - -	- - -	- - -	8	4	59	59	122	140	95
Other and unknown Hispanic or Latino	- - -	- - -	- - -	15	3	18	35	58	48	24
Not Hispanic or Latino:[2]										
White	- - -	- - -	- - -	490	779	2,358	4,050	5,821	5,922	5,590
Black or African American	- - -	- - -	- - -	128	132	306	340	506	631	577

See footnotes at end of table.

This table will be updated on the Web. Go to www.cdc.gov/nchs/hus.htm.

Table 5 (page 2 of 2). Live births, by plurality, and detailed race and Hispanic origin of mother: United States, selected years 1970–2004

[Data are based on birth certificates]

- - - Data not available.

[1]Starting with 2003 data, estimates are not shown for Asian or Pacific Islander subgroups during the transition from single race to multiple race reporting. See Appendix II, Race, Birth File.

[2]Prior to 1993, data from states lacking an Hispanic-origin item on the birth certificate were excluded. See Appendix II, Hispanic origin. Data for non-Hispanic white and non-Hispanic black women for years prior to 1989 are not nationally representative and are provided for comparison with Hispanic data.

NOTES: The race groups, white, black, American Indian or Alaska Native, and Asian or Pacific Islander, include persons of Hispanic and non-Hispanic origin. Persons of Hispanic origin may be of any race. Starting with 2003 data, some states reported multiple-race data. The multiple-race data for these states were bridged to the single-race categories of the 1977 Office of Management and Budget standards for comparability with other states. See Appendix II, Race. Interpretation of trend data should take into consideration expansion of reporting areas and immigration. Data for additional years are available. See Appendix III.

SOURCES: Centers for Disease Control and Prevention, National Center for Health Statistics, National Vital Statistics System, Birth File. Martin JA, Hamilton BE, Sutton PD, Ventura SJ, Menacker F, Kirmeyer S. Births: Final Data for 2004. National vital statistics reports. vol 55 no 1. Hyattsville, MD: National Center for Health Statistics. 2006; Births: Final data for each data year 1997–2003. National vital statistics reports. Hyattsville, MD; Final natality statistics for each data year 1970–1996. Monthly vital statistics report. Hyattsville, MD.

This table will be updated on the Web. Go to www.cdc.gov/nchs/hus.htm.

Table 6. Twin and higher order multiple births, by race, Hispanic origin, and age of mother: United States, selected years 1971–2004

[Data are based on birth certificates]

Plurality of birth and race, Hispanic origin, and age of mother	*1971*	*1975*	*1980*	*1985*	*1990*	*1995*	*1997*	*2000*	*2002*	*2003*	*2004*
Twin births	Number per 1,000 live births										
All races	17.8	18.8	18.9	20.5	22.6	24.8	26.8	29.3	31.1	31.5	32.2
White	17.0	18.1	18.1	19.9	22.1	24.6	26.7	29.2	31.0	31.4	32.1
Black or African American	22.5	22.9	24.0	25.2	26.5	28.2	30.0	33.1	34.4	34.4	35.1
American Indian or Alaska Native	15.6	15.3	16.7	15.8	17.9	20.6	20.6	21.6	23.2	24.3	24.7
Asian or Pacific Islander[1]	11.9	17.5	14.1	14.7	16.4	17.3	19.2	20.7	25.7	25.7	26.5
Chinese	11.1	15.4	11.6	14.1	16.2	18.5	19.8	21.8	27.6	---	---
Japanese	12.5	17.1	13.8	16.3	18.6	24.4	22.7	24.3	34.2	---	---
Filipino	11.6	17.0	12.4	12.3	15.1	17.7	17.5	19.1	22.9	---	---
Hawaiian	*12.4	24.8	14.8	15.0	16.6	16.9	16.7	16.5	23.2	---	---
Other Asian or Pacific Islander	*	*	15.5	15.4	16.6	16.0	19.4	20.8	25.5	---	---
Hispanic or Latino[2]	---	---	16.8	17.6	18.0	18.7	19.5	20.2	20.7	21.3	21.5
Mexican	---	---	16.7	17.7	17.4	17.8	18.5	19.1	19.2	19.8	19.9
Puerto Rican	---	---	18.7	20.1	20.8	22.8	23.0	25.1	28.8	28.5	28.7
Cuban	---	---	14.2	20.1	20.2	25.0	28.6	27.6	28.7	31.3	37.6
Central and South American	---	---	17.4	16.2	17.6	18.6	20.6	20.8	22.1	23.2	23.6
Other and unknown Hispanic or Latino	---	---	15.2	15.7	19.4	21.2	21.1	23.4	23.8	25.4	23.5
Not Hispanic or Latino:[2]											
White	---	---	18.3	20.2	22.9	26.2	28.8	32.2	34.8	35.2	36.3
Black or African American	---	---	24.2	24.9	26.7	28.3	30.0	33.4	34.7	34.7	35.6
Age of mother:											
Under 20 years	11.6	12.7	12.8	13.0	14.3	14.2	15.0	15.8	15.8	15.3	15.7
20–24 years	16.2	17.6	17.4	18.3	19.2	19.9	20.4	22.0	22.4	22.4	22.8
25–29 years	19.8	20.9	20.5	21.6	23.5	24.8	26.3	28.2	29.0	29.6	30.2
30–34 years	23.7	24.5	23.5	25.5	27.6	30.6	33.7	36.5	38.9	39.2	40.1
35–39 years	27.3	25.8	25.3	26.3	30.2	35.7	39.3	43.5	47.7	47.8	48.5
40–44 years	22.3	23.3	23.0	20.5	24.7	32.3	38.6	45.2	52.5	51.3	53.7
45–49 years	*18.1	*	*	*18.9	*23.8	101.9	133.2	153.1	189.7	189.2	195.4
50–54 years	---	---	---	---	---	---	347.2	313.7	384.0	374.6	379.7
Triplet and higher order multiple births	Number per 100,000 live births										
All races	29.1	33.9	37.0	51.2	72.8	127.5	173.6	180.5	184.0	187.4	176.9
White	28.4	35.3	37.6	54.2	80.2	145.4	195.9	205.1	206.0	208.7	196.3
Black or African American	35.4	30.4	37.1	41.2	46.9	58.4	88.3	83.7	102.6	108.4	*98.2
American Indian or Alaska Native	*	*	*	*	*	*53.7	*	*	*54.3	*76.7	*50.1
Asian or Pacific Islander	*	*	*	*22.0	43.1	59.9	103.1	117.2	108.1	111.7	140.5
Hispanic or Latino[2]	---	---	25.4	28.4	39.5	52.2	72.7	80.8	84.1	85.9	76.4
Not Hispanic or Latino:[2]											
White	---	---	39.0	55.3	89.8	170.0	230.8	246.3	250.4	255.0	243.4
Black or African American	---	---	42.6	39.1	46.2	57.8	90.0	83.7	102.2	109.5	99.7
Age of mother:											
Under 20 years	9.1	10.9	14.8	13.8	15.9	17.6	20.7	23.2	21.5	12.8	20.6
20–24 years	25.4	28.1	31.4	35.0	32.4	35.3	46.8	44.2	50.0	48.4	41.7
25–29 years	43.7	45.4	42.8	66.3	73.9	118.3	151.0	163.3	153.5	158.9	158.7
30–34 years	36.4	53.5	58.3	71.2	126.3	217.2	293.6	307.3	297.7	309.1	285.0
35–39 years	35.7	45.1	47.6	70.0	156.8	285.3	403.2	368.5	406.0	409.5	375.3
40–44 years	*	*	*	*	*57.6	273.6	315.4	415.5	393.6	330.7	364.6
45–49 years	*	*	*	*	*	*1,466.8	2,100.2	1,586.6	2,010.0	1,919.6	1,235.2
50–54 years	---	---	---	---	---	---	*	*9,019.6	*	*	*

- - - Data not available.

* Rates preceded by an asterisk are based on fewer than 50 births. Rates based on fewer than 20 births are considered unreliable and are not shown.

[1]Starting with 2003 data, estimates are not shown for Asian or Pacific Islander subgroups during the transition from single race to multiple race reporting. See Appendix II, Race, Birth File.

[2]Prior to 1993, data from states lacking an Hispanic-origin item on the birth certificate were excluded. See Appendix II, Hispanic origin. Data for non-Hispanic white and non-Hispanic black women for years prior to 1989 are not nationally representative and are provided for comparison with Hispanic data.

NOTES: The race groups, white, black, American Indian or Alaska Native, and Asian or Pacific Islander, include persons of Hispanic and non-Hispanic origin. Persons of Hispanic origin may be of any race. Starting with 2003 data, some states reported multiple-race data. The multiple-race data for these states were bridged to the single-race categories of the 1977 Office of Management and Budget standards for comparability with other states. See Appendix II, Race. Interpretation of trend data should take into consideration expansion of reporting areas and immigration. Data for additional years are available. See Appendix III.

SOURCES: Centers for Disease Control and Prevention, National Center for Health Statistics, National Vital Statistics System, Birth File; Martin JA, Park MM. Trends in Twin and Triplet Births: 1980–97. National vital statistics reports. Vol 47 no 24. Hyattsville, MD: National Center for Health Statistics. 1999.

This table will be updated on the Web. Go to www.cdc.gov/nchs/hus.htm.

Table 7. Prenatal care for live births, by detailed race and Hispanic origin of mother: United States, selected years 1970–2004

[Data are based on birth certificates]

Prenatal care, race, and Hispanic origin of mother	1970	1975	1980	1985	1990	1995	2000	2002	2003[1]	43 reporting areas: 2003[2]	43 reporting areas: 2004[1]
Prenatal care began during 1st trimester						Percent of live births[3]					
All races	68.0	72.4	76.3	76.2	75.8	81.3	83.2	83.7	84.1	84.0	83.9
White	72.3	75.8	79.2	79.3	79.2	83.6	85.0	85.4	85.7	85.5	85.4
Black or African American	44.2	55.5	62.4	61.5	60.6	70.4	74.3	75.2	75.9	76.1	76.4
American Indian or Alaska Native	38.2	45.4	55.8	57.5	57.9	66.7	69.3	69.8	70.8	70.6	69.9
Asian or Pacific Islander[4]	- - -	- - -	73.7	74.1	75.1	79.9	84.0	84.8	85.4	85.4	85.6
Chinese	71.8	76.7	82.6	82.0	81.3	85.7	87.6	87.2	- - -	- - -	- - -
Japanese	78.1	82.7	86.1	84.7	87.0	89.7	91.0	90.5	- - -	- - -	- - -
Filipino	60.6	70.6	77.3	76.5	77.1	80.9	84.9	85.4	- - -	- - -	- - -
Hawaiian	- - -	- - -	68.8	67.7	65.8	75.9	79.9	78.1	- - -	- - -	- - -
Other Asian or Pacific Islander	- - -	- - -	67.4	69.9	71.9	77.0	82.5	83.9	- - -	- - -	- - -
Hispanic or Latino[5]	- - -	- - -	60.2	61.2	60.2	70.8	74.4	76.7	77.5	77.3	77.5
Mexican	- - -	- - -	59.6	60.0	57.8	69.1	72.9	75.7	76.5	76.9	77.2
Puerto Rican	- - -	- - -	55.1	58.3	63.5	74.0	78.5	79.9	81.2	80.3	79.9
Cuban	- - -	- - -	82.7	82.5	84.8	89.2	91.7	92.0	92.1	86.5	86.6
Central and South American	- - -	- - -	58.8	60.6	61.5	73.2	77.6	78.7	79.2	78.1	77.6
Other and unknown Hispanic or Latino	- - -	- - -	66.4	65.8	66.4	74.3	75.8	76.7	77.0	77.5	78.1
Not Hispanic or Latino:[5]											
White	- - -	- - -	81.2	81.4	83.3	87.1	88.5	88.6	89.0	89.1	88.9
Black or African American	- - -	- - -	60.8	60.2	60.7	70.4	74.3	75.2	75.9	76.2	76.5
Prenatal care began during 3rd trimester or no prenatal care											
All races	7.9	6.0	5.1	5.7	6.1	4.2	3.9	3.6	3.5	3.6	3.6
White	6.3	5.0	4.3	4.8	4.9	3.5	3.3	3.1	3.0	3.1	3.2
Black or African American	16.6	10.5	8.9	10.2	11.3	7.6	6.7	6.2	6.0	5.9	5.7
American Indian or Alaska Native	28.9	22.4	15.2	12.9	12.9	9.5	8.6	8.0	7.6	7.7	7.9
Asian or Pacific Islander[4]	- - -	- - -	6.5	6.5	5.8	4.3	3.3	3.1	3.1	3.1	3.0
Chinese	6.5	4.4	3.7	4.4	3.4	3.0	2.2	2.1	- - -	- - -	- - -
Japanese	4.1	2.7	2.1	3.1	2.9	2.3	1.8	2.1	- - -	- - -	- - -
Filipino	7.2	4.1	4.0	4.8	4.5	4.1	3.0	2.8	- - -	- - -	- - -
Hawaiian	- - -	- - -	6.7	7.4	8.7	5.1	4.2	4.7	- - -	- - -	- - -
Other Asian or Pacific Islander	- - -	- - -	9.3	8.2	7.1	5.0	3.8	3.5	- - -	- - -	- - -
Hispanic or Latino[5]	- - -	- - -	12.0	12.4	12.0	7.4	6.3	5.5	5.3	5.3	5.4
Mexican	- - -	- - -	11.8	12.9	13.2	8.1	6.9	5.8	5.6	5.5	5.5
Puerto Rican	- - -	- - -	16.2	15.5	10.6	5.5	4.5	4.1	3.7	3.9	3.9
Cuban	- - -	- - -	3.9	3.7	2.8	2.1	1.4	1.3	1.3	2.9	2.9
Central and South American	- - -	- - -	13.1	12.5	10.9	6.1	5.4	4.9	4.7	4.9	5.1
Other and unknown Hispanic or Latino	- - -	- - -	9.2	9.4	8.5	6.0	5.9	5.3	5.4	5.6	5.5
Not Hispanic or Latino:[5]											
White	- - -	- - -	3.5	4.0	3.4	2.5	2.3	2.2	2.1	2.1	2.2
Black or African American	- - -	- - -	9.7	10.9	11.2	7.6	6.7	6.2	6.0	5.9	5.7

- - - Data not available.

[1]Reporting areas that have adopted the 2003 revision of the U.S. Standard Certificate of Live Birth are excluded because prenatal care data based on the 2003 revision are not comparable with data based on the 1989 and earlier revisions of the U.S. Standard Certificate of Live Birth. In 2003, Pennsylvania and Washington adopted the 2003 revision; in 2004, Florida, Idaho, Kentucky, New Hampshire, New York State (excluding New York City), South Carolina, and Tennessee adopted the 2003 Revision. See Appendix II, Prenatal care.

[2]Data for 2003 are limited to the 43 reporting areas using the 1989 revision of the U.S. Standard Certificate of Live Birth in 2004 and are provided for comparison with 2004.

[3]Excludes live births where trimester when prenatal care began is unknown.

[4]Starting with 2003 data, estimates are not shown for Asian or Pacific Islander subgroups during the transition from single race to multiple race reporting. See Appendix II, Race; Birth File.

[5]Prior to 1993, data from states lacking an Hispanic-origin item on the birth certificate were excluded. See Appendix II, Hispanic origin. Data for non-Hispanic white and non-Hispanic black women for years prior to 1989 are not nationally representative and are provided for comparison with Hispanic data.

NOTES: Data are based on the 1989 and earlier revisions of the U.S. Standard Certificate of Live Birth. Data for 1970 and 1975 exclude births that occurred in states not reporting prenatal care. The race groups, white, black, American Indian or Alaska Native, and Asian or Pacific Islander, include persons of Hispanic and non-Hispanic origin. Persons of Hispanic origin may be of any race. Starting with 2003 data, some states reported multiple-race data. The multiple-race data for these states were bridged to the single-race categories of the 1977 Office of Management and Budget standards for comparability with other states. See Appendix II, Race. Interpretation of trend data should take into consideration changes in reporting areas and immigration. Data for additional years are available. See Appendix III.

SOURCES: Centers for Disease Control and Prevention, National Center for Health Statistics, National Vital Statistics System, Birth File. Martin JA, Hamilton BE, Sutton PD, Ventura SJ, Menacker F, Kirmeyer S. Births: Final Data for 2004. National vital statistics reports. vol 55 no 1. Hyattsville, MD: National Center for Health Statistics. 2006; Births: Final data for each data year 1997–2003. National vital statistics reports. Hyattsville, MD; Final natality statistics for each data year 1970–1996. Monthly vital statistics report. Hyattsville, MD.

This table will be updated on the Web. Go to www.cdc.gov/nchs/hus.htm.

Table 8 (page 1 of 3). Early prenatal care by race and Hispanic origin of mother, geographic division, and state: United States, average annual 1996–1998, 1999–2001, and 2002–2004

[Data are based on birth certificates]

Geographic division and state	All races			Not Hispanic or Latino: White			Not Hispanic or Latino: Black or African American		
	1996–1998	1999–2001	2002–2004	1996–1998	1999–2001	2002–2004	1996–1998	1999–2001	2002–2004
	Percent of live births with early prenatal care (beginning in the 1st trimester)								
United States[1]	82.4	83.2	83.8	87.7	88.5	88.9	72.4	74.3	76.1
New England[1]	88.1	89.5	89.2	90.6	92.0	91.9	77.8	80.7	80.1
Connecticut	88.4	89.1	88.1	91.9	92.9	92.4	79.4	82.1	80.3
Maine	89.3	88.7	87.9	89.7	89.0	88.4	84.3	80.1	76.4
Massachusetts	87.4	89.5	89.8	90.4	92.4	92.4	76.3	79.3	80.0
New Hampshire[1]	89.5	90.8	- - -	89.9	91.6	- - -	77.2	75.7	- - -
Rhode Island	89.6	91.1	90.2	92.0	93.5	92.8	80.0	84.7	81.2
Vermont	87.6	88.5	89.8	87.8	88.8	90.2	*73.6	78.3	72.1
Middle Atlantic[1]	81.7	82.0	- - -	88.2	88.4	- - -	68.3	69.7	- - -
New Jersey	81.6	80.6	79.8	89.5	89.3	88.9	64.5	63.8	63.5
New York[1]	85.4	85.0	- - -	89.1	88.9	- - -	70.5	70.6	- - -
New York City	73.5	75.5	79.2	83.1	85.2	88.0	69.4	71.0	73.5
Pennsylvania[1]	84.3	85.3	- - -	87.9	88.4	- - -	68.7	72.4	- - -
East North Central	83.4	84.0	85.4	87.5	88.2	89.0	70.1	71.7	74.2
Illinois	82.2	82.9	85.3	89.3	89.9	90.9	69.5	71.4	74.2
Indiana	80.1	80.6	81.2	82.6	83.6	84.5	65.4	68.2	69.2
Michigan	84.2	84.2	85.9	88.3	88.8	89.7	71.0	69.7	71.9
Ohio	85.3	86.8	87.8	87.8	89.0	89.8	72.7	76.3	78.8
Wisconsin	84.3	84.0	84.9	88.0	87.8	88.5	67.5	69.5	74.0
West North Central	85.2	86.0	86.6	88.0	89.0	89.5	72.4	75.3	77.5
Iowa	87.3	88.1	88.7	88.7	89.5	90.3	74.1	77.2	77.1
Kansas	85.6	86.5	87.0	89.1	90.0	90.1	76.0	78.5	79.3
Minnesota	84.0	84.6	86.1	87.4	88.7	90.2	65.0	66.7	72.2
Missouri	85.9	87.5	88.2	88.4	89.7	90.1	73.4	78.0	80.3
Nebraska	84.1	83.6	83.2	87.0	87.0	86.7	72.0	69.9	71.9
North Dakota	85.0	86.2	86.4	87.1	88.9	89.2	76.8	76.9	82.6
South Dakota	82.2	80.1	78.0	86.0	84.3	83.1	70.5	67.6	63.5
South Atlantic[1]	84.3	84.6	84.3	89.5	89.9	90.3	74.3	76.0	77.3
Delaware	83.2	85.4	85.6	88.2	89.9	89.9	73.0	78.2	81.2
District of Columbia	67.6	73.9	76.8	89.4	90.7	90.8	62.7	68.6	71.5
Florida[1]	83.6	83.9	- - -	88.6	89.1	- - -	72.6	74.0	- - -
Georgia	85.8	86.8	84.2	91.0	91.7	90.4	78.6	80.8	79.1
Maryland	88.3	85.7	83.4	92.9	91.4	90.7	79.8	77.4	75.5
North Carolina	84.0	84.7	84.3	90.0	91.0	90.7	73.4	75.9	76.3
South Carolina[1]	80.4	79.7	- - -	87.5	86.4	- - -	69.0	70.4	- - -
Virginia	84.9	85.2	85.4	90.0	90.3	90.5	73.4	75.7	77.6
West Virginia	82.6	85.8	85.9	83.2	86.5	86.4	67.1	72.5	75.0
East South Central[1]	83.0	83.7	- - -	87.9	88.5	- - -	70.7	73.1	- - -
Alabama	82.1	82.8	83.7	88.7	89.7	90.0	69.7	71.7	75.5
Kentucky[1]	85.6	86.7	- - -	86.8	87.9	- - -	75.9	78.7	- - -
Mississippi	79.8	81.8	84.4	89.0	89.4	90.8	69.3	73.3	77.2
Tennessee[1]	83.7	83.4	- - -	87.7	87.7	- - -	72.0	73.0	- - -
West South Central	78.9	79.9	81.2	85.8	86.9	87.2	72.1	74.5	76.1
Arkansas	76.1	79.5	81.1	80.7	83.6	84.6	63.8	69.5	73.3
Louisiana	81.5	83.1	84.5	89.1	90.4	90.8	71.2	73.4	75.9
Oklahoma	78.6	78.9	77.6	81.9	82.7	81.7	68.0	71.0	70.4
Texas	78.6	79.5	81.1	86.8	87.6	88.1	74.8	76.7	77.4
Mountain[1]	78.1	77.7	77.5	84.8	85.2	85.3	71.3	71.8	72.6
Arizona	74.7	76.4	76.5	84.4	86.9	87.5	71.5	74.6	78.2
Colorado	82.2	80.7	79.5	87.5	87.8	86.2	76.4	74.3	71.2
Idaho[1]	78.7	81.1	- - -	81.6	83.5	- - -	72.2	75.9	- - -
Montana	82.5	83.2	83.8	84.9	86.1	86.7	75.9	86.5	85.2
Nevada	76.1	75.1	75.6	83.3	84.5	84.6	66.8	67.6	70.0
New Mexico	69.2	68.1	69.1	77.8	75.7	76.8	62.3	64.6	68.2
Utah	83.2	79.7	79.9	86.4	83.7	83.7	67.2	60.0	60.3
Wyoming	81.9	82.9	85.5	83.8	84.4	87.0	69.7	78.3	86.1
Pacific[1]	81.7	84.0	86.3	86.8	88.1	89.4	79.0	81.4	83.4
Alaska	80.9	80.0	80.2	83.4	83.6	84.0	82.3	83.1	83.7
California	81.6	84.5	87.0	87.7	89.7	90.6	79.0	81.8	83.5
Hawaii	84.3	85.1	82.7	90.1	90.3	86.7	89.5	91.2	90.3
Oregon	80.4	81.2	81.1	83.1	84.2	84.4	78.4	76.4	75.6
Washington[1]	83.2	82.9	- - -	86.0	86.0	- - -	77.0	75.8	- - -

See footnotes at end of table.

This table will be updated on the Web. Go to www.cdc.gov/nchs/hus.htm.

Table 8 (page 2 of 3). Early prenatal care by race and Hispanic origin of mother, geographic division, and state: United States, average annual 1996–1998, 1999–2001, and 2002–2004

[Data are based on birth certificates]

Geographic division and state	Hispanic or Latino[2]			American Indian or Alaska Native[3]			Asian or Pacific Islander[3]		
	1996–1998	1999–2001	2002–2004	1996–1998	1999–2001	2002–2004	1996–1998	1999–2001	2002–2004
	Percent of live births with early prenatal care (beginning in the 1st trimester)								
United States[1]	73.4	74.9	77.1	68.2	69.4	69.9	82.2	83.9	85.3
New England[1]	77.4	80.4	81.1	75.8	81.0	84.1	82.2	85.4	86.1
Connecticut	78.2	78.8	76.9	75.2	82.1	85.4	85.9	87.5	87.7
Maine	80.2	80.6	80.5	72.9	76.2	78.0	81.5	86.8	82.1
Massachusetts	75.9	80.2	83.0	71.1	82.3	88.5	81.0	84.7	86.1
New Hampshire[1]	77.3	80.4	- - -	86.2	81.9	- - -	84.6	85.3	- - -
Rhode Island	82.6	86.7	86.8	81.5	81.9	80.9	81.5	83.8	81.8
Vermont	82.8	82.2	79.4	*79.3	*82.4	*85.7	75.7	85.6	86.9
Middle Atlantic[1]	70.7	71.6	- - -	74.2	77.1	- - -	77.8	78.5	- - -
New Jersey	71.0	68.6	67.9	71.8	73.8	67.9	83.2	83.3	84.8
New York[1]	73.9	73.3	- - -	72.5	74.8	- - -	81.9	82.7	- - -
New York City	69.3	72.4	77.0	77.5	77.5	84.7	72.9	73.2	77.0
Pennsylvania[1]	71.5	73.5	- - -	78.2	82.4	- - -	78.5	81.1	- - -
East North Central	72.4	72.6	77.0	72.6	75.2	75.7	82.1	83.4	86.0
Illinois	72.6	74.0	79.6	75.1	77.8	81.4	85.2	85.0	88.1
Indiana	65.9	63.1	64.5	68.1	74.2	70.9	81.8	81.0	83.5
Michigan	73.2	71.6	77.9	73.9	75.6	79.4	85.6	87.0	88.2
Ohio	76.8	76.7	78.7	79.4	80.4	80.9	86.0	88.7	90.3
Wisconsin	71.3	69.6	70.7	69.3	72.7	71.2	62.3	65.8	70.0
West North Central	67.8	69.7	73.4	66.9	66.3	65.8	73.2	78.2	81.2
Iowa	71.0	73.3	75.5	69.9	74.7	75.9	82.0	83.7	87.6
Kansas	65.9	69.4	74.1	77.7	80.4	82.0	82.5	85.4	86.2
Minnesota	61.7	63.2	69.6	62.1	62.2	64.0	61.2	69.5	74.5
Missouri	76.8	78.2	79.7	76.9	77.3	80.4	84.2	87.8	88.4
Nebraska	67.6	68.1	70.0	67.5	68.3	68.5	82.1	80.7	83.7
North Dakota	73.8	77.5	80.5	70.1	66.8	66.9	78.4	86.3	87.2
South Dakota	72.2	68.5	63.9	64.3	61.8	57.7	74.8	80.1	72.3
South Atlantic[1]	78.1	77.3	70.4	73.9	73.7	80.6	85.4	86.6	86.1
Delaware	68.7	72.3	72.0	*76.2	78.1	87.1	84.0	89.2	90.1
District of Columbia	64.1	70.8	70.5	*83.3	*61.9	*	73.2	77.9	81.7
Florida[1]	81.4	81.4	- - -	69.4	64.2	- - -	87.1	87.8	- - -
Georgia	76.0	77.9	71.0	82.9	81.7	83.5	87.3	90.2	88.6
Maryland	81.4	77.3	68.1	84.0	82.6	78.7	89.5	87.0	84.9
North Carolina	68.5	69.1	69.9	72.5	76.5	80.2	81.9	83.5	85.0
South Carolina[1]	65.9	61.7	- - -	76.1	77.4	- - -	76.0	79.5	- - -
Virginia	72.8	71.6	71.1	81.0	80.2	82.1	83.7	85.7	85.5
West Virginia	76.5	67.4	74.2	*84.2	*74.4	*69.2	82.2	80.4	86.1
East South Central[1]	66.7	60.8	- - -	75.7	78.6	- - -	83.4	84.6	- - -
Alabama	62.5	55.7	53.1	80.0	79.4	81.4	83.4	86.7	87.4
Kentucky[1]	74.0	68.6	- - -	79.4	85.2	- - -	84.6	87.2	- - -
Mississippi	77.1	73.4	77.0	72.8	75.8	72.2	80.1	83.0	85.9
Tennessee[1]	64.5	58.5	- - -	73.8	78.2	- - -	84.0	83.1	- - -
West South Central	71.3	72.5	75.6	70.4	70.9	72.5	85.6	87.3	88.1
Arkansas	59.8	66.2	70.6	68.4	74.0	75.4	73.4	78.6	82.4
Louisiana	83.8	85.0	83.7	78.0	80.7	84.4	83.7	85.7	88.3
Oklahoma	68.6	66.7	64.6	69.3	69.4	70.2	81.7	80.7	80.3
Texas	71.4	72.6	76.0	74.1	74.6	79.4	86.6	88.4	89.0
Mountain[1]	65.3	65.0	66.6	60.9	63.8	64.9	78.0	78.9	79.1
Arizona	64.1	65.7	66.8	61.0	65.9	68.0	82.4	84.5	84.2
Colorado	68.3	65.5	67.6	71.9	68.3	67.6	80.0	82.6	80.8
Idaho[1]	61.2	66.9	- - -	59.3	67.5	- - -	78.2	80.4	- - -
Montana	76.7	79.3	80.1	66.4	65.6	66.1	79.7	80.4	83.7
Nevada	64.0	61.8	64.1	70.3	67.4	68.6	78.5	79.2	80.2
New Mexico	66.2	65.5	66.7	55.6	58.8	59.2	74.3	75.0	76.1
Utah	64.5	61.3	64.1	59.0	55.3	56.7	69.8	64.7	65.7
Wyoming	71.1	73.5	79.6	65.1	71.8	70.9	84.4	82.2	84.7
Pacific[1]	76.6	80.3	84.3	72.7	72.5	73.0	83.5	85.5	87.1
Alaska	78.1	80.8	78.2	75.7	71.3	70.3	75.2	76.4	75.1
California	77.0	81.0	84.8	71.8	73.9	76.0	84.2	86.5	88.5
Hawaii	83.0	83.7	81.1	82.9	83.4	81.2	82.3	83.4	81.2
Oregon	66.6	69.2	70.2	66.2	68.7	68.9	80.2	81.8	81.7
Washington[1]	70.8	71.8	- - -	72.1	72.0	- - -	80.5	81.6	- - -

See footnotes at end of table.

This table will be updated on the Web. Go to www.cdc.gov/nchs/hus.htm.

Table 8 (page 3 of 3). Early prenatal care by race and Hispanic origin of mother, geographic division, and state: United States, average annual 1996–1998, 1999–2001, and 2002–2004

[Data are based on birth certificates]

- - - Data not available.
* Percents preceded by an asterisk are based on fewer than 50 births. Percents not shown are based on fewer than 20 births.
[1]Reporting areas that have adopted the 2003 revision of the U.S. Standard Certificate of Live Birth are excluded for 2002–2004 because prenatal care data based on the 2003 revision are not comparable with data based on the 1989 revision of the U.S. Standard Certificate of Live Birth. In 2003, Pennsylvania and Washington adopted the 2003 revision; in 2004, Florida, Idaho, Kentucky, New Hampshire, New York State (excluding New York City), South Carolina, and Tennessee adopted the 2003 revision. See Appendix II, Prenatal Care.
[2]Persons of Hispanic origin may be of any race. See Appendix II, Hispanic origin.
[3]Includes persons of Hispanic and non-Hispanic origin.

NOTES: Data are based on the 1989 revision of the U.S. Standard Certificate of Live Birth. Starting with 2003 data, some states reported multiple-race data. The multiple-race data for these states were bridged to the single-race categories of the 1977 Office of Management and Budget standards for comparability with other states. See Appendix II, Race.

SOURCE: Centers for Disease Control and Prevention, National Center for Health Statistics, National Vital Statistics System, Birth File.

This table will be updated on the Web. Go to www.cdc.gov/nchs/hus.htm.

Table 9. Teenage childbearing, by detailed race and Hispanic origin of mother: United States, selected years 1970–2004

[Data are based on birth certificates]

Maternal age, race, and Hispanic origin of mother	1970	1975	1980	1985	1990	1995	2000	2001	2002	2003	2004
Age of mother under 18 years					Percent of live births						
All races	6.3	7.6	5.8	4.7	4.7	5.3	4.1	3.8	3.6	3.4	3.4
White	4.8	6.0	4.5	3.7	3.6	4.3	3.5	3.3	3.1	3.0	3.0
Black or African American	14.8	16.3	12.5	10.6	10.1	10.8	7.8	7.3	6.9	6.6	6.4
American Indian or Alaska Native	7.5	11.2	9.4	7.6	7.2	8.7	7.3	6.8	6.6	6.6	6.4
Asian or Pacific Islander[1]	- - -	- - -	1.5	1.6	2.1	2.2	1.5	1.3	1.1	1.1	1.1
Chinese	1.1	0.4	0.3	0.3	0.4	0.3	0.2	0.2	0.2	- - -	- - -
Japanese	2.0	1.7	1.0	0.9	0.8	0.8	0.6	0.5	0.6	- - -	- - -
Filipino	3.7	2.4	1.6	1.6	2.0	2.2	1.6	1.5	1.2	- - -	- - -
Hawaiian	- - -	- - -	6.6	5.7	6.5	7.6	5.7	4.9	4.5	- - -	- - -
Other Asian or Pacific Islander	- - -	- - -	1.2	1.8	2.4	2.5	1.7	1.5	1.3	- - -	- - -
Hispanic or Latino[2]	- - -	- - -	7.4	6.4	6.6	7.6	6.3	5.8	5.6	5.4	5.4
Mexican	- - -	- - -	7.7	6.9	6.9	8.0	6.6	6.2	6.0	5.8	5.8
Puerto Rican	- - -	- - -	10.0	8.5	9.1	10.8	7.8	7.4	6.9	6.9	6.8
Cuban	- - -	- - -	3.8	2.2	2.7	2.8	3.1	2.7	2.7	2.4	2.4
Central and South American	- - -	- - -	2.4	2.4	3.2	4.1	3.3	3.1	2.8	2.8	2.8
Other and unknown Hispanic or Latino	- - -	- - -	6.5	7.0	8.0	9.0	7.6	6.8	6.5	6.3	6.3
Not Hispanic or Latino:[2]											
White	- - -	- - -	4.0	3.2	3.0	3.4	2.6	2.3	2.2	2.1	2.0
Black or African American	- - -	- - -	12.7	10.7	10.2	10.8	7.8	7.3	6.9	6.6	6.5
Age of mother 18–19 years											
All races	11.3	11.3	9.8	8.0	8.1	7.9	7.7	7.5	7.1	6.9	6.8
White	10.4	10.3	9.0	7.1	7.3	7.2	7.1	6.9	6.6	6.4	6.4
Black or African American	16.6	16.9	14.5	12.9	13.0	12.4	11.9	11.5	11.1	10.7	10.7
American Indian or Alaska Native	12.8	15.2	14.6	12.4	12.3	12.7	12.4	12.5	11.9	11.6	11.5
Asian or Pacific Islander[1]	- - -	- - -	3.9	3.4	3.7	3.5	3.0	3.0	2.7	2.4	2.3
Chinese	3.9	1.7	1.0	0.6	0.8	0.6	0.7	0.8	0.7	- - -	- - -
Japanese	4.1	3.3	2.3	1.9	2.0	1.7	1.4	1.2	1.1	- - -	- - -
Filipino	7.1	5.0	4.0	3.7	4.1	4.1	3.7	3.6	3.3	- - -	- - -
Hawaiian	- - -	- - -	13.3	12.3	11.9	11.5	11.7	11.3	10.2	- - -	- - -
Other Asian or Pacific Islander	- - -	- - -	3.8	3.5	3.9	3.8	3.2	3.1	2.8	- - -	- - -
Hispanic or Latino[2]	- - -	- - -	11.6	10.1	10.2	10.3	9.9	9.7	9.3	8.9	8.9
Mexican	- - -	- - -	12.0	10.6	10.7	10.8	10.4	10.3	9.8	9.5	9.4
Puerto Rican	- - -	- - -	13.3	12.4	12.6	12.7	12.2	11.8	10.9	11.0	10.8
Cuban	- - -	- - -	9.2	4.9	5.0	4.9	4.4	4.8	5.5	5.5	5.4
Central and South American	- - -	- - -	6.0	5.8	5.9	6.5	6.5	6.3	5.7	5.6	5.6
Other and unknown Hispanic or Latino	- - -	- - -	10.8	10.5	11.1	11.1	11.3	10.5	10.2	9.6	9.9
Not Hispanic or Latino:[2]											
White	- - -	- - -	8.5	6.5	6.6	6.4	6.1	5.9	5.6	5.4	5.4
Black or African American	- - -	- - -	14.7	12.9	13.0	12.4	12.0	11.6	11.1	10.8	10.8

- - - Data not available.

[1]Starting with 2003 data, estimates are not shown for Asian or Pacific Islander subgroups during the transition from single race to multiple race reporting. See Appendix II, Race, Birth File.

[2]Prior to 1993, data from states lacking an Hispanic-origin item on the birth certificate were excluded. See Appendix II, Hispanic origin. Data for non-Hispanic white and non-Hispanic black women for years prior to 1989 are not nationally representative and are provided for comparison with Hispanic data.

NOTES: The race groups, white, black, American Indian or Alaska Native, and Asian or Pacific Islander, include persons of Hispanic and non-Hispanic origin. Persons of Hispanic origin may be of any race. Starting with 2003 data, some states reported multiple-race data. The multiple-race data for these states were bridged to the single-race categories of the 1977 Office of Management and Budget standards for comparability with other states. See Appendix II, Race. Interpretation of trend data should take into consideration expansion of reporting areas and immigration. Data for additional years are available. See Appendix III.

SOURCES: Centers for Disease Control and Prevention, National Center for Health Statistics, National Vital Statistics System, Birth File.

This table will be updated on the Web. Go to www.cdc.gov/nchs/hus.htm.

Table 10. Nonmarital childbearing by detailed race and Hispanic origin of mother, and maternal age: United States, selected years 1970–2004

[Data are based on birth certificates]

Race, Hispanic origin of mother, and maternal age	1970	1975	1980	1985	1990	1995	2000	2001	2002	2003	2004
	Live births per 1,000 unmarried women 15–44 years of age[1]										
All races and origins	26.4	24.5	29.4	32.8	43.8	44.3	44.0	43.8	43.7	44.9	46.1
White[2]	13.9	12.4	18.1	22.5	32.9	37.0	38.2	38.5	38.9	40.4	41.6
Black or African American[2]	95.5	84.2	81.1	77.0	90.5	74.5	70.5	68.2	66.2	66.3	67.2
Asian or Pacific Islander	- - -	- - -	- - -	- - -	- - -	- - -	20.9	21.2	21.3	22.2	23.6
Hispanic or Latino[3]	- - -	- - -	- - -	- - -	89.6	88.7	87.2	87.8	87.9	92.2	95.7
White, not Hispanic or Latino	- - -	- - -	- - -	- - -	24.4	28.1	28.0	27.8	27.8	28.6	29.4
	Percent of live births to unmarried mothers										
All races and origins	10.7	14.3	18.4	22.0	28.0	32.2	33.2	33.5	34.0	34.6	35.8
White	5.5	7.1	11.2	14.7	20.4	25.3	27.1	27.7	28.5	29.4	30.5
Black or African American	37.5	49.5	56.1	61.2	66.5	69.9	68.5	68.4	68.2	68.2	68.8
American Indian or Alaska Native	22.4	32.7	39.2	46.8	53.6	57.2	58.4	59.7	59.7	61.3	62.3
Asian or Pacific Islander[4]	- - -	- - -	7.3	9.5	13.2	16.3	14.8	14.9	14.9	15.0	15.5
Chinese	3.0	1.6	2.7	3.0	5.0	7.9	7.6	8.4	9.0	- - -	- - -
Japanese	4.6	4.6	5.2	7.9	9.6	10.8	9.5	9.2	10.3	- - -	- - -
Filipino	9.1	6.9	8.6	11.4	15.9	19.5	20.3	20.4	20.0	- - -	- - -
Hawaiian	- - -	- - -	32.9	37.3	45.0	49.0	50.0	50.6	50.4	- - -	- - -
Other Asian or Pacific Islander	- - -	- - -	5.4	8.5	12.6	16.2	13.8	13.7	13.5	- - -	- - -
Hispanic or Latino[3]	- - -	- - -	23.6	29.5	36.7	40.8	42.7	42.5	43.5	45.0	46.4
Mexican	- - -	- - -	20.3	25.7	33.3	38.1	40.7	40.8	42.1	43.7	45.2
Puerto Rican	- - -	- - -	46.3	51.1	55.9	60.0	59.6	58.9	59.1	59.8	61.0
Cuban	- - -	- - -	10.0	16.1	18.2	23.8	27.3	27.2	29.8	31.4	33.2
Central and South American	- - -	- - -	27.1	34.9	41.2	44.1	44.7	44.3	44.8	46.0	47.6
Other and unknown Hispanic or Latino	- - -	- - -	22.4	31.1	37.2	44.0	46.2	44.2	44.4	46.7	46.6
Not Hispanic or Latino:[3]											
White	- - -	- - -	9.5	12.4	16.9	21.2	22.1	22.5	23.0	23.6	24.5
Black or African American	- - -	- - -	57.2	62.0	66.7	70.0	68.7	68.6	68.4	68.5	69.3
	Number of live births, in thousands										
Live births to unmarried mothers	399	448	666	828	1,165	1,254	1,347	1,349	1,366	1,416	1,470
Maternal age	Percent distribution of live births to unmarried mothers										
Under 20 years	50.1	52.1	40.8	33.8	30.9	30.9	28.0	26.6	25.4	24.3	23.7
20–24 years	31.8	29.9	35.6	36.3	34.7	34.5	37.4	38.2	38.6	38.8	38.5
25 years and over	18.1	18.0	23.5	29.9	34.4	34.7	34.6	35.2	35.9	36.9	37.8

- - - Data not available.

[1]Rates computed by relating births to unmarried mothers, regardless of age of mother, to unmarried women 15–44 years of age. Population data for unmarried American Indian or Alaska Native women are not available for rate calculations. Prior to 2000, population data for unmarried Asian or Pacific Islander women were not available for rate calculations.

[2]For 1970 and 1975, birth rates are by race of child.

[3]Prior to 1993, data from states lacking an Hispanic-origin item on the birth certificate were excluded. See Appendix II, Hispanic origin. Data for non-Hispanic white and non-Hispanic black women for years prior to 1989 are not nationally representative and are provided for comparison with Hispanic data.

[4]Starting with 2003 data, estimates are not shown for Asian or Pacific Islander subgroups during the transition from single race to multiple race reporting. See Appendix II, Race, Birth File.

NOTES: National estimates for 1970 and 1975 for unmarried mothers are based on births occurring in states reporting marital status of mother. Changes in reporting procedures for marital status occurred in some states during the 1990s. Interpretation of trend data should also take into consideration expansion of reporting areas and immigration. See Appendix II, Marital status. The race groups, white, black, American Indian or Alaska Native, and Asian or Pacific Islander, include persons of Hispanic and non-Hispanic origin. Persons of Hispanic origin may be of any race. Starting with 2003 data, some states reported multiple-race data. The multiple-race data for these states were bridged to the single-race categories of the 1977 Office of Management and Budget standards for comparability with other states. See Appendix II, Race. Starting with *Health, United States, 2003*, rates for 1991–1999 were revised using intercensal population estimates based on the 2000 census. Rates for 2000 were computed using the 2000 census counts and starting with 2001, rates were computed using 2000-based postcensal estimates. Data for additional years are available. See Appendix III.

SOURCES: Centers for Disease Control and Prevention, National Center for Health Statistics, National Vital Statistics System, Birth File. Martin JA, Hamilton BE, Sutton PD, Ventura SJ, Menacker F, Kirmeyer S. Births: Final Data for 2004. National vital statistics reports. vol 55 no 1. Hyattsville, MD: National Center for Health Statistics. 2006; Hamilton BE, Sutton PD, Ventura SJ. Revised birth and fertility rates for the 1990s and new rates for Hispanic populations, 2000 and 2001: United States. National vital statistics reports. vol 51 no 12. Hyattsville, MD: National Center for Health Statistics. 2003; Births: Final data for each data year 1997–2003. National vital statistics reports. Hyattsville, MD; Final natality statistics for each data year 1993–1996. Monthly vital statistics report. Hyattsville, MD; Ventura SJ. Births to unmarried mothers: United States, 1980–1992. Vital Health Stat 21(53). 1995.

This table will be updated on the Web. Go to www.cdc.gov/nchs/hus.htm.

Table 11. Maternal education for live births, by detailed race and Hispanic origin of mother: United States, selected years 1970–2004

[Data are based on birth certificates]

Education, race, and Hispanic origin of mother	1970	1975	1980	1985	1990	1995	2000	2002	2003[1]	43 reporting areas 2003[2]	43 reporting areas 2004[1]
Less than 12 years of education					Percent of live births[3]						
All races	30.8	28.6	23.7	20.6	23.8	22.6	21.7	21.5	21.6	22.1	22.2
White	27.1	25.1	20.8	17.8	22.4	21.6	21.4	21.6	21.8	22.5	22.7
Black or African American	51.2	45.3	36.4	32.6	30.2	28.7	25.5	24.4	24.0	23.9	23.8
American Indian or Alaska Native	60.5	52.7	44.2	39.0	36.4	33.0	31.6	30.8	30.5	30.2	30.1
Asian or Pacific Islander[4]	- - -	- - -	21.0	19.4	20.0	16.1	11.6	10.3	9.9	10.0	9.3
Chinese	23.0	16.5	15.2	15.5	15.8	12.9	11.7	11.3	- - -	- - -	- - -
Japanese	11.8	9.1	5.0	4.8	3.5	2.6	2.1	2.2	- - -	- - -	- - -
Filipino	26.4	22.3	16.4	13.9	10.3	8.0	6.2	5.3	- - -	- - -	- - -
Hawaiian	- - -	- - -	20.7	18.7	19.3	17.6	16.7	14.3	- - -	- - -	- - -
Other Asian or Pacific Islander	- - -	- - -	27.6	24.3	26.8	21.2	13.5	11.6	- - -	- - -	- - -
Hispanic or Latino[5]	- - -	- - -	51.1	44.5	53.9	52.1	48.9	48.1	47.5	48.7	48.4
Mexican	- - -	- - -	62.8	59.0	61.4	58.6	55.0	54.2	53.6	53.1	52.5
Puerto Rican	- - -	- - -	55.3	46.6	42.7	38.6	33.4	31.5	29.9	31.7	31.6
Cuban	- - -	- - -	24.1	21.1	17.8	14.4	11.9	11.8	11.5	13.4	13.0
Central and South American	- - -	- - -	41.2	37.0	44.2	41.7	37.2	35.8	35.3	38.0	39.1
Other and unknown Hispanic or Latino	- - -	- - -	40.1	36.5	33.3	33.8	31.4	31.7	30.1	28.3	29.4
Not Hispanic or Latino:[5]											
White	- - -	- - -	18.1	15.7	15.2	13.3	12.2	11.7	11.5	11.0	11.0
Black or African American	- - -	- - -	37.3	33.4	30.0	28.6	25.3	24.3	23.8	23.5	23.4
16 years or more of education											
All races	8.6	11.4	14.0	16.7	17.5	21.4	24.7	25.9	26.6	26.7	26.9
White	9.6	12.7	15.5	18.6	19.3	23.1	26.3	27.3	27.9	27.8	28.0
Black or African American	2.8	4.3	6.2	7.0	7.2	9.5	11.7	12.7	13.4	13.8	13.7
American Indian or Alaska Native	2.7	2.2	3.5	3.7	4.4	6.2	7.8	8.7	8.5	8.3	8.6
Asian or Pacific Islander[4]	- - -	- - -	30.8	30.3	31.0	35.0	42.8	45.7	47.1	46.8	48.6
Chinese	34.0	37.8	41.5	35.2	40.3	49.0	55.6	57.3	- - -	- - -	- - -
Japanese	20.7	30.6	36.8	38.1	44.1	46.2	51.1	53.5	- - -	- - -	- - -
Filipino	28.1	36.6	37.1	35.2	34.5	36.7	40.5	43.3	- - -	- - -	- - -
Hawaiian	- - -	- - -	7.9	6.5	6.8	9.7	13.5	14.6	- - -	- - -	- - -
Other Asian or Pacific Islander	- - -	- - -	29.2	30.2	27.3	30.5	40.7	44.4	- - -	- - -	- - -
Hispanic or Latino[5]	- - -	- - -	4.2	6.0	5.1	6.1	7.6	8.3	8.7	7.8	8.0
Mexican	- - -	- - -	2.2	3.0	3.3	4.0	5.1	5.5	5.9	5.9	6.1
Puerto Rican	- - -	- - -	3.0	4.6	6.5	8.7	10.4	11.8	12.9	11.7	12.0
Cuban	- - -	- - -	11.6	15.0	20.4	26.5	31.0	30.5	31.3	34.5	35.4
Central and South American	- - -	- - -	6.1	8.1	8.6	10.3	14.1	15.5	16.0	14.1	14.2
Other and unknown Hispanic or Latino	- - -	- - -	5.5	7.2	8.5	10.5	12.5	13.2	14.4	14.5	14.0
Not Hispanic or Latino:[5]											
White	- - -	- - -	16.6	19.4	22.6	27.7	32.5	34.3	35.5	36.4	37.0
Black or African American	- - -	- - -	5.8	6.7	7.3	9.5	11.7	12.7	13.4	13.9	13.8

- - - Data not available.

[1]Reporting areas that have adopted the 2003 revision of the U.S. Standard Certificate of Live Birth are excluded because maternal education data based on the 2003 revision are not comparable with data based on the 1989 and earlier revisions of the U.S. Standard Certificate of Live Birth. In 2003, Pennsylvania and Washington adopted the 2003 revision; in 2004, Florida, Idaho, Kentucky, New Hampshire, New York State (excluding New York City), South Carolina, and Tennessee adopted the 2003 revision. See Appendix II, Education.

[2]Data for 2003 are limited to the 43 reporting areas using the 1989 revision of the U.S. Standard Certificate of Live Birth in 2004 and are provided for comparison with 2004.

[3]Excludes live births for whom education of mother is unknown.

[4]Starting with 2003 data, estimates are not shown for Asian or Pacific Islander subgroups during the transition from single race to multiple race reporting. See Appendix II, Race, Birth File.

[5]Prior to 1993, data are shown only for states with an Hispanic-origin item and education of mother item on the birth certificate. See Appendix II, Education; Hispanic origin. Data for non-Hispanic white and non-Hispanic black women for years prior to 1989 are not nationally representative and are provided for comparison with Hispanic data.

NOTES: Data are based on the 1989 and earlier revisions of the U.S. Standard Certificate of Live Birth. Maternal education groups shown in this table generally represent the group at highest risk for unfavorable birth outcomes (less than 12 years of education) and the group at lowest risk (16 years or more of education). In 1992–2002, education of mother was reported on the birth certificate by all 50 states and the District of Columbia. See Appendix II, Education. Prior to 1992, data from states lacking an education of mother item were excluded. The race groups, white, black, American Indian or Alaska Native, and Asian or Pacific Islander, include persons of Hispanic and non-Hispanic origin. Persons of Hispanic origin may be of any race. Starting with 2003 data, some states reported multiple-race data. The multiple-race data for these states were bridged to the single-race categories of the 1977 Office of Management and Budget standards for comparability with other states. See Appendix II, Race. Interpretation of trend data should take into consideration changes in reporting areas and immigration. Data for additional years are available. See Appendix III.

SOURCE: Centers for Disease Control and Prevention, National Center for Health Statistics, National Vital Statistics System, Birth File.

This table will be updated on the Web. Go to www.cdc.gov/nchs/hus.htm.

Table 12. Mothers who smoked cigarettes during pregnancy, by detailed race, Hispanic origin, age, and education of mother: United States, selected years, 1989–2004

[Data are based on birth certificates]

Characteristic of mother	*1989*	*1990*	*1995*	*2000*	*2002*	*2003*[1]	*42 reporting areas* *2003*[2]	*42 reporting areas* *2004*[1]
Race of mother	Percent of mothers who smoked[3,4]							
All races	19.5	18.4	13.9	12.2	11.4	10.7	10.4	10.2
White	20.4	19.4	15.0	13.2	12.3	11.6	11.1	11.0
Black or African American	17.1	15.9	10.6	9.1	8.7	8.1	8.3	8.2
American Indian or Alaska Native	23.0	22.4	20.9	20.0	19.7	18.1	18.2	18.2
Asian or Pacific Islander[5]	5.7	5.5	3.4	2.8	2.5	2.2	2.2	2.2
Chinese	2.7	2.0	0.8	0.6	0.5	- - -	- - -	- - -
Japanese	8.2	8.0	5.2	4.2	4.0	- - -	- - -	- - -
Filipino	5.1	5.3	3.4	3.2	2.9	- - -	- - -	- - -
Hawaiian	19.3	21.0	15.9	14.4	13.7	- - -	- - -	- - -
Other Asian or Pacific Islander	4.2	3.8	2.7	2.3	2.1	- - -	- - -	- - -
Hispanic origin and race of mother[6]								
Hispanic or Latino	8.0	6.7	4.3	3.5	3.0	2.7	2.7	2.6
Mexican	6.3	5.3	3.1	2.4	2.2	2.0	2.1	2.0
Puerto Rican	14.5	13.6	10.4	10.3	9.0	7.9	8.5	8.5
Cuban	6.9	6.4	4.1	3.3	2.8	2.4	5.8	6.4
Central and South American	3.6	3.0	1.8	1.5	1.3	1.1	1.1	1.2
Other and unknown Hispanic or Latino	12.1	10.8	8.2	7.4	6.5	6.6	6.9	6.4
Not Hispanic or Latino:								
White	21.7	21.0	17.1	15.6	15.0	14.3	13.8	13.8
Black or African American	17.2	15.9	10.6	9.2	8.8	8.3	8.4	8.4
Age of mother[3]								
Under 15 years	7.7	7.5	7.3	7.1	5.8	5.3	5.1	4.1
15–19 years	22.2	20.8	16.8	17.8	16.7	15.4	14.9	14.2
15–17 years	19.0	17.6	14.6	15.0	13.4	11.9	11.5	10.5
18–19 years	23.9	22.5	18.1	19.2	18.2	17.1	16.5	16.0
20–24 years	23.5	22.1	17.1	16.8	16.7	16.1	15.5	15.5
25–29 years	19.0	18.0	12.8	10.5	9.9	9.4	9.0	9.2
30–34 years	15.7	15.3	11.4	8.0	7.1	6.5	6.2	6.1
35–39 years	13.6	13.3	12.0	9.1	7.8	6.8	6.7	6.3
40–54 years[7]	13.2	12.3	10.1	9.5	8.4	8.0	7.8	7.2
Education of mother[8]	Percent of mothers 20 years of age and over who smoked[3,4]							
0–8 years	18.9	17.5	11.0	7.9	6.8	6.2	5.7	5.5
9–11 years	42.2	40.5	32.0	28.2	26.8	25.5	24.2	23.7
12 years	22.8	21.9	18.3	16.6	16.0	15.2	14.9	14.9
13–15 years	13.7	12.8	10.6	9.1	8.8	8.5	8.3	8.4
16 years or more	5.0	4.5	2.7	2.0	1.7	1.6	1.5	1.5

- - - Data not available.

[1]Reporting areas that have adopted the 2003 revision of the U.S. Standard Certificate of Live Birth are excluded because maternal tobacco use and education data based on the 2003 revision are not comparable with data based on the 1989 and earlier revisions of the U.S. Standard Certificate of Live Birth. In 2003, Pennsylvania and Washington adopted the 2003 revision; in 2004 Florida, Idaho, Kentucky, New Hampshire, New York State (excluding New York City), South Carolina, and Tennessee adopted the 2003 revision. In addition, California did not require reporting of tobacco use during pregnancy. See Appendix II, Cigarette smoking.

[2]Data for 2003 are limited to the 42 reporting areas using the 1989 revision of the U.S. Standard Certificate of Live Birth in 2004 and are provided for comparison with 2004.

[3]Data from states that did not require the reporting of mother's tobacco use during pregnancy on the birth certificate are not included. Reporting area for tobacco use increased from 43 states and the District of Columbia (DC) in 1989 to 49 states and DC in 2000–2002. See Appendix II, Cigarette smoking.

[4]Excludes live births for whom smoking status of mother is unknown.

[5]Maternal tobacco use during pregnancy was not reported on the birth certificates of California, which in 2004 accounted for 30% of the births to Asian or Pacific Islander mothers. Starting with 2003 data, estimates are not shown for Asian or Pacific Islander subgroups during the transition from single race to multiple race reporting. See Appendix II, Race, Birth File.

[6]Data from states that did not require the reporting of Hispanic origin of mother on the birth certificate are not included. Reporting of Hispanic origin increased from 47 states in 1989 to include all 50 states and DC by 1993. See Appendix II, Hispanic origin.

[7]Prior to 1997, data are for live births to mothers 45–49 years of age.

[8]Data from states that did not require the reporting of mother's education on the birth certificate are not included. See Appendix II, Education.

NOTES: Data are based on the 1989 revision of the U.S. Standard Certificate of Live Birth. The race groups, white, black, American Indian or Alaska Native, and Asian or Pacific Islander, include persons of Hispanic and non-Hispanic origin. Persons of Hispanic origin may be of any race. Starting with 2003 data, some states reported multiple-race data. The multiple-race data for these states were bridged to the single-race categories of the 1977 Office of Management and Budget standards for comparability with other states. See Appendix II, Race. Interpretation of trend data should take into consideration changes in reporting areas and immigration. Data for additional years are available. See Appendix III.

SOURCES: Centers for Disease Control and Prevention, National Center for Health Statistics, National Vital Statistics System, Birth File.

This table will be updated on the Web. Go to www.cdc.gov/nchs/hus.htm.

Table 13. Low-birthweight live births, by detailed race, Hispanic origin, and smoking status of mother: United States, selected years 1970–2004

[Data are based on birth certificates]

Birthweight, race and Hispanic origin of mother, and smoking status of mother	*1970*	*1975*	*1980*	*1985*	*1990*	*1995*	*1999*	*2000*	*2002*	*2003*	*2004*
Low birthweight (less than 2,500 grams)					Percent of live births[1]						
All races	7.93	7.38	6.84	6.75	6.97	7.32	7.62	7.57	7.82	7.93	8.08
White	6.85	6.27	5.72	5.65	5.70	6.22	6.57	6.55	6.80	6.94	7.07
Black or African American	13.90	13.19	12.69	12.65	13.25	13.13	13.11	12.99	13.29	13.37	13.44
American Indian or Alaska Native	7.97	6.41	6.44	5.86	6.11	6.61	7.15	6.76	7.23	7.37	7.45
Asian or Pacific Islander[2]	---	---	6.68	6.16	6.45	6.90	7.45	7.31	7.78	7.78	7.89
Chinese	6.67	5.29	5.21	4.98	4.69	5.29	5.19	5.10	5.52	---	---
Japanese	9.03	7.47	6.60	6.21	6.16	7.26	7.95	7.14	7.57	---	---
Filipino	10.02	8.08	7.40	6.95	7.30	7.83	8.30	8.46	8.61	---	---
Hawaiian	---	---	7.23	6.49	7.24	6.84	7.69	6.76	8.14	---	---
Other Asian or Pacific Islander	---	---	6.83	6.19	6.65	7.05	7.76	7.67	8.16	---	---
Hispanic or Latino[3]	---	---	6.12	6.16	6.06	6.29	6.38	6.41	6.55	6.69	6.79
Mexican	---	---	5.62	5.77	5.55	5.81	5.94	6.01	6.16	6.28	6.44
Puerto Rican	---	---	8.95	8.69	8.99	9.41	9.30	9.30	9.68	10.01	9.82
Cuban	---	---	5.62	6.02	5.67	6.50	6.80	6.49	6.50	7.04	7.72
Central and South American	---	---	5.76	5.68	5.84	6.20	6.38	6.34	6.53	6.70	6.70
Other and unknown Hispanic or Latino	---	---	6.96	6.83	6.87	7.55	7.63	7.84	7.87	8.01	7.78
Not Hispanic or Latino:[3]											
White	---	---	5.69	5.61	5.61	6.20	6.64	6.60	6.91	7.04	7.20
Black or African American	---	---	12.71	12.62	13.32	13.21	13.23	13.13	13.39	13.55	13.74
Cigarette smoker[4]	---	---	---	---	11.25	12.18	12.06	11.88	12.15	12.40	12.54
Nonsmoker[4]	---	---	---	---	6.14	6.79	7.21	7.19	7.48	7.66	7.79
Very low birthweight (less than 1,500 grams)											
All races	1.17	1.16	1.15	1.21	1.27	1.35	1.45	1.43	1.46	1.45	1.48
White	0.95	0.92	0.90	0.94	0.95	1.06	1.15	1.14	1.17	1.17	1.20
Black or African American	2.40	2.40	2.48	2.71	2.92	2.97	3.14	3.07	3.13	3.07	3.07
American Indian or Alaska Native	0.98	0.95	0.92	1.01	1.01	1.10	1.26	1.16	1.28	1.30	1.28
Asian or Pacific Islander[2]	---	---	0.92	0.85	0.87	0.91	1.08	1.05	1.12	1.09	1.14
Chinese	0.80	0.52	0.66	0.57	0.51	0.67	0.68	0.77	0.74	---	---
Japanese	1.48	0.89	0.94	0.84	0.73	0.87	0.86	0.75	0.97	---	---
Filipino	1.08	0.93	0.99	0.86	1.05	1.13	1.41	1.38	1.31	---	---
Hawaiian	---	---	1.05	1.03	0.97	0.94	1.41	1.39	1.55	---	---
Other Asian or Pacific Islander	---	---	0.96	0.91	0.92	0.91	1.09	1.04	1.17	---	---
Hispanic or Latino[3]	---	---	0.98	1.01	1.03	1.11	1.14	1.14	1.17	1.16	1.20
Mexican	---	---	0.92	0.97	0.92	1.01	1.04	1.03	1.06	1.06	1.13
Puerto Rican	---	---	1.29	1.30	1.62	1.79	1.86	1.93	1.96	2.01	1.96
Cuban	---	---	1.02	1.18	1.20	1.19	1.49	1.21	1.15	1.37	1.30
Central and South American	---	---	0.99	1.01	1.05	1.13	1.15	1.20	1.20	1.17	1.19
Other and unknown Hispanic or Latino	---	---	1.01	0.96	1.09	1.28	1.32	1.42	1.44	1.28	1.27
Not Hispanic or Latino:[3]											
White	---	---	0.87	0.91	0.93	1.04	1.15	1.14	1.17	1.18	1.20
Black or African American	---	---	2.47	2.67	2.93	2.98	3.18	3.10	3.15	3.12	3.15
Cigarette smoker[4]	---	---	---	---	1.73	1.85	1.91	1.91	1.88	1.92	1.88
Nonsmoker[4]	---	---	---	---	1.18	1.31	1.43	1.40	1.45	1.44	1.47

- - - Data not available.

[1]Excludes live births with unknown birthweight. Percent based on live births with known birthweight.

[2]Starting with 2003 data, estimates are not shown for Asian or Pacific Islander subgroups during the transition from single race to multiple race reporting. See Appendix II, Race, Birth File.

[3]Prior to 1993, data from states lacking an Hispanic-origin item on the birth certificate were excluded. See Appendix II, Hispanic origin. Data for non-Hispanic white and non-Hispanic black women for years prior to 1989 are not nationally representative and are provided for comparison with Hispanic data.

[4]Percent based on live births with known smoking status of mother and known birthweight. Data from states that did not require the reporting of mother's tobacco use during pregnancy on the birth certificate are not included. Reporting area for tobacco use increased from 43 states and the District of Columbia (DC) in 1989 to 49 states and DC in 2000–2002. Data for 2003 and 2004 exclude states that implemented the 2003 revision of the U.S. Standard Certificate of Live Birth: Pennsylvania and Washington (in 2003), Florida, Idaho, Kentucky, New Hampshire, New York State (excluding New York City), Pennsylvania, South Carolina, Tennessee, and Washington (in 2004). Tobacco use data based on the 2003 revision are not comparable with data based on the 1989 revision of the U.S. Standard Certificate of Live Birth. California has never required reporting of tobacco use during pregnancy. See Appendix II, Cigarette smoking.

NOTES: The race groups, white, black, American Indian or Alaska Native, and Asian or Pacific Islander, include persons of Hispanic and non-Hispanic origin. Persons of Hispanic origin may be of any race. Starting with 2003 data, some states reported multiple-race data. The multiple-race data for these states were bridged to the single-race categories of the 1977 Office of Management and Budget standards for comparability with other states. See Appendix II, Race. Interpretation of trend data should take into consideration expansion of reporting areas and immigration. Data for additional years are available. See Appendix III.

SOURCES: Centers for Disease Control and Prevention, National Center for Health Statistics, National Vital Statistics System, Birth File.

This table will be updated on the Web. Go to www.cdc.gov/nchs/hus.htm.

Table 14 (page 1 of 2). Low-birthweight live births among mothers 20 years of age and over, by detailed race, Hispanic origin, and education of mother: United States, selected years 1989–2004

[Data are based on birth certificates]

Education, race, and Hispanic origin of mother	1989	1990	1995	2000	2002	2003[1]	43 reporting areas	
							2003[2]	2004[1]
Less than 12 years of education	Percent of live births weighing less than 2,500 grams[3]							
All races	9.0	8.6	8.4	8.2	8.2	8.4	8.2	8.3
White	7.3	7.0	7.1	7.1	7.1	7.3	7.1	7.2
Black or African American	17.0	16.5	16.0	14.8	15.0	15.2	15.3	15.3
American Indian or Alaska Native	7.3	7.4	8.0	7.2	8.4	8.0	8.0	8.7
Asian or Pacific Islander[4]	6.6	6.4	6.7	7.2	7.4	7.5	7.6	7.7
Chinese	5.4	5.2	5.3	5.3	4.4	- - -	- - -	- - -
Japanese	4.0	10.6	11.0	6.8	4.7	- - -	- - -	- - -
Filipino	6.9	7.2	7.5	8.6	9.0	- - -	- - -	- - -
Hawaiian	11.0	10.7	9.8	9.4	7.8	- - -	- - -	- - -
Other Asian or Pacific Islander	6.8	6.4	6.7	7.5	8.1	- - -	- - -	- - -
Hispanic or Latino[5]	6.0	5.7	5.8	6.0	6.0	6.2	6.2	6.2
Mexican	5.3	5.2	5.4	5.6	5.7	5.9	5.9	6.0
Puerto Rican	11.3	10.3	10.5	10.9	10.4	11.2	11.0	10.5
Cuban	9.4	7.9	9.2	8.4	7.5	7.9	9.7	12.1
Central and South American	5.8	5.8	6.2	6.2	6.2	6.4	6.5	6.4
Other and unknown Hispanic or Latino	8.2	8.0	7.7	8.6	7.8	8.1	8.9	7.7
Not Hispanic or Latino:[5]								
White	8.4	8.3	8.9	9.0	9.3	9.5	9.4	9.6
Black or African American	17.6	16.7	16.2	15.2	15.3	15.7	15.9	16.1
12 years of education								
All races	7.1	7.1	7.6	7.9	8.2	8.4	8.3	8.4
White	5.7	5.8	6.4	6.8	7.0	7.2	7.2	7.3
Black or African American	13.4	13.1	13.3	13.0	13.4	13.5	13.5	13.7
American Indian or Alaska Native	5.6	6.1	6.5	6.7	7.1	7.2	7.2	7.2
Asian or Pacific Islander[4]	6.4	6.5	7.0	7.4	7.9	7.8	7.8	7.7
Chinese	5.1	4.9	5.7	5.6	5.2	- - -	- - -	- - -
Japanese	7.4	6.2	7.4	7.2	7.1	- - -	- - -	- - -
Filipino	6.8	7.6	7.7	8.1	8.7	- - -	- - -	- - -
Hawaiian	7.0	6.7	6.6	6.8	8.3	- - -	- - -	- - -
Other Asian or Pacific Islander	6.5	6.7	7.1	7.7	8.2	- - -	- - -	- - -
Hispanic or Latino[5]	5.9	6.0	6.1	6.2	6.5	6.5	6.5	6.7
Mexican	5.2	5.5	5.6	5.8	6.1	6.1	6.1	6.4
Puerto Rican	8.8	8.3	8.7	8.8	9.3	9.8	10.1	9.8
Cuban	5.3	5.2	6.7	6.5	6.0	6.4	7.2	8.3
Central and South American	5.7	5.8	5.9	6.0	6.4	6.6	6.6	6.8
Other and unknown Hispanic or Latino	6.1	6.6	7.1	7.3	7.7	7.4	7.8	7.7
Not Hispanic or Latino:[5]								
White	5.7	5.7	6.5	6.9	7.3	7.5	7.5	7.6
Black or African American	13.6	13.2	13.4	13.1	13.5	13.7	13.7	13.9
13 years or more of education								
All races	5.5	5.4	6.0	6.6	7.0	7.1	7.1	7.2
White	4.6	4.6	5.3	5.8	6.2	6.4	6.4	6.5
Black or African American	11.2	11.1	11.4	11.6	12.0	12.0	12.0	12.2
American Indian or Alaska Native	5.6	4.7	5.7	6.5	7.0	7.3	7.4	6.5
Asian or Pacific Islander[4]	6.1	6.0	6.6	7.0	7.6	7.6	7.6	7.8
Chinese	4.5	4.4	5.1	4.8	5.7	- - -	- - -	- - -
Japanese	6.6	6.0	7.1	7.0	7.7	- - -	- - -	- - -
Filipino	7.2	7.0	7.6	8.3	8.4	- - -	- - -	- - -
Hawaiian	6.3	4.7	5.0	4.5	7.2	- - -	- - -	- - -
Other Asian or Pacific Islander	6.1	6.2	6.7	7.4	7.9	- - -	- - -	- - -
Hispanic or Latino[5]	5.5	5.5	5.9	6.2	6.6	6.8	6.8	6.8
Mexican	5.1	5.2	5.6	5.8	6.2	6.3	6.3	6.6
Puerto Rican	7.4	7.4	7.9	7.9	8.9	9.1	9.3	8.9
Cuban	4.9	5.0	5.6	5.9	6.4	6.9	7.5	8.1
Central and South American	5.2	5.6	5.8	6.3	6.5	6.8	6.8	6.7
Other and unknown Hispanic or Latino	5.4	5.2	6.1	6.6	7.0	7.6	7.8	6.9
Not Hispanic or Latino:[5]								
White	4.6	4.5	5.2	5.8	6.2	6.4	6.3	6.5
Black or African American	11.2	11.1	11.5	11.7	12.1	12.1	12.1	12.3

See footnotes at end of table.

This table will be updated on the Web. Go to www.cdc.gov/nchs/hus.htm.

Table 14 (page 2 of 2). Low-birthweight live births among mothers 20 years of age and over, by detailed race, Hispanic origin, and education of mother: United States, selected years 1989–2004

[Data are based on birth certificates]

[1]Reporting areas that have adopted the 2003 revision of the U.S. Standard Certificate of Live Birth are excluded because maternal education data based on the 2003 revision are not comparable with data based on the 1989 or earlier revisions to the U.S. Standard Certificate of Live Birth. In 2003, Pennsylvania and Washington adopted the 2003 revision; in 2004, Florida, Idaho, Kentucky, New Hampshire, New York State (excluding New York City), South Carolina, and Tennessee adopted the 2003 revision. See Appendix II, Education.
[2]Data for 2003 are limited to the 43 reporting areas using the 1989 revision of the U.S. Standard Certificate of Live Birth in 2004, and are provided for comparison with 2004.
[3]Excludes live births with unknown birthweight. Percent based on live births with known birthweight.
[4]Starting with 2003 data, estimates are not shown for Asian or Pacific Islander subgroups during the transition from single race to multiple race reporting. See Appendix II, Race, Birth File.
[5]Prior to 1993, data shown only for states with an Hispanic-origin item and education of mother item on the birth certificate. See Appendix II, Education; Hispanic origin.

NOTES: Data are based on the 1989 or earlier revisions of the U.S. Standard Certificate of Live Birth. In 1992–2002, education of mother was reported on the birth certificate by all 50 states and the District of Columbia. Prior to 1992, data from states lacking an education of mother item were excluded. Starting with 2003 data, states adopting the 2003 revision of the U. S. Standard Certificate of Live Birth are excluded. See Appendix II, Education. The race groups, white, black, American Indian or Alaska Native, and Asian or Pacific Islander, include persons of Hispanic and non-Hispanic origin. Persons of Hispanic origin may be of any race. Starting with 2003 data, some states reported multiple-race data. The multiple-race data for these states were bridged to the single-race categories of the 1977 Office of Management and Budget standards for comparability with other states. See Appendix II, Race. Interpretation of trend data should take into consideration changes in reporting areas and immigration. Data for additional years are available. See Appendix III.

SOURCE: Centers for Disease Control and Prevention, National Center for Health Statistics, National Vital Statistics System, Birth File.

This table will be updated on the Web. Go to www.cdc.gov/nchs/hus.htm.

Table 15 (page 1 of 3). Low-birthweight live births, by race and Hispanic origin of mother, geographic division, and state: United States, average annual 1996–1998, 1999–2001, and 2002–2004

[Data are based on birth certificates]

Geographic division and state	All races			Not Hispanic or Latino: White			Not Hispanic or Latino: Black or African American		
	1996–1998	*1999–2001*	*2002–2004*	*1996–1998*	*1999–2001*	*2002–2004*	*1996–1998*	*1999–2001*	*2002–2004*
	Percent of live births weighing less than 2,500 grams[1]								
United States	7.49	7.62	7.94	6.46	6.67	7.05	13.13	13.14	13.56
New England	6.78	7.02	7.45	6.06	6.30	6.80	11.79	11.93	12.03
Connecticut	7.43	7.47	7.68	6.16	6.33	6.60	12.82	12.53	12.60
Maine	5.88	6.03	6.42	5.95	6.06	6.41	*13.27	*9.97	*8.57
Massachusetts	6.77	7.11	7.64	6.13	6.43	6.98	11.12	11.44	11.86
New Hampshire	5.44	6.36	6.44	5.31	6.04	6.51	*	11.88	10.19
Rhode Island	7.28	7.27	8.17	6.46	6.52	7.50	11.35	12.55	11.52
Vermont	6.32	5.90	6.63	6.22	5.79	6.67	*	*	*
Middle Atlantic	7.73	7.82	8.06	6.27	6.56	6.86	13.02	12.73	13.02
New Jersey	7.84	7.94	8.13	6.26	6.54	7.03	13.86	13.45	13.42
New York	7.77	7.75	7.98	6.19	6.47	6.68	12.32	11.97	12.50
Pennsylvania	7.57	7.84	8.14	6.36	6.68	6.97	13.86	13.87	13.86
East North Central	7.64	7.76	8.05	6.47	6.63	7.03	13.73	13.81	14.06
Illinois	7.96	7.99	8.28	6.44	6.59	7.13	14.22	14.03	14.45
Indiana	7.76	7.62	7.86	7.06	7.04	7.29	13.68	12.85	13.33
Michigan	7.72	7.95	8.17	6.35	6.43	6.90	13.51	14.47	14.21
Ohio	7.66	7.93	8.38	6.64	6.95	7.36	13.34	13.36	13.83
Wisconsin	6.40	6.59	6.80	5.58	5.82	6.06	13.21	13.28	13.49
West North Central	6.69	6.78	7.12	6.20	6.27	6.63	12.91	12.47	12.62
Iowa	6.38	6.23	6.74	6.11	5.97	6.57	12.66	12.58	11.50
Kansas	6.96	6.99	7.22	6.49	6.66	6.92	13.20	12.36	12.95
Minnesota	5.84	6.17	6.34	5.61	5.79	5.86	11.42	10.61	10.51
Missouri	7.68	7.64	8.10	6.65	6.68	7.18	13.48	13.22	13.76
Nebraska	6.60	6.73	7.04	6.32	6.37	6.86	11.58	12.81	12.32
North Dakota	6.15	6.26	6.46	6.17	6.23	6.26	*11.69	*	*10.25
South Dakota	5.73	6.15	6.90	5.72	6.02	6.74	*10.36	*11.42	*8.08
South Atlantic	8.45	8.57	8.87	6.75	7.00	7.38	13.09	13.07	13.51
Delaware	8.54	8.84	9.45	6.50	7.28	7.85	14.41	13.71	14.36
District of Columbia	13.60	12.37	11.19	6.15	6.56	5.91	16.28	15.17	14.09
Florida	7.98	8.10	8.49	6.77	6.92	7.29	12.30	12.42	13.02
Georgia	8.62	8.72	9.08	6.58	6.85	7.29	12.83	12.82	13.42
Maryland	8.68	8.88	9.13	6.39	6.70	7.14	13.37	13.12	13.16
North Carolina	8.80	8.87	9.00	7.08	7.39	7.64	13.82	13.72	14.16
South Carolina	9.30	9.69	10.08	6.99	7.30	7.77	13.60	14.29	15.01
Virginia	7.77	7.85	8.13	6.28	6.52	6.80	12.49	12.39	12.82
West Virginia	8.10	8.28	8.96	7.95	8.11	8.80	12.94	13.20	13.52
East South Central	8.98	9.32	9.71	7.42	7.77	8.21	13.48	13.97	14.71
Alabama	9.26	9.56	10.09	7.33	7.58	8.18	13.34	13.87	14.63
Kentucky	7.94	8.26	8.69	7.49	7.73	8.25	12.73	13.69	13.82
Mississippi	10.03	10.55	11.40	7.34	7.72	8.50	13.31	14.03	15.31
Tennessee	8.89	9.21	9.23	7.46	7.96	8.08	14.07	14.12	14.37
West South Central	7.77	7.90	8.30	6.73	6.95	7.43	13.29	13.42	14.04
Arkansas	8.57	8.66	8.92	7.31	7.48	7.78	13.41	13.60	14.54
Louisiana	10.05	10.25	10.69	6.98	7.36	7.76	14.49	14.40	14.91
Oklahoma	7.27	7.55	7.92	6.80	7.23	7.63	12.63	12.93	13.48
Texas	7.30	7.43	7.88	6.54	6.68	7.23	12.51	12.76	13.45
Mountain	7.34	7.34	7.56	7.08	7.08	7.32	13.70	13.37	13.68
Arizona	6.80	6.95	7.00	6.63	6.73	6.94	12.88	13.19	12.09
Colorado	8.75	8.43	8.94	8.34	8.02	8.71	14.48	14.39	14.98
Idaho	6.02	6.43	6.48	5.84	6.31	6.39	*	*	*8.87
Montana	6.56	6.65	7.10	6.28	6.69	6.94	*	*	*15.63
Nevada	7.57	7.45	7.86	7.28	7.38	7.51	13.78	12.69	13.87
New Mexico	7.63	7.87	8.21	7.68	7.85	8.01	13.46	13.37	14.99
Utah	6.65	6.60	6.55	6.44	6.43	6.32	15.06	12.49	13.76
Wyoming	8.76	8.32	8.67	8.69	8.15	8.57	*15.82	*14.29	*
Pacific	6.07	6.13	6.50	5.47	5.59	5.98	11.73	11.56	11.96
Alaska	5.78	5.70	5.93	5.30	5.03	4.98	12.00	10.64	9.52
California	6.15	6.20	6.56	5.61	5.72	6.13	11.90	11.73	12.14
Hawaii	7.34	7.74	8.26	5.35	5.60	6.47	9.79	10.77	11.47
Oregon	5.39	5.52	5.99	5.14	5.32	5.92	10.71	10.64	10.67
Washington	5.63	5.74	6.04	5.25	5.40	5.61	10.32	10.30	10.83

See footnotes at end of table.

This table will be updated on the Web. Go to www.cdc.gov/nchs/hus.htm.

Table 15 (page 2 of 3). Low-birthweight live births, by race and Hispanic origin of mother, geographic division, and state: United States, average annual 1996–1998, 1999–2001, and 2002–2004

[Data are based on birth certificates]

Geographic division and state	Hispanic or Latino[2]			American Indian or Alaska Native[3]			Asian or Pacific Islander[3]		
	1996–1998	1999–2001	2002–2004	1996–1998	1999–2001	2002–2004	1996–1998	1999–2001	2002–2004
	Percent of live births weighing less than 2,500 grams[1]								
United States	6.38	6.42	6.68	6.69	7.08	7.35	7.24	7.42	7.82
New England	8.28	8.17	8.31	8.17	7.54	8.18	7.19	7.39	7.83
Connecticut	8.94	8.60	8.41	*10.94	*8.09	8.97	7.73	7.59	7.96
Maine	*5.74	*4.91	*5.46	*	*	*	*5.03	*5.42	7.85
Massachusetts	8.03	8.28	8.46	*6.37	*6.84	*6.13	6.95	7.38	7.66
New Hampshire	*6.48	5.89	5.35	*	*	*	*8.30	5.83	6.08
Rhode Island	7.68	7.07	8.24	*10.49	*10.67	12.37	8.30	8.78	10.83
Vermont	*	*	*	*	*	*	*	*	*6.52
Middle Atlantic	7.71	7.49	7.59	8.21	8.96	8.60	7.32	7.38	7.85
New Jersey	7.30	7.19	7.22	12.20	10.04	10.67	7.52	7.67	7.86
New York	7.65	7.41	7.48	7.40	8.44	6.84	7.24	7.24	7.84
Pennsylvania	9.34	8.95	9.11	7.31	9.41	11.03	7.26	7.38	7.91
East North Central	6.33	6.40	6.42	6.51	7.04	7.24	7.52	7.85	8.17
Illinois	6.11	6.38	6.41	7.70	9.05	8.63	8.02	8.37	8.23
Indiana	7.00	6.10	6.19	*10.98	*6.89	*9.54	6.50	7.42	7.59
Michigan	6.48	6.37	6.41	6.12	7.24	6.50	7.25	7.72	8.22
Ohio	7.38	7.23	7.18	7.20	8.39	10.04	7.43	7.36	8.67
Wisconsin	6.56	6.29	6.10	5.71	5.97	6.29	6.81	7.02	7.45
West North Central	6.09	6.06	6.12	6.12	6.65	7.17	7.04	7.42	7.51
Iowa	6.21	5.83	6.16	8.48	*7.36	8.72	7.63	7.72	7.11
Kansas	5.95	6.00	6.14	6.40	6.36	7.08	7.49	7.34	7.15
Minnesota	6.13	5.98	5.85	6.21	6.92	7.18	6.66	7.48	7.41
Missouri	6.24	5.98	6.39	7.87	8.95	6.53	7.18	6.89	7.83
Nebraska	6.08	6.49	6.05	6.36	6.32	7.11	7.94	7.91	7.70
North Dakota	*5.88	*6.89	*6.42	5.66	6.21	7.15	*	*	*6.56
South Dakota	*6.14	*6.07	7.12	5.58	6.25	7.14	*	*9.37	*12.89
South Atlantic	6.37	6.30	6.61	9.00	9.22	9.86	7.54	7.75	8.16
Delaware	7.76	6.62	7.06	*	*	*	8.04	8.98	9.61
District of Columbia	6.73	6.99	8.20	*	*	*	*8.43	*8.79	7.36
Florida	6.55	6.49	6.90	7.35	7.08	7.68	7.98	8.51	8.57
Georgia	5.36	5.66	5.94	*7.21	9.79	8.48	7.51	7.67	8.40
Maryland	6.29	6.80	7.09	*8.48	9.95	11.07	7.15	7.37	7.67
North Carolina	6.14	6.21	6.22	10.22	10.33	11.16	7.61	8.05	7.79
South Carolina	5.99	6.57	6.46	*9.40	10.20	*9.11	7.56	7.10	8.97
Virginia	6.68	5.96	6.31	*6.94	*9.23	*10.13	7.30	7.15	7.95
West Virginia	*	*	*8.26	*	*	*	*6.58	*7.94	*8.24
East South Central	6.53	6.73	6.51	7.73	7.61	8.12	7.60	7.84	7.99
Alabama	6.51	6.68	6.93	*7.60	*8.25	11.50	7.94	7.59	8.52
Kentucky	7.14	7.18	7.13	*10.38	*	*9.93	6.78	7.68	7.35
Mississippi	5.26	6.92	6.79	*6.59	8.42	6.00	6.00	7.75	7.58
Tennessee	6.56	6.57	5.97	*7.88	*7.13	*7.43	8.40	8.03	8.22
West South Central	6.61	6.73	7.05	6.20	6.57	6.96	7.50	7.75	8.09
Arkansas	6.34	5.92	5.96	*5.97	7.95	8.41	7.40	8.80	6.78
Louisiana	6.04	6.70	7.25	8.02	8.41	10.31	8.37	7.92	8.55
Oklahoma	6.13	6.03	6.55	6.07	6.34	6.53	7.02	7.19	7.13
Texas	6.63	6.76	7.08	6.34	6.76	7.54	7.45	7.74	8.19
Mountain	7.22	7.21	7.35	6.72	7.14	7.28	8.57	8.33	8.87
Arizona	6.52	6.67	6.67	6.57	7.12	6.84	7.54	7.69	8.20
Colorado	8.71	8.23	8.46	8.16	8.60	9.82	9.92	10.10	10.14
Idaho	6.95	6.78	6.73	7.07	7.82	7.07	*5.97	7.62	6.51
Montana	7.69	7.02	8.11	7.43	6.77	7.71	*8.97	*6.42	*8.76
Nevada	6.26	6.21	6.61	6.23	7.80	6.73	9.17	7.88	9.41
New Mexico	7.69	7.93	8.38	6.27	6.88	7.18	9.26	8.28	7.62
Utah	7.55	7.33	7.06	7.44	6.58	7.64	7.50	7.18	7.94
Wyoming	8.33	7.86	8.60	7.51	8.93	10.62	*	*17.06	*
Pacific	5.55	5.59	5.94	6.10	6.38	6.59	6.95	7.10	7.49
Alaska	6.48	6.09	5.62	5.73	5.83	6.08	6.43	7.05	6.79
California	5.53	5.59	5.95	5.85	6.27	6.54	6.84	6.98	7.33
Hawaii	7.08	7.63	8.41	*7.37	*6.11	*	7.95	8.29	8.79
Oregon	5.72	5.51	5.28	5.72	6.79	7.35	6.45	6.08	7.12
Washington	5.53	5.31	5.67	7.09	7.14	7.03	6.12	6.41	6.88

See footnotes at end of table.

This table will be updated on the Web. Go to www.cdc.gov/nchs/hus.htm.

[Data are based on birth certificates]

* Percents preceded by an asterisk are based on fewer than 50 births. Percents not shown are based on fewer than 20 births.
[1]Excludes live births with unknown birthweight.
[2]Persons of Hispanic origin may be of any race. See Appendix II, Hispanic origin.
[3]Includes persons of Hispanic and non-Hispanic origin.

NOTES: For information on very low birthweight live births, see Table 36 in Martin JA, Hamilton BE, Sutton PD, Ventura SJ, Menacker F, Kirmeyer S. Births: Final Data for 2004. National vital statistics reports. Hyattsville, MD: National Center for Health Statistics. 2006. Starting with 2003 data, some states reported multiple-race data. The multiple-race data for these states were bridged to the single-race categories of the 1977 Office of Management and Budget standards for comparability with other states. See Appendix II, Race.

SOURCE: Centers for Disease Control and Prevention, National Center for Health Statistics, National Vital Statistics System, Birth File.

This table will be updated on the Web. Go to www.cdc.gov/nchs/hus.htm.

Table 16 (page 1 of 2). Legal abortions and legal abortion ratios, by selected patient characteristics: United States, selected years 1973–2003

[Data are based on reporting by state health departments and by hospitals and other medical facilities]

Characteristic	*1973*	*1975*	*1980*	*1985*	*1990*	*1995*	*1999*[1]	*2000*[2]	*2001*[2]	*2002*[2]	*2003*[3]
	Number of legal abortions reported in thousands										
Centers for Disease Control and Prevention	616	855	1,298	1,329	1,429	1,211	862	857	853	854	848
Alan Guttmacher Institute[4]	745	1,034	1,554	1,589	1,609	1,359	1,315	1,313	1,303	1,293	1,287
	Abortions per 100 live births[5]										
Total	19.6	27.2	35.9	35.4	34.4	31.1	25.6	24.5	24.6	24.6	24.1
Age											
Under 15 years	123.7	119.3	139.7	137.6	81.8	66.4	70.9	70.8	74.4	75.3	83.0
15–19 years	53.9	54.2	71.4	68.8	51.1	39.9	37.5	36.1	36.6	36.8	37.4
20–24 years	29.4	28.9	39.5	38.6	37.8	34.8	31.6	30.0	30.4	30.3	30.0
25–29 years	20.7	19.2	23.7	21.7	21.8	22.0	20.8	19.8	20.0	20.0	19.5
30–34 years	28.0	25.0	23.7	19.9	19.0	16.4	15.2	14.5	14.7	14.8	14.4
35–39 years	45.1	42.2	41.0	33.6	27.3	22.3	19.3	18.1	18.0	18.0	17.3
40 years and over	68.4	66.8	80.7	62.3	50.6	38.5	32.9	30.1	30.4	31.0	29.3
Race											
White[6]	32.6	27.7	33.2	27.7	25.8	20.3	17.7	16.7	16.5	16.4	16.5
Black or African American[7]	42.0	47.6	54.3	47.2	53.7	53.1	52.9	50.3	49.1	49.5	49.1
Hispanic origin[8]											
Hispanic or Latino	---	---	---	---	---	27.1	26.1	22.5	23.0	23.3	22.8
Not Hispanic or Latino	---	---	---	---	---	27.9	25.2	23.3	23.2	23.7	23.4
Marital status											
Married	7.6	9.6	10.5	8.0	8.7	7.6	7.0	6.5	6.5	6.5	6.3
Unmarried	139.8	161.0	147.6	117.4	86.3	64.5	60.4	57.0	57.2	57.0	53.8
Previous live births[9]											
0	43.7	38.4	45.7	45.1	36.0	28.6	24.3	22.6	26.4	23.3	22.7
1	23.5	22.0	20.2	21.6	22.7	22.0	20.6	19.4	18.0	19.4	19.0
2	36.8	36.8	29.5	29.9	31.5	30.6	29.0	27.4	25.5	27.9	27.1
3	46.9	47.7	29.8	18.2	30.1	30.7	29.8	28.5	26.4	29.1	28.3
4 or more[10]	44.7	43.5	24.3	21.5	26.6	23.7	24.2	23.7	21.9	23.6	23.4
	Percent distribution[11]										
Total	100.0	100.0	100.0	100.0	100.0	100.0	100.0	100.0	100.0	100.0	100.0
Period of gestation											
Under 9 weeks	36.1	44.6	51.7	50.3	51.6	54.0	57.6	58.1	59.1	60.5	60.5
9–10 weeks	29.4	28.4	26.2	26.6	25.3	23.1	20.2	19.8	19.0	18.4	18.0
11–12 weeks	17.9	14.9	12.2	12.5	11.7	10.9	10.2	10.2	10.0	9.6	9.7
13–15 weeks	6.9	5.0	5.1	5.9	6.4	6.3	6.2	6.2	6.2	6.0	6.2
16–20 weeks	8.0	6.1	3.9	3.9	4.0	4.3	4.3	4.3	4.3	4.1	4.2
21 weeks and over	1.7	1.0	0.9	0.8	1.0	1.4	1.5	1.4	1.4	1.4	1.4
Previous induced abortions											
0	—	81.9	67.6	60.1	57.1	55.1	53.7	54.7	55.5	55.3	55.3
1	—	14.9	23.5	25.7	26.9	26.9	27.1	26.4	25.8	25.8	25.7
2	—	2.5	6.6	9.8	10.1	10.9	11.5	11.3	11.0	11.3	11.2
3 or more	---	0.7	2.3	4.4	5.9	7.1	7.7	7.6	7.7	7.6	7.8

See footnotes at end of table.

This table will be updated on the Web. Go to www.cdc.gov/nchs/hus.htm.

Table 16 (page 2 of 2). Legal abortions and legal abortion ratios, by selected patient characteristics: United States, selected years 1973–2003

[Data are based on reporting by state health departments and by hospitals and other medical facilities]

- - - Data not available.
[1]In 1998 and 1999, Alaska, California, New Hampshire, and Oklahoma did not report abortion data to CDC. For comparison, in 1997, the 48 corresponding reporting areas reported about 900,000 legal abortions.
[2]In 2000, 2001, and 2002, Alaska, California, and New Hampshire did not report abortion data to CDC.
[3]In 2003, California, New Hampshire, and West Virginia did not report abortion data to CDC.
[4]No surveys were conducted in 1983, 1986, 1989, 1990, 1993, 1994, 1997, 1998, 2001, 2002, or 2003. Data for these years were estimated by interpolation.
[5]For calculation of ratios by each characteristic, abortions with characteristic unknown were distributed in proportion to abortions with characteristic known.
[6]For 1989 and later years, white race includes women of Hispanic ethnicity.
[7]Before 1989, black race includes races other than white.
[8]Reporting area increased from 20–22 states, the District of Columbia (DC), and New York City (NYC) in 1991–1995 to 27 states, DC, and NYC, with 12 additional states reporting to CDC, but with more than 15% unknowns, and thus excluded from analysis, for 2002 and 2003. California, Florida, Illinois, and Arizona, states with large Hispanic populations, do not report Hispanic ethnicity.
[9]For 1973–1975, data indicate number of living children.
[10]For 1975, data refer to four previous live births, not four or more. For five or more previous live births, the ratio is 47.3.
[11]For calculation of percent distribution by each characteristic, abortions with characteristic unknown were excluded.

NOTES: The number of areas reporting adequate data (less than or equal to 15% missing) for each characteristic varies from year to year. See Appendix I, Abortion Surveillance. For methodological differences between these two data sources, see Appendix I, Abortion Surveillance; Alan Guttmacher Institute Abortion Provider Survey. Data for additional years are available. See Appendix III.

SOURCES: Centers for Disease Control and Prevention, National Center for Chronic Disease Prevention and Health Promotion: Abortion Surveillance, 1973, 1975, 1979–1980. Atlanta, GA: Public Health Service, 1975, 1977, 1983; CDC MMWR Surveillance Summaries. Abortion Surveillance, United States, 1984 and 1985, Vol. 38, No. SS–2, 1989; 1990, Vol. 42, No. SS–6, 1993; 1995, Vol. 47, No. SS–2, 1998; 1997, Vol. 49, No. SS–11, 2000; 1998, Vol. 51, No. SS–3, 2002; 1999, Vol. 51, No. SS–9, 2002; 2000, Vol. 52, No. SS–12, 2003; 2001, Vol. 53, No. SS–9, 2004; 2002, Vol. 54, No. SS–7, 2005; 2003, Vol. 55, No. SS–11. Alan Guttmacher Institute Abortion Provider Survey. Finer LB, Henshaw SK. Abortion incidence and services in the United States in 2000. Perspect Sex Reprod Health 2003;35(1)6–15. Finer LB, Henshaw SK. Estimates of U.S. abortion incidence, 2001–2003. The Alan Guttmacher Institute. August 2006, available from: www.guttmacher.org/pubs/2006/08/03/ab_incidence.pdf.

This table will be updated on the Web. Go to www.cdc.gov/nchs/hus.htm.

Table 17 (page 1 of 4). Contraceptive use in the past month among women 15–44 years of age, by age, race, Hispanic origin, and method of contraception: United States, selected years 1982–2002

[Data are based on household interviews of samples of women of childbearing age]

Race, Hispanic origin, and year[1]	15–44	15–19	20–24	25–34	35–44
	Number of women in population in thousands				
All women:[2]					
1982	54,099	9,521	10,629	19,644	14,305
1988	57,900	9,179	9,413	21,726	17,582
1995	60,201	8,961	9,041	20,758	21,440
2002	61,561	9,834	9,840	19,522	22,365
Not Hispanic or Latino:					
White only:					
1982	41,279	7,010	8,081	14,945	11,243
1988	42,575	6,531	6,630	15,929	13,486
1995	42,154	5,865	6,020	14,471	15,798
2002	39,498	6,069	5,938	12,073	15,418
Black or African American only:					
1982	6,825	1,383	1,456	2,392	1,593
1988	7,408	1,362	1,322	2,760	1,965
1995	8,060	1,334	1,305	2,780	2,641
2002	8,250	1,409	1,396	2,587	2,857
Hispanic or Latino:[3]					
1982	4,393	886	811	1,677	1,018
1988	5,557	999	1,003	2,104	1,451
1995	6,702	1,150	1,163	2,450	1,940
2002	9,107	1,521	1,632	3,249	2,705
	Percent of women in population using contraception				
All women:[2]					
1982	55.7	24.2	55.8	66.7	61.6
1988	60.3	32.1	59.0	66.3	68.3
1995	64.2	29.8	63.5	71.1	72.3
2002	61.9	31.5	60.7	68.6	69.9
Not Hispanic or Latino:					
White only:					
1982	57.3	23.6	58.7	67.8	63.5
1988	63.0	34.0	62.6	67.7	71.5
1995	66.2	30.5	65.4	72.9	73.6
2002	64.6	35.0	66.3	69.9	71.4
Black or African American only:					
1982	51.6	29.8	52.3	63.5	52.0
1988	56.8	35.7	61.8	63.5	58.7
1995	62.3	36.1	67.6	66.8	68.3
2002	57.6	32.9	50.8	67.9	63.8
Hispanic or Latino:[3]					
1982	50.6	*	*36.8	67.2	59.0
1988	50.4	*18.3	40.8	67.4	54.3
1995	59.0	26.1	50.6	69.2	70.8
2002	59.0	20.4	57.4	66.2	72.9

See footnotes at end of table.

Table 17 (page 2 of 4). Contraceptive use in the past month among women 15–44 years of age, by age, race, Hispanic origin, and method of contraception: United States, selected years 1982–2002

[Data are based on household interviews of samples of women of childbearing age]

Method of contraception and year	Age in years				
	15–44	15–19	20–24	25–34	35–44
	Percent of contracepting women				
Female sterilization					
1982	23.2	–	*4.5	22.1	43.5
1988	27.6	*	*4.6	25.0	47.6
1995	27.8	*	4.0	23.8	45.0
2002	27.0	–	3.6	21.7	45.8
Male sterilization					
1982	10.9	*	*3.6	10.1	19.9
1988	11.7	*	*	10.2	20.8
1995	10.9	–	*	7.8	19.5
2002	10.2	–	*	7.2	18.2
Implant[4]					
1982	. . .	. . .	. . .	. . .	. . .
1988	. . .	. . .	. . .	. . .	. . .
1995	1.3	*	3.7	*1.3	*
2002	1.2	*	*	*1.9	*
Injectable[4]					
1982	. . .	. . .	. . .	. . .	. . .
1988	. . .	. . .	. . .	. . .	. . .
1995	3.0	9.7	6.1	2.9	*0.8
2002	5.4	13.9	10.2	5.3	*1.8
Birth control pill					
1982	28.0	63.9	55.1	25.7	*3.7
1988	30.8	58.8	68.2	32.6	4.3
1995	27.0	43.8	52.1	33.4	8.7
2002	31.0	53.8	52.5	34.8	15.0
Intrauterine device					
1982	7.1	*	*4.2	9.7	6.9
1988	2.0	–	*	2.1	3.1
1995	0.8	–	*	*0.8	1.1
2002	2.2	*	1.8	3.7	*
Diaphragm					
1982	8.1	*6.0	10.2	10.3	4.0
1988	5.7	*	*3.7	7.3	6.0
1995	1.9	*	*	1.7	2.8
2002	0.6	–	*	*	*
Condom					
1982	12.0	20.8	10.7	11.4	11.3
1988	14.6	32.8	14.5	13.7	11.2
1995	23.4	45.8	33.7	23.7	15.3
2002	23.8	44.6	36.0	23.1	15.6
Periodic abstinence-calendar rhythm					
1982	3.3	2.0	3.1	3.3	3.7
1988	1.7	*	1.1	1.8	2.0
1995	3.3	*	*1.5	3.7	3.9
2002	2.0	*	*2.3	*1.7	*2.4
Periodic abstinence-natural family planning					
1982	0.6	–	*	0.9	*
1988	0.6	–	*	0.7	0.7
1995	*0.5	–	*	*0.7	*
2002	*0.4	–	-	*	*
Withdrawal					
1982	2.0	2.9	3.0	1.8	1.3
1988	2.2	3.0	3.4	2.8	0.8
1995	6.1	13.2	7.1	6.0	4.5
2002	8.8	15.0	11.9	10.7	4.7
Other methods[5]					
1982	4.9	2.6	5.4	4.8	5.3
1988	3.2	*	1.8	3.8	3.5
1995	3.2	*	3.2	3.1	3.4
2002	1.7	*	*	*1.5	*1.8

See footnotes at end of table.

Table 17 (page 3 of 4). Contraceptive use in the past month among women 15–44 years of age, by age, race, Hispanic origin, and method of contraception: United States, selected years 1982–2002

[Data are based on household interviews of samples of women of childbearing age]

Method of contraception and year	Not Hispanic or Latino[1]		Hispanic or Latino[3]
	White only	Black or African American only	
	Percent of contracepting women		
Female sterilization			
1982	22.0	30.0	23.0
1988	25.6	37.8	31.7
1995	24.5	39.9	36.6
2002	23.9	39.2	33.8
Male sterilization			
1982	13.0	*1.5	*
1988	14.3	*0.9	*
1995	13.7	*1.8	*4.0
2002	12.9	*	4.7
Implant[4]			
1982	. . .	. . .	. . .
1988	. . .	. . .	. . .
1995	*1.0	*2.4	*2.0
2002	*0.8	*	*3.1
Injectable[4]			
1982	. . .	. . .	. . .
1988	. . .	. . .	. . .
1995	2.4	5.4	4.7
2002	4.2	9.4	7.3
Birth control pill			
1982	26.4	37.9	30.2
1988	29.5	38.2	33.4
1995	28.7	23.7	23.0
2002	34.9	23.1	22.1
Intrauterine device			
1982	5.8	9.3	19.2
1988	1.5	3.2	*5.0
1995	0.7	*	*
2002	1.7	*	5.3
Diaphragm			
1982	9.2	*3.2	*
1988	6.6	*2.0	*
1995	2.3	*	*
2002	*	*	–
Condom			
1982	13.1	6.3	*6.9
1988	15.2	10.1	13.7
1995	22.5	24.9	21.2
2002	21.7	29.6	24.1
Periodic abstinence-calendar rhythm			
1982	3.2	2.9	3.9
1988	1.6	1.9	*
1995	3.3	*1.7	3.2
2002	2.3	*	*
Periodic abstinence-natural family planning			
1982	0.7	0.3	–
1988	0.7	*	*
1995	0.7	*	*
2002	*	*	*
Withdrawal			
1982	2.1	1.3	2.6
1988	2.0	1.4	4.5
1995	6.4	3.3	5.7
2002	9.5	4.9	6.3
Other methods[5]			
1982	4.6	7.3	5.0
1988	3.0	4.4	2.6
1995	3.3	3.8	*2.2
2002	*1.7	*1.9	*1.2

See footnotes at end of table.

Table 17 (page 4 of 4). Contraceptive use in the past month among women 15–44 years of age, by age, race, Hispanic origin, and method of contraception: United States, selected years 1982–2002

[Data are based on household interviews of samples of women of childbearing age]

– Quantity zero.
- - - Data not available.
. . . Data not applicable.
* Estimates are considered unreliable. Data preceded by an asterisk have a relative standard error of 20%–30%. Data not shown have an RSE greater than 30%.
[1]Starting with 1995 data, race-specific estimates are tabulated according to 1997 Revisions to the Standards for the Classification of Federal Data on Race and Ethnicity and are not strictly comparable with estimates for earlier years. Starting with 1995 data, race-specific estimates are for persons who reported only one racial group. Prior to data year 1995, data were tabulated according to the 1977 Standards. Estimates for single-race categories prior to 1995 included persons who reported one race or, if they reported more than one race, identified one race as best representing their race. See Appendix II, Race.
[2]Includes women of other or unknown race not shown separately.
[3]Persons of Hispanic origin may be of any race. See Appendix II, Hispanic origin.
[4]Data collected starting with the 1995 survey.
[5]In 2002, includes female condom, foam, cervical cap, Today Sponge®, suppository or insert, jelly or cream, and other methods. See Appendix II, Contraception, for the list of other methods reported in previous surveys.

NOTES: Survey collects up to four methods of contraception used in the month of interview. Percents may not add to the total because more than one method could have been used in the month of interview. These data replace estimates of most effective method used and may differ from previous editions of *Health, United States*. Standard errors for selected years are available in the spreadsheet version of this table. Available from: www.cdc.gov/nchs/hus.htm.

SOURCE: Centers for Disease Control and Prevention, National Center for Health Statistics, National Survey of Family Growth.

Table 18. Breastfeeding among mothers 15–44 years of age, by year of baby's birth, and selected characteristics of mother: United States, average annual 1986–1988 through 1999–2001

[Data are based on household interviews of samples of women of childbearing age]

Selected characteristics of mother	*1986–1988*	*1989–1991*	*1992–1994*	*1995–1998*	*1999–2001*
			Percent of babies breastfed		
Total	54.1	53.3	57.6	64.4	66.5
Age at baby's birth					
Under 20 years	28.4	34.7	41.0	49.5	47.3
20–24 years	48.2	44.3	50.0	55.9	59.3
25–29 years	58.2	56.4	57.4	68.1	63.5
30–44 years	68.6	66.0	70.2	72.8	80.0
Race and Hispanic origin[1]					
Not Hispanic or Latino:					
White	59.1	58.4	61.7	66.5	68.7
Black or African American	22.3	22.4	26.1	47.9	45.3
Hispanic or Latino	55.6	57.0	63.8	71.2	76.0
Education[2]					
No high school diploma or GED	31.8	36.5	44.6	50.6	46.6
High school diploma or GED	47.4	45.5	51.1	55.9	61.6
Some college, no bachelor's degree	62.2	61.4	64.3	70.1	75.6
Bachelor's degree or higher	78.4	80.6	82.5	82.0	81.3
Geographic region[3]					
Northeast	51.3	53.5	56.5	61.6	66.9
Midwest	52.3	49.6	51.7	61.7	61.9
South	44.6	43.6	48.6	58.1	60.9
West	71.4	69.5	77.3	78.1	78.9
			Percent of babies who were breastfed 3 months or more		
Total	34.6	31.8	33.6	45.8	48.4
Age at baby's birth					
Under 20 years	18.5	*10.5	*11.7	30.0	30.0
20–24 years	26.1	24.1	25.1	36.6	41.8
25–29 years	36.9	32.3	35.6	46.3	43.7
30–44 years	50.1	46.8	46.7	57.5	62.4
Race and Hispanic origin[1]					
Not Hispanic or Latino:					
White	37.7	35.2	36.6	47.8	49.7
Black or African American	11.6	11.5	13.3	29.6	33.7
Hispanic or Latino	38.2	33.9	35.0	49.7	54.3
Education[2]					
No high school diploma or GED	21.8	17.6	25.2	33.9	37.0
High school diploma or GED	28.2	28.0	27.4	36.9	43.1
Some college, no bachelor's degree	38.7	33.1	38.7	49.6	52.8
Bachelor's degree or higher	55.0	56.1	59.3	64.5	64.1
Geographic region[3]					
Northeast	29.9	37.2	36.4	48.2	48.8
Midwest	30.3	31.5	30.1	42.0	42.8
South	27.7	20.1	26.2	38.9	44.4
West	52.4	42.9	45.3	58.2	59.2

* Estimates are considered unreliable. Data preceded by an asterisk have a relative standard error of 20%–30%.

[1] Persons of Hispanic origin may be of any race. All race-specific estimates are tabulated according to the 1997 Revisions to the Standards for the Classification of Federal Data on Race and Ethnicity and are for persons who reported only one racial group. See Appendix II, Race.

[2] Educational attainment is presented only for women 22–44 years of age. Education is as of year of interview. GED stands for General Educational Development high school equivalency diploma. See Appendix II, Education.

[3] See Appendix II, Geographic region and division.

NOTES: Data are based on single births to mothers 15–44 years of age at interview, including those births that occurred when the mothers were younger than 15 years of age. Data on breastfeeding during 1986–1994 are based on responses to questions in the National Survey of Family Growth (NSFG) Cycle 5, conducted in 1995. Data for 1995–2001 are based on the NSFG Cycle 6 conducted in 2002. See Appendix I, National Survey of Family Growth. Standard errors are available in the spreadsheet version of this table. Available from: www.cdc.gov/nchs/hus.htm. Data for additional years are available. See Appendix III.

SOURCE: Centers for Disease Control and Prevention, National Center for Health Statistics, National Survey of Family Growth, Cycle 5 (1995), Cycle 6 (2002).

Table 19 (page 1 of 3). Infant, neonatal, and postneonatal mortality rates, by detailed race and Hispanic origin of mother: United States, selected years 1983–2004

[Data are based on linked birth and death certificates for infants]

Race and Hispanic origin of mother	1983[1]	1985[1]	1990[1]	1995[2]	2000[2]	2002[2]	2003[2]	2004[2]
				Infant[3] deaths per 1,000 live births				
All mothers	10.9	10.4	8.9	7.6	6.9	7.0	6.8	6.8
White	9.3	8.9	7.3	6.3	5.7	5.8	5.7	5.7
Black or African American	19.2	18.6	16.9	14.6	13.5	13.8	13.5	13.2
American Indian or Alaska Native	15.2	13.1	13.1	9.0	8.3	8.6	8.7	8.4
Asian or Pacific Islander[4]	8.3	7.8	6.6	5.3	4.9	4.8	4.8	4.7
Chinese	9.5	5.8	4.3	3.8	3.5	3.0	- - -	- - -
Japanese	*5.6	*6.0	*5.5	*5.3	*4.5	*4.9	- - -	- - -
Filipino	8.4	7.7	6.0	5.6	5.7	5.7	- - -	- - -
Hawaiian	11.2	*9.9	*8.0	*6.5	9.0	9.6	- - -	- - -
Other Asian or Pacific Islander	8.1	8.5	7.4	5.5	4.8	4.7	- - -	- - -
Hispanic or Latino[5,6]	9.5	8.8	7.5	6.3	5.6	5.6	5.6	5.5
Mexican	9.1	8.5	7.2	6.0	5.4	5.4	5.5	5.5
Puerto Rican	12.9	11.2	9.9	8.9	8.2	8.2	8.2	7.8
Cuban	7.5	8.5	7.2	5.3	4.6	3.7	4.6	4.6
Central and South American	8.5	8.0	6.8	5.5	4.6	5.1	5.0	4.6
Other and unknown Hispanic or Latino	10.6	9.5	8.0	7.4	6.9	7.1	6.7	6.7
Not Hispanic or Latino:								
White[6]	9.2	8.6	7.2	6.3	5.7	5.8	5.7	5.7
Black or African American[6]	19.1	18.3	16.9	14.7	13.6	13.9	13.6	13.6
				Neonatal[3] deaths per 1,000 live births				
All mothers	7.1	6.8	5.7	4.9	4.6	4.7	4.6	4.5
White	6.1	5.8	4.6	4.1	3.8	3.9	3.9	3.8
Black or African American	12.5	12.3	11.1	9.6	9.1	9.3	9.2	8.9
American Indian or Alaska Native	7.5	6.1	6.1	4.0	4.4	4.6	4.5	4.3
Asian or Pacific Islander[4]	5.2	4.8	3.9	3.4	3.4	3.4	3.4	3.2
Chinese	5.5	3.3	2.3	2.3	2.5	2.4	- - -	- - -
Japanese	*3.7	*3.1	*3.5	*3.3	*2.6	*3.7	- - -	- - -
Filipino	5.6	5.1	3.5	3.4	4.1	4.1	- - -	- - -
Hawaiian	*7.0	*5.7	*4.3	*4.0	*6.2	*5.6	- - -	- - -
Other Asian or Pacific Islander	5.0	5.4	4.4	3.7	3.4	3.3	- - -	- - -
Hispanic or Latino[5,6]	6.2	5.7	4.8	4.1	3.8	3.8	3.9	3.8
Mexican	5.9	5.4	4.5	3.9	3.6	3.6	3.8	3.7
Puerto Rican	8.7	7.6	6.9	6.1	5.8	5.8	5.7	5.3
Cuban	*5.0	6.2	5.3	*3.6	*3.2	*3.2	3.4	*2.8
Central and South American	5.8	5.6	4.4	3.7	3.3	3.5	3.6	3.4
Other and unknown Hispanic or Latino	6.4	5.6	5.0	4.8	4.6	5.1	4.7	4.7
Not Hispanic or Latino:								
White[6]	5.9	5.6	4.5	4.0	3.8	3.9	3.8	3.7
Black or African American[6]	12.0	11.9	11.0	9.6	9.2	9.3	9.3	9.1
				Postneonatal[3] deaths per 1,000 live births				
All mothers	3.8	3.6	3.2	2.6	2.3	2.3	2.2	2.3
White	3.2	3.1	2.7	2.2	1.9	1.9	1.9	1.9
Black or African American	6.7	6.3	5.9	5.0	4.3	4.5	4.3	4.3
American Indian or Alaska Native	7.7	7.0	7.0	5.1	3.9	4.0	4.2	4.2
Asian or Pacific Islander[4]	3.1	2.9	2.7	1.9	1.4	1.4	1.4	1.5
Chinese	4.0	*2.5	*2.0	*1.5	*1.0	*0.7	- - -	- - -
Japanese	*	*2.9	*	*	*	*	- - -	- - -
Filipino	*2.8	2.7	2.5	2.2	1.6	1.7	- - -	- - -
Hawaiian	*4.2	*4.3	*3.8	*	*	*4.0	- - -	- - -
Other Asian or Pacific Islander	3.0	3.0	3.0	1.9	1.4	1.4	- - -	- - -
Hispanic or Latino[5,6]	3.3	3.2	2.7	2.1	1.8	1.8	1.7	1.7
Mexican	3.2	3.2	2.7	2.1	1.8	1.8	1.7	1.7
Puerto Rican	4.2	3.5	3.0	2.8	2.4	2.4	2.5	2.5
Cuban	*2.5	*2.3	*1.9	*1.7	*	*	*	*1.7
Central and South American	2.6	2.4	2.4	1.9	1.4	1.6	1.4	1.2
Other and unknown Hispanic or Latino	4.2	3.9	3.0	2.6	2.3	2.0	1.9	2.0
Not Hispanic or Latino:								
White[6]	3.2	3.0	2.7	2.2	1.9	1.9	1.9	2.0
Black or African American[6]	7.0	6.4	5.9	5.0	4.4	4.6	4.3	4.5

See footnotes at end of table.

Table 19 (page 2 of 3). Infant, neonatal, and postneonatal mortality rates, by detailed race and Hispanic origin of mother: United States, selected years 1983–2004

[Data are based on linked birth and death certificates for infants]

Race and Hispanic origin of mother	1983–1985[1,7]	1986–1988[1,7]	1989–1991[1,7]	1995–1997[2,7]	1999–2001[2,7]	2002–2004[2,7]
	Infant[3] deaths per 1,000 live births					
All mothers	10.6	9.8	9.0	7.4	6.9	6.9
White	9.0	8.2	7.4	6.1	5.7	5.7
Black or African American	18.7	17.9	17.1	14.1	13.6	13.5
American Indian or Alaska Native	13.9	13.2	12.6	9.2	9.1	8.6
Asian or Pacific Islander[4]	8.3	7.3	6.6	5.1	4.8	4.8
Chinese	7.4	5.8	5.1	3.3	3.2	- - -
Japanese	6.0	6.9	5.3	4.9	4.0	- - -
Filipino	8.2	6.9	6.4	5.7	5.7	- - -
Hawaiian	11.3	11.1	9.0	7.0	7.8	- - -
Other Asian or Pacific Islander	8.6	7.6	7.0	5.4	4.9	- - -
Hispanic or Latino[5,6]	9.2	8.3	7.5	6.1	5.6	5.6
Mexican	8.8	7.9	7.2	5.9	5.4	5.5
Puerto Rican	12.3	11.1	10.4	8.5	8.4	8.1
Cuban	8.0	7.3	6.2	5.3	4.5	4.3
Central and South American	8.2	7.5	6.6	5.3	4.8	4.9
Other and unknown Hispanic or Latino	9.8	9.0	8.2	7.1	6.7	6.8
Not Hispanic or Latino:						
White[6]	8.8	8.1	7.3	6.1	5.7	5.7
Black or African American[6]	18.5	17.9	17.2	14.2	13.7	13.7
	Neonatal[3] deaths per 1,000 live births					
All mothers	6.9	6.3	5.7	4.8	4.6	4.6
White	5.9	5.2	4.7	4.0	3.8	3.8
Black or African American	12.2	11.7	11.1	9.4	9.2	9.2
American Indian or Alaska Native	6.7	5.9	5.9	4.4	4.5	4.5
Asian or Pacific Islander[4]	5.2	4.5	3.9	3.3	3.2	3.3
Chinese	4.3	3.3	2.7	2.1	2.1	- - -
Japanese	3.4	4.4	3.0	2.8	2.6	- - -
Filipino	5.3	4.5	4.0	3.7	4.0	- - -
Hawaiian	7.4	7.1	4.8	4.5	4.9	- - -
Other Asian or Pacific Islander	5.5	4.7	4.2	3.5	3.3	- - -
Hispanic or Latino[5,6]	6.0	5.3	4.8	4.0	3.8	3.9
Mexican	5.7	5.0	4.5	3.8	3.6	3.7
Puerto Rican	8.3	7.2	7.0	5.7	5.9	5.6
Cuban	5.9	5.3	4.6	3.7	3.1	3.1
Central and South American	5.7	4.9	4.4	3.7	3.3	3.5
Other and unknown Hispanic or Latino	6.1	5.8	5.2	4.6	4.4	4.9
Not Hispanic or Latino:						
White[6]	5.7	5.1	4.6	4.0	3.8	3.8
Black or African American[6]	11.8	11.4	11.1	9.4	9.2	9.2
	Postneonatal[3] deaths per 1,000 live births					
All mothers	3.7	3.5	3.3	2.5	2.3	2.2
White	3.1	3.0	2.7	2.1	1.9	1.9
Black or African American	6.4	6.2	6.0	4.7	4.4	4.4
American Indian or Alaska Native	7.2	7.3	6.7	4.8	4.5	4.1
Asian or Pacific Islander[4]	3.1	2.8	2.6	1.8	1.6	1.4
Chinese	3.1	2.5	2.4	1.2	1.1	- - -
Japanese	2.6	2.5	2.2	2.1	*1.4	- - -
Filipino	2.9	2.4	2.3	2.1	1.7	- - -
Hawaiian	3.9	4.0	4.1	*2.5	2.9	- - -
Other Asian or Pacific Islander	3.1	2.9	2.8	1.9	1.6	- - -
Hispanic or Latino[5,6]	3.2	3.0	2.7	2.1	1.8	1.7
Mexican	3.2	2.9	2.7	2.1	1.8	1.7
Puerto Rican	4.0	3.9	3.4	2.8	2.5	2.4
Cuban	2.2	2.0	1.6	1.5	1.4	1.2
Central and South American	2.5	2.6	2.2	1.7	1.5	1.4
Other and unknown Hispanic or Latino	3.7	3.2	3.0	2.5	2.3	2.0
Not Hispanic or Latino:						
White[6]	3.1	3.0	2.7	2.2	1.9	1.9
Black or African American[6]	6.7	6.5	6.1	4.8	4.5	4.5

See footnotes at end of table.

Table 19 (page 3 of 3). Infant, neonatal, and postneonatal mortality rates, by detailed race and Hispanic origin of mother: United States, selected years 1983–2004

[Data are based on linked birth and death certificates for infants]

- - - Data not available.
* Estimates are considered unreliable. Rates preceded by an asterisk are based on fewer than 50 deaths in the numerator. Rates not shown are based on fewer than 20 deaths in the numerator.
[1]Rates based on unweighted birth cohort data.
[2]Rates based on a period file using weighted data. See Appendix I, National Vital Statistics System (NVSS), Linked Birth/Infant Death Data Set.
[3]Infant (under 1 year of age), neonatal (under 28 days), and postneonatal (28 days–11 months).
[4]Starting with 2003 data, estimates are not shown for Asian or Pacific Islander subgroups during the transition from single race to multiple race reporting. See Appendix II, Race, Birth file.
[5]Persons of Hispanic origin may be of any race.
[6]Prior to 1995, data shown only for states with an Hispanic-origin item on their birth certificates. See Appendix II, Hispanic origin.
[7]Average annual mortality rate.

NOTES: The race groups white, black, American Indian or Alaska Native, and Asian or Pacific Islander include persons of Hispanic and non-Hispanic origin. Starting with 2003 data, some states reported multiple-race data. The multiple-race data for these states were bridged to the single-race categories of the 1977 Office of Management and Budget standards for comparability with other states. See Appendix II, Race. National linked files do not exist for 1992–1994. Data for additional years are available. See Appendix III.

SOURCE: Centers for Disease Control and Prevention, National Center for Health Statistics, National Vital Statistics System, Linked Birth/Infant Death Data Set.

Table 20 (page 1 of 2). Infant mortality rates among mothers 20 years of age and over, by education, detailed race, and Hispanic origin of mother: United States, selected years 1983–2004

[Data are based on linked birth and death certificates for infants]

Education, race, and Hispanic origin of mother	*1983*[1]	*1985*[1]	*1990*[1]	*1995*[2]	*2000*[2]	*2002*[2]	*2003*[2,3]	*43 reporting areas* *2003*[2,4]	*43 reporting areas* *2004*[2,3]
	Infant deaths per 1,000 live births								
Less than 12 years of education									
All mothers	15.0	14.3	10.8	8.9	7.9	7.9	7.8	7.5	7.5
White	12.5	12.2	9.0	7.6	6.8	6.7	6.7	6.5	6.5
Black or African American	23.4	21.5	19.5	17.0	14.7	15.6	14.8	14.6	14.4
American Indian or Alaska Native	14.5	17.3	14.3	12.7	10.1	8.6	8.7	8.9	10.6
Asian or Pacific Islander[5]	9.7	8.0	6.6	5.7	5.9	4.5	6.3	5.8	5.7
Hispanic or Latino[6,7]	10.9	10.4	7.3	6.0	5.4	5.3	5.5	5.4	5.4
Mexican	8.7	10.0	7.0	5.8	5.2	5.0	5.4	5.3	5.4
Puerto Rican	15.3	11.8	10.1	10.6	9.6	10.1	8.8	8.1	7.8
Cuban	*14.5	*	*	*	*	*	*	*	*
Central and South American	9.8	8.7	7.0	5.1	4.9	5.7	5.4	5.2	4.8
Other and unknown Hispanic or Latino	9.2	11.2	9.9	7.3	7.6	6.0	6.0	*6.7	*6.4
Not Hispanic or Latino:[7]									
White	12.8	12.5	10.9	9.9	9.2	9.4	9.1	9.0	9.0
Black or African American	24.7	21.6	19.7	17.3	15.0	15.9	15.3	15.1	15.2
12 years of education									
All mothers	10.2	9.9	8.8	7.8	7.3	7.6	7.4	7.4	7.4
White	8.7	8.5	7.1	6.4	6.0	6.3	6.1	6.1	6.1
Black or African American	17.8	17.6	16.0	14.7	13.3	13.6	13.4	13.5	13.3
American Indian or Alaska Native	15.5	10.9	13.4	7.9	7.8	8.8	9.3	9.1	8.1
Asian or Pacific Islander[5]	10.0	8.0	7.5	5.5	5.0	5.3	5.9	5.9	4.9
Hispanic or Latino[6,7]	8.4	9.1	7.0	5.9	5.0	5.4	5.5	5.5	5.3
Mexican	6.9	9.3	6.8	5.7	4.9	5.2	5.3	5.3	5.3
Puerto Rican	9.5	11.1	8.5	6.5	7.2	8.1	7.5	7.4	7.4
Cuban	*6.9	*9.2	*8.0	*	*	*	4.6	*	*
Central and South American	8.7	7.5	6.5	6.1	4.2	4.6	5.4	5.4	4.7
Other and unknown Hispanic or Latino	8.8	8.3	7.4	6.5	5.8	7.2	5.3	5.9	6.2
Not Hispanic or Latino:[7]									
White	8.7	8.2	7.1	6.5	6.3	6.7	6.3	6.3	6.6
Black or African American	17.8	18.3	16.1	14.8	13.5	13.7	13.6	13.7	13.6
13 years or more of education									
All mothers	8.1	7.7	6.4	5.4	5.0	5.0	5.0	5.0	5.0
White	7.2	6.6	5.4	4.7	4.2	4.2	4.3	4.3	4.2
Black or African American	15.3	15.8	13.7	11.9	11.4	11.1	11.2	11.1	11.7
American Indian or Alaska Native	12.5	*8.5	6.8	5.9	6.7	7.3	7.0	6.9	6.0
Asian or Pacific Islander[5]	6.6	6.2	5.1	4.4	3.9	4.0	3.8	3.8	3.8
Hispanic or Latino[6,7]	9.0	6.4	5.7	5.0	4.5	4.5	4.8	4.9	4.7
Mexican	*8.3	*5.8	5.5	5.2	4.5	4.7	4.8	4.9	4.6
Puerto Rican	10.9	*7.1	7.3	6.3	6.5	5.4	6.4	6.6	6.7
Cuban	*	*6.3	*5.3	*5.3	*4.9	*3.0	*4.6	*	*
Central and South American	*7.1	*6.6	5.6	3.7	3.7	4.2	3.9	3.9	4.7
Other and unknown Hispanic or Latino	11.6	*6.2	5.4	5.2	4.2	3.9	5.4	5.4	*3.6
Not Hispanic or Latino:[7]									
White	7.0	6.6	5.4	4.6	4.2	4.2	4.2	4.3	4.1
Black or African American	14.8	15.1	13.7	12.0	11.5	11.2	11.3	11.2	11.9

See footnotes at end of table.

Table 20 (page 2 of 2). Infant mortality rates among mothers 20 years of age and over, by education, detailed race, and Hispanic origin of mother: United States, selected years 1983–2004

[Data are based on linked birth and death certificates for infants]

Education, race, and Hispanic origin of mother	Average annual mortality rate					43 reporting areas
	1983–1985[1]	1986–1988[1]	1989–1991[1]	1995–1997[2]	1999–2001[2]	2002–2004[2,3]
	Infant deaths per 1,000 live births					
Less than 12 years of education						
All mothers	14.6	13.8	11.1	8.6	7.9	7.5
White	12.4	11.4	9.2	7.3	6.7	6.5
Black or African American	21.8	21.1	20.3	16.0	14.5	14.9
American Indian or Alaska Native	15.2	16.8	13.8	11.4	11.3	9.1
Asian or Pacific Islander[5]	9.5	8.2	6.9	5.8	5.6	5.3
Hispanic or Latino[6,7]	10.6	9.9	7.5	5.8	5.3	5.4
Mexican	9.5	8.3	7.1	5.6	5.2	5.3
Puerto Rican	14.1	12.8	11.7	9.5	8.9	8.3
Cuban	*10.5	*9.4	*8.2	*6.7	*	*
Central and South American	8.6	9.2	6.8	5.4	4.8	5.1
Other and unknown Hispanic or Latino	10.1	10.6	10.0	7.0	6.8	6.8
Not Hispanic or Latino:[7]						
White	12.6	11.8	11.0	9.6	9.1	9.1
Black or African American	22.6	21.6	20.6	16.3	14.8	15.5
12 years of education						
All mothers	10.0	9.6	8.9	7.6	7.3	7.5
White	8.5	8.0	7.2	6.3	6.0	6.2
Black or African American	17.7	17.1	16.4	14.1	13.4	13.5
American Indian or Alaska Native	13.4	11.6	12.3	8.5	8.8	8.7
Asian or Pacific Islander[5]	9.3	7.9	7.5	5.6	5.5	5.4
Hispanic or Latino[6,7]	9.1	8.3	6.8	5.8	5.1	5.4
Mexican	7.8	8.2	6.5	5.6	4.9	5.2
Puerto Rican	10.8	10.1	8.6	7.6	8.1	7.5
Cuban	8.6	6.6	7.6	5.4	*3.5	*
Central and South American	8.7	7.4	6.3	5.5	4.6	4.9
Other and unknown Hispanic or Latino	8.8	7.7	7.0	6.6	6.0	6.5
Not Hispanic or Latino:[7]						
White	8.3	7.9	7.3	6.4	6.2	6.5
Black or African American	17.9	17.4	16.5	14.2	13.6	13.7
13 years or more of education						
All mothers	7.8	7.2	6.4	5.3	5.1	5.0
White	6.9	6.2	5.5	4.5	4.3	4.3
Black or African American	15.3	14.9	13.7	11.6	11.5	11.3
American Indian or Alaska Native	10.4	8.4	8.1	6.6	6.9	6.7
Asian or Pacific Islander[5]	6.7	5.9	5.1	4.1	3.9	3.9
Hispanic or Latino[6,7]	7.4	7.0	5.8	5.0	4.6	4.7
Mexican	7.6	6.4	5.7	5.1	4.7	4.7
Puerto Rican	8.1	6.9	7.8	6.4	6.2	6.2
Cuban	5.5	5.9	4.2	4.3	4.4	*5.8
Central and South American	7.2	7.6	5.4	4.0	3.9	4.3
Other and unknown Hispanic or Latino	7.9	7.5	5.6	5.3	4.2	4.3
Not Hispanic or Latino:[7]						
White	6.8	6.1	5.4	4.5	4.2	4.2
Black or African American	14.7	14.9	13.8	11.7	11.6	11.4

* Estimates are considered unreliable. Rates preceded by an asterisk are based on fewer than 50 deaths in the numerator. Rates not shown are based on fewer than 20 deaths in the numerator.
[1]Rates based on unweighted birth cohort data.
[2]Rates based on a period file using weighted data. See Appendix I, National Vital Statistics System (NVSS), Linked Birth/Infant Death Data Set.
[3]Data are excluded for states which implemented the 2003 revision of the U.S. Standard Certificate of Live Birth. Maternal education data based on the 2003 revision are not comparable with data based on the 1989 and earlier revisions of the U.S. Standard Certificate of Live Birth. Data for 2003 and 2001–2003 exclude Pennsylvania and Washington. Data for 2004 and 2002–2004 exclude Florida, Idaho, Kentucky, New Hampshire, New York State (excluding New York City), Pennsylvania, South Carolina, Tennessee, and Washington.
[4]Data for 2003, with 43 reporting areas, are presented for comparison with data for 2004.
[5]Asian or Pacific Islander births occurred disproportionately in the states not reporting maternal education on the birth certificate prior to 1992. Starting with 1992 data, maternal education was reported by all 50 states and the District of Columbia. See Appendix II, Education.
[6]Persons of Hispanic origin may be of any race.
[7]Prior to 1995, data shown only for states with an Hispanic-origin item and education of mother on their birth certificates. See Appendix II, Education; Hispanic origin.

NOTES: Infants are under 1 year of age. Prior to 1995, data are shown only for states reporting education of mother on their birth certificates. See Appendix II, Education. The race groups white, black, American Indian or Alaska Native, and Asian or Pacific Islander include persons of Hispanic and non-Hispanic origin. Starting with 2003 data, some states reported multiple-race data. The multiple-race data for these states were bridged to the single-race categories of the 1977 Office of Management and Budget standards for comparability with other states. See Appendix II, Race. National linked files do not exist for 1992–1994. Some data have been revised and differ from previous editions of *Health, United States*. Data for additional years are available. See Appendix III.

SOURCE: Centers for Disease Control and Prevention, National Center for Health Statistics, National Vital Statistics System, Linked Birth/Infant Death Data Set.

Table 21. Infant mortality rates by birthweight: United States, selected years 1983–2004

[Data are based on linked birth and death certificates for infants]

Birthweight	1983[1]	1985[1]	1990[1]	1995[2]	2000[2]	2002[2]	2003[2]	2004[2]
	Infant deaths per 1,000 live births[3]							
All birthweights	10.9	10.4	8.9	7.6	6.9	7.0	6.8	6.8
Less than 2,500 grams	95.9	93.9	78.1	65.3	60.2	60.3	59.4	57.9
Less than 1,500 grams	400.6	387.7	317.6	270.7	246.9	253.2	253.1	245.2
Less than 500 grams	890.3	895.9	898.2	904.9	847.9	863.6	866.2	850.1
500–999 grams	584.2	559.2	440.1	351.0	313.8	321.5	319.0	314.6
1,000–1,499 grams	162.3	145.4	97.9	69.6	60.9	57.7	56.9	55.7
1,500–1,999 grams	58.4	54.0	43.8	33.5	28.7	26.9	28.0	27.4
2,000–2,499 grams	22.5	20.9	17.8	13.7	11.9	11.7	11.0	11.1
2,500 grams or more	4.7	4.3	3.7	3.0	2.5	2.4	2.3	2.3
2,500–2,999 grams	8.8	7.9	6.7	5.5	4.6	4.5	4.1	4.2
3,000–3,499 grams	4.4	4.3	3.7	2.9	2.4	2.3	2.2	2.1
3,500–3,999 grams	3.2	3.0	2.6	2.0	1.7	1.6	1.6	1.5
4,000 grams or more	3.3	3.2	2.4	2.0	1.6	1.5	1.6	1.5
4,000–4,499 grams	2.9	2.9	2.2	1.8	1.5	1.4	1.3	1.4
4,500–4,999 grams	3.9	3.8	2.5	2.2	2.1	2.0	2.4	1.5
5,000 grams or more[4]	14.4	14.7	9.8	8.5	*6.1	*5.1	*6.4	*4.9

* Estimates are considered unreliable. Rates preceded by an asterisk are based on fewer than 50 deaths in the numerator.
[1]Rates based on unweighted birth cohort data.
[2]Rates based on a period file using weighted data; unknown birthweight imputed when period of gestation is known and proportionately distributed when period of gestation is unknown. See Appendix I, National Vital Statistics System (NVSS), Linked Birth/Infant Death Data Set.
[3]For calculation of birthweight-specific infant mortality rates, unknown birthweight has been distributed in proportion to known birthweight separately for live births (denominator) and infant deaths (numerator).
[4]In 1989, a birthweight-gestational age consistency check instituted for the natality file resulted in a decrease in the number of deaths to infants coded with birthweights of 5,000 grams or more and a discontinuity in the mortality trend for infants weighing 5,000 grams or more at birth. Starting with 1989 data, the rates are believed to be more accurate.

NOTES: National linked files do not exist for 1992–1994. Data for additional years are available. See Appendix III.

SOURCE: Centers for Disease Control and Prevention, National Center for Health Statistics, National Vital Statistics System, Linked Birth/Infant Death Data Set.

Table 22. Infant mortality rates, fetal mortality rates, and perinatal mortality rates, by race: United States, selected years 1950–2005

[Data are based on death certificates, fetal death records, and birth certificates]

Race and year	Infant[1]	Neonatal[1] Under 28 days	Neonatal[1] Under 7 days	Postneonatal[1]	Fetal mortality rate[2]	Late fetal mortality rate[3]	Perinatal mortality rate[4]
All races	Deaths per 1,000 live births						
1950[5]	29.2	20.5	17.8	8.7	18.4	14.9	32.5
1960[5]	26.0	18.7	16.7	7.3	15.8	12.1	28.6
1970	20.0	15.1	13.6	4.9	14.0	9.5	23.0
1980	12.6	8.5	7.1	4.1	9.1	6.2	13.2
1990	9.2	5.8	4.8	3.4	7.5	4.3	9.1
1995	7.6	4.9	4.0	2.7	7.0	3.6	7.6
1999	7.1	4.7	3.8	2.3	6.7	3.4	7.1
2000	6.9	4.6	3.7	2.3	6.6	3.3	7.0
2001	6.8	4.5	3.6	2.3	6.5	3.3	6.9
2002	7.0	4.7	3.7	2.3	6.4	3.2	6.9
2003	6.9	4.6	3.7	2.2	6.2	3.0	6.7
2004	6.8	4.5	3.6	2.3	---	---	---
2005	6.9	4.5	3.6	2.3	---	---	---
Race of child:[6] White							
1950[5]	26.8	19.4	17.1	7.4	16.6	13.3	30.1
1960[5]	22.9	17.2	15.6	5.7	13.9	10.8	26.2
1970	17.8	13.8	12.5	4.0	12.3	8.6	21.0
1980	11.0	7.5	6.2	3.5	8.1	5.7	11.9
Race of mother:[7] White							
1980	10.9	7.4	6.1	3.5	8.1	5.7	11.8
1990	7.6	4.8	3.9	2.8	6.4	3.8	7.7
1995	6.3	4.1	3.3	2.2	5.9	3.3	6.5
1999	5.8	3.9	3.1	1.9	5.7	3.0	6.1
2000	5.7	3.8	3.0	1.9	5.6	2.9	5.9
2001	5.7	3.8	3.0	1.9	5.5	2.9	5.9
2002	5.8	3.9	3.1	1.9	5.5	2.8	5.9
2003	5.7	3.9	3.1	1.8	5.2	2.7	5.8
2004	5.7	3.8	3.0	1.9	---	---	---
2005	5.7	3.8	3.0	1.9	---	---	---
Race of child:[6] Black or African American							
1950[5]	43.9	27.8	23.0	16.1	32.1	---	---
1960[5]	44.3	27.8	23.7	16.5	---	---	---
1970	32.6	22.8	20.3	9.9	23.2	---	34.5
1980	21.4	14.1	11.9	7.3	14.4	8.9	20.7
Race of mother:[7] Black or African American							
1980	22.2	14.6	12.3	7.6	14.7	9.1	21.3
1990	18.0	11.6	9.7	6.4	13.3	6.7	16.4
1995	15.1	9.8	8.2	5.3	12.7	5.7	13.8
1999	14.6	9.8	7.9	4.8	12.6	5.4	13.2
2000	14.1	9.4	7.6	4.7	12.4	5.4	13.0
2001	14.0	9.2	7.6	4.8	12.1	5.3	12.8
2002	14.4	9.5	7.8	4.8	11.9	5.2	12.8
2003	14.0	9.4	7.5	4.6	12.0	5.1	12.4
2004	13.8	9.1	7.3	4.7	---	---	---
2005	13.7	9.1	7.3	4.7	---	---	---

- - - Data not available.
[1]Infant (under 1 year of age), neonatal (under 28 days), early neonatal (under 7 days), and postneonatal (28 days–11 months).
[2]Number of fetal deaths of 20 weeks or more gestation per 1,000 live births plus fetal deaths.
[3]Number of fetal deaths of 28 weeks or more gestation (late fetal deaths) per 1,000 live births plus late fetal deaths.
[4]Number of late fetal deaths plus infant deaths within 7 days of birth per 1,000 live births plus late fetal deaths.
[5]Includes births and deaths of persons who were not residents of the 50 states and the District of Columbia.
[6]Infant deaths, live births, and fetal deaths are tabulated by race of child. See Appendix II, Race.
[7]Infant deaths are tabulated by race of decedent; fetal deaths and live births are tabulated by race of mother. See Appendix II, Race.

NOTES: Infant mortality rates in this table are based on infant deaths from the mortality file (numerator) and live births from the natality file (denominator). Inconsistencies in reporting race for the same infant between the birth and death certificate can result in underestimated infant mortality rates for races other than white or black. Infant mortality rates for minority population groups are available from the Linked Birth/Infant Death Data Set and are presented in Tables 19–20 and 23–24. Data for additional years are available. See Appendix III.

SOURCE: Centers for Disease Control and Prevention, National Center for Health Statistics, National Vital Statistics System: Kung H-C, Hoyert DL, Xu JQ, Murphy SL. Deaths: Final data for 2005. National vital statistics reports. vol 56 no 10. Hyattsville, MD: National Center for Health Statistics. 2008 and unpublished numbers.

Table 23 (page 1 of 3). Infant mortality rates, by race and Hispanic origin of mother, geographic division, and state: United States, average annual 1989–1991, 1999–2001, and 2002–2004

[Data are based on linked birth and death certificates for infants]

Geographic division and state	*All races*			*Not Hispanic or Latino*					
				White			*Black or African American*		
	1989–1991[1]	*1999–2001*[2]	*2002–2004*[2]	*1989–1991*[1]	*1999–2001*[2]	*2002–2004*[2]	*1989–1991*[1]	*1999–2001*[2]	*2002–2004*[2]
	Infant[3] deaths per 1,000 live births								
United States	9.0	6.9	6.9	7.3	5.7	5.7	17.2	13.7	13.7
New England[4]	7.3	5.4	5.2	6.2	4.5	4.3	15.1	12.1	11.0
Connecticut	7.9	6.2	5.8	5.9	4.7	4.4	17.0	13.3	12.1
Maine	6.6	5.3	5.0	6.2	5.3	4.9	*	*	*
Massachusetts	7.0	4.9	4.8	5.9	4.1	3.9	14.2	11.1	10.2
New Hampshire[4]	7.1	5.2	4.9	7.2	4.5	4.8	*	*	*
Rhode Island	8.7	6.3	6.4	7.5	4.6	5.4	*13.6	*13.0	*11.6
Vermont	6.6	5.9	4.7	6.3	5.7	4.7	*	*	*
Middle Atlantic	9.2	6.5	6.4	6.6	5.0	5.0	18.5	12.8	12.4
New Jersey	8.4	6.4	5.6	6.1	4.4	3.8	17.8	14.0	12.2
New York	9.5	6.2	6.1	6.3	4.8	4.7	18.4	11.4	11.7
Pennsylvania	9.2	7.2	7.4	7.2	5.7	6.0	19.1	15.0	13.9
East North Central	9.8	7.9	7.6	7.7	6.3	6.1	19.1	16.0	15.9
Illinois	10.7	8.2	7.5	7.6	6.1	5.9	20.5	16.4	15.5
Indiana	9.4	7.8	7.8	8.4	7.0	6.9	17.3	14.5	15.0
Michigan	10.5	8.1	8.1	7.7	5.9	6.2	20.7	16.7	16.8
Ohio	9.0	7.8	7.7	7.7	6.6	6.3	16.2	14.9	15.6
Wisconsin	8.4	6.8	6.4	7.4	5.7	5.1	17.0	16.8	17.6
West North Central	8.5	6.7	6.4	7.4	5.8	5.7	17.5	14.5	13.1
Iowa	8.2	5.9	5.4	7.8	5.5	5.1	15.8	15.8	*10.4
Kansas	8.5	7.1	7.0	7.8	6.7	6.6	15.4	14.1	14.1
Minnesota	7.3	5.7	4.9	6.4	5.0	4.4	18.5	11.4	8.7
Missouri	9.7	7.4	7.9	8.0	5.9	6.7	18.0	16.0	14.8
Nebraska	8.1	6.9	6.3	7.2	6.1	5.5	18.3	13.2	16.2
North Dakota	8.0	8.0	6.5	7.3	7.0	5.9	*	*	*
South Dakota	9.5	7.1	7.1	7.5	6.2	5.8	*	*	*
South Atlantic	10.4	8.0	8.0	7.6	6.0	6.1	17.2	13.8	13.9
Delaware	11.2	9.2	8.9	8.2	6.8	7.1	20.1	16.3	15.0
District of Columbia	20.3	13.0	11.4	*8.2	*	*3.8	23.9	16.9	15.5
Florida	9.4	7.1	7.3	7.2	5.6	5.8	16.2	12.8	13.1
Georgia	11.9	8.4	8.7	8.4	6.0	6.3	17.9	13.5	13.6
Maryland	9.1	8.0	8.1	6.3	5.1	5.5	15.0	13.6	13.6
North Carolina	10.7	8.7	8.4	8.0	6.7	6.1	16.9	15.1	15.4
South Carolina	11.8	9.3	9.0	8.4	6.3	6.2	17.2	15.2	14.4
Virginia	9.9	7.2	7.5	7.4	5.5	5.8	18.0	13.0	13.9
West Virginia	9.1	7.4	8.0	8.8	7.3	7.7	*15.7	*10.0	*13.6
East South Central	10.4	8.7	8.7	8.1	6.6	6.8	16.5	14.9	14.8
Alabama	11.4	9.5	8.8	8.6	6.8	6.7	16.8	15.2	13.5
Kentucky	8.7	6.8	6.9	8.1	6.5	6.5	14.4	10.5	11.6
Mississippi	11.5	10.4	10.3	7.9	6.9	6.9	15.2	14.6	14.7
Tennessee	10.2	8.5	9.0	7.8	6.5	7.0	18.2	16.0	17.3
West South Central[4]	8.4	6.7	7.1	7.2	6.1	6.5	14.2	12.2	13.0
Arkansas	9.8	8.2	8.5	8.1	7.5	7.6	15.2	12.2	13.2
Louisiana[4]	10.2	9.4	9.9	7.5	6.5	7.2	14.3	13.7	14.0
Oklahoma[4]	8.0	8.1	8.0	7.3	7.6	7.5	12.7	14.3	13.8
Texas	7.9	5.9	6.4	6.9	5.4	5.9	14.1	10.9	12.2
Mountain	8.4	6.3	6.1	7.9	5.8	5.6	16.9	13.3	13.2
Arizona	8.8	6.8	6.6	8.2	6.3	6.0	17.3	16.5	11.1
Colorado	8.7	6.2	6.1	8.0	5.7	5.1	16.7	12.7	16.3
Idaho	8.9	6.9	6.1	8.9	6.6	6.1	*	*	*
Montana	9.0	6.6	6.4	8.0	5.9	5.8	*	*	*
Nevada	8.6	6.2	6.0	7.8	5.2	5.8	16.9	11.9	13.0
New Mexico	8.4	6.6	6.1	8.1	6.9	6.5	*17.2	*14.7	*
Utah	7.0	5.0	5.3	6.8	4.8	4.8	*	*	*
Wyoming	8.4	6.6	7.0	8.0	6.4	6.8	*	*	*
Pacific	7.7	5.5	5.4	7.0	4.8	4.8	15.4	11.3	11.1
Alaska	9.2	7.0	6.4	7.2	5.3	5.1	*	*	*
California	7.6	5.4	5.3	6.9	4.7	4.6	15.4	11.6	11.3
Hawaii	7.0	7.1	6.9	5.5	6.4	4.6	*13.6	*	*15.0
Oregon	8.0	5.5	5.6	7.4	5.4	5.6	21.3	*7.5	*10.1
Washington	8.0	5.3	5.6	7.4	4.9	5.1	15.1	10.3	9.2

See footnotes at end of table.

Table 23 (page 2 of 3). Infant mortality rates, by race and Hispanic origin of mother, geographic division, and state: United States, average annual 1989–1991, 1999–2001, and 2002–2004

[Data are based on linked birth and death certificates for infants]

Geographic division and state	Hispanic or Latino[5]			American Indian or Alaska Native[6]			Asian or Pacific Islander[6]		
	1989–1991[1]	1999–2001[2]	2002–2004[2]	1989–1991[1]	1999–2001[2]	2002–2004[2]	1989–1991[1]	1999–2001[2]	2002–2004[2]
	Infant[3] deaths per 1,000 live births								
United States	7.5	5.6	5.6	12.6	9.1	8.6	6.6	4.8	4.8
New England[7]	8.1	6.6	6.7	*	*	*	5.8	4.1	3.6
Connecticut	7.9	7.5	7.1	*	*	*	*	*	*
Maine	*	*	*	*	*	*	*	*	*
Massachusetts	8.3	5.5	6.6	*	*	*	5.7	3.8	3.5
New Hampshire[7]	---	*	*	*	*	*	*	*	*
Rhode Island	*7.2	*7.9	*6.3	*	*	*	*	*	*
Vermont	*	*	*	*	*	*	*	*	*
Middle Atlantic	9.1	6.3	5.8	*11.6	*6.5	*10.8	6.4	3.6	4.0
New Jersey	7.5	6.3	5.8	*	*	*	5.6	3.7	4.2
New York	9.4	5.8	5.5	*15.2	*	*11.0	6.4	3.6	3.8
Pennsylvania	10.9	9.0	7.5	*	*	*	7.8	*3.7	4.7
East North Central	8.7	6.8	6.4	11.6	9.2	7.5	6.1	5.8	5.0
Illinois	9.2	6.9	6.0	*	*	*	6.0	6.7	4.6
Indiana	*7.2	6.8	6.9	*	*	*	*	*	*5.4
Michigan	7.9	6.5	7.3	*10.7	*	*	*6.1	6.0	5.0
Ohio	8.0	7.5	7.9	*	*	*	*4.8	*4.2	*4.7
Wisconsin	*7.3	6.4	6.0	*11.9	*10.1	*9.7	*6.7	*5.0	*6.5
West North Central	9.3	6.6	6.2	17.1	11.2	10.5	7.4	6.1	4.9
Iowa	*11.9	*6.6	*5.8	*	*	*	*	*	*
Kansas	8.7	6.3	6.2	*	*	*	*	*	*6.2
Minnesota	*8.4	6.8	5.0	17.3	*10.8	*8.8	*5.1	7.4	*3.6
Missouri	*9.1	*5.7	8.2	*	*	*	*9.1	*	*6.8
Nebraska	*8.8	7.6	6.2	*18.2	*17.3	*	*	*	*
North Dakota	*	*	*	*13.8	*15.2	*8.7	*	*	*
South Dakota	*	*	*	19.9	11.7	13.5	*	*	*
South Atlantic	7.4	5.3	5.6	12.7	8.5	9.6	6.8	5.2	5.3
Delaware	*	*8.2	*6.2	*	*	*	*	*	*
District of Columbia	*8.8	*8.5	*7.9	*	*	*	*	*	*
Florida	7.1	5.0	5.1	*	*	*8.3	*6.2	4.9	6.0
Georgia	9.0	5.1	6.2	*	*	*	*8.2	6.2	5.8
Maryland	7.2	6.1	5.7	*	*	*	7.5	*4.8	4.2
North Carolina	*7.5	5.9	6.6	12.2	11.6	11.1	*6.3	6.9	*5.2
South Carolina	*	*4.4	6.4	*	*	*	*	*	*7.8
Virginia	7.6	4.9	5.2	*	*	*	6.0	4.6	4.8
West Virginia	*	*	*	*	*	*	*	*	*
East South Central	*5.9	6.2	6.5	*	*10.0	*11.6	*7.7	*5.6	6.1
Alabama	*	*7.0	7.9	*	*	*	*	*	*
Kentucky	*	*	*6.2	*	*	*	*	*	*
Mississippi	*	*	*	*	*	*	*	*	*
Tennessee	*	6.3	6.0	*	*	*	*	*5.8	*6.2
West South Central[7]	7.0	5.1	5.5	8.4	8.2	7.6	6.7	4.2	4.5
Arkansas	*	*4.2	6.0	*	*	*	*	*	*
Louisiana[7]	---	*5.3	*5.1	*	*	*	*	*	*7.0
Oklahoma[7]	---	4.9	6.1	7.8	8.4	7.8	*	*	*
Texas	7.0	5.1	5.5	*	*	*	6.8	3.9	4.2
Mountain	7.9	6.2	6.1	11.6	9.0	8.1	8.1	5.7	6.2
Arizona	8.0	6.3	6.5	11.4	9.3	8.3	*8.5	*5.2	6.7
Colorado	8.5	6.1	6.7	*16.5	*	*	*7.8	*6.2	*6.4
Idaho	*7.2	8.1	6.2	*	*	*	*	*	*
Montana	*	*	*	16.7	*11.7	*8.4	*	*	*
Nevada	7.0	5.5	4.5	*	*15.8	*	*	*5.4	*5.2
New Mexico	7.8	6.3	5.5	9.8	7.1	7.0	*	*	*
Utah	*7.0	5.9	6.6	*10.0	*	*	*10.7	*7.0	*7.3
Wyoming	*	*	*	*	*	*	*	*	*
Pacific	7.1	5.2	5.1	14.6	9.3	8.7	6.5	4.9	4.8
Alaska	*	*	*	15.7	11.9	9.4	*	*	*
California	7.0	5.1	5.0	11.0	7.9	6.3	6.4	4.5	4.2
Hawaii	10.7	*6.6	7.1	*	*	*	7.1	7.2	7.3
Oregon	8.5	6.4	4.6	*15.7	*9.5	*11.1	*8.4	*4.0	*5.3
Washington	7.6	4.9	5.4	19.6	8.9	10.5	6.2	4.4	5.2

See footnotes at end of table.

Table 23 (page 3 of 3). Infant mortality rates, by race and Hispanic origin of mother, geographic division, and state: United States, average annual 1989–1991, 1999–2001, and 2002–2004

[Data are based on linked birth and death certificates for infants]

* Estimates are considered unreliable. Rates preceded by an asterisk are based on fewer than 50 deaths in the numerator. Rates not shown are based on fewer than 20 deaths in the numerator.
- - - Data not available.
[1]Rates based on unweighted birth cohort data.
[2]Rates based on period file using weighted data. See Appendix I, National Vital Statistics System (NVSS), Linked Birth/Infant Death Data Set.
[3]Under 1 year of age.
[4]Rates for white and black are substituted for non-Hispanic white and non-Hispanic black for Louisiana for 1989, Oklahoma for 1989–1990, and New Hampshire for 1989–1991.
[5]Persons of Hispanic origin may be of any race. See Appendix II, Hispanic origin.
[6]Includes persons of Hispanic origin.
[7]Rates for Hispanic origin exclude data from states not reporting Hispanic origin on the birth certificate for 1 or more years in a 3-year period.

NOTES: Starting with 2003 data, some states reported multiple-race data. The multiple-race data for these states were bridged to the single-race categories of the 1977 Office of Management and Budget standards for comparability with other states. See Appendix II, Race. National linked files do not exist for 1992–1994.

SOURCE: Centers for Disease Control and Prevention, National Center for Health Statistics, National Vital Statistics System, Linked Birth/Infant Death Data Set.

Table 24 (page 1 of 3). Neonatal mortality rates, by race and Hispanic origin of mother, geographic division, and state: United States, average annual 1989–1991, 1999–2001, and 2002–2004

[Data are based on linked birth and death certificates for infants]

Geographic division and state	All races			Not Hispanic or Latino: White			Not Hispanic or Latino: Black or African American		
	1989–1991[1]	1999–2001[2]	2002–2004[2]	1989–1991[1]	1999–2001[2]	2002–2004[2]	1989–1991[1]	1999–2001[2]	2002–2004[2]
	Neonatal[3] deaths per 1,000 live births								
United States	5.7	4.6	4.6	4.6	3.8	3.8	11.1	9.2	9.2
New England[4]	5.1	4.1	3.9	4.2	3.4	3.2	11.0	9.2	8.0
Connecticut	5.7	4.7	4.2	4.2	3.6	3.3	12.5	9.8	8.1
Maine	4.5	4.0	3.8	4.2	3.9	3.8	*	*	*
Massachusetts	4.9	3.8	3.7	4.1	3.2	2.9	10.4	8.6	7.8
New Hampshire[4]	4.3	3.6	3.6	4.4	3.1	3.4	*	*	*
Rhode Island	6.4	4.9	4.7	5.3	3.6	3.7	*9.8	*9.5	*8.6
Vermont	4.1	3.6	3.5	3.9	3.7	3.5	*	*	*
Middle Atlantic	6.3	4.6	4.5	4.6	3.6	3.6	12.3	8.8	8.6
New Jersey	5.8	4.5	4.1	4.5	3.2	2.7	11.4	9.5	8.7
New York	6.5	4.4	4.3	4.3	3.4	3.4	12.6	8.0	8.1
Pennsylvania	6.2	5.1	5.3	4.9	4.1	4.2	12.5	10.0	9.8
East North Central	6.3	5.3	5.2	4.9	4.3	4.2	12.1	10.6	10.6
Illinois	7.0	5.6	5.1	5.1	4.3	4.2	12.7	10.8	9.9
Indiana	6.0	5.1	5.2	5.2	4.6	4.6	11.5	9.0	10.1
Michigan	6.9	5.6	5.6	4.9	4.0	4.3	14.0	11.5	11.4
Ohio	5.5	5.3	5.2	4.8	4.4	4.2	9.8	10.2	10.6
Wisconsin	5.1	4.5	4.4	4.6	3.8	3.5	9.1	10.2	11.4
West North Central	5.0	4.3	4.3	4.5	3.7	3.8	10.2	9.8	8.7
Iowa	4.8	3.7	3.4	4.5	3.4	3.3	*10.5	*10.4	*6.3
Kansas	4.9	4.7	4.6	4.6	4.3	4.3	8.3	9.7	9.7
Minnesota	4.3	3.7	3.3	3.9	3.2	3.2	10.7	7.3	4.8
Missouri	6.0	4.9	5.4	5.0	3.8	4.5	10.6	11.0	10.1
Nebraska	4.5	4.7	4.2	4.2	4.2	3.8	*9.8	*8.3	11.9
North Dakota	5.0	5.1	4.8	4.7	4.6	4.5	*	*	*
South Dakota	5.1	4.0	3.9	4.5	3.7	3.5	*	*	*
South Atlantic	6.9	5.5	5.5	4.9	4.0	3.9	11.7	9.7	9.7
Delaware	7.5	6.5	6.5	5.8	4.6	5.3	12.4	12.4	10.9
District of Columbia	14.1	9.7	8.0	*5.2	*	*	16.7	12.8	10.5
Florida	6.2	4.7	4.8	4.7	3.6	3.6	10.5	8.5	8.7
Georgia	7.9	5.7	5.8	5.5	4.0	4.0	12.0	9.3	9.3
Maryland	5.9	5.8	5.8	3.9	3.6	3.9	10.2	10.0	9.8
North Carolina	7.3	6.3	5.8	5.3	4.7	4.0	11.9	11.0	11.1
South Carolina	7.7	6.4	6.3	5.4	4.1	4.2	11.3	10.8	10.4
Virginia	6.8	4.9	5.2	4.8	3.7	3.8	13.0	9.2	9.9
West Virginia	5.8	4.9	4.9	5.6	4.8	4.6	*9.7	*	*
East South Central	6.6	5.5	5.4	5.0	4.1	3.9	10.6	9.6	9.6
Alabama	7.5	5.9	5.4	5.7	4.1	4.0	11.1	9.8	8.6
Kentucky	5.0	4.4	4.1	4.6	4.2	3.8	8.9	6.6	6.8
Mississippi	7.1	6.4	6.2	4.9	4.0	3.9	9.5	9.2	9.1
Tennessee	6.5	5.5	5.7	4.9	4.1	4.1	11.8	10.6	12.2
West South Central[4]	5.0	4.1	4.5	4.2	3.7	3.9	8.4	7.5	8.3
Arkansas	5.4	4.7	5.2	4.5	4.1	4.6	8.5	7.4	8.2
Louisiana[4]	6.3	6.1	6.2	4.8	4.1	4.2	8.5	8.8	9.0
Oklahoma[4]	4.4	4.8	4.7	4.1	4.8	4.3	6.3	7.8	9.4
Texas	4.7	3.6	4.1	4.1	3.2	3.7	8.5	6.7	7.8
Mountain	4.8	4.1	4.1	4.4	3.7	3.7	10.1	8.9	8.7
Arizona	5.3	4.4	4.3	4.9	4.1	4.0	11.0	11.2	7.0
Colorado	5.0	4.3	4.3	4.7	3.8	3.5	10.9	10.0	11.6
Idaho	5.3	4.6	3.9	5.2	4.3	3.9	*	*	*
Montana	4.6	3.8	3.7	4.2	3.5	3.6	*	*	*
Nevada	4.3	3.6	3.8	3.8	2.8	3.7	*8.3	*6.1	7.9
New Mexico	5.0	3.8	3.9	4.8	4.0	4.1	*	*	*
Utah	3.7	3.3	3.6	3.6	3.2	3.3	*	*	*
Wyoming	3.9	4.2	4.6	3.8	4.1	4.6	*	*	*
Pacific	4.6	3.6	3.6	4.0	3.2	3.1	9.2	7.3	7.1
Alaska	4.1	3.4	2.9	3.7	3.3	*2.4	*	*	*
California	4.6	3.6	3.5	4.1	3.1	3.0	9.2	7.5	7.2
Hawaii	4.3	5.0	4.9	3.5	*4.9	*3.8	*	*	*
Oregon	4.4	3.7	3.8	4.0	3.6	3.8	*11.6	*	*
Washington	4.3	3.3	3.6	3.8	3.1	3.2	9.7	6.4	5.9

See footnotes at end of table.

Table 24 (page 2 of 3). Neonatal mortality rates, by race and Hispanic origin of mother, geographic division, and state: United States, average annual 1989–1991, 1999–2001, and 2002–2004

[Data are based on linked birth and death certificates for infants]

Geographic division and state	Hispanic or Latino[5]			American Indian or Alaska Native[6]			Asian or Pacific Islander[6]		
	1989–1991[1]	1999–2001[2]	2002–2004[2]	1989–1991[1]	1999–2001[2]	2002–2004[2]	1989–1991[1]	1999–2001[2]	2002–2004[2]
	Neonatal[3] deaths per 1,000 live births								
United States	4.8	3.8	3.9	5.9	4.5	4.5	3.9	3.2	3.3
New England[7]	5.5	5.0	5.2	*	*	*	4.4	2.9	2.8
Connecticut	5.3	5.8	5.6	*	*	*	*	*	*
Maine	*	*	*	*	*	*	*	*	*
Massachusetts	5.8	4.2	5.0	*	*	*	*3.9	*2.5	*2.8
New Hampshire[7]	- - -	*	*	*	*	*	*	*	*
Rhode Island	*4.9	*5.7	*5.0	*	*	*	*	*	*
Vermont	*	*	*	*	*	*	*	*	*
Middle Atlantic	6.2	4.3	4.1	*	*	*6.2	4.1	2.4	2.9
New Jersey	5.1	4.3	4.1	*	*	*	*3.4	2.3	3.1
New York	6.4	4.1	3.8	*	*	*	4.1	2.5	2.6
Pennsylvania	7.3	5.7	5.3	*	*	*	*5.2	*2.4	3.6
East North Central	5.9	4.8	4.5	*6.2	*5.2	*4.2	3.6	4.2	3.8
Illinois	6.4	4.8	4.2	*	*	*	3.9	4.9	3.3
Indiana	*4.7	5.2	4.9	*	*	*	*	*	*5.1
Michigan	5.2	4.3	5.0	*	*	*	*	*4.2	3.7
Ohio	*5.4	5.7	5.5	*	*	*	*	*	*4.0
Wisconsin	*3.9	4.2	4.5	*	*	*	*	*3.9	*5.0
West North Central	5.3	4.8	4.1	6.1	5.3	5.2	4.6	4.3	3.1
Iowa	*	*4.7	*4.0	*	*	*	*	*	*
Kansas	*5.4	4.2	4.0	*	*	*	*	*	*
Minnesota	*	4.8	*3.3	*4.9	*5.4	*	*3.2	5.2	*1.9
Missouri	*	*4.3	6.0	*	*	*	*	*	*5.2
Nebraska	*	*5.8	*3.6	*	*	*	*	*	*
North Dakota	*	*	*	*	*	*	*	*	*
South Dakota	*	*	*	*8.2	*4.5	*6.3	*	*	*
South Atlantic	5.2	3.7	3.9	7.4	6.2	6.4	4.6	3.8	3.9
Delaware	*	*	*	*	*	*	*	*	*
District of Columbia	*	*	*	*	*	*	*	*	*
Florida	5.1	3.5	3.6	*	*	*	*4.4	3.6	4.2
Georgia	*5.7	3.4	4.3	*	*	*	*5.3	*4.7	4.3
Maryland	*4.7	4.7	3.8	*	*	*	*4.5	*3.5	*3.4
North Carolina	*5.5	4.4	4.4	*7.7	*9.0	*8.4	*	*5.0	*3.8
South Carolina	*	*3.4	*4.4	*	*	*	*	*	*
Virginia	*4.8	3.4	4.1	*	*	*	*4.1	*3.2	3.8
West Virginia	*	*	*	*	*	*	*	*	*
East South Central	*	3.8	4.2	*	*	*	*	*4.3	*4.1
Alabama	*	*3.8	*5.0	*	*	*	*	*	*
Kentucky	*	*	*3.7	*	*	*	*	*	*
Mississippi	*	*	*	*	*	*	*	*	*
Tennessee	*	*4.2	4.2	*	*	*	*	*	*
West South Central[7]	4.2	3.2	3.7	4.3	3.8	3.7	4.1	2.8	3.0
Arkansas	*	*	*4.1	*	*	*	*	*	*
Louisiana[7]	- - -	*	*	*	*	*	*	*	*
Oklahoma[7]	- - -	*2.8	3.9	*3.7	3.9	3.8	*	*	*
Texas	4.2	3.2	3.7	*	*	*	4.0	2.5	2.7
Mountain	4.7	4.2	4.2	5.8	4.5	4.1	4.6	3.4	4.3
Arizona	5.0	4.2	4.5	5.4	5.0	4.1	*	*	*4.0
Colorado	4.4	4.5	4.9	*	*	*	*	*4.1	*4.6
Idaho	*	*5.9	*4.2	*	*	*	*	*	*
Montana	*	*	*	*7.6	*6.6	*	*	*	*
Nevada	*4.1	3.7	2.8	*	*	*	*	*	*3.7
New Mexico	4.9	3.8	3.6	4.9	*2.8	*4.1	*	*	*
Utah	*3.6	3.8	4.6	*	*	*	*	*	*5.4
Wyoming	*	*	*	*	*	*	*	*	*
Pacific	4.5	3.5	3.5	6.5	4.0	4.2	3.7	3.2	3.2
Alaska	*	*	*	*5.7	*4.2	*4.2	*	*	*
California	4.4	3.5	3.5	6.3	*4.0	*3.5	3.6	2.9	2.9
Hawaii	*6.6	*4.5	*4.8	*	*	*	4.2	4.9	4.9
Oregon	6.5	4.5	3.4	*	*	*	*5.3	*2.9	*3.5
Washington	4.9	3.3	3.9	*8.5	*3.5	*4.8	*2.7	3.1	3.2

See footnotes at end of table.

Table 24 (page 3 of 3). Neonatal mortality rates, by race and Hispanic origin of mother, geographic division, and state: United States, average annual 1989–1991, 1999–2001, and 2002–2004

[Data are based on linked birth and death certificates for infants]

* Estimates are considered unreliable. Rates preceded by an asterisk are based on fewer than 50 deaths in the numerator. Rates not shown are based on fewer than 20 deaths in the numerator.
- - - Data not available.
[1]Rates based on unweighted birth cohort data.
[2]Rates based on period file using weighted data. See Appendix I, National Vital Statistics System (NVSS), Linked Birth/Infant Death Data Set.
[3]Infants under 28 days of age.
[4]Rates for white and black are substituted for non-Hispanic white and non-Hispanic black for Louisiana for 1989, Oklahoma for 1989–1990, and New Hampshire for 1989–1991.
[5]Persons of Hispanic origin may be of any race. See Appendix II, Hispanic origin.
[6]Includes persons of Hispanic origin.
[7]Rates for Hispanic origin exclude data from states not reporting Hispanic origin on the birth certificate for 1 or more years in a 3-year period.

NOTES: Starting with 2003 data, some states reported multiple-race data. The multiple-race data for these states were bridged to the single-race categories of the 1977 Office of Management and Budget standards for comparability with other states. See Appendix II, Race. National linked files do not exist for 1992–1994.

SOURCE: Centers for Disease Control and Prevention, National Center for Health Statistics, National Vital Statistics System, Linked Birth/Infant Death Data Set.

Table 25. Infant mortality rates and international rankings: Selected countries and territories, selected years 1960–2004

[Data are based on reporting by countries]

Country[2]	1960	1970	1980	1990	2000	2002	2003	2004	International rankings[1] 1960	International rankings[1] 2004
	Infant[3] deaths per 1,000 live births									
Australia	20.2	17.9	10.7	8.2	5.2	5.0	4.8	4.7	5	20
Austria	37.5	25.9	14.3	7.8	4.8	4.1	4.5	4.5	24	18
Belgium	23.9	21.1	12.1	6.5	4.8	4.4	4.3	4.3	11	16
Bulgaria	45.1	27.3	20.2	14.8	13.3	13.3	12.0	11.7	30	36
Canada	27.3	18.8	10.4	6.8	5.3	5.4	5.3	5.3	15	24
Chile	120.3	82.2	33.0	16.0	11.7	7.8	7.8	8.4	36	33
Costa Rica	67.8	65.4	20.3	15.3	10.2	11.2	10.1	9.0	33	34
Cuba	37.3	38.7	19.6	10.7	7.2	6.5	6.3	5.8	23	27
Czech Republic	20.0	20.2	16.9	10.8	4.1	4.2	3.9	3.7	4	8
Denmark	21.5	14.2	8.4	7.5	5.3	4.4	4.4	4.4	8	17
England and Wales	22.4	18.5	12.0	7.9	5.6	5.2	5.3	5.0	9	23
Finland	21.0	13.2	7.6	5.6	3.8	3.0	3.1	3.3	6	6
France	27.5	18.2	10.0	7.3	4.4	4.1	4.0	3.9	16	9
Germany[4]	35.0	22.5	12.4	7.0	4.4	4.2	4.2	4.1	22	11
Greece	40.1	29.6	17.9	9.7	5.9	5.1	4.8	4.1	25	11
Hong Kong	41.5	19.2	11.2	5.9	2.9	2.4	2.3	2.5	26	2
Hungary	47.6	35.9	23.2	14.8	9.2	7.2	7.3	6.6	31	28
Ireland	29.3	19.5	11.1	8.2	6.2	5.0	5.1	4.9	18	21
Israel[5]	31.0	18.9	15.6	9.9	5.4	5.4	4.9	4.5	20	18
Italy	43.9	29.6	14.6	8.2	4.5	4.5	4.2	4.1	29	11
Japan	30.7	13.1	7.5	4.6	3.2	3.0	3.0	2.8	19	3
Netherlands	17.9	12.7	8.6	7.1	5.1	5.0	4.8	4.1	2	11
New Zealand	22.6	16.7	13.0	8.4	6.3	6.2	5.2	5.7	10	26
Northern Ireland	27.2	22.9	13.4	7.5	5.1	4.7	5.2	5.5	14	25
Norway	18.9	12.7	8.1	6.9	3.8	3.5	3.4	3.2	3	5
Poland	54.8	36.7	25.5	19.3	8.1	7.5	7.0	6.8	32	29
Portugal	77.5	55.5	24.3	11.0	5.5	5.0	4.1	4.0	35	10
Puerto Rico	43.3	27.9	18.5	13.4	9.9	9.8	9.8	8.1	27	32
Romania	75.7	49.4	29.3	26.9	18.6	17.3	16.7	16.8	34	37
Russian Federation[6]	- - -	- - -	22.0	17.6	15.2	13.2	12.4	11.5	- - -	35
Scotland	26.4	19.6	12.1	7.7	5.7	5.3	5.1	4.9	13	21
Singapore	34.8	21.4	11.7	6.7	2.5	2.9	2.5	2.0	21	1
Slovakia	28.6	25.7	20.9	12.0	8.6	7.6	7.9	6.8	17	29
Spain	43.7	28.1	12.3	7.6	3.9	4.1	3.6	3.5	28	7
Sweden	16.6	11.0	6.9	6.0	3.4	3.3	3.1	3.1	1	4
Switzerland	21.1	15.1	9.1	6.8	4.9	5.0	4.3	4.2	7	15
United States	26.0	20.0	12.6	9.2	6.9	7.0	6.9	6.8	12	29

- - - Data not available.

[1]Rankings are from lowest to highest infant mortality rates (IMR). Countries with the same IMR receive the same rank. The country with the next highest IMR is assigned the rank it would have received had the lower-ranked countries not been tied, i.e., skip a rank. Some of the variation in IMRs is due to differences among countries in distinguishing between fetal and infant deaths.

[2]Refers to countries, territories, cities, or geographic areas with at least 1 million population and with complete counts of live births and infant deaths according to the United Nations Demographic Yearbook.

[3]Under 1 year of age.

[4]Rates for 1990 and earlier years were calculated by combining information from the Federal Republic of Germany and the German Democratic Republic.

[5]Includes data for East Jerusalem and Israeli residents in certain other territories under occupation by Israeli military forces since June 1967.

[6]Excludes infants born alive after less than 28 weeks gestation, of less than 1,000 grams in weight and 35 centimeters in length, who die within 7 days of birth.

NOTE: Some rates for selected countries and selected years were revised and differ from previous editions of *Health, United States*. Data for additional years are available. See Appendix III.

SOURCES: Organisation for Economic Co-operation and Development (OECD): OECD Health Data 2006, A Comparative Analysis of 30 Countries, www.oecd.org/els/health/; United Nations: 2000 Demographic Yearbook, United Nations Publication, Sales No. E/F.02.XIII.1, New York, 2002; World Health Organization Statistical Information System (WHOSIS), www3.who.int/whosis/; United States and Puerto Rico: Centers for Disease Control and Prevention, National Center for Health Statistics. Vital Statistics of the United States, vol. II, mortality part A (selected years). Public Health Service. Washington, DC; Sweden: Statistics Sweden; Costa Rica: Dirección General de Estadísticas y Censos. Elaboración y estimación, Centro Centroamericano de Población, Universidad de Costa Rica, http://ccp.ucr.ac.cr/observa/index1.htm; Russian Federation: Goskomstat, www.gks.ru/eng/; Israel: Central Bureau Statistics of Israel, www.cbs.gov.il/engindex.htm.

Table 26 (page 1 of 2). Life expectancy at birth and at 65 years of age, by sex: Selected countries and territories, selected years 1980–2003

[Data are based on reporting by countries]

Country	Male							Female						
	1980	1990	1995	2000	2002	2003	2003	1980	1990	1995	2000	2002	2003	2003
At birth	Life expectancy in years						Rank	Life expectancy in years						Rank
Australia	71.0	73.9	75.0	76.6	77.4	77.8	5	78.1	80.1	80.8	82.0	82.6	82.8	6
Austria	69.0	72.2	73.3	75.1	75.8	75.9	18	76.1	78.8	79.9	81.1	81.7	81.6	15
Belgium	70.0	72.7	73.4	75.1	75.6	75.9	18	76.8	79.4	80.7	81.4	81.7	81.7	13
Bulgaria	68.5	68.3	67.4	68.5	68.9	68.9	34	73.9	75.0	74.9	75.1	75.6	75.9	35
Canada	71.7	74.4	75.1	76.7	77.2	77.4	7	78.9	80.8	81.1	81.9	82.1	82.4	9
Chile	- - -	71.1	71.8	72.6	72.9	72.9	29	- - -	76.9	77.8	78.6	78.9	79.0	30
Costa Rica	71.9	74.7	74.0	75.4	76.2	76.2	16	77.0	79.1	78.6	80.2	81.0	81.0	19
Cuba	72.2	74.6	75.4	74.7	74.7	75.4	24	- - -	76.9	77.7	79.0	79.2	79.8	28
Czech Republic[1]	66.8	67.6	69.7	71.7	72.1	72.1	30	73.9	75.4	76.6	78.4	78.7	78.7	32
Denmark	71.2	72.0	72.7	74.5	74.8	76.5	13	77.3	77.7	77.8	79.3	79.5	79.9	27
England and Wales	70.8	73.1	74.3	75.6	76.2	76.5	13	76.8	78.6	79.5	80.3	80.7	80.9	20
Finland	69.2	70.9	72.8	74.2	74.9	75.1	25	77.6	78.9	80.2	81.0	81.5	81.8	11
France	70.2	72.8	73.9	75.3	75.8	75.9	18	78.4	80.9	81.8	82.7	83.0	82.9	5
Germany[2]	69.6	72.0	73.3	75.0	75.4	75.7	23	76.1	78.4	79.7	81.0	81.2	81.4	16
Greece	72.2	74.6	75.0	75.6	76.4	76.5	13	76.8	79.5	80.3	80.6	80.7	81.3	17
Hong Kong	71.6	74.6	76.0	78.0	78.6	78.5	1	77.9	80.3	81.5	83.9	84.5	84.3	2
Hungary	65.5	65.1	65.3	67.4	68.4	68.4	35	72.7	73.7	74.5	75.9	76.7	76.7	34
Ireland	70.1	72.1	72.9	73.4	75.2	75.8	21	75.6	77.6	78.4	79.1	80.3	80.7	22
Israel	72.2	75.1	75.5	76.7	77.5	77.5	6	75.8	78.5	79.5	81.1	81.4	81.7	13
Italy	70.6	73.6	74.9	76.6	76.8	76.8	12	77.4	80.1	81.3	82.5	82.9	82.5	7
Japan	73.4	75.9	76.4	77.7	78.3	78.4	2	78.8	81.9	82.9	84.6	85.2	85.3	1
Netherlands	72.5	73.8	74.6	75.5	76.0	76.2	16	79.2	80.9	80.4	80.5	80.7	80.9	20
New Zealand	70.0	72.4	74.4	76.3	76.3	77.0	10	76.3	78.3	79.7	81.1	81.1	81.3	17
Northern Ireland	68.3	72.1	73.5	74.8	75.6	75.8	21	75.0	78.0	78.9	79.8	80.4	80.6	23
Norway	72.3	73.4	74.8	76.0	76.4	77.1	9	79.2	79.8	80.8	81.4	81.5	82.0	10
Poland	66.0	66.7	67.6	69.7	70.4	70.5	32	74.4	76.3	76.4	77.9	78.8	78.8	31
Portugal	67.7	70.4	71.6	73.2	73.8	74.2	27	75.2	77.4	78.7	80.0	80.5	80.5	25
Puerto Rico	70.8	69.1	69.6	71.1	71.6	71.8	31	76.9	77.2	78.9	80.1	80.5	80.6	23
Romania	66.6	66.6	65.5	67.8	67.4	67.7	36	71.9	73.1	73.5	74.8	74.8	75.1	36
Russian Federation	61.4	63.8	58.3	59.2	58.9	58.6	37	73.0	74.4	71.7	72.4	72.0	71.8	37
Scotland	69.0	71.1	72.1	73.1	73.5	73.8	28	75.2	76.7	77.7	78.6	78.9	79.1	29
Singapore	69.8	73.1	74.2	76.1	76.5	77.4	7	74.7	77.6	78.6	80.1	81.1	81.8	11
Slovakia[1]	66.8	66.6	68.4	69.2	69.8	69.9	33	74.3	75.4	76.3	77.4	77.7	77.8	33
Spain	72.5	73.3	74.3	75.7	76.1	76.9	11	78.6	80.3	81.5	82.5	83.5	83.6	3
Sweden	72.8	74.8	76.2	77.4	77.7	77.9	4	78.8	80.4	81.4	82.0	82.1	82.5	7
Switzerland	72.8	74.0	75.3	76.9	77.8	78.0	3	79.6	80.7	81.7	82.6	83.0	83.1	4
United States	70.0	71.8	72.5	74.1	74.5	74.8	26	77.4	78.8	78.9	79.5	79.9	80.1	26

See footnotes at end of table.

Table 26 (page 2 of 2). Life expectancy at birth and at 65 years of age, by sex: Selected countries and territories, selected years 1980–2003

[Data are based on reporting by countries]

Country	Male							Female						
	1980	*1990*	*1995*	*2000*	*2002*	*2003*	*2003*	*1980*	*1990*	*1995*	*2000*	*2002*	*2003*	*2003*
At 65 years	Life expectancy in years						Rank	Life expectancy in years						Rank
Australia	13.7	15.2	15.7	16.9	17.4	17.6	4	17.9	19.0	19.5	20.4	20.8	21.0	4
Austria	12.9	14.3	14.9	16.0	16.3	16.3	19	16.3	17.8	18.6	19.4	19.7	19.9	13
Belgium	13.0	14.3	14.8	15.5	15.8	15.8	22	16.9	18.5	19.1	19.5	19.7	19.7	15
Bulgaria	12.7	12.9	12.8	12.8	13.1	13.8	32	14.7	15.4	15.4	15.4	15.8	15.9	34
Canada	14.5	15.7	16.0	16.8	17.2	17.4	6	18.9	19.9	20.0	20.4	20.6	20.8	6
Chile	- - -	14.6	14.9	15.3	15.4	15.4	28	- - -	17.6	18.1	18.6	18.8	18.7	27
Costa Rica	16.1	17.1	16.7	17.2	17.8	17.7	3	18.1	19.3	18.6	19.6	20.5	20.0	12
Cuba	- - -	- - -	- - -	16.7	16.8	16.9	12	- - -	- - -	- - -	19.0	19.3	19.3	22
Czech Republic[1]	11.2	11.6	12.7	13.7	14.0	13.9	30	14.3	15.2	16.0	17.1	17.4	17.3	31
Denmark	13.6	14.0	14.1	15.2	15.4	15.5	27	17.6	17.8	17.5	18.3	18.3	18.6	28
England and Wales	12.9	14.1	14.8	15.8	16.3	16.5	18	16.9	17.9	18.3	19.0	19.2	19.4	21
Finland	12.5	13.7	14.5	15.5	15.8	15.8	22	16.5	17.7	18.6	19.3	19.6	19.6	18
France	13.6	15.5	16.1	16.7	17.0	17.1	8	18.2	19.8	20.6	21.2	21.4	21.4	3
Germany[2]	13.0	14.0	14.7	15.7	16.2	16.1	20	16.7	17.6	18.5	19.4	19.7	19.6	18
Greece	14.6	15.7	16.1	16.3	16.7	16.8	13	16.8	18.0	18.4	18.3	18.7	18.9	24
Hong Kong	13.9	15.3	16.2	17.3	17.8	17.9	2	13.9	18.8	19.5	21.5	22.0	21.7	2
Hungary	11.6	12.0	12.1	12.7	13.1	13.0	35	14.6	15.3	15.8	16.5	17.0	16.9	32
Ireland	12.6	13.3	13.6	14.6	15.3	15.7	25	15.7	16.9	17.3	17.8	18.6	18.9	24
Israel	14.4	15.9	16.0	16.9	17.3	17.3	7	15.8	17.8	18.0	19.3	19.7	19.7	15
Italy	13.3	15.1	15.8	16.5	16.6	16.6	17	17.1	18.8	19.6	20.4	20.6	20.6	8
Japan	14.6	16.2	16.5	17.5	18.0	18.0	1	17.7	20.0	20.9	22.4	23.0	23.0	1
Netherlands	13.7	14.4	14.7	15.3	15.6	15.8	22	18.0	18.9	19.0	19.2	19.3	19.5	20
New Zealand	13.2	14.7	15.6	16.7	16.7	17.1	8	17.0	18.3	19.1	20.0	20.0	20.1	10
Northern Ireland	11.9	13.7	14.4	15.3	15.9	16.1	20	15.8	17.5	18.0	18.5	18.9	19.1	23
Norway	14.3	14.6	15.1	16.0	16.2	16.7	16	18.0	18.5	19.1	19.7	19.7	20.1	10
Poland	12.0	12.7	12.9	13.6	14.0	13.9	30	15.5	16.9	16.6	17.3	17.9	17.9	30
Portugal	12.9	13.9	14.6	15.3	15.6	15.6	26	16.5	17.0	17.8	18.7	19.0	18.9	24
Puerto Rico	- - -	- - -	- - -	- - -	- - -	- - -	- - -	- - -	- - -	- - -	- - -	- - -	- - -	- - -
Romania	12.6	13.3	12.9	13.5	13.0	13.1	34	14.2	15.3	15.4	15.9	15.8	15.9	34
Russian Federation	11.6	12.1	10.9	11.1	10.9	10.7	36	15.6	15.9	15.1	15.2	15.1	14.9	36
Scotland	12.3	13.1	13.8	14.7	15.1	15.2	29	16.2	16.7	17.3	17.8	18.1	18.2	29
Singapore	12.6	14.5	14.6	15.8	16.0	17.0	10	15.4	16.9	17.3	19.0	19.2	19.7	15
Slovakia[1]	12.3	12.2	12.7	12.9	13.3	13.3	33	15.4	15.7	16.1	16.5	17.0	16.9	32
Spain	14.8	15.4	16.0	16.6	16.8	16.8	13	17.9	19.0	19.8	20.4	20.7	20.7	7
Sweden	14.3	15.3	16.0	16.7	16.9	17.0	10	17.9	19.0	19.6	20.0	20.0	20.3	9
Switzerland	14.4	15.3	16.1	16.9	17.5	17.5	5	17.9	19.4	20.2	20.7	21.0	21.0	4
United States	14.1	15.1	15.6	16.3	16.6	16.8	13	18.3	18.9	18.9	19.2	19.5	19.8	14

- - - Data not available.

[1]In 1993, Czechoslovakia was divided into two nations, the Czech Republic and Slovakia. Data for years prior to 1993 are from the Czech and Slovak regions of Czechoslovakia.

[2]Until 1990, estimates refer to the Federal Republic of Germany; from 1995 onwards, data refer to Germany after reunification.

NOTES: Rankings are from highest to lowest life expectancy (LE) for the most recent year available. Since calculation of LE estimates varies among countries, comparisons among them and their interpretation should be made with caution. See Appendix II, Life expectancy. Countries with the same LE receive the same rank. The country with the next lower LE is assigned the rank it would have received had the higher-ranked countries not been tied, i.e., skip a rank. Some estimates for selected countries and selected years were revised and differ from the previous editions of *Health, United States.* Data for additional years are available. See Appendix III.

SOURCES: Organisation for Economic Co-operation and Development (OECD) Health Data 2006, A Comparative Analysis of 30 Countries, www.oecd.org/els/health/; European health for all database, World Health Organization Regional Office for Europe, www.who.dk/hfadb; Centers for Disease Control and Prevention, National Center for Health Statistics. Vital statistics of the United States (selected years). Public Health Service. Washington, DC. www.cdc.gov/nchs/fastats/lifexpec.htm; Puerto Rico: Commonwealth of Puerto Rico, Department of Health, Auxiliary Secretariat for Planning, Evaluation, Statistics, and Information Systems: Unpublished data; England and Wales, Northern Ireland, and Scotland: Government Actuary's Department, London www.gad.gov.uk; Hong Kong: Government of Hong Kong, Special Administrative Region, Department of Health, http://info.gov.hk/dh/index.htm; Costa Rica: Instituto Nacional de Estadística y Censos (INEC) y Centro Centroamericano de Población (CCP) http://ccp.ucr.ac.cr/observa/series/serie3.htm; Chile: Instituto Nacional de Estadísticas, Departamento de Demografía. Gobierno de Chile. Ministerio de Salud Departamento de Estadísticas e Información de Salud; Puerto Rico (1999–2001): Pan American Health Organization, Special Program for Health Analysis. Regional Initiative for Health Basic Data, Technical Information Health System, Washington, DC 2006. Cuba and Singapore (2000–2001): WHO Statistical Information System (WHOSIS) www3.who.int/whosis/core/core_select.cfm.

Table 27. Life expectancy at birth, at 65 years of age, and at 75 years of age, by race and sex: United States, selected years 1900–2004

[Data are based on death certificates]

Specified age and year	All races			White			Black or African American[1]		
	Both sexes	Male	Female	Both sexes	Male	Female	Both sexes	Male	Female
	Remaining life expectancy in years								
At birth									
1900[2,3]	47.3	46.3	48.3	47.6	46.6	48.7	33.0	32.5	33.5
1950[3]	68.2	65.6	71.1	69.1	66.5	72.2	60.8	59.1	62.9
1960[3]	69.7	66.6	73.1	70.6	67.4	74.1	63.6	61.1	66.3
1970	70.8	67.1	74.7	71.7	68.0	75.6	64.1	60.0	68.3
1980	73.7	70.0	77.4	74.4	70.7	78.1	68.1	63.8	72.5
1990	75.4	71.8	78.8	76.1	72.7	79.4	69.1	64.5	73.6
1995	75.8	72.5	78.9	76.5	73.4	79.6	69.6	65.2	73.9
1996	76.1	73.1	79.1	76.8	73.9	79.7	70.2	66.1	74.2
1997	76.5	73.6	79.4	77.1	74.3	79.9	71.1	67.2	74.7
1998	76.7	73.8	79.5	77.3	74.5	80.0	71.3	67.6	74.8
1999	76.7	73.9	79.4	77.3	74.6	79.9	71.4	67.8	74.7
2000	77.0	74.3	79.7	77.6	74.9	80.1	71.9	68.3	75.2
2001	77.2	74.4	79.8	77.7	75.0	80.2	72.2	68.6	75.5
2002	77.3	74.5	79.9	77.7	75.1	80.3	72.3	68.8	75.6
2003	77.5	74.8	80.1	78.0	75.3	80.5	72.7	69.0	76.1
2004	77.8	75.2	80.4	78.3	75.7	80.8	73.1	69.5	76.3
At 65 years									
1950[3]	13.9	12.8	15.0	- - -	12.8	15.1	13.9	12.9	14.9
1960[3]	14.3	12.8	15.8	14.4	12.9	15.9	13.9	12.7	15.1
1970	15.2	13.1	17.0	15.2	13.1	17.1	14.2	12.5	15.7
1980	16.4	14.1	18.3	16.5	14.2	18.4	15.1	13.0	16.8
1990	17.2	15.1	18.9	17.3	15.2	19.1	15.4	13.2	17.2
1995	17.4	15.6	18.9	17.6	15.7	19.1	15.6	13.6	17.1
1996	17.5	15.7	19.0	17.6	15.8	19.1	15.8	13.9	17.2
1997	17.7	15.9	19.2	17.8	16.0	19.3	16.1	14.2	17.6
1998	17.8	16.0	19.2	17.8	16.1	19.3	16.1	14.3	17.4
1999	17.7	16.1	19.1	17.8	16.1	19.2	16.0	14.3	17.3
2000	18.0	16.2	19.3	18.0	16.3	19.4	16.2	14.2	17.7
2001	18.1	16.4	19.4	18.2	16.5	19.5	16.4	14.4	17.9
2002	18.2	16.6	19.5	18.2	16.6	19.5	16.6	14.6	18.0
2003	18.4	16.8	19.8	18.5	16.9	19.8	17.0	14.9	18.5
2004	18.7	17.1	20.0	18.7	17.2	20.0	17.1	15.2	18.6
At 75 years									
1980	10.4	8.8	11.5	10.4	8.8	11.5	9.7	8.3	10.7
1990	10.9	9.4	12.0	11.0	9.4	12.0	10.2	8.6	11.2
1995	11.0	9.7	11.9	11.1	9.7	12.0	10.2	8.8	11.1
1996	11.1	9.8	12.0	11.1	9.8	12.0	10.3	9.0	11.2
1997	11.2	9.9	12.1	11.2	9.9	12.1	10.7	9.3	11.5
1998	11.3	10.0	12.2	11.3	10.0	12.2	10.5	9.2	11.3
1999	11.2	10.0	12.1	11.2	10.0	12.1	10.4	9.2	11.1
2000	11.4	10.1	12.3	11.4	10.1	12.3	10.7	9.2	11.6
2001	11.5	10.2	12.4	11.5	10.2	12.3	10.8	9.3	11.7
2002	11.5	10.3	12.4	11.5	10.3	12.3	10.9	9.5	11.7
2003	11.8	10.5	12.6	11.7	10.5	12.6	11.4	9.8	12.4
2004	11.9	10.7	12.8	11.9	10.7	12.8	11.4	9.9	12.2

- - - Data not available.

[1]Data shown for 1900–1960 are for the nonwhite population.

[2]Death registration area only. The death registration area increased from 10 states and the District of Columbia (DC) in 1900 to the coterminous United States in 1933. See Appendix II, Registration area.

[3]Includes deaths of persons who were not residents of the 50 states and DC.

NOTES: Populations for computing life expectancy for 1991–1999 are 1990-based postcensal estimates of U.S. resident population. See Appendix I, Population Census and Population Estimates. In 1997, life table methodology was revised to construct complete life tables by single years of age that extend to age 100 (Anderson RN. Method for constructing complete annual U.S. life tables. National Center for Health Statistics. Vital Health Stat 2(129). 1999). Previously, abridged life tables were constructed for 5-year age groups ending with 85 years and over. Life table values for 2000 and later years were computed using a slight modification of the new life table method due to a change in the age detail of populations received from the U.S. Census Bureau. In 2003, seven states reported multiple-race data. In 2004, 15 states reported multiple-race data. The multiple-race data for these states were bridged to the single-race categories of the 1977 Office of Management and Budget Standards for comparability with other states. See Appendix II, Race. Data for additional years are available. See Appendix III.

SOURCES: Centers for Disease Control and Prevention, National Center for Health Statistics, National Vital Statistics System; Grove RD, Hetzel AM. Vital statistics rates in the United States, 1940–1960. Washington, DC: U.S. Government Printing Office, 1968; Arias, E. United States life tables, 2004. National vital statistics reports; Hyattsville, MD: National Center for Health Statistics. 2006, forthcoming.

This table will be updated on the Web. Go to www.cdc.gov/nchs/hus.htm.

Table 28 (page 1 of 2). Age-adjusted death rates, by race, Hispanic origin, geographic division, and state: United States, average annual 1979–1981, 1989–1991, and 2002–2004

[Data are based on death certificates]

Geographic division and state	All persons			White	Black or African American	American Indian or Alaska Native	Asian or Pacific Islander	Hispanic or Latino[1]	White, not Hispanic or Latino
	1979–1981	1989–1991	2002–2004	2002–2004	2002–2004	2002–2004	2002–2004	2002–2004	2002–2004
	Age-adjusted death rate per 100,000 population[2]								
United States	1,022.8	942.2	826.5	811.0	1,059.7	671.2	460.9	613.9	820.3
New England	979.9	882.4	767.9	769.4	843.2	*	364.2	516.7	768.5
Connecticut	961.5	857.5	736.6	731.2	845.1	*	304.3	562.4	728.2
Maine	1,002.9	918.7	824.2	823.5	790.9	*	509.4	*	822.5
Massachusetts	982.6	884.8	773.2	777.6	842.9	*	375.7	514.8	777.8
New Hampshire	982.3	891.7	765.3	769.3	677.1	*	269.9	427.7	760.7
Rhode Island	990.8	889.6	784.4	784.4	902.6	*	465.9	452.0	786.8
Vermont	990.2	908.6	756.9	760.5	*	*	*	*	762.4
Middle Atlantic	1,059.1	967.8	793.7	787.2	918.0	*	380.5	565.9	790.0
New Jersey	1,047.5	956.0	787.6	771.7	1,012.7	*	365.5	503.5	785.8
New York	1,051.8	973.7	758.6	763.2	812.1	*	388.9	578.8	760.6
Pennsylvania	1,076.4	963.4	845.8	825.9	1,106.8	*	363.0	656.2	825.0
East North Central	1,048.0	957.9	848.7	824.2	1,114.6	*	373.5	521.9	826.9
Illinois	1,063.7	973.8	830.9	798.9	1,126.1	*	372.8	476.9	809.9
Indiana	1,048.3	962.0	882.2	868.0	1,120.7	*	338.9	515.6	871.7
Michigan	1,050.2	966.0	849.0	816.2	1,104.9	*	373.0	689.3	811.9
Ohio	1,070.6	967.4	884.1	863.7	1,116.2	*	330.2	620.2	862.3
Wisconsin	956.4	879.1	774.2	760.9	1,044.0	*	480.9	402.1	763.8
West North Central	951.6	876.6	797.9	783.8	1,096.4	*	433.6	561.4	780.7
Iowa	919.9	848.2	757.1	755.2	1,006.8	*	405.0	530.4	756.2
Kansas	940.1	867.2	821.0	811.3	1,114.2	*	342.8	552.4	805.8
Minnesota	892.9	825.2	715.3	709.3	879.4	1,169.1	491.9	461.6	702.8
Missouri	1,033.7	952.4	895.8	874.9	1,144.1	*	431.4	687.3	875.1
Nebraska	930.6	867.9	782.6	773.5	1,063.6	1,114.8	390.2	576.3	772.2
North Dakota	922.4	818.4	737.3	718.3	*	1,409.8	*	*	697.5
South Dakota	941.9	846.4	770.1	728.7	*	1,542.0	*	455.7	729.4
South Atlantic	1,033.1	951.3	844.5	806.1	1,073.1	*	367.5	573.4	820.3
Delaware	1,069.7	1,001.9	838.6	807.9	1,062.5	*	339.0	680.8	807.7
District of Columbia	1,243.1	1,255.3	991.6	610.7	1,234.7	*	413.5	137.0	656.0
Florida	960.8	870.9	775.0	754.8	1,002.0	*	333.3	609.4	779.0
Georgia	1,094.3	1,037.4	938.2	892.7	1,123.9	*	335.5	355.9	900.8
Maryland	1,063.3	985.2	841.2	787.1	1,067.4	*	363.9	301.9	797.6
North Carolina	1,050.4	986.0	895.3	855.1	1,092.4	869.4	355.2	294.2	860.5
South Carolina	1,104.6	1,030.0	925.4	874.1	1,093.9	*	397.2	357.3	877.2
Virginia	1,054.0	963.1	837.2	804.5	1,060.7	*	433.1	451.9	808.3
West Virginia	1,100.3	1,031.5	982.8	983.7	1,112.3	*	*	349.1	986.4
East South Central	1,079.3	1,031.6	981.8	951.3	1,163.9	*	406.6	380.7	954.3
Alabama	1,091.2	1,037.9	992.8	954.1	1,156.6	*	342.5	332.6	958.3
Kentucky	1,088.9	1,024.5	968.3	962.4	1,128.5	*	397.5	687.3	962.7
Mississippi	1,108.7	1,071.4	1,010.6	949.6	1,166.3	*	465.0	242.5	953.6
Tennessee	1,045.5	1,011.8	969.5	942.2	1,185.2	*	425.4	309.4	946.0
West South Central	1,036.8	974.9	894.9	870.6	1,151.7	*	418.2	691.5	897.9
Arkansas	1,017.0	996.3	939.9	915.2	1,160.1	*	500.7	237.1	923.9
Louisiana	1,132.6	1,074.6	994.5	925.4	1,201.5	*	463.5	437.6	934.8
Oklahoma	1,025.6	961.4	961.0	957.5	1,153.9	*	443.1	666.4	961.7
Texas	1,014.9	947.6	853.5	837.4	1,122.7	*	408.6	701.6	868.0
Mountain	961.8	878.2	796.9	794.2	956.4	867.9	472.3	731.6	795.2
Arizona	951.5	873.5	782.2	776.5	951.4	885.7	421.4	742.9	776.9
Colorado	941.1	856.1	770.9	774.4	876.3	474.6	429.2	761.0	768.8
Idaho	936.7	856.6	777.1	777.8	745.1	979.4	427.3	593.5	780.0
Montana	1,013.6	890.2	816.4	797.3	*	1,260.4	469.8	697.9	797.0
Nevada	1,077.4	1,017.4	909.1	910.5	1,130.3	713.2	600.4	527.5	939.2
New Mexico	967.1	891.9	805.3	802.3	823.7	849.6	315.8	788.3	792.5
Utah	924.9	823.2	775.2	779.3	840.1	800.7	465.7	604.1	783.2
Wyoming	1,016.1	897.4	835.8	829.4	774.4	1,258.3	*	787.2	829.4

See footnotes at end of table.

This table will be updated on the Web. Go to www.cdc.gov/nchs/hus.htm.

Table 28 (page 2 of 2). Age-adjusted death rates, by race, Hispanic origin, geographic division, and state: United States, average annual 1979–1981, 1989–1991, and 2002–2004

[Data are based on death certificates]

Geographic division and state	All persons 1979–1981	All persons 1989–1991	All persons 2002–2004	White 2002–2004	Black or African American 2002–2004	American Indian or Alaska Native 2002–2004	Asian or Pacific Islander 2002–2004	Hispanic or Latino[1] 2002–2004	White, not Hispanic or Latino 2002–2004
	Age-adjusted death rate per 100,000 population[2]								
Pacific	966.5	900.1	748.4	765.8	1,007.3	*	511.6	592.9	788.4
Alaska	1,087.4	944.6	789.2	739.6	764.4	1,154.5	506.2	583.8	743.1
California	975.5	911.0	742.2	759.5	1,023.7	*	480.7	592.8	788.5
Hawaii	801.2	752.2	646.8	694.6	474.0	*	632.3	1,304.6	700.3
Oregon	953.9	893.0	805.3	809.9	939.2	*	470.2	434.5	817.5
Washington	947.7	869.4	765.9	772.5	883.3	909.3	504.8	515.3	776.7

* Data for states with population under 10,000 in the middle year of a 3-year period or fewer than 50 deaths for the 3-year period are considered unreliable and are not shown. Data for American Indian or Alaska Native category in states with more than 10% misclassification of American Indian or Alaska Native deaths on death certificates or without information on misclassification are also not shown (Support Services International, Inc. Methodology for adjusting IHS mortality data for miscoding race-ethnicity of American Indian or Alaska Native on state death certificates. Report submitted to Indian Health Service. 1996). Division death rates for American Indians or Alaska Natives are not shown when any state within the division does not meet reliability criteria.

[1]Caution should be used when comparing death rates by Hispanic origin and race among states. Estimates of death rates may be affected by several factors including possible misreporting of race and Hispanic origin on the death certificate, migration patterns between United States and country of origin for persons who were born outside the United States, and possible biases in population estimates. See Appendix I, National Vital Statistics System, Mortality File and Appendix II, Hispanic origin; Race.

[2]Average annual death rates, age-adjusted using the year 2000 standard population. Prior to 2001, age-adjusted rates were calculated using standard million proportions based on rounded population numbers. Starting with 2001 data, unrounded population numbers are used to calculate age-adjusted rates. See Appendix II, Age adjustment. Denominators for rates are resident population estimates for the middle year of each 3-year period, multiplied by 3. See Appendix I, Population Census and Population Estimates.

NOTES: The race groups, white, black, American Indian or Alaska Native, and Asian or Pacific Islander, include persons of Hispanic and non-Hispanic origin. Persons of Hispanic origin may be of any race. Death rates for the American Indian or Alaska Native and Asian or Pacific Islander populations are known to be underestimated. See Appendix II, Race, for a discussion of sources of bias in death rates by race and Hispanic origin. In 2003, seven states reported multiple-race data. In 2004, 15 states reported multiple-race data. The multiple-race data for these states were bridged to the single-race categories of the 1977 Office of Management and Budget Standards for comparability with other states. See Appendix II, Race.

SOURCES: Centers for Disease Control and Prevention, National Center for Health Statistics, National Vital Statistics System; numerator data from annual mortality files; denominator data from state population estimates prepared by the U.S. Census Bureau 1980 from April 1, 1980 MARS Census File; 1990 from April 1, 1990 MARS Census File; 2003 from bridged-race Vintage 2003 file. Estimates of the July 1, 2003, resident populations of the United States by state and county, race, age, sex, and Hispanic origin, prepared under a collaborative arrangement with the U.S. Census Bureau. Available from: www.cdc.gov/nchs/about/major/dvs/popbridge/popbridge.htm. 2005.

This table will be updated on the Web. Go to www.cdc.gov/nchs/hus.htm.

Table 29 (page 1 of 4). Age-adjusted death rates for selected causes of death, by sex, race, and Hispanic origin: United States, selected years 1950–2004

[Data are based on death certificates]

Sex, race, Hispanic origin, and cause of death[1]	*1950*[2,3]	*1960*[2,3]	*1970*[3]	*1980*[3]	*1990*	*2000*[4]	*2002*	*2003*	*2004*
All persons				Age-adjusted death rate per 100,000 population[5]					
All causes	1,446.0	1,339.2	1,222.6	1,039.1	938.7	869.0	845.3	832.7	800.8
Diseases of heart	586.8	559.0	492.7	412.1	321.8	257.6	240.8	232.3	217.0
Ischemic heart disease	- - -	- - -	- - -	345.2	249.6	186.8	170.8	162.9	150.2
Cerebrovascular diseases	180.7	177.9	147.7	96.2	65.3	60.9	56.2	53.5	50.0
Malignant neoplasms	193.9	193.9	198.6	207.9	216.0	199.6	193.5	190.1	185.8
Trachea, bronchus, and lung	15.0	24.1	37.1	49.9	59.3	56.1	54.9	54.1	53.2
Colon, rectum, and anus	- - -	30.3	28.9	27.4	24.5	20.8	19.7	19.1	18.0
Prostate[6]	28.6	28.7	28.8	32.8	38.4	30.4	27.9	26.5	25.4
Breast[7]	31.9	31.7	32.1	31.9	33.3	26.8	25.6	25.3	24.4
Chronic lower respiratory diseases	- - -	- - -	- - -	28.3	37.2	44.2	43.5	43.3	41.1
Influenza and pneumonia	48.1	53.7	41.7	31.4	36.8	23.7	22.6	22.0	19.8
Chronic liver disease and cirrhosis	11.3	13.3	17.8	15.1	11.1	9.5	9.4	9.3	9.0
Diabetes mellitus	23.1	22.5	24.3	18.1	20.7	25.0	25.4	25.3	24.5
Human immunodeficiency virus (HIV) disease	- - -	- - -	- - -	- - -	10.2	5.2	4.9	4.7	4.5
Unintentional injuries	78.0	62.3	60.1	46.4	36.3	34.9	36.9	37.3	37.7
Motor vehicle-related injuries	24.6	23.1	27.6	22.3	18.5	15.4	15.7	15.3	15.2
Suicide[8]	13.2	12.5	13.1	12.2	12.5	10.4	10.9	10.8	10.9
Homicide[8]	5.1	5.0	8.8	10.4	9.4	5.9	6.1	6.0	5.9
Male									
All causes	1,674.2	1,609.0	1,542.1	1,348.1	1,202.8	1,053.8	1,013.7	994.3	955.7
Diseases of heart	697.0	687.6	634.0	538.9	412.4	320.0	297.4	286.6	267.9
Ischemic heart disease	- - -	- - -	- - -	459.7	328.2	241.4	220.4	209.9	194.1
Cerebrovascular diseases	186.4	186.1	157.4	102.2	68.5	62.4	56.5	54.1	50.4
Malignant neoplasms	208.1	225.1	247.6	271.2	280.4	248.9	238.9	233.3	227.7
Trachea, bronchus, and lung	24.6	43.6	67.5	85.2	91.1	76.7	73.2	71.7	70.1
Colon, rectum, and anus	- - -	31.8	32.3	32.8	30.4	25.1	23.7	22.9	21.5
Prostate	28.6	28.7	28.8	32.8	38.4	30.4	27.9	26.5	25.4
Chronic lower respiratory diseases	- - -	- - -	- - -	49.9	55.4	55.8	53.5	52.3	49.5
Influenza and pneumonia	55.0	65.8	54.0	42.1	47.8	28.9	27.0	26.1	23.7
Chronic liver disease and cirrhosis	15.0	18.5	24.8	21.3	15.9	13.4	12.9	13.0	12.5
Diabetes mellitus	18.8	19.9	23.0	18.1	21.7	27.8	28.6	28.9	28.2
Human immunodeficiency virus (HIV) disease	- - -	- - -	- - -	- - -	18.5	7.9	7.4	7.1	6.6
Unintentional injuries	101.8	85.5	87.4	69.0	52.9	49.3	51.5	51.8	52.1
Motor vehicle-related injuries	38.5	35.4	41.5	33.6	26.5	21.7	22.1	21.6	21.4
Suicide[8]	21.2	20.0	19.8	19.9	21.5	17.7	18.4	18.0	18.0
Homicide[8]	7.9	7.5	14.3	16.6	14.8	9.0	9.4	9.4	9.2
Female									
All causes	1,236.0	1,105.3	971.4	817.9	750.9	731.4	715.2	706.2	679.2
Diseases of heart	484.7	447.0	381.6	320.8	257.0	210.9	197.2	190.3	177.3
Ischemic heart disease	- - -	- - -	- - -	263.1	193.9	146.5	133.6	127.2	116.7
Cerebrovascular diseases	175.8	170.7	140.0	91.7	62.6	59.1	55.2	52.3	48.9
Malignant neoplasms	182.3	168.7	163.2	166.7	175.7	167.6	163.1	160.9	157.4
Trachea, bronchus, and lung	5.8	7.5	13.1	24.4	37.1	41.3	41.6	41.3	40.9
Colon, rectum, and anus	- - -	29.1	26.5	23.8	20.6	17.7	16.7	16.2	15.3
Breast	31.9	31.7	32.1	31.9	33.3	26.8	25.6	25.3	24.4
Chronic lower respiratory diseases	- - -	- - -	- - -	14.9	26.6	37.4	37.4	37.8	36.0
Influenza and pneumonia	41.9	43.8	32.7	25.1	30.5	20.7	19.9	19.4	17.3
Chronic liver disease and cirrhosis	7.8	8.7	11.9	9.9	7.1	6.2	6.3	6.0	5.8
Diabetes mellitus	27.0	24.7	25.1	18.0	19.9	23.0	23.0	22.5	21.7
Human immunodeficiency virus (HIV) disease	- - -	- - -	- - -	- - -	2.2	2.5	2.5	2.4	2.4
Unintentional injuries	54.0	40.0	35.1	26.1	21.5	22.0	23.5	24.1	24.5
Motor vehicle-related injuries	11.5	11.7	14.9	11.8	11.0	9.5	9.6	9.3	9.3
Suicide[8]	5.6	5.6	7.4	5.7	4.8	4.0	4.2	4.2	4.5
Homicide[8]	2.4	2.6	3.7	4.4	4.0	2.8	2.8	2.6	2.5

See footnotes at end of table.

This table will be updated on the Web. Go to www.cdc.gov/nchs/hus.htm.

Table 29 (page 2 of 4). Age-adjusted death rates for selected causes of death, by sex, race, and Hispanic origin: United States, selected years 1950–2004

[Data are based on death certificates]

Sex, race, Hispanic origin, and cause of death[1]	1950[2,3]	1960[2,3]	1970[3]	1980[3]	1990	2000[4]	2002	2003	2004
	Age-adjusted death rate per 100,000 population[5]								
White[9]									
All causes	1,410.8	1,311.3	1,193.3	1,012.7	909.8	849.8	829.0	817.0	786.3
Diseases of heart	584.8	559.0	492.2	409.4	317.0	253.4	236.7	228.2	213.3
Ischemic heart disease	---	---	---	347.6	249.7	185.6	169.8	161.7	149.2
Cerebrovascular diseases	175.5	172.7	143.5	93.2	62.8	58.8	54.2	51.4	48.0
Malignant neoplasms	194.6	193.1	196.7	204.2	211.6	197.2	191.7	188.5	184.4
Trachea, bronchus, and lung	15.2	24.0	36.7	49.2	58.6	56.2	55.3	54.5	53.6
Colon, rectum, and anus	---	30.9	29.2	27.4	24.1	20.3	19.2	18.6	17.6
Prostate[6]	28.4	27.7	27.4	30.5	35.5	27.8	25.7	24.4	23.4
Breast[7]	32.4	32.0	32.5	32.1	33.2	26.3	25.0	24.7	23.9
Chronic lower respiratory diseases	---	---	---	29.3	38.3	46.0	45.4	45.4	43.2
Influenza and pneumonia	44.8	50.4	39.8	30.9	36.4	23.5	22.6	21.9	19.6
Chronic liver disease and cirrhosis	11.5	13.2	16.6	13.9	10.5	9.6	9.6	9.5	9.2
Diabetes mellitus	22.9	21.7	22.9	16.7	18.8	22.8	23.1	23.0	22.3
Human immunodeficiency virus (HIV) disease	---	---	---	---	8.3	2.8	2.6	2.5	2.3
Unintentional injuries	77.0	60.4	57.8	45.3	35.5	35.1	37.5	38.2	38.8
Motor vehicle-related injuries	24.4	22.9	27.1	22.6	18.5	15.6	16.0	15.7	15.6
Suicide[8]	13.9	13.1	13.8	13.0	13.4	11.3	12.0	11.8	12.0
Homicide[8]	2.6	2.7	4.7	6.7	5.5	3.6	3.7	3.7	3.6
Black or African American[9]									
All causes	1,722.1	1,577.5	1,518.1	1,314.8	1,250.3	1,121.4	1,083.3	1,065.9	1,027.3
Diseases of heart	586.7	548.3	512.0	455.3	391.5	324.8	308.4	300.2	280.6
Ischemic heart disease	---	---	---	334.5	267.0	218.3	203.0	195.0	179.8
Cerebrovascular diseases	233.6	235.2	197.1	129.1	91.6	81.9	76.3	74.3	69.9
Malignant neoplasms	176.4	199.1	225.3	256.4	279.5	248.5	238.8	233.3	227.2
Trachea, bronchus, and lung	11.1	23.7	41.3	59.7	72.4	64.0	61.9	60.8	59.8
Colon, rectum, and anus	---	22.8	26.1	28.3	30.6	28.2	26.8	26.4	24.7
Prostate[6]	30.9	41.2	48.5	61.1	77.0	68.1	62.0	57.4	55.5
Breast[7]	25.3	27.9	28.9	31.7	38.1	34.5	34.0	34.0	32.2
Chronic lower respiratory diseases	---	---	---	19.2	28.1	31.6	31.2	30.1	28.2
Influenza and pneumonia	76.7	81.1	57.2	34.4	39.4	25.6	24.0	23.3	22.3
Chronic liver disease and cirrhosis	9.0	13.6	28.1	25.0	16.5	9.4	8.5	8.4	7.9
Diabetes mellitus	23.5	30.9	38.8	32.7	40.5	49.5	49.5	49.2	48.0
Human immunodeficiency virus (HIV) disease	---	---	---	---	26.7	23.3	22.5	21.3	20.4
Unintentional injuries	79.9	74.0	78.3	57.6	43.8	37.7	36.9	36.1	36.3
Motor vehicle-related injuries	26.0	24.2	31.1	20.2	18.8	15.7	15.0	14.9	14.8
Suicide[8]	4.5	5.0	6.2	6.5	7.1	5.5	5.3	5.2	5.3
Homicide[8]	28.3	26.0	44.0	39.0	36.3	20.5	21.0	21.0	20.1
American Indian or Alaska Native[9]									
All causes	---	---	---	867.0	716.3	709.3	677.4	685.0	650.0
Diseases of heart	---	---	---	240.6	200.6	178.2	157.4	160.2	148.0
Ischemic heart disease	---	---	---	173.6	139.1	129.1	114.0	114.1	106.5
Cerebrovascular diseases	---	---	---	57.8	40.7	45.0	37.5	34.6	35.3
Malignant neoplasms	---	---	---	113.7	121.8	127.8	125.4	119.3	124.9
Trachea, bronchus, and lung	---	---	---	20.7	30.9	32.3	33.1	31.3	36.0
Colon, rectum, and anus	---	---	---	9.5	12.0	13.4	14.2	11.8	12.1
Prostate[6]	---	---	---	20.7	17.8	19.6	15.2	17.8	16.0
Breast[7]	---	---	---	10.8	13.7	13.6	13.8	14.0	14.8
Chronic lower respiratory diseases	---	---	---	14.2	25.4	32.8	30.1	31.7	28.5
Influenza and pneumonia	---	---	---	44.4	36.1	22.3	20.4	24.1	17.6
Chronic liver disease and cirrhosis	---	---	---	45.3	24.1	24.3	22.8	22.6	22.7
Diabetes mellitus	---	---	---	29.6	34.1	41.5	43.2	43.7	39.2
Human immunodeficiency virus (HIV) disease	---	---	---	---	1.8	2.2	2.2	2.5	2.9
Unintentional injuries	---	---	---	99.0	62.6	51.3	53.8	56.4	53.1
Motor vehicle-related injuries	---	---	---	54.5	32.5	27.3	28.8	28.1	26.0
Suicide[8]	---	---	---	11.9	11.7	9.8	10.2	10.0	12.2
Homicide[8]	---	---	---	15.5	10.4	6.8	8.4	7.3	7.0

See footnotes at end of table.

This table will be updated on the Web. Go to www.cdc.gov/nchs/hus.htm.

Table 29 (page 3 of 4). Age-adjusted death rates for selected causes of death, by sex, race, and Hispanic origin: United States, selected years 1950–2004

[Data are based on death certificates]

Sex, race, Hispanic origin, and cause of death[1]	*1950*[2,3]	*1960*[2,3]	*1970*[3]	*1980*[3]	*1990*	*2000*[4]	*2002*	*2003*	*2004*
Asian or Pacific Islander[9]			Age-adjusted death rate per 100,000 population[5]						
All causes	---	---	---	589.9	582.0	506.4	474.4	465.7	443.9
Diseases of heart	---	---	---	202.1	181.7	146.0	134.6	127.6	117.8
Ischemic heart disease	---	---	---	168.2	139.6	109.6	98.6	92.8	84.1
Cerebrovascular diseases	---	---	---	66.1	56.9	52.9	47.7	45.2	41.3
Malignant neoplasms	---	---	---	126.1	134.2	121.9	113.6	113.5	110.5
Trachea, bronchus, and lung	---	---	---	28.4	30.2	28.1	25.6	26.9	26.2
Colon, rectum, and anus	---	---	---	16.4	14.4	12.7	12.5	12.1	11.3
Prostate[6]	---	---	---	10.2	16.8	12.5	10.2	10.9	11.4
Breast[7]	---	---	---	11.9	13.7	12.3	12.8	12.6	12.7
Chronic lower respiratory diseases	---	---	---	12.9	19.4	18.6	15.8	16.2	14.7
Influenza and pneumonia	---	---	---	24.0	31.4	19.7	17.5	17.3	16.0
Chronic liver disease and cirrhosis	---	---	---	6.1	5.2	3.5	3.2	3.0	3.2
Diabetes mellitus	---	---	---	12.6	14.6	16.4	17.4	17.3	16.6
Human immunodeficiency virus (HIV) disease	---	---	---	---	2.2	0.6	0.8	0.7	0.7
Unintentional injuries	---	---	---	27.0	23.9	17.9	17.9	18.0	16.7
Motor vehicle-related injuries	---	---	---	13.9	14.0	8.6	8.4	8.4	7.8
Suicide[8]	---	---	---	7.8	6.7	5.5	5.4	5.6	5.8
Homicide[8]	---	---	---	5.9	5.0	3.0	2.9	2.9	2.5
Hispanic or Latino[9,10]									
All causes	---	---	---	---	692.0	665.7	629.3	621.2	586.7
Diseases of heart	---	---	---	---	217.1	196.0	180.5	173.2	158.4
Ischemic heart disease	---	---	---	---	173.3	153.2	138.3	130.0	119.2
Cerebrovascular diseases	---	---	---	---	45.2	46.4	41.3	40.5	38.2
Malignant neoplasms	---	---	---	---	136.8	134.9	128.4	126.6	121.9
Trachea, bronchus, and lung	---	---	---	---	26.5	24.8	23.7	23.2	22.4
Colon, rectum, and anus	---	---	---	---	14.7	14.1	13.7	13.4	12.6
Prostate[6]	---	---	---	---	23.3	21.6	21.6	20.2	19.1
Breast[7]	---	---	---	---	19.5	16.9	15.5	16.1	15.6
Chronic lower respiratory diseases	---	---	---	---	19.3	21.1	20.6	20.2	18.4
Influenza and pneumonia	---	---	---	---	29.7	20.6	19.2	18.4	17.1
Chronic liver disease and cirrhosis	---	---	---	---	18.3	16.5	15.4	14.7	14.0
Diabetes mellitus	---	---	---	---	28.2	36.9	35.6	35.0	32.1
Human immunodeficiency virus (HIV) disease	---	---	---	---	16.3	6.7	5.8	5.9	5.3
Unintentional injuries	---	---	---	---	34.6	30.1	30.7	30.6	29.8
Motor vehicle-related injuries	---	---	---	---	19.5	14.7	15.2	15.1	14.4
Suicide[8]	---	---	---	---	7.8	5.9	5.7	5.6	5.9
Homicide[8]	---	---	---	---	16.2	7.5	7.3	7.7	7.2

See footnotes at end of table.

This table will be updated on the Web. Go to www.cdc.gov/nchs/hus.htm.

Table 29 (page 4 of 4). Age-adjusted death rates for selected causes of death, by sex, race, and Hispanic origin: United States, selected years 1950–2004

[Data are based on death certificates]

Sex, race, Hispanic origin, and cause of death[1]	*1950*[2,3]	*1960*[2,3]	*1970*[3]	*1980*[3]	*1990*	*2000*[4]	*2002*	*2003*	*2004*
White, not Hispanic or Latino[10]	Age-adjusted death rate per 100,000 population[5]								
All causes	---	---	---	---	914.5	855.5	837.5	826.1	797.1
Diseases of heart	---	---	---	---	319.7	255.5	239.2	230.9	216.3
Ischemic heart disease	---	---	---	---	251.9	186.6	171.0	163.3	150.9
Cerebrovascular diseases	---	---	---	---	63.5	59.0	54.6	51.7	48.3
Malignant neoplasms	---	---	---	---	215.4	200.6	195.6	192.4	188.6
Trachea, bronchus, and lung	---	---	---	---	60.3	58.2	57.5	56.7	56.0
Colon, rectum, and anus	---	---	---	---	24.6	20.5	19.5	18.8	17.9
Prostate[6]	---	---	---	---	36.1	28.0	25.8	24.6	23.6
Breast[7]	---	---	---	---	33.9	26.8	25.6	25.2	24.5
Chronic lower respiratory diseases	---	---	---	---	39.2	47.2	46.9	47.0	44.9
Influenza and pneumonia	---	---	---	---	36.5	23.5	22.6	22.0	19.6
Chronic liver disease and cirrhosis	---	---	---	---	9.9	9.0	9.0	9.0	8.7
Diabetes mellitus	---	---	---	---	18.3	21.8	22.2	22.1	21.5
Human immunodeficiency virus (HIV) disease	---	---	---	---	7.4	2.2	2.1	2.0	1.9
Unintentional injuries	---	---	---	---	35.0	35.3	38.0	38.8	39.7
Motor vehicle-related injuries	---	---	---	---	18.2	15.6	16.0	15.5	15.6
Suicide[8]	---	---	---	---	13.8	12.0	12.9	12.7	12.9
Homicide[8]	---	---	---	---	4.0	2.8	2.8	2.7	2.7

- - - Data not available.

[1]Underlying cause of death code numbers are based on the applicable revision of the *International Classification of Diseases* (ICD) for data years shown. For the period 1980–1998, causes were coded using ICD–9 codes that are most nearly comparable with the 113 cause list for ICD–10. See Appendix II, Cause of death; Tables IV and V.

[2]Includes deaths of persons who were not residents of the 50 states and the District of Columbia.

[3]Underlying cause of death was coded according to the Sixth Revision of the International Classification of Diseases (ICD) in 1950, Seventh Revision in 1960, Eighth Revision in 1970, and Ninth Revision in 1980–1998. See Appendix II, Cause of death; Tables IV and V.

[4]Starting with 1999 data, cause of death is coded according to ICD–10. See Appendix II, Cause of death, Table V; Comparability ratio, Table VI.

[5]Age-adjusted rates are calculated using the year 2000 standard population. Prior to 2003, age-adjusted rates were calculated using standard million proportions based on rounded population numbers. Starting with 2003 data, unrounded population numbers are used to calculate age-adjusted rates. See Appendix II, Age adjustment.

[6]Rate for male population only.

[7]Rate for female population only.

[8]Figures for 2001 include September 11-related deaths for which death certificates were filed as of October 24, 2002. See Appendix II, Cause of death; Table V for terrorism-related ICD–10 codes.

[9]The race groups, white, black, Asian or Pacific Islander, and American Indian or Alaska Native, include persons of Hispanic and non-Hispanic origin. Persons of Hispanic origin may be of any race. Death rates for the American Indian or Alaska Native and Asian or Pacific Islander populations are known to be underestimated. See Appendix II, Race, for a discussion of sources of bias in death rates by race and Hispanic origin.

[10]Prior to 1997, excludes data from states lacking an Hispanic-origin item on the death certificate. See Appendix II, Hispanic origin.

NOTES: Starting with *Health, United States, 2003*, rates for 1991–1999 were revised using intercensal population estimates based on the 2000 census. Rates for 2000 were revised based on 2000 census counts. Rates for 2001 and later years were computed using 2000-based postcensal estimates. See Appendix I, Population Census and Population Estimates. In 2003, seven states reported multiple-race data. In 2004, 15 states reported multiple-race data. The multiple-race data for these states were bridged to the single-race categories of the 1977 Office of Management and Budget Standards for comparability with other states. See Appendix II, Race. Data for additional years are available. See Appendix III.

SOURCES: Centers for Disease Control and Prevention, National Center for Health Statistics, National Vital Statistics System; Grove RD, Hetzel AM. Vital statistics rates in the United States, 1940–1960. Washington, DC: U.S. Government Printing Office. 1968; numerator data from National Vital Statistics System, annual mortality files; denominator data from national population estimates for race groups from Table 1 and unpublished Hispanic population estimates for 1985–1996 prepared by the Housing and Household Economic Statistics Division, U.S. Census Bureau; additional mortality tables are available from: www.cdc.gov/nchs/datawh/statab/unpubd/mortabs.htm; Miniño AM, Heron M, Murphy SL, Kochanek KD. Deaths: Final data for 2004. Health E-Stats. Hyattsville, MD: National Center for Health Statistics. 2006.

This table will be updated on the Web. Go to www.cdc.gov/nchs/hus.htm.

Table 30 (page 1 of 4). Years of potential life lost before age 75 for selected causes of death, by sex, race, and Hispanic origin: United States, selected years 1980–2004

[Data are based on death certificates]

Sex, race, Hispanic origin, and cause of death[2]	Crude	Age-adjusted[1]					
	2004	1980	1990	2000[3]	2002	2003	2004
All persons	Years lost before age 75 per 100,000 population under 75 years of age						
All causes	7,411.4	10,448.4	9,085.5	7,578.1	7,499.6	7,466.9	7,270.6
Diseases of heart	1,165.4	2,238.7	1,617.7	1,253.0	1,212.7	1,187.9	1,128.9
Ischemic heart disease	748.0	1,729.3	1,153.6	841.8	792.0	765.1	720.6
Cerebrovascular diseases	203.1	357.5	259.6	223.3	208.1	203.6	198.1
Malignant neoplasms	1,601.2	2,108.8	2,003.8	1,674.1	1,622.7	1,586.9	1,543.4
Trachea, bronchus, and lung	421.9	548.5	561.4	443.1	423.4	412.2	402.8
Colorectal	132.2	190.0	164.7	141.9	141.0	133.8	127.3
Prostate[4]	54.6	84.9	96.8	63.6	60.1	58.6	55.8
Breast[5]	319.4	463.2	451.6	332.6	316.8	313.7	302.1
Chronic lower respiratory diseases	179.4	169.1	187.4	188.1	184.5	183.9	173.7
Influenza and pneumonia	80.5	160.2	141.5	87.1	82.7	90.8	79.1
Chronic liver disease and cirrhosis	158.2	300.3	196.9	164.1	160.5	159.6	153.9
Diabetes mellitus	184.5	134.4	155.9	178.4	184.3	184.6	178.4
Human immunodeficiency virus (HIV) disease	141.5	---	383.8	174.6	161.8	153.3	143.4
Unintentional injuries	1,098.7	1,543.5	1,162.1	1,026.5	1,079.2	1,084.6	1,098.0
Motor vehicle-related injuries	569.7	912.9	716.4	574.3	585.8	569.6	567.6
Suicide[6]	353.9	392.0	393.1	334.5	346.7	343.3	353.0
Homicide[6]	265.3	425.5	417.4	266.5	274.4	274.3	264.8
Male							
All causes	9,208.4	13,777.2	11,973.5	9,572.2	9,470.0	9,416.4	9,143.1
Diseases of heart	1,590.1	3,352.1	2,356.0	1,766.0	1,706.9	1,664.2	1,583.4
Ischemic heart disease	1,075.8	2,715.1	1,766.3	1,255.4	1,179.6	1,138.8	1,070.5
Cerebrovascular diseases	218.8	396.7	286.6	244.6	227.6	225.9	219.6
Malignant neoplasms	1,673.6	2,360.8	2,214.6	1,810.8	1,754.2	1,711.4	1,663.3
Trachea, bronchus, and lung	493.0	821.1	764.8	554.9	520.5	504.6	490.3
Colorectal	150.5	214.9	194.3	167.3	168.2	157.7	149.7
Prostate	54.6	84.9	96.8	63.6	60.1	58.6	55.8
Chronic lower respiratory diseases	186.1	235.1	224.8	206.0	200.7	199.5	188.4
Influenza and pneumonia	93.5	202.5	180.0	102.8	97.3	106.4	93.6
Chronic liver disease and cirrhosis	221.0	415.0	283.9	236.9	226.6	229.4	219.0
Diabetes mellitus	213.4	140.4	170.4	203.8	217.2	218.2	212.6
Human immunodeficiency virus (HIV) disease	201.6	---	686.2	258.9	237.0	223.7	205.1
Unintentional injuries	1,563.4	2,342.7	1,715.1	1,475.6	1,542.2	1,537.7	1,547.4
Motor vehicle-related injuries	802.4	1,359.7	1,018.4	796.4	817.2	795.0	789.1
Suicide[6]	557.5	605.6	634.8	539.1	555.7	548.2	553.0
Homicide[6]	422.7	675.0	658.0	410.5	425.0	430.5	414.3
Female							
All causes	5,617.0	7,350.3	6,333.1	5,644.6	5,580.0	5,560.5	5,435.8
Diseases of heart	741.4	1,246.0	948.5	774.6	748.8	739.5	699.9
Ischemic heart disease	420.7	852.1	600.3	457.6	430.2	415.0	391.8
Cerebrovascular diseases	187.4	324.0	235.9	203.9	190.3	183.0	178.1
Malignant neoplasms	1,528.8	1,896.8	1,826.6	1,555.3	1,507.7	1,477.3	1,437.6
Trachea, bronchus, and lung	350.9	310.4	382.2	342.1	335.4	328.1	323.2
Colorectal	114.1	168.7	138.7	118.7	115.9	111.9	106.8
Breast	319.4	463.2	451.6	332.6	316.8	313.7	302.1
Chronic lower respiratory diseases	172.7	114.0	155.9	172.3	170.0	169.9	160.4
Influenza and pneumonia	67.5	122.0	106.2	72.3	69.1	76.0	65.3
Chronic liver disease and cirrhosis	95.6	194.5	115.1	94.5	97.4	92.6	91.3
Diabetes mellitus	155.6	128.5	142.3	154.4	153.1	152.9	146.0
Human immunodeficiency virus (HIV) disease	81.4	---	87.8	92.0	88.1	84.1	82.7
Unintentional injuries	634.7	755.3	607.4	573.2	610.3	624.6	641.1
Motor vehicle-related injuries	337.3	470.4	411.6	348.5	349.8	339.2	341.1
Suicide[6]	150.5	184.2	153.3	129.1	136.6	136.6	150.9
Homicide[6]	108.1	181.3	174.3	118.9	119.6	112.9	110.2

See footnotes at end of table.

This table will be updated on the Web. Go to www.cdc.gov/nchs/hus.htm.

Table 30 (page 2 of 4). Years of potential life lost before age 75 for selected causes of death, by sex, race, and Hispanic origin: United States, selected years 1980–2004

[Data are based on death certificates]

Sex, race, Hispanic origin, and cause of death[2]	Crude	Age-adjusted[1]					
	2004	1980	1990	2000[3]	2002	2003	2004
White[7]		Years lost before age 75 per 100,000 population under 75 years of age					
All causes	6,994.5	9,554.1	8,159.5	6,949.5	6,936.6	6,910.6	6,743.7
Diseases of heart	1,104.2	2,100.8	1,490.3	1,149.4	1,111.8	1,081.3	1,031.0
Ischemic heart disease	746.5	1,682.7	1,113.4	805.3	759.5	731.5	690.4
Cerebrovascular diseases	175.4	300.7	213.1	187.1	173.5	166.7	165.4
Malignant neoplasms	1,617.6	2,035.9	1,929.3	1,627.8	1,582.8	1,546.5	1,502.0
Trachea, bronchus, and lung	437.2	529.9	544.2	436.3	418.5	407.9	398.3
Colorectal	130.2	186.8	157.8	134.1	134.0	125.5	120.5
Prostate[4]	50.2	74.8	86.6	54.3	51.3	50.5	48.4
Breast[5]	308.3	460.2	441.7	315.6	297.5	295.0	282.1
Chronic lower respiratory diseases	189.2	165.4	182.3	185.3	183.5	184.2	174.3
Influenza and pneumonia	74.5	130.8	116.9	77.7	75.1	82.2	71.5
Chronic liver disease and cirrhosis	166.3	257.3	175.8	162.7	162.9	162.3	157.2
Diabetes mellitus	166.6	115.7	133.7	155.6	160.3	160.3	155.2
Human immunodeficiency virus (HIV) disease	73.9	- - -	309.0	94.7	84.7	82.1	74.5
Unintentional injuries	1,125.9	1,520.4	1,139.7	1,031.8	1,101.6	1,117.7	1,134.9
Motor vehicle-related injuries	582.3	939.9	726.7	586.1	604.0	588.5	587.6
Suicide[6]	385.9	414.5	417.7	362.0	380.1	375.0	386.0
Homicide[6]	154.7	271.7	234.9	156.6	159.7	159.3	157.0
Black or African American[7]							
All causes	11,305.3	17,873.4	16,593.0	12,897.1	12,401.0	12,304.0	11,922.4
Diseases of heart	1,816.1	3,619.9	2,891.8	2,275.2	2,212.8	2,205.7	2,090.5
Ischemic heart disease	944.4	2,305.1	1,676.1	1,300.1	1,218.7	1,182.6	1,119.0
Cerebrovascular diseases	391.3	883.2	656.4	507.0	474.1	479.6	452.0
Malignant neoplasms	1,814.1	2,946.1	2,894.8	2,294.7	2,196.6	2,163.9	2,107.3
Trachea, bronchus, and lung	441.9	776.0	811.3	593.0	561.9	542.1	529.3
Colorectal	166.5	232.3	241.8	222.4	213.7	214.4	196.6
Prostate[4]	100.4	200.3	223.5	171.0	160.3	154.3	143.0
Breast[5]	438.9	524.2	592.9	500.0	495.9	490.6	477.7
Chronic lower respiratory diseases	178.1	203.7	240.6	232.7	222.8	212.3	201.8
Influenza and pneumonia	130.7	384.9	330.8	161.2	146.7	157.5	141.2
Chronic liver disease and cirrhosis	131.1	644.0	371.8	185.6	161.3	158.9	148.4
Diabetes mellitus	324.6	305.3	361.5	383.4	396.7	396.0	378.8
Human immunodeficiency virus (HIV) disease	591.6	- - -	1,014.7	763.3	720.6	670.1	637.8
Unintentional injuries	1,116.2	1,751.5	1,392.7	1,152.8	1,129.3	1,082.1	1,095.5
Motor vehicle-related injuries	564.2	750.2	699.5	580.8	558.5	536.2	543.8
Suicide[6]	205.8	238.0	261.4	208.7	196.5	199.5	200.6
Homicide[6]	977.3	1,580.8	1,612.9	941.6	962.2	965.0	918.7
American Indian or Alaska Native[7]							
All causes	7,832.0	13,390.9	9,506.2	7,758.2	8,278.0	8,541.6	8,405.4
Diseases of heart	818.8	1,819.9	1,391.0	1,030.1	959.9	1,099.3	975.8
Ischemic heart disease	511.1	1,208.2	901.8	709.3	648.4	708.1	628.3
Cerebrovascular diseases	138.5	269.3	223.3	198.1	201.7	190.7	171.4
Malignant neoplasms	880.4	1,101.3	1,141.1	995.7	1,066.0	997.2	1,068.4
Trachea, bronchus, and lung	202.6	181.1	268.1	227.8	226.3	223.9	264.1
Colorectal	74.8	78.8	82.4	93.8	115.7	85.5	92.1
Prostate[4]	25.0	66.7	42.0	44.5	36.3	34.7	37.1
Breast[5]	163.5	205.5	213.4	174.1	187.1	146.8	186.0
Chronic lower respiratory diseases	117.9	89.3	129.0	151.8	137.0	163.6	148.6
Influenza and pneumonia	104.3	307.9	206.3	124.0	100.9	171.8	116.1
Chronic liver disease and cirrhosis	421.8	1,190.3	535.1	519.4	495.8	504.6	480.5
Diabetes mellitus	263.2	305.5	292.3	305.6	344.7	355.2	323.5
Human immunodeficiency virus (HIV) disease	84.8	- - -	70.1	68.4	79.9	80.7	93.8
Unintentional injuries	1,809.6	3,541.0	2,183.9	1,700.1	1,764.6	1,818.4	1,732.9
Motor vehicle-related injuries	1,043.5	2,102.4	1,301.5	1,032.2	1,089.3	1,081.8	968.3
Suicide[6]	551.0	515.0	495.9	403.1	420.8	418.2	511.6
Homicide[6]	328.3	628.9	434.2	278.5	366.5	323.1	304.7

See footnotes at end of table.

This table will be updated on the Web. Go to www.cdc.gov/nchs/hus.htm.

Table 30 (page 3 of 4). Years of potential life lost before age 75 for selected causes of death, by sex, race, and Hispanic origin: United States, selected years 1980–2004

[Data are based on death certificates]

Sex, race, Hispanic origin, and cause of death[2]	Crude	Age-adjusted[1]					
	2004	1980	1990	2000[3]	2002	2003	2004
Asian or Pacific Islander[7]		Years lost before age 75 per 100,000 population under 75 years of age					
All causes	3,340.2	5,378.4	4,705.2	3,811.1	3,635.5	3,657.5	3,452.1
Diseases of heart	440.8	952.8	702.2	567.9	539.4	534.3	474.9
Ischemic heart disease	274.5	697.7	486.6	381.1	352.0	354.7	303.4
Cerebrovascular diseases	154.5	266.9	233.5	199.4	186.5	192.9	167.5
Malignant neoplasms	890.6	1,218.6	1,166.4	1,033.8	990.3	959.1	949.9
Trachea, bronchus, and lung	158.4	238.2	204.7	185.8	173.8	173.9	176.0
Colorectal	82.8	115.9	105.1	91.6	92.8	94.4	87.7
Prostate[4]	11.6	17.0	32.4	18.8	20.8	14.6	15.1
Breast[5]	193.0	222.2	216.5	200.8	188.4	192.3	193.4
Chronic lower respiratory diseases	32.0	56.4	72.8	56.5	44.8	45.1	36.5
Influenza and pneumonia	32.8	79.3	74.0	48.6	38.0	47.7	36.1
Chronic liver disease and cirrhosis	37.6	85.6	72.4	44.8	40.0	36.8	38.3
Diabetes mellitus	70.8	83.1	74.0	77.0	76.4	79.9	78.3
Human immunodeficiency virus (HIV) disease	22.5	- - -	77.0	19.9	24.8	22.3	21.9
Unintentional injuries	425.0	742.7	636.6	425.7	431.1	429.6	415.0
Motor vehicle-related injuries	263.1	472.6	445.5	263.4	269.7	269.6	254.4
Suicide[6]	186.9	217.1	200.6	168.6	162.7	172.1	175.5
Homicide[6]	103.9	201.1	205.8	113.1	127.5	120.6	98.8
Hispanic or Latino[7,8]							
All causes	5,146.5	- - -	7,963.3	6,037.6	5,865.9	5,910.0	5,654.0
Diseases of heart	499.9	- - -	1,082.0	821.3	796.9	767.7	733.1
Ischemic heart disease	302.6	- - -	756.6	564.6	540.1	501.3	483.3
Cerebrovascular diseases	131.7	- - -	238.0	207.8	193.4	187.3	187.9
Malignant neoplasms	721.6	- - -	1,232.2	1,098.2	1,052.9	1,056.5	1,013.7
Trachea, bronchus, and lung	82.9	- - -	193.7	152.1	150.5	144.9	136.3
Colorectal	60.5	- - -	100.2	101.4	96.7	100.1	91.2
Prostate[4]	18.5	- - -	47.7	42.9	44.1	43.4	38.8
Breast[5]	150.0	- - -	299.3	230.7	205.1	218.4	203.4
Chronic lower respiratory diseases	44.2	- - -	78.8	68.5	69.0	67.1	64.1
Influenza and pneumonia	56.5	- - -	130.1	76.0	65.5	76.4	67.8
Chronic liver disease and cirrhosis	151.0	- - -	329.1	252.1	237.9	221.8	212.5
Diabetes mellitus	122.2	- - -	177.8	215.6	207.1	214.0	192.3
Human immunodeficiency virus (HIV) disease	131.5	- - -	600.1	209.4	179.1	175.4	154.9
Unintentional injuries	978.5	- - -	1,190.6	920.1	958.1	961.5	917.6
Motor vehicle-related injuries	604.3	- - -	740.8	540.2	569.6	563.6	547.7
Suicide[6]	209.5	- - -	256.2	188.5	185.6	188.3	200.3
Homicide[6]	376.3	- - -	720.8	335.1	330.2	345.0	328.8

See footnotes at end of table.

This table will be updated on the Web. Go to www.cdc.gov/nchs/hus.htm.

Table 30 (page 4 of 4). Years of potential life lost before age 75 for selected causes of death, by sex, race, and Hispanic origin: United States, selected years 1980–2004

[Data are based on death certificates]

Sex, race, Hispanic origin, and cause of death[2]	Crude	Age-adjusted[1]					
	2004	1980	1990	2000[3]	2002	2003	2004
White, not Hispanic or Latino[8]	Years lost before age 75 per 100,000 population under 75 years of age						
All causes	7,304.9	---	8,022.5	6,960.5	6,997.9	6,961.6	6,832.9
Diseases of heart	1,219.5	---	1,504.0	1,175.1	1,143.8	1,114.7	1,064.9
Ischemic heart disease	831.7	---	1,127.2	824.7	781.3	755.8	713.8
Cerebrovascular diseases	182.4	---	210.1	183.0	169.4	162.8	161.1
Malignant neoplasms	1,790.5	---	1,974.1	1,668.4	1,629.7	1,590.6	1,549.7
Trachea, bronchus, and lung	508.0	---	566.8	460.3	443.7	433.5	425.1
Colorectal	143.7	---	162.1	136.2	137.6	127.7	123.4
Prostate[4]	56.7	---	89.2	54.9	51.7	51.0	49.2
Breast[5]	337.3	---	451.5	322.3	305.9	301.8	290.0
Chronic lower respiratory diseases	217.8	---	188.1	193.8	193.3	194.2	184.1
Influenza and pneumonia	77.5	---	112.3	76.4	75.8	82.1	71.3
Chronic liver disease and cirrhosis	166.8	---	162.4	150.9	152.1	153.2	148.3
Diabetes mellitus	174.1	---	131.2	150.2	155.8	154.9	152.0
Human immunodeficiency virus (HIV) disease	60.5	---	271.2	76.0	67.8	65.4	59.7
Unintentional injuries	1,143.3	---	1,114.7	1,041.4	1,117.4	1,135.8	1,170.6
Motor vehicle-related injuries	570.5	---	715.7	588.8	603.3	585.3	588.6
Suicide[6]	418.4	---	433.0	389.2	413.9	408.1	419.8
Homicide[6]	105.9	---	162.0	113.2	114.8	109.6	110.3

--- Data not available.

* Rates based on fewer than 20 deaths are considered unreliable and are not shown.

[1]Age-adjusted rates are calculated using the year 2000 standard population. Prior to 2003, age-adjusted rates were calculated using standard million proportions based on rounded population numbers. Starting with 2003 data, unrounded population numbers are used to calculate age-adjusted rates. See Appendix II, Age adjustment.

[2]Underlying cause of death code numbers are based on the applicable revision of the *International Classification of Diseases* (ICD) for data years shown. For the period 1980–1998, causes were coded using ICD–9 codes that are most nearly comparable with the 113 cause list for ICD–10. See Appendix II, Cause of death; Tables IV and V.

[3]Starting with 1999 data, cause of death is coded according to ICD–10. See Appendix II, Cause of death, Table V; Comparability ratio, Table VI.

[4]Rate for male population only.

[5]Rate for female population only.

[6]Figures for 2001 include September 11-related deaths for which death certificates were filed as of October 24, 2002. See Appendix II, Cause of death; Table V for terrorism-related ICD–10 codes.

[7]The race groups, white, black, Asian or Pacific Islander, and American Indian or Alaska Native, include persons of Hispanic and non-Hispanic origin. Persons of Hispanic origin may be of any race. Death rates for the American Indian or Alaska Native and Asian or Pacific Islander populations are known to be underestimated. See Appendix II, Race, for a discussion of sources of bias in death rates by race and Hispanic origin.

[8]Prior to 1997, excludes data from states lacking an Hispanic-origin item on the death certificate. See Appendix II, Hispanic origin.

NOTES: Starting with *Health, United States, 2003*, rates for 1991–1999 were revised using intercensal population estimates based on the 2000 census. Rates for 2000 were revised based on 2000 census counts. Rates for 2001 and later years were computed using 2000-based postcensal estimates. See Appendix I, Population Census and Population Estimates. See Appendix II, Years of potential life lost (YPLL) for definition and method of calculation. In 2003, seven states reported multiple-race data. In 2004, 15 states reported multiple-race data. The multiple-race data for these states were bridged to the single-race categories of the 1977 Office of Management and Budget Standards for comparability with other states. See Appendix II, Race. Data for additional years are available. See Appendix III.

SOURCES: Centers for Disease Control and Prevention, National Center for Health Statistics, National vital statistics system; numerator data from annual mortality files; denominator data from national population estimates for race groups from Table 1 and unpublished Hispanic population estimates for 1990–1996 prepared by the Housing and Household Economic Statistics Division, U.S. Census Bureau.

This table will be updated on the Web. Go to www.cdc.gov/nchs/hus.htm.

Table 31 (page 1 of 4). Leading causes of death and numbers of deaths, by sex, race, and Hispanic origin: United States, 1980 and 2004

[Data are based on death certificates]

Sex, race, Hispanic origin, and rank order	1980 Cause of death	1980 Deaths	2004 Cause of death	2004 Deaths
All persons				
. . .	All causes	1,989,841	All causes	2,397,615
1	Diseases of heart	761,085	Diseases of heart	652,486
2	Malignant neoplasms	416,509	Malignant neoplasms	553,888
3	Cerebrovascular diseases	170,225	Cerebrovascular diseases	150,074
4	Unintentional injuries	105,718	Chronic lower respiratory diseases	121,987
5	Chronic obstructive pulmonary diseases	56,050	Unintentional injuries	112,012
6	Pneumonia and influenza	54,619	Diabetes mellitus	73,138
7	Diabetes mellitus	34,851	Alzheimer's disease	65,965
8	Chronic liver disease and cirrhosis	30,583	Influenza and pneumonia	59,664
9	Atherosclerosis	29,449	Nephritis, nephrotic syndrome and nephrosis	42,480
10	Suicide	26,869	Septicemia	33,373
Male				
. . .	All causes	1,075,078	All causes	1,181,668
1	Diseases of heart	405,661	Diseases of heart	321,973
2	Malignant neoplasms	225,948	Malignant neoplasms	286,830
3	Unintentional injuries	74,180	Unintentional injuries	72,050
4	Cerebrovascular diseases	69,973	Cerebrovascular diseases	58,800
5	Chronic obstructive pulmonary diseases	38,625	Chronic lower respiratory diseases	58,646
6	Pneumonia and influenza	27,574	Diabetes mellitus	35,267
7	Suicide	20,505	Influenza and pneumonia	26,861
8	Chronic liver disease and cirrhosis	19,768	Suicide	25,566
9	Homicide	18,779	Nephritis, nephrotic syndrome and nephrosis	20,370
10	Diabetes mellitus	14,325	Alzheimer's disease	18,974
Female				
. . .	All causes	914,763	All causes	1,215,947
1	Diseases of heart	355,424	Diseases of heart	330,513
2	Malignant neoplasms	190,561	Malignant neoplasms	267,058
3	Cerebrovascular diseases	100,252	Cerebrovascular diseases	91,274
4	Unintentional injuries	31,538	Chronic lower respiratory diseases	63,341
5	Pneumonia and influenza	27,045	Alzheimer's disease	46,991
6	Diabetes mellitus	20,526	Unintentional injuries	39,962
7	Atherosclerosis	17,848	Diabetes mellitus	37,871
8	Chronic obstructive pulmonary diseases	17,425	Influenza and pneumonia	32,803
9	Chronic liver disease and cirrhosis	10,815	Nephritis, nephrotic syndrome and nephrosis	22,110
10	Certain conditions originating in the perinatal period	9,815	Septicemia	18,362
White				
. . .	All causes	1,738,607	All causes	2,056,643
1	Diseases of heart	683,347	Diseases of heart	565,703
2	Malignant neoplasms	368,162	Malignant neoplasms	478,134
3	Cerebrovascular diseases	148,734	Cerebrovascular diseases	127,868
4	Unintentional injuries	90,122	Chronic lower respiratory diseases	112,914
5	Chronic obstructive pulmonary diseases	52,375	Unintentional injuries	95,890
6	Pneumonia and influenza	48,369	Alzheimer's disease	61,087
7	Diabetes mellitus	28,868	Diabetes mellitus	58,087
8	Atherosclerosis	27,069	Influenza and pneumonia	52,430
9	Chronic liver disease and cirrhosis	25,240	Nephritis, nephrotic syndrome and nephrosis	33,691
10	Suicide	24,829	Suicide	29,251
Black or African American				
. . .	All causes	233,135	All causes	287,315
1	Diseases of heart	72,956	Diseases of heart	74,225
2	Malignant neoplasms	45,037	Malignant neoplasms	62,499
3	Cerebrovascular diseases	20,135	Cerebrovascular diseases	18,118
4	Unintentional injuries	13,480	Diabetes mellitus	12,834
5	Homicide	10,172	Unintentional injuries	12,670
6	Certain conditions originating in the perinatal period	6,961	Homicide	8,135
7	Pneumonia and influenza	5,648	Nephritis, nephrotic syndrome and nephrosis	7,834
8	Diabetes mellitus	5,544	Chronic lower respiratory diseases	7,400
9	Chronic liver disease and cirrhosis	4,790	Human immunodeficiency virus (HIV) disease	7,271
10	Nephritis, nephrotic syndrome, and nephrosis	3,416	Septicemia	6,010

See footnotes at end of table.

This table will be updated on the Web. Go to www.cdc.gov/nchs/hus.htm.

Table 31 (page 2 of 4). Leading causes of death and numbers of deaths, by sex, race, and Hispanic origin: United States, 1980 and 2004

[Data are based on death certificates]

Sex, race, Hispanic origin, and rank order	1980 Cause of death	1980 Deaths	2004 Cause of death	2004 Deaths
American Indian or Alaska Native				
...	All causes	6,923	All causes	13,124
1	Diseases of heart	1,494	Diseases of heart	2,598
2	Unintentional injuries	1,290	Malignant neoplasms	2,392
3	Malignant neoplasms	770	Unintentional injuries	1,520
4	Chronic liver disease and cirrhosis	410	Diabetes mellitus	746
5	Cerebrovascular diseases	322	Cerebrovascular diseases	581
6	Pneumonia and influenza	257	Chronic liver disease and cirrhosis	577
7	Homicide	217	Chronic lower respiratory diseases	486
8	Diabetes mellitus	210	Suicide	404
9	Certain conditions originating in the perinatal period	199	Influenza and pneumonia	291
10	Suicide	181	Nephritis, nephrotic syndrome and nephrosis	247
Asian or Pacific Islander				
...	All causes	11,071	All causes	40,533
1	Diseases of heart	3,265	Malignant neoplasms	10,863
2	Malignant neoplasms	2,522	Diseases of heart	9,960
3	Cerebrovascular diseases	1,028	Cerebrovascular diseases	3,507
4	Unintentional injuries	810	Unintentional injuries	1,932
5	Pneumonia and influenza	342	Diabetes mellitus	1,471
6	Suicide	249	Influenza and pneumonia	1,243
7	Certain conditions originating in the perinatal period	246	Chronic lower respiratory diseases	1,187
8	Diabetes mellitus	227	Suicide	765
9	Homicide	211	Nephritis, nephrotic syndrome and nephrosis	708
10	Chronic obstructive pulmonary diseases	207	Alzheimer's disease	534
Hispanic or Latino				
...	---	---	All causes	122,416
1	---	---	Diseases of heart	27,788
2	---	---	Malignant neoplasms	24,522
3	---	---	Unintentional injuries	10,408
4	---	---	Cerebrovascular diseases	6,781
5	---	---	Diabetes mellitus	5,999
6	---	---	Chronic liver disease and cirrhosis	3,383
7	---	---	Homicide	3,271
8	---	---	Chronic lower respiratory diseases	3,107
9	---	---	Influenza and pneumonia	2,912
10	---	---	Certain conditions originating in the perinatal period	2,681
White male				
...	All causes	933,878	All causes	1,007,266
1	Diseases of heart	364,679	Diseases of heart	278,914
2	Malignant neoplasms	198,188	Malignant neoplasms	247,450
3	Unintentional injuries	62,963	Unintentional injuries	61,267
4	Cerebrovascular diseases	60,095	Chronic lower respiratory diseases	53,622
5	Chronic obstructive pulmonary diseases	35,977	Cerebrovascular diseases	49,296
6	Pneumonia and influenza	23,810	Diabetes mellitus	28,629
7	Suicide	18,901	Influenza and pneumonia	23,348
8	Chronic liver disease and cirrhosis	16,407	Suicide	23,081
9	Diabetes mellitus	12,125	Alzheimer's disease	17,605
10	Atherosclerosis	10,543	Nephritis, nephrotic syndrome and nephrosis	16,349
Black or African American male				
...	All causes	130,138	All causes	145,970
1	Diseases of heart	37,877	Diseases of heart	36,222
2	Malignant neoplasms	25,861	Malignant neoplasms	32,443
3	Unintentional injuries	9,701	Unintentional injuries	8,603
4	Cerebrovascular diseases	9,194	Cerebrovascular diseases	7,644
5	Homicide	8,274	Homicide	6,839
6	Certain conditions originating in the perinatal period	3,869	Diabetes mellitus	5,565
7	Pneumonia and influenza	3,386	Human immunodeficiency virus (HIV) disease	4,769
8	Chronic liver disease and cirrhosis	3,020	Chronic lower respiratory diseases	4,046
9	Chronic obstructive pulmonary diseases	2,429	Nephritis, nephrotic syndrome and nephrosis	3,537
10	Diabetes mellitus	2,010	Influenza and pneumonia	2,775

See footnotes at end of table.

This table will be updated on the Web. Go to www.cdc.gov/nchs/hus.htm.

Table 31 (page 3 of 4). Leading causes of death and numbers of deaths, by sex, race, and Hispanic origin: United States, 1980 and 2004

[Data are based on death certificates]

Sex, race, Hispanic origin, and rank order	1980 Cause of death	1980 Deaths	2004 Cause of death	2004 Deaths
American Indian or Alaska Native male				
. . .	All causes	4,193	All causes	7,134
1	Unintentional injuries	946	Diseases of heart	1,437
2	Diseases of heart	917	Malignant neoplasms	1,241
3	Malignant neoplasms	408	Unintentional injuries	1,010
4	Chronic liver disease and cirrhosis	239	Diabetes mellitus	365
5	Cerebrovascular diseases	163	Chronic liver disease and cirrhosis	323
6	Homicide	162	Suicide	306
7	Pneumonia and influenza	148	Cerebrovascular diseases	246
8	Suicide	147	Chronic lower respiratory diseases	235
9	Certain conditions originating in the perinatal period	107	Homicide	181
10	Diabetes mellitus	86	Influenza and pneumonia	142
Asian or Pacific Islander male				
. . .	All causes	6,809	All causes	21,298
1	Diseases of heart	2,174	Malignant neoplasms	5,696
2	Malignant neoplasms	1,485	Diseases of heart	5,400
3	Unintentional injuries	556	Cerebrovascular diseases	1,614
4	Cerebrovascular diseases	521	Unintentional injuries	1,170
5	Pneumonia and influenza	227	Chronic lower respiratory diseases	743
6	Suicide	159	Diabetes mellitus	708
7	Chronic obstructive pulmonary diseases	158	Influenza and pneumonia	596
8	Homicide	151	Suicide	524
9	Certain conditions originating in the perinatal period	128	Nephritis, nephrotic syndrome and nephrosis	372
10	Diabetes mellitus	103	Homicide	256
Hispanic or Latino male				
. . .	- - -	- - -	All causes	68,544
1	- - -	- - -	Diseases of heart	14,983
2	- - -	- - -	Malignant neoplasms	13,002
3	- - -	- - -	Unintentional injuries	7,796
4	- - -	- - -	Cerebrovascular diseases	3,207
5	- - -	- - -	Diabetes mellitus	2,855
6	- - -	- - -	Homicide	2,782
7	- - -	- - -	Chronic liver disease and cirrhosis	2,376
8	- - -	- - -	Suicide	1,840
9	- - -	- - -	Chronic lower respiratory diseases	1,631
10	- - -	- - -	Certain conditions originating in the perinatal period	1,538
White female				
. . .	All causes	804,729	All causes	1,049,377
1	Diseases of heart	318,668	Diseases of heart	286,789
2	Malignant neoplasms	169,974	Malignant neoplasms	230,684
3	Cerebrovascular diseases	88,639	Cerebrovascular diseases	78,572
4	Unintentional injuries	27,159	Chronic lower respiratory diseases	59,292
5	Pneumonia and influenza	24,559	Alzheimer's disease	43,482
6	Diabetes mellitus	16,743	Unintentional injuries	34,623
7	Atherosclerosis	16,526	Diabetes mellitus	29,458
8	Chronic obstructive pulmonary diseases	16,398	Influenza and pneumonia	29,082
9	Chronic liver disease and cirrhosis	8,833	Nephritis, nephrotic syndrome and nephrosis	17,342
10	Certain conditions originating in the perinatal period	6,512	Septicemia	14,692
Black or African American female				
. . .	All causes	102,997	All causes	141,345
1	Diseases of heart	35,079	Diseases of heart	38,003
2	Malignant neoplasms	19,176	Malignant neoplasms	30,056
3	Cerebrovascular diseases	10,941	Cerebrovascular diseases	10,474
4	Unintentional injuries	3,779	Diabetes mellitus	7,269
5	Diabetes mellitus	3,534	Nephritis, nephrotic syndrome and nephrosis	4,297
6	Certain conditions originating in the perinatal period	3,092	Unintentional injuries	4,067
7	Pneumonia and influenza	2,262	Chronic lower respiratory diseases	3,354
8	Homicide	1,898	Septicemia	3,320
9	Chronic liver disease and cirrhosis	1,770	Alzheimer's disease	3,085
10	Nephritis, nephrotic syndrome, and nephrosis	1,722	Influenza and pneumonia	2,925

See footnotes at end of table.

This table will be updated on the Web. Go to www.cdc.gov/nchs/hus.htm.

Table 31 (page 4 of 4). Leading causes of death and numbers of deaths, by sex, race, and Hispanic origin: United States, 1980 and 2004

[Data are based on death certificates]

Sex, race, Hispanic origin, and rank order	1980		2004	
	Cause of death	Deaths	Cause of death	Deaths
American Indian or Alaska Native female				
. . .	All causes	2,730	All causes	5,990
1	Diseases of heart	577	Diseases of heart	1,161
2	Malignant neoplasms	362	Malignant neoplasms	1,151
3	Unintentional injuries	344	Unintentional injuries	510
4	Chronic liver disease and cirrhosis	171	Diabetes mellitus	381
5	Cerebrovascular diseases	159	Cerebrovascular diseases	335
6	Diabetes mellitus	124	Chronic liver disease and cirrhosis	254
7	Pneumonia and influenza	109	Chronic lower respiratory diseases	251
8	Certain conditions originating in the perinatal period	92	Influenza and pneumonia	149
9	Nephritis, nephrotic syndrome, and nephrosis	56	Nephritis, nephrotic syndrome and nephrosis	135
10	Homicide	55	Septicemia	98
Asian or Pacific Islander female				
. . .	All causes	4,262	All causes	19,235
1	Diseases of heart	1,091	Malignant neoplasms	5,167
2	Malignant neoplasms	1,037	Diseases of heart	4,560
3	Cerebrovascular diseases	507	Cerebrovascular diseases	1,893
4	Unintentional injuries	254	Diabetes mellitus	763
5	Diabetes mellitus	124	Unintentional injuries	762
6	Certain conditions originating in the perinatal period	118	Influenza and pneumonia	647
7	Pneumonia and influenza	115	Chronic lower respiratory diseases	444
8	Congenital anomalies	104	Alzheimer's disease	344
9	Suicide	90	Nephritis, nephrotic syndrome and nephrosis	336
10	Homicide	60	Essential (primary) hypertension and hypertensive renal disease	312
Hispanic or Latino female				
. . .	- - -	- - -	All causes	53,872
1	- - -	- - -	Diseases of heart	12,805
2	- - -	- - -	Malignant neoplasms	11,520
3	- - -	- - -	Cerebrovascular diseases	3,574
4	- - -	- - -	Diabetes mellitus	3,144
5	- - -	- - -	Unintentional injuries	2,612
6	- - -	- - -	Influenza and pneumonia	1,509
7	- - -	- - -	Chronic lower respiratory diseases	1,476
8	- - -	- - -	Alzheimer's disease	1,291
9	- - -	- - -	Certain conditions originating in the perinatal period	1,143
10	- - -	- - -	Nephritis, nephrotic syndrome and nephrosis	1,095

. . . Category not applicable.
- - - Data not available.

NOTES: For cause of death codes based on the *International Classification of Diseases, 9th Revision* (ICD–9) in 1980 and ICD–10 in 2002, see Appendix II, Cause of death; Tables IV and V. In 2003, seven states reported multiple-race data. In 2004, 15 states reported multiple-race data. The multiple-race data for these states were bridged to the single-race categories of the 1977 Office of Management and Budget standards for comparability with other states. See Appendix II, Race.

SOURCES: Centers for Disease Control and Prevention, National Center for Health Statistics, National Vital Statistics System; *Vital statistics of the United States, Vol II, mortality, part A*, 1980. Washington, DC: Public Health Service. 1985; 2004 annual mortality file.

This table will be updated on the Web. Go to www.cdc.gov/nchs/hus.htm.

Table 32 (page 1 of 2). Leading causes of death and numbers of deaths, by age: United States, 1980 and 2004

[Data are based on death certificates]

Age and rank order	1980 Cause of death	1980 Deaths	2004 Cause of death	2004 Deaths
Under 1 year				
. . .	All causes	45,526	All causes	27,936
1	Congenital anomalies	9,220	Congenital malformations, deformations and chromosomal abnormalities	5,622
2	Sudden infant death syndrome	5,510	Disorders related to short gestation and low birth weight, not elsewhere classified	4,642
3	Respiratory distress syndrome	4,989	Sudden infant death syndrome	2,246
4	Disorders relating to short gestation and unspecified low birthweight	3,648	Newborn affected by maternal complications of pregnancy	1,715
5	Newborn affected by maternal complications of pregnancy	1,572	Unintentional injuries	1,052
6	Intrauterine hypoxia and birth asphyxia	1,497	Newborn affected by complications of placenta, cord and membranes	1,042
7	Unintentional injuries	1,166	Respiratory distress of newborn	875
8	Birth trauma	1,058	Bacterial sepsis of newborn	827
9	Pneumonia and influenza	1,012	Neonatal hemorrhage	616
10	Newborn affected by complications of placenta, cord, and membranes	985	Diseases of circulatory system	593
1–4 years				
. . .	All causes	8,187	All causes	4,785
1	Unintentional injuries	3,313	Unintentional injuries	1,641
2	Congenital anomalies	1,026	Congenital malformations, deformations and chromosomal abnormalities	569
3	Malignant neoplasms	573	Malignant neoplasms	399
4	Diseases of heart	338	Homicide	377
5	Homicide	319	Diseases of heart	187
6	Pneumonia and influenza	267	Influenza and pneumonia	119
7	Meningitis	223	Septicemia	84
8	Meningococcal infection	110	Certain conditions originating in the perinatal period	61
9	Certain conditions originating in the perinatal period	84	In situ neoplasms, benign neoplasms and neoplasms of uncertain or unknown behavior	53
10	Septicemia	71	Chronic lower respiratory diseases	48
5–14 years				
. . .	All causes	10,689	All causes	6,834
1	Unintentional injuries	5,224	Unintentional injuries	2,666
2	Malignant neoplasms	1,497	Malignant neoplasms	1,019
3	Congenital anomalies	561	Congenital malformations, deformations and chromosomal abnormalities	389
4	Homicide	415	Homicide	329
5	Diseases of heart	330	Suicide	285
6	Pneumonia and influenza	194	Diseases of heart	245
7	Suicide	142	Chronic lower respiratory diseases	120
8	Benign neoplasms	104	In situ neoplasms, benign neoplasms and neoplasms of uncertain or unknown behavior	84
9	Cerebrovascular diseases	95	Influenza and pneumonia	82
10	Chronic obstructive pulmonary diseases	85	Cerebrovascular diseases	77
15–24 years				
. . .	All causes	49,027	All causes	33,421
1	Unintentional injuries	26,206	Unintentional injuries	15,449
2	Homicide	6,537	Homicide	5,085
3	Suicide	5,239	Suicide	4,316
4	Malignant neoplasms	2,683	Malignant neoplasms	1,709
5	Diseases of heart	1,223	Diseases of heart	1,038
6	Congenital anomalies	600	Congenital malformations, deformations and chromosomal abnormalities	483
7	Cerebrovascular diseases	418	Cerebrovascular diseases	211
8	Pneumonia and influenza	348	Human immunodeficiency virus (HIV) disease	191
9	Chronic obstructive pulmonary diseases	141	Influenza and pneumonia	185
10	Anemias	133	Chronic lower respiratory diseases	179

See footnotes at end of table.

This table will be updated on the Web. Go to www.cdc.gov/nchs/hus.htm.

Table 32 (page 2 of 2). Leading causes of death and numbers of deaths, by age: United States, 1980 and 2004

[Data are based on death certificates]

Age and rank order	1980 Cause of death	1980 Deaths	2004 Cause of death	2004 Deaths
25–44 years				
. . .	All causes	108.658	All causes	126.230
1	Unintentional injuries	26.722	Unintentional injuries	29.503
2	Malignant neoplasms	17.551	Malignant neoplasms	18.356
3	Diseases of heart	14.513	Diseases of heart	16.088
4	Homicide	10.983	Suicide	11.712
5	Suicide	9.855	Homicide	7.479
6	Chronic liver disease and cirrhosis	4.782	Human immunodeficiency virus (HIV) disease	6.294
7	Cerebrovascular diseases	3.154	Chronic liver disease and cirrhosis	3.108
8	Diabetes mellitus	1.472	Cerebrovascular diseases	2.928
9	Pneumonia and influenza	1.467	Diabetes mellitus	2.625
10	Congenital anomalies	817	Influenza and pneumonia	1.194
45–64 years				
. . .	All causes	425.338	All causes	442.394
1	Diseases of heart	148.322	Malignant neoplasms	146.476
2	Malignant neoplasms	135.675	Diseases of heart	101.169
3	Cerebrovascular diseases	19.909	Unintentional injuries	26,593
4	Unintentional injuries	18.140	Diabetes mellitus	16.347
5	Chronic liver disease and cirrhosis	16.089	Cerebrovascular diseases	16.147
6	Chronic obstructive pulmonary diseases	11.514	Chronic lower respiratory diseases	15.265
7	Diabetes mellitus	7.977	Chronic liver disease and cirrhosis	14.065
8	Suicide	7.079	Suicide	10.917
9	Pneumonia and influenza	5.804	Nephritis, nephrotic syndrome and nephrosis	6.030
10	Homicide	4.019	Septicemia	5.996
65 years and over				
. . .	All causes	1,341,848	All causes	1,755,669
1	Diseases of heart	595,406	Diseases of heart	533,302
2	Malignant neoplasms	258,389	Malignant neoplasms	385,847
3	Cerebrovascular diseases	146,417	Cerebrovascular diseases	130,538
4	Pneumonia and influenza	45,512	Chronic lower respiratory diseases	105,197
5	Chronic obstructive pulmonary diseases	43,587	Alzheimer's disease	65,313
6	Atherosclerosis	28,081	Diabetes mellitus	53,956
7	Diabetes mellitus	25,216	Influenza and pneumonia	52,760
8	Unintentional injuries	24,844	Nephritis, nephrotic syndrome and nephrosis	35,105
9	Nephritis, nephrotic syndrome, and nephrosis	12,968	Unintentional injuries	35,020
10	Chronic liver disease and cirrhosis	9,519	Septicemia	25,644

. . . Category not applicable.

NOTES: For cause of death codes based on the *International Classification of Diseases, 9th Revision* (ICD–9) in 1980 and ICD–10 in 2002, see Appendix II, Cause of death; Tables IV and V.

SOURCES: Centers for Disease Control and Prevention, National Center for Health Statistics, National Vital Statistics System; *Vital statistics of the United States, Vol II, mortality, part A*, 1980. Washington, DC: Public Health Service. 1985; 2004 annual mortality file.

This table will be updated on the Web. Go to www.cdc.gov/nchs/hus.htm.

Table 33 (page 1 of 3). Age-adjusted death rates, by race, sex, region, and urbanization level: United States, average annual 1996–1998, 1999–2001, and 2002–2004

[Data are based on the National Vital Statistics System]

Sex, region, and urbanization level[1]	All races			White			Black or African American		
	1996–1998	*1999–2001*	*2002–2004*	*1996–1998*	*1999–2001*	*2002–2004*	*1996–1998*	*1999–2001*	*2002–2004*
Both sexes	Age-adjusted death rate per 100,000 standard population[2]								
All regions:									
Metropolitan counties:									
Large:									
Central	894.5	869.0	809.5	858.8	836.7	783.4	1,164.2	1,133.6	1,060.9
Fringe	839.3	833.0	789.1	828.0	823.7	782.7	1,059.6	1,040.8	975.7
Medium	865.6	859.0	821.7	846.5	842.2	807.2	1,152.4	1,137.3	1,077.7
Small	887.8	887.9	852.5	866.5	868.8	834.4	1,173.1	1,164.3	1,116.9
Nonmetropolitan counties:									
Micropolitan	913.0	907.1	880.0	892.1	890.0	863.3	1,208.2	1,174.9	1,139.6
Nonmicropolitan	933.0	923.2	901.1	909.6	902.8	880.8	1,191.6	1,162.8	1,133.3
Northeast:									
Metropolitan counties:									
Large:									
Central	909.6	861.7	788.4	881.4	838.6	772.1	1,052.4	1,001.1	916.1
Fringe	827.8	814.0	760.2	823.3	810.8	760.5	1,000.0	986.6	905.8
Medium	851.9	836.2	787.4	842.2	828.6	781.4	1,076.6	1,040.8	955.0
Small	852.0	849.5	800.1	847.8	846.5	796.6	1,106.9	1,072.4	1,030.0
Nonmetropolitan counties:									
Micropolitan	878.4	854.4	816.5	877.9	855.7	817.3	*	*	*
Nonmicropolitan	893.6	877.4	832.4	892.0	876.3	831.7	*	*	*
Midwest:									
Metropolitan counties:									
Large:									
Central	951.7	939.6	875.1	880.7	868.9	808.2	1,213.7	1,205.9	1,126.4
Fringe	856.4	856.1	809.5	845.9	846.3	801.2	1,121.2	1,123.1	1,070.3
Medium	876.1	873.5	829.7	857.0	856.1	813.8	1,168.9	1,151.6	1,080.5
Small	860.8	861.5	817.3	847.4	850.8	804.8	1,178.9	1,146.9	1,123.4
Nonmetropolitan counties:									
Micropolitan	868.8	865.2	826.8	863.9	863.0	824.4	1,222.0	1,103.5	1,059.7
Nonmicropolitan	867.6	852.7	823.8	858.2	845.9	815.7	1,388.1	1,058.9	1,118.8
South:									
Metropolitan counties:									
Large:									
Central	938.1	926.8	881.0	864.9	859.1	819.3	1,241.9	1,212.8	1,152.3
Fringe	845.3	845.6	808.9	821.9	826.2	794.5	1,071.4	1,048.4	979.7
Medium	891.8	892.4	863.1	852.1	855.8	830.2	1,172.6	1,164.4	1,110.6
Small	943.6	950.5	925.1	907.5	917.9	896.5	1,183.2	1,180.0	1,128.5
Nonmetropolitan counties:									
Micropolitan	974.1	973.3	958.6	933.5	939.3	928.5	1,218.9	1,194.3	1,159.3
Nonmicropolitan	1,005.3	1,003.0	991.6	975.9	978.5	970.3	1,188.4	1,171.2	1,139.7
West:									
Metropolitan counties:									
Large:									
Central	819.2	792.4	737.9	829.4	804.1	755.1	1,107.9	1,077.7	1,019.0
Fringe	818.6	803.6	767.8	823.2	810.1	775.9	1,060.8	1,006.2	1,007.2
Medium	814.7	800.5	769.5	826.9	815.8	787.3	1,045.4	996.3	950.9
Small	827.6	815.7	785.9	826.6	815.7	787.8	973.5	990.7	899.7
Nonmetropolitan counties:									
Micropolitan	861.0	851.8	827.7	860.4	854.7	829.0	*	*	*
Nonmicropolitan	867.1	847.4	821.1	845.9	828.6	801.7	*	*	*

See footnotes at end of table.

This table will be updated on the Web. Go to www.cdc.gov/nchs/hus.htm.

 Age-adjusted death rates, by race, sex, region, and urbanization level: United States, average annual 1996–1998, 1999–2001, and 2002–2004

[Data are based on the National Vital Statistics System]

Sex, region, and urbanization level[1]	All races 1996–1998	All races 1999–2001	All races 2002–2004	White 1996–1998	White 1999–2001	White 2002–2004	Black or African American 1996–1998	Black or African American 1999–2001	Black or African American 2002–2004
Male	Age-adjusted death rate per 100,000 standard population[2]								
All regions:									
Metropolitan counties:									
Large:									
Central	1,108.6	1,057.6	975.1	1,060.6	1,015.2	941.4	1,503.8	1,436.1	1,329.6
Fringe	1,025.2	998.7	928.4	1,010.9	987.3	920.9	1,329.0	1,281.1	1,174.3
Medium	1,069.9	1,038.5	982.3	1,045.4	1,017.7	963.1	1,469.0	1,409.2	1,324.1
Small	1,104.6	1,079.2	1,023.3	1,077.4	1,056.1	1,001.3	1,497.6	1,449.1	1,373.8
Nonmetropolitan counties:									
Micropolitan	1,139.9	1,108.6	1,057.0	1,113.5	1,087.5	1,036.0	1,547.8	1,475.9	1,411.2
Nonmicropolitan	1,172.3	1,132.9	1,087.4	1,143.3	1,108.3	1,063.1	1,529.0	1,457.3	1,410.0
Northeast:									
Metropolitan counties:									
Large:									
Central	1,142.0	1,065.3	961.2	1,102.8	1,034.5	939.2	1,374.4	1,280.7	1,156.2
Fringe	1,018.1	985.3	899.3	1,012.6	982.3	900.8	1,263.0	1,219.0	1,088.4
Medium	1,061.6	1,018.1	946.0	1,049.9	1,009.7	939.3	1,351.2	1,262.4	1,157.2
Small	1,062.7	1,034.1	958.1	1,057.9	1,032.3	955.0	1,376.8	1,280.7	1,212.9
Nonmetropolitan counties:									
Micropolitan	1,093.5	1,042.5	981.0	1,093.7	1,045.6	983.5	*	*	*
Nonmicropolitan	1,096.9	1,056.9	988.9	1,096.1	1,056.6	989.7	*	*	*
Midwest:									
Metropolitan counties:									
Large:									
Central	1,192.6	1,155.5	1,063.3	1,101.0	1,064.6	978.1	1,559.8	1,525.5	1,414.9
Fringe	1,051.7	1,030.0	949.9	1,038.7	1,018.7	940.9	1,399.4	1,372.7	1,266.9
Medium	1,089.0	1,063.2	989.5	1,065.3	1,043.8	972.4	1,470.0	1,394.4	1,285.1
Small	1,076.0	1,057.3	990.5	1,059.7	1,045.0	976.7	1,463.9	1,401.9	1,342.0
Nonmetropolitan counties:									
Micropolitan	1,092.0	1,063.4	1,001.2	1,086.0	1,062.0	1,000.0	1,551.8	1,315.8	1,181.8
Nonmicropolitan	1,094.7	1,050.5	1,000.3	1,083.0	1,043.3	991.8	1,788.2	1,225.3	1,344.1
South:									
Metropolitan counties:									
Large:									
Central	1,172.0	1,130.9	1,061.9	1,074.6	1,042.9	983.1	1,616.0	1,542.6	1,446.9
Fringe	1,030.8	1,009.7	950.9	1,000.5	984.8	932.5	1,351.1	1,297.8	1,190.4
Medium	1,106.6	1,081.2	1,032.8	1,053.0	1,033.8	990.4	1,517.1	1,466.2	1,388.1
Small	1,185.9	1,160.8	1,114.5	1,138.6	1,118.6	1,077.5	1,526.9	1,487.0	1,405.5
Nonmetropolitan counties:									
Micropolitan	1,228.0	1,198.9	1,154.0	1,175.1	1,154.7	1,113.2	1,577.6	1,519.8	1,458.1
Nonmicropolitan	1,275.7	1,240.6	1,203.8	1,239.3	1,210.2	1,176.7	1,530.4	1,478.0	1,425.9
West:									
Metropolitan counties:									
Large:									
Central	996.3	949.8	880.4	1,006.7	962.4	899.9	1,383.8	1,323.2	1,244.7
Fringe	981.1	947.0	899.5	988.0	954.5	909.1	1,228.8	1,171.2	1,155.7
Medium	987.4	952.8	916.8	1,003.1	969.3	930.4	1,230.6	1,165.1	1,118.8
Small	1,003.7	970.5	927.3	1,001.7	971.6	928.7	1,178.9	1,088.1	1,057.5
Nonmetropolitan counties:									
Micropolitan	1,037.8	1,012.6	975.9	1,036.0	1,013.6	973.3	*	*	*
Nonmicropolitan	1,048.7	1,010.9	966.4	1,023.0	986.8	940.0	*	*	*

See footnotes at end of table.

This table will be updated on the Web. Go to www.cdc.gov/nchs/hus.htm.

Table 33 (page 3 of 3). Age-adjusted death rates, by race, sex, region, and urbanization level: United States, average annual 1996–1998, 1999–2001, and 2002–2004

[Data are based on the National Vital Statistics System]

Sex, region, and urbanization level[1]	All races			White			Black or African American		
	1996–1998	1999–2001	2002–2004	1996–1998	1999–2001	2002–2004	1996–1998	1999–2001	2002–2004
Female	Age-adjusted death rate per 100,000 standard population[2]								
All regions:									
Metropolitan counties:									
Large:									
Central	738.9	730.1	683.2	711.3	703.8	661.5	934.4	929.3	874.1
Fringe	705.7	711.1	680.8	696.3	702.7	674.7	875.9	876.4	832.2
Medium	716.8	724.6	696.3	701.9	710.6	684.6	932.0	945.4	899.2
Small	731.2	745.7	720.3	713.7	729.1	704.5	951.9	966.5	933.1
Nonmetropolitan counties:									
Micropolitan	745.9	754.8	739.2	728.8	740.2	725.1	975.6	968.3	945.9
Nonmicropolitan	750.6	759.5	748.2	731.4	741.9	730.6	951.5	953.0	934.6
Northeast:									
Metropolitan counties:									
Large:									
Central	748.4	719.6	662.9	725.6	699.1	648.0	848.3	823.6	758.9
Fringe	696.3	692.6	655.0	692.4	689.3	654.1	827.2	828.1	774.9
Medium	709.1	707.5	668.6	701.4	700.9	663.3	883.4	877.0	800.9
Small	706.7	717.3	679.6	703.2	713.8	676.2	919.9	930.0	894.5
Nonmetropolitan counties:									
Micropolitan	725.0	717.5	689.8	724.3	718.1	689.6	*	*	*
Nonmicropolitan	741.8	738.5	702.5	740.1	737.4	700.9	*	*	*
Midwest:									
Metropolitan counties:									
Large:									
Central	784.1	786.2	736.5	729.7	730.9	683.6	974.4	984.5	922.5
Fringe	722.9	733.8	703.0	714.5	725.1	695.4	924.6	948.2	922.9
Medium	728.9	739.6	709.1	713.6	724.3	694.7	955.1	972.7	920.8
Small	710.8	721.4	689.3	700.0	712.2	678.2	963.1	952.5	952.1
Nonmetropolitan counties:									
Micropolitan	711.2	721.2	694.2	707.3	718.6	691.3	998.7	948.8	954.0
Nonmicropolitan	696.1	700.0	680.6	688.9	693.9	673.2	1,123.8	955.4	947.4
South:									
Metropolitan counties:									
Large:									
Central	768.6	776.3	743.5	712.1	721.7	692.4	988.2	989.8	949.3
Fringe	705.7	719.6	695.3	686.1	702.4	682.3	882.4	881.0	830.9
Medium	731.2	746.6	727.3	700.1	716.0	699.5	938.9	958.2	918.5
Small	771.0	795.0	778.8	740.9	767.1	754.2	956.5	974.2	937.8
Nonmetropolitan counties:									
Micropolitan	788.4	803.8	802.9	754.8	774.5	778.1	977.3	975.7	952.0
Nonmicropolitan	803.4	821.3	821.7	778.3	799.5	802.7	946.7	955.0	935.9
West:									
Metropolitan counties:									
Large:									
Central	682.6	670.1	624.1	691.8	679.9	638.5	906.0	899.3	846.1
Fringe	696.3	693.8	664.4	699.2	699.1	670.9	920.1	876.5	881.3
Medium	680.5	681.3	652.4	691.6	696.1	672.2	890.3	855.7	806.9
Small	687.3	691.3	668.5	687.2	690.7	670.7	789.8	886.6	740.9
Nonmetropolitan counties:									
Micropolitan	712.6	715.1	697.6	713.8	720.0	701.3	*	*	*
Nonmicropolitan	710.4	704.0	688.5	694.2	690.7	675.6	*	*	*

* Estimates of death rates for the black population in nonmetropolitan counties in the Northeast and West may be unreliable, possibly due to anomalies in population estimates for the black population in nonmetropolitan counties in these regions.

[1]Urbanization levels are for county of residence of decedent. The levels were developed by NCHS using information from the Office of Management and Budget, Department of Agriculture, and Census Bureau. More information on this six-level urban-rural classification scheme is available from: www.cdc.gov/nchs/r&d/rdc_urbanrural.htm. See Appendix II, Urbanization.

[2]Average annual death rates are age-adjusted using the year 2000 standard population. In earlier editions of *Health, United States*, age-adjusted rates were calculated using standard million proportions based on rounded population numbers. Starting with *Health, United States 2006*, unrounded population numbers are used to calculate age-adjusted rates. See Appendix II, Age adjustment. Denominators for rates are population estimates for the middle year of each 3-year period multiplied by 3. The 1997 population estimates used to compute rates for 1996–1998 are intercensal population estimates based on the 2000 census. The 2000 population estimates used to compute rates for 1999–2001 are based on the 2000 census. The 2003 population estimates used to compute rates for 2002–2004 are postcensal population estimates based on the 2000 census. See Appendix I, Population Census and Population Estimates.

NOTE: The race groups, white and black, include persons of Hispanic and non-Hispanic origin. Starting with 2003 data, some states reported multiple-race data. The multiple-race data for these states were bridged to the single-race categories of the 1977 Office of Management and Budget standards for comparability with other states. In 2003, California, Hawaii, Idaho, Maine, Montana, New York, and Wisconsin reported multiple-race data. In 2004, 15 states reported multiple-race data. In addition to the seven states listed above, Michigan, Minnesota, New Hampshire, New Jersey, Oklahoma, South Dakota, Washington, and Wyoming reported multiple-race data. See Appendix II, Race. Data have been revised and differ from previous editions of *Health, United States*.

SOURCE: Centers for Disease Control and Prevention, National Center for Health Statistics, National Vital Statistics System, Compressed Mortality File.

This table will be updated on the Web. Go to www.cdc.gov/nchs/hus.htm.

Table 34 (page 1 of 2). Age-adjusted death rates among persons 25–64 years of age for selected causes of death, by sex and educational attainment: Selected states, 1994–2004

[Data are based on death certificates]

	Years of educational attainment[1]								
	Both sexes			Male			Female		
Cause of death[2] and year	*Less than 12*	*12*	*13 or more*	*Less than 12*	*12*	*13 or more*	*Less than 12*	*12*	*13 or more*
	Age-adjusted death rate per 100,000 population[3]								
All causes									
1994	594.6	506.4	254.8	793.6	707.1	323.5	397.3	342.9	182.1
1995	604.7	512.5	251.9	801.1	713.2	316.8	408.6	348.1	183.5
1996	579.6	492.5	241.8	763.9	669.6	300.7	396.6	344.2	180.3
1997	554.1	473.4	232.7	719.7	634.4	283.4	387.2	337.5	180.2
1998	561.6	465.8	223.9	727.6	627.1	271.9	395.6	330.9	174.3
1999	585.3	474.5	219.1	763.7	636.7	264.2	409.9	337.3	172.6
2000	591.0	484.5	216.7	780.2	641.8	260.8	409.0	347.7	171.9
2001	576.6	480.9	214.6	745.8	631.2	257.3	407.1	348.6	171.5
2002	575.1	490.9	211.3	726.1	650.2	253.5	416.6	350.7	168.8
2003[4]	669.9	490.9	211.7	826.8	650.9	252.5	496.8	349.4	171.0
2004[4]	667.2	477.1	208.3	838.7	618.8	250.7	486.2	344.9	166.7
Chronic and noncommunicable diseases									
1994	440.5	380.7	193.7	561.9	504.4	228.4	325.0	286.8	155.5
1995	445.1	384.0	192.1	563.4	507.3	224.4	332.1	290.0	156.3
1996	432.7	375.3	189.0	550.6	486.9	222.1	321.2	287.7	153.4
1997	419.0	368.8	187.4	527.0	474.1	219.0	316.0	284.6	153.8
1998	425.2	362.9	180.9	534.4	470.2	211.3	321.3	277.9	148.6
1998 comparability-modified[5]	429.5	366.5	182.7	539.7	474.9	213.4	324.5	280.7	150.1
1999[6]	447.0	369.8	177.2	563.0	477.6	205.5	337.2	283.6	147.4
2000	446.2	377.6	175.7	567.2	481.5	202.9	334.3	292.3	147.2
2001	436.5	370.7	171.1	545.1	468.2	195.7	331.7	290.3	145.5
2002	432.0	374.4	168.6	528.9	478.2	193.9	334.9	288.5	142.6
2003[4]	502.7	373.4	167.6	603.6	478.5	191.8	396.7	286.4	142.7
2004[4]	498.4	358.6	162.9	611.0	449.3	188.0	385.7	279.1	137.6
Injuries									
1994	95.8	73.4	31.9	149.4	119.2	45.7	38.9	31.7	17.9
1995	96.6	74.3	31.6	149.4	120.3	45.3	40.0	32.1	17.8
1996	92.3	73.0	32.0	139.8	116.2	45.7	40.6	32.7	18.4
1997	92.7	73.5	31.9	138.8	116.4	45.5	41.1	33.4	18.4
1998	93.9	73.8	31.2	139.4	116.6	44.4	43.8	33.7	18.3
1998 comparability-modified[5]	95.4	75.0	31.7	141.6	118.4	45.1	44.5	34.2	18.6
1999[6]	95.5	75.5	30.6	145.1	118.9	43.3	42.6	34.4	18.1
2000	100.4	76.7	30.3	155.1	119.2	43.1	43.7	35.3	17.9
2001[7]	97.9	80.7	33.2	147.0	122.7	47.6	44.8	38.6	19.3
2002	99.6	85.2	32.2	143.3	129.6	45.5	49.2	41.0	19.2
2003[4]	116.6	88.3	33.5	162.9	133.7	46.8	60.5	42.6	20.6
2004[4]	120.5	90.1	35.0	170.5	132.4	48.9	61.5	45.7	22.0
Communicable diseases									
1994	57.5	51.6	28.9	81.5	82.8	49.1	32.5	23.7	8.4
1995	62.1	53.4	27.9	87.3	84.7	46.7	35.8	25.2	8.9
1996	53.7	43.3	20.2	72.5	65.6	32.6	33.8	23.0	8.0
1997	41.6	30.1	12.9	53.1	42.9	18.4	29.3	18.7	7.6
1998	41.5	28.2	11.4	52.8	39.4	15.7	29.6	18.4	7.0
1998 comparability-modified[5]	35.6	24.2	9.8	45.3	33.8	13.5	25.4	15.8	6.0
1999[6]	42.1	28.5	10.8	54.8	39.5	15.1	29.4	18.8	6.6
2000	43.5	29.4	10.3	56.9	40.4	14.3	30.3	19.5	6.4
2001	41.4	28.7	9.9	52.9	39.4	13.6	29.7	19.0	6.3
2002	42.7	30.5	10.2	53.0	41.6	13.8	31.8	20.4	6.7
2003[4]	49.6	28.3	10.2	59.3	37.8	13.5	38.7	19.8	7.2
2004[4]	47.4	27.6	10.0	56.2	36.4	13.3	38.0	19.3	6.8

See footnotes at end of table.

This table will be updated on the Web. Go to www.cdc.gov/nchs/hus.htm.

Table 34 (page 2 of 2). Age-adjusted death rates among persons 25–64 years of age for selected causes of death, by sex and educational attainment: Selected states, 1994–2004

[Data are based on death certificates]

Cause of death[2] and year	Both sexes: Less than 12	Both sexes: 12	Both sexes: 13 or more	Male: Less than 12	Male: 12	Male: 13 or more	Female: Less than 12	Female: 12	Female: 13 or more
	Years of educational attainment[1]								
	Age-adjusted death rate per 100,000 population[3]								
HIV disease:									
1994	36.2	36.5	21.4	54.7	63.0	39.7	16.8	12.3	2.9
1995	39.7	38.0	20.6	59.0	64.4	37.8	19.0	13.7	3.5
1996	31.9	27.7	13.1	45.4	45.4	23.8	17.2	11.2	2.4
1997	19.4	14.3	5.8	26.3	23.0	10.1	11.8	6.2	1.6
1998	17.3	11.7	4.3	23.4	18.3	7.5	10.6	5.6	1.1
1998 comparability-modified[5]	18.7	12.7	4.7	25.3	19.8	8.1	11.5	6.1	1.2
1999[6]	19.0	13.1	4.6	26.1	20.1	7.9	11.7	6.6	1.4
2000	19.8	13.2	4.1	26.9	19.8	7.1	12.6	7.1	1.2
2001	18.4	12.5	3.8	25.0	18.6	6.4	11.6	6.8	1.2
2002	18.2	12.6	3.8	23.4	18.6	6.3	12.6	6.9	1.3
2003[4]	19.6	10.6	3.4	23.9	15.5	5.8	14.5	5.8	1.2
2004[4]	17.9	10.0	3.3	21.6	14.6	5.5	13.9	5.5	1.2
Other communicable diseases:									
1994	21.2	15.1	7.5	26.8	19.7	9.4	15.7	11.4	5.5
1995	22.4	15.5	7.2	28.2	20.3	8.8	16.8	11.5	5.5
1996	21.8	15.7	7.2	27.2	20.2	8.8	16.7	11.9	5.6
1997	22.2	15.9	7.1	26.8	19.9	8.2	17.6	12.5	6.0
1998	24.2	16.5	7.1	29.4	21.1	8.2	19.0	12.8	5.9
1998 comparability-modified[5]	19.4	13.2	5.7	23.5	16.9	6.6	15.2	10.2	4.7
1999[6]	23.1	15.4	6.2	28.8	19.4	7.2	17.6	12.2	5.3
2000	23.7	16.2	6.2	30.0	20.6	7.2	17.7	12.4	5.1
2001	22.9	16.2	6.1	27.9	20.8	7.1	18.1	12.2	5.1
2002	24.5	17.9	6.4	29.6	23.0	7.5	19.1	13.5	5.4
2003[4]	30.1	17.8	6.8	35.4	22.3	7.7	24.2	13.9	6.0
2004[4]	29.4	17.6	6.7	34.6	21.8	7.8	24.1	13.8	5.6

[1]Educational attainment for the numerator is based on the death certificate item highest grade completed. Educational attainment for the denominator is based on answers to the Current Population Survey question, What is the highest level of school completed or highest degree received? (Kominski R, Adams A. Educational Attainment in the United States: March 1993 and 1992, U.S. Census Bureau, Current Population Reports, P20–476, Washington, DC. 1994.)

[2]Underlying cause of death was coded according to the Ninth Revision of the *International Classification of Diseases* (ICD) in 1994–1998 and the Tenth Revision starting in 1999. See Appendix II, Cause of death; Tables IV and V.

[3]Age-adjusted to the 2000 standard population using four age groups: 25–34, 35–44, 45–54, and 55–64 years. Prior to 2003, age-adjusted rates were calculated using standard million proportions based on rounded population numbers. Starting with 2003 data, unrounded population numbers are used to calculate age-adjusted rates. See Appendix II, Age adjustment, Table I. Death records that are missing information about decedent's education are not included. Percent with no stated education averages 2–9% for causes of death in this table. Age-adjusted death rates for 1994–2000 were calculated using 1990-based postcensal population estimates in the denominator. Starting with 2001 data, rates were computed using 2000-based postcensal estimates. See Appendix I, Population Census and Population Estimates.

[4]Reporting areas that have adopted the 2003 revision of the U.S. Standard Certificate of Death are excluded because educational attainment data based on the 2003 revision are not comparable with data based on the 1989 revision of the U.S. Standard Certificate of Death. Starting with 2003 data, data from California, Idaho, Montana, and New York are excluded. In addition to these four states, starting with 2004 data, Connecticut, Georgia, Michigan, New Hampshire, New Jersey, Oklahoma, Rhode Island, South Dakota, Washington, and Wyoming have adopted the 2003 revision and therefore are excluded. Because of different education profiles of the excluded states compared with the remaining reporting areas, 2003 and subsequent years are not directly comparable to earlier years. See Appendix II, Education.

[5]Calculated by multiplying the 1998 rate by its comparability ratio to adjust for differences between ICD–9 and ICD–10. See Appendix II, Cause of death; Comparability ratio, Table VI.

[6]Starting with 1999 data, cause of death is coded according to ICD–10. To estimate change between 1998 and 1999, compare the 1999 rate with the comparability-modified rate for 1998. See Appendix II, Cause of death, Table V; Comparability ratio, Table VI.

[7]Figures include September 11, 2001-related deaths for which death certificates were filed as of October 24, 2002. See Appendix II, Cause of death, Table V for terrorism-related ICD–10 codes.

NOTES: Based on data from 36–47 states and the District of Columbia. Death rates for age groups 65 years and over are not shown because reporting quality of educational attainment on the death certificate is poorer among older decedents. See Appendix II, Education, for information about reporting states and sources of bias in death rates by educational attainment. Injury data for 1999–2003 were revised and may differ from previous editions of *Health, United States*.
Starting with 2003 data, some states reported multiple-race data. The multiple-race data for these states were bridged to the single-race categories of the 1977 Office of Management and Budget standards for comparability with other states. In 2003, California, Hawaii, Idaho, Maine, Montana, New York, and Wisconsin reported multiple-race data. In 2004, 15 states reported multiple-race data. In addition to the seven states listed above, Michigan, Minnesota, New Hampshire, New Jersey, Oklahoma, South Dakota, Washington, and Wyoming reported multiple-race data. See Appendix II, Race.

SOURCES: Centers for Disease Control and Prevention, National Center for Health Statistics, National Vital Statistics System; numerator data from annual mortality files; denominator data from unpublished population estimates prepared by the Housing and Household Economic Statistics Division, U.S. Census Bureau.

This table will be updated on the Web. Go to www.cdc.gov/nchs/hus.htm.

Table 35 (page 1 of 4). Death rates for all causes, by sex, race, Hispanic origin, and age: United States, selected years 1950–2004

[Data are based on death certificates]

Sex, race, Hispanic origin, and age	1950[1]	1960[1]	1970	1980	1990	2000	2003	2004
All persons	Deaths per 100,000 resident population							
All ages, age-adjusted[2]	1,446.0	1,339.2	1,222.6	1,039.1	938.7	869.0	832.7	800.8
All ages, crude	963.8	954.7	945.3	878.3	863.8	854.0	841.9	816.5
Under 1 year	3,299.2	2,696.4	2,142.4	1,288.3	971.9	736.7	700.0	685.2
1–4 years	139.4	109.1	84.5	63.9	46.8	32.4	31.5	29.9
5–14 years	60.1	46.6	41.3	30.6	24.0	18.0	17.0	16.8
15–24 years	128.1	106.3	127.7	115.4	99.2	79.9	81.5	80.1
25–34 years	178.7	146.4	157.4	135.5	139.2	101.4	103.6	102.1
35–44 years	358.7	299.4	314.5	227.9	223.2	198.9	201.6	193.5
45–54 years	853.9	756.0	730.0	584.0	473.4	425.6	433.2	427.0
55–64 years	1,901.0	1,735.1	1,658.8	1,346.3	1,196.9	992.2	940.9	910.3
65–74 years	4,104.3	3,822.1	3,582.7	2,994.9	2,648.6	2,399.1	2,255.0	2,164.6
75–84 years	9,331.1	8,745.2	8,004.4	6,692.6	6,007.2	5,666.5	5,463.1	5,275.1
85 years and over	20,196.9	19,857.5	16,344.9	15,980.3	15,327.4	15,524.4	14,593.3	13,823.5
Male								
All ages, age-adjusted[2]	1,674.2	1,609.0	1,542.1	1,348.1	1,202.8	1,053.8	994.3	955.7
All ages, crude	1,106.1	1,104.5	1,090.3	976.9	918.4	853.0	840.3	817.6
Under 1 year	3,728.0	3,059.3	2,410.0	1,428.5	1,082.8	806.5	777.4	753.7
1–4 years	151.7	119.5	93.2	72.6	52.4	35.9	35.1	32.4
5–14 years	70.9	55.7	50.5	36.7	28.5	20.9	19.8	19.2
15–24 years	167.9	152.1	188.5	172.3	147.4	114.9	116.5	114.7
25–34 years	216.5	187.9	215.3	196.1	204.3	138.6	141.4	139.5
35–44 years	428.8	372.8	402.6	299.2	310.4	255.2	255.0	243.6
45–54 years	1,067.1	992.2	958.5	767.3	610.3	542.8	552.2	543.5
55–64 years	2,395.3	2,309.5	2,282.7	1,815.1	1,553.4	1,230.7	1,165.5	1,128.8
65–74 years	4,931.4	4,914.4	4,873.8	4,105.2	3,491.5	2,979.6	2,771.7	2,644.8
75–84 years	10,426.0	10,178.4	10,010.2	8,816.7	7,888.6	6,972.6	6,641.8	6,394.3
85 years and over	21,636.0	21,186.3	17,821.5	18,801.1	18,056.6	17,501.4	15,794.0	15,031.1
Female								
All ages, age-adjusted[2]	1,236.0	1,105.3	971.4	817.9	750.9	731.4	706.2	679.2
All ages, crude	823.5	809.2	807.8	785.3	812.0	855.0	843.4	815.4
Under 1 year	2,854.6	2,321.3	1,863.7	1,141.7	855.7	663.4	619.1	613.4
1–4 years	126.7	98.4	75.4	54.7	41.0	28.7	27.8	27.3
5–14 years	48.9	37.3	31.8	24.2	19.3	15.0	14.0	14.3
15–24 years	89.1	61.3	68.1	57.5	49.0	43.1	44.4	43.6
25–34 years	142.7	106.6	101.6	75.9	74.2	63.5	64.6	63.5
35–44 years	290.3	229.4	231.1	159.3	137.9	143.2	148.5	143.5
45–54 years	641.5	526.7	517.2	412.9	342.7	312.5	318.4	314.3
55–64 years	1,404.8	1,196.4	1,098.9	934.3	878.8	772.2	732.7	707.4
65–74 years	3,333.2	2,871.8	2,579.7	2,144.7	1,991.2	1,921.2	1,823.0	1,761.4
75–84 years	8,399.6	7,633.1	6,677.6	5,440.1	4,883.1	4,814.7	4,675.5	4,521.8
85 years and over	19,194.7	19,008.4	15,518.0	14,746.9	14,274.3	14,719.2	14,062.5	13,280.3
White male[3]								
All ages, age-adjusted[2]	1,642.5	1,586.0	1,513.7	1,317.6	1,165.9	1,029.4	973.9	936.9
All ages, crude	1,089.5	1,098.5	1,086.7	983.3	930.9	887.8	877.6	854.2
Under 1 year	3,400.5	2,694.1	2,113.2	1,230.3	896.1	667.6	658.7	631.6
1–4 years	135.5	104.9	83.6	66.1	45.9	32.6	31.5	29.4
5–14 years	67.2	52.7	48.0	35.0	26.4	19.8	18.4	17.9
15–24 years	152.4	143.7	170.8	167.0	131.3	105.8	108.9	108.3
25–34 years	185.3	163.2	176.6	171.3	176.1	124.1	128.8	127.0
35–44 years	380.9	332.6	343.5	257.4	268.2	233.6	237.6	229.1
45–54 years	984.5	932.2	882.9	698.9	548.7	496.9	509.2	504.0
55–64 years	2,304.4	2,225.2	2,202.6	1,728.5	1,467.2	1,163.3	1,102.3	1,065.9
65–74 years	4,864.9	4,848.4	4,810.1	4,035.7	3,397.7	2,905.7	2,707.3	2,584.0
75–84 years	10,526.3	10,299.6	10,098.8	8,829.8	7,844.9	6,933.1	6,620.6	6,384.8
85 years and over	22,116.3	21,750.0	18,551.7	19,097.3	18,268.3	17,716.4	16,037.9	15,250.7

See footnotes at end of table.

This table will be updated on the Web. Go to www.cdc.gov/nchs/hus.htm.

Table 35 (page 2 of 4). Death rates for all causes, by sex, race, Hispanic origin, and age: United States, selected years 1950–2004

[Data are based on death certificates]

Sex, race, Hispanic origin, and age	*1950*[1]	*1960*[1]	*1970*	*1980*	*1990*	*2000*	*2003*	*2004*
Black or African American male[3]				Deaths per 100,000 resident population				
All ages, age-adjusted[2]	1,909.1	1,811.1	1,873.9	1,697.8	1,644.5	1,403.5	1,319.1	1,269.4
All ages, crude	1,257.7	1,181.7	1,186.6	1,034.1	1,008.0	834.1	813.7	792.6
Under 1 year	---	5,306.8	4,298.9	2,586.7	2,112.4	1,567.6	1,410.0	1,414.2
1–4 years[4]	1,412.6	208.5	150.5	110.5	85.8	54.5	53.7	48.6
5–14 years	95.1	75.1	67.1	47.4	41.2	28.2	26.8	26.0
15–24 years	289.7	212.0	320.6	209.1	252.2	181.4	171.3	164.3
25–34 years	503.5	402.5	559.5	407.3	430.8	261.0	256.2	252.3
35–44 years	878.1	762.0	956.6	689.8	699.6	453.0	426.7	397.0
45–54 years	1,905.0	1,624.8	1,777.5	1,479.9	1,261.0	1,017.7	991.4	954.9
55–64 years	3,773.2	3,316.4	3,256.9	2,873.0	2,618.4	2,080.1	2,011.2	1,960.8
65–74 years	5,310.3	5,798.7	5,803.2	5,131.1	4,946.1	4,253.5	3,981.3	3,818.3
75–84 years[5]	10,101.9	8,605.1	9,454.9	9,231.6	9,129.5	8,486.0	8,067.0	7,710.3
85 years and over	---	14,844.8	12,222.3	16,098.8	16,954.9	16,791.0	14,903.4	14,452.5
American Indian or Alaska Native male[3]								
All ages, age-adjusted[2]	---	---	---	1,111.5	916.2	841.5	797.0	758.1
All ages, crude	---	---	---	597.1	476.4	415.6	457.6	453.8
Under 1 year	---	---	---	1,598.1	1,056.6	700.2	911.5	1,076.0
1–4 years	---	---	---	82.7	77.4	44.9	57.3	55.3
5–14 years	---	---	---	43.7	33.4	20.2	29.3	24.1
15–24 years	---	---	---	311.1	219.8	136.2	153.1	136.5
25–34 years	---	---	---	360.6	256.1	179.1	185.3	188.8
35–44 years	---	---	---	556.8	365.4	295.2	338.1	321.2
45–54 years	---	---	---	871.3	619.9	520.0	583.6	543.5
55–64 years	---	---	---	1,547.5	1,211.3	1,090.4	1,058.3	1,067.3
65–74 years	---	---	---	2,968.4	2,461.7	2,478.3	2,237.3	2,196.8
75–84 years	---	---	---	5,607.0	5,389.2	5,351.2	4,644.0	4,584.2
85 years and over	---	---	---	12,635.2	11,243.9	10,725.8	9,583.8	7,923.8
Asian or Pacific Islander male[3]								
All ages, age-adjusted[2]	---	---	---	786.5	716.4	624.2	562.7	534.7
All ages, crude	---	---	---	375.3	334.3	332.9	330.0	321.1
Under 1 year	---	---	---	816.5	605.3	529.4	496.9	443.1
1–4 years	---	---	---	50.9	45.0	23.3	24.8	20.7
5–14 years	---	---	---	23.4	20.7	12.9	14.6	14.7
15–24 years	---	---	---	80.8	76.0	55.2	56.3	53.9
25–34 years	---	---	---	83.5	79.6	55.0	53.8	50.9
35–44 years	---	---	---	128.3	130.8	104.9	95.9	91.3
45–54 years	---	---	---	342.3	287.1	249.7	242.6	241.9
55–64 years	---	---	---	881.1	789.1	642.4	565.5	545.3
65–74 years	---	---	---	2,236.1	2,041.4	1,661.0	1,472.8	1,363.4
75–84 years	---	---	---	5,389.5	5,008.6	4,328.2	4,041.0	3,766.3
85 years and over	---	---	---	13,753.6	12,446.3	12,125.3	10,391.7	10,118.2
Hispanic or Latino male[3,6]								
All ages, age-adjusted[2]	---	---	---	---	886.4	818.1	748.1	706.8
All ages, crude	---	---	---	---	411.6	331.3	330.7	321.1
Under 1 year	---	---	---	---	921.8	637.1	665.5	636.5
1–4 years	---	---	---	---	53.8	31.5	33.8	30.2
5–14 years	---	---	---	---	26.0	17.9	18.4	16.7
15–24 years	---	---	---	---	159.3	107.7	112.9	115.3
25–34 years	---	---	---	---	234.0	120.2	118.1	109.2
35–44 years	---	---	---	---	341.8	211.0	189.8	184.2
45–54 years	---	---	---	---	533.9	439.0	436.4	417.8
55–64 years	---	---	---	---	1,123.7	965.7	920.8	874.0
65–74 years	---	---	---	---	2,368.2	2,287.9	2,115.7	1,994.3
75–84 years	---	---	---	---	5,369.1	5,395.3	4,948.5	4,791.6
85 years and over	---	---	---	---	12,272.1	13,086.2	11,029.2	9,932.8

See footnotes at end of table.

This table will be updated on the Web. Go to www.cdc.gov/nchs/hus.htm.

Table 35 (page 3 of 4). Death rates for all causes, by sex, race, Hispanic origin, and age: United States, selected years 1950–2004

[Data are based on death certificates]

Sex, race, Hispanic origin, and age	1950[1]	1960[1]	1970	1980	1990	2000	2003	2004
White, not Hispanic or Latino male[6]				Deaths per 100,000 resident population				
All ages, age-adjusted[2]	- - -	- - -	- - -	- - -	1,170.9	1,035.4	984.0	949.0
All ages, crude	- - -	- - -	- - -	- - -	985.9	978.5	979.1	957.4
Under 1 year	- - -	- - -	- - -	- - -	865.4	658.7	647.2	625.2
1–4 years	- - -	- - -	- - -	- - -	43.8	32.4	30.2	29.0
5–14 years	- - -	- - -	- - -	- - -	25.7	20.0	18.1	17.9
15–24 years	- - -	- - -	- - -	- - -	123.4	103.5	105.9	104.8
25–34 years	- - -	- - -	- - -	- - -	165.3	123.0	129.9	130.9
35–44 years	- - -	- - -	- - -	- - -	257.1	233.9	243.8	235.7
45–54 years	- - -	- - -	- - -	- - -	544.5	497.7	513.2	510.5
55–64 years	- - -	- - -	- - -	- - -	1,479.7	1,170.9	1,110.5	1,076.4
65–74 years	- - -	- - -	- - -	- - -	3,434.5	2,930.5	2,738.5	2,617.9
75–84 years	- - -	- - -	- - -	- - -	7,920.4	6,977.8	6,692.2	6,461.5
85 years and over	- - -	- - -	- - -	- - -	18,505.4	17,853.2	16,234.4	15,489.2
White female[3]								
All ages, age-adjusted[2]	1,198.0	1,074.4	944.0	796.1	728.8	715.3	693.1	666.9
All ages, crude	803.3	800.9	812.6	806.1	846.9	912.3	902.3	871.9
Under 1 year	2,566.8	2,007.7	1,614.6	962.5	690.0	550.5	520.7	513.6
1–4 years	112.2	85.2	66.1	49.3	36.1	25.5	25.5	24.4
5–14 years	45.1	34.7	29.9	22.9	17.9	14.1	13.1	13.0
15–24 years	71.5	54.9	61.6	55.5	45.9	41.1	43.2	42.4
25–34 years	112.8	85.0	84.1	65.4	61.5	55.1	58.0	56.8
35–44 years	235.8	191.1	193.3	138.2	117.4	125.7	132.9	129.5
45–54 years	546.4	458.8	462.9	372.7	309.3	281.4	287.2	285.4
55–64 years	1,293.8	1,078.9	1,014.9	876.2	822.7	730.9	693.7	671.8
65–74 years	3,242.8	2,779.3	2,470.7	2,066.6	1,923.5	1,868.3	1,780.6	1,723.6
75–84 years	8,481.5	7,696.6	6,698.7	5,401.7	4,839.1	4,785.3	4,671.6	4,514.4
85 years and over	19,679.5	19,477.7	15,980.2	14,979.6	14,400.6	14,890.7	14,240.6	13,450.9
Black or African American female[3]								
All ages, age-adjusted[2]	1,545.5	1,369.7	1,228.7	1,033.3	975.1	927.6	885.6	855.3
All ages, crude	1,002.0	905.0	829.2	733.3	747.9	733.0	717.9	700.3
Under 1 year	- - -	4,162.2	3,368.8	2,123.7	1,735.5	1,279.8	1,132.2	1,149.9
1–4 years[4]	1,139.3	173.3	129.4	84.4	67.6	45.3	39.7	40.9
5–14 years	72.8	53.8	43.8	30.5	27.5	20.0	18.9	21.1
15–24 years	213.1	107.5	111.9	70.5	68.7	58.3	54.0	53.7
25–34 years	393.3	273.2	231.0	150.0	159.5	121.8	113.5	112.3
35–44 years	758.1	568.5	533.0	323.9	298.6	271.9	270.0	256.0
45–54 years	1,576.4	1,177.0	1,043.9	768.2	639.4	588.3	582.3	564.1
55–64 years	3,089.4	2,510.9	1,986.2	1,561.0	1,452.6	1,227.2	1,178.8	1,128.6
65–74 years	4,000.2	4,064.2	3,860.9	3,057.4	2,865.7	2,689.6	2,487.2	2,386.1
75–84 years[5]	8,347.0	6,730.0	6,691.5	6,212.1	5,688.3	5,696.5	5,385.5	5,300.0
85 years and over	- - -	13,052.6	10,706.6	12,367.2	13,309.5	13,941.3	13,616.7	12,896.9
American Indian or Alaska Native female[3]								
All ages, age-adjusted[2]	- - -	- - -	- - -	662.4	561.8	604.5	592.1	557.9
All ages, crude	- - -	- - -	- - -	380.1	330.4	346.1	387.7	380.0
Under 1 year	- - -	- - -	- - -	1,352.6	688.7	492.2	676.2	715.4
1–4 years	- - -	- - -	- - -	87.5	37.8	39.8	43.0	53.4
5–14 years	- - -	- - -	- - -	33.5	25.5	17.7	17.9	20.2
15–24 years	- - -	- - -	- - -	90.3	69.0	58.9	61.5	64.6
25–34 years	- - -	- - -	- - -	178.5	102.3	84.8	88.7	102.9
35–44 years	- - -	- - -	- - -	286.0	156.4	171.9	196.0	191.6
45–54 years	- - -	- - -	- - -	491.4	380.9	284.9	364.4	340.0
55–64 years	- - -	- - -	- - -	837.1	805.9	772.1	785.0	704.0
65–74 years	- - -	- - -	- - -	1,765.5	1,679.4	1,899.8	1,710.7	1,700.9
75–84 years	- - -	- - -	- - -	3,612.9	3,073.2	3,850.0	3,834.3	3,533.4
85 years and over	- - -	- - -	- - -	8,567.4	8,201.1	9,118.2	7,920.2	7,093.7

See footnotes at end of table.

This table will be updated on the Web. Go to www.cdc.gov/nchs/hus.htm.

Table 35 (page 4 of 4). Death rates for all causes, by sex, race, Hispanic origin, and age: United States, selected years 1950–2004

[Data are based on death certificates]

Sex, race, Hispanic origin, and age	1950[1]	1960[1]	1970	1980	1990	2000	2003	2004
Asian or Pacific Islander female[3]				Deaths per 100,000 resident population				
All ages, age-adjusted[2]	---	---	---	425.9	469.3	416.8	392.7	375.5
All ages, crude	---	---	---	222.5	234.3	262.3	279.2	274.6
Under 1 year	---	---	---	755.8	518.2	434.3	427.5	392.2
1–4 years	---	---	---	35.4	32.0	20.0	20.1	22.0
5–14 years	---	---	---	21.5	13.0	11.7	11.5	9.7
15–24 years	---	---	---	32.3	28.8	22.4	28.8	24.1
25–34 years	---	---	---	45.4	37.5	27.6	29.9	26.8
35–44 years	---	---	---	89.7	69.9	65.6	58.2	54.2
45–54 years	---	---	---	214.1	182.7	155.5	150.8	145.8
55–64 years	---	---	---	440.8	483.4	390.9	359.2	339.9
65–74 years	---	---	---	1,027.7	1,089.2	996.4	989.9	933.2
75–84 years	---	---	---	2,833.6	3,127.9	2,882.4	2,681.8	2,558.2
85 years and over	---	---	---	7,923.3	10,254.0	9,052.2	8,329.2	8,125.8
Hispanic or Latino female[3,6]								
All ages, age-adjusted[2]	---	---	---	---	537.1	546.0	515.8	485.9
All ages, crude	---	---	---	---	285.4	274.6	279.3	269.7
Under 1 year	---	---	---	---	746.6	553.6	552.4	535.1
1–4 years	---	---	---	---	42.1	27.5	26.3	24.3
5–14 years	---	---	---	---	17.3	13.4	12.8	12.0
15–24 years	---	---	---	---	40.6	31.7	35.5	31.8
25–34 years	---	---	---	---	62.9	43.4	43.0	40.9
35–44 years	---	---	---	---	109.3	100.5	95.5	88.2
45–54 years	---	---	---	---	253.3	223.8	219.1	208.3
55–64 years	---	---	---	---	607.5	548.4	527.9	511.3
65–74 years	---	---	---	---	1,453.8	1,423.2	1,342.9	1,297.2
75–84 years	---	---	---	---	3,351.3	3,624.5	3,506.4	3,329.6
85 years and over	---	---	---	---	10,098.7	11,202.8	10,128.1	9,253.0
White, not Hispanic or Latino female[6]								
All ages, age-adjusted[2]	---	---	---	---	734.6	721.5	702.1	677.5
All ages, crude	---	---	---	---	903.6	1,007.3	1,007.6	977.7
Under 1 year	---	---	---	---	655.3	530.9	502.5	500.7
1–4 years	---	---	---	---	34.0	24.4	24.9	24.4
5–14 years	---	---	---	---	17.6	13.9	12.9	13.0
15–24 years	---	---	---	---	46.0	42.6	44.3	44.3
25–34 years	---	---	---	---	60.6	56.8	61.2	60.3
35–44 years	---	---	---	---	116.8	128.1	138.0	136.0
45–54 years	---	---	---	---	312.1	285.0	293.1	292.9
55–64 years	---	---	---	---	834.5	742.1	705.0	683.8
65–74 years	---	---	---	---	1,940.2	1,891.0	1,807.9	1,752.0
75–84 years	---	---	---	---	4,887.3	4,819.3	4,720.5	4,571.1
85 years and over	---	---	---	---	14,533.1	14,971.7	14,377.2	13,609.6

- - - Data not available.

[1]Includes deaths of persons who were not residents of the 50 states and the District of Columbia.

[2]Age-adjusted rates are calculated using the year 2000 standard population. Prior to 2003, age-adjusted rates were calculated using standard million proportions based on rounded population numbers. Starting with 2003 data, unrounded population numbers are used to calculate age-adjusted rates. See Appendix II, Age adjustment.

[3]The race groups, white, black, Asian or Pacific Islander, and American Indian or Alaska Native, include persons of Hispanic and non-Hispanic origin. Persons of Hispanic origin may be of any race. Death rates for the American Indian or Alaska Native and Asian or Pacific Islander populations are known to be underestimated. See Appendix II, Race, for a discussion of sources of bias in death rates by race and Hispanic origin.

[4]In 1950, rate is for the age group under 5 years.

[5]In 1950, rate is for the age group 75 years and over.

[6]Prior to 1997, excludes data from states lacking an Hispanic-origin item on the death certificate. See Appendix II, Hispanic origin.

NOTES: Starting with *Health, United States, 2003*, rates for 1991–1999 were revised using intercensal population estimates based on the 2000 census. Rates for 2000 were revised based on 2000 census counts. Rates for 2001 and later years were computed using 2000-based postcensal estimates. See Appendix I, Population Census and Population Estimates. In 2003, seven states reported multiple-race data. In 2004, 15 states reported multiple-race data. The multiple-race data for these states were bridged to the single-race categories of the 1977 Office of Management and Budget standards for comparability with other states. See Appendix II, Race. Data for additional years are available. See Appendix III.

SOURCES: Centers for Disease Control and Prevention, National Center for Health Statistics, National Vital Statistics System; Grove RD, Hetzel AM. Vital statistics rates in the United States, 1940–1960. Washington, DC: U.S. Government Printing Office, 1968; numerator data from National Vital Statistics System, annual mortality files; denominator data from national population estimates for race groups from Table 1 and unpublished Hispanic population estimates for 1985–1996 prepared by the Housing and Household Economic Statistics Division, U.S. Census Bureau; additional mortality tables are available from: www.cdc.gov/nchs/datawh/statab/unpubd/mortabs.htm; Miniño AM, Heron M, Murphy SL, Kochanek KD. Deaths: Final data for 2004. Health E-Stats. Hyattsville, MD: National Center for Health Statistics. 2006.

This table will be updated on the Web. Go to www.cdc.gov/nchs/hus.htm.

Table 36 (page 1 of 3). Death rates for diseases of heart, by sex, race, Hispanic origin, and age: United States, selected years 1950–2004

[Data are based on death certificates]

Sex, race, Hispanic origin, and age	1950[1,2]	1960[1,2]	1970[2]	1980[2]	1990	2000[3]	2003	2004
	Deaths per 100,000 resident population							
All persons								
All ages, age-adjusted[4]	586.8	559.0	492.7	412.1	321.8	257.6	232.3	217.0
All ages, crude	355.5	369.0	362.0	336.0	289.5	252.6	235.6	222.2
Under 1 year	3.5	6.6	13.1	22.8	20.1	13.0	11.0	10.3
1–4 years	1.3	1.3	1.7	2.6	1.9	1.2	1.2	1.2
5–14 years	2.1	1.3	0.8	0.9	0.9	0.7	0.6	0.6
15–24 years	6.8	4.0	3.0	2.9	2.5	2.6	2.7	2.5
25–34 years	19.4	15.6	11.4	8.3	7.6	7.4	8.2	7.9
35–44 years	86.4	74.6	66.7	44.6	31.4	29.2	30.7	29.3
45–54 years	308.6	271.8	238.4	180.2	120.5	94.2	92.5	90.2
55–64 years	808.1	737.9	652.3	494.1	367.3	261.2	233.2	218.8
65–74 years	1,839.8	1,740.5	1,558.2	1,218.6	894.3	665.6	585.0	541.6
75–84 years	4,310.1	4,089.4	3,683.8	2,993.1	2,295.7	1,780.3	1,611.1	1,506.3
85 years and over	9,150.6	9,317.8	7,891.3	7,777.1	6,739.9	5,926.1	5,278.4	4,895.9
Male								
All ages, age-adjusted[4]	697.0	687.6	634.0	538.9	412.4	320.0	286.6	267.9
All ages, crude	423.4	439.5	422.5	368.6	297.6	249.8	235.0	222.8
Under 1 year	4.0	7.8	15.1	25.5	21.9	13.3	12.1	10.9
1–4 years	1.4	1.4	1.9	2.8	1.9	1.4	1.1	1.1
5–14 years	2.0	1.4	0.9	1.0	0.9	0.8	0.7	0.6
15–24 years	6.8	4.2	3.7	3.7	3.1	3.2	3.4	3.2
25–34 years	22.9	20.1	15.2	11.4	10.3	9.6	10.5	10.5
35–44 years	118.4	112.7	103.2	68.7	48.1	41.4	42.8	40.9
45–54 years	440.5	420.4	376.4	282.6	183.0	140.2	136.2	132.3
55–64 years	1,104.5	1,066.9	987.2	746.8	537.3	371.7	331.7	312.8
65–74 years	2,292.3	2,291.3	2,170.3	1,728.0	1,250.0	898.3	785.3	723.8
75–84 years	4,825.0	4,742.4	4,534.8	3,834.3	2,968.2	2,248.1	2,030.3	1,893.6
85 years and over	9,659.8	9,788.9	8,426.2	8,752.7	7,418.4	6,430.0	5,621.5	5,239.3
Female								
All ages, age-adjusted[4]	484.7	447.0	381.6	320.8	257.0	210.9	190.3	177.3
All ages, crude	288.4	300.6	304.5	305.1	281.8	255.3	236.2	221.6
Under 1 year	2.9	5.4	10.9	20.0	18.3	12.5	9.8	9.7
1–4 years	1.2	1.1	1.6	2.5	1.9	1.0	1.3	1.2
5–14 years	2.2	1.2	0.8	0.9	0.8	0.5	0.5	0.6
15–24 years	6.7	3.7	2.3	2.1	1.8	2.1	2.1	1.7
25–34 years	16.2	11.3	7.7	5.3	5.0	5.2	5.7	5.2
35–44 years	55.1	38.2	32.2	21.4	15.1	17.2	18.6	17.7
45–54 years	177.2	127.5	109.9	84.5	61.0	49.8	50.2	49.6
55–64 years	510.0	429.4	351.6	272.1	215.7	159.3	141.9	131.5
65–74 years	1,419.3	1,261.3	1,082.7	828.6	616.8	474.0	417.5	388.6
75–84 years	3,872.0	3,582.7	3,120.8	2,497.0	1,893.8	1,475.1	1,331.1	1,245.6
85 years and over	8,796.1	9,016.8	7,591.8	7,350.5	6,478.1	5,720.9	5,126.7	4,741.5
White male[5]								
All ages, age-adjusted[4]	700.2	694.5	640.2	539.6	409.2	316.7	282.9	264.6
All ages, crude	433.0	454.6	438.3	384.0	312.7	265.8	249.5	236.5
45–54 years	423.6	413.2	365.7	269.8	170.6	130.7	125.3	122.2
55–64 years	1,081.7	1,056.0	979.3	730.6	516.7	351.8	313.2	294.4
65–74 years	2,308.3	2,297.9	2,177.2	1,729.7	1,230.5	877.8	761.1	703.2
75–84 years	4,907.3	4,839.9	4,617.6	3,883.2	2,983.4	2,247.0	2,030.1	1,897.1
85 years and over	9,950.5	10,135.8	8,818.0	8,958.0	7,558.7	6,560.8	5,747.2	5,348.4
Black or African American male[5]								
All ages, age-adjusted[4]	639.4	615.2	607.3	561.4	485.4	392.5	364.3	342.1
All ages, crude	346.2	330.6	330.3	301.0	256.8	211.1	206.0	196.7
45–54 years	622.5	514.0	512.8	433.4	328.9	247.2	248.1	240.0
55–64 years	1,433.1	1,236.8	1,135.4	987.2	824.0	631.2	580.9	560.2
65–74 years	2,139.1	2,281.4	2,237.8	1,847.2	1,632.9	1,268.8	1,195.5	1,096.6
75–84 years[6]	4,106.1	3,533.6	3,783.4	3,578.8	3,107.1	2,597.6	2,426.6	2,235.5
85 years and over	- - -	6,037.9	5,367.6	6,819.5	6,479.6	5,633.5	4,850.3	4,637.3

See footnotes at end of table.

This table will be updated on the Web. Go to www.cdc.gov/nchs/hus.htm.

Table 36 (page 2 of 3). Death rates for diseases of heart, by sex, race, Hispanic origin, and age: United States, selected years 1950–2004

[Data are based on death certificates]

Sex, race, Hispanic origin, and age	1950[1,2]	1960[1,2]	1970[2]	1980[2]	1990	2000[3]	2003	2004
	Deaths per 100,000 resident population							
American Indian or Alaska Native male[5]								
All ages, age-adjusted[4]	---	---	---	320.5	264.1	222.2	203.2	182.7
All ages, crude	---	---	---	130.6	108.0	90.1	98.5	91.4
45–54 years	---	---	---	238.1	173.8	108.5	116.7	94.1
55–64 years	---	---	---	496.3	411.0	285.0	293.5	260.7
65–74 years	---	---	---	1,009.4	839.1	748.2	655.6	590.0
75–84 years	---	---	---	2,062.2	1,788.8	1,655.7	1,309.9	1,252.1
85 years and over	---	---	---	4,413.7	3,860.3	3,318.3	3,266.5	2,812.6
Asian or Pacific Islander male[5]								
All ages, age-adjusted[4]	---	---	---	286.9	220.7	185.5	158.3	146.5
All ages, crude	---	---	---	119.8	88.7	90.6	86.3	81.4
45–54 years	---	---	---	112.0	70.4	61.1	62.7	56.6
55–64 years	---	---	---	306.7	226.1	182.6	152.9	138.9
65–74 years	---	---	---	852.4	623.5	482.5	398.3	347.7
75–84 years	---	---	---	2,010.9	1,642.2	1,354.7	1,145.1	1,047.0
85 years and over	---	---	---	5,923.0	4,617.8	4,154.2	3,524.6	3,416.7
Hispanic or Latino male[5,7]								
All ages, age-adjusted[4]	---	---	---	---	270.0	238.2	206.8	193.9
All ages, crude	---	---	---	---	91.0	74.7	72.2	70.2
45–54 years	---	---	---	---	116.4	84.3	79.6	77.6
55–64 years	---	---	---	---	363.0	264.8	235.6	224.6
65–74 years	---	---	---	---	829.9	684.8	625.0	572.2
75–84 years	---	---	---	---	1,971.3	1,733.2	1,543.5	1,489.0
85 years and over	---	---	---	---	4,711.9	4,897.5	3,874.5	3,496.8
White, not Hispanic or Latino male[7]								
All ages, age-adjusted[4]	---	---	---	---	413.6	319.9	286.9	268.7
All ages, crude	---	---	---	---	336.5	297.5	282.9	269.1
45–54 years	---	---	---	---	172.8	134.3	129.8	126.9
55–64 years	---	---	---	---	521.3	356.3	317.7	298.8
65–74 years	---	---	---	---	1,243.4	885.1	767.3	709.5
75–84 years	---	---	---	---	3,007.7	2,261.9	2,049.9	1,915.1
85 years and over	---	---	---	---	7,663.4	6,606.6	5,821.0	5,430.9
White female[5]								
All ages, age-adjusted[4]	478.0	441.7	376.7	315.9	250.9	205.6	185.4	172.9
All ages, crude	289.4	306.5	313.8	319.2	298.4	274.5	253.8	238.3
45–54 years	141.9	103.4	91.4	71.2	50.2	40.9	41.1	40.7
55–64 years	460.2	383.0	317.7	248.1	192.4	141.3	125.2	117.2
65–74 years	1,400.9	1,229.8	1,044.0	796.7	583.6	445.2	392.0	365.4
75–84 years	3,925.2	3,629.7	3,143.5	2,493.6	1,874.3	1,452.4	1,315.2	1,229.1
85 years and over	9,084.7	9,280.8	7,839.9	7,501.6	6,563.4	5,801.4	5,193.6	4,810.4
Black or African American female[5]								
All ages, age-adjusted[4]	536.9	488.9	435.6	378.6	327.5	277.6	253.8	236.5
All ages, crude	287.6	268.5	261.0	249.7	237.0	212.6	200.0	188.3
45–54 years	525.3	360.7	290.9	202.4	155.3	125.0	124.1	121.2
55–64 years	1,210.2	952.3	710.5	530.1	442.0	332.8	304.7	276.0
65–74 years	1,659.4	1,680.5	1,553.2	1,210.3	1,017.5	815.2	712.0	656.5
75–84 years[6]	3,499.3	2,926.9	2,964.1	2,707.2	2,250.9	1,913.1	1,699.6	1,622.9
85 years and over	---	5,650.0	5,003.8	5,796.5	5,766.1	5,298.7	4,976.5	4,534.7

See footnotes at end of table.

This table will be updated on the Web. Go to www.cdc.gov/nchs/hus.htm.

Table 36 (page 3 of 3). Death rates for diseases of heart, by sex, race, Hispanic origin, and age: United States, selected years 1950–2004

[Data are based on death certificates]

Sex, race, Hispanic origin, and age	1950[1,2]	1960[1,2]	1970[2]	1980[2]	1990	2000[3]	2003	2004
	Deaths per 100,000 resident population							
American Indian or Alaska Native female[5]								
All ages, age-adjusted[4]	---	---	---	175.4	153.1	143.6	127.5	119.9
All ages, crude	---	---	---	80.3	77.5	71.9	75.9	73.6
45–54 years	---	---	---	65.2	62.0	40.2	45.4	49.5
55–64 years	---	---	---	193.5	197.0	149.4	153.4	116.9
65–74 years	---	---	---	577.2	492.8	391.8	390.3	317.4
75–84 years	---	---	---	1,364.3	1,050.3	1,044.1	950.3	894.1
85 years and over	---	---	---	2,893.3	2,868.7	3,146.3	2,284.1	2,449.1
Asian or Pacific Islander female[5]								
All ages, age-adjusted[4]	---	---	---	132.3	149.2	115.7	104.2	96.1
All ages, crude	---	---	---	57.0	62.0	65.0	68.2	65.1
45–54 years	---	---	---	28.6	17.5	15.9	*14.8	13.7
55–64 years	---	---	---	92.9	99.0	68.8	60.3	50.7
65–74 years	---	---	---	313.3	323.9	229.6	207.2	205.6
75–84 years	---	---	---	1,053.2	1,130.9	866.2	769.7	697.4
85 years and over	---	---	---	3,211.0	4,161.2	3,367.2	3,020.0	2,817.1
Hispanic or Latino female[5,7]								
All ages, age-adjusted[4]	---	---	---	---	177.2	163.7	145.8	130.0
All ages, crude	---	---	---	---	79.4	71.5	69.6	64.1
45–54 years	---	---	---	---	43.5	28.2	27.0	27.0
55–64 years	---	---	---	---	153.2	111.2	102.1	93.1
65–74 years	---	---	---	---	460.4	366.3	330.6	305.5
75–84 years	---	---	---	---	1,259.7	1,169.4	1,067.0	962.7
85 years and over	---	---	---	---	4,440.3	4,605.8	3,962.5	3,421.2
White, not Hispanic or Latino female[7]								
All ages, age-adjusted[4]	---	---	---	---	252.6	206.8	187.1	175.1
All ages, crude	---	---	---	---	320.0	304.9	285.1	269.1
45–54 years	---	---	---	---	50.2	41.9	42.4	42.2
55–64 years	---	---	---	---	193.6	142.9	126.6	118.9
65–74 years	---	---	---	---	584.7	448.5	394.8	368.6
75–84 years	---	---	---	---	1,890.2	1,458.9	1,324.0	1,241.2
85 years and over	---	---	---	---	6,615.2	5,822.7	5,232.2	4,862.4

- - - Data not available.
[1]Includes deaths of persons who were not residents of the 50 states and the District of Columbia.
[2]Underlying cause of death was coded according to the Sixth Revision of the International Classification of Diseases (ICD) in 1950, Seventh Revision in 1960, Eighth Revision in 1970, and Ninth Revision in 1980–1998. See Appendix II, Cause of death; Tables IV and V.
[3]Starting with 1999 data, cause of death is coded according to ICD–10. See Appendix II, Cause of death, Table V; Comparability ratio, Table VI.
[4]Age-adjusted rates are calculated using the year 2000 standard population. Prior to 2003, age-adjusted rates were calculated using standard million proportions based on rounded population numbers. Starting with 2003 data, unrounded population numbers are used to calculate age-adjusted rates. See Appendix II, Age adjustment.
[5]The race groups, white, black, Asian or Pacific Islander, and American Indian or Alaska Native, include persons of Hispanic and non-Hispanic origin. Persons of Hispanic origin may be of any race. Death rates for the American Indian or Alaska Native and Asian or Pacific Islander populations are known to be underestimated. See Appendix II, Race, for a discussion of sources of bias in death rates by race and Hispanic origin.
[6]In 1950, rate is for the age group 75 years and over.
[7]Prior to 1997, excludes data from states lacking an Hispanic-origin item on the death certificate. See Appendix II, Hispanic origin.

NOTES: Starting with *Health, United States, 2003*, rates for 1991–1999 were revised using intercensal population estimates based on the 2000 census. Rates for 2000 were revised based on 2000 census counts. Rates for 2001 and later years were computed using 2000-based postcensal estimates. See Appendix I, Population Census and Population Estimates. For the period 1980–1998, diseases of heart was coded using ICD–9 codes that are most nearly comparable with diseases of heart codes in the 113 cause list for ICD–10. See Appendix II, Cause of death; Table V. Age groups were selected to minimize the presentation of unstable age-specific death rates based on small numbers of deaths and for consistency among comparison groups. In 2003, seven states reported multiple-race data. In 2004, 15 states reported multiple-race data. The multiple-race data for these states were bridged to the single-race categories of the 1977 Office of Management and Budget standards for comparability with other states. See Appendix II, Race. Data for additional years are available. See Appendix III.

SOURCES: Centers for Disease Control and Prevention, National Center for Health Statistics, National Vital Statistics System; numerator data from annual mortality files; denominator data from national population estimates for race groups from Table 1 and unpublished Hispanic population estimates for 1985–1996 prepared by the Housing and Household Economic Statistics Division, U.S. Census Bureau; additional mortality tables are available from: www.cdc.gov/nchs/datawh/statab/unpubd/mortabs.htm; Miniño AM, Heron M, Murphy SL, Kochanek KD. Deaths: Final data for 2004. Health E-Stats. Hyattsville, MD: National Center for Health Statistics. 2006.

This table will be updated on the Web. Go to www.cdc.gov/nchs/hus.htm.

Table 37 (page 1 of 3). Death rates for cerebrovascular diseases, by sex, race, Hispanic origin, and age: United States, selected years 1950–2004

[Data are based on death certificates]

Sex, race, Hispanic origin, and age	1950[1,2]	1960[1,2]	1970[2]	1980[2]	1990	2000[3]	2003	2004
All persons	Deaths per 100,000 resident population							
All ages, age-adjusted[4]	180.7	177.9	147.7	96.2	65.3	60.9	53.5	50.0
All ages, crude	104.0	108.0	101.9	75.0	57.8	59.6	54.2	51.1
Under 1 year	5.1	4.1	5.0	4.4	3.8	3.3	2.5	3.1
1–4 years	0.9	0.8	1.0	0.5	0.3	0.3	0.3	0.3
5–14 years	0.5	0.7	0.7	0.3	0.2	0.2	0.2	0.2
15–24 years	1.6	1.8	1.6	1.0	0.6	0.5	0.5	0.5
25–34 years	4.2	4.7	4.5	2.6	2.2	1.5	1.5	1.4
35–44 years	18.7	14.7	15.6	8.5	6.4	5.8	5.5	5.4
45–54 years	70.4	49.2	41.6	25.2	18.7	16.0	15.0	14.9
55–64 years	194.2	147.3	115.8	65.1	47.9	41.0	35.6	34.3
65–74 years	554.7	469.2	384.1	219.0	144.2	128.6	112.9	107.8
75–84 years	1,499.6	1,491.3	1,254.2	786.9	498.0	461.3	410.7	386.2
85 years and over	2,990.1	3,680.5	3,014.3	2,283.7	1,628.9	1,589.2	1,370.1	1,245.9
Male								
All ages, age-adjusted[4]	186.4	186.1	157.4	102.2	68.5	62.4	54.1	50.4
All ages, crude	102.5	104.5	94.5	63.4	46.7	46.9	42.9	40.7
Under 1 year	6.4	5.0	5.8	5.0	4.4	3.8	2.8	3.4
1–4 years	1.1	0.9	1.2	0.4	0.3	*	0.3	0.3
5–14 years	0.5	0.7	0.8	0.3	0.2	0.2	0.2	0.2
15–24 years	1.8	1.9	1.8	1.1	0.7	0.5	0.5	0.5
25–34 years	4.2	4.5	4.4	2.6	2.1	1.5	1.6	1.4
35–44 years	17.5	14.6	15.7	8.7	6.8	5.8	5.8	5.6
45–54 years	67.9	52.2	44.4	27.2	20.5	17.5	16.7	16.7
55–64 years	205.2	163.8	138.7	74.6	54.3	47.2	40.8	39.5
65–74 years	589.6	530.7	449.5	258.6	166.6	145.0	127.8	121.1
75–84 years	1,543.6	1,555.9	1,361.6	866.3	551.1	490.8	431.4	402.9
85 years and over	3,048.6	3,643.1	2,895.2	2,193.6	1,528.5	1,484.3	1,236.0	1,118.1
Female								
All ages, age-adjusted[4]	175.8	170.7	140.0	91.7	62.6	59.1	52.3	48.9
All ages, crude	105.6	111.4	109.0	85.9	68.4	71.8	65.1	61.2
Under 1 year	3.7	3.2	4.0	3.8	3.1	2.7	2.2	2.8
1–4 years	0.7	0.7	0.7	0.5	0.3	0.4	0.3	*
5–14 years	0.4	0.6	0.6	0.3	0.2	0.2	0.1	0.2
15–24 years	1.5	1.6	1.4	0.8	0.6	0.5	0.5	0.5
25–34 years	4.3	4.9	4.7	2.6	2.2	1.5	1.4	1.4
35–44 years	19.9	14.8	15.6	8.4	6.1	5.7	5.3	5.1
45–54 years	72.9	46.3	39.0	23.3	17.0	14.5	13.4	13.1
55–64 years	183.1	131.8	95.3	56.8	42.2	35.3	30.9	29.5
65–74 years	522.1	415.7	333.3	188.7	126.7	115.1	100.5	96.6
75–84 years	1,462.2	1,441.1	1,183.1	740.1	466.2	442.1	396.8	374.9
85 years and over	2,949.4	3,704.4	3,081.0	2,323.1	1,667.6	1,632.0	1,429.4	1,303.4
White male[5]								
All ages, age-adjusted[4]	182.1	181.6	153.7	98.7	65.5	59.8	51.7	48.1
All ages, crude	100.5	102.7	93.5	63.1	46.9	48.4	44.2	41.8
45–54 years	53.7	40.9	35.6	21.7	15.4	13.6	12.9	12.8
55–64 years	182.2	139.0	119.9	64.0	45.7	39.7	33.3	32.4
65–74 years	569.7	501.0	420.0	239.8	152.9	133.8	117.3	110.8
75–84 years	1,556.3	1,564.8	1,361.6	852.7	539.2	480.0	422.4	393.7
85 years and over	3,127.1	3,734.8	3,018.1	2,230.8	1,545.4	1,490.7	1,247.0	1,129.3
Black or African American male[5]								
All ages, age-adjusted[4]	228.8	238.5	206.4	142.0	102.2	89.6	79.5	74.9
All ages, crude	122.0	122.9	108.8	73.0	53.0	46.1	43.2	41.5
45–54 years	211.9	166.1	136.1	82.1	68.4	49.5	46.9	44.8
55–64 years	522.8	439.9	343.4	189.7	141.7	115.4	112.1	107.4
65–74 years	783.6	899.2	780.1	472.3	326.9	268.5	237.4	235.2
75–84 years[6]	1,504.9	1,475.2	1,445.7	1,066.3	721.5	659.2	588.9	551.0
85 years and over	- - -	2,700.0	1,963.1	1,873.2	1,421.5	1,458.8	1,180.3	1,061.0

See footnotes at end of table.

This table will be updated on the Web. Go to www.cdc.gov/nchs/hus.htm.

Table 37 (page 2 of 3). Death rates for cerebrovascular diseases, by sex, race, Hispanic origin, and age: United States, selected years 1950–2004

[Data are based on death certificates]

Sex, race, Hispanic origin, and age	1950[1,2]	1960[1,2]	1970[2]	1980[2]	1990	2000[3]	2003	2004
	Deaths per 100,000 resident population							
American Indian or Alaska Native male[5]								
All ages, age-adjusted[4]	- - -	- - -	- - -	66.4	44.3	46.1	34.9	35.0
All ages, crude	- - -	- - -	- - -	23.1	16.0	16.8	15.6	15.6
45–54 years	- - -	- - -	- - -	*	*	13.3	15.5	14.0
55–64 years	- - -	- - -	- - -	72.0	39.8	48.6	30.7	29.9
65–74 years	- - -	- - -	- - -	170.5	120.3	144.7	101.4	109.4
75–84 years	- - -	- - -	- - -	523.9	325.9	373.3	280.7	312.0
85 years and over	- - -	- - -	- - -	1,384.7	949.8	834.9	596.9	559.5
Asian or Pacific Islander male[5]								
All ages, age-adjusted[4]	- - -	- - -	- - -	71.4	59.1	58.0	48.5	44.2
All ages, crude	- - -	- - -	- - -	28.7	23.3	27.2	26.0	24.3
45–54 years	- - -	- - -	- - -	17.0	15.6	15.0	14.7	19.2
55–64 years	- - -	- - -	- - -	59.9	51.8	49.3	42.2	36.8
65–74 years	- - -	- - -	- - -	197.9	167.9	135.6	128.3	102.6
75–84 years	- - -	- - -	- - -	619.5	483.9	438.7	355.7	350.8
85 years and over	- - -	- - -	- - -	1,399.0	1,196.6	1,415.6	1,093.0	969.0
Hispanic or Latino male[5,7]								
All ages, age-adjusted[4]	- - -	- - -	- - -	- - -	46.5	50.5	43.0	41.5
All ages, crude	- - -	- - -	- - -	- - -	15.6	15.8	14.9	15.0
45–54 years	- - -	- - -	- - -	- - -	20.0	18.1	18.1	17.5
55–64 years	- - -	- - -	- - -	- - -	49.2	48.8	43.5	42.9
65–74 years	- - -	- - -	- - -	- - -	126.4	136.1	113.9	114.4
75–84 years	- - -	- - -	- - -	- - -	356.6	392.9	337.1	323.3
85 years and over	- - -	- - -	- - -	- - -	866.3	1,029.9	837.4	778.9
White, not Hispanic or Latino male[7]								
All ages, age-adjusted[4]	- - -	- - -	- - -	- - -	66.3	59.9	51.9	48.2
All ages, crude	- - -	- - -	- - -	- - -	50.6	53.9	49.7	47.0
45–54 years	- - -	- - -	- - -	- - -	14.9	13.0	12.1	12.1
55–64 years	- - -	- - -	- - -	- - -	45.1	38.7	32.1	31.1
65–74 years	- - -	- - -	- - -	- - -	154.5	133.1	116.9	110.0
75–84 years	- - -	- - -	- - -	- - -	547.3	482.3	426.0	396.9
85 years and over	- - -	- - -	- - -	- - -	1,578.7	1,505.9	1,264.2	1,145.3
White female[5]								
All ages, age-adjusted[4]	169.7	165.0	135.5	89.0	60.3	57.3	50.5	47.2
All ages, crude	103.3	110.1	109.8	88.6	71.6	76.9	69.5	65.3
45–54 years	55.0	33.8	30.5	18.6	13.5	11.2	10.0	10.1
55–64 years	156.9	103.0	78.1	48.6	35.8	30.2	25.8	25.1
65–74 years	498.1	383.3	303.2	172.5	116.1	107.3	92.1	89.0
75–84 years	1,471.3	1,444.7	1,176.8	728.8	456.5	434.2	389.9	366.8
85 years and over	3,017.9	3,795.7	3,167.6	2,362.7	1,685.9	1,646.7	1,442.1	1,315.7
Black or African American female[5]								
All ages, age-adjusted[4]	238.4	232.5	189.3	119.6	84.0	76.2	69.8	65.5
All ages, crude	128.3	127.7	112.2	77.8	60.7	58.3	54.8	51.9
45–54 years	248.9	166.2	119.4	61.8	44.1	38.1	36.0	33.9
55–64 years	567.7	452.0	272.4	138.4	96.9	76.4	71.8	65.0
65–74 years	754.4	830.5	673.5	361.7	236.7	190.9	175.3	166.8
75–84 years[6]	1,496.7	1,413.1	1,338.3	917.5	595.0	549.2	498.3	489.5
85 years and over	- - -	2,578.9	2,210.5	1,891.6	1,495.2	1,556.5	1,414.2	1,270.7

See footnotes at end of table.

This table will be updated on the Web. Go to www.cdc.gov/nchs/hus.htm.

Table 37 (page 3 of 3). Death rates for cerebrovascular diseases, by sex, race, Hispanic origin, and age: United States, selected years 1950–2004

[Data are based on death certificates]

Sex, race, Hispanic origin, and age	1950[1,2]	1960[1,2]	1970[2]	1980[2]	1990	2000[3]	2003	2004
American Indian or Alaska Native female[5]				Deaths per 100,000 resident population				
All ages, age-adjusted[4]	---	---	---	51.2	38.4	43.7	34.2	35.1
All ages, crude	---	---	---	22.0	19.3	21.5	19.9	21.3
45–54 years	---	---	---	*	*	14.4	14.6	10.8
55–64 years	---	---	---	*	40.7	37.9	26.0	24.5
65–74 years	---	---	---	128.3	100.5	79.5	94.8	110.9
75–84 years	---	---	---	404.2	282.0	391.1	304.7	258.8
85 years and over	---	---	---	1,095.5	776.2	931.5	569.1	710.1
Asian or Pacific Islander female[5]								
All ages, age-adjusted[4]	---	---	---	60.8	54.9	49.1	42.6	38.9
All ages, crude	---	---	---	26.4	24.3	28.7	28.8	27.0
45–54 years	---	---	---	20.3	19.7	13.3	12.6	10.5
55–64 years	---	---	---	43.7	42.1	33.3	30.8	28.1
65–74 years	---	---	---	136.1	124.0	102.8	95.6	78.1
75–84 years	---	---	---	446.6	396.6	386.0	330.2	312.5
85 years and over	---	---	---	1,545.2	1,395.0	1,246.6	1,042.4	979.9
Hispanic or Latino female[5,7]								
All ages, age-adjusted[4]	---	---	---	---	43.7	43.0	38.1	35.4
All ages, crude	---	---	---	---	20.1	19.4	18.6	17.9
45–54 years	---	---	---	---	15.2	12.4	11.7	11.8
55–64 years	---	---	---	---	38.5	31.9	27.8	27.7
65–74 years	---	---	---	---	102.6	95.2	86.0	83.0
75–84 years	---	---	---	---	308.5	311.3	302.8	272.2
85 years and over	---	---	---	---	1,055.3	1,108.9	902.3	830.4
White, not Hispanic or Latino female[7]								
All ages, age-adjusted[4]	---	---	---	---	61.0	57.6	50.8	47.7
All ages, crude	---	---	---	---	77.2	85.5	78.2	73.7
45–54 years	---	---	---	---	13.2	10.9	9.7	9.8
55–64 years	---	---	---	---	35.7	29.9	25.5	24.7
65–74 years	---	---	---	---	116.9	107.6	92.1	89.0
75–84 years	---	---	---	---	461.9	438.3	393.6	371.6
85 years and over	---	---	---	---	1,714.7	1,661.6	1,461.3	1,335.1

- - - Data not available.

* Rates based on fewer than 20 deaths are considered unreliable and are not shown.

[1]Includes deaths of persons who were not residents of the 50 states and the District of Columbia.

[2]Underlying cause of death was coded according to the Sixth Revision of the International Classification of Diseases (ICD) in 1950, Seventh Revision in 1960, Eighth Revision in 1970, and Ninth Revision in 1980–1998. See Appendix II, Cause of death; Tables IV and V.

[3]Starting with 1999 data, cause of death is coded according to ICD–10. See Appendix II, Cause of death, Table V; Comparability ratio, Table VI.

[4]Age-adjusted rates are calculated using the year 2000 standard population. Prior to 2003, age-adjusted rates were calculated using standard million proportions based on rounded population numbers. Starting with 2003 data, unrounded population numbers are used to calculate age-adjusted rates. See Appendix II, Age adjustment.

[5]The race groups, white, black, Asian or Pacific Islander, and American Indian or Alaska Native, include persons of Hispanic and non-Hispanic origin. Persons of Hispanic origin may be of any race. Death rates for the American Indian or Alaska Native and Asian or Pacific Islander populations are known to be underestimated. See Appendix II, Race, for a discussion of sources of bias in death rates by race and Hispanic origin.

[6]In 1950, rate is for the age group 75 years and over.

[7]Prior to 1997, excludes data from states lacking an Hispanic-origin item on the death certificate. See Appendix II, Hispanic origin.

NOTES: Starting with *Health, United States, 2003*, rates for 1991–1999 were revised using intercensal population estimates based on the 2000 census. Rates for 2000 were revised based on 2000 census counts. Rates for 2001 and later years were computed using 2000-based postcensal estimates. See Appendix I, Population Census and Population Estimates. For the period 1980–1998, cerebrovascular diseases was coded using ICD–9 codes that are most nearly comparable with cerebrovascular diseases codes in the 113 cause list for ICD–10. See Appendix II, Cause of death; Table V. Age groups were selected to minimize the presentation of unstable age-specific death rates based on small numbers of deaths and for consistency among comparison groups. In 2003, seven states reported multiple-race data. In 2004, 15 states reported multiple-race data. The multiple-race data for these states were bridged to the single-race categories of the 1977 Office of Management and Budget standards for comparability with other states. See Appendix II, Race. Data for additional years are available. See Appendix III.

SOURCES: Centers for Disease Control and Prevention, National Center for Health Statistics, National Vital Statistics System; Grove RD, Hetzel AM. Vital statistics rates in the United States, 1940–1960. Washington, DC: U.S. Government Printing Office. 1968; numerator data from National Vital Statistics System, annual mortality files; denominator data from national population estimates for race groups from Table 1 and unpublished Hispanic population estimates for 1985–1996 prepared by the Housing and Household Economic Statistics Division, U.S. Census Bureau; additional mortality tables are available from: www.cdc.gov/nchs/datawh/statab/unpubd/mortabs.htm; Miniño AM, Heron M, Murphy SL, Kochanek KD. Deaths: Final data for 2004. Health E-Stats. Hyattsville, MD: National Center for Health Statistics. 2006.

This table will be updated on the Web. Go to www.cdc.gov/nchs/hus.htm.

Table 38 (page 1 of 4). Death rates for malignant neoplasms, by sex, race, Hispanic origin, and age: United States, selected years 1950–2004

[Data are based on death certificates]

Sex, race, Hispanic origin, and age	1950[1,2]	1960[1,2]	1970[2]	1980[2]	1990	2000[3]	2003	2004
	Deaths per 100,000 resident population							
All persons								
All ages, age-adjusted[4]	193.9	193.9	198.6	207.9	216.0	199.6	190.1	185.8
All ages, crude	139.8	149.2	162.8	183.9	203.2	196.5	191.5	188.6
Under 1 year	8.7	7.2	4.7	3.2	2.3	2.4	1.9	1.8
1–4 years	11.7	10.9	7.5	4.5	3.5	2.7	2.5	2.5
5–14 years	6.7	6.8	6.0	4.3	3.1	2.5	2.6	2.5
15–24 years	8.6	8.3	8.3	6.3	4.9	4.4	4.0	4.1
25–34 years	20.0	19.5	16.5	13.7	12.6	9.8	9.4	9.1
35–44 years	62.7	59.7	59.5	48.6	43.3	36.6	35.0	33.4
45–54 years	175.1	177.0	182.5	180.0	158.9	127.5	122.2	119.0
55–64 years	390.7	396.8	423.0	436.1	449.6	366.7	343.0	333.4
65–74 years	698.8	713.9	754.2	817.9	872.3	816.3	770.3	755.1
75–84 years	1,153.3	1,127.4	1,169.2	1,232.3	1,348.5	1,335.6	1,302.5	1,280.4
85 years and over	1,451.0	1,450.0	1,320.7	1,594.6	1,752.9	1,819.4	1,698.2	1,653.3
Male								
All ages, age-adjusted[4]	208.1	225.1	247.6	271.2	280.4	248.9	233.3	227.7
All ages, crude	142.9	162.5	182.1	205.3	221.3	207.2	201.3	198.4
Under 1 year	9.7	7.7	4.4	3.7	2.4	2.6	1.7	1.8
1–4 years	12.5	12.4	8.3	5.2	3.7	3.0	2.8	2.6
5–14 years	7.4	7.6	6.7	4.9	3.5	2.7	2.8	2.7
15–24 years	9.7	10.2	10.4	7.8	5.7	5.1	4.6	4.8
25–34 years	17.7	18.8	16.3	13.4	12.6	9.2	8.9	8.6
35–44 years	45.6	48.9	53.0	44.0	38.5	32.7	30.8	29.1
45–54 years	156.2	170.8	183.5	188.7	162.5	130.9	127.4	124.3
55–64 years	413.1	459.9	511.8	520.8	532.9	415.8	386.8	376.7
65–74 years	791.5	890.5	1,006.8	1,093.2	1,122.2	1,001.9	931.7	907.6
75–84 years	1,332.6	1,389.4	1,588.3	1,790.5	1,914.4	1,760.6	1,695.4	1,662.1
85 years and over	1,668.3	1,741.2	1,720.8	2,369.5	2,739.9	2,710.7	2,413.8	2,349.5
Female								
All ages, age-adjusted[4]	182.3	168.7	163.2	166.7	175.7	167.6	160.9	157.4
All ages, crude	136.8	136.4	144.4	163.6	186.0	186.2	182.0	179.1
Under 1 year	7.6	6.8	5.0	2.7	2.2	2.3	2.1	1.9
1–4 years	10.8	9.3	6.7	3.7	3.2	2.5	2.1	2.4
5–14 years	6.0	6.0	5.2	3.6	2.8	2.2	2.4	2.2
15–24 years	7.6	6.5	6.2	4.8	4.1	3.6	3.4	3.4
25–34 years	22.2	20.1	16.7	14.0	12.6	10.4	9.9	9.6
35–44 years	79.3	70.0	65.6	53.1	48.1	40.4	39.1	37.7
45–54 years	194.0	183.0	181.5	171.8	155.5	124.2	117.1	113.8
55–64 years	368.2	337.7	343.2	361.7	375.2	321.3	302.3	293.2
65–74 years	612.3	560.2	557.9	607.1	677.4	663.6	635.3	627.1
75–84 years	1,000.7	924.1	891.9	903.1	1,010.3	1,058.5	1,040.1	1,023.5
85 years and over	1,299.7	1,263.9	1,096.7	1,255.7	1,372.1	1,456.4	1,381.9	1,340.1
White male[5]								
All ages, age-adjusted[4]	210.0	224.7	244.8	265.1	272.2	243.9	230.1	224.4
All ages, crude	147.2	166.1	185.1	208.7	227.7	218.1	213.1	209.9
25–34 years	17.7	18.8	16.2	13.6	12.3	9.2	8.9	8.6
35–44 years	44.5	46.3	50.1	41.1	35.8	30.9	29.9	28.2
45–54 years	150.8	164.1	172.0	175.4	149.9	123.5	119.9	117.5
55–64 years	409.4	450.9	498.1	497.4	508.2	401.9	375.6	364.9
65–74 years	798.7	887.3	997.0	1,070.7	1,090.7	984.3	922.7	896.3
75–84 years	1,367.6	1,413.7	1,592.7	1,779.7	1,883.2	1,736.0	1,683.6	1,652.7
85 years and over	1,732.7	1,791.4	1,772.2	2,375.6	2,715.1	2,693.7	2,412.1	2,348.9
Black or African American male[5]								
All ages, age-adjusted[4]	178.9	227.6	291.9	353.4	397.9	340.3	308.8	301.2
All ages, crude	106.6	136.7	171.6	205.5	221.9	188.5	178.3	176.2
25–34 years	18.0	18.4	18.8	14.1	15.7	10.1	10.3	10.0
35–44 years	55.7	72.9	81.3	73.8	64.3	48.4	41.7	38.4
45–54 years	211.7	244.7	311.2	333.0	302.6	214.2	207.0	197.0
55–64 years	490.8	579.7	689.2	812.5	859.2	626.4	583.8	569.2
65–74 years	636.5	938.5	1,168.9	1,417.2	1,613.9	1,363.8	1,221.5	1,209.7
75–84 years[6]	853.5	1,053.3	1,624.8	2,029.6	2,478.3	2,351.8	2,144.2	2,087.2
85 years and over	- - -	1,155.2	1,387.0	2,393.9	3,238.3	3,264.8	2,825.5	2,748.8

See footnotes at end of table.

This table will be updated on the Web. Go to www.cdc.gov/nchs/hus.htm.

Table 38 (page 2 of 4). Death rates for malignant neoplasms, by sex, race, Hispanic origin, and age: United States, selected years 1950–2004

[Data are based on death certificates]

Sex, race, Hispanic origin, and age	1950[1,2]	1960[1,2]	1970[2]	1980[2]	1990	2000[3]	2003	2004
	Deaths per 100,000 resident population							
American Indian or Alaska Native male[5]								
All ages, age-adjusted[4]	- - -	- - -	- - -	140.5	145.8	155.8	139.9	147.1
All ages, crude	- - -	- - -	- - -	58.1	61.4	67.0	70.3	78.9
25–34 years	- - -	- - -	- - -	*	*	*	*	*
35–44 years	- - -	- - -	- - -	*	22.8	21.4	19.0	18.1
45–54 years	- - -	- - -	- - -	86.9	86.9	70.3	81.9	86.3
55–64 years	- - -	- - -	- - -	213.4	246.2	255.6	222.7	268.6
65–74 years	- - -	- - -	- - -	613.0	530.6	648.0	565.4	642.0
75–84 years	- - -	- - -	- - -	936.4	1,038.4	1,152.5	995.2	1,060.0
85 years and over	- - -	- - -	- - -	1,471.2	1,654.4	1,584.2	1,459.1	1,134.1
Asian or Pacific Islander male[5]								
All ages, age-adjusted[4]	- - -	- - -	- - -	165.2	172.5	150.8	137.2	136.3
All ages, crude	- - -	- - -	- - -	81.9	82.7	85.2	84.2	85.9
25–34 years	- - -	- - -	- - -	6.3	9.2	7.4	7.6	5.9
35–44 years	- - -	- - -	- - -	29.4	27.7	26.1	21.7	23.6
45–54 years	- - -	- - -	- - -	108.2	92.6	78.5	77.0	77.2
55–64 years	- - -	- - -	- - -	298.5	274.6	229.2	196.1	198.7
65–74 years	- - -	- - -	- - -	581.2	687.2	559.4	498.1	496.8
75–84 years	- - -	- - -	- - -	1,147.6	1,229.9	1,086.1	1,056.9	1,021.6
85 years and over	- - -	- - -	- - -	1,798.7	1,837.0	1,823.2	1,545.6	1,552.4
Hispanic or Latino male[5,7]								
All ages, age-adjusted[4]	- - -	- - -	- - -	- - -	174.7	171.7	156.5	151.2
All ages, crude	- - -	- - -	- - -	- - -	65.5	61.3	61.5	60.9
25–34 years	- - -	- - -	- - -	- - -	8.0	6.9	6.8	6.4
35–44 years	- - -	- - -	- - -	- - -	22.5	20.1	18.2	18.6
45–54 years	- - -	- - -	- - -	- - -	96.6	79.4	81.1	77.4
55–64 years	- - -	- - -	- - -	- - -	294.0	253.1	246.5	239.0
65–74 years	- - -	- - -	- - -	- - -	655.5	651.2	617.6	585.8
75–84 years	- - -	- - -	- - -	- - -	1,233.4	1,306.4	1,163.9	1,174.2
85 years and over	- - -	- - -	- - -	- - -	2,019.4	2,049.7	1,668.6	1,508.8
White, not Hispanic or Latino male[7]								
All ages, age-adjusted[4]	- - -	- - -	- - -	- - -	276.7	247.7	234.6	229.2
All ages, crude	- - -	- - -	- - -	- - -	246.2	244.4	241.8	239.2
25–34 years	- - -	- - -	- - -	- - -	12.8	9.7	9.4	9.3
35–44 years	- - -	- - -	- - -	- - -	36.8	32.3	31.9	29.9
45–54 years	- - -	- - -	- - -	- - -	153.9	127.2	123.8	121.9
55–64 years	- - -	- - -	- - -	- - -	520.6	412.0	384.8	374.6
65–74 years	- - -	- - -	- - -	- - -	1,109.0	1,002.1	942.0	917.5
75–84 years	- - -	- - -	- - -	- - -	1,906.6	1,750.2	1,707.8	1,677.3
85 years and over	- - -	- - -	- - -	- - -	2,744.4	2,714.1	2,441.7	2,387.1
White female[5]								
All ages, age-adjusted[4]	182.0	167.7	162.5	165.2	174.0	166.9	160.2	157.0
All ages, crude	139.9	139.8	149.4	170.3	196.1	199.4	194.6	191.7
25–34 years	20.9	18.8	16.3	13.5	11.9	10.1	9.4	9.0
35–44 years	74.5	66.6	62.4	50.9	46.2	38.2	37.3	35.8
45–54 years	185.8	175.7	177.3	166.4	150.9	120.1	112.1	109.2
55–64 years	362.5	329.0	338.6	355.5	368.5	319.7	299.8	290.8
65–74 years	616.5	562.1	554.7	605.2	675.1	665.6	638.9	630.8
75–84 years	1,026.6	939.3	903.5	905.4	1,011.8	1,063.4	1,046.3	1,033.1
85 years and over	1,348.3	1,304.9	1,126.6	1,266.8	1,372.3	1,459.1	1,386.5	1,348.9

See footnotes at end of table.

This table will be updated on the Web. Go to www.cdc.gov/nchs/hus.htm.

Table 38 (page 3 of 4). Death rates for malignant neoplasms, by sex, race, Hispanic origin, and age: United States, selected years 1950–2004

[Data are based on death certificates]

Sex, race, Hispanic origin, and age	1950[1,2]	1960[1,2]	1970[2]	1980[2]	1990	2000[3]	2003	2004
Black or African American female[5]				Deaths per 100,000 resident population				
All ages, age-adjusted[4]	174.1	174.3	173.4	189.5	205.9	193.8	187.7	182.5
All ages, crude	111.8	113.8	117.3	136.5	156.1	151.8	151.4	148.9
25–34 years	34.3	31.0	20.9	18.3	18.7	13.5	13.9	13.9
35–44 years	119.8	102.4	94.6	73.5	67.4	58.9	55.4	54.2
45–54 years	277.0	254.8	228.6	230.2	209.9	173.9	167.2	160.9
55–64 years	484.6	442.7	404.8	450.4	482.4	391.0	380.4	369.4
65–74 years	477.3	541.6	615.8	662.4	773.2	753.1	714.6	706.2
75–84 years[6]	605.3	696.3	763.3	923.9	1,059.9	1,124.0	1,116.9	1,083.6
85 years and over	- - -	728.9	791.5	1,159.9	1,431.3	1,527.7	1,475.3	1,387.7
American Indian or Alaska Native female[5]								
All ages, age-adjusted[4]	- - -	- - -	- - -	94.0	106.9	108.3	105.6	108.6
All ages, crude	- - -	- - -	- - -	50.4	62.1	61.3	68.2	73.0
25–34 years	- - -	- - -	- - -	*	*	*	*	*
35–44 years	- - -	- - -	- - -	36.9	31.0	23.7	24.3	27.4
45–54 years	- - -	- - -	- - -	96.9	104.5	59.7	75.7	72.0
55–64 years	- - -	- - -	- - -	198.4	213.3	200.9	195.8	211.8
65–74 years	- - -	- - -	- - -	350.8	438.9	458.3	411.2	480.7
75–84 years	- - -	- - -	- - -	446.4	554.3	714.0	784.4	707.3
85 years and over	- - -	- - -	- - -	786.5	843.7	983.2	686.0	724.6
Asian or Pacific Islander female[5]								
All ages, age-adjusted[4]	- - -	- - -	- - -	93.0	103.0	100.7	96.7	92.0
All ages, crude	- - -	- - -	- - -	54.1	60.5	72.1	75.6	73.8
25–34 years	- - -	- - -	- - -	9.5	7.3	8.1	7.2	6.6
35–44 years	- - -	- - -	- - -	38.7	29.8	28.9	25.8	24.2
45–54 years	- - -	- - -	- - -	99.8	93.9	78.2	77.6	77.0
55–64 years	- - -	- - -	- - -	174.7	196.2	176.5	166.7	159.1
65–74 years	- - -	- - -	- - -	301.9	346.2	357.4	361.5	344.2
75–84 years	- - -	- - -	- - -	522.1	641.4	650.1	616.9	578.4
85 years and over	- - -	- - -	- - -	800.0	971.7	988.5	907.9	872.9
Hispanic or Latino female[5,7]								
All ages, age-adjusted[4]	- - -	- - -	- - -	- - -	111.9	110.8	105.9	101.4
All ages, crude	- - -	- - -	- - -	- - -	60.7	58.5	59.1	57.7
25–34 years	- - -	- - -	- - -	- - -	9.7	7.8	7.4	7.5
35–44 years	- - -	- - -	- - -	- - -	34.8	30.7	28.0	25.4
45–54 years	- - -	- - -	- - -	- - -	100.5	84.7	80.2	73.5
55–64 years	- - -	- - -	- - -	- - -	205.4	192.5	185.9	183.0
65–74 years	- - -	- - -	- - -	- - -	404.8	410.0	379.7	380.7
75–84 years	- - -	- - -	- - -	- - -	663.0	716.5	702.1	663.6
85 years and over	- - -	- - -	- - -	- - -	1,022.7	1,056.5	1,014.8	937.0

See footnotes at end of table.

This table will be updated on the Web. Go to www.cdc.gov/nchs/hus.htm.

Table 38 (page 4 of 4). Death rates for malignant neoplasms, by sex, race, Hispanic origin, and age: United States, selected years 1950–2004

[Data are based on death certificates]

Sex, race, Hispanic origin, and age	1950[1,2]	1960[1,2]	1970[2]	1980[2]	1990	2000[3]	2003	2004
White, not Hispanic or Latino female[7]								
	Deaths per 100,000 resident population							
All ages, age-adjusted[4]	- - -	- - -	- - -	- - -	177.5	170.0	163.8	160.9
All ages, crude	- - -	- - -	- - -	- - -	210.6	220.6	217.6	215.3
25–34 years	- - -	- - -	- - -	- - -	11.9	10.5	9.3	9.3
35–44 years	- - -	- - -	- - -	- - -	47.0	38.9	38.6	37.5
45–54 years	- - -	- - -	- - -	- - -	154.9	123.0	115.1	112.9
55–64 years	- - -	- - -	- - -	- - -	379.5	328.9	308.9	299.8
65–74 years	- - -	- - -	- - -	- - -	688.5	681.0	657.6	649.8
75–84 years	- - -	- - -	- - -	- - -	1,027.2	1,075.3	1,062.4	1,052.0
85 years and over	- - -	- - -	- - -	- - -	1,385.7	1,468.7	1,399.1	1,364.5

- - - Data not available.

* Rates based on fewer than 20 deaths are considered unreliable and are not shown.

[1]Includes deaths of persons who were not residents of the 50 states and the District of Columbia.

[2]Underlying cause of death was coded according to the Sixth Revision of the International Classification of Diseases (ICD) in 1950, Seventh Revision in 1960, Eighth Revision in 1970, and Ninth Revision in 1980–1998. See Appendix II, Cause of death; Tables IV and V.

[3]Starting with 1999 data, cause of death is coded according to ICD–10. See Appendix II, Cause of death, Table V; Comparability ratio, Table VI.

[4]Age-adjusted rates are calculated using the year 2000 standard population. Prior to 2003, age-adjusted rates were calculated using standard million proportions based on rounded population numbers. Starting with 2003 data, unrounded population numbers are used to calculate age-adjusted rates. See Appendix II, Age adjustment.

[5]The race groups, white, black, Asian or Pacific Islander, and American Indian or Alaska Native, include persons of Hispanic and non-Hispanic origin. Persons of Hispanic origin may be of any race. Death rates for the American Indian or Alaska Native and Asian or Pacific Islander populations are known to be underestimated. See Appendix II, Race, for a discussion of sources of bias in death rates by race and Hispanic origin.

[6]In 1950, rate is for the age group 75 years and over.

[7]Prior to 1997, excludes data from states lacking an Hispanic-origin item on the death certificate. See Appendix II, Hispanic origin.

NOTES: Starting with *Health, United States, 2003*, rates for 1991–1999 were revised using intercensal population estimates based on the 2000 census. Rates for 2000 were revised based on 2000 census counts. Rates for 2001 and later years were computed using 2000-based postcensal estimates. See Appendix I, Population Census and Population Estimates. See Appendix II, Cause of death; Tables IV and V. Age groups were selected to minimize the presentation of unstable age-specific death rates based on small numbers of deaths and for consistency among comparison groups. In 2003, seven states reported multiple-race data. In 2004, 15 states reported multiple-race data. The multiple-race data for these states were bridged to the single-race categories of the 1977 Office of Management and Budget standards for comparability with other states. See Appendix II, Race. Data for additional years are available. See Appendix III.

SOURCES: Centers for Disease Control and Prevention, National Center for Health Statistics, National Vital Statistics System; Grove RD, Hetzel AM. Vital statistics rates in the United States, 1940–1960. Washington, DC: U.S. Government Printing Office. 1968; numerator data from National Vital Statistics System, annual mortality files; denominator data from national population estimates for race groups from Table 1 and unpublished Hispanic population estimates for 1985–1996 prepared by the Housing and Household Economic Statistics Division, U.S. Census Bureau; additional mortality tables are available from: www.cdc.gov/nchs/datawh/statab/unpubd/mortabs.htm; Miniño AM, Heron M, Murphy SL, Kochanek KD. Deaths: Final data for 2004. Health E-Stats. Hyattsville, MD: National Center for Health Statistics. 2006.

This table will be updated on the Web. Go to www.cdc.gov/nchs/hus.htm.

Table 39 (page 1 of 3). Death rates for malignant neoplasms of trachea, bronchus, and lung, by sex, race, Hispanic origin, and age: United States, selected years 1950–2004

[Data are based on death certificates]

Sex, race, Hispanic origin, and age	*1950[1,2]*	*1960[1,2]*	*1970[2]*	*1980[2]*	*1990*	*2000[3]*	*2003*	*2004*
	Deaths per 100,000 resident population							
All persons								
All ages, age-adjusted[4]	15.0	24.1	37.1	49.9	59.3	56.1	54.1	53.2
All ages, crude	12.2	20.3	32.1	45.8	56.8	55.3	54.4	53.8
Under 25 years	0.1	0.0	0.1	0.0	0.0	0.0	0.0	0.0
25–34 years	0.8	1.0	0.9	0.6	0.7	0.5	0.4	0.4
35–44 years	4.5	6.8	11.0	9.2	6.8	6.1	5.6	5.5
45–54 years	20.4	29.6	43.4	54.1	46.8	31.6	30.3	29.9
55–64 years	48.7	75.3	109.1	138.2	160.6	122.4	111.0	106.9
65–74 years	59.7	108.1	164.5	233.3	288.4	284.2	269.3	265.5
75–84 years	55.8	91.5	163.2	240.5	333.3	370.8	377.8	373.6
85 years and over	42.3	65.6	101.7	176.0	242.5	302.1	298.9	297.5
Male								
All ages, age-adjusted[4]	24.6	43.6	67.5	85.2	91.1	76.7	71.7	70.1
All ages, crude	19.9	35.4	53.4	68.6	75.1	65.5	62.9	62.0
Under 25 years	0.0	0.0	0.1	0.1	0.0	*	*	*
25–34 years	1.1	1.4	1.3	0.8	0.9	0.5	0.4	0.4
35–44 years	7.1	10.5	16.1	11.9	8.5	6.9	6.1	5.8
45–54 years	35.0	50.6	67.5	76.0	59.7	38.5	36.5	35.8
55–64 years	83.8	139.3	189.7	213.6	222.9	154.0	136.7	131.7
65–74 years	98.7	204.3	320.8	403.9	430.4	377.9	346.6	337.6
75–84 years	82.6	167.1	330.8	488.8	572.9	532.2	525.1	517.3
85 years and over	62.5	107.7	194.0	368.1	513.2	521.2	475.1	466.8
Female								
All ages, age-adjusted[4]	5.8	7.5	13.1	24.4	37.1	41.3	41.3	40.9
All ages, crude	4.5	6.4	11.9	24.3	39.4	45.4	46.1	45.9
Under 25 years	0.1	0.0	0.0	*	*	*	*	*
25–34 years	0.5	0.5	0.5	0.5	0.5	0.5	0.4	0.3
35–44 years	1.9	3.2	6.1	6.5	5.2	5.3	5.1	5.2
45–54 years	5.8	9.2	21.0	33.7	34.5	25.0	24.4	24.2
55–64 years	13.6	15.4	36.8	72.0	105.0	93.3	87.1	83.9
65–74 years	23.3	24.4	43.1	102.7	177.6	206.9	204.8	205.0
75–84 years	32.9	32.8	52.4	94.1	190.1	265.6	279.4	277.0
85 years and over	28.2	38.8	50.0	91.9	138.1	212.8	221.0	221.3
White male[5]								
All ages, age-adjusted[4]	25.1	43.6	67.1	83.8	89.0	75.7	71.1	69.4
All ages, crude	20.8	36.4	54.6	70.2	77.8	69.4	66.9	65.9
45–54 years	35.1	49.2	63.3	70.9	55.2	35.7	34.1	33.3
55–64 years	85.4	139.2	186.8	205.6	213.7	150.8	133.1	127.6
65–74 years	101.5	207.5	325.0	401.0	422.1	374.9	347.1	338.1
75–84 years	85.5	170.4	336.7	493.5	572.2	529.9	524.6	517.5
85 years and over	67.4	109.4	199.6	374.1	516.3	522.4	478.5	472.2
Black or African American male[5]								
All ages, age-adjusted[4]	17.8	42.6	75.4	107.6	125.4	101.1	92.4	90.0
All ages, crude	12.1	28.1	47.7	66.6	73.7	58.3	54.9	54.3
45–54 years	34.4	68.4	115.4	133.8	114.9	70.7	63.6	62.5
55–64 years	68.3	146.8	234.3	321.1	358.6	223.5	210.0	206.9
65–74 years	53.8	168.3	300.5	472.3	585.4	488.8	427.1	410.4
75–84 years[6]	36.2	107.3	271.6	472.9	645.4	642.5	622.2	611.1
85 years and over	- - -	82.8	137.0	311.3	499.5	562.8	502.5	481.8
American Indian or Alaska Native male[5]								
All ages, age-adjusted[4]	- - -	- - -	- - -	31.7	47.5	42.9	37.6	44.1
All ages, crude	- - -	- - -	- - -	14.2	20.0	18.1	19.4	23.7
45–54 years	- - -	- - -	- - -	*	26.6	14.5	17.1	19.8
55–64 years	- - -	- - -	- - -	72.0	97.8	86.0	79.2	88.1
65–74 years	- - -	- - -	- - -	202.8	194.3	184.8	186.0	236.7
75–84 years	- - -	- - -	- - -	*	356.2	367.9	284.9	320.0
85 years and over	- - -	- - -	- - -	*	*	*	*	*

See footnotes at end of table.

This table will be updated on the Web. Go to www.cdc.gov/nchs/hus.htm.

Table 39 (page 2 of 3). Death rates for malignant neoplasms of trachea, bronchus, and lung, by sex, race, Hispanic origin, and age: United States, selected years 1950–2004

[Data are based on death certificates]

Sex, race, Hispanic origin, and age	1950[1,2]	1960[1,2]	1970[2]	1980[2]	1990	2000[3]	2003	2004
	Deaths per 100,000 resident population							
Asian or Pacific Islander male[5]								
All ages, age-adjusted[4]	---	---	---	43.3	44.2	40.9	37.9	37.1
All ages, crude	---	---	---	22.1	20.7	22.7	22.7	23.1
45–54 years	---	---	---	33.3	18.8	17.2	17.5	17.3
55–64 years	---	---	---	94.4	74.4	61.4	50.4	51.1
65–74 years	---	---	---	174.3	215.8	183.2	157.5	166.2
75–84 years	---	---	---	301.3	307.5	323.2	333.3	313.1
85 years and over	---	---	---	*	421.3	378.0	328.4	289.2
Hispanic or Latino male[5,7]								
All ages, age-adjusted[4]	---	---	---	---	44.1	39.0	34.5	33.4
All ages, crude	---	---	---	---	16.2	13.3	12.8	12.7
45–54 years	---	---	---	---	21.5	14.8	12.6	12.6
55–64 years	---	---	---	---	80.7	58.6	55.4	50.0
65–74 years	---	---	---	---	195.5	167.3	161.8	151.7
75–84 years	---	---	---	---	313.4	327.5	277.3	279.7
85 years and over	---	---	---	---	420.7	368.8	290.9	287.2
White, not Hispanic or Latino male[7]								
All ages, age-adjusted[4]	---	---	---	---	91.1	77.9	73.6	72.1
All ages, crude	---	---	---	---	84.7	78.9	77.3	76.5
45–54 years	---	---	---	---	57.8	37.7	36.5	35.8
55–64 years	---	---	---	---	221.0	157.7	139.4	134.2
65–74 years	---	---	---	---	431.4	387.3	359.6	351.4
75–84 years	---	---	---	---	580.4	537.7	537.0	530.6
85 years and over	---	---	---	---	520.9	527.3	486.8	480.3
White female[5]								
All ages, age-adjusted[4]	5.9	6.8	13.1	24.5	37.6	42.3	42.3	41.9
All ages, crude	4.7	5.9	12.3	25.6	42.4	49.9	50.7	50.4
45–54 years	5.7	9.0	20.9	33.0	34.6	24.8	23.8	24.1
55–64 years	13.7	15.1	37.2	71.9	105.7	96.1	89.8	86.1
65–74 years	23.7	24.8	42.9	104.6	181.3	213.2	212.2	212.5
75–84 years	34.0	32.7	52.6	95.2	194.6	272.7	286.6	283.8
85 years and over	29.3	39.1	50.6	92.4	138.3	215.9	224.4	225.3
Black or African American female[5]								
All ages, age-adjusted[4]	4.5	6.8	13.7	24.8	36.8	39.8	40.2	39.9
All ages, crude	2.8	4.3	9.4	18.3	28.1	30.8	32.0	32.1
45–54 years	7.5	11.3	23.9	43.4	41.3	32.9	33.4	30.7
55–64 years	12.9	17.9	33.5	79.9	117.9	95.3	91.0	89.0
65–74 years	14.0	18.1	46.1	88.0	164.3	194.1	190.0	186.2
75–84 years[6]	*	31.3	49.1	79.4	148.1	224.3	248.0	256.3
85 years and over	---	34.2	44.8	85.8	134.9	185.9	194.8	196.5
American Indian or Alaska Native female[5]								
All ages, age-adjusted[4]	---	---	---	11.7	19.3	24.8	26.4	29.7
All ages, crude	---	---	---	6.0	11.2	14.0	16.4	19.3
45–54 years	---	---	---	*	22.9	12.1	15.1	13.2
55–64 years	---	---	---	*	53.7	52.6	42.5	54.8
65–74 years	---	---	---	*	78.5	151.5	147.8	186.4
75–84 years	---	---	---	*	111.8	136.3	190.1	181.1
85 years and over	---	---	---	*	*	*	*	144.9

See footnotes at end of table.

This table will be updated on the Web. Go to www.cdc.gov/nchs/hus.htm.

Table 39 (page 3 of 3). Death rates for malignant neoplasms of trachea, bronchus, and lung, by sex, race, Hispanic origin, and age: United States, selected years 1950–2004

[Data are based on death certificates]

Sex, race, Hispanic origin, and age	1950[1,2]	1960[1,2]	1970[2]	1980[2]	1990	2000[3]	2003	2004
Asian or Pacific Islander female[5]	Deaths per 100,000 resident population							
All ages, age-adjusted[4]	- - -	- - -	- - -	15.4	18.9	18.4	18.7	18.0
All ages, crude	- - -	- - -	- - -	8.4	10.5	12.6	14.1	14.1
45–54 years	- - -	- - -	- - -	13.5	11.3	9.9	11.4	11.1
55–64 years	- - -	- - -	- - -	24.6	38.3	30.4	28.0	29.2
65–74 years	- - -	- - -	- - -	62.4	71.6	77.0	76.3	84.7
75–84 years	- - -	- - -	- - -	117.7	137.9	135.0	142.6	130.1
85 years and over	- - -	- - -	- - -	*	172.9	175.3	180.6	145.7
Hispanic or Latino female[5,7]								
All ages, age-adjusted[4]	- - -	- - -	- - -	- - -	14.1	14.7	14.8	14.3
All ages, crude	- - -	- - -	- - -	- - -	7.2	7.2	7.8	7.6
45–54 years	- - -	- - -	- - -	- - -	8.7	7.1	7.9	6.2
55–64 years	- - -	- - -	- - -	- - -	25.1	22.2	22.4	22.1
65–74 years	- - -	- - -	- - -	- - -	66.8	66.0	61.2	63.1
75–84 years	- - -	- - -	- - -	- - -	94.3	112.3	119.6	108.9
85 years and over	- - -	- - -	- - -	- - -	118.2	137.5	137.5	144.8
White, not Hispanic or Latino female[7]								
All ages, age-adjusted[4]	- - -	- - -	- - -	- - -	39.0	44.1	44.3	44.1
All ages, crude	- - -	- - -	- - -	- - -	46.2	56.4	58.1	58.1
45–54 years	- - -	- - -	- - -	- - -	36.6	26.4	25.6	26.2
55–64 years	- - -	- - -	- - -	- - -	111.3	102.2	95.7	92.0
65–74 years	- - -	- - -	- - -	- - -	186.4	222.9	223.9	224.6
75–84 years	- - -	- - -	- - -	- - -	199.1	279.2	295.1	293.5
85 years and over	- - -	- - -	- - -	- - -	139.0	218.0	227.4	228.4

0.0 Quantity more than zero but less than 0.05.
* Rates based on fewer than 20 deaths are considered unreliable and are not shown.
- - - Data not available.
[1]Includes deaths of persons who were not residents of the 50 states and the District of Columbia.
[2]Underlying cause of death was coded according to the Sixth Revision of the International Classification of Diseases (ICD) in 1950, Seventh Revision in 1960, Eighth Revision in 1970, and Ninth Revision in 1980–1998. See Appendix II, Cause of death; Tables IV and V.
[3]Starting with 1999 data, cause of death is coded according to ICD–10. See Appendix II, Cause of death, Table V; Comparability ratio, Table VI.
[4]Age-adjusted rates are calculated using the year 2000 standard population. Prior to 2003, age-adjusted rates were calculated using standard million proportions based on rounded population numbers. Starting with 2003 data, unrounded population numbers are used to calculate age-adjusted rates. See Appendix II, Age adjustment.
[5]The race groups, white, black, Asian or Pacific Islander, and American Indian or Alaska Native, include persons of Hispanic and non-Hispanic origin. Persons of Hispanic origin may be of any race. Death rates for the American Indian or Alaska Native and Asian or Pacific Islander populations are known to be underestimated. See Appendix II, Race, for a discussion of sources of bias in death rates by race and Hispanic origin.
[6]In 1950, rate is for the age group 75 years and over.
[7]Prior to 1997, excludes data from states lacking an Hispanic-origin item on the death certificate. See Appendix II, Hispanic origin.

NOTES: Starting with *Health, United States, 2003*, rates for 1991–1999 were revised using intercensal population estimates based on the 2000 census. Rates for 2000 were revised based on 2000 census counts. Rates for 2001 and later years were computed using 2000-based postcensal estimates. See Appendix I, Population Census and Population Estimates. For the period 1980–1998, lung cancer was coded using ICD–9 codes that are most comparable with lung cancer codes in the 113 cause list for ICD–10. See Appendix II, Cause of death; Table V. Age groups were selected to minimize the presentation of unstable age-specific death rates based on small numbers of deaths and for consistency among comparison groups. In 2003, seven states reported multiple-race data. In 2004, 15 states reported multiple-race data. The multiple-race data for these states were bridged to the single-race categories of the 1977 Office of Management and Budget standards for comparability with other states. See Appendix II, Race. Data for additional years are available. See Appendix III.

SOURCES: Centers for Disease Control and Prevention, National Center for Health Statistics, National Vital Statistics System; Grove RD, Hetzel AM. Vital statistics rates in the United States, 1940–1960. Washington, DC: U.S. Government Printing Office. 1968; numerator data from National Vital Statistics System, annual mortality files; denominator data from national population estimates for race groups from Table 1 and unpublished Hispanic population estimates for 1985–1996 prepared by the Housing and Household Economic Statistics Division, U.S. Census Bureau; additional mortality tables are available from: www.cdc.gov/nchs/datawh/statab/unpubd/mortabs.htm; Miniño AM, Heron M, Murphy SL, Kochanek KD. Deaths: Final data for 2004. Health E-Stats. Hyattsville, MD: National Center for Health Statistics. 2006.

This table will be updated on the Web. Go to www.cdc.gov/nchs/hus.htm.

Table 40 (page 1 of 2). Death rates for malignant neoplasm of breast among females, by race, Hispanic origin, and age: United States, selected years 1950–2004

[Data are based on death certificates]

Race, Hispanic origin, and age	1950[1,2]	1960[1,2]	1970[2]	1980[2]	1990	2000[3]	2003	2004
	Deaths per 100,000 resident population							
All females								
All ages, age-adjusted[4]	31.9	31.7	32.1	31.9	33.3	26.8	25.3	24.4
All ages, crude	24.7	26.1	28.4	30.6	34.0	29.2	28.2	27.5
Under 25 years	*	*	*	*	*	*	*	*
25–34 years	3.8	3.8	3.9	3.3	2.9	2.3	2.1	2.0
35–44 years	20.8	20.2	20.4	17.9	17.8	12.4	12.2	11.3
45–54 years	46.9	51.4	52.6	48.1	45.4	33.0	30.4	29.3
55–64 years	69.9	70.8	77.6	80.5	78.6	59.3	56.6	55.8
65–74 years	95.0	90.0	93.8	101.1	111.7	88.3	82.6	81.6
75–84 years	139.8	129.9	127.4	126.4	146.3	128.9	123.7	119.5
85 years and over	195.5	191.9	157.1	169.3	196.8	205.7	189.4	178.6
White[5]								
All ages, age-adjusted[4]	32.4	32.0	32.5	32.1	33.2	26.3	24.7	23.9
All ages, crude	25.7	27.2	29.9	32.3	35.9	30.7	29.3	28.6
35–44 years	20.8	19.7	20.2	17.3	17.1	11.3	11.1	10.1
45–54 years	47.1	51.2	53.0	48.1	44.3	31.2	28.4	27.0
55–64 years	70.9	71.8	79.3	81.3	78.5	57.9	54.9	54.3
65–74 years	96.3	91.6	95.9	103.7	113.3	89.3	82.6	82.2
75–84 years	143.6	132.8	129.6	128.4	148.2	130.2	124.6	121.3
85 years and over	204.2	199.7	161.9	171.7	198.0	205.5	189.4	179.7
Black or African American[5]								
All ages, age-adjusted[4]	25.3	27.9	28.9	31.7	38.1	34.5	34.0	32.2
All ages, crude	16.4	18.7	19.7	22.9	29.0	27.9	28.5	27.5
35–44 years	21.0	24.8	24.4	24.1	25.8	20.9	20.8	20.5
45–54 years	46.5	54.4	52.0	52.7	60.5	51.5	48.9	48.0
55–64 years	64.3	63.2	64.7	79.9	93.1	80.9	81.1	78.2
65–74 years	67.0	72.3	77.3	84.3	112.2	98.6	100.1	95.1
75–84 years[6]	81.0	87.5	101.8	114.1	140.5	139.8	141.0	127.4
85 years and over	---	92.1	112.1	149.9	201.5	238.7	222.4	196.9
American Indian or Alaska Native[5]								
All ages, age-adjusted[4]	---	---	---	10.8	13.7	13.6	14.0	14.8
All ages, crude	---	---	---	6.1	8.6	8.7	9.4	10.7
35–44 years	---	---	---	*	*	*	*	*
45–54 years	---	---	---	*	23.9	14.4	14.1	20.6
55–64 years	---	---	---	*	*	40.0	31.2	31.9
65–74 years	---	---	---	*	*	42.5	38.5	43.1
75–84 years	---	---	---	*	*	71.8	96.5	83.4
85 years and over	---	---	---	*	*	*	*	*
Asian or Pacific Islander[5]								
All ages, age-adjusted[4]	---	---	---	11.9	13.7	12.3	12.6	12.7
All ages, crude	---	---	---	8.2	9.3	10.2	11.0	11.2
35–44 years	---	---	---	10.4	8.4	8.1	7.6	7.4
45–54 years	---	---	---	23.4	26.4	22.3	20.1	21.4
55–64 years	---	---	---	35.7	33.8	31.3	33.8	32.7
65–74 years	---	---	---	*	38.5	34.7	40.7	38.4
75–84 years	---	---	---	*	48.0	37.5	41.4	41.8
85 years and over	---	---	---	*	*	68.2	64.7	74.4
Hispanic or Latino[5,7]								
All ages, age-adjusted[4]	---	---	---	---	19.5	16.9	16.1	15.6
All ages, crude	---	---	---	---	11.5	9.7	9.8	9.6
35–44 years	---	---	---	---	11.7	8.7	9.1	7.7
45–54 years	---	---	---	---	32.8	23.9	21.0	19.5
55–64 years	---	---	---	---	45.8	39.1	38.8	38.2
65–74 years	---	---	---	---	64.8	54.9	48.4	52.1
75–84 years	---	---	---	---	67.2	74.9	70.8	69.1
85 years and over	---	---	---	---	102.8	105.8	114.8	108.8

See footnotes at end of table.

This table will be updated on the Web. Go to www.cdc.gov/nchs/hus.htm.

Table 40 (page 2 of 2). Death rates for malignant neoplasm of breast among females, by race, Hispanic origin, and age: United States, selected years 1950–2004

[Data are based on death certificates]

Race, Hispanic origin, and age	1950[1,2]	1960[1,2]	1970[2]	1980[2]	1990	2000[3]	2003	2004
White, not Hispanic or Latino[7]				Deaths per 100,000 resident population				
All ages, age-adjusted[4]	- - -	- - -	- - -	- - -	33.9	26.8	25.2	24.5
All ages, crude	- - -	- - -	- - -	- - -	38.5	33.8	32.6	32.0
35–44 years	- - -	- - -	- - -	- - -	17.5	11.6	11.3	10.4
45–54 years	- - -	- - -	- - -	- - -	45.2	31.7	29.1	27.7
55–64 years	- - -	- - -	- - -	- - -	80.6	59.2	56.0	55.6
65–74 years	- - -	- - -	- - -	- - -	115.7	91.4	85.1	84.4
75–84 years	- - -	- - -	- - -	- - -	151.4	132.2	127.1	124.2
85 years and over	- - -	- - -	- - -	- - -	201.5	208.3	192.3	182.4

* Rates based on fewer than 20 deaths are considered unreliable and are not shown.
0.0 Quantity more than zero but less than 0.05.
- - - Data not available.
[1]Includes deaths of persons who were not residents of the 50 states and the District of Columbia.
[2]Underlying cause of death was coded according to the Sixth Revision of the International Classification of Diseases (ICD) in 1950, Seventh Revision in 1960, Eighth Revision in 1970, and Ninth Revision in 1980–1998. See Appendix II, Cause of death; Tables IV and V.
[3]Starting with 1999 data, cause of death is coded according to ICD–10. See Appendix II, Cause of death, Table V; Comparability ratio, Table VI.
[4]Age-adjusted rates are calculated using the year 2000 standard population. Prior to 2003, age-adjusted rates were calculated using standard million proportions based on rounded population numbers. Starting with 2003 data, unrounded population numbers are used to calculate age-adjusted rates. See Appendix II, Age adjustment.
[5]The race groups, white, black, Asian or Pacific Islander, and American Indian or Alaska Native, include persons of Hispanic and non-Hispanic origin. Persons of Hispanic origin may be of any race. Death rates for the American Indian or Alaska Native and Asian or Pacific Islander populations are known to be underestimated. See Appendix II, Race, for a discussion of sources of bias in death rates by race and Hispanic origin.
[6]In 1950, rate is for the age group 75 years and over.
[7]Prior to 1997, excludes data from states lacking an Hispanic-origin item on the death certificate. See Appendix II, Hispanic origin.

NOTES: Starting with *Health, United States, 2003*, rates for 1991–1999 were revised using intercensal population estimates based on the 2000 census. Rates for 2000 were revised based on 2000 census counts. Rates for 2001 and 2002 were computed using 2000-based postcensal estimates. See Appendix I, Population Census and Population Estimates. Age groups were selected to minimize the presentation of unstable age-specific death rates based on small numbers of deaths and for consistency among comparison groups. In 2003, seven states reported multiple-race data. In 2004, 15 states reported multiple-race data. The multiple-race data for these states were bridged to the single-race categories of the 1977 Office of Management and Budget standards for comparability with other states. See Appendix II, Race. Data for additional years are available. See Appendix III.

SOURCES: Centers for Disease Control and Prevention, National Center for Health Statistics, National Vital Statistics System; numerator data from annual mortality files; denominator data from national population estimates for race groups from Table 1 and unpublished Hispanic population estimates for 1985–1996 prepared by the Housing and Household Economic Statistics Division, U.S. Census Bureau; additional mortality tables are available from: www.cdc.gov/nchs/datawh/statab/unpubd/mortabs.htm; Miniño AM, Heron M, Murphy SL, Kochanek KD. Deaths: Final data for 2004. Health E-Stats. Hyattsville, MD: National Center for Health Statistics. 2006.

This table will be updated on the Web. Go to www.cdc.gov/nchs/hus.htm.

Table 41 (page 1 of 3). Death rates for chronic lower respiratory diseases, by sex, race, Hispanic origin, and age: United States, selected years 1980–2004

[Data are based on death certificates]

Sex, race, Hispanic origin, and age	*1980*[1]	*1990*	*1995*	*2000*[2]	*2002*	*2003*	*2004*
			Deaths per 100,000 resident population				
All persons							
All ages, age-adjusted[3]	28.3	37.2	40.1	44.2	43.5	43.3	41.1
All ages, crude	24.7	34.9	38.6	43.4	43.3	43.5	41.5
Under 1 year.	1.6	1.4	1.1	0.9	1.0	0.8	0.9
1–4 years	0.4	0.4	0.2	0.3	0.4	0.3	0.3
5–14 years	0.2	0.3	0.4	0.3	0.3	0.3	0.3
15–24 years	0.3	0.5	0.7	0.5	0.5	0.5	0.4
25–34 years	0.5	0.7	0.9	0.7	0.8	0.7	0.6
35–44 years	1.6	1.6	1.9	2.1	2.2	2.1	2.0
45–54 years	9.8	9.1	8.7	8.6	8.7	8.7	8.4
55–64 years	42.7	48.9	46.8	44.2	42.4	43.3	40.4
65–74 years	129.1	152.5	159.6	169.4	163.0	163.2	153.8
75–84 years	224.4	321.1	349.3	386.1	386.7	383.0	366.7
85 years and over	274.0	433.3	520.1	648.6	637.6	635.1	601.7
Male							
All ages, age-adjusted[3]	49.9	55.5	54.8	55.8	53.5	52.3	49.5
All ages, crude	35.1	40.8	41.4	43.5	42.9	42.4	40.6
Under 1 year.	1.9	1.6	1.4	1.2	1.1	1.1	1.2
1–4 years	0.5	0.5	0.2	0.4	0.6	0.5	0.4
5–14 years	0.2	0.4	0.5	0.4	0.4	0.4	0.4
15–24 years	0.4	0.5	0.7	0.6	0.6	0.5	0.5
25–34 years	0.6	0.7	0.9	0.8	0.8	0.8	0.7
35–44 years	1.7	1.7	1.7	1.9	2.2	1.9	2.0
45–54 years	12.1	9.4	8.8	9.0	9.1	9.1	8.8
55–64 years	59.9	58.6	52.3	47.8	45.2	46.5	43.1
65–74 years	210.0	204.0	195.6	195.2	184.8	183.6	172.1
75–84 years	437.4	500.0	483.8	488.5	480.8	464.9	445.6
85 years and over	583.4	815.1	889.8	967.9	894.8	865.9	811.1
Female							
All ages, age-adjusted[3]	14.9	26.6	31.8	37.4	37.4	37.8	36.0
All ages, crude	15.0	29.2	36.0	43.2	43.7	44.4	42.5
Under 1 year.	1.3	1.2	*	*	*	*	*
1–4 years	*	*	*	0.3	0.3	*	*
5–14 years	0.3	0.3	0.2	0.3	0.3	0.2	0.2
15–24 years	0.3	0.5	0.6	0.4	0.4	0.4	0.3
25–34 years	0.5	0.7	0.9	0.7	0.7	0.6	0.5
35–44 years	1.5	1.5	2.2	2.2	2.3	2.3	2.1
45–54 years	7.7	8.8	8.7	8.3	8.2	8.2	8.1
55–64 years	27.6	40.3	41.9	41.0	39.8	40.3	38.0
65–74 years	67.1	112.3	130.8	148.2	144.9	146.0	138.4
75–84 years	98.7	214.2	265.3	319.2	324.1	328.3	313.6
85 years and over	138.7	286.0	377.7	518.5	526.0	533.0	507.4
White male[4]							
All ages, age-adjusted[3]	51.6	56.6	55.9	57.2	54.9	53.8	51.1
All ages, crude	37.9	44.3	45.5	48.3	47.8	47.4	45.5
35–44 years	1.2	1.3	1.4	1.6	1.8	1.7	1.7
45–54 years	11.4	8.6	8.1	8.4	8.8	8.9	8.5
55–64 years	60.0	58.7	52.7	48.6	46.0	47.6	43.8
65–74 years	218.4	208.1	200.0	201.4	192.3	191.6	180.6
75–84 years	459.8	513.5	497.9	503.6	495.2	478.5	462.4
85 years and over	611.2	847.0	918.3	997.4	923.4	894.4	837.7
Black or African American male[4]							
All ages, age-adjusted[3]	34.0	47.6	47.4	47.5	46.3	44.4	40.9
All ages, crude	19.3	25.2	24.4	24.3	24.1	23.3	22.0
35–44 years	5.8	5.3	4.3	4.8	5.7	4.0	4.0
45–54 years	19.7	18.8	16.9	15.0	14.4	13.3	13.9
55–64 years	66.6	67.4	60.5	54.6	52.3	50.5	50.1
65–74 years	142.0	184.5	178.7	176.9	158.0	155.1	140.4
75–84 years	229.8	390.9	370.0	370.3	392.2	382.2	336.3
85 years and over	271.6	498.0	624.1	693.1	645.4	601.6	566.3

See footnotes at end of table.

This table will be updated on the Web. Go to www.cdc.gov/nchs/hus.htm.

Table 41 (page 2 of 3). Death rates for chronic lower respiratory diseases, by sex, race, Hispanic origin, and age: United States, selected years 1980–2004

[Data are based on death certificates]

Sex, race, Hispanic origin, and age	*1980[1]*	*1990*	*1995*	*2000[2]*	*2002*	*2003*	*2004*
American Indian or Alaska Native male[4]				Deaths per 100,000 resident population			
All ages, age-adjusted[3]	23.0	38.3	35.6	43.7	35.9	40.3	32.2
All ages, crude	8.4	13.8	12.3	15.3	14.3	17.3	14.9
35–44 years	*	*	*	*	*	*	*
45–54 years	*	*	*	*	*	*	*
55–64 years	*	*	36.5	46.4	34.5	43.8	40.5
65–74 years	*	135.7	132.1	111.3	126.1	125.9	121.9
75–84 years	*	363.8	307.3	416.6	348.9	387.0	300.0
85 years and over	*	*	*	770.7	500.3	563.8	362.9
Asian or Pacific Islander male[4]							
All ages, age-adjusted[3]	21.5	29.8	28.9	28.3	25.0	25.2	22.6
All ages, crude	8.7	11.3	11.8	12.6	12.0	12.5	11.2
35–44 years	*	*	*	*	*	*	*
45–54 years	*	*	*	4.8	2.6	*	*
55–64 years	*	22.1	15.7	8.8	11.5	12.7	9.6
65–74 years	70.6	91.4	87.9	71.3	58.5	58.4	46.8
75–84 years	155.7	258.6	240.6	254.3	235.9	234.9	199.8
85 years and over	472.4	615.2	650.4	670.7	582.5	590.7	596.1
Hispanic or Latino male[4,5]							
All ages, age-adjusted[3]	- - -	28.6	31.8	28.8	27.2	27.1	23.8
All ages, crude	- - -	8.4	8.9	8.0	8.1	8.2	7.6
35–44 years	- - -	*	1.1	0.9	1.0	1.0	1.4
45–54 years	- - -	4.1	3.9	3.4	3.8	3.2	2.8
55–64 years	- - -	17.2	19.1	18.2	17.5	16.6	13.7
65–74 years	- - -	81.0	82.4	72.4	69.2	68.1	68.4
75–84 years	- - -	252.4	292.0	250.3	243.3	231.2	206.4
85 years and over	- - -	613.9	689.0	671.1	602.4	646.5	518.4
White, not Hispanic or Latino male[5]							
All ages, age-adjusted[3]	- - -	57.9	56.6	58.5	56.5	55.4	52.8
All ages, crude	- - -	48.5	50.2	55.1	55.1	54.9	53.0
35–44 years	- - -	1.4	1.4	1.7	2.0	1.8	1.8
45–54 years	- - -	9.0	8.4	8.9	9.3	9.5	9.2
55–64 years	- - -	61.3	54.6	50.8	48.3	50.0	46.3
65–74 years	- - -	213.4	204.3	208.8	200.4	200.2	188.5
75–84 years	- - -	523.7	501.7	513.6	506.7	491.0	476.6
85 years and over	- - -	860.6	922.6	1,008.6	935.4	903.6	852.5
White female[4]							
All ages, age-adjusted[3]	15.5	27.8	33.3	39.5	39.7	40.3	38.4
All ages, crude	16.4	32.8	40.8	49.7	50.5	51.5	49.3
35–44 years	1.3	1.2	1.7	1.8	2.0	2.1	1.9
45–54 years	7.6	8.3	8.4	7.9	8.1	8.1	7.9
55–64 years	28.7	41.9	44.0	43.2	42.4	42.9	40.8
65–74 years	71.0	118.8	139.0	159.6	157.0	158.6	151.1
75–84 years	104.0	226.3	279.5	339.1	345.4	352.0	335.5
85 years and over	144.2	298.4	395.5	544.8	554.5	562.8	536.5
Black or African American female[4]							
All ages, age-adjusted[3]	9.1	16.6	20.2	22.7	22.6	22.0	20.9
All ages, crude	6.8	12.6	15.5	17.6	17.7	17.3	16.6
35–44 years	3.4	3.8	5.4	4.7	4.6	4.6	3.9
45–54 years	9.3	14.0	12.8	13.4	11.6	11.9	11.5
55–64 years	20.8	33.4	34.7	35.3	31.5	32.4	28.5
65–74 years	32.7	64.7	78.7	82.9	82.0	83.3	74.9
75–84 years	41.1	96.0	132.7	158.4	167.4	153.2	158.6
85 years and over	63.2	133.0	185.8	255.0	262.0	256.4	241.8

See footnotes at end of table.

This table will be updated on the Web. Go to www.cdc.gov/nchs/hus.htm.

Table 41 (page 3 of 3). Death rates for chronic lower respiratory diseases, by sex, race, Hispanic origin, and age: United States, selected years 1980–2004

[Data are based on death certificates]

Sex, race, Hispanic origin, and age	1980[1]	1990	1995	2000[2]	2002	2003	2004
			Deaths per 100,000 resident population				
American Indian or Alaska Native female[4]							
All ages, age-adjusted[3]	7.7	16.8	22.8	26.2	26.4	26.1	26.1
All ages, crude	3.8	8.7	11.5	13.4	15.1	15.6	15.9
35–44 years	*	*	*	*	*	*	*
45–54 years	*	*	*	*	*	*	*
55–64 years	*	*	38.8	31.6	34.1	39.0	35.2
65–74 years	*	56.4	79.5	136.8	119.1	101.2	104.8
75–84 years	*	116.7	191.3	175.8	194.8	217.2	247.3
85 years and over	*	*	*	362.2	353.4	296.2	224.6
Asian or Pacific Islander female[4]							
All ages, age-adjusted[3]	5.8	11.0	12.1	11.7	9.3	9.9	9.3
All ages, crude	2.6	5.2	6.3	6.8	6.0	6.5	6.3
35–44 years	*	*	*	*	*	*	*
45–54 years	*	*	3.6	*	*	*	*
55–64 years	*	15.2	9.6	6.2	4.9	6.0	4.1
65–74 years	*	26.5	29.2	29.2	24.6	24.8	20.3
75–84 years	*	80.6	113.2	88.9	77.0	77.2	75.8
85 years and over	*	232.5	227.8	299.5	219.1	253.8	252.7
Hispanic or Latino female[4,5]							
All ages, age-adjusted[3]	- - -	13.4	16.9	16.3	16.2	15.8	14.9
All ages, crude	- - -	6.3	7.7	7.2	7.6	7.7	7.4
35–44 years	- - -	*	1.4	1.3	1.4	1.0	0.7
45–54 years	- - -	4.9	4.6	3.3	3.1	3.8	3.4
55–64 years	- - -	14.4	12.9	10.8	10.6	9.3	10.9
65–74 years	- - -	36.6	43.1	38.0	41.5	41.5	38.3
75–84 years	- - -	101.1	125.0	136.0	129.8	129.6	125.7
85 years and over	- - -	269.0	402.6	387.8	385.5	365.6	326.3
White, not Hispanic or Latino female[5]							
All ages, age-adjusted[3]	- - -	28.5	34.0	40.7	41.2	41.8	40.0
All ages, crude	- - -	35.7	44.7	56.2	57.7	59.0	56.7
35–44 years	- - -	1.2	1.7	1.9	2.1	2.2	2.1
45–54 years	- - -	8.5	8.5	8.3	8.6	8.5	8.4
55–64 years	- - -	43.7	46.2	45.8	45.1	45.7	43.5
65–74 years	- - -	122.8	143.0	167.6	165.5	167.6	160.1
75–84 years	- - -	231.9	284.5	347.2	355.7	363.5	347.2
85 years and over	- - -	302.1	393.7	548.7	559.8	569.5	544.3

* Rates based on fewer than 20 deaths are considered unreliable and are not shown.
- - - Data not available.
[1]For the period 1980–1998, underlying cause of death was coded according to the Ninth Revision of the International Classification of Diseases (ICD), using ICD–9 codes for chronic lower respiratory diseases (CLRD) that are most nearly comparable with CLRD codes in the 113 cause list for ICD–10. See Appendix II, Cause of death; Tables IV and V.
[2]Starting with 1999 data, cause of death is coded according to ICD–10. See Appendix II, Cause of death, Table V; Comparability ratio, Table VI.
[3]Age-adjusted rates are calculated using the year 2000 standard population. Prior to 2003, age-adjusted rates were calculated using standard million proportions based on rounded population numbers. Starting with 2003 data, unrounded population numbers are used to calculate age-adjusted rates. See Appendix II, Age adjustment.
[4]The race groups, white, black, Asian or Pacific Islander, and American Indian or Alaska Native, include persons of Hispanic and non-Hispanic origin. Persons of Hispanic origin may be of any race. Death rates for the American Indian or Alaska Native and Asian or Pacific Islander populations are known to be underestimated. See Appendix II, Race, for a discussion of sources of bias in death rates by race and Hispanic origin.
[5]Prior to 1997, excludes data from states lacking an Hispanic-origin item on the death certificate. See Appendix II, Hispanic origin.

NOTES: Starting with *Health, United States, 2003*, rates for 1991–1999 were revised using intercensal population estimates based on the 2000 census. Rates for 2000 were revised based on 2000 census counts. Rates for 2001 and later years were computed using 2000-based postcensal estimates. See Appendix I, Population Census and Population Estimates. Age groups were selected to minimize the presentation of unstable age-specific death rates based on small numbers of deaths and for consistency among comparison groups. In 2003, seven states reported multiple-race data. In 2004, 15 states reported multiple-race data. The multiple-race data for these states were bridged to the single-race categories of the 1977 Office of Management and Budget standards for comparability with other states. See Appendix II, Race. Data for additional years are available. See Appendix III.

SOURCES: Centers for Disease Control and Prevention, National Center for Health Statistics, National Vital Statistics System; numerator data from annual mortality files; denominator data from national population estimates for race groups from Table 1 and unpublished Hispanic population estimates for 1985–1996 prepared by the Housing and Household Economic Statistics Division, U.S. Census Bureau; additional mortality tables are available from: www.cdc.gov/nchs/datawh/statab/unpubd/mortabs.htm; Miniño AM, Heron M, Murphy SL, Kochanek KD. Deaths: Final data for 2004. Health E-Stats. Hyattsville, MD: National Center for Health Statistics. 2006.

This table will be updated on the Web. Go to www.cdc.gov/nchs/hus.htm.

Table 42 (page 1 of 2). Death rates for human immunodeficiency virus (HIV) disease, by sex, race, Hispanic origin, and age: United States, selected years 1987–2004

[Data are based on death certificates]

Sex, race, Hispanic origin, and age[1]	1987[2]	1990	1995	2000[3]	2002	2003	2004
All persons			Deaths per 100,000 resident population				
All ages, age-adjusted[4]	5.6	10.2	16.2	5.2	4.9	4.7	4.5
All ages, crude	5.6	10.1	16.2	5.1	4.9	4.7	4.4
Under 1 year	2.3	2.7	1.5	*	*	*	*
1–4 years	0.7	0.8	1.3	*	*	*	*
5–14 years	0.1	0.2	0.5	0.1	0.1	0.1	0.1
15–24 years	1.3	1.5	1.7	0.5	0.4	0.4	0.5
25–34 years	11.7	19.7	28.3	6.1	4.6	4.0	3.7
35–44 years	14.0	27.4	44.2	13.1	12.7	12.0	10.9
45–54 years	8.0	15.2	26.0	11.0	11.2	10.9	10.6
55–64 years	3.5	6.2	10.9	5.1	5.1	5.4	5.4
65–74 years	1.3	2.0	3.6	2.2	2.2	2.4	2.4
75–84 years	0.8	0.7	0.7	0.7	0.8	0.7	0.8
85 years and over	*	*	*	*	*	*	*
Male							
All ages, age-adjusted[4]	10.4	18.5	27.3	7.9	7.4	7.1	6.6
All ages, crude	10.2	18.5	27.6	7.9	7.4	7.1	6.6
Under 1 year	2.2	2.4	1.7	*	*	*	*
1–4 years	0.7	0.8	1.2	*	*	*	*
5–14 years	0.2	0.3	0.5	0.1	*	*	*
15–24 years	2.2	2.2	2.0	0.5	0.4	0.4	0.5
25–34 years	20.7	34.5	45.5	8.0	5.9	5.1	4.5
35–44 years	26.3	50.2	75.5	19.8	18.8	17.5	15.7
45–54 years	15.5	29.1	46.2	17.8	17.7	17.2	16.3
55–64 years	6.8	12.0	19.7	8.7	8.5	9.1	9.0
65–74 years	2.4	3.7	6.4	3.8	3.9	4.0	4.0
75–84 years	1.2	1.1	1.3	1.3	1.4	1.5	1.4
85 years and over	*	*	*	*	*	*	*
Female							
All ages, age-adjusted[4]	1.1	2.2	5.3	2.5	2.5	2.4	2.4
All ages, crude	1.1	2.2	5.3	2.5	2.5	2.4	2.4
Under 1 year	2.5	3.0	1.2	*	*	*	*
1–4 years	0.7	0.8	1.5	*	*	*	*
5–14 years	*	0.2	0.5	0.1	*	*	*
15–24 years	0.3	0.7	1.4	0.4	0.4	0.4	0.4
25–34 years	2.8	4.9	10.9	4.2	3.3	2.8	2.8
35–44 years	2.1	5.2	13.3	6.5	6.7	6.5	6.2
45–54 years	0.8	1.9	6.6	4.4	4.8	4.8	5.2
55–64 years	0.5	1.1	2.8	1.8	1.9	2.1	2.0
65–74 years	0.5	0.8	1.4	0.8	0.8	1.0	1.0
75–84 years	0.5	0.4	0.3	0.3	0.3	0.3	0.5
85 years and over	*	*	*	*	*	*	*
All ages, age-adjusted[4]							
White male	8.7	15.7	20.4	4.6	4.3	4.2	3.8
Black or African American male	26.2	46.3	89.0	35.1	33.3	31.3	29.2
American Indian or Alaska Native male	*	3.3	10.5	3.5	3.4	3.5	4.3
Asian or Pacific Islander male	2.5	4.3	6.0	1.2	1.5	1.1	1.2
Hispanic or Latino male[5]	18.8	28.8	40.8	10.6	9.1	9.2	8.2
White, not Hispanic or Latino male[5]	10.7	14.1	17.9	3.8	3.5	3.4	3.1
White female	0.6	1.1	2.5	1.0	0.9	0.9	0.9
Black or African American female	4.6	10.1	24.4	13.2	13.4	12.8	13.0
American Indian or Alaska Native female	*	*	2.5	1.0	*	1.5	1.5
Asian or Pacific Islander female	*	*	0.6	0.2	*	*	*
Hispanic or Latino female[5]	2.1	3.8	8.8	2.9	2.6	2.7	2.4
White, not Hispanic or Latino female[5]	0.5	0.7	1.7	0.7	0.6	0.6	0.6

See footnotes at end of table.

This table will be updated on the Web. Go to www.cdc.gov/nchs/hus.htm.

Table 42 (page 2 of 2). Death rates for human immunodeficiency virus (HIV) disease, by sex, race, Hispanic origin, and age: United States, selected years 1987–2004

[Data are based on death certificates]

Sex, race, Hispanic origin, and age[1]	1987[2]	1990	1995	2000[3]	2002	2003	2004
Age 25–44 years				Deaths per 100,000 resident population			
All persons	12.7	23.2	36.3	9.8	8.9	8.2	7.5
White male	19.2	35.0	46.1	8.8	7.7	7.2	6.3
Black or African American male	60.2	102.0	179.4	55.4	49.9	44.8	39.9
American Indian or Alaska Native male	*	7.7	28.5	5.5	8.3	6.4	8.6
Asian or Pacific Islander male	4.1	8.1	12.1	1.9	1.8	1.9	1.7
Hispanic or Latino male[5]	36.8	59.3	73.9	14.3	11.5	10.3	9.3
White, not Hispanic or Latino male[5]	23.3	31.6	41.2	7.4	6.6	6.2	5.5
White female	1.2	2.3	5.9	2.1	1.8	1.8	1.6
Black or African American female	11.6	23.6	53.6	26.7	25.9	23.6	23.1
American Indian or Alaska Native female	*	*	*	*	*	*	*
Asian or Pacific Islander female	*	*	1.2	*	*	*	*
Hispanic or Latino female[5]	4.9	8.9	17.2	4.6	3.8	3.8	3.1
White, not Hispanic or Latino female[5]	1.0	1.5	4.2	1.6	1.3	1.3	1.3
Age 45–64 years							
All persons	5.8	11.1	19.9	8.7	8.7	8.7	8.5
White male	9.9	18.6	26.0	8.1	7.8	7.9	7.5
Black or African American male	27.3	53.0	133.2	71.6	70.7	68.1	66.0
American Indian or Alaska Native male	*	*	*	*	*	*	7.2
Asian or Pacific Islander male	*	6.5	9.1	2.1	3.4	2.1	2.4
Hispanic or Latino male[5]	25.8	37.9	67.1	23.3	20.3	22.5	19.4
White, not Hispanic or Latino male[5]	12.6	16.9	22.4	6.5	6.4	6.2	6.0
White female	0.5	0.9	2.4	1.3	1.4	1.4	1.4
Black or African American female	2.6	7.5	27.0	19.6	21.4	21.8	22.7
American Indian or Alaska Native female	*	*	*	*	*	*	*
Asian or Pacific Islander female	*	*	*	*	*	*	*
Hispanic or Latino female[5]	*	3.1	12.6	5.8	5.7	5.3	5.0
White, not Hispanic or Latino female[5]	0.5	0.7	1.5	0.9	0.9	0.9	0.9

* Rates based on fewer than 20 deaths are considered unreliable and are not shown.

[1]The race groups, white, black, Asian or Pacific Islander, and American Indian or Alaska Native, include persons of Hispanic and non-Hispanic origin. Persons of Hispanic origin may be of any race. Death rates for the American Indian or Alaska Native and Asian or Pacific Islander populations are known to be underestimated. See Appendix II, Race, for a discussion of sources of bias in death rates by race and Hispanic origin.

[2]Categories for the coding and classification of human immunodeficiency virus (HIV) disease were introduced in the United States in 1987. For the period 1987–1998, underlying cause of death was coded according to the Ninth Revision of the International Classification of Diseases (ICD). See Appendix II, Cause of death; Human immunodeficiency virus (HIV) disease; Tables IV and V.

[3]Starting with 1999 data, cause of death is coded according to ICD–10. To estimate change between 1998 and 1999, compare the 1999 rate with the comparability-modified rate for 1998. Additional years of data available in spreadsheet version of this table. Available from: www.cdc.gov/nchs/hus.htm; See Appendix II, Cause of death, Table V; Comparability ratio, Table VI.

[4]Age-adjusted rates are calculated using the year 2000 standard population. Prior to 2003, age-adjusted rates were calculated using standard million proportions based on rounded population numbers. Starting with 2003 data, unrounded population numbers are used to calculate age-adjusted rates. See Appendix II, Age adjustment.

[5]Prior to 1997, excludes data from states lacking an Hispanic-origin item on the death certificate. See Appendix II, Hispanic origin.

NOTES: Starting with *Health, United States, 2003*, rates for 1991–1999 were revised using intercensal population estimates based on the 2000 census. Rates for 2000 were revised based on 2000 census counts. Rates for 2001 and 2002 were computed using 2000-based postcensal estimates. See Appendix I, Population Census and Population Estimates. In 2003, seven states reported multiple-race data. In 2004, 15 states reported multiple-race data. The multiple-race data for these states were bridged to the single-race categories of the 1977 Office of Management and Budget standards for comparability with other states. See Appendix II, Race. Data for additional years are available. See Appendix III.

SOURCES: Centers for Disease Control and Prevention, National Center for Health Statistics, National Vital Statistics System; numerator data from annual mortality files; denominator data from national population estimates for race groups from Table 1 and unpublished Hispanic population estimates for 1987–1996 prepared by the Housing and Household Economic Statistics Division, U.S. Census Bureau; additional mortality tables are available from: www.cdc.gov/nchs/datawh/statab/unpubd/mortabs.htm; Miniño AM, Heron M, Murphy SL, Kochanek KD. Deaths: Final data for 2004. Health E-Stats. Hyattsville, MD: National Center for Health Statistics. 2006.

This table will be updated on the Web. Go to www.cdc.gov/nchs/hus.htm.

Table 43. Maternal mortality for complications of pregnancy, childbirth, and the puerperium, by race, Hispanic origin, and age: United States, selected years 1950–2004

[Data are based on death certificates]

Race, Hispanic origin, and age	1950[1,2]	1960[1,2]	1970[2]	1980[2]	1990[2]	2000[3]	2002	2003[4]	2004[4]
				Number of deaths					
All persons	2,960	1,579	803	334	343	396	357	495	540
White	1,873	936	445	193	177	240	190	280	300
Black or African American	1,041	624	342	127	153	137	148	183	214
American Indian or Alaska Native	---	---	---	3	4	6	–	7	4
Asian or Pacific Islander	---	---	---	11	9	13	19	25	22
Hispanic or Latino[5]	---	---	---	---	47	81	62	92	80
White, not Hispanic or Latino[5]	---	---	---	---	125	160	128	188	225
				Deaths per 100,000 live births					
All persons									
All ages, age-adjusted[6]	73.7	32.1	21.5	9.4	7.6	8.2	7.6	9.7	11.3
All ages, crude	83.3	37.1	21.5	9.2	8.2	9.8	8.9	12.1	13.1
Under 20 years	70.7	22.7	18.9	7.6	7.5	*	6.7	6.2	6.6
20–24 years	47.6	20.7	13.0	5.8	6.1	7.4	5.8	7.7	10.8
25–29 years	63.5	29.8	17.0	7.7	6.0	7.9	7.5	8.7	11.0
30–34 years	107.7	50.3	31.6	13.6	9.5	10.0	9.3	10.9	11.8
35 years and over[7]	222.0	104.3	81.9	36.3	20.7	22.7	18.4	33.1	28.2
White									
All ages, age-adjusted[6]	53.1	22.4	14.4	6.7	5.1	6.2	4.8	6.9	7.5
All ages, crude	61.1	26.0	14.3	6.6	5.4	7.5	6.0	8.7	9.3
Under 20 years	44.9	14.8	13.8	5.8	*	*	*	*	*
20–24 years	35.7	15.3	8.4	4.2	3.9	5.6	3.4	5.3	6.5
25–29 years	45.0	20.3	11.1	5.4	4.8	5.9	4.6	6.9	6.9
30–34 years	75.9	34.3	18.7	9.3	5.0	7.1	6.7	6.8	9.0
35 years and over[7]	174.1	73.9	59.3	25.5	12.6	18.0	13.3	23.8	22.0
Black or African American									
All ages, age-adjusted[6]	---	92.0	65.5	24.9	21.7	20.1	22.9	25.5	32.3
All ages, crude	---	103.6	60.9	22.4	22.4	22.0	24.9	30.5	34.7
Under 20 years	---	54.8	32.3	13.1	*	*	*	*	*
20–24 years	---	56.9	41.9	13.9	14.7	15.3	14.9	15.8	27.9
25–29 years	---	92.8	65.2	22.4	14.9	21.8	27.1	20.7	38.6
30–34 years	---	150.6	117.8	44.0	44.2	34.8	28.4	46.1	40.4
35 years and over[7]	---	299.5	207.5	100.6	79.7	62.8	62.9	104.1	79.2
Hispanic or Latino[5,8]									
All ages, age-adjusted[6]	---	---	---	---	7.4	9.0	6.0	8.6	7.3
All ages, crude	---	---	---	---	7.9	9.9	7.1	10.1	8.5
White, not Hispanic or Latino[5]									
All ages, age-adjusted[6]	---	---	---	---	4.4	5.5	4.4	6.3	7.8
All ages, crude	---	---	---	---	4.8	6.8	5.6	8.1	9.8

--- Data not available.
– Quantity zero.
* Rates based on fewer than 20 deaths are considered unreliable and are not shown.
[1]Includes deaths of persons who were not residents of the 50 states and the District of Columbia.
[2]Underlying cause of death was coded according to the Sixth Revision of the International Classification of Diseases (ICD) in 1950, Seventh Revision in 1960, Eighth Revision in 1970, and Ninth Revision in 1980–1998. See Appendix II, Cause of death; Tables IV and V.
[3]Starting with 1999 data, cause of death is coded according to ICD–10. Major changes in the classification and coding of maternal deaths account for an increase in the number of maternal deaths under ICD–10. See Appendix II, Cause of death, Table V; Comparability ratio, Table VI; *International Classification of Diseases* (ICD); Maternal death.
[4]Increases are due to methodological changes in reporting and data processing. See Appendix II, Maternal death.
[5]Prior to 1997, excludes data from states lacking an Hispanic-origin item on the death certificate. See Appendix II, Hispanic origin.
[6]Rates are age-adjusted to the 1970 distribution of live births by mother's age in the United States. See Appendix II, Age adjustment.
[7]Rates computed by relating deaths of women 35 years and over to live births to women 35–49 years. See Appendix II, Rate: Death and related rates.
[8]Age-specific maternal mortality rates are not calculated because rates based on fewer than 20 deaths are considered unreliable.

NOTES: The race groups, white, black, Asian or Pacific Islander, and American Indian or Alaska Native, include persons of Hispanic and non-Hispanic origin. Persons of Hispanic origin may be of any race. For 1950 and 1960, rates were based on live births by race of child; for all other years, rates are based on live births by race of mother. See Appendix II, Race. Rates are not calculated for American Indian or Alaska Native and Asian or Pacific Islander mothers because rates based on fewer than 20 deaths are considered unreliable. Data for additional years are available. See Appendix III.

SOURCES: Centers for Disease Control and Prevention, National Center for Health Statistics, National Vital Statistics System; numerator data from annual mortality files; denominator data from annual natality files; Miniño AM, Heron M, Murphy SL, Kochanek KD. Deaths: Final data for 2004. Health E-Stats. Hyattsville, MD: National Center for Health Statistics. 2006.

This table will be updated on the Web. Go to www.cdc.gov/nchs/hus.htm.

Table 44 (page 1 of 4). Death rates for motor vehicle-related injuries, by sex, race, Hispanic origin, and age: United States, selected years 1950–2004

[Data are based on death certificates]

Sex, race, Hispanic origin, and age	*1950*[1,2]	*1960*[1,2]	*1970*[2]	*1980*[2]	*1990*	*2000*[3]	*2003*	*2004*
All persons				Deaths per 100,000 resident population				
All ages, age-adjusted[4]	24.6	23.1	27.6	22.3	18.5	15.4	15.3	15.2
All ages, crude	23.1	21.3	26.9	23.5	18.8	15.4	15.4	15.3
Under 1 year	8.4	8.1	9.8	7.0	4.9	4.4	3.6	3.5
1–14 years	9.8	8.6	10.5	8.2	6.0	4.3	4.0	4.0
1–4 years	11.5	10.0	11.5	9.2	6.3	4.2	3.9	4.0
5–14 years	8.8	7.9	10.2	7.9	5.9	4.3	4.0	4.1
15–24 years	34.4	38.0	47.2	44.8	34.1	26.9	26.6	26.3
15–19 years	29.6	33.9	43.6	43.0	33.1	26.0	25.7	25.2
20–24 years	38.8	42.9	51.3	46.6	35.0	28.0	27.5	27.5
25–34 years	24.6	24.3	30.9	29.1	23.6	17.3	17.1	17.6
35–44 years	20.3	19.3	24.9	20.9	16.9	15.3	15.7	15.1
45–64 years	25.2	23.0	26.5	18.0	15.7	14.3	14.6	14.7
45–54 years	22.2	21.4	25.5	18.6	15.6	14.2	14.9	15.1
55–64 years	29.0	25.1	27.9	17.4	15.9	14.4	14.2	14.1
65 years and over	43.1	34.7	36.2	22.5	23.1	21.4	21.0	20.4
65–74 years	39.1	31.4	32.8	19.2	18.6	16.5	16.2	16.1
75–84 years	52.7	41.8	43.5	28.1	29.1	25.7	24.9	24.5
85 years and over	45.1	37.9	34.2	27.6	31.2	30.4	28.8	26.1
Male								
All ages, age-adjusted[4]	38.5	35.4	41.5	33.6	26.5	21.7	21.6	21.4
All ages, crude	35.4	31.8	39.7	35.3	26.7	21.3	21.4	21.3
Under 1 year	9.1	8.6	9.3	7.3	5.0	4.6	3.9	3.8
1–14 years	12.3	10.7	13.0	10.0	7.0	4.9	4.7	4.5
1–4 years	13.0	11.5	12.9	10.2	6.9	4.7	4.4	4.2
5–14 years	11.9	10.4	13.1	9.9	7.0	5.0	4.8	4.7
15–24 years	56.7	61.2	73.2	68.4	49.5	37.4	36.9	36.4
15–19 years	46.3	51.7	64.1	62.6	45.5	33.9	33.3	32.5
20–24 years	66.7	73.2	84.4	74.3	53.3	41.2	40.4	40.4
25–34 years	40.8	40.1	49.4	46.3	35.7	25.5	25.5	25.8
35–44 years	32.5	29.9	37.7	31.7	24.7	22.0	22.5	21.9
45–64 years	37.7	33.3	38.9	26.5	21.9	20.2	20.9	21.1
45–54 years	33.6	31.6	37.2	27.6	22.0	20.4	21.5	21.9
55–64 years	43.1	35.6	40.9	25.4	21.7	19.8	20.0	19.8
65 years and over	66.6	52.1	54.4	33.9	32.1	29.5	28.5	28.2
65–74 years	59.1	45.8	47.3	27.3	24.2	21.7	21.3	21.3
75–84 years	85.0	66.0	68.2	44.3	41.2	35.6	34.3	34.7
85 years and over	78.1	62.7	63.1	56.1	64.5	57.5	50.0	44.2
Female								
All ages, age-adjusted[4]	11.5	11.7	14.9	11.8	11.0	9.5	9.3	9.3
All ages, crude	10.9	11.0	14.7	12.3	11.3	9.7	9.5	9.5
Under 1 year	7.6	7.5	10.4	6.7	4.9	4.2	3.3	3.2
1–14 years	7.2	6.3	7.9	6.3	4.9	3.7	3.3	3.5
1–4 years	10.0	8.4	10.0	8.1	5.6	3.8	3.5	3.7
5–14 years	5.7	5.4	7.2	5.7	4.7	3.6	3.2	3.4
15–24 years	12.6	15.1	21.6	20.8	17.9	15.9	15.8	15.7
15–19 years	12.9	16.0	22.7	22.8	20.0	17.5	17.8	17.5
20–24 years	12.2	14.0	20.4	18.9	16.0	14.2	13.9	13.8
25–34 years	9.3	9.2	13.0	12.2	11.5	8.8	8.5	9.1
35–44 years	8.5	9.1	12.9	10.4	9.2	8.8	8.9	8.3
45–64 years	12.6	13.1	15.3	10.3	10.1	8.7	8.6	8.6
45–54 years	10.9	11.6	14.5	10.2	9.6	8.2	8.5	8.5
55–64 years	14.9	15.2	16.2	10.5	10.8	9.5	8.8	8.8
65 years and over	21.9	20.3	23.1	15.0	17.2	15.8	15.6	14.9
65–74 years	20.6	19.0	21.6	13.0	14.1	12.3	11.9	11.7
75–84 years	25.2	23.0	27.2	18.5	21.9	19.2	18.7	17.7
85 years and over	22.1	22.0	18.0	15.2	18.3	19.3	19.5	17.9
White male[5]								
All ages, age-adjusted[4]	37.9	34.8	40.4	33.8	26.3	21.8	21.9	21.8
All ages, crude	35.1	31.5	39.1	35.9	26.7	21.6	22.0	21.9
Under 1 year	9.1	8.8	9.1	7.0	4.8	4.2	3.9	3.3
1–14 years	12.4	10.6	12.5	9.8	6.6	4.8	4.7	4.6
15–24 years	58.3	62.7	75.2	73.8	52.5	39.6	39.2	39.4
25–34 years	39.1	38.6	47.0	46.6	35.4	25.1	25.9	25.8
35–44 years	30.9	28.4	35.2	30.7	23.7	21.8	22.6	22.2
45–64 years	36.2	31.7	36.5	25.2	20.6	19.7	20.6	20.7
65 years and over	67.1	52.1	54.2	32.7	31.4	29.4	28.8	28.5

See footnotes at end of table.

This table will be updated on the Web. Go to www.cdc.gov/nchs/hus.htm.

Table 44 (page 2 of 4). Death rates for motor vehicle-related injuries, by sex, race, Hispanic origin, and age: United States, selected years 1950–2004

[Data are based on death certificates]

Sex, race, Hispanic origin, and age	1950[1,2]	1960[1,2]	1970[2]	1980[2]	1990	2000[3]	2003	2004
Black or African American male[5]				Deaths per 100,000 resident population				
All ages, age-adjusted[4]	34.8	39.6	51.0	34.2	29.9	24.4	22.7	22.7
All ages, crude	37.2	33.1	44.3	31.1	28.1	22.5	21.1	21.2
Under 1 year	- - -	*	10.6	7.8	*	6.7	*	*
1–14 years[6]	10.4	11.2	16.3	11.4	8.9	5.5	4.8	4.8
15–24 years	42.5	46.4	58.1	34.9	36.1	30.2	27.9	26.4
25–34 years	54.4	51.0	70.4	44.9	39.5	32.6	29.0	31.8
35–44 years	46.7	43.6	59.5	41.2	33.5	27.2	26.4	24.7
45–64 years	54.6	47.8	61.7	39.5	33.3	27.1	26.1	26.9
65 years and over	52.6	48.2	53.4	42.4	36.3	32.1	28.9	28.6
American Indian or Alaska Native male[5]								
All ages, age-adjusted[4]	- - -	- - -	- - -	78.9	48.3	35.8	35.2	34.5
All ages, crude	- - -	- - -	- - -	74.6	47.6	33.6	35.9	33.7
1–14 years	- - -	- - -	- - -	15.1	11.6	7.8	9.8	6.8
15–24 years	- - -	- - -	- - -	126.1	75.2	56.8	60.2	47.4
25–34 years	- - -	- - -	- - -	107.0	78.2	49.8	45.5	46.7
35–44 years	- - -	- - -	- - -	82.8	57.0	36.3	43.6	37.8
45–64 years	- - -	- - -	- - -	77.4	45.9	32.0	36.0	38.3
65 years and over	- - -	- - -	- - -	97.0	43.0	48.5	25.4	42.3
Asian or Pacific Islander male[5]								
All ages, age-adjusted[4]	- - -	- - -	- - -	19.0	17.9	10.6	10.3	9.3
All ages, crude	- - -	- - -	- - -	17.1	15.8	9.8	9.4	8.8
1–14 years	- - -	- - -	- - -	8.2	6.3	2.5	2.4	2.6
15–24 years	- - -	- - -	- - -	27.2	25.7	17.0	18.3	15.3
25–34 years	- - -	- - -	- - -	18.8	17.0	10.4	8.2	8.4
35–44 years	- - -	- - -	- - -	13.1	12.2	6.9	6.8	7.4
45–64 years	- - -	- - -	- - -	13.7	15.1	10.1	9.7	9.0
65 years and over	- - -	- - -	- - -	37.3	33.6	21.1	20.1	17.0
Hispanic or Latino male[5,7]								
All ages, age-adjusted[4]	- - -	- - -	- - -	- - -	29.5	21.3	22.0	20.9
All ages, crude	- - -	- - -	- - -	- - -	29.2	20.1	21.1	20.2
1–14 years	- - -	- - -	- - -	- - -	7.2	4.4	4.9	4.7
15–24 years	- - -	- - -	- - -	- - -	48.2	34.7	37.2	38.3
25–34 years	- - -	- - -	- - -	- - -	41.0	24.9	27.6	25.4
35–44 years	- - -	- - -	- - -	- - -	28.0	21.6	22.1	20.8
45–64 years	- - -	- - -	- - -	- - -	28.9	21.7	20.4	19.6
65 years and over	- - -	- - -	- - -	- - -	35.3	28.9	29.2	26.1
White, not Hispanic or Latino male[7]								
All ages, age-adjusted[4]	- - -	- - -	- - -	- - -	25.7	21.7	21.6	21.7
All ages, crude	- - -	- - -	- - -	- - -	26.0	21.5	21.8	22.0
1–14 years	- - -	- - -	- - -	- - -	6.4	4.9	4.6	4.5
15–24 years	- - -	- - -	- - -	- - -	52.3	40.3	39.1	39.1
25–34 years	- - -	- - -	- - -	- - -	34.0	24.7	24.9	25.5
35–44 years	- - -	- - -	- - -	- - -	23.1	21.6	22.4	22.2
45–64 years	- - -	- - -	- - -	- - -	19.8	19.3	20.4	20.7
65 years and over	- - -	- - -	- - -	- - -	31.1	29.3	28.6	28.5
White female[5]								
All ages, age-adjusted[4]	11.4	11.7	14.9	12.2	11.2	9.8	9.5	9.5
All ages, crude	10.9	11.2	14.8	12.8	11.6	10.0	9.8	9.8
Under 1 year	7.8	7.5	10.2	7.1	4.7	3.5	3.0	3.2
1–14 years	7.2	6.2	7.5	6.2	4.8	3.7	3.2	3.4
15–24 years	12.6	15.6	22.7	23.0	19.5	17.1	17.2	16.8
25–34 years	9.0	9.0	12.7	12.2	11.6	8.9	8.6	9.4
35–44 years	8.1	8.9	12.3	10.6	9.2	8.9	9.0	8.4
45–64 years	12.7	13.1	15.1	10.4	9.9	8.7	8.5	8.7
65 years and over	22.2	20.8	23.7	15.3	17.4	16.2	15.8	15.3

See footnotes at end of table.

This table will be updated on the Web. Go to www.cdc.gov/nchs/hus.htm.

Table 44 (page 3 of 4). Death rates for motor vehicle-related injuries, by sex, race, Hispanic origin, and age: United States, selected years 1950–2004

[Data are based on death certificates]

Sex, race, Hispanic origin, and age	1950[1,2]	1960[1,2]	1970[2]	1980[2]	1990	2000[3]	2003	2004
Black or African American female[5]				Deaths per 100,000 resident population				
All ages, age-adjusted[4]	9.3	10.4	14.1	8.5	9.6	8.4	8.3	8.1
All ages, crude	10.2	9.7	13.4	8.3	9.4	8.2	8.0	7.9
Under 1 year	- - -	8.1	11.9	*	7.0	*	*	*
1–14 years[6]	7.2	6.9	10.2	6.3	5.3	3.9	3.5	4.0
15–24 years	11.6	9.9	13.4	8.0	9.9	11.7	9.6	10.9
25–34 years	10.8	9.8	13.3	10.6	11.1	9.4	8.7	8.7
35–44 years	11.1	11.0	16.1	8.3	9.4	8.2	8.9	8.3
45–64 years	11.8	12.7	16.7	9.2	10.7	9.0	8.9	8.8
65 years and over	14.3	13.2	15.7	9.5	13.5	10.4	12.4	9.6
American Indian or Alaska Native female[5]								
All ages, age-adjusted[4]	- - -	- - -	- - -	32.0	17.5	19.5	20.8	17.8
All ages, crude	- - -	- - -	- - -	32.0	17.3	18.6	19.8	17.3
1–14 years	- - -	- - -	- - -	15.0	8.1	6.5	6.3	7.3
15–24 years	- - -	- - -	- - -	42.3	31.4	30.3	27.7	27.0
25–34 years	- - -	- - -	- - -	52.5	18.8	22.3	24.5	21.6
35–44 years	- - -	- - -	- - -	38.1	18.2	22.0	18.7	21.4
45–64 years	- - -	- - -	- - -	32.6	17.6	17.8	22.6	10.4
65 years and over	- - -	- - -	- - -	*	*	24.0	32.3	30.0
Asian or Pacific Islander female[5]								
All ages, age-adjusted[4]	- - -	- - -	- - -	9.3	10.4	6.7	6.8	6.3
All ages, crude	- - -	- - -	- - -	8.2	9.0	5.9	6.4	6.0
1–14 years	- - -	- - -	- - -	7.4	3.6	2.3	1.7	*
15–24 years	- - -	- - -	- - -	7.4	11.4	6.0	9.7	9.0
25–34 years	- - -	- - -	- - -	7.3	7.3	4.5	4.5	4.5
35–44 years	- - -	- - -	- - -	8.6	7.5	4.9	4.5	5.0
45–64 years	- - -	- - -	- - -	8.5	11.8	6.4	7.5	6.3
65 years and over	- - -	- - -	- - -	18.6	24.3	18.5	16.2	14.9
Hispanic or Latino female[5,7]								
All ages, age-adjusted[4]	- - -	- - -	- - -	- - -	9.6	7.9	8.0	7.7
All ages, crude	- - -	- - -	- - -	- - -	8.9	7.2	7.3	7.1
1–14 years	- - -	- - -	- - -	- - -	4.8	3.9	3.0	3.4
15–24 years	- - -	- - -	- - -	- - -	11.6	10.6	11.9	11.1
25–34 years	- - -	- - -	- - -	- - -	9.4	6.5	6.6	7.3
35–44 years	- - -	- - -	- - -	- - -	8.0	7.3	8.0	6.4
45–64 years	- - -	- - -	- - -	- - -	11.4	8.3	8.4	8.1
65 years and over	- - -	- - -	- - -	- - -	14.9	13.4	13.1	12.3

See footnotes at end of table.

This table will be updated on the Web. Go to www.cdc.gov/nchs/hus.htm.

Table 44 (page 4 of 4). Death rates for motor vehicle-related injuries, by sex, race, Hispanic origin, and age: United States, selected years 1950–2004

[Data are based on death certificates]

Sex, race, Hispanic origin, and age	*1950[1,2]*	*1960[1,2]*	*1970[2]*	*1980[2]*	*1990*	*2000[3]*	*2003*	*2004*
White, not Hispanic or Latino female[7]			Deaths per 100,000 resident population					
All ages, age-adjusted[4]	---	---	---	---	11.3	10.0	9.7	9.8
All ages, crude	---	---	---	---	11.7	10.3	10.2	10.2
1–14 years	---	---	---	---	4.7	3.5	3.2	3.4
15–24 years	---	---	---	---	20.4	18.4	18.3	18.0
25–34 years	---	---	---	---	11.7	9.3	9.0	9.8
35–44 years	---	---	---	---	9.3	9.0	9.1	8.7
45–64 years	---	---	---	---	9.7	8.7	8.5	8.6
65 years and over	---	---	---	---	17.5	16.3	15.9	15.5

- - - Data not available.
* Rates based on fewer than 20 deaths are considered unreliable and are not shown.
[1]Includes deaths of persons who were not residents of the 50 states and the District of Columbia.
[2]Underlying cause of death was coded according to the Sixth Revision of the International Classification of Diseases (ICD) in 1950, Seventh Revision in 1960, Eighth Revision in 1970, and Ninth Revision in 1980–1998. See Appendix II, Cause of death; Tables IV and V.
[3]Starting with 1999 data, cause of death is coded according to ICD–10. See Appendix II, Cause of death, Table V; Comparability ratio, Table VI.
[4]Age-adjusted rates are calculated using the year 2000 standard population. Prior to 2003, age-adjusted rates were calculated using standard million proportions based on rounded population numbers. Starting with 2003 data, unrounded population numbers are used to calculate age-adjusted rates. See Appendix II, Age adjustment.
[5]The race groups, white, black, Asian or Pacific Islander, and American Indian or Alaska Native, include persons of Hispanic and non-Hispanic origin. Persons of Hispanic origin may be of any race. Death rates for the American Indian or Alaska Native and Asian or Pacific Islander populations are known to be underestimated. See Appendix II, Race, for a discussion of sources of bias in death rates by race and Hispanic origin.
[6]In 1950, rate is for the age group under 15 years.
[7]Prior to 1997, excludes data from states lacking an Hispanic-origin item on the death certificate. See Appendix II, Hispanic origin.

NOTES: Starting with *Health, United States, 2003*, rates for 1991–1999 were revised using intercensal population estimates based on the 2000 census. Rates for 2000 were revised based on 2000 census counts. Rates for 2001 and later years were computed using 2000-based postcensal estimates. See Appendix I, Population Census and Population Estimates. Age groups were selected to minimize the presentation of unstable age-specific death rates based on small numbers of deaths and for consistency among comparison groups. For additional injury-related statistics, see Web-based Injury Statistics Query and Reporting System, available from: www.cdc.gov/ncipc/wisqars. In 2003, seven states reported multiple-race data. In 2004, 15 states reported multiple-race data. The multiple-race data for these states were bridged to the single-race categories of the 1977 Office of Management and Budget standards for comparability with other states. See Appendix II, Race. Data for additional years are available. See Appendix III.

SOURCES: Centers for Disease Control and Prevention, National Center for Health Statistics, National Vital Statistics System; Grove RD, Hetzel AM. Vital statistics rates in the United States, 1940–1960. Washington, DC: U.S. Government Printing Office. 1968; numerator data from National Vital Statistics System, annual mortality files; denominator data from national population estimates for race groups from Table 1 and unpublished Hispanic population estimates for 1985–1996 prepared by the Housing and Household Economic Statistics Division, U.S. Census Bureau; additional mortality tables are available from: www.cdc.gov/nchs/datawh/statab/unpubd/mortabs.htm; Miniño AM, Heron M, Murphy SL, Kochanek KD. Deaths: Final data for 2004. Health E-Stats. Hyattsville, MD: National Center for Health Statistics. 2006.

This table will be updated on the Web. Go to www.cdc.gov/nchs/hus.htm.

Table 45 (page 1 of 4). Death rates for homicide, by sex, race, Hispanic origin, and age: United States, selected years 1950–2004

[Data are based on death certificates]

Sex, race, Hispanic origin, and age	1950[1,2]	1960[1,2]	1970[2]	1980[2]	1990	2000[3]	2003	2004
All persons				Deaths per 100,000 resident population				
All ages, age-adjusted[4]	5.1	5.0	8.8	10.4	9.4	5.9	6.0	5.9
All ages, crude	5.0	4.6	8.1	10.6	9.9	6.0	6.1	5.9
Under 1 year	4.4	4.8	4.3	5.9	8.4	9.2	8.5	8.0
1–14 years	0.6	0.6	1.1	1.5	1.8	1.3	1.2	1.2
1–4 years	0.6	0.7	1.9	2.5	2.5	2.3	2.4	2.4
5–14 years	0.5	0.5	0.9	1.2	1.5	0.9	0.8	0.8
15–24 years	5.8	5.6	11.3	15.4	19.7	12.6	13.0	12.2
15–19 years	3.9	3.9	7.7	10.5	16.9	9.5	9.5	9.3
20–24 years	8.5	7.7	15.6	20.2	22.2	16.0	16.5	15.0
25–44 years	8.9	8.5	14.9	17.5	14.7	8.7	9.1	8.9
25–34 years	9.3	9.2	16.2	19.3	17.4	10.4	11.3	11.2
35–44 years	8.4	7.8	13.5	14.9	11.6	7.1	7.0	6.8
45–64 years	5.0	5.3	8.7	9.0	6.3	4.0	4.1	4.1
45–54 years	5.9	6.1	10.0	11.0	7.5	4.7	4.9	4.8
55–64 years	3.9	4.1	7.1	7.0	5.0	3.0	2.8	3.0
65 years and over	3.0	2.7	4.6	5.5	4.0	2.4	2.4	2.3
65–74 years	3.2	2.8	4.9	5.7	3.8	2.4	2.4	2.4
75–84 years	2.5	2.3	4.0	5.2	4.3	2.4	2.5	2.2
85 years and over	2.3	2.4	4.2	5.3	4.6	2.4	2.2	2.1
Male								
All ages, age-adjusted[4]	7.9	7.5	14.3	16.6	14.8	9.0	9.4	9.2
All ages, crude	7.7	6.8	13.1	17.1	15.9	9.3	9.7	9.4
Under 1 year	4.5	4.7	4.5	6.3	8.8	10.4	10.0	8.0
1–14 years	0.6	0.6	1.2	1.6	2.0	1.5	1.4	1.4
1–4 years	0.5	0.7	1.9	2.7	2.7	2.5	2.5	2.5
5–14 years	0.6	0.5	1.0	1.2	1.7	1.1	1.0	1.0
15–24 years	8.6	8.4	18.2	24.0	32.5	20.9	21.8	20.4
15–19 years	5.5	5.7	12.1	15.9	27.8	15.5	15.9	15.3
20–24 years	13.5	11.8	25.6	32.2	36.9	26.7	27.6	25.4
25–44 years	13.8	12.8	24.4	28.9	23.5	13.3	14.3	14.1
25–34 years	14.4	13.9	26.8	31.9	27.7	16.7	18.5	18.5
35–44 years	13.2	11.7	21.7	24.5	18.6	10.3	10.4	10.1
45–64 years	8.1	8.1	14.8	15.2	10.2	6.0	6.1	6.2
45–54 years	9.5	9.4	16.8	18.4	11.9	6.9	7.4	7.3
55–64 years	6.3	6.4	12.1	11.8	8.0	4.6	4.2	4.6
65 years and over	4.8	4.3	7.7	8.8	5.8	3.3	3.4	3.2
65–74 years	5.2	4.6	8.5	9.2	5.8	3.4	3.4	3.6
75–84 years	3.9	3.7	5.9	8.1	5.7	3.2	3.3	2.6
85 years and over	2.5	3.6	7.4	7.5	6.7	3.3	3.2	2.7
Female								
All ages, age-adjusted[4]	2.4	2.6	3.7	4.4	4.0	2.8	2.6	2.5
All ages, crude	2.4	2.4	3.4	4.5	4.2	2.8	2.6	2.5
Under 1 year	4.2	4.9	4.1	5.6	8.0	7.9	6.9	7.9
1–14 years	0.6	0.5	1.0	1.4	1.6	1.1	1.0	1.1
1–4 years	0.7	0.7	1.9	2.2	2.3	2.1	2.3	2.2
5–14 years	0.5	0.4	0.7	1.1	1.2	0.7	0.5	0.6
15–24 years	3.0	2.8	4.6	6.6	6.2	3.9	3.7	3.5
15–19 years	2.4	1.9	3.2	4.9	5.4	3.1	2.6	3.0
20–24 years	3.7	3.8	6.2	8.2	7.0	4.7	4.8	4.0
25–44 years	4.2	4.3	5.8	6.4	6.0	4.0	3.8	3.6
25–34 years	4.5	4.6	6.0	6.9	7.1	4.1	3.9	3.7
35–44 years	3.8	4.0	5.7	5.7	4.8	4.0	3.6	3.4
45–64 years	1.9	2.5	3.1	3.4	2.8	2.1	2.1	2.1
45–54 years	2.3	2.9	3.7	4.1	3.2	2.5	2.5	2.4
55–64 years	1.4	2.0	2.5	2.8	2.3	1.6	1.5	1.6
65 years and over	1.4	1.3	2.3	3.3	2.8	1.8	1.7	1.7
65–74 years	1.3	1.3	2.2	3.0	2.2	1.6	1.5	1.4
75–84 years	1.4	1.3	2.7	3.5	3.4	2.0	1.9	1.9
85 years and over	2.1	1.6	2.5	4.3	3.8	2.0	1.8	1.9

See footnotes at end of table.

This table will be updated on the Web. Go to www.cdc.gov/nchs/hus.htm.

Table 45 (page 2 of 4). Death rates for homicide, by sex, race, Hispanic origin, and age: United States, selected years 1950–2004

[Data are based on death certificates]

Sex, race, Hispanic origin, and age	1950[1,2]	1960[1,2]	1970[2]	1980[2]	1990	2000[3]	2003	2004
	Deaths per 100,000 resident population							
White male[5]								
All ages, age-adjusted[4]	3.8	3.9	7.2	10.4	8.3	5.2	5.3	5.3
All ages, crude	3.6	3.6	6.6	10.7	8.8	5.2	5.4	5.3
Under 1 year	4.3	3.8	2.9	4.3	6.4	8.2	8.1	6.9
1–14 years	0.4	0.5	0.7	1.2	1.3	1.2	0.9	1.0
15–24 years	3.2	5.0	7.6	15.1	15.2	9.9	10.6	10.2
25–44 years	5.4	5.5	11.6	17.2	13.0	7.4	7.7	7.7
25–34 years	4.9	5.7	12.5	18.5	14.7	8.4	9.2	9.3
35–44 years	6.1	5.2	10.8	15.2	11.1	6.5	6.3	6.3
45–64 years	4.8	4.6	8.3	9.8	6.9	4.1	4.2	4.3
65 years and over	3.8	3.1	5.4	6.7	4.1	2.5	2.7	2.5
Black or African American male[5]								
All ages, age-adjusted[4]	47.0	42.3	78.2	69.4	63.1	35.4	36.7	35.1
All ages, crude	44.7	35.0	66.0	65.7	68.5	37.2	38.9	37.1
Under 1 year	---	10.3	14.3	18.6	21.4	23.3	17.8	14.2
1–14 years[6]	1.8	1.5	4.4	4.1	5.8	3.1	4.1	3.5
15–24 years	53.8	43.2	98.3	82.6	137.1	85.3	84.6	77.6
25–44 years	92.8	80.5	140.2	130.0	105.4	55.8	61.0	59.6
25–34 years	104.3	86.4	154.5	142.9	123.7	73.9	82.5	81.6
35–44 years	80.0	74.4	124.0	109.3	81.2	38.5	40.2	37.9
45–64 years	46.0	44.6	82.3	70.6	41.4	21.9	22.2	22.0
65 years and over	16.5	17.3	33.3	30.9	25.7	12.8	10.9	11.0
American Indian or Alaska Native male[5]								
All ages, age-adjusted[4]	---	---	---	23.3	16.7	10.7	10.5	11.0
All ages, crude	---	---	---	23.1	16.6	10.7	11.3	11.5
15–24 years	---	---	---	35.4	25.1	17.0	19.7	17.7
25–44 years	---	---	---	39.2	25.7	17.0	14.8	17.8
45–64 years	---	---	---	22.1	14.8	*	9.5	7.5
Asian or Pacific Islander male[5]								
All ages, age-adjusted[4]	---	---	---	9.1	7.3	4.3	4.2	3.7
All ages, crude	---	---	---	8.3	7.9	4.4	4.5	3.9
15–24 years	---	---	---	9.3	14.9	7.8	9.8	7.8
25–44 years	---	---	---	11.3	9.6	4.6	4.5	3.7
45–64 years	---	---	---	10.4	7.0	6.1	4.3	5.1
Hispanic or Latino male[5,7]								
All ages, age-adjusted[4]	---	---	---	---	27.4	11.8	12.1	11.5
All ages, crude	---	---	---	---	31.0	13.4	13.6	13.0
Under 1 year	---	---	---	---	8.7	6.6	7.9	9.1
1–14 years	---	---	---	---	3.1	1.7	1.3	1.5
15–24 years	---	---	---	---	55.4	28.5	30.3	29.6
25–44 years	---	---	---	---	46.4	17.2	17.6	16.6
25–34 years	---	---	---	---	50.9	19.9	21.2	20.3
35–44 years	---	---	---	---	39.3	13.5	12.9	11.8
45–64 years	---	---	---	---	20.5	9.1	8.7	8.5
65 years and over	---	---	---	---	9.4	4.4	6.0	3.7
White, not Hispanic or Latino male[7]								
All ages, age-adjusted[4]	---	---	---	---	5.6	3.6	3.6	3.6
All ages, crude	---	---	---	---	5.8	3.6	3.6	3.6
Under 1 year	---	---	---	---	5.4	8.3	8.0	6.1
1–14 years	---	---	---	---	0.9	1.0	0.8	0.8
15–24 years	---	---	---	---	7.5	4.7	5.0	4.7
25–44 years	---	---	---	---	8.7	5.2	5.1	5.2
25–34 years	---	---	---	---	9.3	5.2	5.2	5.5
35–44 years	---	---	---	---	8.0	5.2	4.9	5.0
45–64 years	---	---	---	---	5.7	3.6	3.7	3.8
65 years and over	---	---	---	---	3.7	2.3	2.4	2.4

See footnotes at end of table.

This table will be updated on the Web. Go to www.cdc.gov/nchs/hus.htm.

Table 45 (page 3 of 4). Death rates for homicide, by sex, race, Hispanic origin, and age: United States, selected years 1950–2004

[Data are based on death certificates]

Sex, race, Hispanic origin, and age	*1950*[1,2]	*1960*[1,2]	*1970*[2]	*1980*[2]	*1990*	*2000*[3]	*2003*	*2004*
White female[5]				Deaths per 100,000 resident population				
All ages, age-adjusted[4]	1.4	1.5	2.3	3.2	2.7	2.1	2.0	1.9
All ages, crude	1.4	1.4	2.1	3.2	2.8	2.1	2.0	1.9
Under 1 year	3.9	3.5	2.9	4.3	5.1	5.0	5.7	6.2
1–14 years	0.4	0.4	0.7	1.1	1.0	0.8	0.7	0.8
15–24 years	1.3	1.5	2.7	4.7	4.0	2.7	2.5	2.5
25–44 years	2.0	2.1	3.3	4.2	3.8	2.9	2.8	2.7
45–64 years	1.5	1.7	2.1	2.6	2.3	1.8	1.8	1.7
65 years and over	1.2	1.2	1.9	2.9	2.2	1.6	1.5	1.6
Black or African American female[5]								
All ages, age-adjusted[4]	11.1	11.4	14.7	13.2	12.5	7.1	6.4	6.3
All ages, crude	11.5	10.4	13.2	13.5	13.4	7.2	6.6	6.4
Under 1 year	---	13.8	10.7	12.8	22.8	22.2	14.2	17.0
1–14 years[6]	1.8	1.2	3.1	3.3	4.7	2.7	2.4	2.8
15–24 years	16.5	11.9	17.7	18.4	18.9	10.7	10.1	8.8
25–44 years	22.5	22.7	25.3	22.6	21.0	11.0	9.8	9.4
45–64 years	6.8	10.3	13.4	10.8	6.5	4.5	4.8	5.1
65 years and over	3.6	3.0	7.4	8.0	9.4	3.5	3.3	2.9
American Indian or Alaska Native female[5]								
All ages, age-adjusted[4]	---	---	---	8.1	4.6	3.0	3.9	3.0
All ages, crude	---	---	---	7.7	4.8	2.9	4.0	3.0
15–24 years	---	---	---	*	*	*	7.2	*
25–44 years	---	---	---	13.7	6.9	5.9	5.4	*
45–64 years	---	---	---	*	*	*	*	*
Asian or Pacific Islander female[5]								
All ages, age-adjusted[4]	---	---	---	3.1	2.8	1.7	1.6	1.3
All ages, crude	---	---	---	3.1	2.8	1.7	1.6	1.4
15–24 years	---	---	---	*	*	*	*	*
25–44 years	---	---	---	4.6	3.8	2.2	1.9	1.5
45–64 years	---	---	---	*	*	2.0	1.5	1.8
Hispanic or Latino female[5,7]								
All ages, age-adjusted[4]	---	---	---	---	4.3	2.8	2.7	2.3
All ages, crude	---	---	---	---	4.7	2.8	2.8	2.4
Under 1 year	---	---	---	---	*	7.4	5.9	7.0
1–14 years	---	---	---	---	1.9	1.0	1.2	1.1
15–24 years	---	---	---	---	8.1	3.7	4.5	3.3
25–44 years	---	---	---	---	6.1	3.7	3.6	3.3
45–64 years	---	---	---	---	3.3	2.9	2.3	1.9
65 years and over	---	---	---	---	*	2.4	1.9	*
White, not Hispanic or Latino female[7]								
All ages, age-adjusted[4]	---	---	---	---	2.5	1.9	1.8	1.8
All ages, crude	---	---	---	---	2.5	1.9	1.8	1.8
Under 1 year	---	---	---	---	4.4	4.1	5.5	5.8
1–14 years	---	---	---	---	0.8	0.8	0.6	0.7
15–24 years	---	---	---	---	3.3	2.3	1.9	2.3
25–44 years	---	---	---	---	3.5	2.7	2.6	2.5
45–64 years	---	---	---	---	2.2	1.6	1.7	1.6
65 years and over	---	---	---	---	2.2	1.6	1.4	1.6

See footnotes at end of table.

This table will be updated on the Web. Go to www.cdc.gov/nchs/hus.htm.

Table 45 (page 4 of 4). Death rates for homicide, by sex, race, Hispanic origin, and age: United States, selected years 1950–2004

[Data are based on death certificates]

- - - Data not available.
* Rates based on fewer than 20 deaths are considered unreliable and are not shown.
[1]Includes deaths of persons who were not residents of the 50 states and the District of Columbia.
[2]Underlying cause of death was coded according to the Sixth Revision of the International Classification of Diseases (ICD) in 1950, Seventh Revision in 1960, Eighth Revision in 1970, and Ninth Revision in 1980–1998. See Appendix II, Cause of death; Tables IV and V.
[3]Starting with 1999 data, cause of death is coded according to ICD–10. See Appendix II, Cause of death, Table V; Comparability ratio, Table VI.
[4]Age-adjusted rates are calculated using the year 2000 standard population. Prior to 2003, age-adjusted rates were calculated using standard million proportions based on rounded population numbers. Starting with 2003 data, unrounded population numbers are used to calculate age-adjusted rates. See Appendix II, Age adjustment.
[5]The race groups, white, black, Asian or Pacific Islander, and American Indian or Alaska Native, include persons of Hispanic and non-Hispanic origin. Persons of Hispanic origin may be of any race. Death rates for the American Indian or Alaska Native and Asian or Pacific Islander populations are known to be underestimated. See Appendix II, Race, for a discussion of sources of bias in death rates by race and Hispanic origin.
[6]In 1950, rate is for the age group under 15 years.
[7]Prior to 1997, excludes data from states lacking an Hispanic-origin item on the death certificate. See Appendix II, Hispanic origin.

NOTES: Starting with *Health, United States, 2003*, rates for 1991–1999 were revised using intercensal population estimates based on the 2000 census. Rates for 2000 were revised based on 2000 census counts. Rates for 2001 and later years were computed using 2000-based postcensal estimates. See Appendix I, Population Census and Population Estimates. Figures for 2001 include September 11-related deaths for which death certificates were filed as of October 24, 2002. For the period 1980–1998, homicide was coded using ICD–9 codes that are most nearly comparable with homicide codes in the 113 cause list for ICD–10. See Appendix II, Cause of death; Table V for terrorism-related ICD–10 codes. Age groups were selected to minimize the presentation of unstable age-specific death rates based on small numbers of deaths and for consistency among comparison groups. For additional injury-related statistics, see Web-based Injury Statistics Query and Reporting System, available from: www.cdc.gov/ncipc/wisqars. In 2003, seven states reported multiple-race data. In 2004, 15 states reported multiple-race data. The multiple-race data for these states were bridged to the single-race categories of the 1977 Office of Management and Budget standards for comparability with other states. See Appendix II, Race. Data for additional years are available. See Appendix III.

SOURCES: Centers for Disease Control and Prevention, National Center for Health Statistics, National Vital Statistics System; Grove RD, Hetzel AM. Vital statistics rates in the United States, 1940–1960. Washington, DC: U.S. Government Printing Office. 1968; numerator data from National Vital Statistics System, annual mortality files; denominator data from national population estimates for race groups from Table 1 and unpublished Hispanic population estimates for 1985–1996 prepared by the Housing and Household Economic Statistics Division, U.S. Census Bureau; additional mortality tables are available from: www.cdc.gov/nchs/datawh/statab/unpubd/mortabs.htm; Miniño AM, Heron M, Murphy SL, Kochanek KD. Deaths: Final data for 2004. Health E-Stats. Hyattsville, MD: National Center for Health Statistics. 2006.

This table will be updated on the Web. Go to www.cdc.gov/nchs/hus.htm.

Table 46 (page 1 of 3). Death rates for suicide, by sex, race, Hispanic origin, and age: United States, selected years 1950–2004

[Data are based on death certificates]

Sex, race, Hispanic origin, and age	1950[1,2]	1960[1,2]	1970[2]	1980[2]	1990	2000[3]	2003	2004
All persons				Deaths per 100,000 resident population				
All ages, age-adjusted[4]	13.2	12.5	13.1	12.2	12.5	10.4	10.8	10.9
All ages, crude	11.4	10.6	11.6	11.9	12.4	10.4	10.8	11.0
Under 1 year	. . .	. . .	. . .	. . .	. . .	. . .	*	*
1–4 years	. . .	. . .	. . .	. . .	. . .	. . .	*	*
5–14 years	0.2	0.3	0.3	0.4	0.8	0.7	0.6	0.7
15–24 years	4.5	5.2	8.8	12.3	13.2	10.2	9.7	10.3
15–19 years	2.7	3.6	5.9	8.5	11.1	8.0	7.3	8.2
20–24 years	6.2	7.1	12.2	16.1	15.1	12.5	12.1	12.5
25–44 years	11.6	12.2	15.4	15.6	15.2	13.4	13.8	13.9
25–34 years	9.1	10.0	14.1	16.0	15.2	12.0	12.7	12.7
35–44 years	14.3	14.2	16.9	15.4	15.3	14.5	14.9	15.0
45–64 years	23.5	22.0	20.6	15.9	15.3	13.5	15.0	15.4
45–54 years	20.9	20.7	20.0	15.9	14.8	14.4	15.9	16.6
55–64 years	26.8	23.7	21.4	15.9	16.0	12.1	13.8	13.8
65 years and over	30.0	24.5	20.8	17.6	20.5	15.2	14.6	14.3
65–74 years	29.6	23.0	20.8	16.9	17.9	12.5	12.7	12.3
75–84 years	31.1	27.9	21.2	19.1	24.9	17.6	16.4	16.3
85 years and over	28.8	26.0	19.0	19.2	22.2	19.6	16.9	16.4
Male								
All ages, age-adjusted[4]	21.2	20.0	19.8	19.9	21.5	17.7	18.0	18.0
All ages, crude	17.8	16.5	16.8	18.6	20.4	17.1	17.6	17.7
Under 1 year	. . .	. . .	. . .	. . .	. . .	. . .	*	*
1–4 years	. . .	. . .	. . .	. . .	. . .	. . .	*	*
5–14 years	0.3	0.4	0.5	0.6	1.1	1.2	0.9	0.9
15–24 years	6.5	8.2	13.5	20.2	22.0	17.1	16.0	16.8
15–19 years	3.5	5.6	8.8	13.8	18.1	13.0	11.6	12.6
20–24 years	9.3	11.5	19.3	26.8	25.7	21.4	20.2	20.8
25–44 years	17.2	17.9	20.9	24.0	24.4	21.3	21.9	21.7
25–34 years	13.4	14.7	19.8	25.0	24.8	19.6	20.6	20.4
35–44 years	21.3	21.0	22.1	22.5	23.9	22.8	23.2	23.0
45–64 years	37.1	34.4	30.0	23.7	24.3	21.3	23.5	23.7
45–54 years	32.0	31.6	27.9	22.9	23.2	22.4	24.4	24.8
55–64 years	43.6	38.1	32.7	24.5	25.7	19.4	22.3	22.1
65 years and over	52.8	44.0	38.4	35.0	41.6	31.1	29.8	29.0
65–74 years	50.5	39.6	36.0	30.4	32.2	22.7	23.4	22.6
75–84 years	58.3	52.5	42.8	42.3	56.1	38.6	35.1	34.8
85 years and over	58.3	57.4	42.4	50.6	65.9	57.5	47.8	45.0
Female								
All ages, age-adjusted[4]	5.6	5.6	7.4	5.7	4.8	4.0	4.2	4.5
All ages, crude	5.1	4.9	6.6	5.5	4.8	4.0	4.3	4.6
Under 1 year	. . .	. . .	. . .	. . .	. . .	. . .	*	*
1–4 years	. . .	. . .	. . .	. . .	. . .	. . .	*	*
5–14 years	0.1	0.1	0.2	0.2	0.4	0.3	0.3	0.5
15–24 years	2.6	2.2	4.2	4.3	3.9	3.0	3.0	3.6
15–19 years	1.8	1.6	2.9	3.0	3.7	2.7	2.7	3.5
20–24 years	3.3	2.9	5.7	5.5	4.1	3.2	3.4	3.6
25–44 years	6.2	6.6	10.2	7.7	6.2	5.4	5.7	6.0
25–34 years	4.9	5.5	8.6	7.1	5.6	4.3	4.6	4.7
35–44 years	7.5	7.7	11.9	8.5	6.8	6.4	6.6	7.1
45–64 years	9.9	10.2	12.0	8.9	7.1	6.2	7.0	7.6
45–54 years	9.9	10.2	12.6	9.4	6.9	6.7	7.7	8.6
55–64 years	9.9	10.2	11.4	8.4	7.3	5.4	5.9	6.1
65 years and over	9.4	8.4	8.1	6.1	6.4	4.0	3.8	3.8
65–74 years	10.1	8.4	9.0	6.5	6.7	4.0	3.8	3.8
75–84 years	8.1	8.9	7.0	5.5	6.3	4.0	4.0	3.9
85 years and over	8.2	6.0	5.9	5.5	5.4	4.2	3.3	3.6
White male[5]								
All ages, age-adjusted[4]	22.3	21.1	20.8	20.9	22.8	19.1	19.6	19.6
All ages, crude	19.0	17.6	18.0	19.9	22.0	18.8	19.5	19.6
15–24 years	6.6	8.6	13.9	21.4	23.2	17.9	16.9	17.9
25–44 years	17.9	18.5	21.5	24.6	25.4	22.9	23.9	23.8
45–64 years	39.3	36.5	31.9	25.0	26.0	23.2	26.1	26.1
65 years and over	55.8	46.7	41.1	37.2	44.2	33.3	32.1	31.2
65–74 years	53.2	42.0	38.7	32.5	34.2	24.3	25.2	24.2
75–84 years	61.9	55.7	45.5	45.5	60.2	41.1	37.5	37.1
85 years and over	61.9	61.3	45.8	52.8	70.3	61.6	51.4	48.4

See footnotes at end of table.

This table will be updated on the Web. Go to www.cdc.gov/nchs/hus.htm.

Table 46 (page 2 of 3). Death rates for suicide, by sex, race, Hispanic origin, and age: United States, selected years 1950–2004

[Data are based on death certificates]

Sex, race, Hispanic origin, and age	1950[1,2]	1960[1,2]	1970[2]	1980[2]	1990	2000[3]	2003	2004
	Deaths per 100,000 resident population							
Black or African American male[5]								
All ages, age-adjusted[4]	7.5	8.4	10.0	11.4	12.8	10.0	9.2	9.6
All ages, crude	6.3	6.4	8.0	10.3	12.0	9.4	8.8	9.0
15–24 years	4.9	4.1	10.5	12.3	15.1	14.2	12.1	12.2
25–44 years	9.8	12.6	16.1	19.2	19.6	14.3	14.3	13.7
45–64 years	12.7	13.0	12.4	11.8	13.1	9.9	9.0	10.1
65 years and over	9.0	9.9	8.7	11.4	14.9	11.5	9.2	11.3
65–74 years	10.0	11.3	8.7	11.1	14.7	11.1	8.3	9.8
75–84 years[6]	*	*	*	10.5	14.4	12.1	11.3	15.0
85 years and over	- - -	*	*	*	*	*	*	*
American Indian or Alaska Native male[5]								
All ages, age-adjusted[4]	- - -	- - -	- - -	19.3	20.1	16.0	16.6	18.7
All ages, crude	- - -	- - -	- - -	20.9	20.9	15.9	17.1	19.5
15–24 years	- - -	- - -	- - -	45.3	49.1	26.2	27.2	30.7
25–44 years	- - -	- - -	- - -	31.2	27.8	24.5	30.1	30.8
45–64 years	- - -	- - -	- - -	*	*	15.4	9.5	16.0
65 years and over	- - -	- - -	- - -	*	*	*	*	*
Asian or Pacific Islander male[5]								
All ages, age-adjusted[4]	- - -	- - -	- - -	10.7	9.6	8.6	8.5	8.4
All ages, crude	- - -	- - -	- - -	8.8	8.7	7.9	8.0	7.9
15–24 years	- - -	- - -	- - -	10.8	13.5	9.1	9.0	9.3
25–44 years	- - -	- - -	- - -	11.0	10.6	9.9	9.2	8.4
45–64 years	- - -	- - -	- - -	13.0	9.7	9.7	10.0	11.1
65 years and over	- - -	- - -	- - -	18.6	16.8	15.4	17.5	15.1
Hispanic or Latino male[5,7]								
All ages, age-adjusted[4]	- - -	- - -	- - -	- - -	13.7	10.3	9.7	9.8
All ages, crude	- - -	- - -	- - -	- - -	11.4	8.4	8.3	8.6
15–24 years	- - -	- - -	- - -	- - -	14.7	10.9	11.2	12.8
25–44 years	- - -	- - -	- - -	- - -	16.2	11.2	10.9	11.0
45–64 years	- - -	- - -	- - -	- - -	16.1	12.0	12.0	11.8
65 years and over	- - -	- - -	- - -	- - -	23.4	19.5	15.6	15.9
White, not Hispanic or Latino male[7]								
All ages, age-adjusted[4]	- - -	- - -	- - -	- - -	23.5	20.2	21.0	21.0
All ages, crude	- - -	- - -	- - -	- - -	23.1	20.4	21.6	21.6
15–24 years	- - -	- - -	- - -	- - -	24.4	19.5	18.2	19.0
25–44 years	- - -	- - -	- - -	- - -	26.4	25.1	26.8	26.8
45–64 years	- - -	- - -	- - -	- - -	26.8	24.0	27.4	27.4
65 years and over	- - -	- - -	- - -	- - -	45.4	33.9	33.1	32.1
White female[5]								
All ages, age-adjusted[4]	6.0	5.9	7.9	6.1	5.2	4.3	4.6	5.0
All ages, crude	5.5	5.3	7.1	5.9	5.3	4.4	4.7	5.1
15–24 years	2.7	2.3	4.2	4.6	4.2	3.1	3.1	3.8
25–44 years	6.6	7.0	11.0	8.1	6.6	6.0	6.4	6.6
45–64 years	10.6	10.9	13.0	9.6	7.7	6.9	7.8	8.5
65 years and over	9.9	8.8	8.5	6.4	6.8	4.3	4.0	4.0
Black or African American female[5]								
All ages, age-adjusted[4]	1.8	2.0	2.9	2.4	2.4	1.8	1.9	1.8
All ages, crude	1.5	1.6	2.6	2.2	2.3	1.7	1.8	1.8
15–24 years	1.8	*	3.8	2.3	2.3	2.2	2.0	2.2
25–44 years	2.3	3.0	4.8	4.3	3.8	2.6	2.8	2.9
45–64 years	2.7	3.1	2.9	2.5	2.9	2.1	2.4	2.2
65 years and over	*	*	2.6	*	1.9	1.3	1.4	*

See footnotes at end of table.

This table will be updated on the Web. Go to www.cdc.gov/nchs/hus.htm.

Table 46 (page 3 of 3). Death rates for suicide, by sex, race, Hispanic origin, and age: United States, selected years 1950–2004

[Data are based on death certificates]

Sex, race, Hispanic origin, and age	1950[1,2]	1960[1,2]	1970[2]	1980[2]	1990	2000[3]	2003	2004
	Deaths per 100,000 resident population							
American Indian or Alaska Native female[5]								
All ages, age-adjusted[4]	---	---	---	4.7	3.6	3.8	3.5	5.9
All ages, crude	---	---	---	4.7	3.7	4.0	3.7	6.2
15–24 years	---	---	---	*	*	*	8.3	10.5
25–44 years	---	---	---	10.7	*	7.2	4.6	9.8
45–64 years	---	---	---	*	*	*	*	*
65 years and over	---	---	---	*	*	*	*	*
Asian or Pacific Islander female[5]								
All ages, age-adjusted[4]	---	---	---	5.5	4.1	2.8	3.1	3.5
All ages, crude	---	---	---	4.7	3.4	2.7	3.1	3.4
15–24 years	---	---	---	*	3.9	2.7	3.4	2.8
25–44 years	---	---	---	5.4	3.8	3.3	3.4	4.1
45–64 years	---	---	---	7.9	5.0	3.2	4.3	4.5
65 years and over	---	---	---	*	8.5	5.2	4.6	6.4
Hispanic or Latino female[5,7]								
All ages, age-adjusted[4]	---	---	---	---	2.3	1.7	1.7	2.0
All ages, crude	---	---	---	---	2.2	1.5	1.5	1.8
15–24 years	---	---	---	---	3.1	2.0	2.2	2.5
25–44 years	---	---	---	---	3.1	2.1	2.0	2.3
45–64 years	---	---	---	---	2.5	2.5	2.4	3.1
65 years and over	---	---	---	---	*	*	*	1.8
White, not Hispanic or Latino female[7]								
All ages, age-adjusted[4]	---	---	---	---	5.4	4.7	5.0	5.4
All ages, crude	---	---	---	---	5.6	4.9	5.3	5.7
15–24 years	---	---	---	---	4.3	3.3	3.3	4.0
25–44 years	---	---	---	---	7.0	6.7	7.2	7.5
45–64 years	---	---	---	---	8.0	7.3	8.3	9.1
65 years and over	---	---	---	---	7.0	4.4	4.2	4.1

. . . Category not applicable.

* Rates based on fewer than 20 deaths are considered unreliable and are not shown.

- - - Data not available.

[1]Includes deaths of persons who were not residents of the 50 states and the District of Columbia.

[2]Underlying cause of death was coded according to the Sixth Revision of the International Classification of Diseases (ICD) in 1950, Seventh Revision in 1960, Eighth Revision in 1970, and Ninth Revision in 1980–1998. See Appendix II, Cause of death; Tables IV and V.

[3]Starting with 1999 data, cause of death is coded according to ICD–10. See Appendix II, Cause of death, Table V; Comparability ratio, Table VI.

[4]Age-adjusted rates are calculated using the year 2000 standard population. Prior to 2003, age-adjusted rates were calculated using standard million proportions based on rounded population numbers. Starting with 2003 data, unrounded population numbers are used to calculate age-adjusted rates. See Appendix II, Age adjustment.

[5]The race groups, white, black, Asian or Pacific Islander, and American Indian or Alaska Native, include persons of Hispanic and non-Hispanic origin. Persons of Hispanic origin may be of any race. Death rates for the American Indian or Alaska Native and Asian or Pacific Islander populations are known to be underestimated. See Appendix II, Race, for a discussion of sources of bias in death rates by race and Hispanic origin.

[6]In 1950, rate is for the age group 75 years and over.

[7]Prior to 1997, excludes data from states lacking an Hispanic-origin item on the death certificate. See Appendix II, Hispanic origin.

NOTES: Starting with *Health, United States, 2003*, rates for 1991–1999 were revised using intercensal population estimates based on the 2000 census. Rates for 2000 were revised based on 2000 census counts. Rates for 2001 and later years were computed using 2000-based postcensal estimates. See Appendix I, Population Census and Population Estimates. Figures for 2001 include September 11-related deaths for which death certificates were filed as of October 24, 2002. See Appendix II, Cause of death; Table V for terrorism-related ICD–10 codes. Age groups were selected to minimize the presentation of unstable age-specific death rates based on small numbers of deaths and for consistency among comparison groups. For additional injury-related statistics, see Web-based Injury Statistics Query and Reporting System, available from:www.cdc.gov/ncipc/wisqars. In 2003, seven states reported multiple-race data. In 2004, 15 states reported multiple-race data. The multiple-race data for these states were bridged to the single-race categories of the 1977 Office of Management and Budget standards for comparability with other states. See Appendix II, Race. Data for additional years are available. See Appendix III.

SOURCES: Centers for Disease Control and Prevention, National Center for Health Statistics, National Vital Statistics System; Grove RD, Hetzel AM. Vital statistics rates in the United States, 1940–1960. Washington, DC: U.S. Government Printing Office. 1968; numerator data from National Vital Statistics System, annual mortality files; denominator data from national population estimates for race groups from Table 1 and unpublished Hispanic population estimates for 1985–1996 prepared by the Housing and Household Economic Statistics Division, U.S. Census Bureau; additional mortality tables are available from: www.cdc.gov/nchs/datawh/statab/unpubd/mortabs.htm; Miniño AM, Heron M, Murphy SL, Kochanek KD. Deaths: Final data for 2004. Health E-Stats. Hyattsville, MD: National Center for Health Statistics. 2006.

This table will be updated on the Web. Go to www.cdc.gov/nchs/hus.htm.

Table 47 (page 1 of 3). Death rates for firearm-related injuries, by sex, race, Hispanic origin, and age: United States, selected years 1970–2004

[Data are based on death certificates]

Sex, race, Hispanic origin, and age	1970[1]	1980[1]	1990	1995	2000[2]	2002	2003	2004
	Deaths per 100,000 resident population							
All persons								
All ages, age-adjusted[3]	14.3	14.8	14.6	13.4	10.2	10.4	10.3	10.0
All ages, crude	13.1	14.9	14.9	13.5	10.2	10.5	10.4	10.1
Under 1 year	*	*	*	*	*	*	*	*
1–14 years	1.6	1.4	1.5	1.6	0.7	0.7	0.7	0.6
1–4 years	1.0	0.7	0.6	0.6	0.3	0.4	0.3	0.3
5–14 years	1.7	1.6	1.9	1.9	0.9	0.8	0.8	0.7
15–24 years	15.5	20.6	25.8	26.7	16.8	16.7	16.6	15.7
15–19 years	11.4	14.7	23.3	24.1	12.9	12.1	12.1	12.0
20–24 years	20.3	26.4	28.1	29.2	20.9	21.3	21.1	19.3
25–44 years	20.9	22.5	19.3	16.9	13.1	13.7	13.4	13.1
25–34 years	22.2	24.3	21.8	19.6	14.5	15.4	15.5	15.0
35–44 years	19.6	20.0	16.3	14.3	11.9	12.1	11.5	11.3
45–64 years	17.6	15.2	13.6	11.7	10.0	10.6	10.7	10.5
45–54 years	18.1	16.4	13.9	12.0	10.5	10.8	11.2	11.0
55–64 years	17.0	13.9	13.3	11.3	9.4	10.2	10.1	9.8
65 years and over	13.8	13.5	16.0	14.1	12.2	12.4	11.8	11.5
65–74 years	14.5	13.8	14.4	12.8	10.6	10.9	10.4	10.2
75–84 years	13.4	13.4	19.4	16.3	13.9	14.4	13.5	13.3
85 years and over	10.2	11.6	14.7	14.4	14.2	12.5	12.5	11.9
Male								
All ages, age-adjusted[3]	24.8	25.9	26.1	23.8	18.1	18.6	18.4	17.7
All ages, crude	22.2	25.7	26.2	23.6	17.8	18.4	18.3	17.6
Under 1 year	*	*	*	*	*	*	*	*
1–14 years	2.3	2.0	2.2	2.3	1.1	1.0	1	0.9
1–4 years	1.2	0.9	0.7	0.8	0.4	0.5	0.3	0.4
5–14 years	2.7	2.5	2.9	2.9	1.4	1.2	1.2	1.1
15–24 years	26.4	34.8	44.7	46.5	29.4	29.3	29.2	27.5
15–19 years	19.2	24.5	40.1	41.6	22.4	21.1	21.2	20.7
20–24 years	35.1	45.2	49.1	51.5	37.0	37.6	37.1	34.2
25–44 years	34.1	38.1	32.6	28.4	22.0	23.1	22.9	22.3
25–34 years	36.5	41.4	37.0	33.2	24.9	26.5	27.1	26.1
35–44 years	31.6	33.2	27.4	23.6	19.4	20.1	19.1	18.7
45–64 years	31.0	25.9	23.4	20.0	17.1	18.1	18.3	17.8
45–54 years	30.7	27.3	23.2	20.1	17.6	18.2	18.8	18.3
55–64 years	31.3	24.5	23.7	19.8	16.3	18.0	17.7	17.1
65 years and over	29.7	29.7	35.3	30.7	26.4	26.9	25.4	24.8
65–74 years	29.5	27.8	28.2	25.1	20.3	21.3	20.3	19.7
75–84 years	31.0	33.0	46.9	37.8	32.2	32.9	30.2	29.8
85 years and over	26.2	34.9	49.3	47.1	44.7	38.9	37.8	35.9
Female								
All ages, age-adjusted[3]	4.8	4.7	4.2	3.8	2.8	2.8	2.7	2.7
All ages, crude	4.4	4.7	4.3	3.8	2.8	2.8	2.7	2.7
Under 1 year	*	*	*	*	*	*	*	*
1–14 years	0.8	0.7	0.8	0.8	0.3	0.5	0.3	0.3
1–4 years	0.9	0.5	0.5	0.5	*	0.3	0.3	0.3
5–14 years	0.8	0.7	1.0	0.9	0.4	0.5	0.3	0.3
15–24 years	4.8	6.1	6.0	5.9	3.5	3.5	3.3	3.2
15–19 years	3.5	4.6	5.7	5.6	2.9	2.7	2.4	2.9
20–24 years	6.4	7.7	6.3	6.1	4.2	4.2	4.2	3.5
25–44 years	8.3	7.4	6.1	5.5	4.2	4.1	3.8	3.8
25–34 years	8.4	7.5	6.7	5.8	4.0	4.0	3.6	3.7
35–44 years	8.2	7.2	5.4	5.2	4.4	4.2	4.0	3.9
45–64 years	5.4	5.4	4.5	3.9	3.4	3.4	3.4	3.7
45–54 years	6.4	6.2	4.9	4.2	3.6	3.6	3.8	4.0
55–64 years	4.2	4.6	4.0	3.5	3.0	3.1	2.9	3.1
65 years and over	2.4	2.5	3.1	2.8	2.2	2.0	2.1	2.0
65–74 years	2.8	3.1	3.6	3.0	2.5	2.3	2.2	2.2
75–84 years	1.7	1.7	2.9	2.8	2.0	2.1	2.2	2.3
85 years and over	*	1.3	1.3	1.8	1.7	1.1	1.3	1.0
White male[4]								
All ages, age-adjusted[3]	19.7	22.1	22.0	20.1	15.9	16.2	16.0	15.4
All ages, crude	17.6	21.8	21.8	19.9	15.6	16.1	16.0	15.5
1–14 years	1.8	1.9	1.9	1.9	1.0	0.8	0.7	0.7
15–24 years	16.9	28.4	29.5	30.8	19.6	19.4	19.2	18.4
25–44 years	24.2	29.5	25.7	23.2	18.0	18.5	18.1	17.6
25–34 years	24.3	31.1	27.8	25.2	18.1	18.5	18.8	18.2
35–44 years	24.1	27.1	23.3	21.2	17.9	18.5	17.5	17.1
45–64 years	27.4	23.3	22.8	19.5	17.4	18.7	19.0	18.4
65 years and over	29.9	30.1	36.8	32.2	28.2	28.9	27.4	26.5

See footnotes at end of table.

This table will be updated on the Web. Go to www.cdc.gov/nchs/hus.htm.

Table 47 (page 2 of 3). Death rates for firearm-related injuries, by sex, race, Hispanic origin, and age: United States, selected years 1970–2004

[Data are based on death certificates]

Sex, race, Hispanic origin, and age	*1970*[1]	*1980*[1]	*1990*	*1995*	*2000*[2]	*2002*	*2003*	*2004*
Black or African American male[4]			Deaths per 100,000 resident population					
All ages, age-adjusted[3]	70.8	60.1	56.3	49.2	34.2	36.0	35.6	34.5
All ages, crude	60.8	57.7	61.9	52.9	36.1	37.8	37.8	36.4
1–14 years	5.3	3.0	4.4	4.4	1.8	1.8	2.1	2.0
15–24 years	97.3	77.9	138.0	138.7	89.3	87.1	87.6	80.7
25–44 years	126.2	114.1	90.3	70.2	54.1	60.6	60.5	59.2
25–34 years	145.6	128.4	108.6	92.3	74.8	85.6	87.2	83.6
35–44 years	104.2	92.3	66.1	46.3	34.3	36.9	34.8	35.1
45–64 years	71.1	55.6	34.5	28.3	18.4	18.6	18.1	18.3
65 years and over	30.6	29.7	23.9	21.8	13.8	14.2	12.1	14.6
American Indian or Alaska Native male[4]								
All ages, age-adjusted[3]	- - -	24.0	19.4	19.4	13.1	14.8	14.1	14.2
All ages, crude	- - -	27.5	20.5	20.9	13.2	15.3	14.7	15.0
15–24 years	- - -	55.3	49.1	40.9	26.9	30.0	27.6	25.7
25–44 years	- - -	43.9	25.4	31.2	16.6	21.7	21.8	23.5
45–64 years	- - -	*	*	14.2	12.2	12.4	10.5	9.5
65 years and over	- - -	*	*	*	*	*	*	*
Asian or Pacific Islander male[4]								
All ages, age-adjusted[3]	- - -	7.8	8.8	9.2	6.0	5.5	5.4	4.8
All ages, crude	- - -	8.2	9.4	10.0	6.2	5.7	5.7	5.0
15–24 years	- - -	10.8	21.0	24.3	9.3	11.7	10.5	8.8
25–44 years	- - -	12.8	10.9	10.6	8.1	6.3	6.9	5.7
45–64 years	- - -	10.4	8.1	8.2	7.4	5.8	5.7	6.1
65 years and over	- - -	*	*	*	*	*	*	4.2
Hispanic or Latino male[4,5]								
All ages, age-adjusted[3]	- - -	- - -	27.6	23.8	13.6	13.4	13.6	13.1
All ages, crude	- - -	- - -	29.9	26.2	14.2	14.2	14.6	13.9
1–14 years	- - -	- - -	2.6	2.8	1.0	0.9	0.8	0.7
15–24 years	- - -	- - -	55.5	61.7	30.8	32.1	32.8	32.4
25–44 years	- - -	- - -	42.7	31.4	17.3	17.6	18.6	17.6
25–34 years	- - -	- - -	47.3	36.4	20.3	21.2	22.8	21.3
35–44 years	- - -	- - -	35.4	24.2	13.2	12.9	13.3	12.9
45–64 years	- - -	- - -	21.4	17.2	12.0	9.9	10.3	9.9
65 years and over	- - -	- - -	19.1	16.5	12.2	12.3	10.6	10.0
White, not Hispanic or Latino male[5]								
All ages, age-adjusted[3]	- - -	- - -	20.6	18.6	15.5	16.0	15.6	15.1
All ages, crude	- - -	- - -	20.4	18.5	15.7	16.3	16.0	15.6
1–14 years	- - -	- - -	1.6	1.6	1.0	0.7	0.7	0.7
15–24 years	- - -	- - -	24.1	23.5	16.2	15.6	15.2	14.3
25–44 years	- - -	- - -	23.3	21.4	17.9	18.4	17.7	17.4
25–34 years	- - -	- - -	24.7	22.5	17.2	17.4	17.3	16.9
35–44 years	- - -	- - -	21.6	20.4	18.4	19.3	18.1	17.8
45–64 years	- - -	- - -	22.7	19.5	17.8	19.4	19.8	19.2
65 years and over	- - -	- - -	37.4	32.5	29.0	29.8	28.4	27.6
White female[4]								
All ages, age-adjusted[3]	4.0	4.2	3.8	3.5	2.7	2.7	2.6	2.7
All ages, crude	3.7	4.1	3.8	3.5	2.7	2.7	2.6	2.7
15–24 years	3.4	5.1	4.8	4.5	2.8	2.6	2.5	2.6
25–44 years	6.9	6.2	5.3	4.9	3.9	3.8	3.6	3.6
45–64 years	5.0	5.1	4.5	4.0	3.5	3.6	3.7	3.9
65 years and over	2.2	2.5	3.1	2.8	2.4	2.2	2.1	2.2

See footnotes at end of table.

This table will be updated on the Web. Go to www.cdc.gov/nchs/hus.htm.

Table 47 (page 3 of 3). Death rates for firearm-related injuries, by sex, race, Hispanic origin, and age: United States, selected years 1970–2004

[Data are based on death certificates]

Sex, race, Hispanic origin, and age	*1970*[1]	*1980*[1]	*1990*	*1995*	*2000*[2]	*2002*	*2003*	*2004*
Black or African American female[4]				Deaths per 100,000 resident population				
All ages, age-adjusted[3]	11.1	8.7	7.3	6.2	3.9	4.1	3.8	3.6
All ages, crude	10.0	8.8	7.8	6.5	4.0	4.2	3.9	3.7
15–24 years	15.2	12.3	13.3	13.2	7.6	8.1	7.4	6.9
25–44 years	19.4	16.1	12.4	9.8	6.5	6.7	6.1	5.7
45–64 years	10.2	8.2	4.8	4.1	3.1	3.0	2.7	3.0
65 years and over	4.3	3.1	3.1	2.6	1.3	1.2	1.8	*
American Indian or Alaska Native female[4]								
All ages, age-adjusted[3]	- - -	5.8	3.3	3.8	2.9	3.1	2.4	2.7
All ages, crude	- - -	5.8	3.4	4.1	2.9	3.4	2.6	2.9
15–24 years	- - -	*	*	*	*	*	*	*
25–44 years	- - -	10.2	*	7.0	5.5	*	*	*
45–64 years	- - -	*	*	*	*	*	*	*
65 years and over	- - -	*	*	*	*	*	*	*
Asian or Pacific Islander female[4]								
All ages, age-adjusted[3]	- - -	2.0	1.9	2.0	1.1	1.1	1.1	0.9
All ages, crude	- - -	2.1	2.1	2.1	1.2	1.2	1.2	1.0
15–24 years	- - -	*	*	3.9	*	*	2.1	*
25–44 years	- - -	3.2	2.7	2.7	1.5	1.7	1.3	1.4
45–64 years	- - -	*	*	*	*	*	1.5	1.3
65 years and over	- - -	*	*	*	*	*	*	*
Hispanic or Latino female[4,5]								
All ages, age-adjusted[3]	- - -	- - -	3.3	3.1	1.8	1.6	1.6	1.5
All ages, crude	- - -	- - -	3.6	3.3	1.8	1.6	1.7	1.5
15–24 years	- - -	- - -	6.9	6.1	2.9	2.8	3.5	2.6
25–44 years	- - -	- - -	5.1	4.7	2.5	2.4	2.2	2.2
45–64 years	- - -	- - -	2.4	2.4	2.2	1.6	1.5	1.5
65 years and over	- - -	- - -	*	*	*	*	*	*
White, not Hispanic or Latino female[5]								
All ages, age-adjusted[3]	- - -	- - -	3.7	3.4	2.8	2.8	2.7	2.8
All ages, crude	- - -	- - -	3.7	3.5	2.9	2.8	2.7	2.9
15–24 years	- - -	- - -	4.3	4.1	2.7	2.5	2.2	2.5
25–44 years	- - -	- - -	5.1	4.8	4.2	4.1	3.9	3.9
45–64 years	- - -	- - -	4.6	4.1	3.6	3.8	3.9	4.1
65 years and over	- - -	- - -	3.2	2.8	2.4	2.3	2.2	2.3

* Rates based on fewer than 20 deaths are considered unreliable and are not shown.
- - - Data not available.
[1]Underlying cause of death was coded according to the Eighth Revision in 1970 and Ninth Revision in 1980–1998. See Appendix II, Cause of death; Tables IV and V.
[2]Starting with 1999 data, cause of death is coded according to ICD–10. See Appendix II, Cause of death, Table V; Comparability ratio, Table VI.
[3]Age-adjusted rates are calculated using the year 2000 standard population. Prior to 2003, age-adjusted rates were calculated using standard million proportions based on rounded population numbers. Starting with 2003 data, unrounded population numbers are used to calculate age-adjusted rates. See Appendix II, Age adjustment.
[4]The race groups, white, black, Asian or Pacific Islander, and American Indian or Alaska Native, include persons of Hispanic and non-Hispanic origin. Persons of Hispanic origin may be of any race. Death rates for the American Indian or Alaska Native and Asian or Pacific Islander populations are known to be underestimated. See Appendix II, Race, for a discussion of sources of bias in death rates by race and Hispanic origin.
[5]Prior to 1997, excludes data from states lacking an Hispanic-origin item on the death certificate. See Appendix II, Hispanic origin.

NOTES: Starting with *Health, United States, 2003*, rates for 1991–1999 were revised using intercensal population estimates based on the 2000 census. Rates for 2000 were revised based on 2000 census counts. Rates for 2001 and later years were computed using 2000-based postcensal estimates. See Appendix I, Population Census and Population Estimates. Age groups were selected to minimize the presentation of unstable age-specific death rates based on small numbers of deaths and for consistency among comparison groups. For additional injury-related statistics, see Web-based Injury Statistics Query and Reporting System, available from: www.cdc.gov/ncipc/wisqars. In 2003, seven states reported multiple-race data. In 2004, 15 states reported multiple-race data. The multiple-race data for these states were bridged to the single-race categories of the 1977 Office of Management and Budget standards for comparability with other states. See Appendix II, Race. Data for additional years are available. See Appendix III.

SOURCES: Centers for Disease Control and Prevention, National Center for Health Statistics, National Vital Statistics System; numerator data from annual mortality files; denominator data from national population estimates for race groups from Table 1 and unpublished Hispanic population estimates for 1985–1996 prepared by the Housing and Household Economic Statistics Division, U.S. Census Bureau; additional mortality tables are available from: www.cdc.gov/nchs/datawh/statab/unpubd/mortabs.htm; Miniño AM, Heron M, Murphy SL, Kochanek KD. Deaths: Final data for 2004. Health E-Stats. Hyattsville, MD: National Center for Health Statistics. 2006.

This table will be updated on the Web. Go to www.cdc.gov/nchs/hus.htm.

Table 48. Deaths from selected occupational diseases among persons 15 years of age and over: United States, selected years 1980–2004

[Data are based on death certificates]

Cause of death[1]	*1980*[2]	*1985*	*1990*	*1995*	*2000*[3]	*2002*	*2003*	*2004*
Underlying and nonunderlying cause of death	Number of death certificates with cause of death code(s) mentioned							
Angiosarcoma of liver[4]	- - -	- - -	- - -	- - -	16	23	24	21
Malignant mesothelioma[5]	699	715	874	897	2,531	2,573	2,625	2,657
Pneumoconiosis[6]	4,151	3,783	3,644	3,151	2,859	2,715	2,635	2,524
Coal workers' pneumoconiosis	2,576	2,615	1,990	1,413	949	858	772	703
Asbestosis	339	534	948	1,169	1,486	1,467	1,464	1,460
Silicosis	448	334	308	242	151	146	177	165
Other (including unspecified)	814	321	413	343	290	263	236	214
Underlying cause of death	Number of deaths							
Angiosarcoma of liver[4]	- - -	- - -	- - -	- - -	15	20	20	21
Malignant mesothelioma[5]	531	573	725	780	2,384	2,429	2,476	2,504
Pneumoconiosis	1,581	1,355	1,335	1,117	1,142	1,094	1,101	1,013
Coal workers' pneumoconiosis	982	958	734	533	389	354	318	292
Asbestosis	101	139	302	355	558	529	583	542
Silicosis	207	143	150	114	71	89	102	76
Other (including unspecified)	291	115	149	115	124	122	98	103

- - - Data not available.

[1]Cause-of-death titles for selected occupational diseases and corresponding code numbers according to the *International Classification of Diseases*, Ninth and Tenth Revisions. See Appendix II, Cause of death; Table IV.

Cause of death	*ICD–9 code*	*ICD–10 code*
Angiosarcoma of liver	- - -	C22.3
Malignant mesothelioma	158.8,158.9,163	C45
Pneumoconiosis	500–505	J60–J66
Coal workers' pneumoconiosis	500	J60
Asbestosis	501	J61
Silicosis	502	J62
Other (including unspecified)	503–505	J63–J66

[2]For the period 1980–1998, underlying cause of death was coded according to the Ninth Revision of the International Classification of Diseases (ICD). See Appendix II, Cause of death; Tables IV and V.
[3]Starting with 1999 data, ICD–10 was introduced for coding cause of death. Discontinuities exist between 1998 and 1999 due to ICD–10 coding and classification changes. Caution should be exercised in interpreting trends for the causes of death in this table, especially for those with major ICD–10 changes (e.g., malignant mesothelioma). See Appendix II, *International Classification of Diseases* (ICD).
[4]Prior to 1999, there was no discrete code for this condition.
[5]Prior to 1999, the combined ICD–9 categories of malignant neoplasm of peritoneum and malignant neoplasm of pleura served as a crude surrogate for malignant mesothelioma category under ICD–10.
[6]For underlying and nonunderlying cause of death, counts for pneumoconiosis subgroups may sum to slightly more than total pneumoconiosis due to the reporting of more than one type of pneumoconiosis on some death certificates.

NOTES: See Appendix I, National Vital Statistics System, Multiple Cause of Death File, for information about tabulating cause-of-death data in this table. Selection of occupational diseases is based on definitions in Mullan RJ, Murthy LI. Occupational sentinel health events: An updated list for physician recognition and public health surveillance. 1991; Am J Ind Med 19(6):775–99. For more detailed information about pneumoconiosis deaths, see *Work-Related Lung Disease Surveillance Report 2002*, DHHS (NIOSH) Publication Number 2003–111 available from: www.cdc.gov/niosh/publistd.html. Data for additional years are available. See Appendix III.

SOURCE: Centers for Disease Control and Prevention, National Center for Health Statistics, National Vital Statistics System; annual mortality files for underlying and multiple cause of death.

This table will be updated on the Web. Go to www.cdc.gov/nchs/hus.htm.

Table 49 (page 1 of 2). Occupational injury deaths and rates, by industry, sex, age, race, and Hispanic origin: United States, selected years 1992–2005

[Data are compiled from various federal, state, and local administrative sources]

Characteristic	*1992*[1]	*1995*	*1999*	*2000*	*2001*[2]	*2002*	*2003*	*2004*	*2005*
					Deaths per 100,000 employed workers[3]				
Total work force	5.2	4.9	4.5	4.3	4.3	4.0	4.0	4.1	4.0
Sex									
Male	---	8.3	7.7	7.4	7.4	6.9	7.0	7.2	6.9
Female	---	0.9	0.7	0.7	0.7	0.7	0.7	0.6	0.6
Age									
16–17 years	---	1.6	1.6	1.6	1.3	1.1	1.2	1.1	1.4
18–19 years	---	3.3	2.7	2.7	2.8	2.2	2.3	2.8	2.9
20–24 years	---	3.8	3.4	3.3	3.2	3.2	3.4	3.1	2.8
25–34 years	---	4.3	3.8	3.8	3.8	3.3	3.4	3.3	3.3
35–44 years	---	4.6	4.1	4.0	4.1	4.0	3.8	3.9	3.6
45–54 years	---	5.2	4.6	4.4	4.5	4.0	4.1	4.3	4.2
55–64 years	---	7.2	6.1	6.1	5.5	5.0	4.8	5.2	5.1
65 years and over	---	14.0	14.6	12.0	12.7	11.5	11.3	11.8	11.3
Race and Hispanic origin[4]									
Hispanic or Latino	---	5.5	5.2	5.6	6.0	5.0	4.5	5.0	4.9
Not Hispanic or Latino	---	4.9	4.4	4.2	4.1	3.9	4.0	4.0	---
White	---	---	---	4.2	4.2	3.9	4.0	4.1	3.9
Black or African American	---	---	---	3.9	3.8	3.5	3.8	3.8	3.9
Industry[5]									
Private sector	---	---	---	---	---	---	4.2	4.4	4.3
Agriculture, forestry, fishing, and hunting	---	---	---	---	---	---	31.3	30.5	32.5
Mining	---	---	---	---	---	---	26.9	28.3	25.6
Utilities	---	---	---	---	---	---	14.3	6.1	3.6
Construction	---	---	---	---	---	---	11.7	12.0	11.1
Manufacturing	---	---	---	---	---	---	2.5	2.8	2.4
Wholesale trade	---	---	---	---	---	---	4.2	4.5	4.6
Retail trade	---	---	---	---	---	---	2.1	2.3	2.4
Transportation and warehousing	---	---	---	---	---	---	17.6	18.0	17.7
Information	---	---	---	---	---	---	1.8	1.7	2.0
Finance, insurance, real estate, and rental and leasing	---	---	---	---	---	---	1.4	1.2	1.0
Professional, scientific, management, and administrative	---	---	---	---	---	---	3.3	3.3	3.5
Educational, health and social services	---	---	---	---	---	---	0.8	0.8	0.8
Arts, entertainment, recreation, accommodation, and food services	---	---	---	---	---	---	2.4	2.2	1.8
Other services (except public administration)	---	---	---	---	---	---	2.8	3.0	3.0
Government[6]	---	---	---	---	---	---	2.7	2.5	2.4
					Number of deaths[7]				
Total work force	6,217	6,275	6,054	5,920	5,915	5,534	5,575	5,764	5,734
Sex									
Male	5,774	5,736	5,612	5,471	5,442	5,092	5,129	5,349	5,328
Female	443	539	442	449	473	442	446	415	406
Age									
Under 16 years	27	26	26	29	20	16	25	13	23
16–17 years	41	42	46	44	33	25	28	25	31
18–19 years	107	130	122	127	122	92	84	103	111
20–24 years	544	486	451	446	441	436	462	421	403
25–34 years	1,556	1,409	1,175	1,163	1,142	1,023	1,018	996	1,017
35–44 years	1,538	1,571	1,510	1,473	1,478	1,403	1,329	1,342	1,243
45–54 years	1,167	1,256	1,333	1,313	1,368	1,253	1,301	1,384	1,389
55–64 years	767	827	816	831	775	784	802	907	933
65 years and over	467	515	565	488	530	495	523	569	578
Unspecified	3	13	10	6	6	7	3	4	6

See footnotes at end of table.

Table 49 (page 2 of 2). Occupational injury deaths and rates, by industry, sex, age, race, and Hispanic origin: United States, selected years 1992–2005

[Data are compiled from various federal, state, and local administrative sources]

Characteristic	1992[1]	1995	1999	2000	2001[2]	2002	2003	2004	2005
Race and Hispanic origin					Number of deaths[8]				
White	5,173	5,120	4,990	---	---	---	---	---	---
Black or African American	624	697	626	---	---	---	---	---	---
Hispanic or Latino	533	619	730	815	895	841	794	902	923
Not Hispanic or Latino	5,684	5,656	5,324	5,105	5,020	4,693	4,781	4,862	4,809
White	4,712	4,599	4,410	4,244	4,175	3,926	3,988	4,066	3,977
Black or African American	618	684	616	575	565	491	543	546	584
American Indian or Alaska Native	36	27	54	33	48	40	42	28	50
Asian[8]	192	188	180	171	173	131	147	168	154
Native Hawaiian or Other Pacific Islander	---	---	---	14	9	9	11	12	9
Multiple races	---	---	---	---	6	4	3	4	---
Other races or not reported	126	158	64	68	44	92	47	38	35
Industry[5]									
Private sector	---	---	---	---	---	---	5,043	5,229	5,214
Agriculture, forestry, fishing, and hunting	---	---	---	---	---	---	709	669	715
Mining	---	---	---	---	---	---	141	152	159
Utilities	---	---	---	---	---	---	32	51	30
Construction	---	---	---	---	---	---	1,131	1,234	1,192
Manufacturing	---	---	---	---	---	---	420	463	393
Wholesale trade	---	---	---	---	---	---	191	205	209
Retail trade	---	---	---	---	---	---	344	377	400
Transportation and warehousing	---	---	---	---	---	---	808	840	885
Information	---	---	---	---	---	---	64	55	65
Finance, insurance, real estate, and rental and leasing	---	---	---	---	---	---	129	116	99
Professional, scientific, management, and administrative	---	---	---	---	---	---	453	452	482
Educational, health and social services	---	---	---	---	---	---	143	157	150
Arts, entertainment, recreation, accommodation, and food services	---	---	---	---	---	---	275	247	213
Other services (except public administration)	---	---	---	---	---	---	194	207	210
Government[6]	---	---	---	---	---	---	532	535	520

- - - Data not available.

[1]1992 and 1993 employment data by demographic characteristics are not available from the Current Population Survey (CPS) for calculation of rates.

[2]2,871 fatalities due to the September 11 terrorist attacks are not included.

[3]Numerator excludes deaths to workers under the age of 16 years. Starting with 2003 data, employment data in denominators are average annual estimates of employed civilians 16 years of age and over from the CPS; in prior years, data also included resident armed forces figures from the U.S. Census Bureau (1992–1998) and the Department of Defense (1999–2002). Starting with 2005 data, rates are taken directly from the U.S. Department of Labor, Bureau of Labor Statistics, Census of Fatal Occupational Injuries, 2005.

[4]Employment data for American Indian or Alaska Native workers and, prior to 2003, Asian or Pacific Islander workers, were not available for the calculation of rates. Employment data for non-Hispanic white and non-Hispanic black workers were not available before the year 2000. In 1999 and earlier years, the race groups white and black included persons of Hispanic and non-Hispanic origin.

[5]Starting with 2003 data, establishments were classified by industry according to the 2002 North American Industry Classification System (NAICS). Prior to 2003, the Standard Industrial Classification (SIC) system was used. Because of substantial differences between these systems, industry data classified by these two systems are not comparable. Industry data for 1992–2002 classified by SIC are available in *Health, United States, 2004*, Table 49 available from: www.cdc.gov/nchs/hus.htm. See Appendix II, Industry of employment.

[6]Includes fatalities to workers employed by governmental organizations, regardless of industry.

[7]Includes fatalities to all workers, regardless of age.

[8]In 1999 and earlier years, category also included Native Hawaiian or Other Pacific Islander.

NOTES: Fatalities and rates are based on revised data and may differ from originally published data from the Census of Fatal Occupational Injuries (CFOI). See Appendix I, Census of Fatal Occupational Injuries. CFOI began collecting fatality data in 1992. For data for prior years, see Centers for Disease Control and Prevention. Fatal Occupational Injuries—United States, 1980–1997. MMWR 2001;50(16):317–20, which reports trend data from the National Traumatic Occupational Fatalities (NTOF) surveillance system. NTOF was established at the National Institute of Occupational Safety and Health (NIOSH) to monitor occupational injury deaths through death certificates. Industry categories presented in this table differ from those shown in previous editions of *Health, United States.* Data for additional years are available. See Appendix III.

SOURCE: Department of Labor, Bureau of Labor Statistics, Census of Fatal Occupational Injuries. Revised annual data.

Table 50. Occupational injuries and illnesses with days away from work, job transfer, or restriction, by industry: United States, 2003–2005

[Data are based on employer records from a sample of business establishments]

Industry	Injuries and illnesses with days away from work, job transfer, or restriction					
	Cases per 100 full-time workers[1]			*Number of cases in thousands*[2]		
	2003	*2004*	*2005*	*2003*	*2004*	*2005*
Total private sector[3]	2.6	2.5	2.4	2,301.9	2,225.0	2,184.8
Agriculture, forestry, fishing, and hunting[4]	3.3	3.7	3.3	29.3	31.5	29.5
Mining	2.0	2.3	2.2	11.2	12.9	13.7
Utilities	2.2	2.5	2.4	12.2	14.1	12.9
Construction	3.6	3.4	3.4	218.0	212.2	222.5
Manufacturing	3.8	3.6	3.5	538.0	519.9	490.8
Wholesale trade	2.8	2.7	2.7	147.4	146.2	146.8
Retail trade	2.7	2.7	2.6	319.6	322.8	314.2
Transportation and warehousing	5.4	4.9	4.6	204.0	190.0	185.6
Information	1.1	1.1	1.1	30.8	31.1	30.9
Finance and insurance	0.4	0.3	0.4	21.3	18.4	19.1
Real estate and rental and leasing	2.1	1.9	2.1	35.6	33.4	37.1
Professional, scientific, and technical services	0.6	0.5	0.6	36.0	32.2	38.4
Management of companies and enterprises	1.6	1.5	1.3	25.1	23.4	20.8
Administrative and support and waste management and remediation services	2.4	2.2	2.0	96.7	94.9	89.5
Educational services	1.2	1.0	1.0	17.9	14.5	14.8
Health care and social assistance	3.1	2.9	2.8	337.9	322.8	318.4
Arts, entertainment, and recreation	2.9	3.1	2.9	34.1	35.2	34.1
Accommodation and food services	2.0	1.7	1.7	135.2	122.5	120.8
Other services, except public administration	1.7	1.6	1.5	51.7	47.0	44.8

[1]Incidence rate calculated as (N/EH) x 200,000, where N = total number of injuries and illnesses, EH = total hours worked by all employees during the calendar year, and 200,000 = base for 100 full-time equivalent employees working 40 hours per week, 50 weeks per year.
[2]Because of rounding, components may not add to total number of cases in private sector.
[3]Totals include data for industries not shown separately. Excludes self-employed, private households, and employees in federal, state, and local government agencies.
[4]Excludes farms with fewer than 11 employees.

NOTES: Starting with 2003 data, the Survey of Occupational Injuries and Illnesses began using the 2002 North American Industry Classification System (NAICS) to classify establishments by industry. Prior to 2003, the survey used the Standard Industrial Classification (SIC) system. Because of substantial differences between these systems, the data measured by these surveys are not directly comparable. See Appendix II, Industry of employment. Data for previous years are presented in *Health, United States, 2004*, Table 50. Available from: www.cdc.gov/nchs/hus.htm. See Appendix I, Survey of Occupational Injuries and Illnesses (SOII).

SOURCE: U.S. Department of Labor, Bureau of Labor Statistics, Survey of Occupational Injuries and Illnesses: Workplace injuries and illnesses, 2003, 2004, and 2005 editions. Summary News Release. 2004, 2005, and 2006. Available from: www.bls.gov/iif/home.htm.

Table 51 (page 1 of 2). Selected notifiable disease rates and number of cases: United States, selected years 1950–2005

[Data are based on reporting by state health departments]

Disease	1950	1960	1970	1980	1990	2000	2003	2004	2005
				Cases per 100,000 population					
Diphtheria	3.83	0.51	0.21	0.00	0.00	0.00	0.00	–	–
Haemophilus influenzae, invasive	- - -	- - -	- - -	- - -	- - -	0.51	0.70	0.72	0.78
Hepatitis A	- - -	- - -	27.87	12.84	12.64	4.91	2.66	1.95	1.53
Hepatitis B	- - -	- - -	4.08	8.39	8.48	2.95	2.61	2.14	1.78
Lyme disease	- - -	- - -	- - -	- - -	- - -	6.53	7.39	6.84	7.94
Meningococcal disease	- - -	- - -	1.23	1.25	0.99	0.83	0.61	0.47	0.42
Mumps	- - -	- - -	55.55	3.86	2.17	0.13	0.08	0.09	0.11
Pertussis (whooping cough)	79.82	8.23	2.08	0.76	1.84	2.88	4.04	8.88	8.72
Poliomyelitis, total	22.02	1.77	0.02	0.00	0.00	–	–	–	–
Paralytic[1]	- - -	1.40	0.02	0.00	0.00	–	–	–	0.00
Rocky Mountain spotted fever	- - -	- - -	0.19	0.52	0.26	0.18	0.38	0.60	0.66
Rubella (German measles)	- - -	- - -	27.75	1.72	0.45	0.06	0.00	–	–
Rubeola (measles)	211.01	245.42	23.23	5.96	11.17	0.03	0.02	0.01	0.02
Salmonellosis, excluding typhoid fever	- - -	3.85	10.84	14.88	19.54	14.51	15.16	14.51	15.43
Shigellosis	15.45	6.94	6.79	8.41	10.89	8.41	8.19	5.03	5.51
Tuberculosis[2]	- - -	30.83	18.28	12.25	10.33	6.01	5.17	4.99	4.80
Sexually transmitted diseases:[3]									
Syphilis[4]	146.02	68.78	45.26	30.51	54.32	11.20	11.79	11.38	11.33
Primary and secondary	16.73	9.06	10.89	12.06	20.26	2.12	2.47	2.72	2.97
Early latent	39.71	10.11	8.08	9.00	22.19	3.35	2.88	2.65	2.78
Late and late latent[5]	70.22	45.91	24.94	9.30	10.32	5.53	6.30	5.89	5.47
Congenital[6]	8.97	2.48	0.97	0.12	1.55	0.21	0.15	0.13	0.11
Chlamydia[7]	- - -	- - -	- - -	- - -	160.19	251.38	301.74	316.51	332.51
Gonorrhea[8]	192.50	145.40	297.22	445.10	276.43	128.67	115.23	112.42	115.64
Chancroid	3.34	0.94	0.70	0.30	1.69	0.03	0.02	0.01	0.01
				Number of cases					
Diphtheria	5,796	918	435	3	4	1	1	–	–
Haemophilus influenzae, invasive	- - -	- - -	- - -	- - -	- - -	1,398	2,013	2,085	2,304
Hepatitis A	- - -	- - -	56,797	29,087	31,441	13,397	7,653	5,683	4,488
Hepatitis B	- - -	- - -	8,310	19,015	21,102	8,036	7,526	6,212	5,119
Lyme disease	- - -	- - -	- - -	- - -	- - -	17,730	21,273	19,804	23,305
Meningococcal disease	- - -	- - -	2,505	2,840	2,451	2,256	1,756	1,361	1,245
Mumps	- - -	- - -	104,953	8,576	5,292	338	231	258	314
Pertussis (whooping cough)	120,718	14,809	4,249	1,730	4,570	7,867	11,647	25,827	25,616
Poliomyelitis, total	33,300	3,190	33	9	6	–	–	–	–
Paralytic[1]	- - -	2,525	31	9	6	–	–	–	1
Rocky Mountain spotted fever	- - -	- - -	380	1,163	651	495	1,091	1,713	1,936
Rubella (German measles)	- - -	- - -	56,552	3,904	1,125	176	7	10	11
Rubeola (measles)	319,124	441,703	47,351	13,506	27,786	86	56	37	66
Salmonellosis, excluding typhoid fever	- - -	6,929	22,096	33,715	48,603	39,574	43,657	42,197	45,322
Shigellosis	23,367	12,487	13,845	19,041	27,077	22,922	23,581	14,627	16,168
Tuberculosis[2]	- - -	55,494	37,137	27,749	25,701	16,377	14,874	14,517	14,097
Sexually transmitted diseases:[3]									
Syphilis[4]	217,558	122,538	91,382	68,832	135,590	31,618	34,289	33,419	33,278
Primary and secondary	23,939	16,145	21,982	27,204	50,578	5,979	7,177	7,980	8,724
Early latent	59,256	18,017	16,311	20,297	55,397	9,465	8,361	7,768	8,176
Late and late latent[5]	113,569	81,798	50,348	20,979	25,750	15,594	18,319	17,300	16,049
Congenital[6]	13,377	4,416	1,953	277	3,865	580	432	371	329
Chlamydia[7]	- - -	- - -	- - -	- - -	323,663	709,452	877,478	929,462	976,445
Gonorrhea[8]	286,746	258,933	600,072	1,004,029	690,042	363,136	335,104	330,132	339,593
Chancroid	4,977	1,680	1,416	788	4,212	78	54	30	17

See footnotes at end of table.

Table 51 (page 2 of 2). Selected notifiable disease rates and number of cases: United States, selected years 1950–2005

[Data are based on reporting by state health departments]

0.00 Rate greater than zero but less than 0.005.
– Quantity zero.
- - - Data not available.
[1]Data for 1986 and subsequent years may be updated due to retrospective case evaluations or late reports.
[2]Case reporting for tuberculosis began in 1953. Data prior to 1975 are not comparable with subsequent years because of changes in reporting criteria effective in 1975. 2005 data were updated through the Division of Tuberculosis Elimination, NCHHSTP, as of May 12, 2005.
[3]Starting with 1991, data include both civilian and military cases. Adjustments to the number of cases reported from state health departments were made for hardcopy forms and for electronic data submissions through June 7, 2006. For 1950, data for Alaska and Hawaii were not included.
[4]Includes stage of syphilis not stated.
[5]Includes cases of unknown duration.
[6]Starting with 1989, data reflect change in case definition introduced in 1988. All cases of congenitally acquired syphilis were reported through 1994; starting with 1995 data, only congenital syphilis for cases less than one year of age were reported. See STD Surveillance Report for congenital syphilis rates per 100,000 live births. In 2005, the rate was 8.0 congenital syphilis cases per 100,000 live births.
[7]Prior to 1994, chlamydia was not notifiable. In 1994–1999, cases for New York were exclusively reported by New York City. Starting with 2000 data, includes cases for the entire state.
[8]Data for 1994 do not include cases from Georgia.

NOTES: The total resident population was used to calculate all rates except sexually transmitted diseases (STD), which used the civilian resident population prior to 1991. STD rates for 1990–2002 have been revised and may differ from previous editions of *Health, United States*. Revised rates are due to revision of population estimates to incorporate bridged single-race estimates. 2004 population estimates were used to calculate 2005 rates. See Appendix I, Population census and Population estimates. Population data from those states where diseases were not notifiable or not available were excluded from the rate calculation. See Appendix I, National Notifiable Diseases Surveillance System, for information on underreporting of notifiable diseases. Data for additional years are available. See Appendix III.

SOURCES: Centers for Disease Control and Prevention. Summary of notifiable diseases, United States, 2005. MMWR 2007;54(53):2–92 and Centers for Disease Control and Prevention. Sexually transmitted disease surveillance, 2005. Atlanta, GA: U.S. Department of Health and Human Services, 2006.

Table 52 (page 1 of 2). Acquired immunodeficiency syndrome (AIDS) cases, by year of diagnosis and selected characteristics: United States, 2001–2005

[Data are based on reporting by state and the District of Columbia health departments]

Sex, race and Hispanic origin, age at diagnosis, and region of residence	Year of diagnosis					
	All years[1]	2001	2002	2003	2004	2005
	Estimated number of cases[2]					
All persons[3]	952,629	38,079	38,408	39,666	39,524	40,608
Male, 13 years and over	761,723	27,908	28,276	28,891	28,817	29,766
Female, 13 years and over	181,802	10,049	10,027	10,704	10,656	10,774
Children, under 13 years	9,101	121	105	71	50	68
Male, 13 years and over						
Hispanic origin and race:						
Not Hispanic or Latino:						
White	346,533	9,352	9,558	9,613	9,714	10,027
Black or African American	278,917	12,696	12,769	12,940	12,843	13,048
Asian or Pacific Islander	6,545	312	352	378	373	389
American Indian or Alaska Native	2,544	126	134	142	127	137
Hispanic or Latino[4]	124,598	5,255	5,274	5,646	5,579	5,949
Age at diagnosis:						
13–14 years	615	40	32	35	48	43
15–24 years	27,413	929	1,049	1,242	1,370	1,581
25–34 years	246,054	6,445	6,236	6,048	6,076	6,060
35–44 years	305,376	11,769	11,970	11,984	11,538	11,502
45–54 years	132,339	6,378	6,589	7,005	6,982	7,716
55–64 years	38,713	1,791	1,894	1,993	2,158	2,274
65 years and over	11,207	557	506	585	644	591
Female, 13 years and over						
Hispanic origin and race:						
Not Hispanic or Latino:						
White	37,390	1,637	1,702	1,629	1,800	1,747
Black or African American	112,999	6,684	6,717	7,237	7,108	7,093
Asian or Pacific Islander	1,060	60	74	84	97	92
American Indian or Alaska Native	662	40	47	44	59	45
Hispanic or Latino[4]	28,843	1,570	1,420	1,633	1,510	1,714
Age at diagnosis:						
13–14 years	447	42	35	44	35	44
15–24 years	12,671	642	673	662	674	701
25–34 years	62,013	2,799	2,650	2,737	2,607	2,470
35–44 years	67,825	3,938	3,790	4,150	3,989	3,954
45–54 years	27,342	1,975	2,110	2,269	2,455	2,637
55–64 years	8,204	490	586	633	695	757
65 years and over	3,297	163	183	210	201	211
Children, under 13 years						
Hispanic origin and race:						
Not Hispanic or Latino:						
White	1,613	13	14	12	6	6
Black or African American	5,631	85	72	46	31	46
Asian or Pacific Islander	54	1	1	–	1	1
American Indian or Alaska Native	32	–	1	–	1	–
Hispanic or Latino[4]	1,738	23	16	11	9	13
Region of residence						
Northeast	300,963	11,273	10,292	10,955	10,452	11,529
Midwest	97,930	3,929	4,126	4,282	4,225	4,862
South	359,725	16,571	17,301	18,014	18,761	18,115
West	194,011	6,306	6,689	6,414	6,086	6,102

See footnotes at end of table.

 Acquired immunodeficiency syndrome (AIDS) cases, by year of diagnosis and selected characteristics: United States, 2001–2005

[Data are based on reporting by state and the District of Columbia health departments]

Sex, race and Hispanic origin, age at diagnosis, and region of residence	All years[1]	2001	2002	2003	2004	2005
	Percent distribution[5]					
All persons[3]	100.0	100.0	100.0	100.0	100.0	100.0
Male, 13 years and over	80.0	73.3	73.6	72.8	72.9	73.3
Female, 13 years and over	19.1	26.4	26.1	27.0	27.0	26.5
Children, under 13 years	1.0	0.3	0.3	0.2	0.1	0.2
Male, 13 years and over						
Hispanic origin and race:						
Not Hispanic or Latino:						
White	36.4	24.6	24.9	24.2	24 6	24.7
Black or African American	29.3	33.3	33.2	32.6	32.5	32.1
Asian or Pacific Islander	0.7	0.8	0.9	1.0	0.9	1.0
American Indian or Alaska Native	0.3	0.3	0.3	0.4	0.3	0.3
Hispanic or Latino[4]	13.1	13.8	13.7	14.2	14.1	14.6
Age at diagnosis:						
13–14 years	0.1	0.1	0.1	0.1	0.1	0.1
15–24 years	2.9	2.4	2.7	3.1	3.5	3.9
25–34 years	25.8	16.9	16.2	15.2	15.4	14.9
35–44 years	32.1	30.9	31.2	30.2	29.2	28.3
45–54 years	13.9	16.7	17.2	17.7	17.7	19.0
55–64 years	4.1	4.7	4.9	5.0	5.5	5.6
65 years and over	1.2	1.5	1.3	1.5	1.6	1.5
Female, 13 years and over						
Hispanic origin and race:						
Not Hispanic or Latino:						
White	3.9	4.3	4.4	4.1	4.6	4.3
Black or African American	11.9	17.6	17.5	18.2	18.0	17.5
Asian or Pacific Islander	0.1	0.2	0.2	0.2	0.2	0.2
American Indian or Alaska Native	0.1	0.1	0.1	0.1	0.1	0.1
Hispanic or Latino[4]	3.0	4.1	3.7	4.1	3.8	4.2
Age at diagnosis:						
13–14 years	0.0	0.1	0.1	0.1	0.1	0.1
15–24 years	1.3	1.7	1.8	1.7	1.7	1.7
25–34 years	6.5	7.4	6.9	6.9	6.6	6.1
35–44 years	7.1	10.3	9.9	10.5	10.1	9.7
45–54 years	2.9	5.2	5.5	5.7	6.2	6.5
55–64 years	0.9	1.3	1.5	1.6	1.8	1.9
65 years and over	0.3	0.4	0.5	0.5	0.5	0.5
Children, under 13 years						
Hispanic origin and race:						
Not Hispanic or Latino:						
White	0.2	0.0	0.0	0.0	0.0	0.0
Black or African American	0.6	0.2	0.2	0.1	0.1	0.1
Asian or Pacific Islander	0.0	0.0	0.0	–	0.0	0.0
American Indian or Alaska Native	0.0	–	0.0	–	0.0	–
Hispanic or Latino[4]	0.2	0.1	0.0	0.0	0.0	0.0
Region of residence						
Northeast	31.6	29.6	26.8	27.6	26.4	28.4
Midwest	10.3	10.3	10.7	10.8	10.7	12.0
South	37.8	43.5	45.0	45.4	47.5	44.6
West	20.4	16.6	17.4	16.2	15.4	15.0

0.0 Rate greater than zero but less than 0.05. – Quantity zero.

[1]Based on cases reported to the Centers for Disease Control and Prevention from the beginning of the epidemic (1981) through June 30, 2006.

[2]Numbers are point estimates that result from adjustments for reporting delays to AIDS case counts. The estimates do not include adjustments for incomplete reporting. Data are provisional. See Appendix I, AIDS Surveillance.

[3]Total for all years includes 3,469 persons of unknown race or multiple races, 3 persons of unknown sex, 1,136 persons of unknown state of residence, and 3 persons who were residents of other areas. All persons totals were calculated independent of values for subpopulations. Consequently, sums of subpopulations may not equal totals for all persons.

[4]Persons of Hispanic origin may be of any race. See Appendix II, Hispanic origin.

[5]Percents may not sum to 100% due to rounding and because persons of unknown race and Hispanic origin are included in totals.

NOTES: See Appendix II, Acquired immunodeficiency syndrome (AIDS), for discussion of AIDS case reporting definitions and other issues affecting interpretation of trends. Data are for the 50 states and the District of Columbia. This table replaces surveillance data by year of report in previous editions of *Health, United States.*

SOURCES: Centers for Disease Control and Prevention, National Center for HIV, STD, and TB Prevention, Division of HIV/AIDS Prevention—Surveillance and Epidemiology; HIV/AIDS Surveillance Report, 2005 (vol. 17 Rev ed.). Atlanta, GA: US Department of Health and Human Services, Centers for Disease Control and Prevention. 2007. Available from: www.cdc.gov/hiv/topics/surveillance/resources/reports/.

Table 53 (page 1 of 3). Age-adjusted cancer incidence rates for selected cancer sites, by sex, race, and Hispanic origin: United States, selected geographic areas, selected years 1990–2004

[Data are based on the Surveillance, Epidemiology, and End Results (SEER) Program's 13 population-based cancer registries]

Site, sex, race, and Hispanic origin	1990	1995	1999	2000	2001	2002	2003	2004	1990–2004 APC[1]
All sites	Number of new cases per 100,000 population[2]								
All persons	475.3	470.0	479.0	471.4	472.8	465.9	452.3	446.6	–0.5[3]
White	482.8	476.4	488.4	483.3	485.6	476.5	462.4	456.4	–0.4[3]
Black or African American	512.2	533.1	529.6	514.6	503.2	510.3	495.4	489.8	–0.7[3]
American Indian or Alaska Native[4]	341.6	360.9	390.8	336.2	351.2	322.7	334.2	353.5	–0.3
Asian or Pacific Islander	334.9	335.6	337.2	330.1	334.8	333.0	319.7	317.8	–0.5[3]
Hispanic or Latino[5]	352.5	354.3	365.4	352.9	352.3	354.3	332.4	336.3	–0.5[3]
White, not Hispanic or Latino[5]	495.1	490.7	505.5	501.8	505.3	495.4	483.1	476.4	–0.3[3]
Male	583.7	562.9	565.7	560.5	558.9	548.3	532.5	523.0	–1.1[3]
White	590.5	562.1	567.8	565.7	566.0	553.1	536.1	527.8	–1.1[3]
Black or African American	685.3	731.9	706.3	692.6	670.9	671.0	645.2	628.2	–1.2[3]
American Indian or Alaska Native[4]	388.3	414.8	451.9	348.7	397.9	343.9	390.4	351.8	–1.0
Asian or Pacific Islander	386.5	393.2	389.9	386.3	380.0	375.3	370.2	360.5	–0.8[3]
Hispanic or Latino[5]	414.9	434.4	437.5	425.0	421.5	422.1	392.9	398.0	–0.7[3]
White, not Hispanic or Latino[5]	606.3	576.4	585.0	585.5	586.2	572.3	557.4	548.1	–1.0[3]
Female	410.9	409.6	421.7	411.1	413.8	409.9	397.5	394.1	–0.1
White	421.0	422.4	437.0	428.6	431.5	425.0	412.6	407.7	0.0
Black or African American	403.4	400.1	413.0	394.6	388.6	402.2	394.1	396.7	–0.2
American Indian or Alaska Native[4]	310.1	326.3	350.3	333.7	321.3	306.8	297.3	358.4	0.4
Asian or Pacific Islander	294.5	293.3	301.4	291.5	305.0	307.1	287.5	291.7	0.0
Hispanic or Latino[5]	318.3	305.0	321.7	310.3	309.4	312.3	294.9	298.0	–0.3
White, not Hispanic or Latino[5]	430.8	436.5	453.7	445.4	450.2	443.0	432.4	426.7	0.2
Lung and bronchus									
Male	95.0	86.8	80.3	77.5	76.7	75.0	74.3	69.3	–2.1[3]
White	94.2	85.0	78.8	76.3	75.9	74.4	73.3	68.1	–2.1[3]
Black or African American	133.6	136.6	120.1	109.6	111.8	108.1	109.2	98.4	–2.3[3]
Asian or Pacific Islander	64.4	59.9	62.2	62.4	56.2	56.6	56.7	57.0	–1.0[3]
Hispanic or Latino[5]	59.2	52.1	44.2	44.3	41.8	47.7	42.9	37.1	–2.3[3]
White, not Hispanic or Latino[5]	97.5	88.4	82.9	80.3	80.5	78.0	77.3	72.5	–1.9[3]
Female	47.2	49.3	50.3	48.5	48.5	48.8	48.8	47.2	0.0
White	48.4	51.7	52.4	50.8	50.7	51.0	51.6	48.8	0.1
Black or African American	52.8	49.7	57.9	54.1	54.1	54.7	53.3	55.9	0.3
Asian or Pacific Islander	28.3	27.3	28.7	26.9	29.2	28.6	27.8	29.4	0.3
Hispanic or Latino[5]	25.8	24.7	25.1	23.7	23.6	23.0	22.0	23.4	–1.2[3]
White, not Hispanic or Latino[5]	50.8	54.9	56.0	54.5	54.5	55.1	56.1	52.8	0.4[3]
Colon and rectum									
Male	72.2	63.1	64.0	62.4	61.2	59.2	57.3	54.8	–1.6[3]
White	72.9	62.5	64.0	62.2	60.7	58.2	56.1	54.0	–1.7[3]
Black or African American	72.7	74.3	73.2	72.4	70.9	70.5	74.1	70.9	–0.4
Asian or Pacific Islander	61.4	58.0	54.0	56.4	55.3	57.1	51.2	47.2	–1.2[3]
Hispanic or Latino[5]	47.5	44.8	49.1	49.1	48.4	43.9	44.8	43.9	–0.5
White, not Hispanic or Latino[5]	75.0	64.0	65.6	63.6	62.2	59.7	57.5	55.3	–1.7[3]
Female	50.2	45.8	46.9	45.9	45.0	44.6	42.6	40.7	–1.0[3]
White	49.8	45.5	46.2	45.5	44.2	43.8	42.2	39.7	–1.1[3]
Black or African American	60.9	54.9	58.0	57.3	55.6	54.5	53.2	51.6	–0.6[3]
Asian or Pacific Islander	38.0	38.3	40.0	36.6	40.1	40.1	35.4	35.2	–0.7
Hispanic or Latino[5]	34.2	31.3	34.2	32.9	31.1	30.9	31.1	30.4	–0.6[3]
White, not Hispanic or Latino[5]	50.9	46.8	47.5	46.8	45.8	45.3	43.5	41.0	–1.0[3]
Prostate									
Male	166.7	165.7	179.2	177.0	177.7	174.9	162.0	159.3	–1.5[3]
White	168.3	160.7	174.3	173.0	175.3	170.9	157.1	155.5	–1.7[3]
Black or African American	217.9	273.0	282.0	284.2	262.2	271.9	243.2	233.9	–1.1
American Indian or Alaska Native[4]	98.4	88.0	94.5	60.9	76.7	75.2	90.9	68.6	–3.2[3]
Asian or Pacific Islander	88.1	102.4	103.8	103.2	104.5	98.7	99.7	96.0	–0.9
Hispanic or Latino[5]	118.1	138.1	147.8	145.5	142.2	143.7	128.6	137.7	–0.3
White, not Hispanic or Latino[5]	172.1	163.3	178.2	177.0	179.9	174.7	161.4	158.4	–1.7[3]
Breast									
Female	129.2	130.6	137.9	133.5	134.3	130.7	121.6	121.0	–0.1
White	134.2	136.1	144.7	140.6	141.7	137.1	126.5	125.4	–0.1
Black or African American	116.5	122.3	123.5	119.1	114.4	119.4	119.7	118.8	0.0
American Indian or Alaska Native[4]	65.3	92.5	80.9	88.8	80.3	70.9	81.6	85.9	–0.2
Asian or Pacific Islander	86.9	86.4	96.5	91.4	97.9	96.9	88.0	92.5	0.8[3]
Hispanic or Latino[5]	88.2	86.7	92.5	93.6	88.0	89.0	81.9	83.9	–0.2
White, not Hispanic or Latino[5]	138.9	142.0	152.1	147.4	149.9	144.6	134.0	132.7	0.1

See footnotes at end of table.

Table 53 (page 2 of 3). Age-adjusted cancer incidence rates for selected cancer sites, by sex, race, and Hispanic origin: United States, selected geographic areas, selected years 1990–2004

[Data are based on the Surveillance, Epidemiology, and End Results (SEER) Program's 13 population-based cancer registries]

Site, sex, race, and Hispanic origin	*1990*	*1995*	*1999*	*2000*	*2001*	*2002*	*2003*	*2004*	*1990–2004 APC*[1]
Cervix uteri	Number of new cases per 100,000 population[2]								
Female	11.9	9.9	9.3	8.8	8.7	8.2	8.1	7.7	–2.7[3]
White	11.2	9.2	9.1	8.9	8.4	8.2	7.8	7.6	–2.4[3]
Black or African American	16.4	14.6	12.9	10.6	10.6	9.7	10.3	9.5	–3.7[3]
Asian or Pacific Islander	12.1	10.9	8.0	7.8	9.4	7.9	7.8	6.8	–4.2[3]
Hispanic or Latino[5]	21.3	17.7	17.0	17.0	14.9	14.3	13.8	12.6	–3.4[3]
White, not Hispanic or Latino[5]	9.7	7.8	7.6	7.0	7.0	6.9	6.4	6.5	–2.5[3]
Corpus uteri[6]									
Female	24.2	24.4	24.2	23.3	24.0	23.3	22.6	22.9	–0.3[3]
White	26.0	26.0	25.8	25.2	25.6	24.2	24.0	24.2	–0.4[3]
Black or African American	16.2	16.9	17.5	16.3	18.7	21.1	18.4	18.2	1.3[3]
Asian or Pacific Islander	12.9	17.0	17.1	15.9	17.0	18.3	16.0	17.8	1.4[3]
Hispanic or Latino[5]	17.3	16.2	16.1	14.9	16.4	16.6	16.6	18.2	0.2
White, not Hispanic or Latino[5]	26.7	27.1	27.1	26.5	26.9	25.2	25.1	24.9	–0.3
Ovary									
Female	15.5	14.5	14.3	14.1	14.0	13.6	13.1	12.6	–1.2[3]
White	16.4	15.4	15.1	15.0	15.2	14.4	13.8	13.2	–1.1[3]
Black or African American	11.2	10.8	10.4	10.5	9.3	9.7	11.1	10.1	–0.6
Asian or Pacific Islander	11.2	10.4	10.8	9.8	9.5	11.6	9.7	9.7	–0.4
Hispanic or Latino[5]	12.2	11.8	10.7	10.7	13.1	13.1	10.5	10.7	–0.4
White, not Hispanic or Latino[5]	16.7	15.8	15.7	15.6	15.6	14.5	14.4	13.6	–1.1[3]
Oral cavity and pharynx									
Male	18.5	16.4	15.3	15.7	14.9	15.5	14.8	14.7	–1.6[3]
White	17.9	16.3	15.3	15.6	15.2	15.6	14.9	15.0	–1.3[3]
Black or African American	25.4	22.1	19.0	19.1	18.1	17.8	16.8	15.6	–2.9[3]
Asian or Pacific Islander	14.8	11.8	11.2	13.1	9.7	12.5	11.3	10.8	–1.7[3]
Hispanic or Latino[5]	10.8	12.1	10.0	8.9	9.2	9.3	7.9	9.5	–2.0[3]
White, not Hispanic or Latino[5]	18.7	16.9	16.0	16.6	16.1	16.6	16.0	15.9	–1.1[3]
Female	7.3	7.0	6.3	6.2	6.6	6.4	5.8	5.9	–1.4[3]
White	7.4	7.1	6.2	6.2	6.6	6.5	5.7	5.9	–1.5[3]
Black or African American	6.4	6.6	5.9	5.3	6.4	6.2	6.6	5.8	–1.0
Asian or Pacific Islander	6.1	5.2	6.2	6.1	5.6	5.8	4.9	5.5	–1.0
Hispanic or Latino[5]	3.9	3.7	4.7	3.6	4.2	3.7	3.4	3.2	–1.5
White, not Hispanic or Latino[5]	7.8	7.5	6.5	6.6	7.0	7.0	6.1	6.3	–1.3[3]
Stomach									
Male	14.6	13.5	12.8	12.5	11.8	11.8	11.5	11.5	–1.9[3]
White	12.8	11.9	11.2	10.7	10.2	10.3	10.0	10.0	–1.9[3]
Black or African American	21.5	18.4	17.0	18.4	17.4	15.7	17.7	15.4	–2.5[3]
Asian or Pacific Islander	26.9	24.1	22.5	22.2	18.9	19.9	18.4	19.1	–2.9[3]
Hispanic or Latino[5]	20.2	19.2	20.4	16.1	15.5	15.8	15.4	15.6	–2.2[3]
White, not Hispanic or Latino[5]	12.1	11.1	10.1	10.0	9.4	9.5	9.1	9.1	–2.1[3]
Female	6.7	6.2	6.6	6.1	5.7	6.1	5.8	5.8	–1.0[3]
White	5.7	5.1	5.5	5.0	4.6	5.0	4.8	4.9	–1.2[3]
Black or African American	9.9	9.8	10.4	8.6	8.9	9.7	9.1	7.2	–1.2
Asian or Pacific Islander	15.3	13.0	12.0	12.8	12.0	10.9	10.7	10.6	–2.8[3]
Hispanic or Latino[5]	10.8	11.0	9.6	10.7	9.9	10.2	9.6	9.6	–0.7[3]
White, not Hispanic or Latino[5]	5.1	4.5	4.9	4.2	3.8	4.2	4.0	4.0	–1.8[3]
Pancreas									
Male	13.0	12.7	12.5	12.8	12.7	12.6	12.2	12.9	–0.1
White	12.7	12.4	12.4	12.6	12.9	12.9	12.1	12.7	0.1
Black or African American	19.3	19.1	18.2	18.1	15.3	13.7	16.6	17.1	–1.4[3]
Asian or Pacific Islander	11.2	10.3	9.2	10.6	9.7	9.7	9.9	11.1	–1.0
Hispanic or Latino[5]	10.7	12.1	9.3	12.1	9.7	10.5	9.5	10.7	–0.3
White, not Hispanic or Latino[5]	12.8	12.4	12.7	12.7	13.2	13.2	12.5	12.9	0.2
Female	10.0	9.9	9.6	9.8	9.8	10.3	10.1	9.9	–0.1
White	9.8	9.6	9.3	9.6	9.5	10.0	10.0	9.7	0.0
Black or African American	12.9	15.5	13.4	12.7	13.3	15.6	14.1	13.6	–0.8
Asian or Pacific Islander	9.7	8.1	8.5	9.1	8.9	8.7	7.9	8.6	0.4
Hispanic or Latino[5]	9.8	8.7	9.7	9.0	9.6	10.4	7.7	8.4	–0.9
White, not Hispanic or Latino[5]	9.7	9.7	9.3	9.7	9.5	10.0	10.4	9.9	0.2

See footnotes at end of table.

Table 53 (page 3 of 3). Age-adjusted cancer incidence rates for selected cancer sites, by sex, race, and Hispanic origin: United States, selected geographic areas, selected years 1990–2004

[Data are based on the Surveillance, Epidemiology, and End Results (SEER) Program's 13 population-based cancer registries]

Site, sex, race, and Hispanic origin	*1990*	*1995*	*1999*	*2000*	*2001*	*2002*	*2003*	*2004*	*1990–2004 APC*[1]
Urinary bladder	Number of new cases per 100,000 population[2]								
Male	37.2	35.3	36.4	36.7	36.4	35.2	36.1	35.5	–0.2[3]
White	40.7	38.8	40.0	40.7	40.5	38.7	39.9	39.3	–0.1
Black or African American	19.6	19.2	21.9	19.9	18.9	20.3	22.2	20.9	0.3
Asian or Pacific Islander	15.6	16.3	17.1	16.5	16.5	18.9	16.9	16.4	1.0[3]
Hispanic or Latino[5]	21.9	17.6	19.1	19.7	20.4	19.3	18.6	17.5	–0.8
White, not Hispanic or Latino[5]	42.3	41.0	42.3	43.2	43.1	41.2	42.6	42.3	0.1
Female	9.5	9.3	9.3	9.0	9.0	9.1	9.0	8.9	–0.4[3]
White	9.9	10.1	10.0	9.9	9.9	10.0	9.7	9.7	–0.1
Black or African American	8.6	7.2	8.7	7.7	7.0	8.2	7.2	8.0	–0.1
Asian or Pacific Islander	5.3	4.4	4.0	4.1	4.5	3.2	4.7	3.7	–0.9
Hispanic or Latino[5]	5.7	5.1	4.5	5.6	5.2	5.8	4.0	5.2	–0.9
White, not Hispanic or Latino[5]	10.3	10.6	10.7	10.4	10.5	10.6	10.6	10.3	0.1
Non-Hodgkin's lymphoma									
Male	22.6	25.0	24.2	23.4	23.8	23.3	23.4	24.0	0.1
White	23.7	26.1	25.2	24.7	24.9	24.6	24.8	25.2	0.1
Black or African American	17.4	21.4	17.9	17.5	17.7	17.8	18.6	21.0	0.2
Asian or Pacific Islander	16.6	16.4	19.0	15.7	17.3	16.0	15.6	15.5	–0.3
Hispanic or Latino[5]	17.4	20.8	17.9	20.0	18.0	19.6	18.3	19.4	0.0
White, not Hispanic or Latino[5]	24.3	26.6	26.1	25.3	25.8	25.2	25.7	26.0	0.2
Female	14.5	15.1	16.1	15.8	15.9	16.1	16.7	16.6	1.1[3]
White	15.4	15.9	17.1	16.8	16.7	17.1	17.6	17.5	1.1[3]
Black or African American	10.2	10.1	11.0	11.8	12.1	11.4	12.8	12.7	2.1[3]
Asian or Pacific Islander	9.1	11.7	11.2	11.1	12.6	11.6	12.2	11.5	1.4[3]
Hispanic or Latino[5]	13.3	12.7	13.9	13.2	14.1	12.8	14.1	14.3	–0.7[3]
White, not Hispanic or Latino[5]	15.7	16.2	17.5	17.2	17.2	17.8	18.1	18.1	1.2[3]
Leukemia									
Male	17.1	17.5	16.4	16.3	16.8	15.9	15.8	15.0	–0.7[3]
White	17.9	18.7	17.4	17.3	18.0	17.2	16.7	15.7	–0.6[3]
Black or African American	16.0	13.1	13.6	13.3	12.4	11.5	13.1	13.9	–0.7
Asian or Pacific Islander	8.5	9.9	10.5	9.9	9.8	8.8	9.9	9.3	–0.2
Hispanic or Latino[5]	12.0	14.5	11.9	12.5	10.8	11.5	11.0	11.5	–0.4
White, not Hispanic or Latino[5]	18.2	19.1	17.8	17.7	18.7	17.7	17.3	16.0	–0.5[3]
Female	9.8	10.1	9.2	9.9	9.9	9.4	9.2	9.3	–0.5[3]
White	10.2	10.7	9.7	10.6	10.6	10.0	9.6	9.7	–0.4
Black or African American	8.4	8.0	7.6	9.2	8.6	7.0	8.0	8.3	–0.7
Asian or Pacific Islander	6.0	6.3	6.2	6.1	5.0	6.2	6.0	6.0	–0.7
Hispanic or Latino[5]	8.4	8.1	7.9	7.5	6.9	8.0	6.6	7.8	–0.8
White, not Hispanic or Latino[5]	10.2	10.9	9.9	10.6	11.0	10.0	10.0	9.8	–0.2

0.0 Annual percent change (APC) is greater than –0.05 but less than 0.05.
[1]Annual percent change (APC) has been calculated by fitting a linear regression model to the natural logarithm of the yearly rates from 1990–2004.
[2]Age adjusted by 5-year age groups to the year 2000 U.S. standard population. Age-adjusted rates are based on at least 25 cases. See Appendix II, Age adjustment.
[3]APC is significantly different from 0 ($p < 0.05$).
[4]Starting with *Health, United States, 2007*, estimates for American Indian or Alaska Native population are based on the Contract Health Service Delivery Area (CHSDA) counties within SEER areas. Estimates for American Indian or Alaska Native are not shown for some sites because of the small number of annual cases.
[5]Starting with *Health, United States, 2007*, Hispanic data exclude cases from Alaska. The race groups, white, black, Asian or Pacific Islander, and American Indian or Alaska Native, include persons of Hispanic and non-Hispanic origin. Persons of Hispanic origin may be of any race. The NAACCR Hispanic Identification Algorithm was used on a combination of variables to classify cases as Hispanic for analytic purposes. See the report, NAACCR Guideline for Enhancing Hispanic-Latino Identification, for more information; available from: seer.cancer.gov/seerstat/variables/seer/yr1973_2004/race_ethnicity/. See Appendix II, Hispanic origin.
[6]Includes corpus uteri only cases and not uterus, not elsewhere specified cases.

NOTES: See Appendix II, Incidence. Estimates are based on 13 SEER areas November 2006 submission and differ from published estimates based on 9 SEER areas or other submission dates. See Appendix I,Surveillance, Epidemiology, and End Results Program (SEER). The site variable distinguishes Kaposi Sarcoma and Mesothelioma as individual cancer sites. As a result, Kaposi Sarcoma and Mesothelioma cases do not contribute to other cancer sites. Numbers have been revised and differ from previous editions of *Health, United States.* Data for additional years are available. See Appendix III.

SOURCE: National Institutes of Health, National Cancer Institute, Surveillance, Epidemiology, and End Results (SEER) Program. Available from: www.seer,cancer.gov.

Table 54. Five-year relative cancer survival rates for selected cancer sites, by race and sex: United States, selected geographic areas, selected years 1975–1977 through 1996–2003

[Data are based on the Surveillance, Epidemiology, and End Results (SEER) Program's 9 population-based cancer registries]

Sex and site	White 1975–1977	White 1981–1983	White 1987–1989	White 1990–1992	White 1993–1995	White 1996–2003	Black or African American 1975–1977	Black or African American 1981–1983	Black or African American 1987–1989	Black or African American 1990–1992	Black or African American 1993–1995	Black or African American 1996–2003
Both sexes						Percent of patients						
All sites	51.0	52.8	57.7	62.4	63.4	67.0	39.8	39.6	43.6	48.2	52.8	57.0
Oral cavity and pharynx	54.6	55.0	56.6	58.7	60.9	62.0	36.4	31.8	34.4	33.3	38.2	40.6
Esophagus	5.6	7.6	11.0	13.6	14.3	17.5	3.1	4.3	6.4	9.4	7.5	10.9
Stomach	14.8	16.9	19.1	19.3	20.7	22.2	16.3	17.2	20.0	24.1	19.8	24.2
Colon	51.6	56.7	61.7	63.9	61.4	65.6	46.3	49.7	53.2	54.2	52.3	54.7
Rectum	49.4	53.8	59.6	61.2	61.7	66.4	44.9	40.6	53.5	52.2	54.8	58.4
Pancreas	2.5	2.8	3.4	4.6	4.2	4.9	2.3	3.7	5.7	3.7	3.7	4.6
Lung and bronchus	12.8	13.9	13.8	14.5	15.1	15.7	11.5	11.7	11.2	10.8	13.0	12.5
Urinary bladder	74.5	79.3	81.4	81.9	82.2	81.3	50.6	60.3	63.3	64.7	61.8	65.0
Non-Hodgkin's lymphoma	48.3	52.8	52.8	52.9	54.4	64.8	48.8	50.4	47.5	42.1	42.0	56.0
Leukemia	35.9	40.2	45.5	48.0	49.3	50.8	33.5	34.3	36.9	37.4	42.0	40.3
Male												
All sites	43.3	47.6	53.3	61.3	62.4	66.6	32.7	34.2	38.8	47.3	53.5	59.2
Oral cavity and pharynx	54.1	53.8	54.4	57.0	59.9	61.2	30.0	26.4	30.1	28.3	32.8	35.0
Esophagus	4.9	6.8	11.4	12.9	14.5	17.1	1.6	3.6	5.0	9.7	7.6	9.4
Stomach	13.7	16.0	16.0	16.4	19.3	20.4	16.4	16.8	17.2	23.1	17.6	22.1
Colon	51.1	57.5	62.5	64.4	61.2	65.8	45.3	45.9	51.6	55.8	51.2	56.1
Rectum	48.4	52.3	59.8	60.4	60.4	65.7	41.7	38.3	49.0	54.1	52.1	57.1
Pancreas	2.7	2.3	3.2	4.3	3.8	5.3	2.7	4.0	5.1	3.2	3.5	3.2
Lung and bronchus	11.5	12.3	12.5	13.0	13.1	13.6	10.7	10.5	11.1	9.6	11.5	10.8
Prostate gland	69.8	75.0	85.4	95.3	96.1	99.0	61.3	63.7	72.2	85.5	91.4	95.3
Urinary bladder	75.6	80.4	83.4	84.1	83.4	82.1	56.8	65.7	68.0	67.6	69.0	68.3
Non-Hodgkin's lymphoma	47.7	52.5	49.2	48.2	50.3	62.8	42.0	49.5	42.6	38.1	35.3	52.1
Leukemia	35.0	40.0	47.4	48.2	50.0	50.8	30.4	33.7	35.0	31.6	41.6	40.6
Female												
All sites	57.8	57.6	62.1	63.5	64.4	67.4	47.2	45.6	48.9	49.2	51.9	54.5
Colon	52.1	56.1	61.0	63.5	61.6	65.5	46.7	52.4	54.5	53.0	53.0	53.7
Rectum	50.5	55.4	59.4	62.2	63.2	67.3	47.4	42.9	58.0	49.8	57.9	59.6
Pancreas	2.3	3.3	3.5	4.9	4.6	4.4	2.0	3.3	6.1	4.0	3.9	5.8
Lung and bronchus	15.9	17.1	15.8	16.6	17.7	18.1	14.0	14.9	11.5	12.8	15.8	14.9
Melanoma of skin	86.7	87.7	91.4	92.1	92.8	94.1	*	*	90.4	*	*	77.5
Breast	75.9	77.7	85.3	86.7	87.9	90.3	62.3	64.1	71.2	71.7	72.8	77.9
Cervix uteri	70.6	69.0	73.6	71.9	74.6	74.3	64.9	61.7	58.2	58.6	64.0	65.8
Corpus uteri[1]	89.2	84.0	85.7	87.2	86.5	86.9	61.8	54.2	59.2	57.0	62.0	62.4
Ovary	36.5	40.3	39.9	42.5	42.7	44.7	43.1	39.3	35.3	37.8	42.8	37.5
Non-Hodgkin's lymphoma	48.9	53.1	57.2	58.7	59.7	67.1	56.1	51.5	53.5	47.7	54.8	61.1

* Data for population groups with fewer than 25 cases are not shown because estimates are considered unreliable.
[1]Includes corpus uteri only cases and not uterus, not elsewhere specified cases.

NOTES: Rates are based on followup of patients through 2004. The rate is the ratio of the observed survival rate for the patient group to the expected survival rate for persons in the general population similar to the patient group with respect to age, sex, race, and calendar year of observation. It estimates the chance of surviving the effects of cancer. The site variable distinguishes Kaposi Sarcoma and Mesothelioma as individual cancer sites. As a result, Kaposi Sarcoma and Mesothelioma cases are excluded from each of the sites shown except all sites combined. The race groups, white and black, include persons of Hispanic and non-Hispanic origin. Due to death certificate race-ethnicity classification and other methodological issues related to developing life tables, survival rates for race-ethnicity groups other than white and black are not calculated. Numbers have been revised and differ from previous editions of *Health, United States*. Data for additional years are available. See Appendix III.

SOURCE: National Institutes of Health, National Cancer Institute, Surveillance, Epidemiology, and End Results (SEER) Program. Available from: www.seer.cancer.gov.

Table 55. Diabetes among adults 20 years of age and over, by sex, age, and race and Hispanic origin: United States, 1988–1994 and 2001–2004

[Data are based on interviews and physical examinations of a sample of the civilian noninstitutionalized population]

Sex, age, and race and Hispanic origin[3]	*Physician-diagnosed and undiagnosed diabetes*[1,2]		*Physician-diagnosed diabetes*[1]		*Undiagnosed diabetes*[2]	
	1988–1994	*2001–2004*	*1988–1994*	*2001–2004*	*1988–1994*	*2001–2004*
20 years and over, age-adjusted[4]			Percent of population			
All persons[5]	8.3	10.2	5.4	7.3	2.9	2.9
Male	8.8	11.8	5.4	7.6	3.4	4.1
Female	7.9	8.8	5.4	7.1	2.5	1.7
Not Hispanic or Latino:						
White only	7.5	8.8	5.0	6.1	2.5	2.6
Black or African American only	12.6	14.5	8.6	11.6	4.0	*2.9
Mexican	14.2	15.0	9.7	11.8	4.5	*3.2
20 years and over, crude						
All persons[5]	7.8	10.0	5.1	7.2	2.7	2.8
Male	7.9	11.2	4.8	7.2	3.0	3.9
Female	7.8	8.9	5.4	7.1	2.4	1.7
Not Hispanic or Latino:						
White only	7.5	9.2	5.0	6.4	2.5	2.8
Black or African American only	10.4	12.7	6.9	10.1	3.4	*2.6
Mexican	9.0	9.3	5.6	7.0	3.4	*
Age						
20–39 years	1.6	2.3	1.1	1.6	*0.6	*
40–59 years	8.8	10.9	5.5	7.9	3.3	3.0
60 years and over	18.9	22.5	12.8	16.2	6.1	6.3

* Estimates are considered unreliable. Data preceded by an asterisk have a relative standard error (RSE) of 20%–30%. Data not shown have an RSE of greater than 30%.
[1]Physician-diagnosed diabetes was obtained by self-report and excludes women who reported having diabetes only during pregnancy.
[2]Undiagnosed diabetes is defined as a fasting blood glucose of at least 126 mg/dL and no reported physician diagnosis. Respondents had fasted for at least 8 hours and less than 24 hours. Estimates in prior editions of *Health, United States* included data from respondents who had fasted for at least 9 hours and less than 24 hours.
[3]Persons of Mexican origin may be of any race. Starting with 1999 data, race-specific estimates are tabulated according to the 1997 Revisions to the Standards for the Classification of Federal Data on Race and Ethnicity and are not strictly comparable with estimates for earlier years. The two non-Hispanic race categories shown in the table conform to the 1997 Standards. Starting with 1999 data, race-specific estimates are for persons who reported only one racial group. Prior to data year 1999, estimates were tabulated according to the 1977 Standards. Estimates for single-race categories prior to 1999 included persons who reported one race or, if they reported more than one race, identified one race as best representing their race. See Appendix II, Hispanic origin; Race.
[4]Estimates are age-adjusted to the year 2000 standard population using three age groups: 20–39 years, 40–59 years, and 60 years and over. Age-adjusted estimates in this table may differ from other age-adjusted estimates based on the same data and presented elsewhere if different age groups are used in the adjustment procedure. See Appendix II, Age adjustment.
[5]Includes all other races and Hispanic origins not shown separately.

NOTES: Standard errors are available in the spreadsheet version of this table. Available from: www.cdc.gov/nchs/hus.htm. Starting with *Health, United States, 2007*, data use a revised weighting scheme. Data have been revised and differ from previous editions of *Health, United States*. Data for additional years are available. See Appendix III.

SOURCE: Centers for Disease Control and Prevention, National Center for Health Statistics, National Health and Nutrition Examination Survey.

Table 56 (page 1 of 2). Severe headache or migraine, low back pain, and neck pain among adults 18 years of age and over, by selected characteristics: United States, 1997, 2004, and 2005

[Data are based on household interviews of a sample of the civilian noninstitutionalized population]

Characteristic	Severe headache or migraine[1] 1997	Severe headache or migraine[1] 2004	Severe headache or migraine[1] 2005	Low back pain[1] 1997	Low back pain[1] 2004	Low back pain[1] 2005	Neck pain[1] 1997	Neck pain[1] 2004	Neck pain[1] 2005
	Percent of adults with pain during past 3 months								
18 years and over, age-adjusted[2,3]	15.8	15.3	15.2	28.2	27.1	28.3	14.7	14.6	14.7
18 years and over, crude[3]	16.0	15.3	15.1	28.1	27.2	28.5	14.6	14.8	14.9
Age									
18–44 years	18.7	18.4	18.4	26.1	23.9	25.0	13.3	12.4	12.8
18–24 years	18.7	18.4	18.0	21.9	19.2	20.4	9.8	8.9	9.2
25–44 years	18.7	18.4	18.5	27.3	25.5	26.6	14.3	13.6	14.0
45–64 years	15.8	15.0	14.3	31.3	30.8	31.6	17.0	18.7	18.1
45–54 years	17.8	16.9	17.2	31.3	29.5	30.3	17.3	18.1	18.0
55–64 years	12.7	12.4	10.2	31.2	32.6	33.5	16.6	19.5	18.2
65 years and over	7.0	6.2	6.4	29.5	30.4	33.0	15.0	14.4	14.9
65–74 years	8.2	7.1	7.4	30.2	28.5	32.1	15.0	13.9	15.8
75 years and over	5.4	5.1	5.2	28.6	32.5	34.1	15.0	15.0	13.9
Sex[2]									
Male	9.9	9.7	9.3	26.5	25.0	26.2	12.6	12.1	12.3
Female	21.4	20.7	20.8	29.6	29.0	30.3	16.6	17.0	16.9
Sex and age									
Male:									
18–44 years	11.9	11.0	11.0	24.8	22.0	23.1	11.6	10.0	10.6
45–54 years	10.3	11.2	10.3	29.4	27.4	29.6	13.9	14.6	15.0
55–64 years	8.8	8.8	7.0	30.7	31.2	30.0	14.6	17.0	15.4
65–74 years	5.0	5.6	4.5	29.0	25.7	28.2	13.6	11.8	13.2
75 years and over	*2.4	3.8	4.5	22.5	29.1	31.1	12.6	13.0	12.0
Female:									
18–44 years	25.4	25.6	25.6	27.3	25.8	26.9	14.9	14.9	14.9
45–54 years	24.9	22.3	23.9	33.1	31.6	30.9	20.6	21.4	20.8
55–64 years	16.3	15.7	13.2	31.7	33.9	36.6	18.4	21.7	20.8
65–74 years	10.7	8.2	9.8	31.1	30.9	35.3	16.1	15.6	18.0
75 years and over	7.4	6.0	5.6	32.4	34.6	36.1	16.5	16.3	15.1
Race[2,4]									
White only	15.9	15.5	15.5	28.7	27.8	28.9	15.1	15.4	15.2
Black or African American only	16.7	15.0	14.1	26.9	24.0	25.7	13.3	10.8	12.1
American Indian or Alaska Native only	18.9	19.1	15.7	33.3	35.3	29.9	16.2	18.8	*11.1
Asian only	11.7	10.1	10.3	21.0	18.3	19.9	9.2	9.0	9.3
Native Hawaiian or Other Pacific Islander only	- - -	*	*	- - -	*	*	- - -	*	*
2 or more races	- - -	24.8	23.8	- - -	34.4	37.8	- - -	19.0	25.3
Hispanic origin and race[2,4]									
Hispanic or Latino	15.5	15.7	15.1	26.4	23.6	27.2	13.9	13.4	14.2
Mexican	14.6	15.8	14.6	25.2	22.1	25.3	12.9	12.7	12.5
Not Hispanic or Latino	15.9	15.5	15.3	28.4	27.6	28.7	14.9	15.0	15.0
White only	16.1	15.8	15.8	29.1	28.7	29.5	15.4	16.0	15.7
Black or African American only	16.8	15.0	14.0	26.9	23.8	25.5	13.3	10.7	12.0
Education[5,6]									
25 years and over:									
No high school diploma or GED	19.2	18.7	17.7	33.6	33.3	33.9	16.5	18.1	16.9
High school diploma or GED	16.0	14.6	15.3	30.2	29.7	30.0	15.5	15.5	15.4
Some college or more	13.8	14.1	13.6	26.9	26.2	28.2	14.6	14.7	15.2

See footnotes at end of table.

Table 56 (page 2 of 2). Severe headache or migraine, low back pain, and neck pain among adults 18 years of age and over, by selected characteristics: United States, 1997, 2004, and 2005

[Data are based on household interviews of a sample of the civilian noninstitutionalized population]

Characteristic	Severe headache or migraine[1]			Low back pain[1]			Neck pain[1]		
	1997	2004	2005	1997	2004	2005	1997	2004	2005
Percent of poverty level[2,7]	Percent of adults with pain during the past 3 months								
Below 100%	23.3	20.8	22.4	35.4	32.9	34.2	18.6	18.6	18.3
100%–less than 200%	18.9	18.8	17.4	30.8	29.8	31.8	16.1	16.0	16.6
200% or more	13.8	13.6	13.5	26.3	25.7	26.7	13.8	13.8	13.8
Hispanic origin and race and percent of poverty level[2,4,7]									
Hispanic or Latino:									
Below 100%	18.9	19.6	19.6	29.5	27.3	29.4	16.4	16.6	17.4
100%–less than 200%	15.7	16.8	13.8	26.8	24.1	27.8	12.9	13.2	14.7
200% or more	13.4	13.3	14.0	24.3	21.9	26.1	13.3	12.1	12.3
Not Hispanic or Latino:									
White only:									
Below 100%	26.2	22.8	25.2	38.9	37.2	38.3	20.5	22.3	21.5
100%–less than 200%	20.1	21.3	20.3	33.3	33.9	35.2	18.0	19.0	19.1
200% or more	14.1	14.1	14.1	27.1	27.0	27.7	14.4	14.9	14.5
Black or African American only:									
Below 100%	22.7	19.4	20.9	34.5	30.9	32.6	17.9	14.3	14.9
100%–less than 200%	17.6	16.5	15.4	27.7	26.3	26.3	14.0	10.7	13.2
200% or more	13.4	12.6	10.8	23.1	20.6	22.4	10.9	9.6	9.9
Geographic region[2]									
Northeast	14.5	13.3	14.8	27.1	27.7	28.2	14.0	14.9	14.4
Midwest	15.6	15.9	16.1	28.7	28.5	29.7	15.3	14.9	15.9
South	17.1	15.8	15.2	27.5	26.0	27.3	13.9	13.6	13.7
West	15.3	15.7	14.3	30.0	27.0	28.8	16.1	15.9	15.4
Location of residence[2]									
Within MSA[8]	15.2	14.6	14.7	27.0	26.2	27.3	14.2	14.1	14.3
Outside MSA[8]	18.1	18.3	17.1	32.5	30.4	32.3	16.4	16.7	16.6

* Estimates are considered unreliable. Data preceded by an asterisk have a relative standard error (RSE) of 20%–30%. Data not shown have an RSE greater than 30%.

- - - Data not available.

[1]In three separate questions, respondents were asked, "During the past 3 months, did you have a severe headache or migraine? ...low back pain? ...neck pain?" Respondents were instructed to report pain that had lasted a whole day or more, and not to report fleeting or minor aches or pains. Persons may be represented in more than one column.

[2]Estimates are age-adjusted to the year 2000 standard population using five age groups: 18–44 years, 45–54 years, 55–64 years, 65–74 years, and 75 years and over. Age-adjusted estimates in this table may differ from other age-adjusted estimates based on the same data and presented elsewhere if different age groups are used in the adjustment procedure. See Appendix II, Age adjustment.

[3]Includes all other races not shown separately and unknown education level.

[4]The race groups, white, black, American Indian or Alaska Native, Asian, Native Hawaiian or Other Pacific Islander, and 2 or more races, include persons of Hispanic and non-Hispanic origin. Persons of Hispanic origin may be of any race. Starting with 1999 data, race-specific estimates are tabulated according to the 1997 Revisions to the Standards for the Classification of Federal Data on Race and Ethnicity and are not strictly comparable with estimates for earlier years. The five single-race categories plus multiple-race categories shown in the table conform to the 1997 Standards. Starting with 1999 data, race-specific estimates are for persons who reported only one racial group; the category 2 or more races includes persons who reported more than one racial group. Prior to 1999, data were tabulated according to the 1977 Standards with four racial groups and the Asian only category included Native Hawaiian or Other Pacific Islander. Estimates for single-race categories prior to 1999 included persons who reported one race or, if they reported more than one race, identified one race as best representing their race. Starting with 2003 data, race responses of other race and unspecified multiple race were treated as missing, and then race was imputed if these were the only race responses. Almost all persons with a race response of other race were of Hispanic origin. See Appendix II, Hispanic origin; Race.

[5]Estimates are for persons 25 years of age and over and are age-adjusted to the year 2000 standard population using five age groups: 25–44 years, 45–54 years, 55–64 years, 65–74 years, and 75 years and over. See Appendix II, Age adjustment.

[6]GED stands for General Educational Development high school equivalency diploma. See Appendix II, Education.

[7]Percent of poverty level is based on family income and family size and composition using U.S. Census Bureau poverty thresholds. Missing family income data were imputed for 27%–31% of persons 18 years of age and over in 1997–1998 and 33%–36% in 1999–2005. See Appendix II, Family Income; Poverty.

[8]MSA is metropolitan statistical area.

NOTES: Standard errors are available in the spreadsheet version of this table. Available from: www.cdc.gov/nchs/hus.htm. Data for additional years are available. See Appendix III.

SOURCE: Centers for Disease Control and Prevention, National Center for Health Statistics, National Health Interview Survey, sample adult questionnaire.

Table 57 (page 1 of 4). Joint pain among adults 18 years of age and over, by selected characteristics: United States, 2002, 2004, and 2005

[Data are based on household interviews of a sample of the civilian noninstitutionalized population]

Characteristic	*Any joint pain*[1]			*Knee pain*[1]			*Shoulder pain*[1]		
	2002	*2004*	*2005*	*2002*	*2004*	*2005*	*2002*	*2004*	*2005*
	Percent of adults reporting joint pain in past 30 days								
18 years and over, age-adjusted[2,3]	29.5	30.8	30.7	16.5	18.2	18.2	8.6	9.2	9.2
18 years and over, crude[3]	29.5	31.1	31.1	16.5	18.4	18.5	8.7	9.4	9.3
Age									
18–44 years	19.3	19.2	19.1	10.5	11.4	11.6	4.9	5.0	4.9
18–24 years	14.2	12.9	14.0	8.3	8.0	8.8	3.4	2.8	2.4
25–44 years	21.0	21.4	20.9	11.2	12.6	12.6	5.4	5.7	5.8
45–64 years	37.5	39.8	39.9	20.4	22.8	23.2	12.3	13.4	12.9
45–54 years	34.3	36.5	35.8	18.4	20.7	20.6	10.5	12.6	11.5
55–64 years	42.3	44.5	45.7	23.4	25.8	26.9	15.1	14.5	14.9
65 years and over	47.2	51.6	50.9	28.6	31.6	30.2	14.1	15.2	16.0
65–74 years	46.0	49.3	49.3	27.6	30.4	29.7	14.0	14.1	15.7
75 years and over	48.7	54.2	52.6	29.7	32.9	30.8	14.1	16.5	16.2
Sex[2]									
Male	28.0	29.3	28.9	15.2	17.1	16.8	8.4	9.4	9.3
Female	30.7	32.2	32.2	17.6	19.2	19.4	8.8	9.0	9.0
Sex and age									
Male:									
18–44 years	20.1	19.5	19.3	10.7	11.5	12.0	5.5	5.5	5.4
45–54 years	31.1	34.0	33.4	16.2	19.0	18.9	9.5	13.1	11.4
55–64 years	37.3	41.2	40.7	20.1	23.5	23.1	13.7	14.7	14.7
65–74 years	41.7	43.3	45.1	24.1	25.6	25.1	13.3	12.7	15.7
75 years and over	43.9	49.8	47.0	25.7	30.9	25.7	11.4	14.6	15.1
Female:									
18–44 years	18.4	18.9	18.9	10.2	11.3	11.2	4.2	4.4	4.5
45–54 years	37.3	38.9	38.2	20.5	22.3	22.3	11.4	12.1	11.5
55–64 years	46.8	47.6	50.4	26.4	27.9	30.5	16.3	14.3	15.1
65–74 years	49.6	54.4	52.9	30.5	34.5	33.6	14.7	15.3	15.7
75 years and over	51.6	57.0	56.2	32.1	34.2	34.0	15.7	17.8	16.9
Race[2,4]									
White only	29.8	31.6	31.3	16.3	18.6	18.5	8.8	9.5	9.5
Black or African American only	30.8	28.1	28.5	20.2	18.2	18.2	8.3	7.7	7.6
American Indian or Alaska Native only	36.7	38.3	34.8	24.5	23.4	15.0	*11.3	*14.2	*8.1
Asian only	18.1	20.0	18.5	8.5	10.8	10.2	3.9	6.3	5.3
Native Hawaiian or Other Pacific Islander only	*	*	*	*	*	*	*	*	*
2 or more races	42.7	37.7	46.2	28.1	20.3	28.6	15.4	13.1	18.9
Hispanic origin and race[2,4]									
Hispanic or Latino	23.4	23.8	24.2	13.6	14.8	14.9	7.6	7.4	8.2
Mexican	24.6	23.3	23.8	14.1	15.0	14.9	8.3	7.7	8.5
Not Hispanic or Latino	30.4	31.9	31.7	17.0	18.9	18.9	8.9	9.5	9.4
White only	30.8	33.1	32.8	16.9	19.4	19.4	9.1	9.9	9.8
Black or African American only	30.8	28.1	28.5	20.1	18.3	18.1	8.3	7.8	7.6
Education[5,6]									
25 years of age and over:									
No high school diploma or GED	33.0	34.0	33.3	19.5	19.9	20.7	10.8	11.8	11.7
High school diploma or GED	32.9	34.2	33.1	18.6	20.3	19.7	10.2	10.4	10.5
Some college or more	31.1	33.2	33.2	16.9	19.3	19.2	8.8	9.5	9.7

See footnotes at end of table.

Table 57 (page 2 of 4). Joint pain among adults 18 years of age and over, by selected characteristics: United States, 2002, 2004, and 2005

[Data are based on household interviews of a sample of the civilian noninstitutionalized population]

Characteristic	Any joint pain[1]			Knee pain[1]			Shoulder pain[1]		
	2002	2004	2005	2002	2004	2005	2002	2004	2005
	Percent of adults reporting joint pain in past 30 days								
Percent of poverty level[2,7]									
Below 100%	31.7	35.7	33.7	19.9	22.7	21.6	11.2	11.3	11.3
100%–less than 200%	31.7	33.9	32.1	19.0	20.9	19.8	10.4	12.0	10.6
200% or more	28.7	31.8	30.0	15.6	18.3	17.5	8.0	9.3	8.6
Hispanic origin and race and percent of poverty level[2,4,7]									
Hispanic or Latino:									
Below 100%	26.8	27.5	24.3	16.1	16.1	15.5	11.5	8.4	11.0
100%–less than 200%	24.5	25.1	24.3	14.4	15.5	15.7	8.2	8.8	8.1
200% or more	21.4	24.4	24.4	11.7	15.3	13.9	5.4	7.0	7.3
Not Hispanic or Latino:									
White only:									
Below 100%	34.2	41.2	38.9	21.3	25.8	24.7	12.4	13.2	13.5
100%–less than 200%	34.9	38.9	36.6	20.3	23.8	22.8	11.6	14.0	12.2
200% or more	29.8	33.5	31.5	15.9	19.2	18.4	8.4	9.8	9.0
Black or African American only:									
Below 100%	31.6	33.8	33.2	20.8	24.8	22.5	9.1	9.7	8.5
100%–less than 200%	34.0	31.4	28.7	23.2	21.6	18.4	10.9	9.4	8.7
200% or more	29.1	26.4	26.4	18.5	16.4	16.0	7.1	7.5	6.8
Geographic region[2]									
Northeast	27.5	29.1	28.6	15.8	16.7	16.7	7.9	7.5	8.1
Midwest	32.1	34.7	34.8	18.4	21.2	21.6	8.6	10.2	10.1
South	29.3	30.1	29.8	16.7	18.0	17.9	9.1	9.5	8.9
West	28.4	29.3	29.2	14.6	16.6	16.3	8.6	9.3	9.6
Location of residence[2]									
Within MSA[8]	28.3	29.6	29.2	16.0	17.3	17.2	8.1	8.8	8.4
Outside MSA[8]	33.9	35.9	36.3	18.7	22.1	22.3	10.8	11.0	12.2

See footnotes at end of table.

Table 57 (page 3 of 4). Joint pain among adults 18 years of age and over, by selected characteristics: United States, 2002, 2004, and 2005

[Data are based on household interviews of a sample of the civilian noninstitutionalized population]

Characteristic	Finger pain[1]			Hip pain[1]		
	2002	2004	2005	2002	2004	2005
	Percent of adults reporting joint pain in past 30 days					
Total, age-adjusted[2,3]	7.5	7.6	7.4	6.6	7.5	7.1
Total, crude[3]	7.5	7.7	7.6	6.6	7.6	7.2
Age						
18–44 years	3.4	3.1	2.8	3.2	3.5	3.2
18–24 years	2.0	1.5	*1.0	1.6	*1.4	2.1
25–44 years	3.9	3.7	3.5	3.8	4.2	3.6
45–64 years	11.0	11.0	11.2	9.1	10.3	9.7
45–54 years	9.1	8.9	9.2	7.8	8.8	7.6
55–64 years	13.9	14.1	14.0	11.0	12.5	12.6
65 years and over	13.9	15.4	15.2	12.9	15.1	14.6
65–74 years	14.4	14.3	14.9	12.6	13.7	13.7
75 years and over	13.3	16.7	15.4	13.3	16.8	15.7
Sex[2]						
Male	5.8	6.0	6.0	5.1	5.5	5.4
Female	8.9	8.9	8.7	8.0	9.2	8.6
Sex and age						
Male:						
18–44 years	3.0	2.8	2.6	2.5	2.5	2.4
45–54 years	6.6	7.2	7.5	5.6	5.9	5.7
55–64 years	10.5	11.1	10.4	8.0	9.2	9.5
65–74 years	11.2	10.2	11.4	10.5	11.1	10.8
75 years and over	10.0	12.2	12.1	10.1	13.1	12.7
Female:						
18–44 years	3.8	3.4	3.0	3.9	4.4	4.0
45–54 years	11.5	10.6	10.9	9.9	11.6	9.5
55–64 years	17.0	16.8	17.4	13.7	15.5	15.4
65–74 years	17.1	17.7	17.9	14.2	15.9	16.2
75 years and over	15.3	19.5	17.5	15.2	19.1	17.5
Race[2,4]						
White only	7.6	8.0	7.8	6.9	7.8	7.4
Black or African American only	6.5	5.1	4.6	5.6	6.1	6.1
American Indian or Alaska Native only	*12.9	*9.1	*13.0	*10.4	*7.9	*
Asian only	*3.2	*4.0	4.1	*2.3	4.0	*2.1
Native Hawaiian or Other Pacific Islander only	*	*	*	*	*	*
2 or more races	12.8	9.2	10.5	10.0	7.7	13.7
Hispanic origin and race[2,4]						
Hispanic or Latino	6.8	6.5	6.0	3.8	4.3	4.1
Mexican	7.8	6.5	7.0	4.0	3.9	4.1
Not Hispanic or Latino	7.6	7.7	7.6	6.9	7.9	7.4
White only	7.8	8.2	8.2	7.3	8.3	7.8
Black or African American only	6.5	5.0	4.7	5.7	6.1	6.2
Education[5,6]						
25 years of age and over:						
No high school diploma or GED	9.5	8.8	8.8	7.3	9.1	8.5
High school diploma or GED	8.3	8.9	8.8	7.3	8.5	7.5
Some college or more	8.2	8.1	8.1	7.5	8.2	7.8

See footnotes at end of table.

Table 57 (page 4 of 4). Joint pain among adults 18 years of age and over, by selected characteristics: United States, 2002, 2004, and 2005

[Data are based on household interviews of a sample of the civilian noninstitutionalized population]

Characteristic	*Finger pain*[1]			*Hip pain*[1]		
	2002	*2004*	*2005*	*2002*	*2004*	*2005*
Percent of poverty level[2,7]	Percent of adults reporting joint pain in past 30 days					
Below 100%	9.8	9.2	7.8	8.5	9.9	9.0
100%–less than 200%	8.9	8.9	8.4	7.5	9.0	8.0
200% or more	6.9	7.7	7.2	6.2	7.5	6.6
Hispanic origin and race and percent of poverty level[2,4,7]						
Hispanic or Latino:						
Below 100%	8.6	8.2	6.1	5.9	4.7	4.5
100%–less than 200%	8.2	6.6	6.2	3.9	4.4	3.9
200% or more	5.5	7.4	5.9	2.5	5.3	4.2
Not Hispanic or Latino:						
White only:						
Below 100%	10.9	11.4	9.6	9.9	13.2	11.7
100%–less than 200%	9.9	10.8	10.0	9.1	11.2	9.8
200% or more	7.3	8.1	7.8	6.7	8.1	7.2
Black or African American only:						
Below 100%	7.9	5.9	5.9	8.1	7.4	7.6
100%–less than 200%	7.4	4.8	5.9	6.4	7.1	6.0
200% or more	5.6	5.7	3.4	4.5	4.8	5.9
Geographic region[2]						
Northeast	6.6	6.5	6.2	5.7	6.5	6.4
Midwest	7.5	8.2	8.5	6.9	8.5	7.9
South	7.6	7.8	7.3	7.0	7.9	7.1
West	8.0	7.5	7.5	6.4	6.7	6.6
Location of residence[2]						
Within MSA[8]	7.2	7.3	7.0	6.2	7.0	6.5
Outside MSA[8]	8.4	8.6	9.1	8.0	9.4	9.3

* Estimates are considered unreliable. Data preceded by an asterisk have a relative standard error (RSE) of 20%–30%. Data not shown have an RSE of greater than 30%.

[1]Starting with 2002 data, respondents were asked, "During the past 30 days, have you had any symptoms of pain, aching, or stiffness in or around a joint?" Respondents were instructed not to include the back or neck. To facilitate their response, respondents were shown a card illustrating the body joints. Respondents reporting more than one type of joint pain were included in each response category. This table shows the most commonly reported joints.

[2]Estimates are age-adjusted to the year 2000 standard population using five age groups: 18–44 years, 45–54 years, 55–64 years, 65–74 years, and 75 years and over. See Appendix II, Age adjustment.

[3]Includes all other races not shown separately and unknown education level.

[4]The race groups, white, black, American Indian or Alaska Native, Asian, Native Hawaiian or Other Pacific Islander, and 2 or more races, include persons of Hispanic and non-Hispanic origin. Persons of Hispanic origin may be of any race. The five single-race categories plus multiple-race categories shown in the table conform to the 1997 Revisions to the Standards for the Classification of Federal Data on Race and Ethnicity. Starting with 2003 data, race responses of other race and unspecified multiple race were treated as missing, and then race was imputed if these were the only race responses. Almost all persons with a race response of other race were of Hispanic origin. See Appendix II, Hispanic origin; Race.

[5]Estimates are for persons 25 years of age and over and are age-adjusted to the year 2000 standard population using five age groups: 25–44 years, 45–54 years, 55–64 years, 65–74 years, and 75 years and over. See Appendix II, Age adjustment.

[6]GED stands for General Educational Development high school equivalency diploma. See Appendix II, Education.

[7]Percent of poverty level is based on family income and family size and composition using U.S. Census Bureau poverty thresholds. Missing family income data were imputed for 34%–36% of persons 18 years of age and over in 2002–2005. See Appendix II, Family Income; Poverty.

[8]MSA is metropolitan statistical area.

NOTES: Standard errors are available in the spreadsheet version of this table. Available from: www.cdc.gov/nchs/hus.htm. Data for additional years are available. See Appendix III.

SOURCE: Centers for Disease Control and Prevention, National Center for Health Statistics, National Health Interview Survey, sample adult questionnaire.

Table 58 (page 1 of 3). Limitation of activity caused by chronic conditions, by selected characteristics: United States, selected years 1997–2005

[Data are based on household interviews of a sample of the civilian noninstitutionalized population]

	Any activity limitation[1]			
Characteristic	1997	2003	2004	2005
All ages	Percent of persons			
All ages, age-adjusted[2,3]	13.3	12.1	11.9	11.7
All ages, crude[2]	12.8	12.1	11.9	11.8
Age				
Under 18 years	6.6	6.9	7.0	7.0
Under 5 years	3.5	3.6	3.5	4.3
5–17 years	7.8	8.1	8.4	8.0
18–44 years	7.0	6.0	6.0	5.7
18–24 years	5.1	4.1	4.4	4.2
25–44 years	7.6	6.6	6.5	6.3
45–54 years	14.2	13.0	12.5	11.9
55–64 years	22.2	21.1	19.9	19.9
65 years and over	38.7	34.6	34.1	33.8
65–74 years	30.0	26.3	25.5	25.2
75 years and over	50.2	44.0	43.9	43.5
Sex[3]				
Male	13.1	11.9	11.8	11.7
Female	13.4	12.2	11.9	11.6
Race[3,4]				
White only	13.1	11.8	11.6	11.5
Black or African American only	17.1	15.3	15.3	14.1
American Indian or Alaska Native only	23.1	21.2	17.1	16.0
Asian only	7.5	6.4	6.4	6.4
Native Hawaiian or Other Pacific Islander only	- - -	*	*	*
2 or more races	- - -	20.2	18.8	19.9
Black or African American; White	- - -	*16.8	*15.8	*10.9
American Indian or Alaska Native; White	- - -	24.8	21.5	26.3
Hispanic origin and race[3,4]				
Hispanic or Latino	12.8	10.2	10.2	10.5
Mexican	12.5	9.7	10.1	11.4
Not Hispanic or Latino	13.5	12.4	12.3	11.9
White only	13.2	12.2	12.1	11.8
Black or African American only	17.0	15.4	15.3	14.2
Percent of poverty level[3,5]				
Below 100%	25.4	23.1	23.0	22.4
100%–less than 200%	17.9	17.0	16.3	16.2
200% or more	10.1	9.2	9.2	9.0
Hispanic origin and race and percent of poverty level[3,4,5]				
Hispanic or Latino:				
Below 100%	19.2	15.5	15.5	15.9
100%–less than 200%	12.7	9.9	10.5	11.0
200% or more	9.2	8.2	7.7	7.9
Not Hispanic or Latino:				
White only:				
Below 100%	27.8	26.2	26.2	25.2
100%–less than 200%	19.2	19.3	18.7	18.5
200% or more	10.4	9.4	9.5	9.3
Black or African American only:				
Below 100%	28.2	26.1	27.1	25.3
100%–less than 200%	19.5	19.0	16.6	15.8
200% or more	10.7	9.7	10.3	9.5
Geographic region[3]				
Northeast	13.0	11.3	11.0	10.6
Midwest	13.1	13.3	12.7	12.8
South	13.9	12.4	12.3	12.0
West	13.0	11.1	11.4	10.9
Location of residence[3]				
Within MSA[6]	12.7	11.2	11.2	11.0
Outside MSA[6]	15.5	15.7	14.9	14.5

See footnotes at end of table.

Table 58 (page 2 of 3). Limitation of activity caused by chronic conditions, by selected characteristics: United States, selected years 1997–2005

[Data are based on household interviews of a sample of the civilian noninstitutionalized population]

Characteristic	ADL limitation[7]				IADL limitation[7]			
	1997	2003	2004	2005	1997	2003	2004	2005
65 years of age and over	Percent of persons							
65 years and over, age-adjusted[2,8]	6.7	6.4	6.1	6.2	13.7	12.2	11.5	12.0
65 years and over, crude[2]	6.4	6.3	6.0	6.1	13.1	12.1	11.5	12.0
65–74 years	3.4	3.1	2.9	3.2	6.9	6.5	5.5	6.4
75 years and over	10.4	9.9	9.5	9.4	21.2	18.4	18.1	18.3
Sex[8]								
Male	5.2	5.2	4.8	4.6	9.1	8.6	8.4	8.1
Female	7.7	7.2	6.9	7.2	16.9	14.6	13.6	14.8
Race[4,8]								
White only	6.3	5.9	5.8	5.7	13.1	11.5	11.0	11.5
Black or African American only	11.7	10.5	8.7	10.3	21.3	19.2	17.0	17.8
American Indian or Alaska Native only	*	*	*	*	*	*	*	*
Asian only	*	*	*8.0	*7.5	*9.1	*11.8	12.3	*11.3
Native Hawaiian or Other Pacific Islander only	- - -	*	*	*	- - -	*	*	*
2 or more races	- - -	*	*	*	- - -	*20.4	*21.4	*
Hispanic origin and race[4,8]								
Hispanic or Latino	10.8	10.3	10.4	10.7	16.3	13.8	14.8	16.9
Mexican	11.4	9.8	10.7	12.0	18.8	15.1	15.3	19.6
Not Hispanic or Latino	6.5	6.1	5.8	5.9	13.6	12.1	11.3	11.8
White only	6.1	5.7	5.5	5.4	13.0	11.4	10.7	11.2
Black or African American only	11.7	10.4	8.7	10.1	21.2	19.0	17.1	17.7
Percent of poverty level[5,8]								
Below 100%	12.5	10.4	10.1	10.4	25.3	21.6	20.9	21.8
100%–less than 200%	7.4	7.0	6.7	6.5	15.8	15.0	13.3	14.7
200% or more	5.3	5.5	5.2	5.4	10.4	9.4	9.1	9.3
Hispanic origin and race and percent of poverty level[4,5,8]								
Hispanic or Latino:								
Below 100%	16.0	*15.2	15.9	16.0	25.5	20.1	24.0	26.2
100%–less than 200%	11.1	*8.4	*10.3	11.3	15.5	12.3	14.4	17.6
200% or more	*6.6	*8.5	*6.6	*7.3	10.2	*11.1	*8.9	11.3
Not Hispanic or Latino:								
White only:								
Below 100%	11.8	8.9	8.2	9.3	24.9	20.7	19.2	20.7
100%–less than 200%	6.6	6.4	6.2	5.7	15.2	14.8	12.7	14.2
200% or more	5.0	5.1	4.9	5.0	10.3	9.0	8.8	8.9
Black or African American only:								
Below 100%	13.5	14.0	13.9	*11.4	27.8	28.3	26.0	24.6
100%–less than 200%	12.4	10.4	*7.4	*8.4	22.4	18.9	17.7	16.3
200% or more	9.8	8.4	*6.3	10.8	15.1	13.9	10.5	14.9

See footnotes at end of table.

Table 58 (page 3 of 3). Limitation of activity caused by chronic conditions, by selected characteristics: United States, selected years 1997–2005

[Data are based on household interviews of a sample of the civilian noninstitutionalized population]

Characteristic	ADL limitation[7]				IADL limitation[7]			
	1997	2003	2004	2005	1997	2003	2004	2005
	Percent of persons							
Geographic region[8]								
Northeast	6.1	6.6	5.6	6.0	12.2	11.4	9.9	10.9
Midwest	5.8	4.7	5.4	5.3	13.1	11.3	11.9	12.0
South	8.2	7.2	6.8	6.8	15.8	13.1	12.7	13.0
West	5.9	6.5	6.1	6.4	12.4	12.1	11.0	11.5
Location of residence[8]								
Within MSA[6]	6.6	6.3	6.3	6.2	13.5	12.0	11.3	11.5
Outside MSA[6]	7.2	6.7	5.3	5.8	14.4	12.8	12.4	14.0

* Estimates are considered unreliable. Data preceded by an asterisk have a relative standard error (RSE) of 20%–30%. Data not shown have an RSE of greater than 30%.

- - - Data not available.

[1]Limitation of activity is assessed by asking respondents a series of questions about limitations in their ability to perform activities usual for their age group because of a physical, mental, or emotional problem(s). The category limitation of activity includes limitations in personal care (ADL), routine needs (IADL), and other limitations due to a chronic condition. See Appendix II, Activities of daily living; Condition; Instrumental activities of daily living; Limitation of activity.

[2]Includes all other races not shown separately.

[3]Estimates are age-adjusted to the year 2000 standard population using six age groups: Under 18 years, 18–44 years, 45–54 years, 55–64 years, 65–74 years, and 75 years and over. Age-adjusted estimates in this table may differ from other age-adjusted estimates based on the same data and presented elsewhere if different age groups are used in the adjustment procedure. See Appendix II, Age adjustment.

[4]The race groups, white, black, American Indian or Alaska Native, Asian, Native Hawaiian or Other Pacific Islander, and 2 or more races, include persons of Hispanic and non-Hispanic origin. Persons of Hispanic origin may be of any race. Starting with 1999 data, race-specific estimates are tabulated according to the 1997 Revisions to the Standards for the Classification of Federal Data on Race and Ethnicity and are not strictly comparable with estimates for earlier years. The five single-race categories plus multiple-race categories shown in the table conform to the 1997 Standards. Starting with 1999 data, race-specific estimates are for persons who reported only one racial group; the category 2 or more races includes persons who reported more than one racial group. Prior to 1999, data were tabulated according to the 1977 Standards with four racial groups and the Asian only category included Native Hawaiian or Other Pacific Islander. Estimates for single-race categories prior to 1999 included persons who reported one race or, if they reported more than one race, identified one race as best representing their race. Starting with 2003 data, race responses of other race and unspecified multiple race were treated as missing, and then race was imputed if these were the only race responses. Almost all persons with a race response of other race were of Hispanic origin. See Appendix II, Hispanic origin; Race.

[5]Percent of poverty level is based on family income and family size and composition using U.S. Census Bureau poverty thresholds. Missing family income data were imputed for 25% of persons in 1997 and 30%–35% in 1999–2005. See Appendix II, Family income; Poverty.

[6]MSA is metropolitan statistical area.

[7]These estimates are for noninstitutionalized older persons. ADL is activities of daily living and IADL is instrumental activities of daily living. Respondents were asked about needing the help of another person with personal care (ADL) and routine needs such as chores and shopping (IADL) because of a physical, mental, or emotional problem(s). See Appendix II, Activities of daily living; Condition; Instrumental activities of daily living.

[8]Estimates are age-adjusted to the year 2000 standard population using two age groups: 65–74 years and 75 years and over. See Appendix II, Age adjustment.

NOTES: Standard errors for selected years are available in the spreadsheet version of this table. Available from: www.cdc.gov/nchs/hus.htm. Data for additional years are available. See Appendix III.

SOURCE: Centers for Disease Control and Prevention, National Center for Health Statistics, National Health Interview Survey, family core questionnaire.

Table 59 (page 1 of 2). Vision and hearing limitations among adults 18 years of age and over, by selected characteristics: United States, selected years 1997–2005

[Data are based on household interviews of a sample of the civilian noninstitutionalized population]

Characteristic	Any trouble seeing, even with glasses or contacts[1]					A lot of trouble hearing or deaf[2]				
	1997	2000	2003	2004	2005	1997	2000	2003	2004	2005
	Percent of adults									
18 years and over, age-adjusted[3,4]	10.0	9.0	8.8	8.8	9.2	3.2	3.2	3.1	3.1	3.5
18 years and over, crude[4]	9.8	8.9	8.7	8.9	9.3	3.1	3.1	3.0	3.1	3.5
Age										
18–44 years	6.2	5.3	5.2	5.1	5.5	1.0	0.9	0.9	0.8	0.9
18–24 years	5.4	4.2	5.1	4.3	5.0	*0.5	*0.7	*	*0.4	*1.0
25–44 years	6.5	5.7	5.2	5.4	5.7	1.2	1.0	1.0	1.0	0.9
45–64 years	12.0	10.7	10.6	10.9	11.2	3.1	3.0	2.8	2.8	3.4
45–54 years	12.2	10.9	10.5	11.2	11.0	2.6	2.3	1.9	2.0	2.3
55–64 years	11.6	10.5	10.7	10.5	11.5	3.9	4.0	4.1	4.0	4.8
65 years and over	18.1	17.4	16.6	16.8	17.4	9.8	10.5	10.5	10.8	11.9
65–74 years	14.2	13.6	13.1	14.1	13.2	6.6	7.4	6.7	7.3	6.4
75 years and over	23.1	21.9	20.6	19.9	22.0	14.1	14.3	14.9	14.8	18.1
Sex[3]										
Male	8.8	7.9	7.3	7.6	7.9	4.2	4.3	4.0	4.1	4.8
Female	11.1	10.1	10.1	10.0	10.5	2.4	2.3	2.3	2.4	2.5
Sex and age										
Male:										
18–44 years	5.3	4.4	4.1	4.4	4.5	1.2	1.1	1.1	0.8	1.2
45–54 years	10.1	8.8	8.6	9.2	8.8	3.6	2.9	2.7	2.7	3.3
55–64 years	10.5	9.5	8.6	9.1	10.5	5.4	6.2	5.4	5.9	7.3
65–74 years	13.2	12.8	11.8	12.0	11.4	9.4	10.8	10.2	10.7	9.5
75 years and over	21.4	20.7	18.1	17.7	20.4	17.7	18.0	17.8	18.9	23.3
Female:										
18–44 years	7.1	6.2	6.2	5.8	6.5	0.9	0.8	0.7	0.9	0.7
45–54 years	14.2	12.8	12.3	13.1	13.2	1.7	1.8	1.2	1.3	1.5
55–64 years	12.6	11.5	12.5	11.7	12.4	2.6	1.9	2.8	2.3	2.6
65–74 years	15.0	14.4	14.1	15.9	14.8	4.4	4.5	3.8	4.5	3.8
75 years and over	24.2	22.7	22.3	21.4	23.0	11.7	12.1	12.9	12.2	14.7
Race[3,5]										
White only	9.7	8.8	8.5	8.8	9.1	3.4	3.4	3.3	3.4	3.8
Black or African American only	12.8	10.6	10.8	10.3	10.9	2.0	1.6	1.7	1.5	1.4
American Indian or Alaska Native only	19.2	16.6	18.9	14.8	*14.9	14.1	*	*	*	*
Asian only	6.2	6.3	6.1	5.1	5.5	*	*2.4	*	*	*2.2
Native Hawaiian or Other Pacific Islander only	- - -	*	*	*	*	- - -	*	*	*	*
2 or more races	- - -	16.2	11.6	11.0	16.4	- - -	*5.7	*	*	*5.8
Hispanic origin and race[3,5]										
Hispanic or Latino	10.0	9.7	9.1	8.8	9.6	1.5	2.3	2.0	1.8	2.8
Mexican	10.2	8.3	9.0	9.0	9.9	1.8	3.0	2.6	1.8	3.3
Not Hispanic or Latino	10.0	9.1	8.8	8.9	9.2	3.3	3.3	3.2	3.2	3.6
White only	9.8	8.9	8.6	8.9	9.1	3.5	3.5	3.4	3.5	3.9
Black or African American only	12.8	10.6	10.7	10.3	10.9	2.0	1.6	1.8	1.5	1.4
Education[6,7]										
25 years of age and over:										
No high school diploma or GED	15.0	12.2	12.6	13.8	13.5	4.8	4.6	4.9	4.8	4.6
High school diploma or GED	10.6	9.5	9.3	10.3	10.3	3.7	3.9	3.5	3.7	4.1
Some college or more	8.9	8.9	8.1	7.9	8.6	2.9	2.8	2.8	3.0	3.5

See footnotes at end of table.

Table 59 (page 2 of 2). Vision and hearing limitations among adults 18 years of age and over, by selected characteristics: United States, selected years 1997–2005

[Data are based on household interviews of a sample of the civilian noninstitutionalized population]

Characteristic	Any trouble seeing, even with glasses or contacts[1]					A lot of trouble hearing or deaf[2]				
	1997	2000	2003	2004	2005	1997	2000	2003	2004	2005
Percent of poverty level[3,8]	Percent of adults									
Below 100%	17.0	12.9	13.7	14.2	16.8	4.5	3.7	3.9	3.9	4.7
100%–less than 200%	12.9	11.6	11.6	12.0	12.5	3.6	4.2	3.6	3.6	4.3
200% or more	8.2	7.8	7.3	7.4	8.4	3.0	2.8	2.8	2.9	3.5
Hispanic origin and race and percent of poverty level[3,5,8]										
Hispanic or Latino:										
Below 100%	12.8	11.0	12.4	11.2	13.7	*1.9	3.3	*3.4	*3.0	4.8
100%–less than 200%	11.2	9.4	10.3	10.8	8.5	*1.5	*2.3	*1.6	*1.2	*3.1
200% or more	7.8	9.7	6.7	6.3	9.3	*1.2	*1.7	*1.4	*1.5	*
Not Hispanic or Latino:										
White only:										
Below 100%	17.9	13.1	14.3	15.8	17.9	5.8	4.5	4.7	4.9	5.8
100%–less than 200%	13.1	12.0	11.8	13.1	13.9	4.3	5.0	4.2	4.5	5.1
200% or more	8.2	7.8	7.3	7.5	8.4	3.2	3.0	3.1	3.1	3.7
Black or African American only:										
Below 100%	17.9	13.6	14.2	15.2	18.2	3.3	*1.6	*2.1	*2.3	*2.0
100%–less than 200%	16.0	12.9	13.0	10.6	12.3	*2.0	*2.0	*2.3	*	*
200% or more	8.5	8.1	8.5	8.4	9.6	*	*	*	*1.3	*
Geographic region[3]										
Northeast	8.6	7.4	7.5	7.0	8.1	2.2	2.4	2.9	2.6	2.9
Midwest	9.5	9.6	9.3	10.0	9.7	3.5	3.5	3.3	3.5	3.7
South	11.4	9.2	9.4	9.2	9.8	3.5	3.3	3.0	3.2	3.7
West	9.7	9.9	8.1	8.6	8.6	3.4	3.5	3.2	3.0	3.8
Location of residence[3]										
Within MSA[9]	9.5	8.5	8.2	8.4	8.6	2.9	3.0	2.7	2.8	3.1
Outside MSA[9]	12.0	11.1	10.7	10.6	11.7	4.5	3.9	4.4	4.2	4.9

* Estimates are considered unreliable. Data preceded by an asterisk have a relative standard error (RSE) of 20%–30%. Data not shown have an RSE greater than 30%.

- - - Data not available.

[1]Respondents were asked, "Do you have any trouble seeing, even when wearing glasses or contact lenses?" In 2005, 0.4% of adults 18 years of age and over identified themselves as blind.

[2]Respondents were asked, "Which statement best describes your hearing without a hearing aid: good, a little trouble, a lot of trouble, or deaf?" In this analysis, a lot of trouble and deaf are combined into one category. In 2005, 0.3% of adults 18 years of age and over identified themselves as deaf.

[3]Estimates are age-adjusted to the year 2000 standard population using five age groups: 18–44 years, 45–54 years, 55–64 years, 65–74 years, and 75 years and over. Age-adjusted estimates in this table may differ from other age-adjusted estimates based on the same data and presented elsewhere if different age groups are used in the adjustment procedure. See Appendix II, Age adjustment.

[4]Includes all other races not shown separately and unknown education level.

[5]The race groups, white, black, American Indian or Alaska Native, Asian, Native Hawaiian or Other Pacific Islander, and 2 or more races, include persons of Hispanic and non-Hispanic origin. Persons of Hispanic origin may be of any race. Starting with 1999 data, race-specific estimates are tabulated according to the 1997 Revisions to the Standards for the Classification of Federal Data on Race and Ethnicity and are not strictly comparable with estimates for earlier years. The five single-race categories plus multiple-race categories shown in the table conform to the 1997 Standards. Starting with 1999 data, race-specific estimates are for persons who reported only one racial group; the category 2 or more races includes persons who reported more than one racial group. Prior to 1999, data were tabulated according to the 1977 Standards with four racial groups and the Asian only category included Native Hawaiian or Other Pacific Islander. Estimates for single-race categories prior to 1999 included persons who reported one race or, if they reported more than one race, identified one race as best representing their race. Starting with 2003 data, race responses of other race and unspecified multiple race were treated as missing, and then race was imputed if these were the only race responses. Almost all persons with a race response of other race were of Hispanic origin. See Appendix II, Hispanic origin; Race.

[6]Estimates are for persons 25 years of age and over and are age-adjusted to the year 2000 standard population using five age groups: 25–44 years, 45–54 years, 55–64 years, 65–74 years, and 75 years and over. See Appendix II, Age adjustment.

[7]GED stands for General Educational Development high school equivalency diploma. See Appendix II, Education.

[8]Percent of poverty level is based on family income and family size and composition using U.S. Census Bureau poverty thresholds. Missing family income data were imputed for 27%–31% of persons 18 years of age and over in 1997–1998 and 33%–36% in 1999–2005. See Appendix II, Family Income; Poverty.

[9]MSA is metropolitan statistical area.

NOTES: Standard errors are available in the spreadsheet version of this table. Available from: www.cdc.gov/nchs/hus.htm. Data for additional years are available. See Appendix III.

SOURCE: Centers for Disease Control and Prevention, National Center for Health Statistics, National Health Interview Survey, sample adult questionnaire.

Table 60 (page 1 of 2). Respondent-assessed health status, by selected characteristics: United States, selected years 1991–2005

[Data are based on household interviews of a sample of the civilian noninstitutionalized population]

Characteristic	1991[1]	1995[1]	1997	2000	2002	2003	2004	2005
	Percent of persons with fair or poor health[2]							
All ages, age-adjusted[3,4]	10.4	10.6	9.2	9.0	9.3	9.2	9.3	9.2
All ages, crude[4]	10.0	10.1	8.9	8.9	9.2	9.2	9.4	9.3
Age								
Under 18 years	2.6	2.6	2.1	1.7	1.9	1.8	1.8	1.8
Under 6 years	2.7	2.7	1.9	1.5	1.6	1.4	1.5	1.6
6–17 years	2.6	2.5	2.1	1.8	2.1	2.0	2.0	1.9
18–44 years	6.1	6.6	5.3	5.1	5.5	5.6	5.7	5.5
18–24 years	4.8	4.5	3.4	3.3	3.6	3.8	3.6	3.3
25–44 years	6.4	7.2	5.9	5.7	6.2	6.3	6.4	6.3
45–54 years	13.4	13.4	11.7	11.9	12.7	12.1	12.3	11.6
55–64 years	20.7	21.4	18.2	17.9	17.9	18.9	17.9	18.3
65 years and over	29.0	28.3	26.7	26.9	26.3	25.5	26.7	26.6
65–74 years	26.0	25.6	23.1	22.5	22.0	22.3	22.4	23.4
75 years and over	33.6	32.2	31.5	32.1	31.3	29.2	31.5	30.2
Sex[3]								
Male	10.0	10.1	8.8	8.8	8.9	8.8	9.0	8.8
Female	10.8	11.1	9.7	9.3	9.6	9.5	9.6	9.5
Race[3,5]								
White only	9.6	9.7	8.3	8.2	8.5	8.5	8.6	8.6
Black or African American only	16.8	17.2	15.8	14.6	14.1	14.7	14.6	14.3
American Indian or Alaska Native only	18.3	18.7	17.3	17.2	13.2	16.3	16.5	13.2
Asian only	7.8	9.3	7.8	7.4	6.7	7.4	8.6	6.8
Native Hawaiian or Other Pacific Islander only	- - -	- - -	- - -	*	*	*	*	*
2 or more races	- - -	- - -	- - -	16.2	12.5	14.7	12.6	14.5
Black or African American; White	- - -	- - -	- - -	*14.5	13.8	21.4	*10.7	8.3
American Indian or Alaska Native; White	- - -	- - -	- - -	18.7	13.5	18.1	12.3	17.2
Hispanic origin and race[3,5]								
Hispanic or Latino	15.6	15.1	13.0	12.8	13.1	13.9	13.3	13.3
Mexican	17.0	16.7	13.1	12.8	13.3	13.7	13.4	14.3
Not Hispanic or Latino	10.0	10.1	8.9	8.7	8.9	8.7	8.9	8.7
White only	9.1	9.1	8.0	7.9	8.2	7.9	8.0	8.0
Black or African American only	16.8	17.3	15.8	14.6	14.0	14.6	14.6	14.4
Percent of poverty level[3,6]								
Below 100%	22.8	23.7	20.8	19.6	20.3	20.4	21.3	20.4
100%–less than 200%	14.7	15.5	13.9	14.1	14.6	14.4	14.4	14.4
200% or more	6.8	6.7	6.1	6.3	6.4	6.1	6.3	6.2
Hispanic origin and race and percent of poverty level[3,5,6]								
Hispanic or Latino:								
Below 100%	23.6	22.7	19.9	18.7	20.8	20.6	20.2	20.2
100%–less than 200%	18.0	16.9	13.5	15.3	15.4	15.5	15.2	15.3
200% or more	9.3	8.7	8.5	8.4	8.7	9.8	8.8	9.2
Not Hispanic or Latino:								
White only:								
Below 100%	21.9	22.8	19.7	18.8	19.1	19.5	20.8	20.1
100%–less than 200%	14.0	14.8	13.3	13.4	14.3	13.9	13.8	13.8
200% or more	6.4	6.2	5.6	5.8	6.0	5.6	5.7	5.7
Black or African American only:								
Below 100%	25.8	27.7	25.3	23.8	24.5	24.4	25.7	23.3
100%–less than 200%	17.0	19.3	19.2	18.2	17.4	18.6	16.7	17.6
200% or more	10.9	9.9	9.7	9.7	8.8	9.1	9.6	9.5

See footnotes at end of table.

Table 60 (page 2 of 2). Respondent-assessed health status, by selected characteristics: United States, selected years 1991–2005

[Data are based on household interviews of a sample of the civilian noninstitutionalized population]

Characteristic	1991[1]	1995[1]	1997	2000	2002	2003	2004	2005
	Percent of persons with fair or poor health[2]							
Geographic region[3]								
Northeast	8.3	9.1	8.0	7.6	8.1	8.2	7.6	7.5
Midwest	9.1	9.7	8.1	8.0	8.3	8.3	8.2	8.3
South	13.1	12.3	10.8	10.7	10.9	10.7	11.2	11.0
West	9.7	10.1	8.8	8.8	8.7	8.4	8.9	8.6
Location of residence[3]								
Within MSA[7]	9.9	10.1	8.7	8.5	8.7	8.6	8.8	8.7
Outside MSA[7]	11.9	12.6	11.1	11.1	11.7	11.5	11.5	11.2

* Estimates are considered unreliable. Data preceded by an asterisk have a relative standard error (RSE) of 20%–30%. Data not shown have an RSE greater than 30%.
- - - Data not available.
[1]Data prior to 1997 are not strictly comparable with data for later years due to the 1997 questionnaire redesign. See Appendix I, National Health Interview Survey.
[2]See Appendix II, Health status, respondent-assessed.
[3]Estimates are age-adjusted to the year 2000 standard population using six age groups: Under 18 years, 18–44 years, 45–54 years, 55–64 years, 65–74 years, and 75 years and over. See Appendix II, Age adjustment.
[4]Includes all other races not shown separately.
[5]The race groups, white, black, American Indian or Alaska Native, Asian, Native Hawaiian or Other Pacific Islander, and 2 or more races, include persons of Hispanic and non-Hispanic origin. Persons of Hispanic origin may be of any race. Starting with 1999 data, race-specific estimates are tabulated according to the 1997 Revisions to the Standards for the Classification of Federal Data on Race and Ethnicity and are not strictly comparable with estimates for earlier years. The five single-race categories plus multiple-race categories shown in the table conform to the 1997 Standards. Starting with 1999 data, race-specific estimates are for persons who reported only one racial group; the category 2 or more races includes persons who reported more than one racial group. Prior to 1999, data were tabulated according to the 1977 Standards with four racial groups and the Asian only category included Native Hawaiian or Other Pacific Islander. Estimates for single-race categories prior to 1999 included persons who reported one race or, if they reported more than one race, identified one race as best representing their race. Starting with 2003 data, race responses of other race and unspecified multiple race were treated as missing, and then race was imputed if these were the only race responses. Almost all persons with a race response of other race were of Hispanic origin. See Appendix II, Hispanic origin; Race.
[6]Percent of poverty level is based on family income and family size and composition using U.S. Census Bureau poverty thresholds. Missing family income data were imputed for 16%–18% of persons in 1991 and 1995, 25%–29% of persons in 1997–1998, and 32%–35% in 1999–2005. See Appendix II, Family income; Poverty.
[7]MSA is metropolitan statistical area.

NOTES: Standard errors for selected years are available in the spreadsheet version of this table. Available from: www.cdc.gov/nchs/hus.htm. Data for additional years are available. See Appendix III.

SOURCE: Centers for Disease Control and Prevention, National Center for Health Statistics, National Health Interview Survey, family core questionnaire.

Table 61 (page 1 of 2). Serious psychological distress among adults 18 years of age and over, by selected characteristics: United States, average annual selected years, 1997–1998 through 2004–2005

[Data are based on household interviews of a sample of the civilian noninstitutionalized population]

Characteristic	*1997–1998*	*2000–2001*	*2002–2003*	*2004–2005*
	Percent of persons with serious psychological distress[1]			
18 years and over, age-adjusted[2,3]	3.2	3.0	3.1	3.0
18 years and over, crude[3]	3.2	3.0	3.1	3.0
Age				
18–44 years	2.9	2.7	2.9	2.8
18–24 years	2.7	2.6	2.8	2.5
25–44 years	3.0	2.8	2.9	2.9
45–64 years	3.7	3.6	4.0	3.7
45–54 years	3.9	3.7	4.2	3.9
55–64 years	3.4	3.4	3.6	3.4
65 years and over	3.1	2.7	2.3	2.5
65–74 years	2.5	2.8	2.3	2.2
75 years and over	3.8	2.5	2.3	2.9
Sex[2]				
Male	2.5	2.4	2.3	2.3
Female	3.8	3.5	3.9	3.7
Race[2,4]				
White only	3.1	2.9	3.0	2.9
Black or African American only	4.0	3.1	3.4	3.6
American Indian or Alaska Native only	7.8	*7.4	*7.1	*3.5
Asian only	2.0	*2.0	*1.9	1.7
Native Hawaiian or Other Pacific Islander only	- - -	*	*	*
2 or more races	- - -	5.5	7.3	7.9
Hispanic origin and race[2,4]				
Hispanic or Latino	5.0	4.0	3.9	3.7
Mexican	5.2	3.4	3.7	3.6
Not Hispanic or Latino	3.0	2.9	3.1	3.0
White only	2.9	2.9	3.0	2.9
Black or African American only	3.9	3.1	3.4	3.6
Percent of poverty level[2,5]				
Below 100%	9.1	7.7	8.6	8.6
100%–less than 200%	5.0	5.0	5.2	5.0
200% or more	1.8	1.9	1.8	1.7
Hispanic origin and race and percent of poverty level[2,4,5]				
Hispanic or Latino:				
Below 100%	8.6	6.9	7.6	6.6
100%–less than 200%	5.4	4.4	3.8	3.9
200% or more	2.9	2.5	2.7	2.4
Not Hispanic or Latino:				
White only:				
Below 100%	9.6	8.9	9.6	10.2
100%–less than 200%	5.2	5.5	6.1	5.6
200% or more	1.8	1.9	1.8	1.7
Black or African American only:				
Below 100%	8.7	6.3	7.1	7.6
100%–less than 200%	4.3	4.3	4.5	4.8
200% or more	1.6	1.5	1.6	1.7

See footnotes at end of table.

Table 61 (page 2 of 2). Serious psychological distress among adults 18 years of age and over, by selected characteristics: United States, average annual selected years, 1997–1998 through 2004–2005

[Data are based on household interviews of a sample of the civilian noninstitutionalized population]

Characteristic	*1997–1998*	*2000–2001*	*2002–2003*	*2004–2005*
Geographic region[2]	Percent of persons with serious psychological distress[1]			
Northeast	2.7	2.5	3.0	2.5
Midwest	2.6	2.8	2.7	2.7
South	3.8	3.2	3.5	3.7
West	3.3	3.2	3.0	2.8
Location of residence[2]				
Within MSA[6]	3.0	2.8	2.9	2.8
Outside MSA[6]	3.9	3.6	3.9	4.0

* Estimates are considered unreliable. Data preceded by an asterisk have a relative standard error (RSE) of 20%–30%. Data not shown have an RSE greater than 30%.

- - - Data not available.

[1]Serious psychological distress is measured by a six-question scale that asks respondents how often they experienced each of six symptoms of psychological distress in the past 30 days. See Appendix II, Serious psychological distress.

[2]Estimates are age-adjusted to the year 2000 standard population using five age groups: 18–44 years, 45–54 years, 55–64 years, 65–74 years, and 75 years and over. See Appendix II, Age adjustment.

[3]Includes all other races not shown separately.

[4]The race groups, white, black, American Indian or Alaska Native, Asian, Native Hawaiian or Other Pacific Islander, and 2 or more races, include persons of Hispanic and non-Hispanic origin. Persons of Hispanic origin may be of any race. Starting with 1999 data, race-specific estimates are tabulated according to the 1997 Revisions to the Standards for the Classification of Federal Data on Race and Ethnicity and are not strictly comparable with estimates for earlier years. The five single-race categories plus multiple-race categories shown in the table conform to the 1997 Standards. Starting with 1999 data, race-specific estimates are for persons who reported only one racial group; the category 2 or more races includes persons who reported more than one racial group. Prior to 1999, data were tabulated according to the 1977 Standards with four racial groups and the Asian only category included Native Hawaiian or Other Pacific Islander. Estimates for single-race categories prior to 1999 included persons who reported one race or, if they reported more than one race, identified one race as best representing their race. Starting with 2003 data, race responses of other race and unspecified multiple race were treated as missing, and then race was imputed if these were the only race responses. Almost all persons with a race response of other race were of Hispanic origin. See Appendix II, Hispanic origin; Race.

[5]Percent of poverty level is based on family income and family size and composition using U.S. Census Bureau poverty thresholds. Missing family income data were imputed for 27%–31% of persons 18 years of age and over in 1997–1998 and 33%–36% in 1999–2005. See Appendix II, Family income; Poverty.

[6]MSA is metropolitan statistical area.

NOTES: Standard errors for selected years are available in the spreadsheet version of this table. Available from: www.cdc.gov/nchs/hus.htm. Data for additional years are available. See Appendix III.

SOURCE: Centers for Disease Control and Prevention, National Center for Health Statistics, National Health Interview Survey, family core questionnaire.

Table 62 (page 1 of 2). Suicidal ideation, suicide attempts, and injurious suicide attempts among students in grades 9–12, by sex, grade level, race, and Hispanic origin: United States, selected years 1991–2005

[Data are based on a national sample of high school students, grades 9–12]

Sex, grade level, race, and Hispanic origin	*1991*	*1993*	*1995*	*1997*	*1999*	*2001*	*2003*	*2005*
	Percent of students who seriously considered suicide [1]							
Total	29.0	24.1	24.1	20.5	19.3	19.0	16.9	16.9
Male								
Total	20.8	18.8	18.3	15.1	13.7	14.2	12.8	12.0
9th grade	17.6	17.7	18.2	16.1	11.9	14.7	11.9	12.2
10th grade	19.5	18.0	16.7	14.5	13.7	13.8	13.2	11.9
11th grade	25.3	20.6	21.7	16.6	13.7	14.1	12.9	11.9
12th grade	20.7	18.3	16.3	13.5	15.6	13.7	13.2	11.6
Not Hispanic or Latino:								
White	21.7	19.1	19.1	14.4	12.5	14.9	12.0	12.4
Black or African American	13.3	15.4	16.7	10.6	11.7	9.2	10.3	7.0
Hispanic or Latino	18.0	17.9	15.7	17.1	13.6	12.2	12.9	11.9
Female								
Total	37.2	29.6	30.4	27.1	24.9	23.6	21.3	21.8
9th grade	40.3	30.9	34.4	28.9	24.4	26.2	22.2	23.9
10th grade	39.7	31.6	32.8	30.0	30.1	24.1	23.8	23.0
11th grade	38.4	28.9	31.1	26.2	23.0	23.6	20.0	21.6
12th grade	30.7	27.3	23.9	23.6	21.2	18.9	18.0	18.0
Not Hispanic or Latino:								
White	38.6	29.7	31.6	26.1	23.2	24.2	21.2	21.5
Black or African American	29.4	24.5	22.2	22.0	18.8	17.2	14.7	17.1
Hispanic or Latino	34.6	34.1	34.1	30.3	26.1	26.5	23.4	24.2
	Percent of students who attempted suicide [1]							
Total	7.3	8.6	8.7	7.7	8.3	8.8	8.5	8.4
Male								
Total	3.9	5.0	5.6	4.5	5.7	6.2	5.4	6.0
9th grade	4.5	5.8	6.8	6.3	6.1	8.2	5.8	6.8
10th grade	3.3	5.9	5.4	3.8	6.2	6.7	5.5	7.6
11th grade	4.1	3.4	5.8	4.4	4.8	4.9	4.6	4.5
12th grade	3.8	4.5	4.7	3.7	5.4	4.4	5.2	4.3
Not Hispanic or Latino:								
White	3.3	4.4	5.2	3.2	4.5	5.3	3.7	5.2
Black or African American	3.3	5.4	7.0	5.6	7.1	7.5	7.7	5.2
Hispanic or Latino	3.7	7.4	5.8	7.2	6.6	8.0	6.1	7.8
Female								
Total	10.7	12.5	11.9	11.6	10.9	11.2	11.5	10.8
9th grade	13.8	14.4	14.9	15.1	14.0	13.2	14.7	14.1
10th grade	12.2	13.1	15.1	14.3	14.8	12.2	12.7	10.8
11th grade	8.7	13.6	11.4	11.3	7.5	11.5	10.0	11.0
12th grade	7.8	9.1	6.6	6.2	5.8	6.5	6.9	6.5
Not Hispanic or Latino:								
White	10.4	11.3	10.4	10.3	9.0	10.3	10.3	9.3
Black or African American	9.4	11.2	10.8	9.0	7.5	9.8	9.0	9.8
Hispanic or Latino	11.6	19.7	21.0	14.9	18.9	15.9	15.0	14.9

See footnotes at end of table.

Table 62 (page 2 of 2). Suicidal ideation, suicide attempts, and injurious suicide attempts among students in grades 9–12, by sex, grade level, race, and Hispanic origin: United States, selected years 1991–2005

[Data are based on a national sample of high school students, grades 9–12]

Sex, grade level, race, and Hispanic origin	*1991*	*1993*	*1995*	*1997*	*1999*	*2001*	*2003*	*2005*
	Percent of students with an injurious suicide attempt[1,2]							
Total	1.7	2.7	2.8	2.6	2.6	2.6	2.9	2.3
Male								
Total	1.0	1.6	2.2	2.0	2.1	2.1	2.4	1.8
9th grade	1.0	2.1	2.3	3.2	2.6	2.6	3.1	2.1
10th grade	0.5	1.3	2.4	1.4	1.8	2.5	2.1	2.2
11th grade	1.5	1.1	2.0	2.6	2.1	1.6	2.0	1.4
12th grade	0.9	1.5	2.2	1.0	1.7	1.5	1.8	1.0
Not Hispanic or Latino:								
White	1.0	1.4	2.1	1.5	1.6	1.7	1.1	1.5
Black or African American	0.4	2.0	2.8	1.8	3.4	3.6	5.2	1.4
Hispanic or Latino	0.5	2.0	2.9	2.1	1.4	2.5	4.2	2.8
Female								
Total	2.5	3.8	3.4	3.3	3.1	3.1	3.2	2.9
9th grade	2.8	3.5	6.3	5.0	3.8	3.8	3.9	4.0
10th grade	2.6	5.1	3.8	3.7	4.0	3.6	3.2	2.4
11th grade	2.1	3.9	2.9	2.8	2.8	2.8	2.9	2.9
12th grade	2.4	2.9	1.3	2.0	1.3	1.7	2.2	2.2
Not Hispanic or Latino:								
White	2.3	3.6	2.9	2.6	2.3	2.9	2.4	2.7
Black or African American	2.9	4.0	3.6	3.0	2.4	3.1	2.2	2.6
Hispanic or Latino	2.7	5.5	6.6	3.8	4.6	4.2	5.7	3.7

[1]Response is for the 12 months preceding the survey.

[2]A suicide attempt that required medical attention.

NOTES: Only youths attending school participated in the survey. Persons of Hispanic origin may be of any race. See Appendix II, Hispanic origin; Race; Suicidal ideation. Standard errors for selected years are available in the spreadsheet version of this table. Available from: www.cdc.gov/nchs/hus.htm.

SOURCE: Centers for Disease Control and Prevention, National Center for Chronic Disease Prevention and Health Promotion, National Youth Risk Behavior Survey (YRBS).

Table 63 (page 1 of 2). Current cigarette smoking among adults 18 years of age and over, by sex, race, and age: United States, selected years 1965–2005

[Data are based on household interviews of a sample of the civilian noninstitutionalized population]

Sex, race, and age	1965[1]	1974[1]	1979[1]	1985[1]	1990[1]	1995[1]	2000	2001	2002	2003	2004	2005
18 years and over, age-adjusted[2]				Percent of persons who are current cigarette smokers[3]								
All persons	41.9	37.0	33.3	29.9	25.3	24.6	23.1	22.6	22.3	21.5	20.8	20.8
Male	51.2	42.8	37.0	32.2	28.0	26.5	25.2	24.6	24.6	23.7	23.0	23.4
Female	33.7	32.2	30.1	27.9	22.9	22.7	21.1	20.7	20.0	19.4	18.7	18.3
White male[4]	50.4	41.7	36.4	31.3	27.6	26.2	25.4	24.8	24.9	23.8	23.0	23.3
Black or African American male[4]	58.8	53.6	43.9	40.2	32.8	29.4	25.7	27.5	26.6	25.3	23.5	25.9
White female[4]	33.9	32.0	30.3	27.9	23.5	23.4	22.0	22.0	21.0	20.1	19.5	19.1
Black or African American female[4]	31.8	35.6	30.5	30.9	20.8	23.5	20.7	18.0	18.3	17.9	16.9	17.1
18 years and over, crude												
All persons	42.4	37.1	33.5	30.1	25.5	24.7	23.2	22.7	22.4	21.6	20.9	20.9
Male	51.9	43.1	37.5	32.6	28.4	27.0	25.6	25.1	25.1	24.1	23.4	23.9
Female	33.9	32.1	29.9	27.9	22.8	22.6	20.9	20.6	19.8	19.2	18.5	18.1
White male[4]	51.1	41.9	36.8	31.7	28.0	26.6	25.7	25.0	25.0	24.0	23.2	23.6
Black or African American male[4]	60.4	54.3	44.1	39.9	32.5	28.5	26.2	27.6	27.0	25.7	23.9	26.5
White female[4]	34.0	31.7	30.1	27.7	23.4	23.1	21.4	21.5	20.6	19.7	19.1	18.7
Black or African American female[4]	33.7	36.4	31.1	31.0	21.2	23.5	20.8	18.1	18.5	18.1	17.3	17.3
All males												
18–24 years	54.1	42.1	35.0	28.0	26.6	27.8	28.1	30.2	32.1	26.3	25.6	28.0
25–34 years	60.7	50.5	43.9	38.2	31.6	29.5	28.9	26.9	27.2	28.7	26.1	27.7
35–44 years	58.2	51.0	41.8	37.6	34.5	31.5	30.2	27.3	29.7	28.1	26.5	26.0
45–64 years	51.9	42.6	39.3	33.4	29.3	27.1	26.4	26.4	24.5	23.9	25.0	25.2
65 years and over	28.5	24.8	20.9	19.6	14.6	14.9	10.2	11.5	10.1	10.1	9.8	8.9
White male[4]												
18–24 years	53.0	40.8	34.3	28.4	27.4	28.4	30.4	32.3	34.3	27.7	26.7	29.7
25–34 years	60.1	49.5	43.6	37.3	31.6	29.9	29.7	28.7	27.7	28.8	26.3	27.7
35–44 years	57.3	50.1	41.3	36.6	33.5	31.2	30.6	27.8	29.7	28.8	26.6	26.3
45–64 years	51.3	41.2	38.3	32.1	28.7	26.3	25.8	25.1	24.4	23.3	24.4	24.5
65 years and over	27.7	24.3	20.5	18.9	13.7	14.1	9.8	10.7	9.3	9.6	9.4	7.9
Black or African American male[4]												
18–24 years	62.8	54.9	40.2	27.2	21.3	*14.6	20.9	21.6	22.7	18.6	18.0	21.6
25–34 years	68.4	58.5	47.5	45.6	33.8	25.1	23.2	23.8	28.9	31.0	21.2	29.8
35–44 years	67.3	61.5	48.6	45.0	42.0	36.3	30.7	29.9	28.3	23.6	28.4	23.3
45–64 years	57.9	57.8	50.0	46.1	36.7	33.9	32.2	34.3	29.8	30.1	29.2	32.4
65 years and over	36.4	29.7	26.2	27.7	21.5	28.5	14.2	21.1	19.4	18.0	14.1	16.8
All females												
18–24 years	38.1	34.1	33.8	30.4	22.5	21.8	24.9	23.2	24.5	21.5	21.5	20.7
25–34 years	43.7	38.8	33.7	32.0	28.2	26.4	22.3	22.7	21.3	21.3	21.0	21.5
35–44 years	43.7	39.8	37.0	31.5	24.8	27.1	26.2	25.7	23.7	24.2	21.6	21.3
45–64 years	32.0	33.4	30.7	29.9	24.8	24.0	21.7	21.4	21.1	20.2	19.8	18.8
65 years and over	9.6	12.0	13.2	13.5	11.5	11.5	9.3	9.1	8.6	8.3	8.1	8.3
White female[4]												
18–24 years	38.4	34.0	34.5	31.8	25.4	24.9	28.5	27.1	26.7	23.6	22.9	22.6
25–34 years	43.4	38.6	34.1	32.0	28.5	27.3	24.9	25.2	23.8	22.5	22.6	23.1
35–44 years	43.9	39.3	37.2	31.0	25.0	27.0	26.6	26.9	24.4	25.2	22.7	22.2
45–64 years	32.7	33.0	30.6	29.7	25.4	24.3	21.4	21.6	21.5	20.1	20.1	18.9
65 years and over	9.8	12.3	13.8	13.3	11.5	11.7	9.1	9.4	8.5	8.4	8.2	8.4
Black or African American female[4]												
18–24 years	37.1	35.6	31.8	23.7	10.0	*8.8	14.2	10.0	17.1	10.8	15.6	14.2
25–34 years	47.8	42.2	35.2	[illegible]	29.1	26.7	15.5	16.8	13.9	17.0	18.3	16.9
35–44 years	42.8	46.4	37.7	40.2	25.5	31.9	30.2	24.0	24.0	23.2	18.9	19.0
45–64 years	25.7	38.9	34.2	33.4	22.6	27.5	25.6	22.6	22.2	23.3	20.9	21.0
65 years and over	7.1	*8.9	*8.5	14.5	11.1	13.3	10.2	9.3	9.4	8.0	6.7	10.0

See footnotes at end of table.

Table 63 (page 2 of 2). Current cigarette smoking among adults 18 years of age and over, by sex, race, and age: United States, selected years 1965–2005

[Data are based on household interviews of a sample of the civilian noninstitutionalized population]

* Estimates are considered unreliable. Data preceded by an asterisk have a relative standard error of 20%–30%.
[1]Data prior to 1997 are not strictly comparable with data for later years due to the 1997 questionnaire redesign. See Appendix I, National Health Interview Survey.
[2]Estimates are age-adjusted to the year 2000 standard population using five age groups: 18–24 years, 25–34 years, 35–44 years, 45–64 years, 65 years and over. Age-adjusted estimates in this table may differ from other age-adjusted estimates based on the same data and presented elsewhere if different age groups are used in the adjustment procedure. See Appendix II, Age adjustment.
[3]Starting with 1993 data, current cigarette smokers were defined as ever smoking 100 cigarettes in their lifetime and smoking now on every day or some days. See Appendix II, Cigarette smoking.
[4]The race groups, white and black, include persons of Hispanic and non-Hispanic origin. Starting with 1999 data, race-specific estimates are tabulated according to the 1997 Revisions to the Standards for the Classification of Federal Data on Race and Ethnicity and are not strictly comparable with estimates for earlier years. The single-race categories shown in the table conform to the 1997 Standards. Starting with 1999 data, race-specific estimates are for persons who reported only one racial group. Prior to 1999, data were tabulated according to the 1977 Standards. Estimates for single-race categories prior to 1999 included persons who reported one race or, if they reported more than one race, identified one race as best representing their race. Starting with 2003 data, race responses of other race and unspecified multiple race were treated as missing, and then race was imputed if these were the only race responses. Almost all persons with a race response of other race were of Hispanic origin. See Appendix II, Hispanic origin; Race. For additional data on cigarette smoking by racial groups, see Table 65.

NOTES: Standard errors for selected years are available in the spreadsheet version of this table. Available from: www.cdc.gov/nchs/hus.htm. For more data on cigarette smoking see the Early Release reports on the National Health Interview Survey home page: www.cdc.gov/nchs/nhis.htm. Data for additional years are available. See Appendix III.

SOURCES: Centers for Disease Control and Prevention, National Center for Health Statistics, National Health Interview Survey. Data are from the core questionnaire (1965) and the following questionnaire supplements: hypertension (1974), smoking (1979), alcohol and health practices (1983), health promotion and disease prevention (1985, 1990–1991), cancer control and cancer epidemiology (1992), and year 2000 objectives (1993–1995). Starting with 1997, data are from the family core and sample adult questionnaires.

Table 64. Age-adjusted prevalence of current cigarette smoking among adults 25 years of age and over, by sex, race, and education level: United States, selected years 1974–2005

[Data are based on household interviews of a sample of the civilian noninstitutionalized population]

Sex, race, and education level	1974[1]	1979[1]	1985[1]	1990[1]	1995[1]	2000	2001	2002	2003	2004	2005
25 years and over, age-adjusted[2]	Percent of persons who are current cigarette smokers[3]										
All persons[4]	36.9	33.1	30.0	25.4	24.5	22.6	22.0	21.4	21.1	20.4	20.3
No high school diploma or GED	43.7	40.7	40.8	36.7	35.6	31.6	30.5	30.5	29.7	29.1	28.2
High school diploma or GED	36.2	33.6	32.0	29.1	29.1	29.2	28.1	27.9	27.8	25.8	27.0
Some college, no bachelor's degree	35.9	33.2	29.5	23.4	22.6	21.7	22.2	21.5	21.1	21.4	21.8
Bachelor's degree or higher	27.2	22.6	18.5	13.9	13.6	10.9	10.8	10.0	10.2	10.0	9.1
All males[4]	42.9	37.3	32.8	28.2	26.4	24.7	23.8	23.5	23.3	22.6	22.7
No high school diploma or GED	52.3	47.6	45.7	42.0	39.7	36.0	34.2	34.0	34.4	33.6	31.7
High school diploma or GED	42.4	38.9	35.5	33.1	32.7	32.1	30.2	31.0	29.9	28.2	29.9
Some college, no bachelor's degree	41.8	36.5	32.9	25.9	23.7	23.3	24.3	23.2	22.7	23.4	24.9
Bachelor's degree or higher	28.3	22.7	19.6	14.5	13.8	11.6	11.2	11.0	11.2	10.8	9.7
White males[4,5]	41.9	36.7	31.7	27.6	25.9	24.7	23.7	23.5	23.2	22.4	22.4
No high school diploma or GED	51.5	47.6	45.0	41.8	38.7	38.2	34.8	35.6	33.6	32.6	31.6
High school diploma or GED	42.0	38.5	34.8	32.9	32.9	32.4	30.3	31.0	29.6	28.9	30.0
Some college, no bachelor's degree	41.6	36.4	32.2	25.4	23.3	23.5	24.5	23.2	23.3	22.9	24.5
Bachelor's degree or higher	27.8	22.5	19.1	14.4	13.4	11.3	11.2	11.1	11.2	10.5	9.3
Black or African American males[4,5]	53.4	44.4	42.1	34.5	31.6	26.4	28.4	27.2	26.3	24.4	26.5
No high school diploma or GED	58.1	49.7	50.5	41.6	41.9	38.2	37.9	37.2	37.4	36.7	35.9
High school diploma or GED	*50.7	48.6	41.8	37.4	36.6	29.0	33.4	31.3	33.4	23.1	30.1
Some college, no bachelor's degree	*45.3	39.2	41.8	28.1	26.4	19.9	24.1	25.6	19.5	24.7	27.4
Bachelor's degree or higher	*41.4	*36.8	*32.0	*20.8	*17.3	14.6	11.3	*10.8	*10.3	11.3	10.0
All females[4]	32.0	29.5	27.5	22.9	22.9	20.5	20.4	19.3	19.1	18.3	18.0
No high school diploma or GED	36.6	34.8	36.5	31.8	31.7	27.1	26.9	26.9	24.9	24.5	24.6
High school diploma or GED	32.2	29.8	29.5	26.1	26.4	26.6	26.4	25.2	25.8	23.7	24.1
Some college, no bachelor's degree	30.1	30.0	26.3	21.0	21.6	20.4	20.4	20.0	19.7	19.7	19.1
Bachelor's degree or higher	25.9	22.5	17.1	13.3	13.3	10.1	10.5	9.0	9.3	9.3	8.5
White females[4,5]	31.7	29.7	27.3	23.3	23.1	21.0	21.3	20.2	19.6	19.0	18.6
No high school diploma or GED	36.8	35.8	36.7	33.4	32.4	28.4	29.2	29.0	25.0	24.4	24.6
High school diploma or GED	31.9	29.9	29.4	26.5	26.8	27.8	28.3	26.8	26.8	24.7	25.9
Some college, no bachelor's degree	30.4	30.7	26.7	21.2	22.2	21.1	21.3	20.5	20.6	21.1	19.5
Bachelor's degree or higher	25.5	21.9	16.5	13.4	13.5	10.2	10.9	9.6	9.4	9.9	9.1
Black or African American females[4,5]	35.6	30.3	32.0	22.4	25.7	21.6	19.1	18.4	18.9	17.1	17.5
No high school diploma or GED	36.1	31.6	39.4	26.3	32.3	31.1	26.3	27.1	26.9	29.2	27.8
High school diploma or GED	40.9	32.6	32.1	24.1	27.8	25.4	21.3	19.5	23.3	21.0	18.2
Some college, no bachelor's degree	32.3	*28.9	23.9	22.7	20.8	20.4	17.4	20.7	17.0	13.9	17.5
Bachelor's degree or higher	*36.3	*43.3	26.6	17.0	17.3	10.8	11.6	*7.7	11.4	*6.9	*6.6

* Estimates are considered unreliable. Data preceded by an asterisk have a relative standard error of 20%–30%.

[1] Data prior to 1997 are not strictly comparable with data for later years due to the 1997 questionnaire redesign. See Appendix I, National Health Interview Survey.

[2] Estimates are age-adjusted to the year 2000 standard population using four age groups: 25–34 years, 35–44 years, 45–64 years, and 65 years and over. See Appendix II, Age adjustment. For age groups where smoking was 0% or 100%, the age-adjustment procedure was modified to substitute the percentage smoking from the next lower education group.

[3] Starting with 1993 data, current cigarette smokers were defined as ever smoking 100 cigarettes in their lifetime and smoking now on every day or some days. For previous definition, see Appendix II, Cigarette smoking.

[4] Includes unknown education level. Education categories shown are for 1997 and subsequent years. GED stands for General Educational Development high school equivalency diploma. In 1974–1995 the following categories based on number of years of school completed were used: less than 12 years, 12 years, 13–15 years, 16 years or more. See Appendix II, Education.

[5] The race groups, white and black, include persons of Hispanic and non-Hispanic origin. Starting with 1999 data, race-specific estimates are tabulated according to the 1997 Revisions to the Standards for the Classification of Federal Data on Race and Ethnicity and are not strictly comparable with estimates for earlier years. The single-race categories shown in the table conform to the 1997 Standards. Starting with 1999 data, race-specific estimates are for persons who reported only one racial group. Prior to 1999, data were tabulated according to the 1977 Standards. Estimates for single-race categories prior to 1999 included persons who reported one race or, if they reported more than one race, identified one race as best representing their race. Starting with 2003 data, race responses of other race and unspecified multiple race were treated as missing, and then race was imputed if these were the only race responses. Almost all persons with a race response of other race were of Hispanic origin. See Appendix II, Hispanic origin; Race. For additional data on cigarette smoking by racial groups, see Table 65.

NOTES: Standard errors for selected years are available in the spreadsheet version of this table. Available from: www.cdc.gov/nchs/hus.htm. For more data on cigarette smoking see the Early Release reports on the National Health Interview Survey home page: www.cdc.gov/nchs/nhis.htm. Data for additional years are available. See Appendix III.

SOURCES: Centers for Disease Control and Prevention, National Center for Health Statistics, National Health Interview Survey. Data are from the following questionnaire supplements: hypertension (1974), smoking (1979), alcohol and health practices (1983), health promotion and disease prevention (1985, 1990–1991), cancer control and cancer epidemiology (1992), and year 2000 objectives (1993–1995). Starting with 1997, data are from the family core and sample adult questionnaires.

Table 65 (page 1 of 2). Current cigarette smoking among adults, by sex, race, Hispanic origin, age, and education level: United States, average annual 1990–1992, 1995–1998, and 2003–2005

[Data are based on household interviews of a sample of the civilian noninstitutionalized population]

Characteristic	Male			Female		
	1990–1992[1]	1995–1998[1]	2003–2005	1990–1992[1]	1995–1998[1]	2003–2005
18 years and over, age-adjusted[2]	Percent of persons who are current cigarette smokers[3]					
All persons[4]	27.9	26.5	23.4	23.7	22.1	18.8
Race[5]						
White only	27.4	26.4	23.4	24.3	22.9	19.6
Black or African American only	33.9	30.7	24.9	23.1	21.8	17.3
American Indian or Alaska Native only	34.2	40.5	32.5	36.7	28.9	24.7
Asian only	24.8	18.1	18.3	6.3	11.0	5.7
Native Hawaiian or Other Pacific Islander only	- - -	- - -	*	- - -	- - -	*
2 or more races	- - -	- - -	29.2	- - -	- - -	26.5
American Indian or Alaska Native; White	- - -	- - -	38.3	- - -	- - -	33.0
Hispanic origin and race[5]						
Hispanic or Latino	25.7	24.4	19.5	15.8	13.7	10.6
Mexican	26.2	24.5	19.7	14.8	12.0	9.3
Not Hispanic or Latino	28.1	26.9	24.1	24.4	23.1	20.1
White only	27.7	26.9	24.3	25.2	24.1	21.4
Black or African American only	33.9	30.7	24.9	23.2	21.9	17.3
18 years and over, crude						
All persons[4]	28.4	27.0	23.8	23.6	22.0	18.6
Race[5]						
White only	27.8	26.8	23.6	24.1	22.6	19.2
Black or African American only	33.2	30.6	25.4	23.3	21.8	17.6
American Indian or Alaska Native only	35.5	39.2	35.4	37.3	31.2	26.3
Asian only	24.9	20.0	18.9	6.3	11.2	6.0
Native Hawaiian or Other Pacific Islander only	- - -	- - -	*	- - -	- - -	*
2 or more races	- - -	- - -	31.2	- - -	- - -	27.2
American Indian or Alaska Native; White	- - -	- - -	39.7	- - -	- - -	33.5
Hispanic origin and race[5]						
Hispanic or Latino	26.5	25.5	20.7	16.6	13.8	10.8
Mexican	27.1	25.2	21.0	15.0	11.6	9.0
Not Hispanic or Latino	28.5	27.2	24.3	24.2	22.9	19.7
White only	28.0	27.0	24.2	24.8	23.5	20.5
Black or African American only	33.3	30.6	25.3	23.3	21.9	17.6
18–24 years:						
Hispanic or Latino	19.3	26.5	20.9	12.8	12.0	10.0
Not Hispanic or Latino:						
White only	28.9	35.5	30.3	28.7	31.6	26.2
Black or African American only	17.7	21.3	18.5	10.8	9.8	13.4
25–34 years:						
Hispanic or Latino	29.9	25.9	20.8	19.2	12.6	9.4
Not Hispanic or Latino:						
White only	32.7	30.5	29.9	30.9	28.5	26.5
Black or African American only	34.6	28.5	27.2	29.2	22.0	17.0
35–44 years:						
Hispanic or Latino	32.1	26.2	22.8	19.9	17.6	12.8
Not Hispanic or Latino:						
White only	32.3	31.5	28.2	27.3	28.1	25.4
Black or African American only	44.1	34.7	25.2	31.3	30.3	20.5
45–64 years:						
Hispanic or Latino	26.6	26.8	21.7	17.1	14.7	12.9
Not Hispanic or Latino:						
White only	28.4	26.8	24.3	26.1	22.3	20.5
Black or African American only	38.0	38.8	31.0	26.1	26.9	21.9
65 years and over:						
Hispanic or Latino	16.1	14.7	9.0	[illegible].6	9.4	5.7
Not Hispanic or Latino:						
White only	14.2	10.6	8.9	12.3	11.6	8.5
Black or African American only	25.2	20.9	16.4	10.7	11.2	8.4

See footnotes at end of table.

Table 65 (page 2 of 2). Current cigarette smoking among adults, by sex, race, Hispanic origin, age, and education level: United States, average annual 1990–1992, 1995–1998, and 2003–2005

[Data are based on household interviews of a sample of the civilian noninstitutionalized population]

Characteristic	Male			Female		
	1990–1992[1]	*1995–1998*[1]	*2003–2005*	*1990–1992*[1]	*1995–1998*[1]	*2003–2005*
Education, Hispanic origin, and race[5,6]	Percent of persons who are current cigarette smokers[3]					
25 years and over, age-adjusted[7]						
No high school diploma or GED:						
Hispanic or Latino	30.2	27.6	21.8	15.8	13.3	9.9
Not Hispanic or Latino:						
White only	46.1	43.9	43.9	40.4	40.7	41.0
Black or African American only	45.4	44.6	37.0	31.3	30.0	28.1
High school diploma or GED:						
Hispanic or Latino	29.6	26.7	18.3	18.4	16.4	11.9
Not Hispanic or Latino:						
White only	32.9	32.8	31.5	28.4	28.8	28.4
Black or African American only	38.2	35.7	29.2	25.4	26.6	20.8
Some college or more:						
Hispanic or Latino	20.4	16.6	15.8	14.3	13.5	11.0
Not Hispanic or Latino:						
White only	19.3	18.3	16.6	18.1	17.2	15.3
Black or African American only	25.6	23.3	18.8	22.8	18.9	13.3

* Estimates are considered unreliable. Data preceded by an asterisk have a relative standard error (RSE) of 20%–30%. Data not shown have an RSE of greater than 30%.

- - - Data not available.

[1]Data prior to 1997 are not strictly comparable with data for later years due to the 1997 questionnaire redesign. See Appendix I, National Health Interview Survey. The column labeled 1995–1998 includes data for 1995, 1997, and 1998 because cigarette smoking data were not collected in 1996.

[2]Estimates are age-adjusted to the year 2000 standard population using five age groups: 18–24 years, 25–34 years, 35–44 years, 45–64 years, and 65 years and over. See Appendix II, Age adjustment. For age groups where smoking is 0% or 100%, the age-adjustment procedure was modified to substitute the percentage smoking from the previous 3-year period.

[3]Starting with 1993 data, current cigarette smokers were defined as ever smoking 100 cigarettes in their lifetime and smoking now on every day or some days. For previous definition, see Appendix II, Cigarette smoking.

[4]Includes all other races not shown separately and unknown education level.

[5]The race groups, white, black, American Indian or Alaska Native (AI/AN), Asian, Native Hawaiian or Other Pacific Islander, and 2 or more races, include persons of Hispanic and non-Hispanic origin. Persons of Hispanic origin may be of any race. Starting with 1999 data, race-specific estimates are tabulated according to the 1997 Revisions to the Standards for the Classification of Federal Data on Race and Ethnicity and are not strictly comparable with estimates for earlier years. The five single-race categories plus multiple-race categories shown in the table conform to the 1997 Standards. Starting with 2002–2004 data, race-specific estimates are for persons who reported only one racial group; the category 2 or more races includes persons who reported more than one racial group. Prior to 1999, data were tabulated according to the 1977 Standards with four racial groups and the Asian only category included Native Hawaiian or Other Pacific Islander. Estimates for single-race categories prior to 1999 included persons who reported one race or, if they reported more than one race, identified one race as best representing their race. Starting with 2003 data, race responses of other race and unspecified multiple race were treated as missing, and then race was imputed if these were the only race responses. Almost all persons with a race response of other race were of Hispanic origin. See Appendix II, Hispanic origin; Race.

[6]Education categories shown are for 1997 and subsequent years. GED stands for General Educational Development high school equivalency diploma. In years prior to 1997, the following categories based on number of years of school completed were used: less than 12 years, 12 years, 13 years or more. See Appendix II, Education.

[7]Estimates are age-adjusted to the year 2000 standard using four age groups: 25–34 years, 35–44 years, 45–64 years, and 65 years and over. See Appendix II, Age adjustment.

NOTES: Standard errors for selected years are available in the spreadsheet version of this table. Available from: www.cdc.gov/nchs/hus.htm. For more data on cigarette smoking see the Early Release reports on the National Health Interview Survey home page available from: www.cdc.gov/nchs/nhis.htm. Data for additional years are available. See Appendix III.

SOURCES: Centers for Disease Control and Prevention, National Center for Health Statistics, National Health Interview Survey. Data are from the following questionnaire supplements: health promotion and disease prevention (1990–1991), cancer control and cancer epidemiology (1992), and year 2000 objectives (1993–1995). Starting with 1997, data are from the family core and sample adult questionnaires.

Table 66 (page 1 of 2). Use of selected substances in the past month among persons 12 years of age and over, by age, sex, race, and Hispanic origin: United States, 2002, 2004, and 2005

[Data are based on household interviews of a sample of the civilian noninstitutionalized population 12 years of age and over]

Age, sex, race, and Hispanic origin	*Any illicit drug*[1]			*Marijuana*			*Nonmedical use of any psychotherapeutic drug*[2]		
	2002	2004	2005	2002	2004	2005	2002	2004	2005
	Percent of population								
12 years and over	8.3	7.9	8.1	6.2	6.1	6.0	2.6	2.5	2.6
Age									
12–13 years	4.2	3.8	3.8	1.4	1.1	0.9	1.7	1.7	1.7
14–15 years	11.2	10.9	8.9	7.6	7.3	5.9	4.0	4.1	2.8
16–17 years	19.8	17.3	17.0	15.7	14.5	13.6	6.2	5.1	5.4
18–25 years	20.2	19.4	20.1	17.3	16.1	16.6	5.4	6.1	6.3
26–34 years	10.5	11.1	11.0	7.7	8.3	8.6	3.6	3.6	3.5
35 years and over	4.6	4.2	4.5	3.1	3.1	3.0	1.6	1.3	1.5
Sex									
Male	10.3	9.9	10.2	8.1	8.0	8.2	2.7	2.6	2.8
Female	6.4	6.1	6.1	4.4	4.3	4.0	2.6	2.4	2.5
Age and sex									
12–17 years	11.6	10.6	9.9	8.2	7.6	6.8	4.0	3.6	3.3
Male	12.3	10.6	10.1	9.1	8.1	7.5	3.6	3.2	3.1
Female	10.9	10.6	9.7	7.2	7.1	6.2	4.3	4.1	3.6
Hispanic origin and race[3]									
Not Hispanic or Latino:									
White only	8.5	8.1	8.1	6.5	6.2	6.1	2.8	2.7	2.8
Black or African American only	9.7	8.7	9.7	7.4	7.0	7.6	2.0	1.6	1.8
American Indian or Alaska Native only	10.1	12.3	12.8	6.7	9.1	9.8	3.2	3.0	5.0
Native Hawaiian or Other Pacific Islander only	7.9	*	8.7	4.4	*	5.7	3.8	4.6	3.3
Asian only	3.5	3.1	3.1	1.8	2.0	1.6	0.7	0.9	1.5
2 or more races	11.4	13.3	12.2	9.0	9.6	10.6	3.5	5.7	2.7
Hispanic or Latino	7.2	7.2	7.6	4.3	5.0	5.1	2.9	2.4	2.5

Age, sex, race, and Hispanic origin	*Alcohol use*			*Binge alcohol use*[4]			*Heavy alcohol use*[5]		
	2002	2004	2005	2002	2004	2005	2002	2004	2005
	Percent of population								
12 years and over	51.0	50.3	51.8	22.9	22.8	22.7	6.7	6.9	6.6
Age									
12–13 years	4.3	4.3	4.2	1.8	2.0	2.0	0.3	0.2	0.2
14–15 years	16.6	16.4	15.1	9.2	9.1	8.0	1.9	1.6	1.7
16–17 years	32.6	32.5	30.1	21.4	22.4	19.7	5.6	6.3	5.3
18–25 years	60.5	60.5	60.9	40.9	41.2	41.9	14.9	15.1	15.3
26–34 years	61.4	60.5	62.5	33.1	32.2	32.9	9.0	9.4	9.6
35 years and over	52.1	51.2	53.3	18.6	18.5	18.3	5.2	5.3	4.7
Sex									
Male	57.4	56.9	58.1	31.2	31.1	30.5	10.8	10.6	10.3
Female	44.9	44.0	45.9	15.1	14.9	15.2	3.0	3.5	3.1
Age and sex									
12–17 years	17.6	17.6	16.5	10.7	11.1	9.9	2.5	2.7	2.4
Male	17.4	17.2	15.9	11.4	11.6	10.4	3.1	3.2	3.0
Female	17.9	18.0	17.2	9.9	10.5	9.4	1.9	2.1	1.8
Hispanic origin and race[3]									
Not Hispanic or Latino:									
White only	55.0	55.2	56.5	23.4	23.8	23.4	7.5	7.9	7.4
Black or African American only	39.9	37.1	40.8	21.0	18.3	20.3	4.4	4.4	4.2
American Indian or Alaska Native only	44.7	36.2	42.4	27.9	25.8	32.8	8.7	7.7	11.5
Native Hawaiian or Other Pacific Islander only	*	*	37.3	25.2	*	25.7	8.3	4.9	5.3
Asian only	37.1	37.4	38.1	12.4	12.4	12.7	2.6	2.7	2.0
2 or more races	49.9	52.4	47.3	19.8	23.5	20.8	7.5	6.9	5.6
Hispanic or Latino	42.8	40.2	42.6	24.8	24.0	23.7	5.9	5.3	5.6

See footnotes at end of table.

Table 66 (page 2 of 2). Use of selected substances in the past month among persons 12 years of age and over, by age, sex, race, and Hispanic origin: United States, 2002, 2004, and 2005

[Data are based on household interviews of a sample of the civilian noninstitutionalized population 12 years of age and over]

Age, sex, race, and Hispanic origin	Any tobacco[6]			Cigarettes			Cigars		
	2002	2004	2005	2002	2004	2005	2002	2004	2005
	Percent of population								
12 years and over	30.4	29.2	29.4	26.0	24.9	24.9	5.4	5.7	5.6
Age									
12–13 years	3.8	3.4	3.0	3.2	2.8	2.4	0.7	0.9	0.7
14–15 years	13.4	13.2	11.3	11.2	10.9	9.2	3.8	3.8	3.3
16–17 years	29.0	27.0	24.8	24.9	22.2	20.6	9.3	9.7	8.6
18–25 years	45.3	44.6	44.3	40.8	39.5	39.0	11.0	12.7	12.0
26–34 years	38.2	37.2	37.7	32.7	32.4	33.0	6.6	6.5	6.8
35 years and over	27.9	26.5	27.0	23.4	22.2	22.3	4.1	4.1	4.2
Sex									
Male	37.0	35.7	35.8	28.7	27.7	27.4	9.4	9.8	9.6
Female	24.3	23.1	23.4	23.4	22.3	22.5	1.7	1.9	1.8
Age and sex									
12–17 years	15.2	14.4	13.1	13.0	11.9	10.8	4.5	4.8	4.2
Male	16.0	15.3	14.2	12.3	11.3	10.7	6.2	6.6	5.8
Female	14.4	13.5	11.9	13.6	12.5	10.8	2.7	2.8	2.5
Hispanic origin and race[3]									
Not Hispanic or Latino:									
White only	32.0	31.4	31.2	26.9	26.4	26.0	5.5	6.0	5.9
Black or African American only	28.8	27.3	28.4	25.3	23.5	24.5	6.8	6.0	6.4
American Indian or Alaska Native only	44.3	33.8	41.7	37.1	31.0	36.0	5.2	4.9	10.6
Native Hawaiian or Other Pacific Islander only	28.8	*	30.3	*	*	28.8	4.1	*	3.7
Asian only	18.6	11.7	14.6	17.7	10.3	13.4	1.1	1.8	1.6
2 or more races	38.1	41.3	33.9	35.0	38.3	30.9	5.5	9.1	7.8
Hispanic or Latino	25.2	23.3	24.5	23.0	21.3	22.1	5.0	4.7	4.3

* Estimates are considered unreliable. Data not shown if the relative standard error is greater than 17.5% of the log transformation of the proportion, the minimum effective sample size is less than 68, the minimum nominal sample size less than 100, or the prevalence close to 0% or 100%.

[1]Any illicit drug includes marijuana/hashish, cocaine (including crack), heroin, hallucinogens (including LSD and PCP), inhalants, or any prescription-type psychotherapeutic drug used nonmedically.

[2]Nonmedical use of prescription-type psychotherapeutic drugs includes the nonmedical use of pain relievers, tranquilizers, stimulants, or sedatives; does not include over-the-counter drugs.

[3]Persons of Hispanic origin may be of any race. Race and Hispanic origin were collected using the 1997 Revisions to the Standards for the Classification of Federal Data on Race and Ethnicity. Single-race categories shown include persons who reported only one racial group. The category 2 or more races includes persons who reported more than one racial group. See Appendix II, Hispanic origin; Race.

[4]Binge alcohol use is defined as drinking five or more drinks on the same occasion on at least one day in the past 30 days. Occasion is defined as at the same time or within a couple of hours of each other. See Appendix II, Binge drinking.

[5]Heavy alcohol use is defined as drinking five or more drinks on the same occasion on each of five or more days in the past 30 days. By definition, all heavy alcohol users are also binge alcohol users.

[6]Any tobacco product includes cigarettes, smokeless tobacco (i.e., chewing tobacco or snuff), cigars, or pipe tobacco.

NOTES: The National Survey on Drug Use & Health (NSDUH), formerly called the National Household Survey on Drug Abuse (NHSDA), began a new baseline in 2002 and cannot be compared with previous years. Because of methodological differences among the National Survey on Drug Use & Health, Monitoring the Future Study (MTF), and Youth Risk Behavior Survey (YRBS), rates of substance use measured by these surveys are not directly comparable. See Appendix I, MTF, NSDUH, and YRBS. Data for additional years are available. See Appendix III.

SOURCE: Substance Abuse and Mental Health Services Administration, Office of Applied Studies, National Survey on Drug Use & Health. Available from: www.oas.samhsa.gov/nsduh.htm.

Table 67 (page 1 of 3). Use of selected substances among high school seniors, tenth-, and eighth-graders, by sex and race: United States, selected years 1980–2006

[Data are based on a survey of high school seniors, tenth-, and eighth-graders in the coterminous United States]

Substance, grade in school, sex, and race	*1980*	*1990*	*1991*	*1995*	*2000*	*2003*	*2004*	*2005*	*2006*
				Percent using substance in the past month					
Cigarettes									
All seniors	30.5	29.4	28.3	33.5	31.4	24.4	25.0	23.2	21.6
Male	26.8	29.1	29.0	34.5	32.8	26.2	25.3	24.8	22.4
Female	33.4	29.2	27.5	32.0	29.7	22.1	24.1	20.7	20.1
White	31.0	32.5	31.8	37.3	36.6	28.2	28.2	27.6	24.7
Black or African American	25.2	12.0	9.4	15.0	13.6	9.0	11.3	10.7	11.0
All tenth-graders	- - -	- - -	20.8	27.9	23.9	16.7	16.0	14.9	14.5
Male	- - -	- - -	20.8	27.7	23.8	16.2	16.2	14.5	13.4
Female	- - -	- - -	20.7	27.9	23.6	17.0	15.7	15.1	15.5
White	- - -	- - -	23.9	31.2	27.3	19.3	18.1	17.6	16.3
Black or African American	- - -	- - -	6.4	12.2	11.3	8.8	9.6	8.7	8.5
All eighth-graders	- - -	- - -	14.3	19.1	14.6	10.2	9.2	9.3	8.7
Male	- - -	- - -	15.5	18.8	14.3	9.6	8.3	8.7	8.1
Female	- - -	- - -	13.1	19.0	14.7	10.6	9.9	9.7	8.9
White	- - -	- -	15.0	21.7	16.4	10.6	9.4	9.4	9.1
Black or African American	- - -	- - -	5.3	8.2	8.4	6.4	7.5	7.1	5.4
Marijuana									
All seniors	33.7	14.0	13.8	21.2	21.6	21.2	19.9	19.8	18.3
Male	37.8	16.1	16.1	24.6	24.7	24.7	23.0	23.6	19.7
Female	29.1	11.5	11.2	17.2	18.3	17.3	16.6	15.8	16.4
White	34.2	15.6	15.0	21.5	22.0	22.8	21.5	21.6	19.2
Black or African American	26.5	5.2	6.5	17.8	17.5	16.1	14.2	14.6	16.7
All tenth-graders	- - -	- - -	8.7	17.2	19.7	17.0	15.9	15.2	14.2
Male	- - -	- - -	10.1	19.2	23.3	19.0	17.4	16.7	15.7
Female	- - -	- - -	7.3	15.0	16.2	15.0	14.2	13.4	12.6
White	- - -	- - -	9.4	17.7	20.1	17.4	15.8	15.7	14.7
Black or African American	- - -	- - -	3.8	15.1	17.0	15.6	17.2	15.3	14.2
All eighth-graders	- - -	- - -	3.2	9.1	9.1	7.5	6.4	6.6	6.5
Male	- - -	- - -	3.8	9.8	10.2	8.5	6.3	7.6	6.7
Female	- - -	- - -	2.6	8.2	7.8	6.4	6.3	5.7	6.0
White	- - -	- - -	3.0	9.0	8.3	7.0	5.5	5.8	5.7
Black or African American	- - -	- - -	2.1	7.0	8.5	7.4	8.1	8.2	6.7
Cocaine									
All seniors	5.2	1.9	1.4	1.8	2.1	2.1	2.3	2.3	2.5
Male	6.0	2.3	1.7	2.2	2.7	2.6	2.9	2.6	3.0
Female	4.3	1.3	0.9	1.3	1.6	1.4	1.7	1.8	2.1
White	5.4	1.8	1.3	1.7	2.2	2.1	2.5	2.4	2.6
Black or African American	2.0	0.5	0.8	0.4	1.0	1.0	0.9	0.7	1.0
All tenth-graders	- - -	- - -	0.7	1.7	1.8	1.3	1.7	1.5	1.5
Male	- - -	- - -	0.7	1.8	2.1	1.3	1.9	1.9	1.6
Female	- - -	- - -	0.6	1.5	1.4	1.3	1.4	1.2	1.3
White	- - -	- - -	0.6	1.7	1.7	1.4	1.7	1.6	1.5
Black or African American	- - -	- - -	0.2	0.4	0.4	0.5	0.4	0.6	0.7
All eighth-graders	- - -	- - -	0.5	1.2	1.2	0.9	0.9	1.0	1.0
Male	- - -	- - -	0.7	1.1	1.3	1.0	0.8	0.9	1.0
Female	- - -	- - -	0.4	1.2	1.1	0.8	1.0	1.0	0.9
White	- - -	- - -	0.4	1.0	1.1	0.8	0.8	0.8	0.8
Black or African American	- - -	- - -	0.4	0.4	0.5	0.5	0.8	0.5	0.4

See footnotes at end of table.

Table 67 (page 2 of 3). Use of selected substances among high school seniors, tenth-, and eighth-graders, by sex and race: United States, selected years 1980–2006

[Data are based on a survey of high school seniors, tenth-, and eighth-graders in the coterminous United States]

Substance, grade in school, sex, and race	1980	1990	1991	1995	2000	2003	2004	2005	2006
	Percent using substance in the past month								
Inhalants									
All seniors	1.4	2.7	2.4	3.2	2.2	1.5	1.5	2.0	1.5
Male	1.8	3.5	3.3	3.9	2.9	2.0	1.7	2.4	1.5
Female	1.0	2.0	1.6	2.5	1.7	1.1	1.3	1.6	1.4
White	1.4	3.0	2.4	3.7	2.1	1.7	1.6	1.9	1.5
Black or African American	1.0	1.5	1.5	1.1	2.1	0.7	1.0	1.2	1.2
All tenth-graders	- - -	- - -	2.7	3.5	2.6	2.2	2.4	2.2	2.3
Male	- - -	- - -	2.9	3.8	3.0	2.3	2.4	1.9	2.2
Female	- - -	- - -	2.6	3.2	2.2	2.2	2.3	2.5	2.4
White	- - -	- - -	2.9	3.9	2.8	2.6	2.6	2.4	2.4
Black or African American	- - -	- - -	2.0	1.2	1.5	0.5	1.4	1.4	1.8
All eighth-graders	- - -	- - -	4.4	6.1	4.5	4.1	4.5	4.2	4.1
Male	- - -	- - -	4.1	5.6	4.1	3.4	4.0	3.1	3.6
Female	- - -	- - -	4.7	6.6	4.8	4.7	5.1	5.3	4.7
White	- - -	- - -	4.5	7.0	4.5	4.3	4.4	4.2	4.2
Black or African American	- - -	- - -	2.3	2.3	2.3	2.3	3.8	3.3	2.7
MDMA (Ecstasy)									
All seniors	- - -	- - -	- - -	- - -	3.6	1.3	1.2	1.0	1.3
Male	- - -	- - -	- - -	- - -	4.1	1.3	1.6	1.0	1.5
Female	- - -	- - -	- - -	- - -	3.1	1.2	0.9	1.0	1.1
White	- - -	- - -	- - -	- - -	3.9	1.3	1.2	1.1	1.4
Black or African American	- - -	- - -	- - -	- - -	1.9	0.6	1.1	1.0	0.6
All tenth-graders	- - -	- - -	- - -	- - -	2.6	1.1	0.8	1.0	1.2
Male	- - -	- - -	- - -	- - -	2.5	1.2	1.0	1.0	1.5
Female	- - -	- - -	- - -	- - -	2.5	1.1	0.6	0.9	0.8
White	- - -	- - -	- - -	- - -	2.5	1.2	0.9	0.9	1.3
Black or African American	- - -	- - -	- - -	- - -	1.8	0.7	0.1	0.2	1.0
All eighth-graders	- - -	- - -	- - -	- - -	1.4	0.7	0.8	0.6	0.7
Male	- - -	- - -	- - -	- - -	1.6	0.7	0.7	0.8	0.5
Female	- - -	- - -	- - -	- - -	1.2	0.7	0.9	0.4	0.8
White	- - -	- - -	- - -	- - -	1.4	0.7	0.6	0.6	0.5
Black or African American	- - -	- - -	- - -	- - -	0.8	0.4	1.2	1.1	0.7
Alcohol[1]									
All seniors	72.0	57.1	54.0	51.3	50.0	47.5	48.0	47.0	45.3
Male	77.4	61.3	58.4	55.7	54.0	51.7	51.1	50.7	47.3
Female	66.8	52.3	49.0	47.0	46.1	43.8	45.1	43.3	43.0
White	75.8	62.2	57.7	54.8	55.3	52.0	52.5	52.3	49.1
Black or African American	47.7	32.9	34.4	37.4	29.3	29.2	29.2	29.0	29.5
All tenth-graders	- - -	- - -	42.8	38.8	41.0	35.4	35.2	33.2	33.8
Male	- - -	- - -	45.5	39.7	43.3	35.3	36.3	32.8	33.8
Female	- - -	- - -	40.3	37.8	38.6	35.3	34.0	33.6	33.8
White	- - -	- - -	45.7	41.3	44.3	38.4	37.3	37.0	36.0
Black or African American	- - -	- - -	30.2	24.9	24.7	24.0	25.4	23.0	22.4
All eighth-graders	- - -	- - -	25.1	24.6	22.4	19.7	18.6	17.1	17.2
Male	- - -	- - -	26.3	25.0	22.5	19.4	17.9	16.2	16.3
Female	- - -	- - -	23.8	24.0	22.0	19.8	19.0	17.9	17.6
White	- - -	- - -	26.0	25.4	23.9	19.9	18.6	17.9	16.5
Black or African American	- - -	- - -	17.8	17.3	15.1	16.5	16.0	14.9	12.4

See footnotes at end of table.

Table 67 (page 3 of 3). Use of selected substances among high school seniors, tenth-, and eighth-graders, by sex and race: United States, selected years 1980–2006

[Data are based on a survey of high school seniors, tenth-, and eighth-graders in the coterminous United States]

Substance, grade in school, sex, and race	*1980*	*1990*	*1991*	*1995*	*2000*	*2003*	*2004*	*2005*	*2006*
Binge drinking[2]					Percent in last 2 weeks				
All seniors	41.2	32.2	29.8	29.8	30.0	27.9	29.2	27.1	25.4
Male	52.1	39.1	37.8	36.9	36.7	34.2	34.3	32.6	28.9
Female	30.5	24.4	21.2	23.0	23.5	22.1	24.2	21.6	21.5
White	44.6	36.2	32.9	32.9	34.4	31.9	33.1	31.8	28.9
Black or African American	17.0	11.6	11.8	15.5	11.0	11.1	11.7	10.9	11.9
All tenth-graders	---	---	22.9	24.0	26.2	22.2	22.0	21.0	21.9
Male	---	---	26.4	26.4	29.8	23.2	23.8	22.0	22.9
Female	---	---	19.5	21.5	22.5	21.2	20.2	19.9	20.9
White	---	---	24.4	25.7	28.5	24.3	23.7	23.5	23.5
Black or African American	---	---	14.4	12.3	12.9	11.7	11.5	11.0	12.2
All eighth-graders	---	---	12.9	14.5	14.1	11.9	11.4	10.5	10.9
Male	---	---	14.3	15.1	14.4	12.2	10.8	10.2	10.5
Female	---	---	11.4	13.9	13.6	11.6	11.8	10.6	10.8
White	---	---	12.6	14.5	14.6	11.4	11.2	10.8	10.1
Black or African American	---	---	9.9	10.0	9.3	10.9	8.6	8.2	8.0

- - - Data not available.

0.0 Quantity more than zero but less than 0.05.

[1]In 1993, the alcohol question was changed to indicate that a drink meant more than a few sips. Data for 1993, available in the spreadsheet version of this table, are based on a half sample. See Appendix II, Alcohol consumption.

[2]Five or more alcoholic drinks in a row at least once in the prior 2-week period. See Appendix II, Binge drinking.

NOTES: Estimates for Hispanic students are not shown due to small sample size. For 2-year estimates for Hispanic students, see Johnson LD, O'Malley PM, Bachman JG, Schulenberg JE. Monitoring the Future national results on adolescent drug use: Overview of key findings, 2005. NIH Pub No. 06–5882, 2006. Bethesda, MD: National Institute on Drug Abuse, available from www.nida.nih.gov/PDF/overview2005.pdf. Because of methodological differences among the National Survey on Drug Use & Health (NSDUH), the Monitoring the Future Study (MTF), and the Youth Risk Behavior Survey (YRBS), rates of substance use measured by these surveys are not directly comparable. See Appendix I, NSDUH, MTF, and YRBS. Data for additional years are available. See Appendix III.

SOURCE: National Institutes of Health, National Institute on Drug Abuse (NIDA), Monitoring the Future Study, annual surveys.

Table 68 (page 1 of 3). Alcohol consumption among adults 18 years of age and over, by selected characteristics: United States, 1997, 2004, and 2005

[Data are based on household interviews of a sample of the civilian noninstitutionalized population]

Characteristic	Both sexes			Male			Female		
	1997	2004	2005	1997	2004	2005	1997	2004	2005
Drinking status[1]	Percent distribution								
18 years and over, age-adjusted[2]									
All	100.0	100.0	100.0	100.0	100.0	100.0	100.0	100.0	100.0
Lifetime abstainer	21.4	24.6	24.4	14.1	17.8	17.9	27.8	30.6	30.1
Former drinker[3]	15.8	14.5	14.3	16.4	14.9	14.6	15.4	14.4	14.1
Infrequent	9.0	8.0	8.2	7.8	6.9	7.1	10.2	9.0	9.2
Regular	6.8	6.5	6.1	8.6	8.0	7.5	5.3	5.4	4.9
Current drinker[3]	62.8	60.8	61.4	69.5	67.3	67.5	56.8	54.9	55.8
Infrequent	13.9	13.3	12.0	10.2	10.0	9.0	17.4	16.4	14.9
Regular	48.5	47.1	48.9	58.7	56.7	58.0	39.2	38.3	40.6
18 years and over, crude									
All	100.0	100.0	100.0	100.0	100.0	100.0	100.0	100.0	100.0
Lifetime abstainer	21.3	24.6	24.3	14.1	17.8	17.9	27.8	30.7	30.2
Former drinker[3]	15.6	14.6	14.3	15.7	14.5	14.3	15.5	14.6	14.4
Infrequent	8.9	8.0	8.2	7.5	6.8	7.0	10.2	9.2	9.3
Regular	6.7	6.5	6.1	8.2	7.8	7.3	5.3	5.4	5.0
Current drinker[3]	63.1	60.8	61.4	70.2	67.6	67.8	56.7	54.6	55.4
Infrequent	14.0	13.3	12.0	10.2	10.0	8.9	17.4	16.3	14.9
Regular	48.8	47.1	49.0	59.4	57.0	58.4	39.1	38.0	40.3
Age	Percent current drinkers among all adults								
All persons:									
18–44 years	68.5	65.7	66.4	73.8	72.4	72.0	63.3	59.2	60.9
18–24 years	61.3	58.0	58.1	65.5	63.6	62.7	57.0	52.5	53.7
25–44 years	70.6	68.3	69.2	76.3	75.4	75.3	65.2	61.5	63.3
45–64 years	62.7	61.7	62.6	69.8	66.4	68.0	55.9	57.4	57.5
45–54 years	66.5	64.4	66.3	73.0	69.1	71.0	60.3	59.9	61.9
55–64 years	56.7	57.9	57.3	64.8	62.4	63.8	49.2	53.9	51.5
65 years and over	42.8	43.6	43.1	52.0	52.8	52.0	36.0	36.9	36.5
65–74 years	47.9	49.5	47.7	56.1	58.1	55.1	41.4	42.4	41.3
75 years and over	36.0	37.0	38.0	45.9	45.8	47.8	29.7	31.4	31.7
Race[2,4]									
White only	65.3	63.6	64.4	71.0	69.4	69.8	60.1	58.2	59.4
Black or African American only	46.7	46.6	46.4	55.5	55.7	56.2	40.0	39.7	38.8
American Indian or Alaska Native only	52.2	48.8	50.0	64.6	50.2	54.1	43.4	46.7	47.7
Asian only	45.7	43.8	42.9	59.8	56.9	53.5	31.6	30.8	32.4
Native Hawaiian or Other Pacific Islander only	---	*	*	---	*	*	---	*	*
2 or more races	---	62.0	51.6	---	68.2	55.7	---	57.3	48.2
Hispanic origin and race[2,4]									
Hispanic or Latino	52.9	49.6	50.8	63.9	63.7	61.8	41.9	35.7	39.7
Mexican	52.7	47.8	48.1	66.3	62.4	61.3	38.7	32.8	34.8
Not Hispanic or Latino	63.3	62.4	62.9	69.3	67.9	68.3	58.0	57.6	58.1
White only	66.7	66.0	67.0	71.7	70.4	71.4	62.2	62.0	63.0
Black or African American only	46.7	46.3	46.0	55.7	55.4	55.8	39.8	39.3	38.5
Geographic region[2]									
Northeast	67.9	67.7	69.0	73.4	73.8	74.2	63.3	62.2	64.6
Midwest	65.7	66.3	66.0	71.6	71.5	71.0	60.3	61.9	61.3
South	55.5	54.2	54.2	63.0	61.5	60.3	48.7	47.5	48.8
West	64.4	59.9	61.6	71.2	67.2	69.8	58.1	52.9	53.6
Location of residence[2]									
Within MSA[5]	63.9	61.3	62.2	70.1	68.0	68.6	58.5	55.4	56.5
Outside MSA[5]	56.5	58.4	56.4	64.6	64.3	61.5	48.8	51.5	50.6

See footnotes at end of table.

Table 68 (page 2 of 3). Alcohol consumption among adults 18 years of age and over, by selected characteristics: United States, 1997, 2004, and 2005

[Data are based on household interviews of a sample of the civilian noninstitutionalized population]

Characteristic	Both sexes 1997	Both sexes 2004	Both sexes 2005	Male 1997	Male 2004	Male 2005	Female 1997	Female 2004	Female 2005
Level of alcohol consumption in past year for current drinkers[6]	Percent distribution of current drinkers[7]								
18 years and over, age-adjusted[2]									
All drinking levels	100.0	100.0	100.0	100.0	100.0	100.0	100.0	100.0	100.0
Light	69.6	69.7	68.1	59.5	60.8	58.2	81.0	79.7	79.2
Moderate	22.5	23.1	24.0	31.8	31.5	33.5	12.0	13.6	13.2
Heavier	7.9	7.2	7.9	8.7	7.7	8.3	7.0	6.7	7.5
18 years and over, crude									
All drinking levels	100.0	100.0	100.0	100.0	100.0	100.0	100.0	100.0	100.0
Light	69.8	69.8	68.3	59.6	60.8	58.4	81.4	79.9	79.4
Moderate	22.3	23.0	23.8	31.7	31.5	33.3	11.7	13.4	13.1
Heavier	7.9	7.3	7.9	8.8	7.8	8.3	6.9	6.7	7.5
Number of days in the past year with five or more drinks	Percent distribution of current drinkers								
18 years and over, crude									
All current drinkers	100.0	100.0	100.0	100.0	100.0	100.0	100.0	100.0	100.0
No days	65.8	67.9	67.4	54.5	57.8	57.3	78.5	79.1	78.6
At least 1 day	34.2	32.1	32.6	45.5	42.2	42.7	21.5	20.9	21.4
1–11 days	18.5	18.2	18.2	22.0	21.5	21.4	14.6	14.5	14.6
12 or more days	15.6	13.9	14.4	23.5	20.7	21.3	6.9	6.4	6.7
Age	Percent of adults with five or more drinks on at least 1 day in the past year among current drinkers								
All persons:									
18 years and over, age-adjusted[2]	32.3	31.1	31.6	43.1	40.5	41.2	20.1	20.5	20.8
18 years and over, crude	34.2	32.1	32.6	45.5	42.2	42.7	21.5	20.9	21.4
18–44 years	42.5	41.8	43.2	54.8	52.3	54.4	28.7	29.5	30.3
18–24 years	51.6	55.9	54.5	61.5	66.8	66.7	40.2	43.1	40.6
25–44 years	40.2	37.6	39.9	53.0	48.0	50.9	25.8	25.5	27.3
45–64 years	25.3	24.3	23.7	36.1	34.3	33.0	12.8	13.5	13.5
45–54 years	28.5	27.1	26.6	40.2	36.7	36.8	15.2	16.8	15.6
55–64 years	19.5	19.7	19.0	28.8	30.5	27.0	8.3	8.4	10.1
65 years and over	11.2	8.9	8.4	17.8	13.9	13.4	4.3	3.7	3.1
65–74 years	13.8	11.6	11.3	21.6	16.7	17.4	5.4	5.9	4.4
75 years and over	6.6	4.7	4.3	10.8	9.1	7.2	*2.5	*	*
Race[2,4]									
White only	33.3	32.5	32.7	44.4	41.9	42.4	20.9	21.9	21.8
Black or African American only	23.9	23.4	24.3	32.0	33.4	34.4	15.0	12.4	13.0
American Indian or Alaska Native only	54.4	33.2	40.9	70.5	43.7	47.8	37.6	*19.5	32.6
Asian only	25.6	18.6	20.8	30.8	25.4	24.4	16.6	*6.1	15.1
Native Hawaiian or Other Pacific Islander only	- - -	*	*	- - -	*	*	- - -	*	*
Hispanic origin and race[2,4]									
Hispanic or Latino	37.0	31.8	32.7	46.6	40.2	43.1	22.4	17.2	16.9
Mexican	39.1	36.6	36.3	50.2	45.3	46.6	20.3	20.1	18.1
Not Hispanic or Latino	31.9	31.1	31.6	42.8	40.8	41.2	20.0	20.8	21.3
White only	33.2	32.8	32.9	44.5	42.5	42.7	21.0	22.5	22.6
Black or African American only	23.7	23.3	24.0	32.0	33.5	33.9	14.5	12.1	13.0

See footnotes at end of table.

Table 68 (page 3 of 3). Alcohol consumption among adults 18 years of age and over, by selected characteristics: United States, 1997, 2004, and 2005

[Data are based on household interviews of a sample of the civilian noninstitutionalized population]

Characteristic	Both sexes			Male			Female		
	1997	2004	2005	1997	2004	2005	1997	2004	2005
	Percent of adults with five or more drinks on at least 1 day in the past year among current drinkers								
Geographic region[2]									
Northeast	31.4	28.6	29.4	43.3	37.8	38.7	19.0	19.1	20.3
Midwest	33.7	35.8	34.6	44.6	46.6	45.6	21.6	24.6	22.7
South	30.9	28.5	29.3	40.6	37.5	38.4	19.3	17.6	18.9
West	33.5	31.4	33.3	44.7	40.3	42.3	20.7	20.7	21.6
Location of residence[2]									
Within MSA[5]	31.7	30.5	31.3	42.4	40.2	41.1	19.9	20.1	20.7
Outside MSA[5]	34.9	36.1	34.0	45.7	43.7	42.4	21.2	24.5	22.0

* Estimates are considered unreliable. Data preceded by an asterisk have a relative standard error (RSE) of 20%–30%. Data not shown have an RSE of greater than 30%.

- - - Data not available.

[1]Drinking status categories are based on self-reported responses to questions about alcohol consumption. Lifetime abstainers had fewer than 12 drinks in their lifetime. Former drinkers had at least 12 drinks in their lifetime and none in the past year. Former infrequent drinkers are former drinkers who had fewer than 12 drinks in any one year. Former regular drinkers are former drinkers who had at least 12 drinks in any one year. Current drinkers had at least 12 drinks in their lifetime and at least one drink in the past year. Current infrequent drinkers are current drinkers who had fewer than 12 drinks in the past year. Current regular drinkers are current drinkers who had at least 12 drinks in the past year. See Appendix II, Alcohol consumption.

[2]Estimates are age-adjusted to the year 2000 standard population using four age groups: 18–24 years, 25–44 years, 45–64 years, and 65 years and over. Age-adjusted estimates in this table may differ from other age-adjusted estimates based on the same data and presented elsewhere if different age groups are used in the adjustment procedure. See Appendix II, Age adjustment.

[3]The totals for current and former drinkers include a small number of adults who did not provide sufficient information on frequency or amount of drinking; therefore, infrequent or regular drinking status could not be determined for these people.

[4]The race groups, white, black, American Indian or Alaska Native, Asian, Native Hawaiian or Other Pacific Islander, and 2 or more races, include persons of Hispanic and non-Hispanic origin. Persons of Hispanic origin may be of any race. Starting with 1999 data, race-specific estimates are tabulated according to the 1997 Revisions to the Standards for the Classification of Federal Data on Race and Ethnicity and are not strictly comparable with estimates for earlier years. The five single-race categories plus multiple-race categories shown in the table conform to the 1997 Standards. Starting with 1999 data, race-specific estimates are for persons who reported only one racial group; the category 2 or more races includes persons who reported more than one racial group. Prior to 1999, data were tabulated according to the 1977 Standards with four racial groups and the Asian only category included Native Hawaiian or Other Pacific Islander. Estimates for single-race categories prior to 1999 included persons who reported one race or, if they reported more than one race, identified one race as best representing their race. Starting with 2003 data, race responses of other race and unspecified multiple race were treated as missing, and then race was imputed if these were the only race responses. Almost all persons with a race response of other race were of Hispanic origin. See Appendix II, Hispanic origin; Race.

[5]MSA is metropolitan statistical area.

[6]Level of alcohol consumption categories are based on self-reported responses to questions about average alcohol consumption and are defined as follows: light drinkers: three drinks or fewer per week; moderate drinkers: more than three drinks and up to 14 drinks per week for men and more than three drinks and up to seven drinks per week for women; heavier drinkers: more than 14 drinks per week for men and more than seven drinks per week for women. (Most drinking guidelines consider more than seven drinks per week to be a heavier level of consumption for women. U.S. Department of Agriculture: Dietary Guidelines for Americans, 2000, 5th edition.)

[7]Percentage based on current drinkers with known frequency and amount of drinking.

NOTES: Standard errors are available in the spreadsheet version of this table. Available from: www.cdc.gov/nchs/hus.htm. For more data on alcohol consumption see the Early Release reports on the National Health Interview Survey home page: www.cdc.gov/nchs/nhis.htm. Data for additional years are available. See Appendix III.

SOURCE: Centers for Disease Control and Prevention, National Center for Health Statistics, National Health Interview Survey, family core and sample adult questionnaires.

Table 69. Selected health conditions and risk factors: United States, 1988–1994 through 2003–2004

[Data are based on interviews and physical examinations of a sample of the civilian noninstitutionalized population]

Health conditions	*1988–1994*	*1999–2000*	*2001–2002*	*2003–2004*
Diabetes[1]	Percent of persons 20 years of age and over			
Total, age-adjusted[2]	8.0	8.5	9.8	10.0
Total, crude	7.8	8.3	9.6	10.3
High serum total cholesterol[3]				
Total, age-adjusted[4]	20.8	18.3	16.5	16.9
Total, crude	19.6	17.8	16.4	17.0
Hypertension[5]				
Total, age-adjusted[4]	25.5	30.0	29.7	32.1
Total, crude	24.1	28.9	28.9	32.5
Overweight (includes Obesity)[6]				
Total, age-adjusted[4]	56.0	64.0	65.3	66.0
Total, crude	54.9	63.6	65.2	66.2
Obesity[7]				
Total, age-adjusted[4]	22.9	30.1	29.9	32.0
Total, crude	22.3	29.9	30.0	32.0
Untreated dental caries[8]				
Total, age-adjusted[4]	27.7	24.3	21.3	27.1
Total, crude	28.2	25.0	21.6	27.6
Overweight[9]	Percent of persons under 20 years of age			
2–5 years	7.2	10.3	10.6	13.9
6–11 years	11.3	15.1	16.3	18.8
12–19 years	10.5	14.8	16.7	17.4
Untreated dental caries[8]				
2–5 years	19.1	23.2	15.8	23.4
6–19 years	23.6	22.7	20.6	25.1

[1]Includes physician-diagnosed and undiagnosed diabetes. Physician-diagnosed diabetes was obtained by self-report and excludes women who reported having diabetes only during pregnancy. Undiagnosed diabetes is defined as a fasting blood glucose of at least 126 mg/dL and no reported physician diagnosis. See related Table 55. Data have been revised and differ from previous editions of *Health, United States.*

[2]Estimates are age-adjusted to the year 2000 standard population using three age groups: 20–39 years, 40–59 years, and 60 years and over. Because of the smaller sample size for fasting tests, age adjustment is to three age groups only. Age-adjusted estimates in this table may differ from other age-adjusted estimates based on the same data and presented elsewhere if different age groups are used in the adjustment procedure. See Appendix II, Age adjustment.

[3]High serum cholesterol is defined as greater than or equal to 240 mg/dL (6.20 mmol/L). Risk levels have been defined by the Third Report of the National Cholesterol Education Program Expert Panel on Detection, Evaluation, and Treatment of High Blood Cholesterol in Adults. National Heart, Lung, and Blood Institute, National Institutes of Health. September 2002. (Available from: www.nhlbi.nih.gov/guidelines/cholesterol/index.htm and summarized in JAMA 2001;285(19):2486–97.) Individuals who take medicine to lower their serum cholesterol levels and whose measured total serum cholesterol levels are below the cut-offs for high cholesterol are not defined as having high cholesterol. See related Table 71.

[4]Age-adjusted to the 2000 standard population using five age groups: 20–34 years, 35–44 years, 45–54 years, 55–64 years, and 65 years and over. Age-adjusted estimates may differ from other age-adjusted estimates based on the same data and presented elsewhere if different age groups are used in the adjustment procedure. See Appendix II, Age adjustment.

[5]Hypertension is defined as having elevated blood pressure and/or taking antihypertensive medication. Elevated blood pressure is defined as having systolic pressure of at least 140 mmHg or diastolic pressure of at least 90 mmHg. Those with elevated blood pressure may be taking prescribed medicine for high blood pressure. Respondents were asked, "Are you now taking prescribed medicine for your high blood pressure?" See Appendix II, Blood pressure, elevated. See related Table 70.

[6]Excludes pregnant women. Overweight is defined as body mass index (BMI) greater than or equal to 25 kilograms/meter^2. See Appendix II, Body mass index. See related Table 74.

[7]Excludes pregnant women. Obesity is defined as body mass index (BMI) greater than or equal to 30 kilograms/meter^2. See Appendix II, Body mass index. See related Table 74.

[8]Untreated dental caries refers to untreated coronal caries, that is, caries on the crown or enamel surface of the tooth. Root caries are not included. For children 2–5 years of age, only dental caries in primary teeth was evaluated. Caries in both permanent and primary teeth was evaluated for children 6–11 years of age. For children 12 years and over and for adults, only dental caries in permanent teeth was evaluated. Excludes edentulous persons (persons without teeth) of all ages. The majority of edentulous persons are 65 years of age and over. Estimates of edentulism among persons 65 years of age and over are 33% in 1988–1994 and 27% in 1999–2004. See Appendix II, Dental caries. See related Table 76.

[9]Overweight is defined as body mass index (BMI) at or above the sex- and age-specific 95th percentile BMI cutoff points from the 2000 CDC Growth Charts: United States. Advance data from vital and health statistics; no 314. Hyattsville, MD: National Center for Health Statistics. 2000. Excludes pregnant girls. See related Table 75.

NOTES:See related Tables 55, 70, 71, 74, 75, and 76. Standard errors for selected years are available in the spreadsheet version of this table. Available from: www.cdc.gov/nchs/hus.htm.

SOURCES: Centers for Disease Control and Prevention, National Center for Health Statistics, National Health and Nutrition Examination Survey.

Table 70 (page 1 of 2). Hypertension and elevated blood pressure among persons 20 years of age and over, by sex, age, race and Hispanic origin, and poverty level: United States, 1988–1994 and 2001–2004

[Data are based on interviews and physical examinations of a sample of the civilian noninstitutionalized population]

Sex, age, race and Hispanic origin[1], and poverty level	*Hypertension*[2,3]		*Elevated blood pressure*[2]	
	1988–1994	*2001–2004*	*1988–1994*	*2001–2004*
20–74 years, age-adjusted[4]	Percent of population			
Both sexes[5]	21.7	26.7	15.4	15.9
Male	23.4	26.9	18.2	16.1
Female	20.0	26.2	12.6	15.5
Not Hispanic or Latino:				
White only, male	22.6	26.0	17.3	14.9
White only, female	18.4	24.1	11.2	14.1
Black or African American only, male	34.3	37.8	27.9	25.1
Black or African American only, female	35.0	40.3	23.5	24.0
Mexican male	23.4	22.1	19.1	14.9
Mexican female	21.0	25.1	16.5	16.8
Percent of poverty level:[6]				
Below 100%	27.5	30.8	19.0	19.5
100%–less than 200%	22.6	30.1	15.8	18.7
200% or more	20.4	25.4	14.6	14.8
20 years and over, age-adjusted[4]				
Both sexes[5]	25.5	30.9	18.5	19.0
Male	26.4	30.3	20.6	18.3
Female	24.4	31.0	16.4	19.2
Not Hispanic or Latino:				
White only, male	25.6	29.3	19.7	17.1
White only, female	23.0	29.0	15.1	17.9
Black or African American only, male	37.5	41.5	30.3	27.8
Black or African American only, female	38.3	44.3	26.4	26.9
Mexican male	26.9	26.1	22.2	17.8
Mexican female	25.0	29.7	20.4	20.5
Percent of poverty level:[6]				
Below 100%	31.7	35.5	22.5	23.1
100%–less than 200%	26.6	34.0	19.3	21.5
200% or more	23.9	29.4	17.5	17.7
20 years and over, crude				
Both sexes[5]	24.1	30.8	17.6	18.7
Male	23.8	29.0	18.7	17.6
Female	24.4	32.5	16.5	19.8
Not Hispanic or Latino:				
White only, male	24.3	29.9	18.7	17.4
White only, female	24.6	32.9	16.4	20.2
Black or African American only, male	31.1	36.7	25.5	24.7
Black or African American only, female	32.5	41.6	22.2	24.4
Mexican male	16.4	15.8	13.9	11.4
Mexican female	15.9	19.0	12.7	12.8
Percent of poverty level:[6]				
Below 100%	25.7	28.3	18.7	18.3
100%–less than 200%	26.7	34.6	19.8	21.6
200% or more	22.2	29.9	16.2	17.8
Male				
20–34 years	7.1	7.0	6.6	6.1
35–44 years	17.1	19.2	15.2	11.9
45–54 years	29.2	35.9	21.9	23.0
55–64 years	40.6	47.5	28.4	25.7
65–74 years	54.4	61.7	39.9	30.2
75 years and over	60.4	67.1	49.7	45.0
Female				
20–34 years	2.9	*2.7	*2.4	
35–44 years	11.2	14.0	6.4	6.8
45–54 years	23.9	35.2	13.7	22.3
55–64 years	42.6	54.4	27.0	29.6
65–74 years	56.2	72.9	38.2	48.3
75 years and over	73.6	82.0	59.9	58.5

See footnotes at end of table.

Table 70 (page 2 of 2). Hypertension and elevated blood pressure among persons 20 years of age and over, by sex, age, race and Hispanic origin, and poverty level: United States, 1988–1994 and 2001–2004

[Data are based on interviews and physical examinations of a sample of the civilian noninstitutionalized population]

* Estimates are considered unreliable. Data preceded by an asterisk have a relative standard error of 20%–30%. Data not shown have an RSE greater than 30%.
[1]Persons of Mexican origin may be of any race. Starting with 1999 data, race-specific estimates are tabulated according to the 1997 Revisions to the Standards for the Classification of Federal Data on Race and Ethnicity and are not strictly comparable with estimates for earlier years. The two non-Hispanic race categories shown in the table conform to the 1997 Standards. Starting with 1999 data, race-specific estimates are for persons who reported only one racial group. Prior to data year 1999, estimates were tabulated according to the 1977 Standards. Estimates for single-race categories prior to 1999 included persons who reported one race or, if they reported more than one race, identified one race as best representing their race. See Appendix II, Hispanic origin; Race.
[2]Hypertension is defined as having elevated blood pressure and/or taking antihypertensive medication. Elevated blood pressure is defined as having systolic pressure of at least 140 mmHg or diastolic pressure of at least 90 mmHg. Those with elevated blood pressure may be taking prescribed medicine for high blood pressure. See Appendix II, Blood pressure, elevated.
[3]Respondents were asked, "Are you now taking prescribed medicine for your high blood pressure?"
[4]Age-adjusted to the 2000 standard population using five age groups: 20–34 years, 35–44 years, 45–54 years, 55–64 years, and 65 years and over (65–74 years for estimates for 20–74 years). Age-adjusted estimates may differ from other age-adjusted estimates based on the same data and presented elsewhere if different age groups are used in the adjustment procedure. See Appendix II, Age adjustment.
[5]Includes persons of all races and Hispanic origins, not just those shown separately.
[6]Poverty level is based on family income and family size. Persons with unknown poverty level are excluded. See Appendix II, Family income; Poverty.

NOTES: Percents are based on the average of blood pressure measurements taken. In 2001–2004, 77% of participants had three blood pressure readings. See *Health, United States, 2003,* Table 66 for a longer trend based on a single blood pressure measurement, which provides comparable data across five time periods (1960–1962 through 1999–2000). Excludes pregnant women. Estimates for persons 20 years and over are used for setting and tracking *Healthy People 2010* objectives. Numbers have been revised and differ from the previous edition of *Health, United States.* Standard errors are available in the spreadsheet version of this table. Available from: www.cdc.gov/nchs/hus.htm. Data for additional years are available. See Appendix III.

SOURCE: Centers for Disease Control and Prevention, National Center for Health Statistics, National Health and Nutrition Examination Survey.

Table 71 (page 1 of 3). Serum total cholesterol levels among persons 20 years of age and over, by sex, age, race and Hispanic origin, and poverty level: United States, selected years 1960–1962 through 2001–2004

[Data are based on physical examinations of a sample of the civilian noninstitutionalized population]

Sex, age, race and Hispanic origin[1], and poverty level	1960–1962	1971–1974	1976–1980[2]	1988–1994	2001–2004
20–74 years, age-adjusted[3]	Percent of population with high serum total cholesterol (greater than or equal to 240 mg/dL)				
Both sexes[4]	33.3	28.6	27.8	19.7	16.5
Male	30.6	27.9	26.4	18.8	16.6
Female	35.6	29.1	28.8	20.5	16.2
Not Hispanic or Latino:					
White only, male	- - -	- - -	26.4	18.7	16.5
White only, female	- - -	- - -	29.6	20.7	16.7
Black or African American only, male[1]	- - -	- - -	25.5	16.4	14.4
Black or African American only, female	- - -	- - -	26.3	19.9	14.3
Mexican male	- - -	- - -	20.3	18.7	17.0
Mexican female	- - -	- - -	20.5	17.7	12.8
Percent of poverty level:[5]					
Below 100%	- - -	24.4	23.5	19.3	18.9
100%–less than 200%	- - -	28.9	26.5	19.4	17.5
200% or more	- - -	28.9	29.0	19.6	16.0
20 years and over, age-adjusted[3]					
Both sexes[4]	- - -	- - -	- - -	20.8	16.7
Male	- - -	- - -	- - -	19.0	16.1
Female	- - -	- - -	- - -	22.0	16.8
Not Hispanic or Latino:					
White only, male	- - -	- - -	- - -	18.8	16.0
White only, female	- - -	- - -	- - -	22.2	17.4
Black or African American only, male	- - -	- - -	- - -	16.9	14.2
Black or African American only, female	- - -	- - -	- - -	21.4	14.8
Mexican male	- - -	- - -	- - -	18.5	16.9
Mexican female	- - -	- - -	- - -	18.7	14.0
Percent of poverty level:[5]					
Below 100%	- - -	- - -	- - -	20.6	19.3
100%–less than 200%	- - -	- - -	- - -	20.6	17.8
200% or more	- - -	- - -	- - -	20.4	15.9
20 years and over, crude					
Both sexes[4]	- - -	- - -	- - -	19.6	16.7
Male	- - -	- - -	- - -	17.7	16.4
Female	- - -	- - -	- - -	21.3	17.0
Not Hispanic or Latino:					
White only, male	- - -	- - -	- - -	18.0	16.5
White only, female	- - -	- - -	- - -	22.5	18.1
Black or African American only, male	- - -	- - -	- - -	14.7	13.8
Black or African American only, female	- - -	- - -	- - -	18.2	13.5
Mexican male	- - -	- - -	- - -	15.4	15.1
Mexican female	- - -	- - -	- - -	14.3	10.8
Percent of poverty level:[5]					
Below 100%	- - -	- - -	- - -	17.6	17.3
100%–less than 200%	- - -	- - -	- - -	19.8	16.4
200% or more	- - -	- - -	- - -	19.5	16.6
Male					
20–34 years	15.1	12.4	11.9	8.2	9.0
35–44 years	33.9	31.8	27.9	19.4	21.2
45–54 years	39.2	37.5	36.9	26.6	23.1
55–64 years	41.6	36.2	36.8	28.0	19.9
65–74 years	38.0	34.7	31.7	21.9	11.0
75 years and over	- - -	- - -	- - -	20.4	9.9
Female					
20–34 years	12.4	10.9	9.8	7.3	9.3
35–44 years	23.1	19.3	20.7	12.3	11.4
45–54 years	46.9	38.7	40.5	26.7	20.0
55–64 years	70.1	53.1	52.9	40.9	27.6
65–74 years	68.5	57.7	51.6	41.3	26.3
75 years and over	- - -	- - -	- - -	38.2	23.8

See footnotes at end of table.

Table 71 (page 2 of 3). Serum total cholesterol levels among persons 20 years of age and over, by sex, age, race and Hispanic origin, and poverty level: United States, selected years 1960–1962 through 2001–2004

[Data are based on physical examinations of a sample of the civilian noninstitutionalized population]

Sex, age, race and Hispanic origin[1], and poverty level	*1960–1962*	*1971–1974*	*1976–1980[2]*	*1988–1994*	*2001–2004*
20–74 years, age-adjusted[3]			Mean serum cholesterol level, mg/dL		
Both sexes[4]	222	216	215	205	202
Male	220	216	213	204	201
Female	224	217	216	205	201
Not Hispanic or Latino:					
White only, male	---	---	213	204	201
White only, female	---	---	216	206	202
Black or African American only, male	---	---	211	201	198
Black or African American only, female	---	---	216	204	198
Mexican male	---	---	209	206	202
Mexican female	---	---	209	204	199
Percent of poverty level:[5]					
Below 100%	---	211	211	203	202
100%–less than 200%	---	217	213	203	202
200% or more	---	217	216	206	202
20 years and over, age-adjusted[3]					
Both sexes[4]	---	---	---	206	202
Male	---	---	---	204	201
Female	---	---	---	207	202
Not Hispanic or Latino:					
White only, male	---	---	---	205	201
White only, female	---	---	---	208	203
Black or African American only, male	---	---	---	202	198
Black or African American only, female	---	---	---	207	199
Mexican male	---	---	---	206	201
Mexican female	---	---	---	206	200
Percent of poverty level:[5]					
Below 100%	---	---	---	205	203
100%–less than 200%	---	---	---	205	202
200% or more	---	---	---	207	202
20 years and over, crude					
Both sexes[4]	---	---	---	204	202
Male	---	---	---	202	201
Female	---	---	---	206	203
Not Hispanic or Latino:					
White only, male	---	---	---	203	201
White only, female	---	---	---	208	205
Black or African American only, male	---	---	---	198	197
Black or African American only, female	---	---	---	201	196
Mexican male	---	---	---	199	198
Mexican female	---	---	---	198	194
Percent of poverty level:[5]					
Below 100%	---	---	---	200	199
100%–less than 200%	---	---	---	202	200
200% or more	---	---	---	205	203
Male					
20–34 years	198	194	192	186	186
35–44 years	227	221	217	206	210
45–54 years	231	229	227	216	213
55–64 years	233	229	229	216	208
65–74 years	230	226	221	212	194
75 years and over	---	---	---	205	194
Female					
20–34 years	194	191	189	184	186
35–44 years	214	207	207	195	198
45–54 years	237	232	232	217	209
55–64 years	262	245	249	235	219
65–74 years	266	250	246	233	219
75 years and over	---	---	---	229	213

See footnotes at end of table.

Table 71 (page 3 of 3). Serum total cholesterol levels among persons 20 years of age and over, by sex, age, race and Hispanic origin, and poverty level: United States, selected years 1960–1962 through 2001–2004

[Data are based on physical examinations of a sample of the civilian noninstitutionalized population]

- - - Data not available.

[1]Persons of Mexican origin may be of any race. Starting with 1999 data, race-specific estimates are tabulated according to the 1997 Revisions to the Standards for the Classification of Federal Data on Race and Ethnicity and are not strictly comparable with estimates for earlier years. The two non-Hispanic race categories shown in the table conform to the 1997 Standards. Starting with 1999 data, race-specific estimates are for persons who reported only one racial group. Prior to data year 1999, estimates were tabulated according to the 1977 Standards. Estimates for single-race categories prior to 1999 included persons who reported one race or, if they reported more than one race, identified one race as best representing their race. See Appendix II, Hispanic origin; Race.

[2]Data for Mexicans are for 1982–1984. See Appendix I, National Health and Nutrition Examination Survey (NHANES).

[3]Age-adjusted to the 2000 standard population using five age groups: 20–34 years, 35–44 years, 45–54 years, 55–64 years, and 65 years and over (65–74 years for estimates for 20–74 years). Age-adjusted estimates may differ from other age-adjusted estimates based on the same data and presented elsewhere if different age groups are used in the adjustment procedure. See Appendix II, Age adjustment.

[4]Includes persons of all races and Hispanic origins, not just those shown separately.

[5]Poverty level is based on family income and family size. Persons with unknown poverty level are excluded. See Appendix II, Family income; Poverty.

NOTES: High serum cholesterol is defined as greater than or equal to 240 mg/dL (6.20 mmol/L). Borderline high serum cholesterol is defined as greater than or equal to 200 mg/dL and less than 240 mg/dL. Risk levels have been defined by the Third Report of the National Cholesterol Education Program Expert Panel on Detection, Evaluation, and Treatment of High Blood Cholesterol in Adults. National Heart, Lung, and Blood Institute, National Institutes of Health. September 2002. (Available from: www.nhlbi.nih.gov/guidelines/cholesterol/index.htm and summarized in JAMA 2001;285(19):2486–97). Individuals who take medicine to lower their serum cholesterol levels and whose measured total serum cholesterol levels are below the cut-offs for high and borderline high cholesterol are not defined as having high or borderline high cholesterol, respectively. Standard errors for selected years are available in the spreadsheet version of this table. Available from: www.cdc.gov/nchs/hus.htm. Data for additional years are available. See Appendix III.

SOURCES: Centers for Disease Control and Prevention, National Center for Health Statistics, National Health and Nutrition Examination Survey, Hispanic Health and Nutrition Examination Survey (1982–1984), and National Health Examination Survey (1960–1962).

Table 72. Mean energy and macronutrient intake among persons 20–74 years of age, by sex and age: United States, 1971–1974 through 2001–2004

[Data are based on dietary recall interviews of a sample of the civilian noninstitutionalized population]

Sex and age	*1971–1974*	*1976–1980*	*1988–1994*	*2001–2004*
	Energy intake in kcals			
Male, age-adjusted[1]	2,450	2,439	2,664	2,693
Male, crude	2,461	2,459	2,692	2,697
20–39 years	2,784	2,753	2,964	2,949
40–59 years	2,303	2,315	2,567	2,649
60–74 years	1,918	1,906	2,104	2,117
Female, age-adjusted[1]	1,542	1,522	1,796	1,886
Female, crude	1,540	1,525	1,804	1,884
20–39 years	1,652	1,643	1,956	2,032
40–59 years	1,510	1,473	1,734	1,836
60–74 years	1,325	1,322	1,520	1,622
	Percent kcals from carbohydrate			
Male, age-adjusted[1]	42.4	42.6	48.3	48.2
Male, crude	42.4	42.7	48.3	48.2
20–39 years	42.2	43.1	48.1	49.5
40–59 years	41.6	41.5	47.8	47.1
60–74 years	44.8	44.1	49.7	47.3
Female, age-adjusted[1]	45.4	46.0	50.7	50.6
Female, crude	45.5	46.1	50.7	50.6
20–39 years	45.8	46.0	50.6	51.4
40–59 years	44.4	45.0	50.0	49.6
60–74 years	46.8	48.6	52.6	51.1
	Percent kcals from total fat			
Male, age-adjusted[1]	36.9	36.7	33.9	33.4
Male, crude	36.9	36.7	33.9	33.4
20–39 years	37.0	36.2	34.0	32.1
40–59 years	36.9	37.2	34.2	34.1
60–74 years	36.4	36.8	32.9	34.9
Female, age-adjusted[1]	36.1	36.0	33.4	33.8
Female, crude	36.0	35.9	33.3	33.8
20–39 years	36.3	36.0	33.6	33.0
40–59 years	36.3	36.4	34.0	34.6
60–74 years	34.9	34.7	31.6	34.0
	Percent kcals from saturated fat			
Male, age-adjusted[1]	13.5	13.2	11.3	10.8
Male, crude	13.5	13.2	11.4	10.8
20–39 years	13.6	13.1	11.5	10.7
40–59 years	13.5	13.4	11.3	10.9
60–74 years	13.3	13.1	10.9	11.0
Female, age-adjusted[1]	13.0	12.5	11.2	10.9
Female, crude	12.9	12.5	11.2	10.9
20–39 years	13.0	12.6	11.4	10.9
40–59 years	13.1	12.6	11.3	11.1
60–74 years	12.4	11.8	10.4	10.6

[1]Age-adjusted to the 2000 standard population using three age groups, 20–39 years, 40–59 years, and 60–74 years. Age-adjusted estimates in this table may differ from other age-adjusted estimates based on the same data and presented elsewhere if different age groups are used in the adjustment procedure. See Appendix II, Age adjustment.

NOTES: Numbers have been revised and differ from previous editions of *Health, United States.* Estimates of energy intake include kilocalories (kcals) from all foods and beverages, including alcoholic beverages, consumed during the preceding 24 hours. Individuals who reported no energy intake were excluded. In 2001–2004, only data collected in the Mobile Examination Center were used to calculate dietary intake. Standard errors are available in the spreadsheet version of this table. Available from: www.cdc.gov/nchs/hus.htm.

SOURCE: Centers for Disease Control and Prevention, National Center for Health Statistics, National Health and Nutrition Examination Survey.

Table 73 (page 1 of 2). Leisure-time physical activity among adults 18 years of age and over, by selected characteristics: United States, 1998, 2004, and 2005

[Data are based on household interviews of a sample of the civilian noninstitutionalized population]

Characteristic	*Inactive*[1]			*Some leisure-time activity*[1]			*Regular leisure-time activity*[1]		
	1998	*2004*	*2005*	*1998*	*2004*	*2005*	*1998*	*2004*	*2005*
	Percent of adults								
18 years and over, age-adjusted[2,3]	40.5	39.5	40.5	30.0	30.4	29.3	29.5	30.2	30.2
18 years and over, crude[3]	40.2	39.4	40.5	30.0	30.4	29.3	29.8	30.2	30.1
Age									
18–44 years	35.2	35.4	35.9	31.4	31.5	30.5	33.5	33.1	33.7
18–24 years	32.8	33.1	33.5	30.1	30.2	29.1	37.1	36.6	37.4
25–44 years	35.9	36.1	36.7	31.8	31.9	31.0	32.4	31.9	32.4
45–64 years	41.2	39.2	41.2	30.6	31.0	29.7	28.2	29.7	29.1
45–54 years	38.9	37.5	39.5	31.4	32.8	30.1	29.8	29.7	30.4
55–64 years	44.9	41.8	43.6	29.3	28.5	29.2	25.8	29.8	27.2
65 years and over	55.4	52.7	53.9	24.7	25.6	24.9	19.9	21.7	21.3
65–74 years	49.1	44.3	47.8	26.5	29.0	27.0	24.4	26.7	25.3
75 years and over	63.3	62.1	60.6	22.4	21.8	22.6	14.3	16.1	16.8
Sex[2]									
Male	37.8	38.1	39.1	28.7	30.5	29.2	33.5	31.4	31.8
Female	42.9	40.6	41.7	31.1	30.3	29.5	26.0	29.1	28.8
Sex and age									
Male:									
18–44 years	32.0	34.0	34.4	30.7	31.6	30.5	37.2	34.4	35.1
45–54 years	37.7	38.3	40.2	29.6	33.4	29.4	32.6	28.3	30.4
55–64 years	44.5	40.7	43.4	26.9	26.9	28.0	28.6	32.4	28.7
65–74 years	45.3	41.7	44.7	23.6	29.1	27.5	31.1	29.2	27.8
75 years and over	57.4	56.8	54.1	21.6	23.1	24.0	20.9	20.1	21.9
Female:									
18–44 years	38.2	36.7	37.3	32.0	31.4	30.5	29.8	31.9	32.2
45–54 years	39.9	36.7	38.8	33.0	32.3	30.8	27.1	31.0	30.3
55–64 years	45.2	42.7	43.8	31.5	29.9	30.3	23.3	27.4	25.9
65–74 years	52.2	46.5	50.4	28.7	28.9	26.5	19.0	24.6	23.1
75 years and over	67.0	65.6	64.8	22.9	21.0	21.7	10.1	13.5	13.6
Race[2,4]									
White only	38.8	38.0	38.6	30.5	30.7	29.9	30.7	31.3	31.6
Black or African American only	52.2	50.5	54.7	25.2	26.1	24.1	22.6	23.3	21.2
American Indian or Alaska Native only	49.2	44.4	42.7	19.0	33.7	29.0	31.8	21.9	28.3
Asian only	39.4	39.1	41.0	35.2	33.4	31.3	25.4	27.5	27.6
Native Hawaiian or Other Pacific Islander only	- - -	*	*	- - -	*	*	- - -	*	*
2 or more races	- - -	28.8	40.7	- - -	38.7	30.9	- - -	32.4	28.4
Hispanic origin and race[2,4]									
Hispanic or Latino	55.5	52.8	56.7	23.4	24.8	23.3	21.1	22.3	20.0
Mexican	56.7	52.4	54.9	23.9	25.5	24.3	19.4	22.1	20.8
Not Hispanic or Latino	38.8	37.5	38.1	30.7	31.1	30.1	30.5	31.4	31.8
White only	36.7	35.3	35.3	31.3	31.6	30.9	32.0	33.1	33.8
Black or African American only	52.2	50.7	54.6	25.1	26.0	24.3	22.6	23.2	21.1
Education[5,6]									
No high school diploma or GED	64.8	63.8	62.9	19.4	21.5	21.5	15.8	14.7	15.7
High school diploma or GED	47.6	48.6	50.2	28.7	28.5	28.1	23.7	22.8	21.6
Some college or more	30.2	28.9	30.7	34.3	34.3	32.4	35.5	36.9	36.8

See footnotes at end of table.

Table 73 (page 2 of 2). Leisure-time physical activity among adults 18 years of age and over, by selected characteristics: United States, 1998, 2004, and 2005

[Data are based on household interviews of a sample of the civilian noninstitutionalized population]

Characteristic	*Inactive*[1]			*Some leisure-time activity*[1]			*Regular leisure-time activity*[1]		
	1998	*2004*	*2005*	*1998*	*2004*	*2005*	*1998*	*2004*	*2005*
Percent of poverty level[2,7]					Percent of adults				
Below 100%	59.4	56.7	58.2	20.5	22.8	22.3	20.1	20.4	19.5
100%–less than 200%	52.2	52.4	52.8	26.2	26.4	25.5	21.6	21.2	21.7
200% or more	34.7	33.4	34.5	32.4	32.6	31.4	33.0	34.0	34.1
Hispanic origin and race and percent of poverty level[2,4,7]									
Hispanic or Latino:									
Below 100%	68.6	63.7	65.9	18.0	20.9	21.1	13.4	15.5	13.0
100%–less than 200%	60.8	59.2	62.7	21.2	23.8	20.4	18.0	17.0	16.9
200% or more	45.6	43.1	48.6	27.6	27.7	26.3	26.8	29.3	25.1
Not Hispanic or Latino:									
White only:									
Below 100%	53.7	51.8	52.1	22.5	23.4	23.5	23.8	24.8	24.4
100%–less than 200%	49.0	48.4	47.6	27.6	27.3	27.5	23.4	24.3	24.9
200% or more	32.7	31.1	31.3	32.9	33.4	32.3	34.4	35.5	36.3
Black or African American only:									
Below 100%	64.3	61.3	65.1	17.4	21.6	18.8	18.3	17.1	16.1
100%–less than 200%	55.6	59.5	60.5	24.4	22.9	23.7	19.9	17.6	15.8
200% or more	46.0	42.4	48.1	28.7	29.2	26.6	25.3	28.4	25.3
Geographic region[2]									
Northeast	39.4	36.1	39.0	31.3	30.6	28.2	29.4	33.3	32.7
Midwest	37.3	34.7	34.3	31.7	34.1	34.3	31.0	31.2	31.4
South	46.9	46.7	47.6	27.1	27.1	25.6	26.0	26.2	26.8
West	33.9	35.3	36.9	31.6	31.6	30.6	34.6	33.2	32.5
Location of residence[2]									
Within MSA[8]	39.3	38.2	39.2	30.6	30.6	29.7	30.0	31.1	31.1
Outside MSA[8]	44.7	44.6	45.7	27.5	29.2	27.9	27.8	26.2	26.5

* Estimates are considered unreliable. Data not shown have a relative standard error of greater than 30%.
- - - Data not available.
[1]All questions related to leisure-time physical activity were phrased in terms of current behavior and lack a specific reference period. Respondents were asked about the frequency and duration of vigorous and light/moderate physical activity during leisure time. Adults classified as inactive reported no sessions of light/moderate or vigorous leisure-time activity of at least 10 minutes duration; adults classified with some leisure-time activity reported at least one session of light/moderate or vigorous physical activity of at least 10 minutes duration but did not meet the definition for regular leisure-time activity; adults classified with regular leisure-time activity reported three or more sessions per week of vigorous activity lasting at least 20 minutes or five or more sessions per week of light/moderate activity lasting at least 30 minutes in duration. See Appendix II, Physical activity, leisure-time.
[2]Estimates are age-adjusted to the year 2000 standard population using five age groups: 18–44 years, 45–54 years, 55–64 years, 65–74 years, and 75 years and over. Age-adjusted estimates in this table may differ from other age-adjusted estimates based on the same data and presented elsewhere if different age groups are used in the adjustment procedure. See Appendix II, Age adjustment.
[3]Includes all other races not shown separately and unknown education level.
[4]The race groups, white, black, American Indian or Alaska Native, Asian, Native Hawaiian or Other Pacific Islander, and 2 or more races, include persons of Hispanic and non-Hispanic origin. Persons of Hispanic origin may be of any race. Starting with 1999 data, race-specific estimates are tabulated according to the 1997 Revisions to the Standards for the Classification of Federal Data on Race and Ethnicity and are not strictly comparable with estimates for earlier years. The five single-race categories plus multiple-race categories shown in the table conform to the 1997 Standards. Starting with 1999 data, race-specific estimates are for persons who reported only one racial group; the category 2 or more races includes persons who reported more than one racial group. Prior to 1999, data were tabulated according to the 1977 Standards with four racial groups and the Asian only category included Native Hawaiian or Other Pacific Islander. Estimates for single-race categories prior to 1999 included persons who reported one race or, if they reported more than one race, identified one race as best representing their race. Starting with 2003 data, race responses of other race and unspecified multiple race were treated as missing, and then race was imputed if these were the only race responses. Almost all persons with a race response of other race were of Hispanic origin. See Appendix II, Hispanic origin; Race.
[5]Estimates are for persons 25 years of age and over and are age-adjusted to the year 2000 standard population using five age groups: 25–44 years, 45–54 years, 55–64 years, 65–74 years, and 75 years and over. See Appendix II, Age adjustment.
[6]GED stands for General Educational Development high school equivalency diploma. See Appendix II, Education.
[7]Percent of poverty level is based on family income and family size and composition using U.S. Census Bureau poverty thresholds. Missing family income data were imputed for 31%–36% of adults 18 years of age and over in 1998–2005. See Appendix II, Family income; Poverty.
[8]MSA is metropolitan statistical area.

NOTES: For more data on leisure-time physical activity, see National Health Interview Survey. Available from: www.cdc.gov/nchs/nhis.htm. Standard errors are available in the spreadsheet version of this table. Available from: www.cdc.gov/nchs/hus.htm. Data for additional years are available. See Appendix III.

SOURCE: Centers for Disease Control and Prevention, National Center for Health Statistics, National Health Interview Survey, family core and sample adult questionnaires.

Table 74 (page 1 of 4). Overweight, obesity, and healthy weight among persons 20 years of age and over, by sex, age, race and Hispanic origin, and poverty level: United States, 1960–1962 through 2001–2004

[Data are based on measured height and weight of a sample of the civilian noninstitutionalized population]

Sex, age, race and Hispanic origin[1], and poverty level	Overweight (includes obesity)[2]				
	1960–1962	1971–1974	1976–1980[3]	1988–1994	2001–2004
20–74 years, age-adjusted[4]	Percent of population				
Both sexes[5]	44.8	47.7	47.4	56.0	66.0
Male	49.5	54.7	52.9	61.0	70.7
Female	40.2	41.1	42.0	51.2	61.4
Not Hispanic or Latino:					
White only, male	---	---	53.8	61.6	71.1
White only, female	---	---	38.7	47.2	57.1
Black or African American only, male	---	---	51.3	58.2	66.8
Black or African American only, female	---	---	62.6	68.5	79.5
Mexican male	---	---	61.6	69.4	75.8
Mexican female	---	---	61.7	69.6	73.2
Percent of poverty level:[6]					
Below 100%	---	49.3	50.0	59.8	63.9
100%–less than 200%	---	50.9	49.0	58.2	66.2
200% or more	---	46.7	46.6	54.5	66.1
20 years and over, age-adjusted[4]					
Both sexes[5]	---	---	---	56.0	66.0
Male	---	---	---	60.9	70.5
Female	---	---	---	51.4	61.6
Not Hispanic or Latino:					
White only, male	---	---	---	61.6	71.0
White only, female	---	---	---	47.5	57.6
Black or African American only, male	---	---	---	57.8	67.0
Black or African American only, female	---	---	---	68.2	79.6
Mexican male	---	---	---	68.9	74.6
Mexican female	---	---	---	68.9	73.0
Percent of poverty level:[6]					
Below 100%	---	---	---	59.6	63.4
100%–less than 200%	---	---	---	58.0	66.2
200% or more	---	---	---	54.8	66.1
20 years and over, crude					
Both sexes[5]	---	---	---	54.9	66.1
Male	---	---	---	59.4	70.4
Female	---	---	---	50.7	61.9
Not Hispanic or Latino:					
White only, male	---	---	---	60.6	71.6
White only, female	---	---	---	47.4	58.7
Black or African American only, male	---	---	---	56.7	66.3
Black or African American only, female	---	---	---	66.0	79.1
Mexican male	---	---	---	63.9	71.8
Mexican female	---	---	---	65.9	71.4
Percent of poverty level:[6]					
Below 100%	---	---	---	56.8	61.4
100%–less than 200%	---	---	---	55.7	65.3
200% or more	---	---	---	54.2	67.1
Male					
20–34 years	42.7	42.8	41.2	47.5	59.0
35–44 years	53.5	63.2	57.2	65.5	72.9
45–54 years	53.9	59.7	60.2	66.1	78.5
55–64 years	52.2	58.5	60.2	70.5	77.3
65–74 years	47.8	54.6	54.2	68.5	76.1
75 years and over	---	---	---	56.5	66.8
Female					
20–34 years	21.2	25.8	27.9	37.0	51.6
35–44 years	37.2	40.5	40.7	49.6	60.1
45–54 years	49.3	49.0	48.7	60.3	67.4
55–64 years	59.9	54.5	53.7	66.3	69.9
65–74 years	60.9	55.9	59.5	60.3	71.5
75 years and over	---	---	---	52.3	63.7

See footnotes at end of table.

Table 74 (page 2 of 4). Overweight, obesity, and healthy weight among persons 20 years of age and over, by sex, age, race and Hispanic origin, and poverty level: United States, 1960–1962 through 2001–2004

[Data are based on measured height and weight of a sample of the civilian noninstitutionalized population]

Sex, age, race and Hispanic origin[1], and poverty level	Obesity[7]				
	1960–1962	1971–1974	1976–1980[3]	1988–1994	2001–2004
20–74 years, age-adjusted[4]	Percent of population				
Both sexes[5]	13.3	14.6	15.1	23.3	32.1
Male	10.7	12.2	12.8	20.6	30.2
Female	15.7	16.8	17.1	26.0	34.0
Not Hispanic or Latino:					
White only, male	- - -	- - -	12.4	20.7	31.0
White only, female	- - -	- - -	15.4	23.3	31.5
Black or African American only, male	- - -	- - -	16.5	21.3	31.2
Black or African American only, female	- - -	- - -	31.0	39.1	51.6
Mexican male	- - -	- - -	15.7	24.4	30.5
Mexican female	- - -	- - -	26.6	36.1	40.3
Percent of poverty level:[6]					
Below 100%	- - -	20.7	21.9	29.2	34.9
100%–less than 200%	- - -	18.4	18.7	26.6	34.6
200% or more	- - -	12.4	12.9	21.4	30.6
20 years and over, age-adjusted[4]					
Both sexes[5]	- - -	- - -	- - -	22.9	31.4
Male	- - -	- - -	- - -	20.2	29.5
Female	- - -	- - -	- - -	25.5	33.2
Not Hispanic or Latino:					
White only, male	- - -	- - -	- - -	20.3	30.2
White only, female	- - -	- - -	- - -	22.9	30.7
Black or African American only, male	- - -	- - -	- - -	20.9	30.8
Black or African American only, female	- - -	- - -	- - -	38.3	51.1
Mexican male	- - -	- - -	- - -	23.8	29.1
Mexican female	- - -	- - -	- - -	35.2	39.4
Percent of poverty level:[6]					
Below 100%	- - -	- - -	- - -	28.1	33.7
100%–less than 200%	- - -	- - -	- - -	26.1	33.6
200% or more	- - -	- - -	- - -	21.1	30.0
20 years and over, crude					
Both sexes[5]	- - -	- - -	- - -	22.3	31.5
Male	- - -	- - -	- - -	19.5	29.5
Female	- - -	- - -	- - -	25.0	33.3
Not Hispanic or Latino:					
White only, male	- - -	- - -	- - -	19.9	30.5
White only, female	- - -	- - -	- - -	22.7	31.2
Black or African American only, male	- - -	- - -	- - -	20.7	30.7
Black or African American only, female	- - -	- - -	- - -	36.7	51.1
Mexican male	- - -	- - -	- - -	20.6	27.8
Mexican female	- - -	- - -	- - -	33.3	38.5
Percent of poverty level:[6]					
Below 100%	- - -	- - -	- - -	25.9	33.0
100%–less than 200%	- - -	- - -	- - -	24.3	32.6
200% or more	- - -	- - -	- - -	20.9	30.7
Male					
20–34 years	9.2	9.7	8.9	14.1	23.2
35–44 years	12.1	13.5	13.5	21.5	33.8
45–54 years	12.5	13.7	16.7	23.2	31.8
55–64 years	9.2	14.1	14.1	27.2	36.0
65–74 years	10.4	10.9	13.2	24.1	32.1
75 years and over	- - -	- - -	- - -	13.2	19.9
Female					
20–34 years	7.2	9.7	11.0	18.5	28.6
35–44 years	14.7	17.7	17.8	25.5	33.3
45–54 years	20.3	18.9	19.6	32.4	38.0
55–64 years	24.4	24.1	22.9	33.7	39.0
65–74 years	23.2	22.0	21.5	26.9	37.9
75 years and over	- - -	- - -	- - -	19.2	23.2

See footnotes at end of table.

Table 74 (page 3 of 4). Overweight, obesity, and healthy weight among persons 20 years of age and over, by sex, age, race and Hispanic origin, and poverty level: United States, 1960–1962 through 2001–2004

[Data are based on measured height and weight of a sample of the civilian noninstitutionalized population]

Sex, age, race and Hispanic origin[1], and poverty level	*Healthy weight[8]*				
	1960–1962	*1971–1974*	*1976–1980[3]*	*1988–1994*	*2001–2004*
	Percent of population				
20–74 years, age-adjusted[4]					
Both sexes[5]	51.2	48.8	49.6	41.7	32.2
Male	48.3	43.0	45.4	37.9	28.1
Female	54.1	54.3	53.7	45.3	36.2
Not Hispanic or Latino:					
White only, male	---	---	45.3	37.4	27.8
White only, female	---	---	56.7	49.2	40.2
Black or African American only, male	---	---	46.6	40.0	31.3
Black or African American only, female	---	---	35.0	28.9	18.9
Mexican male	---	---	37.1	29.8	24.2
Mexican female	---	---	36.4	29.0	26.3
Percent of poverty level:[6]					
Below 100%	---	45.8	45.1	37.3	33.7
100%–less than 200%	---	45.1	47.6	39.2	31.8
200% or more	---	50.2	51.0	43.4	32.4
20 years and over, age-adjusted[4]					
Both sexes[5]	---	---	---	41.6	32.3
Male	---	---	---	37.9	28.3
Female	---	---	---	45.0	36.1
Not Hispanic or Latino:					
White only, male	---	---	---	37.3	28.0
White only, female	---	---	---	48.7	39.8
Black or African American only, male	---	---	---	40.1	30.8
Black or African American only, female	---	---	---	29.2	18.9
Mexican male	---	---	---	30.2	25.3
Mexican female	---	---	---	29.7	26.5
Percent of poverty level:[6]					
Below 100%	---	---	---	37.5	34.3
100%–less than 200%	---	---	---	39.3	31.9
200% or more	---	---	---	43.1	32.4
20 years and over, crude					
Both sexes[5]	---	---	---	42.6	32.2
Male	---	---	---	39.4	28.4
Female	---	---	---	45.7	35.8
Not Hispanic or Latino:					
White only, male	---	---	---	38.2	27.4
White only, female	---	---	---	48.8	38.8
Black or African American only, male	---	---	---	41.5	31.5
Black or African American only, female	---	---	---	31.2	19.3
Mexican male	---	---	---	35.2	28.1
Mexican female	---	---	---	32.4	28.0
Percent of poverty level:[6]					
Below 100%	---	---	---	39.8	36.2
100%–less than 200%	---	---	---	41.5	32.6
200% or more	---	---	---	43.6	31.6
Male					
20–34 years	55.3	54.7	57.1	51.1	38.3
35–44 years	45.2	35.2	41.3	33.4	26.5
45–54 years	44.8	38.5	38.7	33.6	21.2
55–64 years	44.9	38.3	38.7	28.6	22.2
65–74 years	46.2	42.1	42.3	30.1	23.1
75 years and over	---	---	---	40.9	32.1
Female					
20–34 years	67.6	65.8	65.0	57.9	44.2
35–44 years	58.4	56.7	55.6	47.1	38.3
45–54 years	47.6	49.3	48.7	37.2	31.0
55–64 years	38.1	41.1	43.5	31.5	29.2
65–74 years	36.4	40.6	37.8	37.0	27.0
75 years and over	---	---	---	43.0	34.6

See footnotes at end of table.

Table 74 (page 4 of 4). Overweight, obesity, and healthy weight among persons 20 years of age and over, by sex, age, race and Hispanic origin, and poverty level: United States, 1960–1962 through 2001–2004

[Data are based on measured height and weight of a sample of the civilian noninstitutionalized population]

- - - Data not available.

[1]Persons of Mexican origin may be of any race. Starting with 1999 data, race-specific estimates are tabulated according to the 1997 Revisions to the Standards for the Classification of Federal Data on Race and Ethnicity and are not strictly comparable with estimates for earlier years. The two non-Hispanic race categories shown in the table conform to the 1997 Standards. Starting with 1999 data, race-specific estimates are for persons who reported only one racial group. Prior to data year 1999, estimates were tabulated according to the 1977 Standards. Estimates for single-race categories prior to 1999 included persons who reported one race or, if they reported more than one race, identified one race as best representing their race. See Appendix II, Hispanic origin; Race.

[2]Body mass index (BMI) greater than or equal to 25 kilograms/meter^2. See Appendix II, Body mass index.

[3]Data for Mexicans are for 1982–1984. See Appendix I, National Health and Nutrition Examination Survey (NHANES).

[4]Age-adjusted to the 2000 standard population using five age groups: 20–34 years, 35–44 years, 45–54 years, 55–64 years, and 65 years and over (65–74 years for estimates for 20–74 years). Age-adjusted estimates in this table may differ from other age-adjusted estimates based on the same data and presented elsewhere if different age groups are used in the adjustment procedure. See Appendix II, Age adjustment.

[5]Includes persons of all races and Hispanic origins, not just those shown separately.

[6]Poverty level is based on family income and family size. Persons with unknown poverty level are excluded. See Appendix II, Family income; Poverty.

[7]Body mass index (BMI) greater than or equal to 30 kilograms/meter^2.

[8]BMI of 18.5 to less than 25 kilograms/meter^2.

NOTES: Percents do not sum to 100 because the percentage of persons with BMI less than 18.5 kilograms/meter^2 is not shown and the percentage of persons with obesity is a subset of the percent with overweight. Height was measured without shoes; two pounds were deducted from data for 1960–1962 to allow for weight of clothing. Excludes pregnant women. Standard errors for selected years are available in the spreadsheet version of this table. Available from: www.cdc.gov/nchs/hus.htm. Data for additional years are available. See Appendix III.

SOURCES: Centers for Disease Control and Prevention, National Center for Health Statistics, National Health and Nutrition Examination Survey, Hispanic Health and Nutrition Examination Survey (1982–1984), and National Health Examination Survey (1960–1962).

Table 75. Overweight among children and adolescents 6–19 years of age, by age, sex, race and Hispanic origin, and poverty level: United States, 1963–1965 through 2001–2004

[Data are based on physical examinations of a sample of the civilian noninstitutionalized population]

Sex, age, race and Hispanic origin[1], and poverty level	*1963–1965 1966–1970[2]*	*1971–1974*	*1976–1980[3]*	*1988–1994*	*2001–2004*
6–11 years of age			Percent of population		
Both sexes[4]	4.2	4.0	6.5	11.3	17.5
Boys	4.0	*4.3	6.6	11.6	18.7
Not Hispanic or Latino:					
White only	---	---	6.1	10.7	16.9
Black or African American only	---	---	6.8	12.3	17.2
Mexican	---	---	13.3	17.5	25.6
Girls	4.5	*3.6	6.4	11.0	16.3
Not Hispanic or Latino:					
White only	---	---	5.2	*9.8	15.6
Black or African American only	---	---	11.2	17.0	24.8
Mexican	---	---	9.8	15.3	16.6
Percent of poverty level:[5]					
Below 100%	---	---	---	11.4	20.0
100%–less than 200%	---	---	---	11.1	18.4
200% or more	---	---	---	11.1	15.4
12–19 years of age					
Both sexes[4]	4.6	6.1	5.0	10.5	17.0
Boys	4.5	6.1	4.8	11.3	17.9
Not Hispanic or Latino:					
White only	---	---	3.8	11.6	17.9
Black or African American only	---	---	6.1	10.7	17.7
Mexican	---	---	7.7	14.1	20.0
Girls	4.7	6.2	5.3	9.7	16.0
Not Hispanic or Latino:					
White only	---	---	4.6	8.9	14.6
Black or African American only	---	---	10.7	16.3	23.8
Mexican	---	---	8.8	*13.4	17.1
Percent of poverty level:[5]					
Below 100%	---	---	---	15.8	18.2
100%–less than 200%	---	---	---	11.2	17.0
200% or more	---	---	---	7.9	16.3

* Estimates are considered unreliable. Data preceded by an asterisk have a relative standard error of 20%–30%.
- - - Data not available.
[1]Persons of Mexican origin may be of any race. Starting with 1999 data, race-specific estimates are tabulated according to the 1997 Revisions to the Standards for the Classification of Federal Data on Race and Ethnicity and are not strictly comparable with estimates for earlier years. The two non-Hispanic race categories shown in the table conform to the 1997 Standards. Starting with 1999 data, race-specific estimates are for persons who reported only one racial group. Prior to data year 1999, estimates were tabulated according to the 1977 Standards. Estimates for single-race categories prior to 1999 included persons who reported one race or, if they reported more than one race, identified one race as best representing their race. See Appendix II, Hispanic origin; Race.
[2]Data for 1963–1965 are for children 6–11 years of age; data for 1966–1970 are for adolescents 12–17 years of age, not 12–19 years.
[3]Data for Mexicans are for 1982–1984. See Appendix I, National Health and Nutrition Examination Survey (NHANES).
[4]Includes persons of all races and Hispanic origins, not just those shown separately.
[5]Poverty level is based on family income and family size. Persons with unknown poverty level are excluded. See Appendix II, Family income; Poverty.

NOTES: Overweight is defined as body mass index (BMI) at or above the sex- and age-specific 95th percentile BMI cutoff points from the 2000 CDC Growth Charts: United States. Advance data from vital and health statistics; no 314. Hyattsville, MD: National Center for Health Statistics. 2000. Age is at time of examination at mobile examination center. Crude rates, not age-adjusted rates, are shown. Excludes pregnant girls starting with 1971–1974. Pregnancy status not available for 1963–1965 and 1966–1970. Standard errors for selected years are available in the spreadsheet version of this table. Available from: www.cdc.gov/nchs/hus.htm. Data for additional years are available. See Appendix III.

SOURCES: Centers for Disease Control and Prevention, National Center for Health Statistics, National Health and Nutrition Examination Survey, Hispanic Health and Nutrition Examination Survey (1982–1984), and National Health Examination Survey (1963–1965 and 1966–1970).

Table 76 (page 1 of 2). Untreated dental caries, by age, sex, race and Hispanic origin, and poverty level: United States, 1971–1974, 1988–1994, and 2001–2004

[Data are based on dental examinations of a sample of the civilian noninstitutionalized population]

Sex, race and Hispanic origin[1], and poverty level	*2–5 years*			*6–19 years*		
	1971–1974	*1988–1994*	*2001–2004*	*1971–1974*	*1988–1994*	*2001–2004*
	Percent of persons with untreated dental caries					
Total[2]	25.0	19.1	19.5	54.7	23.6	22.9
Sex						
Male	26.4	19.3	20.0	54.9	22.8	23.8
Female	23.6	18.9	19.1	54.5	24.5	21.8
Race and Hispanic origin						
Not Hispanic or Latino:						
White only	23.7	13.8	14.5	51.6	18.8	19.4
Black or African American only	29.0	24.7	24.2	71.0	33.7	28.0
Mexican	- - -	34.9	29.2	- - -	36.5	30.6
Percent of poverty level:[3]						
Below 100%	32.0	30.2	26.1	68.0	38.3	31.5
100%–less than 200%	29.9	24.3	25.4	60.3	28.2	32.6
200% or more	17.8	9.4	12.1	46.2	15.1	14.7
Race, Hispanic origin, and poverty level[3]						
Not Hispanic or Latino:						
White only:						
Below 100% of poverty level	32.1	25.7	19.6	65.9	33.5	29.3
100% or more of poverty level	22.0	11.7	13.8	49.9	16.7	17.6
Black or African American only:						
Below 100% of poverty level	29.1	27.2	26.2	73.9	37.0	33.5
100% or more of poverty level	27.9	22.5	21.8	67.3	31.0	24.1
Mexican:						
Below 100% of poverty level	- - -	38.8	35.0	- - -	46.4	35.9
100% or more of poverty level	- - -	30.3	25.1	- - -	26.4	27.1

Sex, race and Hispanic origin[1], and poverty level	*20–64 years*			*65–74 years*		
	1971–1974	*1988–1994*	*2001–2004*	*1971–1974*	*1988–1994*	*2001–2004*
	Percent of persons with untreated dental caries					
Total[2]	48.0	28.3	25.7	29.7	25.4	16.6
Sex						
Male	50.5	31.5	28.6	32.6	29.8	16.5
Female	45.6	25.3	22.8	27.4	21.5	16.8
Race and Hispanic origin						
Not Hispanic or Latino:						
White only	45.3	23.9	20.7	28.3	22.7	13.5
Black or African American only	67.3	48.5	40.7	41.5	46.7	42.2
Mexican	- - -	40.2	38.4	- - -	43.8	39.8
Percent of poverty level:[3]						
Below 100%	63.5	48.1	44.2	34.3	46.6	44.9
100%–less than 200%	56.2	43.5	38.9	35.6	40.1	26.0
200% or more	42.7	19.6	18.2	26.2	19.2	12.1
Race, Hispanic origin, and poverty level[3]						
Not Hispanic or Latino:						
White only:						
Below 100% of poverty level	60.2	43.7	40.7	33.3	*39.0	*37.6
100% or more of poverty level	44.2	21.8	18.4	28.3	22.7	13.4
Black or African American only:						
Below 100% of poverty level	71.9	60.4	54.4	39.8	49.7	52.8
100% or more of poverty level	65.3	43.9	36.1	41.1	43.8	41.6
Mexican:						
Below 100% of poverty level	- - -	52.7	47.9	- - -	55.5	59.2
100% or more of poverty level	- - -	31.8	34.4	- - -	35.6	33.3

See footnotes at end of table.

Table 76 (page 2 of 2). Untreated dental caries, by age, sex, race and Hispanic origin, and poverty level: United States, 1971–1974, 1988–1994, and 2001–2004

[Data are based on dental examinations of a sample of the civilian noninstitutionalized population]

Sex, race and Hispanic origin[1], and poverty level	75 years and over		
	1971–1974	*1988–1994*	*2001–2004*
	Percent of persons with untreated dental caries		
Total[2]	- - -	30.3	19.4
Sex			
Male	- - -	34.4	21.2
Female	- - -	28.1	18.2
Race and Hispanic origin			
Not Hispanic or Latino:			
White only	- - -	27.8	17.9
Black or African American only	- - -	62.6	*35.2
Mexican	- - -	55.6	44.2
Percent of poverty level:[3]			
Below 100%	- - -	47.1	31.6
100%–less than 200%	- - -	34.5	21.8
200% or more	- - -	23.2	16.4
Race, Hispanic origin, and poverty level[3]			
Not Hispanic or Latino:			
White only:			
Below 100% of poverty level	- - -	38.0	*32.7
100% or more of poverty level	- - -	26.1	16.7
Black or African American only:			
Below 100% of poverty level	- - -	68.6	*52.2
100% or more of poverty level	- - -	60.2	*30.5
Mexican:			
Below 100% of poverty level	- - -	79.4	52.9
100% or more of poverty level	- - -	*	42.3

* Estimates are considered unreliable. Data preceded by an asterisk have a relative standard error (RSE) of 20%–30%. Data not shown have an RSE of greater than 30% or fewer than 30 cases.

- - - Data not available.

[1]Persons of Mexican origin may be of any race. Starting with 1999 data, race-specific estimates are tabulated according to the 1997 Revisions to the Standards for the Classification of Federal Data on Race and Ethnicity and are not strictly comparable with estimates for earlier years. The two non-Hispanic race categories shown in the table conform to the 1997 Standards. Starting with 1999 data, race-specific estimates are for persons who reported only one racial group. Prior to data year 1999, estimates were tabulated according to the 1977 Standards. Estimates for single-race categories prior to 1999 included persons who reported one race or, if they reported more than one race, identified one race as best representing their race. See Appendix II, Hispanic origin; Race.

[2]Includes persons of all races and Hispanic origins, not just those shown separately, and those with unknown poverty level.

[3]Poverty level is based on family income and family size. Persons with unknown poverty level are excluded (4% in 1971–1974, 6% in 1988–1994, and 5% in 2001–2004). See Appendix II, Family income; Poverty.

NOTES: Untreated dental caries refers to untreated coronal caries, that is, caries on the crown or enamel surface of the tooth. Root caries are not included. For children 2–5 years of age, only dental caries in primary teeth was evaluated. Caries in both permanent and primary teeth was evaluated for children 6–11 years of age. For children 12–19 years of age and adults, only dental caries in permanent teeth was evaluated. Excludes edentulous persons (persons without teeth) of all ages. The majority of edentulous persons are 65 years of age and over. Estimates of edentulism among persons 65 years of age and over are 46% in 1971–1974, 33% in 1988–1994, and 26% in 2001–2004. See Appendix II, Dental caries. Standard errors are available in the spreadsheet version of this table. Available from: www.cdc.gov/nchs/hus.htm. Data have been revised and differ from previous editions of *Health, United States.* Data for additional years are available. See Appendix III.

SOURCES: Centers for Disease Control and Prevention, National Center for Health Statistics, National Health and Nutrition Examination Survey.

Table 77 (page 1 of 2). No usual source of health care among children under 18 years of age, by selected characteristics: United States, average annual 1993–1994, 2001–2002, and 2004–2005

[Data are based on household interviews of a sample of the civilian noninstitutionalized population]

Characteristic	Under 18 years			Under 6 years			6–17 years		
	1993–1994[1]	2001–2002	2004–2005	1993–1994[1]	2001–2002	2004–2005	1993–1994[1]	2001–2002	2004–2005
	Percent of children without a usual source of health care[2]								
All children[3]	7.7	6.0	5.4	5.2	4.4	3.3	9.0	6.8	6.4
Race[4]									
White only	7.0	5.2	5.1	4.7	4.0	2.9	8.3	5.8	6.2
Black or African American only	10.3	6.6	6.1	7.6	3.6	*4.5	11.9	8.0	6.8
American Indian or Alaska Native only	*9.3	*	*8.2	*	*	*	*8.7	*	*9.8
Asian only	9.7	11.2	7.7	*3.4	*	*6.3	13.5	13.2	8.3
Native Hawaiian or Other Pacific Islander only	---	*	*	---	*	*	---	*	*
2 or more races	---	7.3	*3.4	---	*7.0	*	---	*7.5	*3.8
Hispanic origin and race[4]									
Hispanic or Latino	14.3	13.5	11.1	9.3	9.2	6.7	17.7	16.0	13.7
Not Hispanic or Latino	6.7	4.4	4.0	4.4	3.2	2.3	7.8	4.9	4.7
White only	5.7	3.4	3.2	3.7	2.7	1.6	6.7	3.7	4.0
Black or African American only	10.2	6.6	6.1	7.7	3.6	*4.4	11.6	8.0	6.8
Percent of poverty level[5]									
Below 100%	13.9	11.7	9.7	9.4	8.2	5.6	16.8	13.7	12.2
100%–less than 200%	9.8	8.9	7.6	6.7	7.0	4.1	11.6	9.9	9.4
200% or more	3.7	3.3	3.2	1.8	2.1	2.1	4.6	3.8	3.7
Hispanic origin and race and percent of poverty level[4,5]									
Hispanic or Latino:									
Below 100%	19.6	18.5	14.3	12.7	12.1	7.8	24.8	22.4	18.6
100%–less than 200%	15.3	16.0	13.0	9.9	11.2	7.6	18.9	18.7	16.2
200% or more	5.0	7.1	6.6	*2.7	*4.5	4.8	6.5	8.6	7.5
Not Hispanic or Latino:									
White only:									
Below 100%	10.2	7.5	7.1	6.5	*	*2.5	12.7	8.2	9.7
100%–less than 200%	8.7	5.4	4.5	6.3	*4.8	*2.1	10.1	5.7	5.8
200% or more	3.4	2.4	2.4	1.6	1.5	1.3	4.2	2.7	2.8
Black or African American only:									
Below 100%	13.7	9.0	6.9	10.9	*4.0	*	15.5	11.5	7.4
100%–less than 200%	9.1	7.3	6.5	*6.0	*5.1	*	10.8	8.4	7.5
200% or more	4.6	4.2	5.1	*	*	*	5.8	5.1	6.0
Health insurance status at the time of interview[6]									
Insured	5.0	3.3	2.9	3.3	2.2	1.9	5.9	3.8	3.3
Private	3.8	2.5	2.2	1.9	1.4	1.2	4.6	3.0	2.7
Medicaid	8.9	5.5	4.3	6.4	4.0	3.2	11.3	6.5	5.0
Uninsured	23.5	29.1	30.3	18.0	25.2	19.9	26.0	30.7	34.1
Health insurance status prior to interview[6]									
Insured continuously all 12 months	4.6	3.0	2.7	3.1	2.0	1.8	5.5	3.4	3.1
Uninsured for any period up to 12 months	15.3	16.7	13.8	10.9	13.8	8.9	18.1	18.4	16.1
Uninsured more than 12 months	27.6	36.5	38.2	21.4	32.1	25.0	30.0	38.1	42.3

See footnotes at end of table.

Table 77 (page 2 of 2). No usual source of health care among children under 18 years of age, by selected characteristics: United States, average annual 1993–1994, 2001–2002, and 2004–2005

[Data are based on household interviews of a sample of the civilian noninstitutionalized population]

Characteristic	Under 18 years			Under 6 years			6–17 years		
	1993–1994[1]	2001–2002	2004–2005	1993–1994[1]	2001–2002	2004–2005	1993–1994[1]	2001–2002	2004–2005
Percent of poverty level and health insurance status prior to interview[5,6]	Percent of children without a usual source of health care[2]								
Below 100%:									
Insured continuously all 12 months	8.6	5.0	4.8	5.8	*2.7	*3.2	10.7	6.4	5.8
Uninsured for any period up to 12 months	21.7	21.2	17.4	18.0	18.5	*10.8	23.7	23.0	20.4
Uninsured more than 12 months	31.2	46.2	45.2	25.5	42.5	28.2	33.4	47.6	51.3
100%–less than 200%:									
Insured continuously all 12 months	5.6	4.0	3.1	3.7	3.3	1.9	6.7	4.4	3.8
Uninsured for any period up to 12 months	14.5	18.7	14.0	*9.7	*15.8	*10.1	18.0	20.2	15.7
Uninsured more than 12 months	27.6	33.8	37.9	21.4	29.9	23.3	30.2	35.3	42.0
200% or more:									
Insured continuously all 12 months	2.8	2.1	2.0	1.4	1.3	1.4	3.5	2.5	2.3
Uninsured for any period up to 12 months	9.1	11.9	11.4	*5.7	*8.4	*7.0	11.4	13.9	13.6
Uninsured more than 12 months	18.3	27.3	31.0	*10.6	*18.8	*23.6	20.9	29.8	33.3
Geographic region									
Northeast	4.1	2.4	2.2	2.9	*2.4	*1.7	4.8	2.4	2.4
Midwest	5.2	4.2	3.6	4.1	3.8	2.3	5.9	4.4	4.3
South	10.9	7.3	6.5	7.3	4.6	4.1	12.7	8.7	7.7
West	8.6	8.8	7.8	5.3	6.3	4.2	10.6	10.1	9.6
Location of residence									
Within MSA[7]	7.7	6.1	5.5	5.0	4.5	3.4	9.2	6.9	6.6
Outside MSA[7]	7.8	5.7	4.6	6.0	3.9	*2.9	8.7	6.5	5.4

* Estimates are considered unreliable. Data preceded by an asterisk have a relative standard error (RSE) of 20%–30%. Data not shown have an RSE of greater than 30%.

- - - Data not available.

[1]Data prior to 1997 are not strictly comparable with data for later years due to the 1997 questionnaire redesign. See Appendix I, National Health Interview Survey.

[2]Persons who report the emergency department as the place of their usual source of care are defined as having no usual source of care. See Appendix II, Usual source of care.

[3]Includes all other races not shown separately and unknown health insurance status.

[4]The race groups, white, black, American Indian or Alaska Native, Asian, Native Hawaiian or Other Pacific Islander, and 2 or more races, include persons of Hispanic and non-Hispanic origin. Persons of Hispanic origin may be of any race. Starting with 1999 data, race-specific estimates are tabulated according to the 1997 Revisions to the Standards for the Classification of Federal Data on Race and Ethnicity and are not strictly comparable with estimates for earlier years. The five single-race categories plus multiple-race categories shown in the table conform to the 1997 Standards. Starting with 1999 data, race-specific estimates are for persons who reported only one racial group; the category 2 or more races includes persons who reported more than one racial group. Prior to 1999, data were tabulated according to the 1977 Standards with four racial groups and the Asian only category included Native Hawaiian or Other Pacific Islander. Estimates for single-race categories prior to 1999 included persons who reported one race or, if they reported more than one race, identified one race as best representing their race. Starting with 2003 data, race responses of other race and unspecified multiple race were treated as missing, and then race was imputed if these were the only race responses. Almost all persons with a race response of other race were of Hispanic origin. See Appendix II, Hispanic origin; Race.

[5]Percent of poverty level is based on family income and family size and composition using U.S. Census Bureau poverty thresholds. Missing family income data were imputed for 14% of children in 1993–1996, 21%–25% in 1997–1998, and 28%–31% in 1999–2005. See Appendix II, Family income; Poverty.

[6]Health insurance categories are mutually exclusive. Persons who reported both Medicaid and private coverage are classified as having private coverage. Medicaid includes other public assistance through 1996. Starting with 1997 data, Medicaid includes state-sponsored health plans and State Children's Health Insurance Program (SCHIP). In addition to private and Medicaid, the insured category also includes military, other government, and Medicare coverage. Persons not covered by private insurance, Medicaid, SCHIP, public assistance (through 1996), state-sponsored or other government-sponsored health plans (starting in 1997), Medicare, or military plans are considered to have no health insurance coverage. Persons with only Indian Health Service coverage are considered to have no health insurance coverage. Health insurance status was unknown for 8%–9% of children in 1993–1996 and about 1% in 1997–2005. See Appendix II, Health insurance coverage.

[7]MSA is metropolitan statistical area.

NOTES: Standard errors are available in the spreadsheet version of this table. Available from: www.cdc.gov/nchs/hus.htm. Data for additional years are available. See Appendix III.

SOURCES: Centers for Disease Control and Prevention, National Center for Health Statistics, National Health Interview Survey, access to care and health insurance supplements (1993–1996). Starting in 1997, data are from the family core and sample child questionnaires.

Table 78 (page 1 of 2). No usual source of health care among adults 18–64 years of age, by selected characteristics: United States, average annual selected years 1993–1994 through 2004–2005

[Data are based on household interviews of a sample of the civilian noninstitutionalized population]

Characteristic	*1993–1994*[1]	*1995–1996*[1]	*1997–1998*	*1999–2000*	*2001–2002*	*2004–2005*
	Percent of adults without a usual source of health care[2]					
18–64 years[3]	18.9	16.9	17.7	17.8	16.4	18.0
Age						
18–44 years	21.7	19.6	21.1	21.6	20.6	22.8
18–24 years	26.6	22.6	27.0	27.2	27.2	29.9
25–44 years	20.3	18.8	19.3	19.9	18.5	20.3
45–64 years	12.8	11.3	11.2	10.9	9.2	10.6
45–54 years	14.1	12.2	12.6	12.0	10.3	11.9
55–64 years	11.1	9.8	9.0	9.2	7.6	8.8
Sex						
Male	23.9	21.4	23.6	24.1	21.6	23.3
Female	14.1	12.6	12.0	11.8	11.4	12.9
Race[4]						
White only	18.4	16.5	17.0	16.7	15.4	17.7
Black or African American only	20.0	18.3	19.4	19.2	16.9	19.3
American Indian or Alaska Native only	19.7	16.5	21.3	19.2	16.3	22.8
Asian only	24.8	21.5	21.7	22.1	20.1	18.8
Native Hawaiian or Other Pacific Islander only	- - -	- - -	- - -	*	*	*
2 or more races	- - -	- - -	- - -	21.0	20.1	18.1
American Indian or Alaska Native; White	- - -		- - -	25.8	18.1	19.1
Hispanic origin and race[4]						
Hispanic or Latino	30.3	27.4	30.4	32.6	32.5	34.0
Mexican	32.4	29.8	35.9	36.5	36.5	37.8
Not Hispanic or Latino	17.7	15.7	16.2	15.8	14.0	15.4
White only	17.1	15.0	15.4	14.9	13.1	14.6
Black or African American only	19.7	18.1	19.3	19.2	16.8	19.0
Percent of poverty level[5]						
Below 100%	29.5	26.1	29.1	29.6	29.3	31.8
100%–less than 200%	25.4	22.9	25.6	27.1	25.6	27.1
200% or more	14.8	13.5	13.9	14.0	12.3	13.4
Hispanic origin and race and percent of poverty level[4,5]						
Hispanic or Latino:						
Below 100%	40.0	34.3	42.8	44.4	46.3	44.5
100%–less than 200%	36.9	32.9	35.4	40.6	40.0	40.7
200% or more	19.0	18.9	20.1	22.7	22.4	24.8
Not Hispanic or Latino:						
White only:						
Below 100%	28.2	23.6	25.0	24.2	23.4	26.8
100%–less than 200%	23.3	20.7	22.4	23.0	20.7	22.8
200% or more	14.3	12.8	13.1	12.8	10.8	11.9
Black or African American only:						
Below 100%	24.7	21.9	23.9	23.7	22.8	28.3
100%–less than 200%	22.3	22.1	25.3	24.4	20.4	22.1
200% or more	15.1	14.0	14.9	15.4	13.2	14.2
Health insurance status at the time of interview[6]						
Insured	13.3	11.4	11.4	10.9	9.1	9.7
Private	13.1	11.3	11.5	11.1	9.0	9.5
Medicaid	16.3	13.0	10.3	9.9	11.1	12.1
Uninsured	43.1	41.8	46.7	49.2	49.1	52.5
Health insurance status prior to interview[6]						
Insured continuously all 12 months	- - -	- - -	10.6	10.3	8.3	8.9
Uninsured for any period up to 12 months	- - -	- - -	30.7	31.2	33.3	34.0
Uninsured more than 12 months	- - -	- - -	51.4	54.8	54.6	57.4

See footnotes at end of table.

Table 78 (page 2 of 2). No usual source of health care among adults 18–64 years of age, by selected characteristics: United States, average annual selected years 1993–1994 through 2004–2005

[Data are based on household interviews of a sample of the civilian noninstitutionalized population]

Characteristic	1993–1994[1]	1995–1996[1]	1997–1998	1999–2000	2001–2002	2004–2005
Percent of poverty level and health insurance status prior to interview[5,6]	Percent of adults without a usual source of health care[2]					
Below 100%:						
Insured continuously all 12 months	- - -	- - -	13.1	11.6	11.5	12.7
Uninsured for any period up to 12 months	- - -	- - -	33.0	31.9	36.5	39.4
Uninsured more than 12 months	- - -	- - -	54.3	57.1	58.8	61.6
100%–less than 200%:						
Insured continuously all 12 months	- - -	- - -	13.0	12.3	11.0	10.7
Uninsured for any period up to 12 months	- - -	- - -	31.1	34.6	35.1	37.1
Uninsured more than 12 months	- - -	- - -	51.1	54.9	54.5	56.0
200% or more:						
Insured continuously all 12 months	- - -	- - -	10.0	9.8	7.6	8.2
Uninsured for any period up to 12 months	- - -	- - -	29.6	29.5	31.5	30.6
Uninsured more than 12 months	- - -	- - -	49.2	53.1	51.7	55.8
Geographic region						
Northeast	14.7	13.4	13.3	12.8	11.9	11.7
Midwest	16.2	14.7	15.1	17.0	14.1	15.4
South	21.8	18.7	20.7	19.7	18.3	21.0
West	21.1	19.9	20.2	20.1	19.9	21.2
Location of residence						
Within MSA[7]	19.3	17.3	17.9	18.1	16.6	18.3
Outside MSA[7]	17.5	15.4	17.0	16.8	15.4	16.6

* Estimates are considered unreliable. Data preceded by an asterisk have a relative standard error (RSE) of 20%–30%. Data not shown have an RSE of greater than 30%.
- - - Data not available.
[1]Data prior to 1997 are not strictly comparable with data for later years due to the 1997 questionnaire redesign. See Appendix I, National Health Interview Survey.
[2]Persons who report the emergency department as the place of their usual source of care are defined as having no usual source of care. See Appendix II, Usual source of care.
[3]Includes all other races not shown separately and unknown health insurance status.
[4]The race groups, white, black, American Indian or Alaska Native, Asian, Native Hawaiian or Other Pacific Islander, and 2 or more races, include persons of Hispanic and non-Hispanic origin. Persons of Hispanic origin may be of any race. Starting with 1999 data, race-specific estimates are tabulated according to the 1997 Revisions to the Standards for the Classification of Federal Data on Race and Ethnicity and are not strictly comparable with estimates for earlier years. The five single-race categories plus multiple-race categories shown in the table conform to the 1997 Standards. Starting with 1999 data, race-specific estimates are for persons who reported only one racial group; the category 2 or more races includes persons who reported more than one racial group. Prior to 1999, data were tabulated according to the 1977 Standards with four racial groups and the Asian only category included Native Hawaiian or Other Pacific Islander. Estimates for single-race categories prior to 1999 included persons who reported one race or, if they reported more than one race, identified one race as best representing their race. Starting with 2003 data, race responses of other race and unspecified multiple race were treated as missing, and then race was imputed if these were the only race responses. Almost all persons with a race response of other race were of Hispanic origin. See Appendix II, Hispanic origin; Race.
[5]Percent of poverty level is based on family income and family size and composition using U.S. Census Bureau poverty thresholds. Missing family income data were imputed for 15%–17% of persons 18–64 years of age in 1993–1996, 25%–29% in 1997–1998, and 31%–34% in 1999–2005. See Appendix II, Family income; Poverty.
[6]Health insurance categories are mutually exclusive. Persons who reported both Medicaid and private coverage are classified as having private coverage. Medicaid includes other public assistance through 1996. Starting with 1997 data, Medicaid includes state-sponsored health plans and State Children's Health Insurance Program (SCHIP). In addition to private and Medicaid, the insured category also includes military, other government, and Medicare coverage. Persons not covered by private insurance, Medicaid, SCHIP, public assistance (through 1996), state-sponsored or other government-sponsored health plans (starting in 1997), Medicare, or military plans are considered to have no health insurance coverage. Persons with only Indian Health Service coverage are considered to have no health insurance coverage. In 1993–1996, health insurance status was unknown for 8%–9% of adults in the sample. In 1997–2005, health insurance status was unknown for 1% of adults. See Appendix II, Health insurance coverage.
[7]MSA is metropolitan statistical area.

NOTES: Standard errors are available in the spreadsheet version of this table. Available from: www.cdc.gov/nchs/hus.htm. For more data on usual source of care, see the National Health Interview Survey home page. Available from: www.cdc.gov/nchs/nhis.htm.

SOURCE: Centers for Disease Control and Prevention, National Center for Health Statistics, National Health Interview Survey, access to care and health insurance supplements (1993–1996). Starting in 1997, data are from the family core and sample adult questionnaires.

Table 79 (page 1 of 2). Reduced access to medical care during the past 12 months due to cost, by selected characteristics: United States, 1997, 2004, and 2005

[Data are based on household interviews of a sample of the civilian noninstitutionalized population]

Characteristic	Did not get medical care due to cost[1]			Delayed medical care due to cost[2]			Did not get prescription drugs due to cost[3]		
	1997	*2004*	*2005*	*1997*	*2004*	*2005*	*1997*	*2004*	*2005*
	Percent								
Total, age-adjusted[4,5]	4.5	5.4	5.2	7.3	7.7	7.4	4.7	7.1	7.2
Total, crude[5]	4.5	5.5	5.3	7.3	7.8	7.5	4.8	7.1	7.2
Age									
Under 18 years	2.2	2.3	2.1	3.7	3.8	3.7	2.2	2.8	2.9
Under 6 years	1.6	1.7	1.5	3.0	3.3	3.0	1.6	2.2	2.5
6–17 years	2.5	2.6	2.4	4.1	4.0	4.1	2.4	3.1	3.1
18–44 years	6.1	7.3	7.3	9.7	10.1	9.8	6.9	9.4	9.8
45–64 years	5.8	7.2	6.8	9.0	10.0	9.4	5.1	8.8	8.7
65 years and over	2.3	2.6	2.4	3.9	4.1	4.0	2.8	5.4	5.1
Sex									
Male	3.8	5.0	4.7	6.4	7.1	6.8	3.9	5.9	5.7
Female	5.2	5.9	5.8	8.1	8.4	8.2	5.6	8.3	8.7
Race[6]									
White only	4.4	5.4	5.1	7.5	7.9	7.6	4.5	6.9	7.0
Black or African American only	5.5	6.4	6.4	6.6	7.7	7.3	7.1	9.4	8.9
American Indian or Alaska Native only	6.7	7.2	6.2	10.0	8.7	9.0	*7.5	9.9	*10.2
Asian only	2.6	[illegible]	2.8	4.0	4.4	3.7	*2.3	2.7	3.2
Native Hawaiian or Other Pacific Islander only	- - -	*	*	- - -	*	*	- - -	*	*
2 or more races	- - -	6.1	8.7	- - -	8.9	11.9	- - -	8.0	13.5
Hispanic origin and race[6]									
Hispanic or Latino	5.7	6.0	6.0	6.9	7.4	7.7	5.5	8.2	8.8
Mexican	5.5	5.6	6.0	6.6	7.0	7.7	5.5	7.9	9.3
Not Hispanic or Latino	4.4	5.4	5.1	7.3	7.8	7.4	4.7	6.9	6.9
White only	4.2	5.3	5.0	7.6	8.0	7.6	4.3	6.7	6.7
Black or African American only	5.6	6.3	6.3	6.6	7.7	7.3	7.1	9.3	8.8
Education[7]									
No high school diploma or GED	8.5	9.3	9.5	10.9	11.0	11.3	8.9	13.5	14.4
High school diploma or GED	5.2	6.8	6.7	8.5	9.1	8.9	5.9	8.9	9.1
Some college or more	4.2	5.6	5.2	7.9	8.6	8.0	4.1	6.8	6.5
Percent of poverty level[8]									
Below 100%	9.8	10.3	10.3	11.6	12.2	12.2	10.3	12.6	14.1
100%–less than 200%	7.4	9.2	9.0	11.2	11.9	11.6	7.9	11.8	11.6
200% or more	2.5	3.4	3.2	5.1	5.7	5.4	2.6	4.6	4.6
Age and percent of poverty level[8]									
Under 18 years of age:									
Below 100%	4.5	3.3	3.7	5.5	5.2	5.4	4.6	4.8	5.7
100%–less than 200%	3.0	3.7	3.6	5.9	6.0	5.9	3.4	4.6	4.2
200% or more	1.1	1.4	1.0	2.2	2.6	2.4	0.8	1.5	1.5
18–44 years:									
Below 100%	12.7	13.5	13.0	14.8	15.3	14.9	13.8	14.6	17.2
100%–less than 200%	10.1	12.6	12.7	14.9	15.8	15.0	11.6	15.4	15.2
200% or more	3.5	4.6	4.6	7.1	7.4	7.3	4.0	6.4	6.6
45–64 years:									
Below 100%	18.3	20.2	20.6	21.9	22.5	22.5	17.7	25.3	25.6
100%–less than 200%	13.8	16.2	15.0	18.5	19.4	18.9	11.7	20.3	18.5
200% or more	2.8	4.3	3.9	5.8	7.1	6.4	2.4	5.1	5.1
65 years and over:									
Below 100%	7.2	6.1	6.1	8.5	8.4	9.0	7.3	11.3	11.7
100%–less than 200%	3.3	4.1	4.3	5.8	5.9	6.3	4.3	8.0	8.7
200% or more	0.9	1.4	1.0	2.2	2.6	2.3	1.2	3.3	2.5

See footnotes at end of table.

Table 79 (page 2 of 2). Reduced access to medical care during the past 12 months due to cost, by selected characteristics: United States, 1997, 2004, and 2005

[Data are based on household interviews of a sample of the civilian noninstitutionalized population]

Characteristic	Did not get medical care due to cost[1]			Delayed medical care due to cost[2]			Did not get prescription drugs due to cost[3]		
	1997	2004	2005	1997	2004	2005	1997	2004	2005
Percent of poverty level and health insurance status prior to interview for persons under 65 years of age[4,8,9]					Percent				
Insured continuously all 12 months	1.8	2.3	2.1	3.9	4.1	3.9	2.2	3.9	4.0
Below 100%	3.6	3.7	3.5	4.8	5.1	5.2	5.2	6.7	7.4
100%–less than 200%	3.4	4.1	4.1	6.4	6.3	5.9	4.3	7.4	6.7
200% or more	1.2	1.7	1.5	3.3	3.5	3.3	1.3	2.8	2.9
Uninsured for any period up to 12 months	14.3	19.6	18.6	22.5	26.5	25.4	14.9	20.9	20.5
Below 100%	18.6	23.3	24.8	23.5	28.4	28.5	20.2	24.8	26.9
100%–less than 200%	15.1	22.4	20.1	24.2	29.2	26.7	15.9	24.6	23.0
200% or more	11.4	16.7	15.3	20.9	24.2	23.5	11.2	17.2	16.7
Uninsured more than 12 months	18.9	22.3	22.2	23.9	26.3	25.7	16.7	21.8	22.7
Below 100%	22.2	24.9	24.5	24.1	26.7	25.9	19.0	24.0	27.0
100%–less than 200%	18.4	22.5	23.7	23.1	25.8	27.0	16.8	21.7	22.2
200% or more	16.4	20.2	19.3	24.7	26.5	24.3	14.5	20.3	19.9
Geographic region									
Northeast	3.5	4.3	3.9	5.7	6.0	5.6	3.4	5.6	5.4
Midwest	4.0	4.4	4.5	7.3	7.7	7.3	4.4	6.0	6.8
South	5.3	6.7	6.5	8.1	8.5	8.4	5.7	8.9	8.9
West	4.7	5.5	5.2	7.2	8.2	7.8	4.8	6.5	6.4
Location of residence									
Within MSA[10]	4.3	5.3	5.1	6.9	7.4	7.3	4.4	6.8	6.8
Outside MSA[10]	5.3	6.2	5.8	8.6	9.1	8.3	6.0	8.3	8.7

* Estimates are considered unreliable. Data preceded by an asterisk have a relative standard error (RSE) of 20%–30%. Data not shown have an RSE of greater than 30%.

- - - Data not available.

[1]Based on persons responding yes to the question, "During the past 12 months was there any time when person needed medical care but did not get it because person couldn't afford it?"

[2]Based on persons responding yes to the question, "During the past 12 months has medical care been delayed because of worry about the cost?"

[3]Based on persons responding yes to the question, "During the past 12 months was there any time when you needed prescription medicine but didn't get it because you couldn't afford it?"

[4]Estimates are age-adjusted to the year 2000 standard population using six age groups: 0–17 years, 18–44 years, 45–54 years, 55–64 years, 65–74 years, and 75 years and over. See Appendix II, Age adjustment.

[5]Includes all other races not shown separately, unknown health insurance status, and unknown education level.

[6]The race groups, white, black, American Indian or Alaska Native, Asian, Native Hawaiian or Other Pacific Islander, and 2 or more races, include persons of Hispanic and non-Hispanic origin. Persons of Hispanic origin may be of any race. Starting with 1999 data, race-specific estimates are tabulated according to the 1997 Revisions to the Standards for the Classification of Federal Data on Race and Ethnicity and are not strictly comparable with estimates for earlier years. The five single-race categories plus multiple-race categories shown in the table conform to the 1997 Standards. Starting with 1999 data, race-specific estimates are for persons who reported only one racial group; the category 2 or more races includes persons who reported more than one racial group. Prior to 1999, data were tabulated according to the 1977 Standards with four racial groups and the Asian only category included Native Hawaiian or Other Pacific Islander. Estimates for single-race categories prior to 1999 included persons who reported one race or, if they reported more than one race, identified one race as best representing their race. Starting with 2003 data, race responses of other race and unspecified multiple race were treated as missing, and then race was imputed if these were the only race responses. Almost all persons with a race response of other race were of Hispanic origin. See Appendix II, Hispanic origin; Race.

[7]Estimates are for persons 25 years of age and over. GED stands for General Educational Development high school equivalency diploma. See Appendix II, Education.

[8]Percent of poverty level is based on family income and family size and composition using U.S. Census Bureau poverty thresholds. Missing family income data were imputed for 25% of persons in 1997 and 33%–34% in 2004–2005. See Appendix II, Family Income; Poverty.

[9]For information on the health insurance categories see Appendix II, Health Insurance Coverage.

[10]MSA is metropolitan statistical area.

NOTES: Standard errors and additional data years are available in the spreadsheet version of this table. Available from: www.cdc.gov/nchs/hus.htm. Data for additional years are available. See Appendix III.

SOURCE: Centers for Disease Control and Prevention, National Center for Health Statistics, National Health Interview Survey, family core, sample child, and sample adult questionnaires.

Table 80. Reduced access to medical care during the past 12 months due to cost, by state: 25 largest states and United States, 1997–1998, 2000–2001, and 2004–2005

[Data are based on household interviews of a sample of the civilian noninstitutionalized population]

State	Did not get medical care due to cost[1]			Delayed medical care due to cost[2]			Did not get prescription drugs due to cost[3]		
	1997–1998	2000–2001	2004–2005	1997–1998	2000–2001	2004–2005	1997–1998	2000–2001	2004–2005
	Percent								
Total, United States	4.4	4.6	5.4	6.9	6.5	7.6	4.5	5.3	7.1
Alabama	4.4	5.3	6.9	6.3	6.5	7.7	6.8	8.3	13.7
Arizona	5.0	4.1	6.0	7.1	6.7	8.1	4.1	4.6	7.5
California	4.2	4.2	4.2	5.8	5.6	5.9	3.9	4.7	5.2
Colorado	3.7	4.5	6.3	5.8	7.5	9.0	3.1	5.5	5.2
Florida	5.8	6.0	6.8	8.7	8.7	9.6	4.8	5.8	8.0
Georgia	4.6	4.8	5.4	7.4	6.9	6.0	4.2	4.0	5.3
Illinois	3.0	3.4	3.5	5.3	5.7	6.1	3.0	4.2	5.8
Indiana	5.2	5.6	6.7	7.8	8.0	9.9	5.1	6.8	8.5
Kentucky	6.5	6.8	8.5	10.1	8.4	10.6	6.3	8.2	11.6
Maryland	5.5	5.4	3.8	6.8	6.3	5.6	5.8	5.2	6.3
Massachusetts	2.4	2.8	3.8	4.3	3.7	6.0	1.7	4.2	5.0
Michigan	3.8	4.3	4.7	6.3	6.0	7.6	3.8	5.1	6.4
Minnesota	3.4	3.1	4.9	7.2	6.1	8.3	3.6	3.9	6.3
Missouri	4.0	4.5	5.1	6.5	5.5	7.4	4.3	5.2	6.8
New Jersey	3.3	3.9	4.2	6.3	5.1	6.0	3.8	3.5	4.6
New York	3.6	3.5	3.8	5.4	5.1	5.0	2.8	3.8	5.3
North Carolina	4.1	4.3	5.1	6.6	7.0	7.4	4.0	5.8	6.4
Ohio	4.6	3.8	4.6	8.2	6.7	8.2	5.0	5.1	7.8
Pennsylvania	3.4	3.4	4.3	5.1	5.0	6.1	4.3	3.5	6.4
South Carolina	5.0	4.3	4.7	6.6	4.9	6.1	5.2	4.4	5.3
Tennessee	4.6	5.2	7.0	9.1	7.6	8.8	8.0	8.5	10.1
Texas	4.8	5.4	7.5	6.9	6.5	9.7	4.7	6.6	11.1
Virginia	3.6	4.4	4.5	5.2	6.2	5.9	4.1	*5.2	6.1
Washington	4.8	5.4	6.2	7.6	8.2	10.5	4.8	6.8	7.2
Wisconsin	2.8	3.1	3.0	5.9	5.1	5.6	*3.0	4.0	4.0

* Estimates are considered unreliable. Data preceded by an asterisk have a relative standard error (RSE) of 20%–30%.
[1]Based on persons responding yes to the question, "During the past 12 months was there any time when person needed medical care but did not get it because person couldn't afford it?"
[2]Based on persons responding yes to the question, "During the past 12 months has medical care been delayed because of worry about the cost?"
[3]Based on persons responding yes to the question, "During the past 12 months was there any time when you needed prescription medicine but didn't get it because you couldn't afford it?"

NOTES: Data are for states with the largest populations in 2004–2005. Standard errors are available in the spreadsheet version of this table. Available from: www.cdc.gov/nchs/hus.htm. See related Table 79.

SOURCE: Centers for Disease Control and Prevention, National Center for Health Statistics, National Health Interview Survey, family core, sample child, and sample adult questionnaires.

Table 81 (page 1 of 2). No health care visits to an office or clinic within the past 12 months among children under 18 years of age, by selected characteristics: United States, average annual 1997–1998, 2001–2002, and 2004–2005

[Data are based on household interviews of a sample of the civilian noninstitutionalized population]

Characteristic	Under 18 years			Under 6 years			6–17 years		
	1997–1998	*2001–2002*	*2004–2005*	*1997–1998*	*2001–2002*	*2004–2005*	*1997–1998*	*2001–2002*	*2004–2005*
	Percent of children without a health care visit[1]								
All children[2]	12.8	12.1	11.6	5.7	6.3	6.2	16.3	14.9	14.1
Race[3]									
White only	12.2	11.5	11.2	5.5	6.4	6.5	15.5	13.9	13.5
Black or African American only	14.3	13.3	11.7	6.5	5.9	4.3	18.1	16.8	15.3
American Indian or Alaska Native only	13.8	*18.6	16.0	*	*	*	*17.6	*23.0	20.1
Asian only	16.3	15.6	17.9	*5.6	*6.8	*11.2	22.1	20.5	20.7
Native Hawaiian or Other Pacific Islander only	---	*	*	---	*	*	---	*	*
2 or more races	---	8.3	10.0	---	*3.3	*	---	12.4	13.7
Hispanic origin and race[3]									
Hispanic or Latino	19.3	18.8	17.8	9.7	9.6	10.1	25.3	24.0	22.3
Not Hispanic or Latino	11.6	10.6	10.1	4.8	5.4	5.2	14.9	13.0	12.3
White only	10.7	9.7	9.1	4.3	5.3	5.1	13.7	11.7	10.9
Black or African American only	14.5	13.4	11.8	6.5	6.0	4.3	18.3	16.8	15.3
Percent of poverty level[4]									
Below 100%	17.6	17.3	15.0	8.1	9.1	7.7	23.6	21.8	19.4
100%–less than 200%	16.2	14.8	15.5	7.2	7.4	8.3	20.8	18.7	19.1
200% or more	9.9	9.6	9.0	4.1	4.8	4.8	12.6	11.7	10.9
Hispanic origin and race and percent of poverty level[3,4]									
Hispanic or Latino:									
Below 100%	23.2	22.1	20.1	11.7	10.4	11.9	31.1	29.4	25.6
100%–less than 200%	20.9	21.3	20.6	9.7	12.3	11.1	28.1	26.2	26.1
200% or more	13.4	13.7	13.1	7.2	6.4	7.1	16.8	17.6	16.2
Not Hispanic or Latino:									
White only:									
Below 100%	14.0	13.2	10.3	*5.6	*8.6	*4.7	19.7	15.6	13.5
100%–less than 200%	14.1	11.8	12.7	6.0	*6.0	7.6	18.0	14.8	15.3
200% or more	9.2	8.8	8.0	3.6	4.5	4.5	11.7	10.5	9.6
Black or African American only:									
Below 100%	15.8	16.1	13.0	7.6	*7.8	*4.6	20.5	20.3	18.0
100%–less than 200%	16.4	13.3	13.1	*7.7	*4.4	*	20.4	17.5	16.1
200% or more	11.8	11.2	9.9	*4.1	*5.4	*3.3	14.8	13.6	12.7
Health insurance status at the time of interview[5]									
Insured	10.4	9.8	9.6	4.5	4.7	5.1	13.4	12.3	11.9
Private	10.4	9.5	9.5	4.3	4.3	5.0	13.1	11.8	11.4
Medicaid	10.1	10.3	9.7	5.0	5.5	5.1	14.4	13.3	12.9
Uninsured	28.8	31.9	30.9	14.6	21.0	20.7	34.9	36.3	34.7
Health insurance status prior to interview[5]									
Insured continuously all 12 months	10.3	9.5	9.6	4.4	4.6	5.0	13.2	12.0	11.9
Uninsured for any period up to 12 months	15.9	17.7	14.1	7.7	10.3	9.4	20.9	21.9	16.3
Uninsured more than 12 months	34.9	41.4	39.4	19.9	30.2	29.1	40.2	45.3	42.6

See footnotes at end of table.

Table 81 (page 2 of 2). No health care visits to an office or clinic within the past 12 months among children under 18 years of age, by selected characteristics: United States, average annual 1997–1998, 2001–2002, and 2004–2005

[Data are based on household interviews of a sample of the civilian noninstitutionalized population]

	Under 18 years			Under 6 years			6–17 years		
Characteristic	*1997–1998*	*2001–2002*	*2004–2005*	*1997–1998*	*2001–2002*	*2004–2005*	*1997–1998*	*2001–2002*	*2004–2005*
Percent of poverty level and health insurance status prior to interview[4,5]	Percent of children without a health care visit[1]								
Below 100%:									
Insured continuously all 12 months.	12.6	11.7	11.7	5.7	6.1	5.8	17.6	14.9	15.7
Uninsured for any period up to 12 months	19.9	21.8	14.5	*9.9	*14.4	*	26.1	26.6	18.6
Uninsured more than 12 months . .	39.9	48.2	44.1	24.9	*28.0	37.7	45.2	55.7	46.3
100%–less than 200%:									
Insured continuously all 12 months.	12.6	10.9	12.1	4.8	4.2	6.1	16.7	14.5	15.4
Uninsured for any period up to 12 months	15.6	18.9	15.9	*8.7	*10.7	*14.5	20.2	23.2	16.4
Uninsured more than 12 months . .	33.7	41.3	42.3	21.3	35.4	27.8	37.9	43.6	46.4
200% or more:									
Insured continuously all 12 months.	8.9	8.6	8.2	3.8	4.2	4.3	11.3	10.6	10.0
Uninsured for any period up to . . . 12 months	12.4	13.8	12.4	*	*6.9	*8.1	16.7	17.7	14.6
Uninsured more than 12 months . .	29.7	32.3	30.3	*10.5	*24.8	*	36.7	34.4	33.4
Geographic region									
Northeast	7.0	6.0	6.9	3.1	3.9	4.1	8.9	6.9	8.2
Midwest	12.2	10.3	9.3	5.9	5.1	5.1	15.3	12.8	11.3
South	14.3	14.0	11.7	5.6	7.0	5.8	18.5	17.4	14.7
West	16.3	16.0	17.3	7.9	8.1	9.7	20.7	20.0	20.9
Location of residence									
Within MSA[6]	12.3	11.7	11.7	5.4	6.1	6.5	15.9	14.5	14.2
Outside MSA[6]	14.6	13.5	11.0	6.9	6.9	4.9	17.9	16.3	13.8

* Estimates are considered unreliable. Data preceded by an asterisk have a relative standard error (RSE) of 20%–30%. Data not shown have an RSE of greater than 30%.
- - - Data not available.
[1]Respondents were asked how many times a doctor or other health care professional was seen in the past 12 months at a doctor's office, clinic, or some other place. Excluded are visits to emergency rooms, hospitalizations, home visits, and telephone calls. Starting with 2000 data, dental visits were also excluded. See Appendix II, Health care contact.
[2]Includes all other races not shown separately and unknown health insurance status.
[3]The race groups, white, black, American Indian or Alaska Native, Asian, Native Hawaiian or Other Pacific Islander, and 2 or more races, include persons of Hispanic and non-Hispanic origin. Persons of Hispanic origin may be of any race. Starting with 1999 data, race-specific estimates are tabulated according to the 1997 Revisions to the Standards for the Classification of Federal Data on Race and Ethnicity and are not strictly comparable with estimates for earlier years. The five single-race categories plus multiple-race categories shown in the table conform to the 1997 Standards. Starting with 1999 data, race-specific estimates are for persons who reported only one racial group; the category 2 or more races includes persons who reported more than one racial group. Prior to 1999, data were tabulated according to the 1977 Standards with four racial groups and the Asian only category included Native Hawaiian or Other Pacific Islander. Estimates for single-race categories prior to 1999 included persons who reported one race or, if they reported more than one race, identified one race as best representing their race. Starting with 2003 data, race responses of other race and unspecified multiple race were treated as missing, and then race was imputed if these were the only race responses. Almost all persons with a race response of other race were of Hispanic origin. See Appendix II, Hispanic origin; Race.
[4]Percent of poverty level is based on family income and family size and composition using U.S. Census Bureau poverty thresholds. Missing family income data were imputed for 21%–25% of children under 18 years of age in 1997–1998 and 28%–31% in 1999–2005. See Appendix II, Family income; Poverty.
[5]Health insurance categories are mutually exclusive. Persons who reported both Medicaid and private coverage are classified as having private coverage. Starting with 1997 data, Medicaid includes state-sponsored health plans and State Children's Health Insurance Program (SCHIP). In addition to private and Medicaid, the insured category also includes military, other government, and Medicare coverage. Persons not covered by private insurance, Medicaid, SCHIP, public assistance (through 1996), state-sponsored or other government-sponsored health plans (starting in 1997), Medicare, or military plans are considered to have no health insurance coverage. Persons with only Indian Health Service coverage are considered to have no health insurance coverage. See Appendix II, Health insurance coverage.
[6]MSA is metropolitan statistical area.

NOTES: In 1997 the National Health Interview Survey questionnaire was redesigned. See Appendix I, National Health Interview Survey. Standard errors for selected years are available in the spreadsheet version of this table. Available from: www.cdc.gov/nchs/hus.htm. Data for additional years are available. See Appendix III.

SOURCE: Centers for Disease Control and Prevention, National Center for Health Statistics, National Health Interview Survey, family core and sample child questionnaires.

Table 82 (page 1 of 3). Health care visits to doctor offices, emergency departments, and home visits within the past 12 months, by selected characteristics: United States, 1997, 2004, and 2005

[Data are based on household interviews of a sample of the civilian noninstitutionalized population]

	Number of health care visits[1]											
	None			*1–3 visits*			*4–9 visits*			*10 or more visits*		
Characteristic	*1997*	*2004*	*2005*	*1997*	*2004*	*2005*	*1997*	*2004*	*2005*	*1997*	*2004*	*2005*
	Percent distribution											
18 years and over, age-adjusted[2,3]	16.5	16.1	15.6	46.2	45.8	46.2	23.6	24.6	24.6	13.7	13.5	13.7
18 years and over, crude[2]	16.5	16.1	15.5	46.5	45.8	46.2	23.5	24.5	24.6	13.5	13.5	13.7
Age												
Under 18 years	11.8	10.6	10.2	54.1	55.3	56.3	25.2	26.2	26.1	8.9	8.0	7.4
Under 6 years	5.0	5.3	5.1	44.9	47.5	47.9	37.0	36.9	37.5	13.0	10.3	9.5
6–17 years	15.3	13.1	12.7	58.7	59.0	60.4	19.3	21.1	20.6	6.8	6.8	6.4
18–44 years	21.7	23.8	23.1	46.7	45.6	46.0	19.0	19.2	18.8	12.6	11.5	12.1
18–24 years	22.0	25.7	24.3	46.8	45.0	44.7	20.0	19.2	19.2	11.2	10.1	11.8
25–44 years	21.6	23.1	22.6	46.7	45.8	46.5	18.7	19.2	18.7	13.0	12.0	12.2
45–64 years	16.9	15.0	14.1	42.9	43.3	43.1	24.7	25.3	26.4	15.5	16.3	16.4
45–54 years	17.9	16.9	15.9	43.9	45.0	45.1	23.4	22.9	23.9	14.8	15.2	15.1
55–64 years	15.3	12.3	11.5	41.3	40.9	40.5	26.7	28.9	29.8	16.7	18.0	18.2
65 years and over	8.9	5.6	5.7	34.7	31.6	31.1	32.5	36.8	36.7	23.8	26.1	26.5
65–74 years	9.8	6.8	6.0	36.9	36.0	34.8	31.6	34.5	35.1	21.6	22.6	24.1
75 years and over	7.7	4.1	5.3	31.8	26.4	26.9	33.8	39.5	38.5	26.6	30.0	29.2
Sex[3]												
Male	21.3	20.9	20.4	47.1	46.6	46.9	20.6	21.6	21.9	11.0	10.9	10.8
Female	11.8	11.5	10.8	45.4	45.0	45.5	26.5	27.5	27.3	16.3	16.0	16.4
Race[3,4]												
White only	16.0	16.0	15.2	46.1	45.4	46.0	23.9	24.8	24.9	14.0	13.8	14.0
Black or African American only	16.8	15.8	16.0	46.1	47.0	47.5	23.2	24.6	23.6	13.9	12.6	12.9
American Indian or Alaska Native only	17.1	17.7	20.5	38.0	41.7	36.6	24.2	25.0	29.4	20.7	15.5	13.4
Asian only	22.8	20.8	21.6	49.1	51.5	49.5	19.7	19.7	20.5	8.3	8.1	8.5
Native Hawaiian or Other Pacific Islander only	- - -	*	*	- - -	*	*	- - -	*	*	- - -	*	*
2 or more races	- - -	13.6	15.6	- - -	42.9	37.9	- - -	26.2	26.7	- - -	17.3	19.9
Hispanic origin and race[3,4]												
Hispanic or Latino	24.9	26.7	24.0	42.3	41.8	42.4	20.3	20.6	21.7	12.5	10.9	11.9
Mexican	28.9	29.7	26.7	40.8	41.0	41.7	18.5	18.9	20.5	11.8	10.4	11.1
Not Hispanic or Latino	15.4	14.2	13.9	46.7	46.5	46.8	24.0	25.2	25.2	13.9	14.1	14.0
White only	14.7	13.5	13.1	46.6	46.1	46.7	24.4	25.7	25.7	14.3	14.7	14.6
Black or African American only	16.9	15.6	16.0	46.1	47.3	47.5	23.1	24.6	23.6	13.8	12.5	12.9
Respondent-assessed health status[3]												
Fair or poor	7.8	8.1	9.2	23.3	22.0	21.9	29.0	28.0	27.1	39.9	41.9	41.9
Good to excellent	17.2	16.9	16.2	48.4	48.0	48.5	23.3	24.4	24.4	11.1	10.7	10.9
Percent of poverty level[3,5]												
Below 100%	20.6	21.1	20.8	37.8	37.7	37.5	22.7	23.5	24.3	18.9	17.7	17.4
100%–less than 200%	20.1	20.9	20.4	43.3	42.5	42.3	21.7	22.3	22.8	14.9	14.4	14.5
200% or more	14.5	13.8	13.3	48.7	48.1	48.7	24.2	25.3	25.2	12.6	12.8	12.8

See footnotes at end of table.

Table 82 (page 2 of 3). Health care visits to doctor offices, emergency departments, and home visits within the past 12 months, by selected characteristics: United States, 1997, 2004, and 2005

[Data are based on household interviews of a sample of the civilian noninstitutionalized population]

Characteristic	Number of health care visits[1]											
	None			1–3 visits			4–9 visits			10 or more visits		
	1997	2004	2005	1997	2004	2005	1997	2004	2005	1997	2004	2005
Hispanic origin and race and percent of poverty level[3,4,5]												
	Percent distribution											
Hispanic or Latino:												
Below 100%	30.2	31.6	28.1	34.8	35.0	37.4	19.9	19.6	19.8	15.0	13.9	14.7
100%–less than 200%	28.7	30.5	27.8	39.7	39.3	39.0	20.4	19.4	22.2	11.2	10.9	11.1
200% or more	18.9	21.5	19.4	48.8	47.0	47.1	20.4	22.2	22.7	11.9	9.2	10.8
Not Hispanic or Latino:												
White only:												
Below 100%	17.0	16.2	16.6	38.3	37.5	36.4	23.9	25.4	27.4	20.9	20.9	19.7
100%–less than 200%	17.3	16.7	17.6	44.1	43.2	42.2	22.2	23.4	23.2	16.3	16.7	17.0
200% or more	13.8	12.7	11.8	48.2	47.4	48.7	24.9	26.1	26.0	13.1	13.8	13.6
Black or African American only:												
Below 100%	17.4	15.9	17.9	38.5	40.9	40.2	23.4	25.7	24.5	20.7	17.5	17.4
100%–less than 200%	18.8	18.1	16.2	43.7	44.5	47.1	22.9	23.8	24.0	14.5	13.7	12.7
200% or more	15.6	14.3	15.2	51.7	51.3	50.4	22.7	24.4	23.4	10.0	10.0	11.0
Health insurance status at the time of interview[6,7]												
Under 65 years:												
Insured	14.3	13.4	12.5	49.0	49.1	49.9	23.6	24.6	24.5	13.1	12.8	13.1
Private	14.7	13.6	12.9	50.6	51.4	51.8	23.1	23.9	24.1	11.6	11.2	11.3
Medicaid	9.8	11.8	10.0	35.5	35.1	38.3	26.5	28.2	25.8	28.2	24.9	25.9
Uninsured	33.7	37.8	37.6	42.8	42.5	42.1	15.3	13.6	14.4	8.2	6.1	5.9
Health insurance status prior to interview[6,7]												
Under 65 years:												
Insured continuously all 12 months	14.1	13.4	12.4	49.2	49.4	50.1	23.6	24.6	24.5	13.0	12.7	12.9
Uninsured for any period up to 12 months	18.9	20.0	18.9	46.0	45.7	45.1	20.8	21.9	22.1	14.4	12.3	13.8
Uninsured more than 12 months	39.0	43.9	43.6	41.4	41.3	40.1	13.2	10.0	12.1	6.4	4.8	4.2
Percent of poverty level and health insurance status prior to interview[5,6,7]												
Under 65 years:												
Below 100%:												
Insured continuously all 12 months	13.8	14.3	12.7	39.7	39.6	40.7	25.2	25.7	25.7	21.4	20.4	21.0
Uninsured for any period up to 12 months	19.7	17.6	19.0	37.6	42.0	37.6	21.9	24.6	23.2	20.9	15.7	20.2
Uninsured more than 12 months	41.2	47.1	46.2	39.9	38.6	35.3	12.2	9.4	14.2	6.6	5.0	4.4
100–less than 200%:												
Insured continuously all 12 months	16.0	15.7	14.9	46.4	45.4	46.1	21.9	23.5	23.6	15.8	15.5	15.4
Uninsured for any period up to 12 months	18.8	21.7	19.3	45.1	45.1	44.9	21.0	22.1	21.7	15.0	11.1	14.1
Uninsured more than 12 months	38.7	45.0	43.6	41.0	39.4	39.4	14.0	9.9	12.5	6.3	5.7	4.5
200% or more:												
Insured continuously all 12 months	13.7	12.6	11.8	51.0	51.3	51.8	23.6	24.7	24.6	11.7	11.5	11.7
Uninsured for any period up to 12 months	17.8	20.3	18.6	50.3	47.5	48.1	20.4	20.4	22.1	11.5	11.9	11.2
Uninsured more than 12 months	36.6	39.7	41.1	43.8	45.4	44.8	13.2	10.9	10.2	6.4	4.1	3.9
Geographic region[3]												
Northeast	13.2	11.6	11.4	45.9	45.5	47.1	26.0	27.5	26.5	14.9	15.4	15.0
Midwest	15.9	13.9	13.8	47.7	47.5	47.4	22.8	25.1	24.7	13.6	13.5	14.0
South	17.2	16.7	16.1	46.1	46.2	46.0	23.3	23.8	24.6	13.5	13.3	13.3
West	19.1	21.3	20.1	44.8	43.8	44.4	22.8	22.7	22.8	13.3	12.2	12.6

See footnotes at end of table.

Table 82 (page 3 of 3). Health care visits to doctor offices, emergency departments, and home visits within the past 12 months, by selected characteristics: United States, 1997, 2004, and 2005

[Data are based on household interviews of a sample of the civilian noninstitutionalized population]

Characteristic	None 1997	None 2004	None 2005	1–3 visits 1997	1–3 visits 2004	1–3 visits 2005	4–9 visits 1997	4–9 visits 2004	4–9 visits 2005	10 or more visits 1997	10 or more visits 2004	10 or more visits 2005
	Number of health care visits[1]											
Location of residence[3]	Percent distribution											
Within MSA[8]	16.2	16.3	15.6	46.4	45.9	46.5	23.7	24.4	24.5	13.7	13.4	13.4
Outside MSA[8]	17.3	15.3	15.4	45.4	45.4	44.7	23.3	25.3	25.2	13.9	14.0	14.7

* Estimates are considered unreliable. Data preceded by an asterisk have a relative standard error (RSE) of 20%–30%. Data not shown have an RSE greater than 30%.

- - - Data not available.

[1]This table presents a summary measure of health care visits to doctor offices, emergency departments, and home visits during a 12-month period. See Appendix II, Emergency department visit; Health care contact; Home visit.

[2]Includes all other races not shown separately and unknown health insurance status.

[3]Estimates are age-adjusted to the year 2000 standard population using six age groups: Under 18 years, 18–44 years, 45–54 years, 55–64 years, 65–74 years, and 75 years and over. See Appendix II, Age adjustment.

[4]The race groups, white, black, American Indian or Alaska Native, Asian, Native Hawaiian or Other Pacific Islander, and 2 or more races, include persons of Hispanic and non-Hispanic origin. Persons of Hispanic origin may be of any race. Starting with 1999 data, race-specific estimates are tabulated according to the 1997 Revisions to the Standards for the Classification of Federal Data on Race and Ethnicity and are not strictly comparable with estimates for earlier years. The five single-race categories plus multiple-race categories shown in the table conform to the 1997 Standards. Starting with 1999 data, race-specific estimates are for persons who reported only one racial group; the category 2 or more races includes persons who reported more than one racial group. Prior to 1999, data were tabulated according to the 1977 Standards with four racial groups and the Asian only category included Native Hawaiian or Other Pacific Islander. Estimates for single-race categories prior to 1999 included persons who reported one race or, if they reported more than one race, identified one race as best representing their race. Starting with 2003 data, race responses of other race and unspecified multiple race were treated as missing, and then race was imputed if these were the only race responses. Almost all persons with a race response of other race were of Hispanic origin. See Appendix II, Hispanic origin; Race.

[5]Percent of poverty level is based on family income and family size and composition using U.S. Census Bureau poverty thresholds. Missing family income data were imputed for 25%–29% of persons in 1997–1998 and 32%–35% in 1999–2005. See Appendix II, Family income; Poverty.

[6]Estimates for persons under 65 years of age are age-adjusted to the year 2000 standard population using four age groups: Under 18 years, 18–44 years, 45–54 years, and 55–64 years of age. See Appendix II, Age adjustment.

[7]Health insurance categories are mutually exclusive. Persons who reported both Medicaid and private coverage are classified as having private coverage. Starting in 1997, Medicaid includes state-sponsored health plans and State Children's Health Insurance Program (SCHIP). In addition to private and Medicaid, the insured category also includes military plans, other government-sponsored health plans, and Medicare, not shown separately. Persons not covered by private insurance, Medicaid, SCHIP, public assistance (through 1996), state-sponsored or other government-sponsored health plans (starting in 1997), Medicare, or military plans are considered to have no health insurance coverage. Persons with only Indian Health Service coverage are considered to have no health insurance coverage. See Appendix II, Health insurance coverage.

[8]MSA is metropolitan statistical area.

NOTES: In 1997, the National Health Interview Survey questionnaire was redesigned. See Appendix I, National Health Interview Survey. Standard errors are available in the spreadsheet version of this table. See www.cdc.gov/nchs/hus.htm. Data for additional years are available. See Appendix III.

SOURCE: Centers for Disease Control and Prevention, National Center for Health Statistics, National Health Interview Survey, family core and sample adult questionnaires.

able 83 (page 1 of 2). Vaccinations of children 19–35 months of age for selected diseases, by race, ispanic origin, poverty level, and residence in metropolitan statistical area (MSA): United States, elected years 1995–2006

)ata are based on telephone interviews of a sample of the civilian noninstitutionalized population supplemented by a survey of immunization oviders for interview participants]

Vaccination and year	All	Race and Hispanic origin[1] — Not Hispanic or Latino: White	Black or African American	American Indian or Alaska Native	Asian[3]	Native Hawaiian or Other Pacific Islander[3]	2 or more races	Hispanic or Latino	Poverty level: Below poverty level	At or above poverty level	Location of residence — Inside MSA[2]: Central city	Remaining area	Outside MSA[2]
	Percent of children 19–35 months of age												
ombined series (4:3:1:3:3:1):[4]													
2002	66	66	62	---	74	---	61	66	62	66	64	68	61
2003	73	74	68	69	76	---	74	71	70	74	72	74	70
2004	76	77	71	67	80	---	77	76	73	77	75	78	74
2005	76	76	76	---	77	---	80	76	74	77	75	78	74
2006	77	78	74	74	76	---	75	77	74	78	77	78	75
TP/DT/DTaP (4 doses or more):[5]													
1995	78	80	74	71	84	---	---	75	71	81	77	79	78
2000	82	84	76	75	85	---	---	79	76	84	80	83	83
2002	82	84	76	*	88	*	78	79	75	84	79	84	80
2003	85	88	80	80	89	*	84	82	80	87	84	86	83
2004	86	88	80	77	90	*	86	84	81	87	84	87	85
2005	86	87	84	*	89	*	86	84	82	87	85	87	85
2006	85	87	81	82	86	*	84	85	81	87	84	86	85
olio (3 doses or more):													
1995	88	89	84	86	90	---	---	87	85	89	87	88	89
2000	90	91	87	90	93	---	---	88	87	90	88	90	91
2002	90	91	87	*	92	95	87	90	88	91	89	91	90
2003	92	93	89	91	91	90	91	90	89	93	91	92	92
2004	92	92	90	87	93	*	92	91	90	92	91	92	92
2005	92	91	91	*	93	*	94	92	90	92	91	93	92
2006	93	93	91	91	92	96	92	93	92	93	93	93	93
leasles, Mumps, Rubella:													
1995	90	91	87	88	95	---	---	88	86	91	90	90	89
2000	91	92	88	87	90	---	---	90	89	91	90	91	91
2002	92	93	90	84	95	94	89	91	90	92	90	93	90
2003	93	93	92	92	96	*	94	93	92	93	93	93	92
2004	93	94	91	89	94	*	94	93	91	94	93	94	92
2005	92	91	92	90	92	90	94	91	89	92	92	92	90
2006	92	93	91	89	95	93	91	92	91	93	93	93	92
lib (3 doses or more):[6]													
1995	91	93	88	93	90	---	---	89	88	93	91	92	92
2000	93	95	93	90	92	---	---	91	90	95	92	94	95
2002	93	94	92	*	95	93	90	92	90	94	92	94	93
2003	94	95	92	89	91	*	93	93	91	95	94	94	94
2004	94	95	91	90	92	*	96	93	92	94	93	94	94
2005	94	94	93	88	89	91	95	94	92	95	93	94	94
2006	93	94	91	94	89	96	92	94	91	94	93	94	92
lepatitis B (3 doses or more):													
1995	68	68	66	52	80	---	---	70	65	69	69	71	59
2000	90	91	89	91	91	---	---	88	87	91	89	90	92
2002	90	91	88	*	94	94	84	90	88	90	89	91	90
2003	92	93	92	90	94	*	93	91	91	93	92	93	93
2004	92	93	91	91	93	*	94	92	91	93	92	93	93
2005	93	93	93	90	93	*	94	93	91	94	92	94	93
2006	93	94	92	95	92	97	92	94	93	94	93	94	93
aricella:[7]													
1998	43	42	42	28	53	---	---	47	41	44	45	45	34
2000	68	66	67	62	77	---	---	70	64	69	69	70	60
2002	81	79	83	71	87	*	79	82	79	81	81	83	75
2003	85	84	85	81	91	*	86	86	84	85	86	86	80
2004	88	87	86	84	91	*	89	89	86	88	88	89	85
2005	88	86	91	82	92	*	90	89	87	88	88	88	86
2006	89	89	89	85	93	90	91	90	89	90	90	90	86

ee footnotes at end of table.

Table 83 (page 2 of 2). Vaccinations of children 19–35 months of age for selected diseases, by race, Hispanic origin, poverty level, and residence in metropolitan statistical area (MSA): United States, selected years 1995–2006

[Data are based on telephone interviews of a sample of the civilian noninstitutionalized population supplemented by a survey of immunization providers for interview participants]

	Race and Hispanic origin[1]								Poverty level		Location of residence		
		Not Hispanic or Latino									Inside MSA[2]		
Vaccination and year	All	White	Black or African American	American Indian or Alaska Native	Asian[3]	Native Hawaiian or Other Pacific Islander[3]	2 or more races	Hispanic or Latino	Below poverty level	At or above poverty level	Central city	Remaining area	Outside MSA[2]
	Percent of children 19–35 months of age												
PCV (3 doses or more):[8]													
2002	41	44	34	33	55	*	38	37	33	43	41	45	32
2003	68	71	62	60	71	*	66	66	62	71	68	71	61
2004	73	75	68	75	76	*	78	70	69	75	72	77	68
2005	83	83	80	*	79	*	87	84	78	84	82	85	78
2006	87	87	83	87	81	*	86	89	85	88	88	88	81

	Not Hispanic or Latino					
	White		Black or African American		Hispanic or Latino	
Vaccination and year	Below poverty level	At or above poverty level	Below poverty level	At or above poverty level	Below poverty level	At or above poverty level
	Percent of children 19–35 months of age					
Combined series (4:3:1:3:3:1):[4]						
2002	59	67	59	62	66	66
2003	69	75	64	72	73	70
2004	72	78	68	75	75	78
2005	70	77	74	80	76	75
2006	70	79	72	77	77	79

- - - Data not available.

* Estimates are considered unreliable. Percents not shown if the unweighted sample size for the numerator was less than 30 or relative standard error greater than 50% or confidence interval half width greater than 10%.

[1]Persons of Hispanic origin may be of any race. Starting with 2002 data, estimates were tabulated using the 1997 Revisions to the Standards for the Classification of Federal Data on Race and Ethnicity. Estimates for earlier years were tabulated using the 1977 Standards on Race and Ethnicity. See Appendix II, Hispanic origin; Race.

[2]Metropolitan statistical area. See Appendix II, Metropolitan statistical area.

[3]Prior to data year 2002, the category Asian included Native Hawaiian and Other Pacific Islander.

[4]The 4:3:1:3:3:1 combined series consists of 4 or more doses of diphtheria and tetanus toxoids and pertussis vaccine (DTP), diphtheria and tetanus toxoids (DT), or diphtheria and tetanus toxoids and acellular pertussis vaccine (DTaP); 3 or more doses of any poliovirus vaccine; 1 or more doses of a measles-containing vaccine (MCV); 3 or more doses of *Haemophilus influenzae* type b vaccine (Hib); 3 or more doses of hepatitis B vaccine; and 1 or more doses of varicella vaccine.

[5]Diphtheria and tetanus toxoids and pertussis vaccine, diphtheria and tetanus toxoids, and diphtheria and tetanus toxoids and acellular pertussis vaccine.

[6]*Haemophilus influenzae* type b vaccine (Hib).

[7]Recommended in 1996. Data collection for varicella began in July 1996.

[8]Pneumococcal conjugate vaccine (PCV). Recommended in 2000. Data collection for PCV began in July 2001.

NOTES: Final estimates from the National Immunization Survey include an adjustment for children with missing immunization provider data. Poverty level is based on family income and family size using U.S. Census Bureau poverty thresholds. In 2006, 5.0% of all children with provider-reported vaccination history data, 10.4% of Hispanic, 2.6% of non-Hispanic white, and 6.6% of non-Hispanic black children were missing information about poverty level and were omitted from the estimates of vaccination coverage by poverty level See Appendix II, Poverty. See Appendix I, National Immunization Survey.
Additional information on childhood immunizations is available from: www.cdc.gov/vaccines/recs/schedules/child-schedule.htm#printable.
Data for additional years are available. See Appendix III.

SOURCE: Centers for Disease Control and Prevention, National Center for Health Statistics and National Immunization Program, National Immunization Survey. Available from: www.cdc.gov/vaccines/stats-surv/imz-coverage.htm#nis and www.cdc.gov/nis/.

Table 84 (page 1 of 2). Vaccination coverage among children 19–35 months of age, by geographic division, state, and selected urban area: United States, selected years 2002–2006

Data are based on telephone interviews of a sample of the civilian noninstitutionalized population supplemented by a survey of immunization roviders for interview participants]

Geographic division and state	*2002*	*2003*	*2004*	*2005*	*2006*
	Percent of children 19–35 months of age with 4:3:1:3:3:1 series[1]				
Jnited States	66	73	76	76	77
Jew England:					
Connecticut	73	89	85	82	82
Maine	62	69	74	76	76
Massachusetts	78	83	84	91	84
New Hampshire	66	76	78	77	76
Rhode Island	81	80	82	80	81
Vermont	58	65	67	63	75
Aiddle Atlantic:					
New Jersey	66	64	74	72	76
New York	67	73	78	74	79
Pennsylvania	68	79	82	77	81
:ast North Central:					
Illinois	58	69	74	77	74
Indiana	59	62	68	70	76
Michigan	72	79	79	81	78
Ohio	64	71	71	78	75
Wisconsin	68	73	78	77	81
Vest North Central:					
Iowa	58	63	76	76	79
Kansas	55	63	66	72	70
Minnesota	62	71	78	78	78
Missouri	60	74	75	73	81
Nebraska	64	68	73	84	75
North Dakota	56	63	71	79	80
South Dakota	62	60	73	80	74
outh Atlantic:					
Delaware	70	66	80	82	80
District of Columbia	68	72	80	72	78
Florida	66	74	85	78	80
Georgia	77	75	82	82	81
Maryland	71	77	76	79	78
North Carolina	70	77	78	82	82
South Carolina	74	80	77	76	80
Virginia	65	80	74	82	77
West Virginia	66	63	76	68	68
ast South Central:					
Alabama	73	79	80	82	79
Kentucky	64	79	77	71	79
Mississippi	64	78	80	79	73
Tennessee	67	74	79	80	77
Vest South Central:					
Arkansas	68	75	81	64	73
Louisiana	62	65	70	74	70
Oklahoma	60	67	71	72	78
Texas	65	70	69	77	75
ountain:					
Arizona	59	68	73	75	71
Colorado	56	63	73	79	76
Idaho	53	61	70	68	69
Montana	49	65	65	65	66
Nevada	65	66	65	63	60
New Mexico	59	71	79	75	72
Utah	61	70	68	68	78
Wyoming	54	57	64	67	64
acific:					
Alaska	56	73	66	68	67
California	67	76	79	74	79
Hawaii	69	79	80	78	79
Oregon	60	70	74	65	73
Washington	52	56	67	66	71

e footnotes at end of table.

Table 84 (page 2 of 2). Vaccination coverage among children 19–35 months of age, by geographic division, state, and selected urban area: United States, selected years 2002–2006

[Data are based on telephone interviews of a sample of the civilian noninstitutionalized population supplemented by a survey of immunization providers for interview participants]

Geographic division and state	2002	2003	2004	2005	2006
	Percent of children 19–35 months of age with 4:3:1:3:3:1 series[1]				
New England:					
Boston, Massachusetts	71	86	79	- - -	81
Middle Atlantic:					
New York City, New York	71	69	77	71	72
Newark, New Jersey	50	64	64	67	68
Philadelphia, Pennsylvania	68	75	75	77	74
East North Central:					
Chicago, Illinois	58	71	71	70	77
Cuyahoga County (Cleveland), Ohio	65	66	78	77	77
Detroit, Michigan	60	64	66	71	65
Franklin County (Columbus), Ohio	69	71	79	81	- - -
Marion County (Indianapolis), Indiana	62	66	74	- - -	77
Milwaukee County (Milwaukee), Wisconsin	60	71	73	74	78
South Atlantic:					
Baltimore, Maryland	69	74	80	77	72
Dade County (Miami), Florida	60	73	73	- - -	80
District of Columbia	68	72	80	72	78
Duval County (Jacksonville), Florida	70	75	69	77	76
Fulton/DeKalb Counties (Atlanta), Georgia	75	71	81	72	75
East South Central:					
Davidson County (Nashville), Tennessee	67	76	88	81	- - -
Shelby County (Memphis), Tennessee	61	69	71	74	74
Jefferson County (Birmingham), Alabama	74	79	81	85	- - -
West South Central:					
Bexar County (San Antonio), Texas	72	75	73	71	75
Dallas County (Dallas), Texas	68	67	67	73	74
El Paso County (El Paso), Texas	61	72	64	69	69
Houston, Texas	56	63	62	77	70
Orleans Parish (New Orleans), Louisiana	53	68	68	- - -	- - -
Mountain:					
Maricopa County (Phoenix), Arizona	62	69	72	76	68
Pacific:					
King County (Seattle), Washington	56	61	74	69	69
Los Angeles County (Los Angeles), California	72	79	77	78	79
San Diego County (San Diego), California	71	75	74	- - -	80
Santa Clara County (Santa Clara), California	75	77	80	- - -	78

- - - Data not available.

* Percents not shown if the unweighted sample size for the numerator was less than 30 or relative standard error greater than 50% or confidence interval half width greater than 10 percentage points.

[1]The 4:3:1:3:3:1 combined series consists of 4 or more doses of diphtheria and tetanus toxoids and pertussis vaccine (DTP), diphtheria and tetanus toxoids (DT), or diphtheria and tetanus toxoids and acellular pertussis vaccine (DTaP); 3 or more doses of any poliovirus vaccine; 1 or more doses of a measles-containing vaccine (MCV); 3 or more doses of *Haemophilus influenzae* type b vaccine (Hib); 3 or more doses of hepatitis B vaccine; and 1 or more doses of varicella vaccine.

NOTES: Urban areas were originally selected because they were at risk for undervaccination. Final estimates from the National Immunization Survey include an adjustment for children with missing immunization provider data. Additional information on childhood immunizations is available from: www.cdc.gov/vaccines/recs/schedules/child-schedule.htm#printable.

SOURCE: Centers for Disease Control and Prevention, National Center for Health Statistics and National Immunization Program, National Immunization Survey. Available from: www.cdc.gov/vaccines/stats-surv/imz-coverage.htm#nis and www.cdc.gov/nis/.

Table 85 (page 1 of 2). Influenza vaccination among adults 18 years of age and over, by selected characteristics: United States, selected years 1989–2005

Data are based on household interviews of a sample of the civilian noninstitutionalized population]

Characteristic	1989	1995	2000	2001	2002	2003	2004	2005
	Percent receiving influenza vaccination during past 12 months[1]							
8 years and over, age-adjusted[2,3]	9.6	23.6	28.7	26.7	28.3	29.2	29.5	21.3
8 years and over, crude[3]	9.1	24.4	28.4	26.4	28.0	29.0	29.4	21.2
Age								
8–49 years	3.4	13.3	17.1	15.0	16.2	16.8	17.9	10.4
0–64 years	10.6	26.9	34.6	32.2	34.0	36.8	35.9	22.9
5 years and over	30.4	57.0	64.4	63.1	65.7	65.5	64.6	59.6
65–74 years	28.0	54.0	61.1	60.7	60.9	60.5	60.1	53.7
75 years and over	34.2	61.2	68.4	65.8	71.3	71.0	69.7	66.3
50 years and over								
Sex								
Male	19.2	40.9	45.9	44.2	45.1	46.8	45.1	34.6
Female	20.6	44.4	49.5	46.9	49.8	50.7	50.2	40.8
Race[4]								
White only	21.0	45.1	49.8	47.7	49.4	50.4	49.8	39.6
Black or African American only	12.5	29.8	33.2	32.7	36.2	35.3	32.8	26.8
American Indian or Alaska Native only	26.2	*35.3	43.6	41.5	*37.6	44.7	51.3	*22.9
Asian only	*9.2	36.9	43.3	35.4	39.5	45.9	41.7	30.6
Native Hawaiian or Other Pacific Islander only	- - -	- - -	*	*	*	*	*	*
or more races	- - -	- - -	50.7	41.5	47.9	53.7	44.5	29.9
Hispanic origin and race[4]								
Hispanic or Latino	13.2	35.1	34.4	32.5	33.7	33.6	36.9	24.4
Mexican	13.0	36.2	33.0	34.3	33.9	32.8	39.2	25.4
Not Hispanic or Latino	20.3	43.8	48.8	46.6	48.7	50.1	48.8	39.1
White only	21.3	46.0	50.6	48.6	50.3	51.8	50.9	41.0
Black or African American only	12.4	30.0	33.2	32.8	36.5	35.4	32.9	26.9
Percent of poverty level[5]								
Below 100%	19.6	41.4	44.1	38.8	41.9	41.8	42.5	35.6
00%–less than 200%	24.0	43.8	50.7	47.2	49.8	50.9	49.9	41.1
00% or more	19.0	43.0	47.6	46.1	47.9	49.4	48.1	37.4
Hispanic origin and race and percent of poverty level[4,5]								
Hispanic or Latino:								
Below 100%	12.7	36.4	35.8	33.0	36.6	31.9	36.3	22.1
100%–less than 200%	20.4	33.0	35.6	35.2	32.6	29.9	33.1	26.8
200% or more	11.9	35.7	33.1	30.6	33.2	36.6	39.2	24.0
Not Hispanic or Latino:								
White only:								
Below 100%	22.3	47.5	48.6	42.7	42.7	45.9	48.1	41.9
100%–less than 200%	26.1	48.1	54.8	51.0	54.2	55.9	55.0	45.9
200% or more	19.9	45.0	49.8	48.5	50.3	51.5	50.2	39.7
Black or African American only:								
Below 100%	14.7	31.3	35.5	34.7	41.8	37.4	32.0	29.6
100%–less than 200%	12.2	30.2	37.9	35.3	39.4	40.9	36.8	28.1
200% or more	12.0	28.7	29.9	30.6	33.3	32.1	31.6	25.2
Geographic region								
Northeast	17.9	41.6	45.9	45.4	47.2	50.5	47.9	38.3
Midwest	20.0	45.1	49.3	47.9	49.6	50.2	49.9	39.8
South	20.2	42.0	46.8	43.3	46.5	48.4	47.3	37.2
West	21.8	43.4	50.1	47.7	48.1	46.4	46.5	36.7
Location of residence								
Within MSA[6]	18.9	42.3	47.1	45.0	47.1	48.8	47.6	37.1
Outside MSA[6]	23.3	45.3	50.2	47.8	49.7	49.3	48.9	40.9

See footnotes at end of table.

Table 85 (page 2 of 2). Influenza vaccination among adults 18 years of age and over, by selected characteristics: United States, selected years 1989–2005

[Data are based on household interviews of a sample of the civilian noninstitutionalized population]

* Estimates are considered unreliable. Data preceded by an asterisk have a relative standard error (RSE) of 20%–30%. Data not shown have an RSE of greater than 30%.
- - - Data not available.
[1]Respondents were asked, "During the past 12 months, have you had a flu shot? A flu shot is usually given in the fall and protects against influenza for the flu season. Estimates exclude 1% of respondents who reported receiving Flu Mist.
[2]Estimates are age-adjusted to the year 2000 standard population using four age groups: 18–49 years, 50–64 years, 65–74 years, and 75 years and over. See Appendix II, Age adjustment.
[3]Includes all other races not shown separately and unknown poverty level in 1989.
[4]The race groups, white, black, American Indian or Alaska Native, Asian, Native Hawaiian or Other Pacific Islander, and 2 or more races, include persons of Hispanic and non-Hispanic origin. Persons of Hispanic origin may be of any race. Starting with 1999 data, race-specific estimates are tabulated according to the 1997 Revisions to the Standards for Federal Data on Race and Ethnicity and are not strictly comparable with estimates for earlier years. The five single-race categories plus multiple-race categories shown in the table conform to the 1997 Standards. Starting with 1999 data, race-specific estimates are for persons who reported only one racial group; the category 2 or more races includes persons who reported more than one racial group. Prior to 1999, data were tabulated according to the 1977 Standards with four racial groups and the Asian only category included Native Hawaiian or Other Pacific Islander. Estimates for single-race categories prior to 1999 included persons who reported one race or, if they reported more than one race, identified one race as best representing their race. Starting with 2003 data, race responses of other race and unspecified multiple race were treated as missing, and then race was imputed if these were the only race responses. Almost all persons with a race response of other race were of Hispanic origin. See Appendix II, Hispanic origin; Race.
[5]Percent of poverty level is based on family income and family size and composition using U.S. Census Bureau poverty thresholds. Poverty level was unknown for 11% of persons 18 years and over in 1989. Missing family income data were imputed for 16% of persons 18 years and over in 1995, 27%–31% in 1997–1998, and 33%–36% in 1999–2005. See Appendix II, Family Income; Poverty.
[6]MSA is metropolitan statistical area.

NOTES: In 2000, the Advisory Committee on Immunization Practices (ACIP) of the Centers for Disease Control and Prevention (CDC) recommended universal influenza vaccination for persons 50 years and over. CDC. Prevention and control of influenza: Recommendations of the Advisory Committee on Immunization Practices (ACIP). MMWR 2000;49(RR03):1–38. Available from www.cdc.gov/mmwr/pdf/rr/rr4903.pdf. Influenza vaccination among adults 19–49 years is recommended for those with other risk factors (medical, occupational, lifestyle, or other indications). Recommended adult immunization schedule United States, October 2006–September 2007. Available from: www.cdc.gov/nip/recs/adult-schedule.pdf. Standard errors for selected years are available in the spreadsheet version of this table. Available from: www.cdc.gov/nchs/hus.htm. Data for additional years are available. See Appendix III.

SOURCE: Centers for Disease Control and Prevention, National Center for Health Statistics, National Health Interview Survey, sample adult questionnaire.

Table 86 (page 1 of 2). Pneumococcal vaccination among adults 18 years of age and over, by selected characteristics: United States, selected years 1989–2005

[Data are based on household interviews of a sample of the civilian noninstitutionalized population]

Characteristic	1989	1995	2000	2001	2002	2003	2004	2005
				Percent ever receiving pneumococcal vaccination[1]				
18 years and over, age-adjusted[2,3]	4.6	11.8	15.4	16.1	16.4	16.4	16.8	16.7
18 years and over, crude[3]	4.4	12.5	15.1	15.7	16.0	16.0	16.5	16.5
Age								
18–49 years	2.1	6.4	5.4	5.9	5.6	5.6	5.7	5.8
50–64 years	4.4	10.3	14.7	15.4	16.3	16.7	17.2	17.1
65 years and over	14.1	32.9	53.1	54.0	56.0	55.6	56.8	56.2
65–74 years	13.1	30.3	48.2	50.3	50.2	49.8	50.4	49.4
75 years and over	15.7	36.7	59.1	58.4	62.8	62.1	64.2	63.9
65 years and over								
Sex								
Male	13.9	32.6	52.1	54.2	55.9	53.7	54.3	53.4
Female	14.3	33.1	53.9	53.8	56.1	57.0	58.7	58.4
Race[4]								
White only	14.9	34.7	55.6	56.7	58.7	57.9	59.1	58.4
Black or African American only	6.5	21.2	30.6	33.9	37.0	36.9	38.6	40.2
American Indian or Alaska Native only	31.2	*46.2	70.1	*50.7	*	*	*42.0	*
Asian only	*	*25.5	40.9	28.1	32.6	35.3	35.1	35.0
Native Hawaiian or Other Pacific Islander only	- - -	- - -	*	*	*	*	*	*
2 or more races	- - -	- - -	55.6	54.0	52.8	*39.3	*48.8	64.8
Hispanic origin and race[4]								
Hispanic or Latino	9.8	21.0	30.4	32.9	27.1	31.0	33.7	27.5
Mexican	12.9	*18.0	32.0	33.8	30.0	33.6	33.3	31.3
Not Hispanic or Latino	14.3	33.8	54.4	55.2	57.7	57.1	58.3	58.1
White only	15.1	35.6	56.8	57.8	60.4	59.6	60.9	60.6
Black or African American only	6.2	20.9	30.6	34.0	37.0	36.9	38.6	40.4
Percent of poverty level[5]								
Below 100%	11.2	26.9	40.6	43.2	42.6	47.7	42.5	46.6
100%–less than 200%	15.1	30.8	51.4	51.0	54.6	56.7	56.1	54.4
200% or more	15.0	36.6	56.2	57.1	59.2	56.5	59.7	58.5
Hispanic origin and race and percent of poverty level[4,5]								
Hispanic or Latino:								
Below 100%	*	*13.7	23.8	25.0	20.1	23.8	31.8	19.8
100%–less than 200%	*11.0	*16.2	32.3	32.4	25.1	26.8	29.0	27.8
200% or more	*10.4	38.3	32.9	39.4	33.5	39.5	39.1	31.8
Not Hispanic or Latino:								
White only:								
Below 100%	13.4	32.3	47.9	53.4	51.5	57.5	50.6	55.3
100%–less than 200%	16.0	34.4	56.1	56.0	59.9	62.1	61.9	60.5
200% or more	15.6	37.2	58.3	59.0	61.8	58.9	61.9	61.3
Black or African American only:								
Below 100%	*5.0	20.6	28.8	30.5	27.8	35.1	27.0	44.4
100%–less than 200%	7.9	18.5	28.1	31.3	40.7	39.6	36.4	35.0
200% or more	*5.2	24.7	34.4	39.0	39.4	35.7	49.1	42.9
Geographic region								
Northeast	10.4	27.2	51.2	52.5	56.9	54.8	56.0	55.8
Midwest	13.7	30.6	52.6	57.3	55.8	57.1	59.5	58.5
South	14.9	34.5	51.3	52.4	54.2	55.1	57.2	57.4
West	17.9	39.8	59.7	54.6	59.3	55.7	53.7	51.4
Location of residence								
Within MSA[6]	13.1	32.7	52.4	53.3	56.3	56.0	56.7	55.1
Outside MSA[6]	17.1	33.9	55.4	56.4	55.3	54.3	57.3	59.8

See footnotes at end of table.

Table 86 (page 2 of 2). Pneumococcal vaccination among adults 18 years of age and over, by selected characteristics: United States, selected years 1989–2005

[Data are based on household interviews of a sample of the civilian noninstitutionalized population]

* Estimates are considered unreliable. Data preceded by an asterisk have a relative standard error (RSE) of 20%–30%. Data not shown have an RSE of greater than 30%.
- - - Data not available.
[1]Respondents were asked, "Have you ever had a pneumonia shot? This shot is usually given only once or twice in a person's lifetime and is different from the flu shot. It is also called the pneumococcal vaccine."
[2]Estimates are age-adjusted to the year 2000 standard population using four age groups: 18–49 years, 50–64 years, 65–74 years, and 75 years and over. See Appendix II, Age adjustment.
[3]Includes all other races not shown separately and unknown poverty level in 1989.
[4]The race groups, white, black, American Indian or Alaska Native, Asian, Native Hawaiian or Other Pacific Islander, and 2 or more races, include persons of Hispanic and non-Hispanic origin. Persons of Hispanic origin may be of any race. Starting with 1999 data, race-specific estimates are tabulated according to the 1997 Revisions to the Standards for Federal Data on Race and Ethnicity and are not strictly comparable with estimates for earlier years. The five single-race categories plus multiple-race categories shown in the table conform to the 1997 Standards. Starting with 1999 data, race-specific estimates are for persons who reported only one racial group; the category 2 or more races includes persons who reported more than one racial group. Prior to 1999, data were tabulated according to the 1977 Standards with four racial groups and the Asian only category included Native Hawaiian or Other Pacific Islander. Estimates for single-race categories prior to 1999 included persons who reported one race or, if they reported more than one race, identified one race as best representing their race. Starting with 2003 data, race responses of other race and unspecified multiple race were treated as missing, and then race was imputed if these were the only race responses. Almost all persons with a race response of other race were of Hispanic origin. See Appendix II, Hispanic origin; Race.
[5]Percent of poverty level is based on family income and family size and composition using U.S. Census Bureau poverty thresholds. Poverty level was unknown for 11% of persons 18 years and over in 1989. Missing family income data were imputed for 16% of persons 18 years of age and over in 1995, 27%–31% in 1997–1998, and 33%–36% in 1999–2005. See Appendix II, Family Income; Poverty.
[6]MSA is metropolitan statistical area.

NOTES: In 1997, the Advisory Committee on Immunization Practices (ACIP) of the Centers for Disease Control and Prevention (CDC) recommended universal pneumonia vaccination for persons 65 years and over. CDC. Prevention of pneumococcal disease: Recommendations of the advisory committee on immunization practices (ACIP). MMWR 1997;46(RR–08);1–24. Available from: www.cdc.gov/mmwr. Pneumococcal vaccination among adults 19–64 years is recommended for those with other risk factors (medical, occupational, lifestyle, or other indications). Recommended adult immunization schedule United States, October 2006–September 2007 Available from: www.cdc.gov/nip/recs/adult-schedule.pdf. Standard errors for selected years are available in the spreadsheet version of this table. Available from: www.cdc.gov/nchs/hus.htm. Data for additional years are available. See Appendix III.

SOURCE: Centers for Disease Control and Prevention, National Center for Health Statistics, National Health Interview Survey, sample adult questionnaire.

Table 87 (page 1 of 2). Use of mammography among women 40 years of age and over, by selected characteristics: United States, selected years 1987–2005

[Data are based on household interviews of a sample of the civilian noninstitutionalized population]

Characteristic	1987	1990	1991	1998	1999	2000	2003	2005
	Percent of women having a mammogram within the past 2 years[1]							
40 years and over, age-adjusted[2,3]	29.0	51.7	54.7	67.0	70.3	70.4	69.5	66.6
40 years and over, crude[2]	28.7	51.4	54.6	66.9	70.3	70.4	69.7	66.8
Age								
40–49 years	31.9	55.1	55.6	63.4	67.2	64.3	64.4	63.5
50–64 years	31.7	56.0	60.3	73.7	76.5	78.7	76.2	71.8
65 years and over	22.8	43.4	48.1	63.8	66.8	67.9	67.7	63.8
65–74 years	26.6	48.7	55.7	69.4	73.9	74.0	74.6	72.5
75 years and over	17.3	35.8	37.8	57.2	58.9	61.3	60.6	54.7
Race[4]								
40 years and over, crude:								
White only	29.6	52.2	55.6	67.4	70.6	71.4	70.1	67.4
Black or African American only	24.0	46.4	48.0	66.0	71.0	67.8	70.4	64.9
American Indian or Alaska Native only	*	43.2	54.5	45.2	63.0	47.4	63.1	72.8
Asian only	*	46.0	45.9	60.2	58.3	53.5	57.6	54.6
Native Hawaiian or Other Pacific Islander only	- - -	- - -	- - -	- - -	*	*	*	*
2 or more races	- - -	- - -	- - -	- - -	70.2	69.2	65.3	63.7
Hispanic origin and race[4]								
40 years and over, crude:								
Hispanic or Latino	18.3	45.2	49.2	60.2	65.7	61.2	65.0	58.8
Not Hispanic or Latino	29.4	51.8	54.9	67.5	70.7	71.1	70.1	67.5
White only	30.3	52.7	56.0	68.0	71.1	72.2	70.5	68.4
Black or African American only	23.8	46.0	47.7	66.0	71.0	67.9	70.5	65.2
Age, Hispanic origin, and race[4]								
40–49 years:								
Hispanic or Latino	*15.3	45.1	44.0	55.2	61.6	54.1	59.4	54.2
Not Hispanic or Latino:								
White only	34.3	57.0	58.1	64.4	68.3	67.2	65.2	65.5
Black or African American only	27.8	48.4	48.0	65.0	69.2	60.9	68.2	62.1
50–64 years:								
Hispanic or Latino	23.0	47.5	61.7	67.2	69.7	66.5	69.4	61.5
Not Hispanic or Latino:								
White only	33.6	58.1	61.5	75.3	77.9	80.6	77.2	73.5
Black or African American only	26.4	48.4	52.4	71.2	75.0	77.7	76.2	71.6
65 years and over:								
Hispanic or Latino	*	41.1	40.9	59.0	67.2	68.3	69.5	63.8
Not Hispanic or Latino:								
White only	24.0	43.8	49.1	64.3	66.8	68.3	68.1	64.7
Black or African American only	14.1	39.7	41.6	60.6	68.1	65.5	65.4	60.5
Age and percent of poverty level[5]								
40 years and over, crude:								
Below 100%	14.6	30.8	35.2	50.1	57.4	54.8	55.4	48.5
100%–less than 200%	20.9	39.1	44.4	56.1	59.5	58.1	60.8	55.3
200% or more	35.2	59.2	62.2	72.6	75.0	75.9	74.3	72.5
40–49 years:								
Below 100%	18.6	32.2	33.0	44.8	51.3	47.4	50.6	42.5
100%–less than 200%	18.4	39.0	43.8	46.9	52.8	43.6	54.0	49.8
200% or more	36.8	60.1	61.2	68.4	71.6	69.9	68.3	69.0
50–64 years:								
Below 100%	14.6	29.9	37.3	52.7	63.3	61.7	58.3	50.4
100%–less than 200%	24.2	39.8	50.2	61.8	64.9	68.3	64.0	58.8
200% or more	37.0	63.3	66.0	78.7	80.2	82.6	80.9	76.8
65 years and over:								
Below 100%	13.1	30.8	35.2	51.9	57.6	54.8	57.0	52.3
100%–less than 200%	19.9	38.6	41.8	57.8	60.2	60.3	62.8	56.2
200% or more	29.7	51.5	57.8	70.1	72.5	75.0	72.6	70.1

See footnotes at end of table.

Table 87 (page 2 of 2). Use of mammography among women 40 years of age and over, by selected characteristics: United States, selected years 1987–2005

[Data are based on household interviews of a sample of the civilian noninstitutionalized population]

Characteristic	1987	1990	1991	1998	1999	2000	2003	2005
Health insurance status at the time of interview[6]	Percent of women having a mammogram within the past 2 years[1]							
40–64 years:								
Insured	---	---	---	72.3	75.5	76.0	75.1	72.6
Private	---	---	---	73.4	76.3	77.1	76.3	74.6
Medicaid	---	---	---	59.7	62.5	61.7	63.5	55.6
Uninsured	---	---	---	40.1	44.8	40.7	41.5	38.1
Health insurance status prior to interview[6]								
40–64 years:								
Insured continuously all 12 months	---	---	---	73.0	76.1	76.8	75.6	73.1
Uninsured for any period up to 12 months	---	---	---	47.6	57.1	53.0	56.0	51.3
Uninsured more than 12 months	---	---	---	36.3	38.9	34.0	37.0	32.9
Age and education[7]								
40 years and over, crude:								
No high school diploma or GED	17.8	36.4	40.0	54.5	56.7	57.7	58.1	52.8
High school diploma or GED	31.3	52.7	55.8	66.7	69.2	69.7	67.8	64.9
Some college or more	37.7	62.8	65.2	72.8	77.3	76.2	75.1	72.7
40–49 years:								
No high school diploma or GED	15.1	38.5	40.8	47.3	48.8	46.8	53.3	51.2
High school diploma or GED	32.6	53.1	52.0	59.1	60.8	59.0	60.8	58.8
Some college or more	39.2	62.3	63.7	68.3	74.4	70.6	68.1	68.3
50–64 years:								
No high school diploma or GED	21.2	41.0	43.6	58.8	62.3	66.5	63.4	56.9
High school diploma or GED	33.8	56.5	60.8	73.3	77.2	76.6	71.8	70.1
Some college or more	40.5	68.0	72.7	79.8	81.2	84.2	82.7	77.0
65 years and over:								
No high school diploma or GED	16.5	33.0	37.7	54.7	56.6	57.4	56.9	50.7
High school diploma or GED	25.9	47.5	54.0	66.8	68.4	71.8	69.7	64.3
Some college or more	32.3	56.7	57.9	71.3	77.1	74.1	75.1	73.0

* Estimates are considered unreliable. Data preceded by an asterisk have a relative standard error (RSE) of 20%–30%. Data not shown have an RSE greater than 30%.

- - - Data not available.

[1]Questions concerning use of mammography differed slightly on the National Health Interview Survey across the years for which data are shown. See Appendix II, Mammography.

[2]Includes all other races not shown separately, unknown poverty level in 1987, unknown health insurance status, and unknown education level.

[3]Estimates are age-adjusted to the year 2000 standard population using four age groups: 40–49 years, 50–64 years, 65–74 years, and 75 years and over. See Appendix II, Age adjustment.

[4]The race groups, white, black, American Indian or Alaska Native, Asian, Native Hawaiian or Other Pacific Islander, and 2 or more races, include persons of Hispanic and non-Hispanic origin. Persons of Hispanic origin may be of any race. Starting with 1999 data, race-specific estimates are tabulated according to the 1997 Revisions to the Standards for the Classification of Federal Data on Race and Ethnicity and are not strictly comparable with estimates for earlier years. The five single-race categories plus multiple-race categories shown in the table conform to the 1997 Standards. Starting with 1999 data, race-specific estimates are for persons who reported only one racial group; the category 2 or more races includes persons who reported more than one racial group. Prior to 1999, data were tabulated according to the 1977 Standards with four racial groups and the Asian only category included Native Hawaiian or Other Pacific Islander. Estimates for single-race categories prior to 1999 included persons who reported one race or, if they reported more than one race, identified one race as best representing their race. Starting with 2003 data, race responses of other race and unspecified multiple race were treated as missing, and then race was imputed if these were the only race responses. Almost all persons with a race response of other race were of Hispanic origin. See Appendix II, Hispanic origin; Race.

[5]Percent of poverty level is based on family income and family size and composition using U.S. Census Bureau poverty thresholds. Poverty level was unknown for 11% of women 40 years of age and over in 1987. Missing family income data were imputed for 19%–23% of women 40 years of age and over in 1990–1994 and 35%–39% in 1998–2005. See Appendix II, Family income; Poverty.

[6]Health insurance categories are mutually exclusive. Persons who reported both Medicaid and private coverage are classified as having private coverage. Starting with 1997 data, Medicaid includes state-sponsored health plans and State Children's Health Insurance Program (SCHIP). In addition to private and Medicaid, the insured category also includes military plans, other government-sponsored health plans, and Medicare, not shown separately. Persons not covered by private insurance, Medicaid, SCHIP, public assistance (through 1996), state-sponsored or other government-sponsored health plans (starting in 1997), Medicare, or military plans are considered to have no health insurance coverage. Persons with only Indian Health Service coverage are considered to have no health insurance coverage. See Appendix II, Health insurance coverage.

[7]Education categories shown are for 1998 and subsequent years. GED stands for General Educational Development high school equivalency diploma. In years prior to 1998 the following categories based on number of years of school completed were used: less than 12 years, 12 years, 13 years or more. See Appendix II, Education.

NOTES: Standard errors are available in the spreadsheet version of this table. Available from: www.cdc.gov/nchs/hus.htm. Data starting in 1997 are not strictly comparable with data for earlier years due to the 1997 questionnaire redesign. See Appendix I, National Health Interview Survey. Data for additional years are available. See Appendix III.

SOURCE: Centers for Disease Control and Prevention, National Center for Health Statistics, National Health Interview Survey. Data are from the following supplements: cancer control (1987), health promotion and disease prevention (1990–1991), and year 2000 objectives (1993–1994). Starting in 1998, data are from the family core and sample adult questionnaires.

Table 88 (page 1 of 2). Use of Pap smears among women 18 years of age and over, by selected characteristics: United States, selected years 1987–2005

[Data are based on household interviews of a sample of the civilian noninstitutionalized population]

Characteristic	1987	1993	1994	1998	1999	2000	2003	2005
	Percent of women having a Pap smear within the past 3 years[1]							
18 years and over, age-adjusted[2,3]	74.1	77.7	76.8	79.3	80.8	81.3	79.2	77.9
18 years and over, crude[2]	74.4	77.7	76.8	79.1	80.8	81.2	79.0	77.8
Age								
18–44 years	83.3	84.6	82.8	84.4	86.8	84.9	83.9	83.6
18–24 years	74.8	78.8	76.6	73.6	76.8	73.5	75.1	74.5
25–44 years	86.3	86.3	84.6	87.6	89.9	88.5	86.8	86.8
45–64 years	70.5	77.2	77.4	81.4	81.7	84.6	81.3	80.6
45–54 years	75.7	82.1	81.9	83.7	83.8	86.3	83.6	83.4
55–64 years	65.2	70.6	71.0	78.0	78.4	82.0	77.8	76.8
65 years and over	50.8	57.6	57.3	59.8	61.0	64.5	60.8	54.9
65–74 years	57.9	64.7	64.9	67.0	70.0	71.6	70.1	66.3
75 years and over	40.4	48.0	47.3	51.2	50.8	56.7	51.1	42.8
Race[4]								
18 years and over, crude:								
White only	74.1	77.3	76.2	78.9	80.6	81.3	78.7	77.7
Black or African American only	80.7	82.7	83.5	84.2	85.7	85.1	84.0	81.1
American Indian or Alaska Native only	85.4	78.1	73.5	74.6	92.2	76.8	84.8	75.2
Asian only	51.9	68.8	66.4	68.5	64.4	66.4	68.3	64.4
Native Hawaiian or Other Pacific Islander only	- - -	- - -	- - -	- - -	*	*	*	*
2 or more races	- - -	- - -	- - -	- - -	86.9	80.0	81.6	86.3
Hispanic origin and race[4]								
18 years and over, crude:								
Hispanic or Latino	67.6	77.2	74.4	75.2	76.3	77.0	75.4	75.5
Not Hispanic or Latino	74.9	77.8	77.0	79.6	81.3	81.7	79.5	78.1
White only	74.7	77.3	76.5	79.3	81.0	81.8	79.3	78.1
Black or African American only	80.9	82.7	83.8	84.2	86.0	85.1	83.8	81.2
Age, Hispanic origin, and race[4]								
18–44 years:								
Hispanic or Latino	73.9	80.9	80.6	76.4	77.0	78.1	75.9	76.5
Not Hispanic or Latino:								
White only	84.5	85.3	82.9	85.7	88.7	86.6	85.8	85.8
Black or African American only	89.1	88.0	89.1	88.9	90.8	88.5	88.6	86.4
45–64 years:								
Hispanic or Latino	57.7	75.8	70.1	78.3	79.5	77.8	77.9	78.4
Not Hispanic or Latino:								
White only	71.2	77.2	77.5	81.7	81.9	85.9	81.4	81.4
Black or African American only	76.2	80.3	82.2	84.1	84.6	85.7	84.7	80.5
65 years and over:								
Hispanic or Latino	41.7	57.1	43.8	59.8	63.7	66.8	64.6	60.0
Not Hispanic or Latino:								
White only	51.8	57.1	58.2	59.7	60.5	64.2	60.7	54.1
Black or African American only	44.8	61.2	59.5	61.7	64.5	67.2	59.6	60.2
Age and percent of poverty level[5]								
18 years and over, crude:								
Below 100%	64.3	70.6	70.5	69.8	73.6	72.0	70.5	68.7
100%–less than 200%	68.2	71.9	70.2	70.6	72.5	73.4	71.4	69.0
200% or more	80.0	82.8	82.9	83.5	84.3	85.0	83.0	82.1
18–44 years:								
Below 100%	77.1	77.2	80.2	77.1	79.7	77.1	77.1	76.2
100%–less than 200%	80.4	83.0	79.3	79.2	84.0	79.4	79.5	78.1
200% or more	86.4	88.4	86.6	87.6	89.0	88.0	86.9	87.2
45–64 years:								
Below 100%	53.6	65.3	65.7	67.6	73.1	73.6	66.0	65.9
100%–less than 200%	60.4	64.4	69.1	69.9	70.4	76.1	71.4	69.7
200% or more	74.9	81.6	82.8	85.1	84.6	87.4	85.1	84.4
65 years and over:								
Below 100%	33.2	46.8	43.8	48.2	51.9	53.7	52.6	44.4
100%–less than 200%	50.4	54.7	50.4	55.1	54.7	61.0	55.4	49.6
200% or more	60.0	62.6	67.4	65.3	66.4	68.8	65.4	59.7

See footnotes at end of table.

Table 88 (page 2 of 2). Use of Pap smears among women 18 years of age and over, by selected characteristics: United States, selected years 1987–2005

[Data are based on household interviews of a sample of the civilian noninstitutionalized population]

Characteristic	*1987*	*1993*	*1994*	*1998*	*1999*	*2000*	*2003*	*2005*
Health insurance status at the time of interview[6]	Percent of women having a Pap smear within the past 3 years[1]							
18–64 years, crude:								
Insured	- - -	84.7	83.8	86.0	87.2	87.8	86.4	85.6
Private	- - -	84.8	83.6	86.5	87.5	88.0	87.0	86.5
Medicaid	- - -	82.7	86.2	83.0	84.2	85.8	82.8	80.9
Uninsured	- - -	69.4	68.6	69.6	73.3	70.4	66.6	67.7
Health insurance status prior to interview[6]								
18–64 years, crude:								
Insured continuously all 12 months	- - -	84.8	83.7	86.3	87.3	88.0	86.6	85.8
Uninsured for any period up to 12 months	- - -	81.8	83.4	81.7	83.5	83.7	81.8	81.3
Uninsured more than 12 months	- - -	65.1	63.6	64.0	68.8	65.1	60.2	62.0
Age and education[7]								
25 years and over, crude:								
No high school diploma or GED	57.1	61.9	60.9	65.0	66.1	69.9	64.9	64.2
High school diploma or GED	76.4	78.2	76.0	77.4	79.3	79.8	75.9	73.9
Some college or more	84.0	84.4	85.2	86.9	87.8	88.0	86.2	84.6
25–44 years:								
No high school diploma or GED	75.1	73.6	73.6	76.8	79.0	79.6	71.7	75.5
High school diploma or GED	85.6	85.4	82.4	83.9	87.6	86.2	84.3	83.1
Some college or more	90.1	89.8	89.1	91.5	93.0	91.4	90.8	90.5
45–64 years:								
No high school diploma or GED	58.0	65.6	66.1	69.2	71.6	75.7	71.4	69.7
High school diploma or GED	72.3	77.6	75.9	81.0	79.8	81.8	77.6	79.1
Some college or more	80.1	83.0	84.7	85.5	85.7	89.1	86.2	84.2
65 years and over:								
No high school diploma or GED	44.0	50.7	47.7	52.4	51.8	56.6	52.5	46.1
High school diploma or GED	55.4	61.6	61.2	60.7	63.7	66.9	61.2	52.5
Some college or more	59.4	62.3	66.5	67.9	68.8	69.8	67.8	63.8

* Estimates are considered unreliable. Data not shown have a relative standard error greater than 30%.
- - - Data not available.
[1]Questions concerning use of Pap smears differed slightly on the National Health Interview Survey across the years for which data are shown. See Appendix II, Pap smear.
[2]Includes all other races not shown separately, unknown poverty level in 1987, unknown health insurance status, and unknown education level.
[3]Estimates are age-adjusted to the year 2000 standard population using five age groups: 18–44 years, 45–54 years, 55–64 years, 65–74 years, and 75 years and over. Age-adjusted estimates in this table may differ from other age-adjusted estimates based on the same data and presented elsewhere if different age groups are used in the adjustment procedure. See Appendix II, Age adjustment.
[4]The race groups, white, black, American Indian or Alaska Native, Asian, Native Hawaiian or Other Pacific Islander, and 2 or more races, include persons of Hispanic and non-Hispanic origin. Persons of Hispanic origin may be of any race. Starting with 1999 data, race-specific estimates are tabulated according to the 1997 Revisions to the Standards for the Classification of Federal Data on Race and Ethnicity and are not strictly comparable with estimates for earlier years. The five single-race categories plus multiple-race categories shown in the table conform to the 1997 Standards. Starting with 1999 data, race-specific estimates are for persons who reported only one racial group; the category 2 or more races includes persons who reported more than one racial group. Prior to 1999, data were tabulated according to the 1977 Standards with four racial groups and the Asian only category included Native Hawaiian or Other Pacific Islander. Estimates for single-race categories prior to 1999 included persons who reported one race or, if they reported more than one race, identified one race as best representing their race. Starting with 2003 data, race responses of other race and unspecified multiple race were treated as missing, and then race was imputed if these were the only race responses. Almost all persons with a race response of other race were of Hispanic origin. See Appendix II, Hispanic origin; Race.
[5]Percent of poverty level is based on family income and family size and composition using U.S. Census Bureau poverty thresholds. Poverty level was unknown for 9% of women 18 years of age and over in 1987. Missing family income data were imputed for 17%–20% of women 18 years of age and over in 1990–1994 and 35%–39% in 1998–2005. See Appendix II, Family income; Poverty.
[6]Health insurance categories are mutually exclusive. Persons who reported both Medicaid and private coverage are classified as having private coverage. Starting with 1997 data, Medicaid includes state-sponsored health plans and State Children's Health Insurance Program (SCHIP). In addition to private and Medicaid, the insured category also includes military plans, other government-sponsored health plans, and Medicare, not shown separately. Persons not covered by private insurance, Medicaid, SCHIP, public assistance (through 1996), state-sponsored or other government-sponsored health plans (starting in 1997), Medicare, or military plans are considered to have no health insurance coverage. Persons with only Indian Health Service coverage are considered to have no health insurance coverage. See Appendix II, Health insurance coverage.
[7]Education categories shown are for 1998 and subsequent years. GED stands for General Educational Development high school equivalency diploma. In years prior to 1998 the following categories based on number of years of school completed were used: less than 12 years, 12 years, 13 years or more. See Appendix II, Education.

NOTES: Standard errors are available in the spreadsheet version of this table. Available from: www.cdc.gov/nchs/hus.htm. Data starting in 1997 are not strictly comparable with data for earlier years due to the 1997 questionnaire redesign. See Appendix I, National Health Interview Survey.

SOURCES: Centers for Disease Control and Prevention, National Center for Health Statistics, National Health Interview Survey. Data are from the following supplements: cancer control (1987), year 2000 objectives (1993–1994). Starting in 1998, data are from the family core and sample adult questionnaires.

Table 89 (page 1 of 3). Emergency department visits within the past 12 months among children under 18 years of age, by selected characteristics: United States, 1997, 2004, and 2005

[Data are based on household interviews of a sample of the civilian noninstitutionalized population]

Characteristic	Under 18 years			Under 6 years			6–17 years		
	1997	2004	2005	1997	2004	2005	1997	2004	2005
	Percent of children with one or more emergency department visits[1]								
All children[2]	19.9	20.9	20.5	24.3	26.2	26.8	17.7	18.4	17.4
Race[3]									
White only	19.4	20.6	19.8	22.6	25.3	25.3	17.8	18.3	17.1
Black or African American only	24.0	23.1	23.8	33.1	31.1	31.6	19.4	19.4	20.0
American Indian or Alaska Native only	*24.1	*17.7	*32.1	*24.3	*	*	*24.0	*16.7	*
Asian only	12.6	15.8	14.6	20.8	*19.4	20.2	8.6	14.3	12.3
Native Hawaiian or Other Pacific Islander only	- - -	*	*	- - -	*	*	- - -	*	*
2 or more races	- - -	27.0	24.8	- - -	35.7	38.3	- - -	21.3	17.1
Hispanic origin and race[3]									
Hispanic or Latino	21.1	20.6	19.5	25.7	26.9	28.0	18.1	16.9	14.5
Not Hispanic or Latino	19.7	21.0	20.7	24.0	26.0	26.5	17.6	18.7	18.0
White only	19.2	20.7	19.9	22.2	24.8	24.5	17.7	18.8	17.9
Black or African American only	23.6	22.8	23.8	32.7	30.7	31.8	19.2	19.1	20.0
Percent of poverty level[4]									
Below 100%	25.1	27.6	27.3	29.5	34.3	33.5	22.2	23.6	23.5
100%–less than 200%	22.0	22.3	21.8	28.0	29.5	30.8	19.0	18.6	17.4
200% or more	17.3	18.5	17.9	20.5	21.9	22.7	15.8	16.9	15.7
Hispanic origin and race and percent of poverty level[3,4]									
Hispanic or Latino:									
Percent of poverty level:									
Below 100%	21.9	23.1	21.8	25.0	29.2	28.4	19.6	19.2	17.4
100%–less than 200%	20.8	20.9	17.8	28.8	26.4	26.1	15.6	17.6	13.1
200% or more	20.4	17.9	18.8	23.4	24.8	29.3	18.7	14.4	13.5
Not Hispanic or Latino:									
White only:									
Percent of poverty level:									
Below 100%	25.5	32.3	34.1	27.2	36.6	37.3	24.4	29.9	32.2
100%–less than 200%	22.3	23.8	22.8	25.8	31.3	30.7	20.7	19.6	19.1
200% or more	17.2	18.3	17.4	20.1	20.9	20.8	15.9	17.2	15.9
Black or African American only:									
Percent of poverty level:									
Below 100%	29.3	29.2	27.1	39.5	37.5	34.8	23.0	24.1	22.6
100%–less than 200%	22.5	21.2	24.1	31.7	27.8	33.3	18.5	18.9	20.3
200% or more	17.7	18.9	20.6	22.6	25.8	27.4	15.9	15.9	17.6
Health insurance status at the time of interview[5]									
Insured	19.8	21.0	20.7	24.4	25.9	26.8	17.5	18.5	17.7
Private	17.5	18.5	17.4	20.9	21.1	21.7	15.9	17.3	15.5
Medicaid	28.2	27.2	28.5	33.0	34.3	35.5	24.1	22.3	23.6
Uninsured	20.2	20.7	18.4	23.0	28.7	26.6	18.9	17.6	15.4
Health insurance status prior to interview[5]									
Insured continuously all 12 months	19.6	20.7	20.5	24.1	25.5	26.7	17.3	18.4	17.3
Uninsured for any period up to 12 months	24.0	27.3	26.0	27.1	37.4	34.4	21.9	22.2	22.4
Uninsured more than 12 months	18.4	16.6	14.4	19.3	21.9	*15.7	18.1	15.0	14.0
Percent of poverty level and health insurance status prior to interview[4,5]									
Below 100%:									
Insured continuously all 12 months	26.3	27.4	28.1	30.9	33.2	34.3	22.8	23.7	23.8
Uninsured for any period up to 12 months	26.5	35.4	31.2	29.7	47.5	39.1	24.4	29.5	*28.2
Uninsured more than 12 months	17.5	*18.9	15.7	*16.0	*	*	18.0	*	*15.6
100%–less than 200%:									
Insured continuously all 12 months	21.8	22.3	22.1	28.0	28.7	31.0	18.6	18.8	17.4
Uninsured for any period up to 12 months	24.5	27.2	27.4	29.7	39.5	41.2	21.0	21.4	21.9
Uninsured more than 12 months	19.5	16.8	14.7	*22.5	*27.3	*	18.6	13.6	*14.5
200% or more:									
Insured continuously all 12 months	17.1	18.5	17.9	20.3	21.7	22.6	15.6	17.1	15.7
Uninsured for any period up to 12 months	20.7	22.2	21.4	21.3	30.0	26.8	20.4	18.1	18.7
Uninsured more than 12 months	17.9	*13.6	*12.6	*19.2	*	*	17.3	*12.6	*

See footnotes at end of table.

Table 89 (page 2 of 3). Emergency department visits within the past 12 months among children under 18 years of age, by selected characteristics: United States, 1997, 2004, and 2005

[Data are based on household interviews of a sample of the civilian noninstitutionalized population]

Characteristic	*Under 18 years* 1997	*Under 18 years* 2004	*Under 18 years* 2005	*Under 6 years* 1997	*Under 6 years* 2004	*Under 6 years* 2005	*6–17 years* 1997	*6–17 years* 2004	*6–17 years* 2005
Geographic region	Percent of children with one or more emergency department visits[1]								
Northeast	18.5	24.2	20.9	20.7	28.6	26.3	17.4	22.2	18.5
Midwest	19.5	21.0	21.8	26.0	25.7	30.1	16.4	18.6	17.8
South	21.8	21.5	21.7	25.6	26.7	27.1	19.9	19.0	18.8
West	18.5	17.6	16.7	23.5	24.2	22.9	15.9	14.3	13.8
Location of residence									
Within MSA[6]	19.7	20.5	20.0	23.9	26.0	25.7	17.4	17.8	17.2
Outside MSA[6]	20.8	23.0	22.4	26.2	27.4	31.8	18.6	21.0	18.2
	Percent of children with two or more emergency department visits[1]								
All children[2]	7.1	8.0	6.8	9.6	9.4	9.8	5.8	7.4	5.4
Race[3]									
White only	6.6	7.8	6.3	8.4	9.2	9.1	5.7	7.0	4.9
Black or African American only	9.6	9.4	9.2	14.9	10.9	12.7	6.9	8.7	7.5
American Indian and Alaska Native only	*	*	*	*	*	*	*	*	*
Asian only	*5.7	*6.3	*4.6	*12.9	*	*	*	*6.9	*3.9
Native Hawaiian and Other Pacific Islander only	---	*	*	---	*	*	---	*	*
2 or more races	---	10.1	*8.6	---	*11.9	*13.2	---	*8.9	*
Hispanic origin and race[3]									
Hispanic or Latino	8.9	8.0	7.7	11.8	10.2	12.1	7.0	6.7	5.2
Not Hispanic or Latino	6.8	8.1	6.6	9.2	9.2	9.2	5.7	7.5	5.4
White only	6.2	7.7	5.9	7.8	8.9	8.2	5.5	7.2	4.9
Black or African American only	9.3	9.4	9.1	14.6	10.7	12.4	6.8	8.8	7.5
Percent of poverty level[4]									
Below 100%	11.1	13.0	11.5	14.5	14.6	16.1	8.9	12.0	8.6
100%–less than 200%	8.3	8.7	7.7	12.2	10.8	12.1	6.3	7.7	5.5
200% or more	5.3	6.3	5.1	6.5	6.9	6.6	4.7	6.0	4.4
Hispanic origin and race and percent of poverty level[3,4]									
Hispanic or Latino:									
Percent of poverty level:									
Below 100%	10.4	9.0	10.2	13.9	10.5	14.0	8.0	8.1	7.6
100%–less than 200%	8.2	7.9	5.8	12.0	9.7	7.6	5.7	6.8	4.8
200% or more	7.6	7.0	7.2	8.4	10.4	14.2	7.1	5.3	3.6
Not Hispanic or Latino:									
White only:									
Percent of poverty level:									
Below 100%	10.7	16.4	13.9	12.2	*16.7	18.8	9.8	16.3	10.9
100%–less than 200%	8.0	8.7	8.0	11.2	11.7	13.3	6.4	7.0	5.4
200% or more	5.0	6.3	4.4	5.8	6.8	5.1	4.6	6.1	4.0
Black or African American only:									
Percent of poverty level:									
Below 100%	12.7	14.3	11.7	19.1	17.4	16.6	8.8	12.4	8.8
100%–less than 200%	9.2	10.4	8.4	*13.5	*11.7	*12.3	*7.2	*10.0	*6.8
200% or more	5.5	5.0	7.3	*8.2	*3.6	*7.8	*4.5	*5.6	7.0
Health insurance status at the time of interview[5]									
Insured	7.0	7.9	6.8	9.6	9.4	9.7	5.7	7.2	5.3
Private	5.2	6.1	5.0	6.8	6.5	6.2	4.5	6.0	4.4
Medicaid	13.1	12.5	11.1	16.2	14.7	15.8	10.4	10.9	7.7
Uninsured	7.7	9.3	7.0	9.8	9.6	11.5	6.6	9.2	5.4
Health insurance status prior to interview[5]									
Insured continuously all 12 months	6.9	7.7	6.7	9.4	9.0	9.7	5.7	7.1	5.2
Uninsured for any period up to 12 months	8.5	12.3	8.9	11.5	14.7	13.6	6.6	11.1	6.9
Uninsured more than 12 months	6.8	*7.3	5.5	*8.6	*8.2	*	6.2	*	5.3

See footnotes at end of table.

Table 89 (page 3 of 3). Emergency department visits within the past 12 months among children under 18 years of age, by selected characteristics: United States, 1997, 2004, and 2005

[Data are based on household interviews of a sample of the civilian noninstitutionalized population]

	Under 18 years			Under 6 years			6–17 years		
Characteristic	1997	2004	2005	1997	2004	2005	1997	2004	2005
Geographic region	Percent of children with two or more emergency department visits[1]								
Northeast	6.2	8.5	6.2	7.6	9.0	8.9	5.4	8.2	5.0
Midwest	6.6	8.1	6.9	10.4	11.2	9.6	4.8	6.6	5.5
South	8.0	9.1	7.9	10.1	10.0	10.8	6.9	8.6	6.3
West	7.1	6.0	5.5	10.0	6.9	9.1	5.6	5.5	3.9
Location of residence									
Within MSA[6]	7.2	7.7	6.7	9.6	8.7	9.5	5.9	7.1	5.2
Outside MSA[6]	6.8	9.7	7.5	9.7	12.4	11.2	5.6	8.4	5.9

* Estimates are considered unreliable. Data preceded by an asterisk have a relative standard error (RSE) of 20%–30%. Data not shown have an RSE of greater than 30%.

\- - - Data not available.

[1]See Appendix II, Emergency department visit.

[2]Includes all other races not shown separately and unknown health insurance status.

[3]The race groups, white, black, American Indian or Alaska Native, Asian, Native Hawaiian or Other Pacific Islander, and 2 or more races, include persons of Hispanic and non-Hispanic origin. Persons of Hispanic origin may be of any race. Starting with 1999 data, race-specific estimates are tabulated according to the 1997 Revisions to the Standards for the Classification of Federal Data on Race and Ethnicity and are not strictly comparable with estimates for earlier years. The five single-race categories plus multiple-race categories shown in the table conform to the 1997 Standards. Starting with 1999 data, race-specific estimates are for persons who reported only one racial group; the category 2 or more races includes persons who reported more than one racial group. Prior to 1999, data were tabulated according to the 1977 Standards with four racial groups and the Asian only category included Native Hawaiian or Other Pacific Islander. Estimates for single-race categories prior to 1999 included persons who reported one race or, if they reported more than one race, identified one race as best representing their race. Starting with 2003 data, race responses of other race and unspecified multiple race were treated as missing, and then race was imputed if these were the only race responses. Almost all persons with a race response of other race were of Hispanic origin. See Appendix II, Hispanic origin; Race.

[4]Percent of poverty level is based on family income and family size and composition using U.S. Census Bureau poverty thresholds. Missing family income data were imputed for 21%–25% of children in 1997–1998 and 28%–31% in 1999–2005. See Appendix II, Family income; Poverty.

[5]Health insurance categories are mutually exclusive. Persons who reported both Medicaid and private coverage are classified as having private coverage. Starting in 1997 Medicaid includes state-sponsored health plans and State Children's Health Insurance Program (SCHIP). In addition to private and Medicaid, the insured category also includes military, other government, and Medicare coverage. Persons not covered by private insurance, Medicaid, SCHIP, public assistance (through 1996), state-sponsored or other government-sponsored health plans (starting in 1997), Medicare, or military plans are considered to have no health insurance coverage. Persons with only Indian Health Service coverage are considered to have no health insurance coverage. See Appendix II, Health insurance coverage.

[6]MSA is metropolitan statistical area.

NOTES: Standard errors are available in the spreadsheet version of this table. Available from: www.cdc.gov/nchs/hus.htm. Data for additional years are available. See Appendix III.

SOURCE: Centers for Disease Control and Prevention, National Center for Health Statistics, National Health Interview Survey, family core and sample child questionnaires.

Table 90 (page 1 of 2). Emergency department visits within the past 12 months among adults 18 years of age and over, by selected characteristics: United States, selected years 1997–2005

[Data are based on household interviews of a sample of the civilian noninstitutionalized population]

Characteristic	*One or more emergency department visits*				*Two or more emergency department visits*			
	1997	*2000*	*2004*	*2005*	*1997*	*2000*	*2004*	*2005*
	Percent of adults with emergency department visits[1]							
18 years and over, age-adjusted[2,3]	19.6	20.2	20.7	20.5	6.7	6.9	7.5	7.1
18 years and over, crude[2]	19.6	20.1	20.6	20.4	6.7	6.8	7.4	7.0
Age								
18–44 years	20.7	20.5	20.9	20.8	6.8	7.0	7.4	7.1
18–24 years	26.3	25.7	24.4	25.3	9.1	8.8	8.6	8.9
25–44 years	19.0	18.8	19.7	19.2	6.2	6.4	7.0	6.5
45–64 years	16.2	17.6	18.1	18.2	5.6	5.6	6.3	6.4
45–54 years	15.7	17.9	17.9	17.6	5.5	5.8	6.4	6.1
55–64 years	16.9	17.0	18.4	19.0	5.7	5.3	6.2	6.8
65 years and over	22.0	23.7	24.5	23.7	8.1	8.6	9.5	8.2
65–74 years	20.3	21.6	20.8	20.8	7.1	7.4	7.5	7.4
75 years and over	24.3	26.2	28.7	27.1	9.3	10.0	11.8	9.1
Sex[3]								
Male	19.1	18.7	19.3	18.6	5.9	5.7	6.5	5.9
Female	20.2	21.6	22.1	22.3	7.5	7.9	8.4	8.2
Race[3,4]								
White only	19.0	19.4	20.0	19.8	6.2	6.4	7.0	6.5
Black or African American only	25.9	26.5	27.0	26.3	11.1	10.8	11.2	11.9
American Indian or Alaska Native only	24.8	30.3	27.8	31.0	13.1	*12.6	*12.6	*11.1
Asian only	11.6	13.6	12.2	15.4	*2.9	*3.8	4.1	*3.8
Native Hawaiian or Other Pacific Islander only	- - -	*	*	*	- - -	*	*	*
2 or more races	- - -	32.5	31.5	25.7	- - -	11.3	14.4	12.8
American Indian or Alaska Native; White	- - -	33.9	32.1	29.3	- - -	*9.4	*15.8	*15.3
Hispanic origin and race[3,4]								
Hispanic or Latino	19.2	18.3	19.2	20.1	7.4	7.0	7.0	7.1
Mexican	17.8	17.4	17.1	17.2	6.4	7.1	5.9	5.8
Not Hispanic or Latino	19.7	20.6	21.1	20.7	6.7	6.9	7.6	7.1
White only	19.1	19.8	20.4	20.1	6.2	6.4	7.0	6.4
Black or African American only	25.9	26.5	27.2	26.2	11.0	10.8	11.3	11.9
Percent of poverty level[3,5]								
Below 100%	28.1	29.0	29.3	29.8	12.8	13.3	13.8	13.7
100%–less than 200%	23.8	23.9	23.6	23.2	9.3	9.6	9.5	9.6
200% or more	17.0	18.0	18.7	18.3	4.9	5.2	6.0	5.3
Hispanic origin and race and percent of poverty level[3,4,5]								
Hispanic or Latino:								
Below 100%	22.1	22.4	22.6	24.0	9.8	9.7	10.0	9.2
100%–less than 200%	19.2	18.1	20.2	18.7	8.1	6.7	7.1	7.1
200% or more	17.6	16.8	16.9	19.6	5.4	6.1	5.4	6.1
Not Hispanic or Latino:								
White only:								
Below 100%	29.5	30.1	30.2	30.8	13.0	13.9	14.1	13.7
100%–less than 200%	24.3	25.5	25.1	24.3	9.1	10.4	10.0	9.8
200% or more	16.8	17.7	18.6	18.1	4.8	5.0	5.9	5.0
Black or African American only:								
Below 100%	34.6	35.4	38.2	35.4	17.5	17.4	19.2	18.3
100%–less than 200%	29.2	28.5	28.5	28.9	12.8	12.2	12.1	14.2
200% or more	19.7	22.6	22.5	21.6	7.2	8.0	8.1	8.5
Health insurance status at the time of interview[6,7]								
18–64 years:								
Insured	18.8	19.5	20.1	20.0	6.1	6.4	6.9	6.6
Private	16.9	17.6	18.0	17.3	4.7	5.1	5.3	4.8
Medicaid	37.6	42.2	36.8	40.1	19.7	21.0	19.8	20.1
Uninsured	20.0	19.3	19.0	19.5	7.5	6.9	7.4	8.0

See footnotes at end of table.

Table 90 (page 2 of 2). Emergency department visits within the past 12 months among adults 18 years of age and over, by selected characteristics: United States, selected years 1997–2005

[Data are based on household interviews of a sample of the civilian noninstitutionalized population]

Characteristic	One or more emergency department visits				Two or more emergency department visits			
	1997	2000	2004	2005	1997	2000	2004	2005
Health insurance status prior to interview[6,7]	Percent of adults with emergency department visits[1]							
18–64 years:								
Insured continuously all 12 months	18.3	19.0	19.6	19.4	5.8	6.1	6.6	6.3
Uninsured for any period up to 12 months	25.5	28.2	25.3	28.0	9.4	10.3	10.3	12.4
Uninsured more than 12 months	18.9	17.3	17.9	18.0	7.1	6.4	7.2	7.0
Percent of poverty level and health insurance status prior to interview[5,6,7]								
18–64 years:								
Below 100%:								
Insured continuously all 12 months	30.2	31.6	32.1	33.6	14.7	15.4	15.9	15.3
Uninsured for any period up to 12 months	34.1	43.7	35.1	39.1	16.1	18.1	*16.2	21.5
Uninsured more than 12 months	20.8	20.5	20.7	20.5	8.1	9.1	9.4	8.5
100%–less than 200%:								
Insured continuously all 12 months	24.5	25.5	24.7	23.7	8.9	10.2	10.3	9.8
Uninsured for any period up to 12 months	28.7	27.7	27.9	28.4	12.3	11.7	11.9	12.7
Uninsured more than 12 months	19.0	17.4	17.8	18.5	8.3	6.4	6.5	7.7
200% or more:								
Insured continuously all 12 months	16.0	17.0	17.6	17.2	4.4	4.7	5.1	4.7
Uninsured for any period up to 12 months	20.2	22.9	20.9	24.0	5.3	7.0	7.5	9.2
Uninsured more than 12 months	17.4	15.6	16.3	15.6	5.3	4.7	6.2	5.4
Geographic region[3]								
Northeast	19.5	20.0	21.9	21.6	6.9	6.2	7.7	7.2
Midwest	19.3	20.1	20.7	21.6	6.2	6.9	7.0	7.2
South	20.9	21.2	21.4	20.7	7.3	7.6	8.1	7.6
West	17.7	18.6	18.6	17.8	6.0	6.3	6.8	6.0
Location of residence[3]								
Within MSA[8]	19.1	19.6	20.3	20.1	6.4	6.6	7.2	6.8
Outside MSA[8]	21.5	22.5	22.6	22.3	7.8	7.8	8.4	8.1

* Estimates are considered unreliable. Data preceded by an asterisk have a relative standard error (RSE) of 20%–30%. Data not shown have an RSE of greater than 30%.

- - - Data not available.

[1]See Appendix II, Emergency department visit.

[2]Includes all other races not shown separately and unknown health insurance status.

[3]Estimates are for persons 18 years of age and over and are age-adjusted to the year 2000 standard population using five age groups: 18–44 years, 45–54 years, 55–64 years, 65–74 years, and 75 years and over. See Appendix II, Age adjustment.

[4]The race groups, white, black, American Indian or Alaska Native, Asian, Native Hawaiian or Other Pacific Islander, and 2 or more races, include persons of Hispanic and non-Hispanic origin. Persons of Hispanic origin may be of any race. Starting with 1999 data, race-specific estimates are tabulated according to the 1997 Revisions to the Standards for the Classification of Federal Data on Race and Ethnicity and are not strictly comparable with estimates for earlier years. The five single-race categories plus multiple-race categories shown in the table conform to the 1997 Standards. Starting with 1999 data, race-specific estimates are for persons who reported only one racial group; the category 2 or more races includes persons who reported more than one racial group. Prior to 1999, data were tabulated according to the 1977 Standards with four racial groups, and the Asian only category included Native Hawaiian or Other Pacific Islander. Estimates for single-race categories prior to 1999 included persons who reported one race or, if they reported more than one race, identified one race as best representing their race. Starting with 2003 data, race responses of other race and unspecified multiple race were treated as missing, and then race was imputed if these were the only race responses. Almost all persons with a race response of other race were of Hispanic origin. See Appendix II, Hispanic origin; Race.

[5]Percent of poverty level is based on family income and family size and composition using U.S. Census Bureau poverty thresholds. Missing family income data were imputed for 27%–31% of persons 18 years of age and over in 1997–1998 and 33%–36% in 1999–2005. See Appendix II, Family income; Poverty.

[6]Estimates for persons 18–64 years of age are age-adjusted to the year 2000 standard population using three age groups: 18–44 years, 45–54 years, and 55–64 years of age. See Appendix II, Age adjustment.

[7]Health insurance categories are mutually exclusive. Persons who reported both Medicaid and private coverage are classified as having private coverage. Starting with 1997 data, Medicaid includes state-sponsored health plans and State Children's Health Insurance Program (SCHIP). In addition to private and Medicaid, the insured category also includes military plans, other government-sponsored health plans, and Medicare, not shown separately. Persons not covered by private insurance, Medicaid, SCHIP, public assistance (through 1996), state-sponsored or other government-sponsored health plans (starting in 1997), Medicare, or military plans are considered to have no health insurance coverage. Persons with only Indian Health Service coverage are considered to have no health insurance coverage. See Appendix II, Health insurance coverage.

[8]MSA is metropolitan statistical area.

NOTES: Standard errors are available in the spreadsheet version of this table. Available from: www.cdc.gov/nchs/hus.htm. Data for additional years are available. See Appendix III.

SOURCE: Centers for Disease Control and Prevention, National Center for Health Statistics, National Health Interview Survey, family core and sample adult questionnaires.

Table 91 (page 1 of 2). Injury-related visits to hospital emergency departments, by sex, age, and intent and mechanism of injury: United States, average annual 1995–1996, 1999–2000, and 2004–2005

[Data are based on reporting by a sample of hospital emergency departments]

Sex, age, and intent and mechanism of injury[1]	1995–1996	1999–2000	2004–2005	1995–1996	1999–2000	2004–2005
Both sexes	Injury-related visits in thousands			Injury-related visits per 10,000 persons		
All ages[2,3]	36,081	39,029	41,664	1,360.9	1,428.1	1,435.8
Male						
All ages[2,3]	20,030	21,286	22,139	1,530.7	1,585.3	1,556.3
Under 18 years[2]	6,238	6,364	6,405	1,720.2	1,722.2	1,711.2
Unintentional injuries[4]	5,478	5,457	5,026	1,510.5	1,476.7	1,342.8
Falls	1,402	1,303	1,530	386.5	352.6	408.7
Struck by or against objects or persons	1,011	1,378	972	278.9	372.8	259.6
Motor vehicle traffic	453	432	401	125.0	116.9	107.1
Cut or pierce	493	455	384	136.0	123.2	102.6
Intentional injuries	290	242	219	80.0	65.6	58.4
18–24 years[2]	2,980	3,096	3,077	2,396.9	2,361.6	2,165.5
Unintentional injuries[4]	2,423	2,416	2,130	1,948.7	1,842.7	1,499.4
Falls	299	307	358	240.8	233.9	251.7
Struck by or against objects or persons	387	405	304	311.0	308.6	213.8
Motor vehicle traffic	347	469	441	279.4	357.5	310.2
Cut or pierce	304	394	261	244.8	300.5	184.0
Intentional injuries	335	322	318	269.2	245.9	224.0
25–44 years[2]	7,245	7,251	6,858	1,767.4	1,796.9	1,647.8
Unintentional injuries[4]	5,757	5,528	4,411	1,404.3	1,370.0	1,059.9
Falls	817	850	842	199.4	210.8	202.4
Struck by or against objects or persons	619	781	532	151.0	193.6	127.7
Motor vehicle traffic	912	848	717	222.6	210.1	172.3
Cut or pierce	860	764	582	209.8	189.4	139.8
Intentional injuries	701	511	500	171.0	126.5	120.1
45–64 years[2]	2,240	2,972	3,852	883.4	1,030.9	1,113.3
Unintentional injuries[4]	1,845	2,325	2,458	727.6	806.7	710.5
Falls	445	582	590	175.6	202.0	170.6
Struck by or against objects or persons	186	232	232	73.3	80.6	67.1
Motor vehicle traffic	244	316	359	96.3	109.6	103.7
Cut or pierce	203	294	334	79.9	101.9	96.5
Intentional injuries	86	99	190	33.8	34.3	55.0
65 years and over[2]	1,327	1,603	1,947	1,000.7	1,158.7	1,312.0
Unintentional injuries[4]	1,009	1,207	1,111	760.6	872.1	748.8
Falls	505	579	653	380.9	418.1	440.2
Struck by or against objects or persons	*39	112	60	*29.4	*80.7	40.5
Motor vehicle traffic	99	114	118	74.7	*82.5	79.4
Cut or pierce	*81	102	62	*61.1	74.0	41.6
Intentional injuries	*	10	33	*	*	*22.1

See footnotes at end of table.

Table 91 (page 2 of 2). Injury-related visits to hospital emergency departments, by sex, age, and intent and mechanism of injury: United States, average annual 1995–1996, 1999–2000, and 2004–2005

[Data are based on reporting by a sample of hospital emergency departments]

Sex, age, and intent and mechanism of injury[1]	*1995–1996*	*1999–2000*	*2004–2005*	*1995–1996*	*1999–2000*	*2004–2005*
Female	Injury-related visits in thousands			Injury-related visits per 10,000 persons		
All ages[2,3]	16,051	17,743	19,524	1,186.4	1,267.4	1,313.3
Under 18 years[2]	4,372	4,443	4,678	1,263.9	1,259.0	1,307.3
Unintentional injuries[4]	3,760	3,722	3,551	1,087.0	1,054.7	992.3
Falls	1,040	1,025	1,183	300.7	290.6	330.5
Struck by or against objects or persons	477	728	487	137.9	206.4	136.0
Motor vehicle traffic	447	430	412	129.3	122.0	115.0
Cut or pierce	253	232	210	73.0	65.7	58.6
Intentional injuries	220	149	231	63.6	42.3	64.7
18–24 years[2]	1,900	2,219	2,440	1,523.4	1,688.1	1,732.5
Unintentional injuries[4]	1,430	1,579	1,557	1,146.7	1,200.9	1,105.7
Falls	268	234	301	214.5	178.0	214.0
Struck by or against objects or persons	134	170	161	107.4	129.6	114.4
Motor vehicle traffic	373	469	480	298.8	357.1	341.1
Cut or pierce	131	156	130	105.3	118.3	92.4
Intentional injuries	239	219	231	191.7	166.8	163.7
25–44 years[2]	5,098	5,584	5,732	1,205.8	1,332.7	1,348.8
Unintentional injuries[4]	3,877	3,976	3,651	916.8	948.9	859.2
Falls	817	947	930	193.3	225.9	218.7
Struck by or against objects or persons	380	382	375	89.8	91.3	88.3
Motor vehicle traffic	872	788	805	206.2	188.0	189.5
Cut or pierce	338	434	326	79.8	103.5	76.7
Intentional injuries	422	425	360	99.8	101.5	84.6
45–64 years[2]	2,369	2,933	3,833	873.7	952.9	1,045.3
Unintentional injuries[4]	1,857	2,180	2,454	685.2	708.2	669.2
Falls	600	749	927	221.5	243.5	252.7
Struck by or against objects or persons	160	192	162	58.8	62.3	44.1
Motor vehicle traffic	343	324	423	126.5	105.2	115.4
Cut or pierce	127	175	177	46.9	56.8	48.2
Intentional injuries	*64	125	143	*23.5	40.5	39.0
65 years and over[2]	2,313	2,564	2,842	1,256.1	1,367.8	1,416.4
Unintentional injuries[4]	1,931	2,013	1,902	1,049.0	1,073.8	947.8
Falls	1,230	1,219	1,298	667.9	650.4	647.0
Struck by or against objects or persons	82	103	116	44.8	54.8	57.6
Motor vehicle traffic	169	132	133	91.6	70.6	66.4
Cut or pierce	*42	72	61	*22.7	*38.3	30.5
Intentional injuries	*	20	12	*	*	*

* Estimates are considered unreliable. Data preceded by an asterisk have a relative standard error (RSE) of 20%–30%. Data not shown have an RSE of greater than 30%.

[1]Intent and mechanism of injury are based on the first-listed external cause of injury code (E code). Intentional injuries include suicide attempts and assaults. See Appendix II, External cause of injury and Table VII for a listing of E codes.

[2]Includes all injury-related visits not shown separately in table including those with undetermined intent (0.6% in 2004–2005), insufficient or no information to code cause of injury (21.8% in 2004–2005), and resulting from adverse effects of medical treatment (4.4% in 2004–2005).

[3]Rates are age adjusted to the year 2000 standard population using six age groups: under 18 years, 18–24 years, 25–44 years, 45–64 years, 65–74 years, and 75 years and over. See Appendix II, Age adjustment.

[4]Includes unintentional injury-related visits with mechanism of injury not shown in table.

NOTES: An emergency department visit was considered injury related if the checkbox for injury was indicated, the physician's diagnosis was injury related (ICD–9–CM 800–999), an external cause of injury code was present (ICD–9–CM E800-E999), or the patient's reason for the visit was injury related. Rates for 1995–2000 were computed using 1990-based postcensal estimates of the civilian noninstitutionalized population as of July 1, adjusted for net underenumeration using the 1990 National Population Adjustment Matrix from the U.S. Census Bureau. Starting with 2001 data, rates were computed using 2000-based postcensal estimates of the civilian noninstitutionalized population as of July 1. The difference between rates for 2000 computed using 1990-based postcensal estimates and rates computed using estimates based on 2000 census counts is minimal. Available from: www.cdc.gov/nchs/about/major/ahcd/census2000.htm. Rates will be overestimated to the extent that visits by institutionalized persons are counted in the numerator (for example, hospital emergency department visits by nursing home residents) and institutionalized persons are omitted from the denominator. Data for additional years are available. See Appendix III.

SOURCE: Centers for Disease Control and Prevention, National Center for Health Statistics, National Hospital Ambulatory Medical Care Survey.

Table 92 (page 1 of 3). Visits to physician offices, hospital outpatient departments, and hospital emergency departments, by selected characteristics: United States, selected years 1995–2005

[Data are based on reporting by a sample of office-based physicians, hospital outpatient departments, and hospital emergency departments]

Age, sex, and race	*All places*[1]				*Physician offices*			
	1995	*2000*	*2003*	*2005*	*1995*	*2000*	*2003*	*2005*
	Number of visits in thousands							
Total	860,859	1,014,848	1,114,504	1,169,333	697,082	823,542	906,023	963,617
Under 18 years	194,644	212,165	223,724	238,389	150,351	163,459	169,392	185,186
18–44 years	285,184	315,774	331,015	324,108	219,065	243,011	251,853	247,568
45–64 years	188,320	255,894	301,558	328,564	159,531	216,783	257,258	283,180
45–54 years	104,891	142,233	164,431	170,674	88,266	119,474	138,634	145,034
55–64 years	83,429	113,661	137,126	157,890	71,264	97,309	118,624	138,146
65 years and over	192,712	231,014	258,206	278,272	168,135	200,289	227,520	247,683
65–74 years	102,605	116,505	120,655	133,334	90,544	102,447	106,424	119,061
75 years and over	90,106	114,510	137,552	144,938	77.591	97,842	121,096	128,623
	Number of visits per 100 persons							
Total, age-adjusted[2]	334	374	391	400	271	304	317	329
Total, crude	329	370	390	402	266	300	317	331
Under 18 years	275	293	307	325	213	226	232	253
18–44 years	264	291	301	294	203	224	229	224
45–64 years	364	422	442	454	309	358	377	391
45–54 years	339	385	406	405	286	323	343	344
55–64 years	401	481	494	523	343	412	428	458
65 years and over	612	706	753	792	534	612	664	705
65–74 years	560	656	667	725	494	577	588	647
75 years and over	683	766	850	865	588	654	748	768
Sex and age								
Male, age-adjusted[2]	290	325	338	352	232	261	273	289
Male, crude	277	314	329	345	220	251	264	283
Under 18 years	273	302	317	338	209	231	241	265
18–44 years	190	203	203	212	139	148	147	158
45–54 years	275	316	335	331	229	260	280	278
55–64 years	351	428	422	468	300	367	365	411
65–74 years	508	614	632	691	445	539	558	619
75 years and over	711	771	881	833	616	670	777	741
Female, age-adjusted[2]	377	420	442	445	309	345	360	367
Female, crude	378	424	449	456	310	348	368	377
Under 18 years	277	285	297	311	217	221	223	240
18–44 years	336	377	397	375	265	298	309	290
45–54 years	400	451	475	476	339	384	403	408
55–64 years	446	529	561	574	382	453	486	501
65–74 years	603	692	696	754	534	609	613	671
75 years and over	666	763	830	886	571	645	730	785
Race and age[3]								
White, age-adjusted[2]	339	380	399	413	282	315	332	347
White, crude	338	381	404	420	281	316	337	355
Under 18 years	295	306	330	348	237	243	260	280
18–44 years	267	301	308	306	211	239	242	242
45–54 years	334	386	409	416	286	330	352	362
55–64 years	397	480	500	534	345	416	439	476
65–74 years	557	641	653	727	496	568	582	656
75 years and over	689	764	844	854	598	658	747	763
Black or African American, age-adjusted	309	353	393	398	204	239	261	270
Black or African American, crude	281	324	365	369	178	214	236	243
Under 18 years	193	264	248	278	100	167	131	162
18–44 years	260	257	329	295	158	149	199	172
45–54 years	387	383	445	422	281	269	315	297
55–64 years	414	495	487	515	294	373	349	374
65–74 years	553	656	761	745	429	512	602	589
75 years and over	534	745	774	982	395	568	608	806

See footnotes at end of table.

Table 92 (page 2 of 3). Visits to physician offices, hospital outpatient departments, and hospital emergency departments, by selected characteristics: United States, selected years 1995–2005

[Data are based on reporting by a sample of office-based physicians, hospital outpatient departments, and hospital emergency departments]

Age, sex, and race	Hospital outpatient departments				Hospital emergency departments			
	1995	2000	2003	2005	1995	2000	2003	2005
	Number of visits in thousands							
Total	67,232	83,289	94,578	90,393	96,545	108,017	113,903	115,323
Under 18 years	17,636	21,076	25,412	24,288	26,657	27,630	28,920	28,915
18–44 years	24,299	26,947	32,714	29,044	41,820	45,816	46,449	47,496
45–64 years	14,811	20,772	23,307	23,202	13,978	18,339	20,992	22,182
45–54 years	8,029	11,558	12,937	12,546	8,595	11,201	12,861	13,094
55–64 years	6,782	9,214	10,370	10,656	5,383	7,138	8,132	9,088
65 years and over	10,486	14,494	13,144	13,859	14,090	16,232	17,542	16,730
65–74 years	6,004	7,515	7,077	7,517	6,057	6,543	7,153	6,756
75 years and over	4,482	6,979	6,067	6,341	8,033	9,690	10,389	9,974
	Number of visits per 100 persons							
Total, age-adjusted[2]	26	31	33	31	37	40	40	40
Total, crude	26	30	33	31	37	39	40	40
Under 18 years	25	29	35	33	38	38	40	39
18–44 years	22	25	30	26	39	42	42	43
45–64 years	29	34	34	32	27	30	31	31
45–54 years	26	31	32	30	28	30	32	31
55–64 years	33	39	37	35	26	30	29	30
65 years and over	33	44	38	39	45	50	51	48
65–74 years	33	42	39	41	33	37	40	37
75 years and over	34	47	38	38	61	65	64	60
Sex and age								
Male, age-adjusted[2]	21	26	27	25	37	38	39	38
Male, crude	21	25	26	25	36	38	38	37
Under 18 years	25	29	34	33	40	41	41	41
18–44 years	14	17	19	16	37	38	37	38
45–54 years	20	26	25	24	26	30	30	29
55–64 years	26	32	29	29	25	30	29	28
65–74 years	29	38	34	34	34	36	41	39
75 years and over	34	42	38	32	61	59	67	60
Female, age-adjusted[2]	31	35	40	37	37	41	42	42
Female, crude	31	35	40	37	37	41	42	42
Under 18 years	25	29	36	33	35	35	38	38
18–44 years	31	33	41	37	40	46	47	48
45–54 years	32	36	39	36	29	31	33	33
55–64 years	38	45	45	41	26	31	30	32
65–74 years	36	46	44	47	32	37	39	35
75 years and over	34	49	37	42	61	69	63	59
Race and age[3]								
White, age-adjusted[2]	23	28	30	28	34	37	38	37
White, crude	23	28	30	28	34	37	37	37
Under 18 years	23	27	32	31	35	36	38	37
18–44 years	20	23	27	24	36	39	39	40
45–54 years	23	28	28	26	25	28	29	28
55–64 years	28	36	33	31	24	28	28	27
65–74 years	29	38	35	36	32	35	36	35
75 years and over	31	44	35	35	60	63	62	56
Black or African American, age-adjusted	48	51	61	58	58	62	71	70
Black or African American, crude	45	48	60	57	58	62	69	69
Under 18 years	39	40	55	*54	53	57	61	63
18–44 years	38	40	54	46	64	68	77	77
45–54 years	55	61	65	63	51	53	65	62
55–64 years	73	70	86	*84	47	52	53	58
65–74 years	*77	85	83	*94	47	59	77	62
75 years and over	66	85	64	*78	73	92	103	98

See footnotes at end of table.

Table 92 (page 3 of 3). Visits to physician offices, hospital outpatient departments, and hospital emergency departments, by selected characteristics: United States, selected years 1995–2005

[Data are based on reporting by a sample of office-based physicians, hospital outpatient departments, and hospital emergency departments]

* Estimates are considered unreliable. Data preceded by an asterisk have a relative standard error of 20%–30%.
[1]All places includes visits to physician offices and hospital outpatient and emergency departments.
[2]Estimates are age-adjusted to the year 2000 standard population using six age groups: under 18 years, 18–44 years, 45–54 years, 55–64 years, 65–74 years, and 75 years and over. See Appendix II, Age adjustment.
[3]Starting with 1999 data, the instruction for the race item on the Patient Record Form was changed so that more than one race could be recorded. In previous years only one race could be checked. Estimates for race in this table are for visits where only one race was recorded. Because of the small number of responses with more than one racial group checked, estimates for visits with multiple races checked are unreliable and are not presented.

NOTES: Rates for 1995–2000 were computed using 1990-based postcensal estimates of the civilian noninstitutionalized population as of July 1 adjusted for net underenumeration using the 1990 National Population Adjustment Matrix from the U.S. Census Bureau. Starting with 2001 data, rates were computed using 2000-based postcensal estimates of the civilian noninstitutionalized population as of July 1. The difference between rates for 2000 computed using 1990-based postcensal estimates and 2000 census counts is minimal. More information is available from: www.cdc.gov/nchs/about/major/ahcd/census2000.htm. Rates will be overestimated to the extent that visits by institutionalized persons are counted in the numerator (for example, hospital emergency department visits by nursing home residents) and institutionalized persons are omitted from the denominator (the civilian noninstitutionalized population). Starting with *Health, United States, 2005*, data for physician offices for 2001 and beyond use a revised weighting scheme. See Appendix I, National Ambulatory Medical Care Survey (NAMCS). Data for additional years are available. See Appendix III.

SOURCES: Centers for Disease Control and Prevention, National Center for Health Statistics, National Ambulatory Medical Care Survey and National Hospital Ambulatory Medical Care Survey.

Table 93 (page 1 of 2). Visits to primary care generalist and specialist physicians, by selected characteristics and type of physician: United States, selected years 1980–2005

[Data are based on reporting by a sample of office-based physicians]

Age, sex, and race	Type of primary care generalist physician[1]: All primary care generalists 1980	1990	2000	2005	General and family practice 1980	1990	2000	2005	Internal medicine 1980	1990	2000	2005
	Percent of all physician office visits											
Total	66.2	63.6	58.9	58.8	33.5	29.9	24.1	22.1	12.1	13.8	15.3	17.4
Under 18 years.	77.8	79.5	79.7	84.0	26.1	26.5	19.9	14.2	2.0	2.9	*	*
18–44 years.	65.3	65.2	62.1	63.5	34.3	31.9	28.2	27.0	8.6	11.8	12.7	18.2
45–64 years.	60.2	55.5	51.2	51.9	36.3	32.1	26.4	25.4	19.5	18.6	20.1	21.9
45–54 years	60.2	55.6	52.3	54.8	37.4	32.0	27.8	26.7	17.1	17.1	18.7	22.1
55–64 years	60.2	55.5	49.9	48.8	35.4	32.1	24.7	24.1	21.8	20.0	21.7	21.6
65 years and over.	61.6	52.6	46.5	43.3	37.5	28.1	20.2	19.3	22.7	23.3	24.5	22.6
65–74 years	61.2	52.7	46.6	43.9	37.4	28.1	19.7	21.7	22.1	23.0	24.5	20.4
75 years and over	62.3	52.4	46.4	42.8	37.6	28.0	20.8	17.0	23.5	23.7	24.5	24.7
Sex and age												
Male:												
Under 18 years	77.3	78.1	77.7	83.3	25.6	24.1	18.3	13.6	2.0	3.0	*	*
18–44 years	50.8	51.8	51.5	58.0	38.0	35.9	34.2	33.8	11.5	15.0	14.4	22.9
45–64 years	55.6	50.6	49.4	53.0	34.4	31.0	28.7	27.0	20.5	19.2	19.8	25.8
65 years and over	58.2	51.2	43.1	39.2	35.6	27.7	19.3	17.1	22.3	23.3	23.8	22.0
Female:												
Under 18 years	78.5	81.1	82.0	84.7	26.6	29.1	21.7	14.8	2.0	2.8	*	*
18–44 years	72.1	71.3	67.2	66.5	32.5	30.0	25.3	23.3	7.3	10.3	11.9	15.7
45–64 years	63.4	58.8	52.5	51.1	37.7	32.8	24.9	24.3	18.9	18.2	20.2	19.1
65 years and over	63.9	53.5	48.9	46.1	38.7	28.3	20.9	20.8	22.9	23.3	25.0	23.0
Race and age[2]												
White:												
Under 18 years	77.6	79.2	78.5	83.8	26.4	27.1	21.2	14.1	2.0	2.3	*	*
18–44 years	64.8	64.4	61.4	62.4	34.5	31.9	29.2	28.1	8.6	10.6	11.0	17.0
45–64 years	59.6	54.2	49.3	51.5	36.0	31.5	27.3	26.1	19.2	17.6	17.1	21.0
65 years and over	61.4	51.9	45.1	42.8	36.6	27.5	20.3	19.8	23.3	23.1	23.0	21.6
Black or African American:												
Under 18 years	79.9	85.5	87.3	83.6	23.7	20.2	*	*	*2.2	9.8	*	*
18–44 years	68.5	68.3	65.0	71.6	31.7	31.9	22.0	20.5	9.0	18.1	20.9	*24.7
45–64 years	66.1	61.6	61.7	51.7	38.6	31.2	23.3	17.2	22.6	26.9	35.9	*28.0
65 years and over	64.6	58.6	52.8	37.8	49.0	28.9	*18.5	*11.2	14.2	28.7	33.4	25.0

See footnotes at end of table.

Table 93 (page 2 of 2). Visits to primary care generalist and specialist physicians, by selected characteristics and type of physician: United States, selected years 1980–2005

[Data are based on reporting by a sample of office-based physicians]

Age, sex, ahd race	*Type of primary care generalist physician*[1]								*Specialty care physicians*			
	Obstetrics and gynecology				*Pediatrics*							
	1980	1990	2000	2005	1980	1990	2000	2005	1980	1990	2000	2005
	Percent of all physician office visits											
Total	9.6	8.7	7.8	6.4	10.9	11.2	11.7	13.0	33.8	36.4	41.1	41.2
Under 18 years	1.3	1.2	*1.1	*1.1	48.5	48.9	57.3	66.2	22.2	20.5	20.3	16.0
18–44 years	21.7	20.8	20.4	17.5	0.7	0.7	*0.9	*0.8	34.7	34.8	37.9	36.5
45–64 years	4.2	4.6	4.5	4.5	*	*	*	*	39.8	44.5	48.8	48.1
45–54 years	5.6	6.3	5.6	5.9	*	*	*	*	39.8	44.4	47.7	45.2
55–64 years	2.9	3.1	3.3	3.0	*	*	*	*	39.8	44.5	50.1	51.2
65 years and over	1.4	1.1	1.5	*1.4	*	*	*	*	38.4	47.4	53.5	56.7
65–74 years	1.7	1.6	2.0	*1.7	*	*	*	*	38.8	47.3	53.4	56.1
75 years and over	1.0	*0.6	*1.0	*1.0	*	*	*	*	37.7	47.6	53.6	57.2
Sex and age												
Male:												
Under 18 years	. . .	. . .	. . .	. . .	49.4	50.7	58.0	67.1	22.7	21.9	22.3	16.7
18–44 years	. . .	. . .	. . .	. . .	1.0	0.7	*1.7	*1.2	49.2	48.2	48.5	42.0
45–64 years	. . .	. . .	. . .	. . .	*	*	*	*	44.4	49.4	50.6	47.0
65 years and over	. . .	. . .	. . .	. . .	*	*	*	*	41.8	48.8	56.9	60.8
Female:												
Under 18 years	2.5	2.3	2.1	*2.4	47.4	46.9	56.5	65.2	21.5	18.9	18.0	15.3
18–44 years	31.7	30.4	29.6	26.8	0.6	0.7	*	*0.6	27.9	28.7	32.8	33.5
45–64 years	6.7	7.7	7.3	7.6	*	*	*	*	36.6	41.2	47.5	48.9
65 years and over	2.1	1.8	2.6	*2.3	*	*	*	*	36.1	46.5	51.1	53.9
Race and age[2]												
White:												
Under 18 years	1.1	1.0	*1.2	*0.9	48.2	48.8	54.7	66.0	22.4	20.8	21.5	16.2
18–44 years	21.0	21.1	20.4	16.5	0.7	0.7	*0.8	*0.8	35.2	35.6	38.6	37.6
45–64 years	4.1	4.8	4.7	4.3	*	*	*	*	40.4	45.8	50.7	48.5
65 years and over	1.4	1.2	1.5	*1.4	*	*	*	*	38.6	48.1	54.9	57.2
Black or African American:												
Under 18 years	2.8	*3.4	*	*	51.2	52.1	75.0	67.2	20.1	14.5	*12.7	*16.4
18–44 years	27.1	17.9	20.7	*25.9	*	*	*	*	31.5	31.7	35.0	28.4
45–64 years	4.8	3.5	*2.4	*6.3	*	*	*	*	33.9	38.4	38.3	48.3
65 years and over	*	*	*	*	*	*	*	*	35.4	41.4	47.2	62.2

* Estimates are considered unreliable. Data preceded by an asterisk have a relative standard error (RSE) of 20%–30%. Data not shown have a RSE of greater than 30%.

. . . Category not applicable.

[1]Type of physician is based on physician's self-designated primary area of practice. Primary care generalist physicians are defined as practitioners in the fields of general and family practice, general internal medicine, general obstetrics and gynecology, and general pediatrics and exclude primary care specialists. Primary care generalists in general and family practice exclude primary care specialities, such as sports medicine and geriatrics. Primary care internal medicine physicians exclude internal medicine specialists, such as allergists, cardiologists, and endocrinologists. Primary care obstetrics and gynecology physicians exclude obstetrics and gynecology specialities, such as gynecological oncology, maternal and fetal medicine, general obstetrics and gynecology critical care medicine, and reproductive endocrinology. Primary care pediatricians exclude pediatric specialists, such as adolescent medicine specialists, neonatologists, pediatric allergists, and pediatric cardiologists. See Appendix II, Physician specialty.

[2]Starting with 1999 data, the instruction for the race item on the Patient Record Form was changed so that more than one race could be recorded. In previous years only one racial category could be checked. Estimates for racial groups presented in this table are for visits where only one race was recorded. Because of the small number of responses with more than one racial group checked, estimates for visits with multiple races checked are unreliable and are not presented.

NOTES: This table presents data on visits to physician offices and excludes visits to other sites, such as hospital outpatient and emergency departments. In 1980 the survey excluded Alaska and Hawaii. Data for all other years include all 50 states and the District of Columbia. Visits with specialty of physician unknown are excluded. Starting with *Health, United States, 2005*, data for 2001 and later years for physician offices use a revised weighting scheme. See Appendix I, National Ambulatory Medical Care Survey (NAMCS). Data for additional years are available. See Appendix III.

SOURCE: Centers for Disease Control and Prevention, National Center for Health Statistics, National Ambulatory Medical Care Survey.

Table 94 (page 1 of 2). Dental visits in the past year, by selected characteristics: United States, 1997, 2004, and 2005

[Data are based on household interviews of a sample of the civilian noninstitutionalized population]

Characteristic	2 years and over			2–17 years			18–64 years			65 years and over[1]		
	1997	2004	2005	1997	2004	2005	1997	2004	2005	1997	2004	2005
	Percent of persons with a dental visit in the past year[2]											
2 years and over[3]	65.1	66.0	65.8	72.7	76.4	76.2	64.1	64.0	63.5	54.8	56.3	57.7
Sex												
Male	62.9	63.7	63.0	72.3	75.1	75.5	60.4	60.5	59.4	55.4	57.1	56.6
Female	67.1	68.1	68.4	73.0	77.7	77.0	67.7	67.4	67.6	54.4	55.8	58.6
Race[4]												
White only	66.4	67.0	66.8	74.0	77.3	77.1	65.7	65.2	64.8	56.8	58.6	59.9
Black or African American only	58.9	59.5	59.8	68.8	72.5	72.9	57.0	56.9	57.0	35.4	33.6	36.0
American Indian or Alaska Native only	55.1	63.4	59.3	66.8	70.3	74.8	49.9	63.4	54.1	*	*32.2	*
Asian only	62.5	66.1	62.5	69.9	73.8	70.1	60.3	64.2	60.2	53.9	58.1	60.0
Native Hawaiian or Other Pacific Islander only	- - -	*	*	- - -	*	*	- - -	*	*	- - -	*	*
2 or more races	- - -	65.3	67.3	- - -	78.0	78.1	- - -	58.4	60.8	- - -	*28.7	*39.7
Black or African American; White	- - -	67.1	66.0	- - -	72.6	75.3	- - -	61.0	51.3	- - -	*	*
American Indian or Alaska Native; White	- - -	55.1	56.2	- - -	78.9	70.9	- - -	49.1	54.4	- - -	*	*
Hispanic origin and race[4]												
Hispanic or Latino	54.0	54.2	53.9	61.0	65.3	66.5	50.8	49.6	48.5	47.8	42.5	43.1
Not Hispanic or Latino	66.4	67.9	67.8	74.7	78.9	78.5	65.7	66.3	66.0	55.2	57.2	58.7
White only	68.0	69.5	69.4	76.4	80.9	80.4	67.5	68.1	67.9	57.2	59.8	61.2
Black or African American only	58.8	59.8	59.7	68.8	72.9	72.7	56.9	57.3	57.0	35.3	33.3	35.5
Percent of poverty level[5]												
Below 100%	50.5	49.6	50.4	62.0	65.5	66.2	46.9	44.5	44.6	31.5	30.7	34.7
100%–less than 200%	50.8	52.6	52.4	62.5	69.0	68.6	48.3	47.6	47.8	40.8	43.2	42.5
200% or more	72.5	73.0	72.6	80.1	82.2	82.0	71.2	71.3	70.5	65.9	66.4	67.8
Hispanic origin and race and percent of poverty level[4,5]												
Hispanic or Latino:												
Below 100%	45.7	47.1	47.4	55.9	61.9	64.4	39.2	38.3	36.3	33.6	29.8	37.1
100%–less than 200%	47.2	47.2	47.6	53.8	59.1	60.2	43.5	41.7	42.3	47.9	37.7	36.2
200% or more	65.1	63.7	61.9	73.7	74.2	73.6	62.3	60.4	58.2	58.8	55.4	51.8
Not Hispanic or Latino:												
White only:												
Below 100%	51.7	51.1	51.5	64.4	68.7	65.0	50.6	48.7	49.6	32.0	33.4	37.9
100%–less than 200%	52.4	54.3	54.5	66.1	73.5	72.5	50.4	50.0	50.9	42.2	45.6	45.7
200% or more	73.8	74.8	74.6	81.3	84.3	84.2	72.7	73.2	72.8	67.0	68.5	69.7
Black or African American only:												
Below 100%	52.8	49.8	52.5	66.1	68.2	71.1	46.2	42.3	44.1	27.7	21.5	24.6
100%–less than 200%	48.7	52.1	51.3	61.2	70.5	70.5	46.3	46.4	45.2	26.9	29.4	26.9
200% or more	67.7	68.2	67.6	77.1	77.7	75.9	66.1	67.0	66.7	49.8	45.0	50.7

See footnotes at end of table.

Table 94 (page 2 of 2). Dental visits in the past year, by selected characteristics: United States, 1997, 2004, and 2005

[Data are based on household interviews of a sample of the civilian noninstitutionalized population]

	2 years and over			2–17 years			18–64 years			65 years and over[1]		
Characteristic	*1997*	*2004*	*2005*	*1997*	*2004*	*2005*	*1997*	*2004*	*2005*	*1997*	*2004*	*2005*
Geographic region	Percent of persons with a dental visit in the past year[2]											
Northeast	69.6	71.6	71.7	77.5	82.0	81.0	69.6	71.0	71.1	55.5	58.4	59.8
Midwest	68.4	69.4	68.6	76.4	78.8	79.0	67.4	68.4	66.8	57.6	57.1	58.7
South	60.2	60.4	60.7	68.0	72.7	72.2	59.4	57.6	58.1	49.0	51.4	52.6
West	65.0	66.7	66.1	71.5	75.4	76.0	62.9	64.0	62.7	61.9	62.5	64.3
Location of residence												
Within MSA[6]	66.7	67.5	67.0	73.6	76.5	76.0	65.7	65.6	64.8	57.6	59.4	60.9
Outside MSA[6]	59.1	59.9	61.0	69.3	76.0	77.0	58.0	57.4	58.5	46.1	46.0	47.5

* Estimates are considered unreliable. Data preceded by an asterisk have a relative standard error (RSE) of 20%–30%. Data not shown have an RSE greater than 30%.

- - - Data not available.

[1]Based on the 1997–2005 National Health Interview Surveys, about 25%–30% of persons 65 years and over were edentulous (having lost all their natural teeth). In 1997–2005 about 68%–70% of older dentate persons compared with 16%–20% of older edentate persons had a dental visit in the past year.

[2]Respondents were asked "About how long has it been since you last saw or talked to a dentist?" See Appendix II, Dental visit.

[3]Includes all other races not shown separately.

[4]The race groups, white, black, American Indian or Alaska Native, Asian, Native Hawaiian or Other Pacific Islander, and 2 or more races, include persons of Hispanic and non-Hispanic origin. Persons of Hispanic origin may be of any race. Starting with 1999 data, race-specific estimates are tabulated according to the 1997 Revisions to the Standards for the Classification of Federal Data on Race and Ethnicity and are not strictly comparable with estimates for earlier years. The five single-race categories plus multiple-race categories shown in the table conform to the 1997 Standards. Starting with 1999 data, race-specific estimates are for persons who reported only one racial group; the category 2 or more races includes persons who reported more than one racial group. Prior to 1999, data were tabulated according to the 1977 Standards with four racial groups, and the Asian only category included Native Hawaiian or Other Pacific Islander. Estimates for single-race categories prior to 1999 included persons who reported one race or, if they reported more than one race, identified one race as best representing their race. Starting with 2003 data, race responses of other race and unspecified multiple race were treated as missing, and then race was imputed if these were the only race responses. Almost all persons with a race response of other race were of Hispanic origin. See Appendix II, Hispanic origin; Race.

[5]Percent of poverty level is based on family income and family size and composition using U.S. Census Bureau poverty thresholds. Missing family income data were imputed for 25%–29% of persons in 1997–1998 and 32%–35% in 1999–2005. See Appendix II, Family income; Poverty.

[6]MSA is metropolitan statistical area.

NOTES: In 1997 the National Health Interview Survey questionnaire was redesigned. See Appendix I, National Health Interview Survey. Standard errors for selected years are available in the spreadsheet version of this table. Available from: www.cdc.gov/nchs/hus.htm. Data for additional years are available. See Appendix III.

SOURCE: Centers for Disease Control and Prevention, National Center for Health Statistics, National Health Interview Survey, sample child and sample adult questionnaires.

Table 95 (page 1 of 3). Selected prescription and nonprescription drugs recorded during physician office visits and hospital outpatient department visits, by sex and age: United States, 1995–1996 and 2004–2005

[Data are based on reporting by a sample of office-based physicians and hospital outpatient departments]

Age group and National Drug Code (NDC) Directory therapeutic class[1] (common reasons for use)	Total		Male		Female	
	1995–1996	2004–2005	1995–1996	2004–2005	1995–1996	2004–2005
All ages	Visits with at least one drug per 100 population[2]					
Drug visits[3]	189.8	239.4	156.5	201.9	221.5	275.2
	Number of drugs per 100 population[4]					
Total number of drugs[5]	400.3	684.2	321.1	568.4	475.6	795.0
Antidepressants (depression and related disorders)	13.8	35.5	9.1	22.8	18.2	47.7
Hypertension control drugs, not otherwise specified (high blood pressure)	6.0	32.1	4.1	28.1	7.8	35.9
Hyperlipidemia (high cholesterol)	5.4	30.8	5.4	31.0	5.4	30.6
Antiasthmatics/bronchodilators (asthma, breathing)	13.1	29.0	11.7	25.6	14.4	32.1
NSAID[6] (pain relief)	19.9	28.8	16.0	24.4	23.7	33.1
Nonnarcotic analgesics (pain relief)	14.4	28.7	13.0	27.3	15.7	30.0
Acid/peptic disorders (gastrointestinal reflux, ulcers)	12.0	25.1	9.8	20.8	14.1	29.2
Blood glucose/sugar regulators (diabetes)	9.5	24.0	8.6	24.4	10.4	23.6
Antihistamines (allergies)	13.7	23.4	10.8	18.3	16.4	28.2
Vitamins/minerals (dietary supplements)	9.2	21.2	3.4	12.6	14.8	29.5
Beta blockers (high blood pressure, heart disease)	5.9	20.0	5.1	17.7	6.7	22.3
ACE inhibitors (high blood pressure, heart disease)	9.6	19.9	9.0	19.5	10.2	20.4
Narcotic analgesics (pain relief)	11.2	19.7	10.3	15.9	12.2	23.3
Diuretics (high blood pressure, heart disease)	10.2	19.5	7.8	15.5	12.6	23.3
Estrogens/progestins (menopause, hot flashes)	. . .	. . .	. . .	. . .	19.8	15.1
Under 18 years	Visits with at least one drug per 100 population[2]					
Drug visits[3]	153.9	178.2	152.3	183.2	155.6	173.0
	Number of drugs per 100 population[4]					
Total number of drugs[5]	261.3	338.4	255.6	350.2	267.3	326.1
Antiasthmatics/bronchodilators (asthma, breathing)	13.4	29.1	14.8	34.2	11.9	23.7
Penicillins (bacterial infections)	37.2	27.5	36.4	29.4	38.0	25.5
Antihistamines (allergies)	17.5	25.1	16.7	23.7	18.4	26.5
Nonnarcotic analgesics (pain relief)	12.1	15.5	10.4	15.7	13.9	15.3
NSAID[6] (pain relief)	7.4	14.6	6.9	15.6	7.9	13.5
Cephalosporins (bacterial infections)	18.1	11.3	18.8	11.6	17.3	10.9
Antitussives/expectorants (cough and cold, congestion)	11.8	11.1	11.0	10.2	12.7	11.9
Erythromycins/lincosamides (infections)	10.2	10.9	11.0	10.1	9.4	11.6
Adrenal corticosteroids (anti-inflammatory)	4.3	10.5	4.7	12.4	3.9	8.6
Nasal corticosteroid inhalants (asthma, breathing, allergies)	3.5	10.1	3.5	10.9	3.5	9.3
Nasal decongestants (congestion)	14.0	9.9	12.4	9.9	15.7	10.0
Anorexiants/CNS stimulants (attention deficit disorder, hyperactivity)	3.9	8.9	5.6	13.8	2.1	3.9
Antidepressants (depression and related disorders)	1.9	7.5	1.9	7.9	1.9	7.0
18–44 years	Visits with at least one drug per 100 population[2]					
Drug visits[3]	136.2	159.9	90.9	109.0	180.4	210.0
	Number of drugs per 100 population[4]					
Total number of drugs[5]	251.0	356.1	168.8	244.7	331.2	466.1
Antidepressants (depression and related disorders)	14.0	29.3	9.3	17.8	18.5	40.5
NSAID[6] (pain relief)	16.7	19.3	14.5	16.5	18.8	22.1
Narcotic analgesics (pain relief)	11.7	17.7	10.8	14.3	12.7	21.0
Antihistamines (allergies)	10.8	17.5	7.5	11.4	14.1	23.6
Vitamins/minerals (dietary supplements)	11.8	15.3	1.1	3.2	22.2	27.3
Antiasthmatics/bronchodilator (asthma, breathing)	6.9	14.0	3.3	8.7	10.3	19.3
Acid/peptic disorders (gastrointestinal reflux, ulcers)	6.6	11.6	5.3	8.3	7.9	14.9
Anticonvulsants (epilepsy, seizure and related disorders)	4.5	10.6	3.8	8.0	5.1	13.3
Nonnarcotic analgesics (pain relief)	6.0	8.7	4.5	6.7	7.4	10.7
Antitussives/expectorants (cough and cold, congestion)	7.7	8.1	5.8	5.9	9.5	10.3
Nasal corticosteroid inhalants (asthma, breathing, allergies)	4.7	8.1	3.3	6.2	6.1	9.9
Antianxiety agents (generalized anxiety and related disorders)	5.8	8.0	4.5	5.3	7.1	10.6
Erythromycins/lincosamides (infections)	7.5	7.9	5.4	6.2	9.5	9.6
Hypertension control drugs, not otherwise specified (high blood pressure)	1.5	7.9	1.0	7.9	2.0	7.8
Contraceptive agents (prevent pregnancy)	. . .	. . .	. . .	. . .	13.4	20.6

See footnotes at end of table.

Table 95 (page 2 of 3). Selected prescription and nonprescription drugs recorded during physician office visits and hospital outpatient department visits, by sex and age: United States, 1995–1996 and 2004–2005

[Data are based on reporting by a sample of office-based physicians and hospital outpatient departments]

Age group and National Drug Code (NDC) Directory therapeutic class[1] (common reasons for use)	*Total*		*Male*		*Female*	
	1995–1996	*2004–2005*	*1995–1996*	*2004–2005*	*1995–1996*	*2004–2005*
45–64 years	Visits with at least one drug per 100 population[2]					
Drug visits[3]	222.4	290.3	185.0	249.6	257.4	328.6
	Number of drugs per 100 population[4]					
Total number of drugs[5]	505.1	912.0	403.2	780.7	600.4	1,035.9
Antidepressants (depression and related disorders)	23.5	59.8	14.9	39.8	31.5	78.6
Hyperlipidemia (high cholesterol)	10.4	53.4	12.0	58.1	8.8	49.0
Hypertension control drugs, not otherwise specified (high blood pressure)	9.4	52.5	6.9	50.6	11.7	54.3
Blood glucose/sugar regulators (diabetes)	17.7	44.4	16.7	49.0	18.7	40.0
NSAID[6] (pain relief)	30.3	41.2	23.9	34.8	36.4	47.3
Acid/peptic disorders (gastrointestinal reflux, ulcers)	19.8	38.4	18.3	33.6	21.3	43.0
Nonnarcotic analgesics (pain relief)	16.3	35.7	15.6	37.3	17.0	34.3
Antiasthmatics/bronchodilators (asthma, breathing)	14.4	34.0	11.4	27.3	17.1	40.3
ACE inhibitors (high blood pressure, heart disease)	16.8	33.4	17.7	35.0	16.0	31.9
Narcotic analgesics (pain relief)	17.5	31.4	17.0	27.7	18.0	34.9
Beta blockers (high blood pressure, heart disease)	10.4	28.5	9.8	27.5	11.0	29.4
Antihistamines (allergies)	13.5	27.3	9.1	19.9	17.7	34.3
Diuretics (high blood pressure, heart disease)	13.6	26.5	11.2	22.3	15.8	30.4
Vitamins/minerals (dietary supplements)	6.4	23.3	4.0	19.0	8.6	27.3
Estrogens/progestins (menopause, hot flashes)	. . .	. . .	. . .	. . .	55.7	30.4
65 years and over	Visits with at least one drug per 100 population[2]					
Drug visits[3]	399.4	515.3	378.1	481.1	414.7	540.5
	Number of drugs per 100 population[4]					
Total number of drugs[5]	1,047.4	1,982.0	956.9	1,820.3	1,112.5	2,101.6
Hypertension control drugs, not otherwise specified (high blood pressure)	29.1	133.3	22.7	120.7	33.8	142.6
Hyperlipidemia (high cholesterol)	24.7	128.1	25.1	135.0	24.5	123.0
Nonnarcotic analgesics (pain relief)	44.9	104.7	49.0	109.3	42.0	101.3
Diuretics (high blood pressure, heart disease)	55.2	95.4	48.5	86.0	60.0	102.4
Beta blockers (high blood pressure, heart disease)	24.9	92.7	22.8	89.5	26.4	95.0
Blood glucose/sugar regulators (diabetes)	37.5	86.4	38.0	95.7	37.1	79.6
Acid/peptic disorders (gastrointestinal reflux, ulcers)	42.2	84.2	36.0	78.8	46.6	88.2
ACE inhibitors (high blood pressure, heart disease)	42.6	81.7	41.2	84.8	43.6	79.4
Vitamins/minerals (dietary supplements)	17.1	69.8	13.1	54.4	20.0	81.2
Calcium channel blockers (high blood pressure, heart disease)	57.3	69.5	52.2	64.0	60.9	73.5
Antiasthmatics/bronchodilators (asthma, breathing)	31.3	65.7	37.1	62.7	27.0	67.9
Antidepressants (depression and related disorders)	23.5	64.7	16.7	38.9	28.5	83.7
NSAID[6] (pain relief)	41.8	63.5	31.9	51.3	49.0	72.5
Anticoagulants/thrombolytics (blood thinning, reduce or prevent blood clots)	20.7	56.8	24.0	65.5	18.3	50.4
Estrogens/progestins (menopause, hot flashes)	. . .	. . .	. . .	. . .	37.1	28.6
65–74 years	Visits with at least one drug per 100 population[2]					
Drug visits[3]	362.8	470.5	323.0	435.7	394.9	499.7
	Number of drugs per 100 population[4]					
Total number of drugs[5]	930.5	1,747.5	804.7	1,632.9	1,032.1	1,843.9
Hyperlipidemia (high cholesterol)	27.3	127.5	27.1	141.7	27.4	115.5
Hypertension control drugs, not otherwise specified (high blood pressure)	24.8	114.6	19.2	103.8	29.3	123.6
Blood glucose/sugar regulators (diabetes)	35.7	87.9	32.4	97.2	38.4	80.1
Nonnarcotic analgesics (pain relief)	38.0	86.0	40.5	93.7	35.9	79.5
Beta blockers (high blood pressure, heart disease)	23.5	78.8	20.4	79.2	26.0	78.4
Acid/peptic disorders (gastrointestinal reflux, ulcers)	38.7	78.0	30.6	73.0	45.2	82.3
ACE inhibitors (high blood pressure, heart disease)	37.1	71.5	35.6	77.9	38.3	66.1
Diuretics (high blood pressure, heart disease)	40.1	71.4	32.4	66.7	46.4	75.3
NSAID[6] (pain relief)	42.0	64.8	31.2	53.0	50.8	74.8
Antiasthmatics/bronchodilators (asthma, breathing)	31.1	63.8	33.0	58.7	29.5	68.1
Antidepressants (depression and related disorders)	22.7	62.9	14.2	40.0	29.6	82.1
Calcium channel blockers (high blood pressure, heart disease)	48.9	61.2	46.2	58.7	51.2	63.2
Vitamins/minerals (dietary supplements)	14.1	56.4	10.1	47.5	17.4	63.9
Anticoagulants/thrombolytics (blood thinning, reduce or prevent blood clots)	14.9	42.1	17.2	50.1	12.9	35.4
Estrogens/progestins (menopause, hot flashes)	. . .	. . .	. . .	. . .	47.5	37.6

See footnotes at end of table.

Table 95 (page 3 of 3). Selected prescription and nonprescription drugs recorded during physician office visits and hospital outpatient department visits, by sex and age: United States, 1995–1996 and 2004–2005

[Data are based on reporting by a sample of office-based physicians and hospital outpatient departments]

Age group and National Drug Code (NDC) Directory therapeutic class[1] (common reasons for use)	Total		Male		Female	
	1995–1996	2004–2005	1995–1996	2004–2005	1995–1996	2004–2005
75 years and over	Visits with at least one drug per 100 population[2]					
Drug visits[3]	449.2	564.7	466.3	539.8	438.7	580.6
	Number of drugs per 100 population[4]					
Total number of drugs[5]	1,206.8	2,240.8	1,200.9	2,062.6	1,210.4	2,354.8
Hypertension control drugs, not otherwise specified (high blood pressure)	35.1	154.0	28.4	142.6	39.2	161.3
Hyperlipidemia (high cholesterol)	21.3	128.7	21.8	126.2	21.0	130.4
Nonnarcotic analgesics (pain relief)	54.4	125.4	62.6	129.4	49.4	122.8
Diuretics (high blood pressure, heart disease)	75.8	122.0	74.5	111.1	76.6	129.0
Beta blockers (high blood pressure, heart disease)	26.8	108.0	26.5	102.9	26.9	111.2
ACE inhibitors (high blood pressure, heart disease)	50.2	93.0	50.2	93.7	50.1	92.5
Acid/peptic disorders (gastrointestinal reflux, ulcers)	47.0	91.1	44.7	86.4	48.3	94.1
Blood glucose/sugar regulators (diabetes)	39.8	84.8	46.9	93.7	35.5	79.1
Vitamins/minerals (dietary supplements)	21.2	84.6	18.0	63.3	23.2	98.2
Calcium channel blockers (high blood pressure, heart disease)	68.6	78.6	61.8	70.7	72.7	83.6
Anticoagulants/thrombolytics (blood thinning, reduce or prevent blood clots)	28.6	73.1	34.9	85.4	24.7	65.2
Antiasthmatics/bronchodilators (asthma, breathing)	31.5	67.7	43.7	67.8	24.0	67.7
Antidepressants (depression and related disorders)	24.6	66.6	20.7	37.5	27.0	85.3
NSAID[6] (pain relief)	41.5	62.0	33.1	49.1	46.7	70.2
Thyroid/antithyroid (hyper- and hypothyroidism)	27.1	61.0	15.1	36.3	34.4	76.7

. . . Category not applicable.

[1]The National Drug Code (NDC) Directory therapeutic class is a general therapeutic or pharmacological classification scheme for drug products reported to the Food and Drug Administration (FDA) under the provisions of the Drug Listing Act. Drugs are classified based on the NDC Directory classifications for 2005 data. See Appendix II, National Drug Code (NDC) Directory therapeutic class; Table XII.

[2]Estimated number of drug visits during the 2-year period divided by the sum of population estimates for both years times 100.

[3]Drug visits are physician office and hospital outpatient department visits in which at least one prescription or nonprescription drug was recorded on the patient record form.

[4]Estimated number of drugs recorded during visits during the 2-year period divided by the sum of population estimates for both years times 100.

[5]Until 2002, up to six prescription and nonprescription medications were recorded on the patient record form. Starting with 2003 data, up to eight prescription and nonprescription medications are recorded on the patient record form. If 2004–2005 data were restricted to six instead of eight drugs, the 2004–2005 total drug rate for all ages would be 6.4% lower. See Appendix II, Drug.

[6]NSAID is nonsteroidal anti-inflammatory drug. Aspirin was not included as an NSAID in this analysis. See Appendix II, National Drug Code (NDC) Directory therapeutic class.

NOTES: Drugs recorded on the patient record form are those prescribed, continued, administered, or provided during a physician office or hospital outpatient department visit. Numbers have been revised and differ from previous editions of *Health, United States.*

SOURCE: Centers for Disease Control and Prevention, National Center for Health Statistics, National Ambulatory Medical Care Survey and National Hospital Ambulatory Medical Care Survey.

Table 96. Prescription drug use in the past month by sex, age, race and Hispanic origin: United States, 1988–1994 and 1999–2002

[Data are based on a sample of the civilian noninstitutionalized population]

	All persons[1]		Not Hispanic or Latino				Mexican[2,3]	
			White only[2]		Black or African American only[2]			
Sex and age	1988–1994	1999–2002	1988–1994	1999–2002	1988–1994	1999–2002	1988–1994	1999–2002
	Percent of population with at least one prescription drug in past month							
Both sexes, age-adjusted[4]	39.1	45.3	41.1	48.9	36.9	40.1	31.7	31.7
Male	32.7	39.9	34.2	43.1	31.1	35.4	27.5	25.8
Female	45.0	50.4	47.6	54.5	41.4	43.8	36.0	37.8
Both sexes, crude	37.8	45.1	41.4	50.9	31.2	36.0	24.0	23.7
Male	30.6	38.7	33.5	43.9	25.5	30.8	20.1	18.8
Female	44.6	51.2	48.9	57.6	36.2	40.6	28.1	28.9
Under 18 years	20.5	24.2	22.9	27.6	14.8	18.6	16.1	15.9
18–44 years	31.3	35.9	34.3	41.3	27.8	28.5	21.1	19.2
45–64 years	54.8	64.1	55.5	66.1	57.5	62.3	48.1	49.3
65 years and over	73.6	84.7	74.0	85.4	74.5	81.1	67.7	72.0
Male:								
Under 18 years	20.4	26.2	22.3	30.6	15.5	19.8	16.3	16.2
18–44 years	21.5	27.1	23.5	31.2	21.1	21.5	14.9	13.0
45–64 years	47.2	55.6	48.1	57.4	48.2	54.0	43.8	36.4
65 years and over	67.2	80.1	67.4	81.0	64.4	78.1	61.3	66.8
Female:								
Under 18 years	20.6	22.0	23.6	24.4	14.2	17.3	16.0	15.6
18–44 years	40.7	44.6	44.7	51.7	33.4	34.2	28.1	26.2
45–64 years	62.0	72.0	62.6	74.7	64.4	69.0	52.2	62.4
65 years and over	78.3	88.1	78.8	88.8	81.3	83.1	73.0	76.3
	Percent of population with three or more prescription drugs in past month							
Both sexes, age-adjusted[4]	11.8	17.7	12.4	18.9	12.6	16.5	9.0	11.2
Male	9.4	14.8	9.9	15.9	10.2	14.4	7.0	9.5
Female	13.9	20.4	14.6	21.7	14.3	18.0	11.0	12.9
Both sexes, crude	11.0	17.6	12.5	20.5	9.2	13.4	4.8	6.1
Male	8.3	13.9	9.5	16.4	7.0	10.9	3.4	4.8
Female	13.6	21.1	15.4	24.5	11.1	15.6	6.4	7.5
Under 18 years	2.4	4.1	3.2	4.9	1.5	2.5	*1.2	2.1
18–44 years	5.7	8.4	6.3	10.1	5.4	6.5	3.0	2.7
45–64 years	20.0	30.8	20.9	31.6	21.9	31.1	16.0	20.7
65 years and over	35.3	51.6	35.0	52.5	41.2	50.1	31.3	39.5
Male:								
Under 18 years	2.6	4.3	3.3	5.2	1.7	3.0	*	1.9
18–44 years	3.6	6.7	4.1	8.4	4.2	4.4	*1.8	*1.7
45–64 years	15.1	23.5	15.8	24.0	18.7	26.3	11.6	18.2
65 years and over	31.3	46.0	30.9	47.0	31.7	48.2	27.6	34.2
Female:								
Under 18 years	2.3	3.9	3.0	4.7	*1.2	*2.0	*1.5	2.2
18–44 years	7.6	10.2	8.5	11.9	6.4	8.3	4.3	4.0
45–64 years	24.7	37.4	25.8	39.1	24.3	35.0	20.3	23.3
65 years and over	38.2	55.7	38.0	56.6	47.7	51.3	34.5	44.0

* Estimates are considered unreliable. Data preceded by an asterisk have a relative standard error (RSE) of 20%–30%. Data not shown have an RSE of greater than 30%.

[1] Includes persons of all races and Hispanic origins, not just those shown separately.

[2] Starting with data year 1999, race-specific estimates are tabulated according to the 1997 Revisions to the Standards for the Classification of Federal Data on Race and Ethnicity and are not strictly comparable with estimates for earlier years. The two non-Hispanic race categories shown in the table conform to the 1997 Standards. Starting with 1999 data, race-specific estimates are for persons who reported only one racial group. Prior to data year 1999, estimates were tabulated according to the 1977 Standards. Estimates for single-race categories prior to 1999 included persons who reported one race or, if they reported more than one race, identified one race as best representing their race. See Appendix II, Hispanic origin; Race.

[3] Persons of Mexican origin may be of any race.

[4] Age-adjusted to the 2000 standard population using four age groups: Under 18 years, 18–44 years, 45–64 years, and 65 years and over. Age-adjusted estimates in this table may differ from other age-adjusted estimates based on the same data and presented elsewhere if different age groups are used in the adjustment procedure. See Appendix II, Age adjustment.

NOTES: Standard errors are available in the spreadsheet version of this table. Available from: www.cdc.gov/nchs/hus.htm. Data for additional years are available. See Appendix III.

SOURCE: Centers for Disease Control and Prevention, National Center for Health Statistics, National Health and Nutrition Examination Survey.

Table 97. Admissions to mental health organizations, by type of service and organization: United States, selected years 1986–2004

[Data are based on inventories of mental health organizations]

Service and organization	1986	1990	2002	2004	1986	1990	2002	2004
24-hour hospital and residential treatment	Admissions in thousands[1]				Admissions per 100,000 civilian population[2]			
All organizations	1,819	2,110	2,158	2,713	759.9	833.0	738.9	910.5
State and county mental hospitals	333	283	234	266	139.1	111.6	80.1	89.1
Private psychiatric hospitals	235	411	477	599	98.0	162.4	163.3	200.9
Nonfederal general hospital psychiatric services[3]	849	962	1,087	1,533	354.8	379.9	372.2	514.6
Department of Veterans Affairs medical centers[4]	180	203	158	- - -	75.1	80.3	54.1	- - -
Residential treatment centers for emotionally disturbed children	25	50	63	61	10.2	19.8	21.6	20.3
All other organizations[5]	198	200	139	255	82.7	79.0	47.6	85.5
Less than 24-hour care[6]								
All organizations	2,955	3,377	4,099	4,667	1,233.4	1,333.3	1,403.2	1,566.6
State and county mental hospitals	68	50	62	130	28.4	19.7	21.2	43.6
Private psychiatric hospitals	132	163	598	447	55.2	64.5	204.7	150.1
Nonfederal general hospital psychiatric services	533	661	681	900	222.4	260.8	233.0	302.2
Department of Veterans Affairs medical centers[4]	133	235	99	- - -	55.3	92.8	33.9	- - -
Residential treatment centers for emotionally disturbed children	67	100	222	194	28.1	39.3	75.8	65.2
All other organizations[5]	2,022	2,168	2,438	2,995	844.0	856.2	834.3	1,005.4

- - - Data not available.

[1]Admissions sometimes are referred to as additions. See Appendix II, Admission.

[2]Civilian population estimates for 2000 and beyond are based on the 2000 census as of July 1; population estimates for 1992–1998 are 1990 postcensal estimates.

[3]These data exclude mental health care provided in nonpsychiatric units of hospitals such as general medical units.

[4]Department of Veterans Affairs Medical Centers (VA general hospital psychiatric services and VA psychiatric outpatient clinics) were dropped from the survey as of 2004.

[5]Includes freestanding psychiatric outpatient clinics, partial care organizations, and multiservice mental health organizations. See Appendix I, Survey of Mental Health Organizations.

[6]Formerly reported as partial care and outpatient treatment, the survey format was changed in 1994 and the reporting of these services was combined due to similarities in the care provided. These data exclude private office-based mental health care.

NOTES: Data for 1990, 1992, 1994, 1998, 2000, and 2002 are revised final estimates and differ from the previous edition of *Health, United States*. Data for additional years are available. See Appendix III.

SOURCES: Substance Abuse and Mental Health Services Administration, Center for Mental Health Services (CMHS). Revised 1990, 1992, 1994, 1998, 2000, and 2002 Estimates from the Survey of Mental Health Organizations. 2004 Survey of Mental Health Organizations, unpublished data.

Table 98 (page 1 of 3). Persons with hospital stays in the past year, by selected characteristics: United States, selected years 1997, 2004, and 2005

[Data are based on household interviews of a sample of the civilian noninstitutionalized population]

Characteristic	One or more hospital stays[1]			Two or more hospital stays[1]		
	1997	2004	2005	1997	2004	2005
	Percent					
1 year and over, age-adjusted[2,3]	7.8	7.4	7.4	1.8	1.8	1.7
1 year and over, crude[2]	7.7	7.4	7.4	1.7	1.8	1.8
Age						
1–17 years	2.8	2.4	2.5	0.5	0.4	0.4
1–5 years	3.9	4.0	3.7	0.7	0.9	0.8
6–17 years	2.3	1.7	2.0	0.4	0.3	0.3
18–44 years	7.4	7.0	6.7	1.2	1.2	1.1
18–24 years	7.9	6.6	6.3	1.3	0.8	1.0
25–44 years	7.3	7.1	6.9	1.2	1.4	1.2
45–64 years	8.2	8.1	8.2	2.2	2.2	2.2
45–54 years	6.9	7.1	7.1	1.7	1.9	1.8
55–64 years	10.2	9.4	9.8	2.9	2.7	2.9
65 years and over	18.0	17.4	17.8	5.4	5.7	5.4
65–74 years	16.1	14.5	14.5	4.8	4.6	4.5
75 years and over	20.4	20.7	21.4	6.2	6.8	6.4
1–64 years						
Total, 1–64 years[2,4]	6.3	5.9	5.9	1.3	1.2	1.2
Sex						
Male	4.5	4.1	4.3	1.0	0.9	1.1
1–17 years	2.9	2.5	2.8	0.6	0.5	0.5
18–44 years	3.6	3.3	3.2	0.6	0.7	0.7
45–54 years	6.0	6.0	6.6	1.4	1.5	1.9
55–64 years	11.1	9.3	10.3	3.0	2.5	3.4
Female	8.0	7.7	7.4	1.6	1.6	1.3
1–17 years	2.6	2.2	2.2	0.5	0.4	0.4
18–44 years	11.2	10.6	10.2	1.8	1.8	1.6
45–54 years	7.6	8.1	7.6	2.0	2.2	1.7
55–64 years	9.4	9.5	9.3	2.9	2.9	2.4
Race[4,5]						
White only	6.2	5.9	5.9	1.2	1.2	1.1
Black or African American only	7.6	6.8	6.6	1.9	1.8	1.8
American Indian or Alaska Native only	7.6	6.7	6.9	*	*1.6	*2.5
Asian only	3.9	3.8	3.9	*0.5	*0.4	*0.5
Native Hawaiian or Other Pacific Islander only	---	*	*	---	*	*
2 or more races	---	6.9	6.0	---	*1.4	*1.9
Hispanic origin and race[4,5]						
Hispanic or Latino	6.8	5.5	5.4	1.3	1.1	1.2
Not Hispanic or Latino	6.2	6.0	6.0	1.3	1.3	1.2
White only	6.1	6.0	6.0	1.2	1.2	1.1
Black or African American only	7.5	6.8	6.6	1.9	1.9	1.7
Percent of poverty level[4,6]						
Below 100%	10.3	9.2	8.8	2.8	2.9	2.5
100%–less than 200%	7.3	6.9	7.4	1.7	1.7	1.9
200% or more	5.3	5.2	5.1	0.9	0.9	0.9
Hispanic origin and race and percent of poverty level[4,5,6]						
Hispanic or Latino:						
Below 100%	9.1	7.2	7.6	2.0	1.7	2.0
100%–less than 200%	5.9	5.3	5.9	1.0	1.1	1.4
200% or more	5.8	5.0	4.2	1.1	0.8	0.7
Not Hispanic or Latino:						
White only:						
Below 100%	10.7	10.1	9.3	3.2	3.3	2.5
100%–less than 200%	7.7	7.7	8.2	1.8	2.0	2.0
200% or more	5.3	5.3	5.2	0.9	0.9	0.9
Black or African American only:						
Below 100%	11.4	11.0	9.4	3.3	3.8	3.1
100%–less than 200%	8.0	7.5	7.7	2.1	2.3	2.0
200% or more	5.5	5.1	5.1	1.2	1.0	1.2

See footnotes at end of table.

Table 98 (page 2 of 3). Persons with hospital stays in the past year, by selected characteristics: United States, selected years 1997, 2004, and 2005

[Data are based on household interviews of a sample of the civilian noninstitutionalized population]

Characteristic	One or more hospital stays[1]			Two or more hospital stays[1]		
	1997	2004	2005	1997	2004	2005
	Percent					
Health insurance status at the time of interview[4,7]						
Insured	6.6	6.3	6.3	1.3	1.3	1.3
Private	5.6	5.4	5.2	1.0	0.9	0.9
Medicaid	16.1	14.0	14.6	4.9	4.8	4.1
Uninsured	4.8	4.1	4.4	1.0	0.8	0.9
Health insurance status prior to interview[4,7]						
Insured continuously all 12 months	6.5	6.2	6.1	1.3	1.3	1.2
Uninsured for any period up to 12 months	8.5	7.6	9.0	1.8	1.6	2.4
Uninsured more than 12 months	3.8	3.1	3.2	0.8	0.6	0.6
Percent of poverty level and health insurance status prior to interview[4,6,7]						
Below 100%:						
Insured continuously all 12 months	12.4	11.5	10.8	3.7	3.9	3.1
Uninsured for any period up to 12 months	13.7	11.5	13.6	3.4	*2.8	4.1
Uninsured more than 12 months	4.9	3.9	3.9	1.0	*1.0	*0.8
100%–less than 200%:						
Insured continuously all 12 months	8.5	8.2	8.4	2.0	2.2	2.2
Uninsured for any period up to 12 months	9.3	8.5	10.7	*1.9	*1.8	3.1
Uninsured more than 12 months	3.8	3.0	3.7	*0.7	*0.6	*0.8
200% or more:						
Insured continuously all 12 months	5.5	5.4	5.3	0.9	0.9	0.9
Uninsured for any period up to 12 months	5.9	5.9	6.8	*1.1	*1.1	1.5
Uninsured more than 12 months	3.0	2.6	2.3	*0.6	*0.5	*0.4
Geographic region[4]						
Northeast	6.0	5.2	5.8	1.2	1.1	1.1
Midwest	6.5	5.9	6.3	1.5	1.3	1.3
South	6.8	6.7	6.3	1.4	1.5	1.4
West	5.4	5.2	4.8	0.8	1.0	0.8
Location of residence[4]						
Within MSA[8]	6.1	5.7	5.7	1.2	1.2	1.2
Outside MSA[8]	7.0	6.9	6.8	1.6	1.6	1.4
65 years and over						
Total 65 years and over[2,9]	18.1	17.5	17.8	5.4	5.7	5.4
65–74 years	16.1	14.5	14.5	4.8	4.6	4.5
75 years and over	20.4	20.7	21.4	6.2	6.8	6.4
Sex[9]						
Male	19.0	18.3	18.6	5.8	5.9	6.0
Female	17.5	16.9	17.3	5.1	5.6	4.9
Hispanic origin and race[5,9]						
Hispanic or Latino	17.3	18.2	17.7	6.2	5.5	5.7
Not Hispanic or Latino	18.2	17.4	17.9	5.4	5.7	5.4
White only	18.3	17.4	17.9	5.4	5.7	5.4
Black or African American only	18.9	18.5	19.0	5.5	5.7	6.3
Percent of poverty level[6,9]						
Below 100%	20.9	19.7	22.1	6.4	7.9	7.9
100%–less than 200%	19.6	18.1	19.2	6.5	5.8	5.9
200% or more	17.1	17.0	16.7	4.9	5.3	4.9
Geographic region[9]						
Northeast	17.2	16.2	16.1	5.1	4.9	4.5
Midwest	18.2	18.8	18.9	5.6	6.3	5.8
South	19.4	18.3	19.7	6.1	6.5	6.3
West	16.5	15.5	15.0	4.4	4.3	4.3

See footnotes at end of table.

Table 98 (page 3 of 3). Persons with hospital stays in the past year, by selected characteristics: United States, selected years 1997, 2004, and 2005

[Data are based on household interviews of a sample of the civilian noninstitutionalized population]

Characteristic	One or more hospital stays[1]			Two or more hospital stays[1]		
	1997	2004	2005	1997	2004	2005
Location of residence[9]	Percent					
Within MSA[8]	17.8	17.1	17.4	5.2	5.6	5.2
Outside MSA[8]	19.1	18.7	19.2	6.3	5.8	6.2

* Estimates are considered unreliable. Data preceded by an asterisk have a relative standard error (RSE) of 20%–30%. Data not shown have an RSE of greater than 30%.
- - - Data not available.
[1]These estimates exclude hospitalizations for institutionalized persons and those who died while hospitalized. See Appendix II, Hospital utilization.
[2]Includes all other races not shown separately and unknown health insurance status.
[3]Estimates for persons 1 year and over are age-adjusted to the year 2000 standard population using six age groups: 1–17 years, 18–44 years, 45–54 years, 55–64 years, 65–74 years, and 75 years of age and over. See Appendix II, Age adjustment.
[4]Estimates are for persons 1–64 years of age and are age-adjusted to the year 2000 standard population using four age groups: 1–17 years, 18–44 years, 45–54 years, and 55–64 years of age. See Appendix II, Age adjustment.
[5]The race groups, white, black, American Indian or Alaska Native, Asian, Native Hawaiian or Other Pacific Islander, and 2 or more races, include persons of Hispanic and non-Hispanic origin. Persons of Hispanic origin may be of any race. Starting with 1999 data, race-specific estimates are tabulated according to the 1997 Revisions to the Standards for Federal Data on Race and Ethnicity and are not strictly comparable with estimates for earlier years. The five single-race categories plus multiple-race categories shown in the table conform to the 1997 Standards. Starting with 1999 data, race-specific estimates are for persons who reported only one racial group; the category 2 or more races includes persons who reported more than one racial group. Prior to 1999, data were tabulated according to the 1977 Standards with four racial groups, and the Asian only category included Native Hawaiian or Other Pacific Islander. Estimates for single-race categories prior to 1999 included persons who reported one race or, if they reported more than one race, identified one race as best representing their race. Starting with 2003 data, race responses of other race and unspecified multiple race were treated as missing, and then race was imputed if these were the only race responses. Almost all persons with a race response of other race were of Hispanic origin. See Appendix II, Hispanic origin; Race.
[6]Percent of poverty level is based on family income and family size and composition using U.S. Census Bureau poverty thresholds. Missing family income data were imputed for 24%–28% of persons 1–64 years of age in 1997–1998 and 30%–33% in 1999–2005; and 36%–41% of persons 65 years of age and over in 1997–1998 and 43%–47% in 1999–2005. See Appendix II, Family income; Poverty.
[7]Health insurance categories are mutually exclusive. Persons who reported both Medicaid and private coverage are classified as having private coverage. Starting with 1997 data, Medicaid includes state-sponsored health plans and State Children's Health Insurance Program (SCHIP). In addition to private and Medicaid, the insured category also includes military, other government, and Medicare coverage. Persons not covered by private insurance, Medicaid, SCHIP, public assistance (through 1996), state-sponsored or other government-sponsored health plans (starting in 1997), Medicare, or military plans are considered to have no health insurance coverage. Persons with only Indian Health Service coverage are considered to have no health insurance coverage. See Appendix II, Health insurance coverage.
[8]MSA is metropolitan statistical area.
[9]Estimates are for persons 65 years of age and over and are age-adjusted to the year 2000 standard population using two age groups: 65–74 years and 75 years and over. See Appendix II, Age adjustment.

NOTES: Standard errors are available in the spreadsheet version of this table. Available from: www.cdc.gov/nchs/hus.htm. Data for additional years are available. See Appendix III.

SOURCE: Centers for Disease Control and Prevention, National Center for Health Statistics, National Health Interview Survey, family core questionnaire.

Table 99 (page 1 of 2). Discharges, days of care, and average length of stay in nonfederal short-stay hospitals, by selected characteristics: United States, selected years 1980–2005

[Data are based on a sample of hospital records]

Characteristic	*1980*[1]	*1985*[1]	*1990*	*1995*	*2000*	*2002*	*2003*	*2004*	*2005*
				Discharges per 1,000 population					
Total, age-adjusted[2]	173.4	151.4	125.2	118.0	113.3	117.3	119.5	118.4	116.2
Total, crude	167.7	148.4	122.3	115.7	112.8	117.5	120.0	119.2	117.4
Age									
Under 18 years	75.6	61.4	46.4	42.4	40.3	43.4	43.6	43.0	41.1
18–44 years	155.3	128.0	102.7	91.4	84.9	90.3	91.3	91.1	89.8
45–54 years	174.8	146.8	112.4	98.5	92.1	95.6	99.5	99.7	96.4
55–64 years	215.4	194.8	163.3	148.3	141.5	146.5	145.7	143.6	140.2
65 years and over	383.7	369.8	334.1	347.7	353.4	357.5	367.9	362.9	359.6
65–74 years	315.8	297.2	261.6	260.0	254.6	254.0	265.1	259.2	262.9
75 years and over	489.3	475.6	434.0	459.1	462.0	466.6	475.2	470.2	458.8
Sex[2]									
Male	153.2	137.3	113.0	104.8	99.1	102.4	104.4	102.6	101.3
Female	195.0	167.3	139.0	131.7	127.7	132.9	135.1	134.9	132.0
Geographic region[2]									
Northeast	162.0	142.6	133.2	133.5	127.5	123.5	127.6	128.8	124.6
Midwest	192.1	158.1	128.8	113.3	110.9	113.6	117.1	114.4	117.5
South	179.7	155.5	132.5	125.2	120.9	126.7	125.8	125.6	120.2
West	150.5	145.7	100.7	96.7	89.4	99.7	103.9	101.2	100.6
				Days of care per 1,000 population					
Total, age-adjusted[2]	1,297.0	997.5	818.9	638.6	557.7	570.9	574.6	568.7	554.2
Total, crude	1,216.7	957.7	784.0	620.2	554.6	571.7	577.8	574.1	562.1
Age									
Under 18 years	341.4	281.2	226.3	184.7	179.0	195.2	195.5	193.2	191.8
18–44 years	818.6	619.2	467.7	351.7	309.4	333.9	339.7	334.9	330.5
45–54 years	1,314.9	967.8	699.7	516.2	437.4	456.7	477.2	491.1	471.1
55–64 years	1,889.4	1,436.9	1,172.3	867.2	729.1	752.2	735.9	735.2	712.4
65 years and over	4,098.3	3,228.0	2,895.6	2,373.7	2,111.9	2,085.1	2,088.3	2,048.6	1,988.3
65–74 years	3,147.0	2,437.3	2,087.8	1,684.7	1,439.0	1,411.9	1,428.9	1,405.2	1,398.5
75 years and over	5,578.8	4,381.3	4,009.1	3,247.8	2,851.9	2,795.0	2,776.1	2,714.9	2,593.9
Sex[2]									
Male	1,239.7	973.3	805.8	623.9	535.9	549.5	546.7	541.1	530.1
Female	1,365.2	1,033.1	840.5	654.9	581.0	596.0	605.2	599.6	582.9
Geographic region[2]									
Northeast	1,400.6	1,113.0	1,026.7	839.0	718.6	690.0	694.4	687.6	663.6
Midwest	1,484.8	1,078.6	830.6	590.9	500.5	502.1	507.9	498.7	495.4
South	1,262.3	957.7	820.4	666.0	592.5	618.6	609.8	614.2	583.0
West	956.9	824.7	575.5	451.1	408.2	454.7	476.4	457.5	469.0
				Average length of stay in days					
Total, age-adjusted[2]	7.5	6.6	6.5	5.4	4.9	4.9	4.8	4.8	4.8
Total, crude	7.3	6.5	6.4	5.4	4.9	4.9	4.8	4.8	4.8
Age									
Under 18 years	4.5	4.6	4.9	4.4	4.4	4.5	4.5	4.5	4.7
18–44 years	5.3	4.8	4.6	3.8	3.6	3.7	3.7	3.7	3.7
45–54 years	7.5	6.6	6.2	5.2	4.8	4.8	4.8	4.9	4.9
55–64 years	8.8	7.4	7.2	5.8	5.2	5.1	5.1	5.1	5.1
65 years and over	10.7	8.7	8.7	6.8	6.0	5.8	5.7	5.6	5.5
65–74 years	10.0	8.2	8.0	6.5	5.7	5.6	5.4	5.4	5.3
75 years and over	11.4	9.2	9.2	7.1	6.2	6.0	5.8	5.8	5.7
Sex[2]									
Male	8.1	7.1	7.1	6.0	5.4	5.4	5.2	5.3	5.2
Female	7.0	6.2	6.0	5.0	4.6	4.5	4.5	4.4	4.4

See footnotes at end of table.

Table 99 (page 2 of 2). Discharges, days of care, and average length of stay in nonfederal short-stay hospitals, by selected characteristics: United States, selected years 1980–2005

[Data are based on a sample of hospital records]

Characteristic	1980[1]	1985[1]	1990	1995	2000	2002	2003	2004	2005
Geographic region[2]	Average length of stay in days								
Northeast	8.6	7.8	7.7	6.3	5.6	5.6	5.4	5.3	5.3
Midwest	7.7	6.8	6.5	5.2	4.5	4.4	4.3	4.4	4.2
South	7.0	6.2	6.2	5.3	4.9	4.9	4.8	4.9	4.8
West	6.4	5.7	5.7	4.7	4.6	4.6	4.6	4.5	4.7

[1]Comparisons of data from 1980–1985 with data from later years should be made with caution as estimates of change may reflect improvements in the survey design rather than true changes in hospital use. See Appendix I, National Hospital Discharge Survey.

[2]Estimates are age-adjusted to the year 2000 standard population using six age groups: under 18 years, 18–44 years, 45–54 years, 55–64 years, 65–74 years, and 75 years and over. See Appendix II, Age adjustment.

NOTES: Excludes newborn infants. Rates are based on the civilian population as of July 1. Starting with *Health, United States, 2003*, rates for 2000 and beyond are based on the 2000 census. Rates for 1990–1999 use population estimates based on the 1990 census adjusted for net underenumeration using the 1990 National Population Adjustment Matrix from the U.S. Census Bureau. Rates for 1990–1999 are not strictly comparable with rates for 2000 and beyond because population estimates for 1990–1999 have not been revised to reflect the 2000 census. See Appendix I, National Hospital Discharge Survey; Population Census and Population Estimates. Data for additional years are available. See Appendix III.

SOURCE: Centers for Disease Control and Prevention, National Center for Health Statistics, National Hospital Discharge Survey.

Table 100 (page 1 of 3). Discharges and days of care in nonfederal short-stay hospitals, by sex, age, and selected first-listed diagnoses: United States, 1990, 2000, and 2005

[Data are based on a sample of hospital records]

Sex, age, and first-listed diagnosis	Discharges 1990	Discharges 2000	Discharges 2005	Days of care 1990	Days of care 2000	Days of care 2005
Both sexes	Number per 1,000 population					
Total, age-adjusted[1,2]	125.2	113.3	116.2	818.9	557.7	554.2
Total, crude[2]	122.3	112.8	117.4	784.0	554.6	562.1
Male						
All ages[1,2]	113.0	99.1	101.3	805.8	535.9	530.1
Under 18 years[2]	46.3	40.9	41.2	233.6	195.6	200.6
Pneumonia	3.7	2.6	2.9	16.7	8.5	9.0
Asthma	3.3	3.5	2.7	9.3	7.4	6.3
Injuries and poisoning	6.8	5.0	4.9	30.1	21.4	*24.0
Fracture, all sites	2.2	1.8	1.6	9.3	7.2	*6.1
18–44 years[2]	57.9	45.0	47.1	351.7	217.5	228.3
HIV infection	*0.3	0.6	0.3	*3.0	*5.4	2.6
Alcohol and drug[3]	3.7	4.0	3.6	33.1	19.1	16.1
Serious mental illness[4]	3.4	*5.3	6.1	47.1	*43.6	*50.3
Diseases of heart	3.0	2.7	2.9	16.3	9.4	11.1
Intervertebral disc disorders	2.6	1.5	1.1	10.7	3.2	2.5
Injuries and poisoning	13.1	7.3	8.0	65.7	33.2	36.7
Fracture, all sites	4.0	2.5	2.7	22.7	12.8	13.4
45–64 years[2]	140.3	112.7	114.9	943.4	570.4	577.3
HIV infection	*0.1	*0.5	0.4	*	*	4.3
Malignant neoplasms	10.6	6.2	5.9	99.1	42.1	39.2
Trachea, bronchus, lung	2.7	0.9	0.8	19.1	5.2	5.9
Diabetes	2.9	3.7	3.1	21.2	22.5	16.4
Alcohol and drug[3]	3.5	3.5	4.0	29.7	15.8	18.6
Serious mental illness[4]	2.5	*4.0	4.7	34.8	*34.6	41.2
Diseases of heart	31.7	26.4	22.4	185.0	101.5	85.1
Ischemic heart disease	22.6	17.7	13.3	128.2	63.8	47.0
Acute myocardial infarction	7.4	5.9	4.3	55.8	27.8	19.8
Heart failure	3.1	3.4	3.9	21.0	17.3	19.1
Cerebrovascular diseases	4.1	3.8	3.3	40.7	19.8	19.5
Pneumonia	3.4	3.4	3.5	27.1	20.3	20.0
Injuries and poisoning	11.6	8.8	10.7	82.6	49.8	59.2
Fracture, all sites	3.3	2.5	2.6	24.2	16.2	14.7
65–74 years[2]	287.8	264.9	274.3	2,251.5	1,489.7	1,450.3
Malignant neoplasms	27.9	17.6	18.6	277.6	121.2	126.7
Large intestine and rectum	3.0	3.0	2.5	34.2	27.3	19.6
Trachea, bronchus, lung	6.4	2.8	2.8	55.7	19.2	21.6
Prostate	5.1	3.7	2.9	33.1	14.0	*9.7
Diabetes	4.4	4.7	5.2	39.8	29.0	29.0
Serious mental illness[4]	2.5	*3.4	2.8	43.8	39.9	27.6
Diseases of heart	69.4	70.6	63.9	487.2	331.9	280.8
Ischemic heart disease	42.0	39.7	34.3	285.2	171.2	148.2
Acute myocardial infarction	14.0	12.5	12.0	122.4	66.5	72.8
Heart failure	11.8	13.6	13.2	93.1	77.6	64.8
Cerebrovascular diseases	13.8	13.2	12.8	114.8	59.0	58.9
Pneumonia	11.2	12.7	14.7	106.9	81.5	75.9
Hyperplasia of prostate	14.4	5.4	3.4	65.0	15.0	8.2
Osteoarthritis	5.5	10.3	12.6	48.5	48.8	48.0
Injuries and poisoning	17.6	17.9	19.4	139.0	105.7	119.1
Fracture, all sites	4.5	4.7	4.5	45.9	29.9	25.0
Fracture of neck of femur (hip)	1.5	*2.0	1.7	*18.1	*15.9	*12.0

See footnotes at end of table.

Table 100 (page 2 of 3). Discharges and days of care in nonfederal short-stay hospitals, by sex, age, and selected first-listed diagnoses: United States, 1990, 2000, and 2005

[Data are based on a sample of hospital records]

Sex, age, and first-listed diagnosis	Discharges			Days of care		
	1990	2000	2005	1990	2000	2005
	Number per 1,000 population					
Male—Con.						
75 years and over[2]	478.5	467.4	476.0	4,231.6	2,888.0	2,745.4
Malignant neoplasms	41.0	21.9	22.7	408.3	165.2	155.8
Large intestine and rectum	5.4	4.2	3.5	80.7	44.1	33.0
Trachea, bronchus, lung	5.4	3.0	3.2	53.4	18.3	21.9
Prostate	9.7	3.2	1.9	65.6	*19.4	*10.1
Diabetes	4.6	6.5	5.3	51.2	43.2	35.4
Serious mental illness[4]	*2.6	2.9	2.0	*40.5	*32.6	*19.3
Diseases of heart	106.2	113.3	102.6	855.7	600.9	490.8
Ischemic heart disease	49.1	53.0	41.0	398.1	276.1	201.3
Acute myocardial infarction	23.1	23.0	17.9	227.5	136.5	117.8
Heart failure	31.8	30.9	31.5	248.6	178.6	158.5
Cerebrovascular diseases	30.2	30.2	24.2	298.3	171.2	132.4
Pneumonia	38.1	36.7	35.8	391.3	228.6	208.7
Hyperplasia of prostate	17.9	6.8	5.2	109.2	21.6	17.1
Osteoarthritis	6.6	7.2	12.6	60.7	28.7	48.0
Injuries and poisoning	31.2	33.6	32.1	341.3	257.7	197.2
Fracture, all sites	13.7	14.4	13.4	145.1	*119.2	91.5
Fracture of neck of femur (hip)	8.5	8.4	7.8	97.8	63.3	54.1
Female						
All ages[1,2]	139.0	127.7	132.0	840.5	581.0	582.9
Under 18 years[2]	46.4	39.6	41.0	218.7	161.5	182.6
Pneumonia	2.9	2.4	2.5	13.7	9.5	8.4
Asthma	2.2	2.4	1.7	6.8	5.5	3.8
Injuries and poisoning	4.3	3.1	3.1	16.7	*12.0	12.0
Fracture, all sites	1.3	0.9	0.9	6.4	2.3	2.6
18–44 years[2]	146.8	124.8	133.1	582.0	401.1	434.2
HIV infection	*	0.3	*0.2	*	*2.1	*
Delivery	69.9	64.5	69.8	195.0	160.2	180.3
Alcohol and drug[3]	1.6	*2.1	2.0	14.1	*10.8	*9.9
Serious mental illness[4]	3.7	*5.4	*6.8	54.3	*41.1	*45.6
Diseases of heart	1.3	1.7	1.7	7.2	6.3	7.6
Intervertebral disc disorders	1.5	1.0	0.9	7.3	2.4	2.0
Injuries and poisoning	6.7	4.3	5.1	36.6	18.1	22.2
Fracture, all sites	1.6	1.0	1.1	10.7	4.5	5.8
45–64 years[2]	131.0	110.2	114.5	886.5	533.6	566.4
HIV infection	*	*	*	*	*	*
Malignant neoplasms	12.7	6.1	6.1	107.4	34.7	38.5
Trachea, bronchus, lung	1.7	0.5	0.7	14.8	3.4	4.3
Breast	2.8	1.3	1.1	12.1	2.6	2.7
Diabetes	2.9	2.9	2.7	25.8	15.0	13.1
Alcohol and drug[3]	1.0	1.5	1.7	8.0	*7.1	7.1
Serious mental illness[4]	4.0	4.6	6.0	60.5	42.7	53.0
Diseases of heart	16.6	14.6	12.0	101.1	59.5	55.9
Ischemic heart disease	9.9	7.8	5.5	57.4	29.5	*24.3
Acute myocardial infarction	2.8	2.0	1.7	21.6	10.0	9.4
Heart failure	2.2	2.9	2.6	16.3	13.6	14.8
Cerebrovascular diseases	3.0	3.5	2.8	32.1	19.5	14.9
Pneumonia	3.3	3.6	3.4	26.1	20.7	18.0
Injuries and poisoning	9.4	7.7	8.7	63.3	41.2	46.0
Fracture, all sites	3.1	2.7	2.4	25.0	13.3	11.9

See footnotes at end of table.

Table 100 (page 3 of 3). Discharges and days of care in nonfederal short-stay hospitals, by sex, age, and selected first-listed diagnoses: United States, 1990, 2000, and 2005

[Data are based on a sample of hospital records]

Sex, age, and first-listed diagnosis	*Discharges*			*Days of care*		
	1990	*2000*	*2005*	*1990*	*2000*	*2005*
Female—Con.	Number per 1,000 population					
65–74 years[2]	241.1	246.1	253.3	1,959.3	1,397.1	1,354.9
Malignant neoplasms	20.9	14.1	12.5	189.8	101.0	82.9
Large intestine and rectum	2.4	1.7	1.8	34.9	15.2	14.0
Trachea, bronchus, lung	2.6	2.4	2.4	26.9	*17.5	17.1
Breast	3.9	2.8	1.3	17.6	*	*4.2
Diabetes	5.8	4.6	4.8	46.8	26.1	22.9
Serious mental illness[4]	3.9	4.0	4.3	62.8	46.3	47.4
Diseases of heart	45.1	52.1	43.0	316.9	256.0	191.1
Ischemic heart disease	24.4	23.3	17.5	153.8	113.9	69.5
Acute myocardial infarction	7.5	8.0	5.3	58.1	52.8	28.1
Heart failure	9.5	12.8	11.0	84.0	69.1	54.6
Cerebrovascular diseases	11.3	12.3	10.3	96.0	59.4	44.8
Pneumonia	8.5	11.3	11.8	79.6	71.4	65.8
Osteoarthritis	7.8	10.0	17.7	74.5	47.2	67.4
Injuries and poisoning	17.8	18.3	18.5	166.2	109.9	114.3
Fracture, all sites	8.4	7.7	8.0	97.3	43.8	43.8
Fracture of neck of femur (hip)	3.6	3.2	3.0	*59.6	21.1	20.8
75 years and over[2]	409.6	458.8	448.4	3,887.1	2,830.8	2,501.4
Malignant neoplasms	22.1	17.6	14.3	257.3	125.7	104.4
Large intestine and rectum	4.6	3.4	2.8	69.8	28.4	26.4
Trachea, bronchus, lung	2.1	1.9	2.0	20.6	14.0	13.6
Breast	3.9	2.5	1.6	22.0	*8.9	*
Diabetes	4.6	6.3	5.5	55.3	34.0	26.7
Serious mental illness[4]	4.2	4.7	3.1	78.4	49.2	29.7
Diseases of heart	84.6	99.1	90.5	672.8	523.4	435.8
Ischemic heart disease	33.7	35.5	26.5	253.2	185.5	119.6
Acute myocardial infarction	13.1	16.5	13.4	125.9	110.7	75.3
Heart failure	28.6	32.5	32.2	240.8	183.4	168.9
Cerebrovascular diseases	29.6	27.6	21.7	302.0	156.8	108.6
Pneumonia	23.5	30.1	28.6	255.8	206.5	168.3
Osteoarthritis	6.2	9.9	12.9	62.2	46.3	51.8
Injuries and poisoning	46.3	44.7	45.9	489.2	275.4	249.3
Fracture, all sites	31.5	30.0	27.9	352.7	190.0	150.7
Fracture of neck of femur (hip)	18.8	17.9	14.9	236.3	125.3	89.3

* Estimates are considered unreliable. Data preceded by an asterisk have a relative standard error (RSE) of 20%–30%. Data not shown have an RSE of greater than 30%.

[1]Estimates are age-adjusted to the year 2000 standard population using six age groups: under 18 years, 18–44 years, 45–54 years, 55–64 years, 65–74 years, and 75 years and over. See Appendix II, Age adjustment.

[2]Includes discharges with first-listed diagnoses not shown in table.

[3]Includes abuse, dependence, and withdrawal. These estimates are for nonfederal short-stay hospitals only and do not include alcohol and drug discharges from other types of facilities or programs such as the Department of Veterans Affairs or day treatment programs.

[4]These estimates are for nonfederal short-stay hospitals only and do not include serious mental illness discharges from other types of facilities or programs such as the Department of Veterans Affairs or long-term hospitals.

NOTES: Excludes newborn infants. Diagnostic categories are based on the *International Classification of Diseases, Ninth Revision, Clinical Modification* (ICD–9–CM). See Appendix II, Diagnosis; Human immunodeficiency virus (HIV) disease; *International Classification of Diseases, Ninth Revision, Clinical Modification*; Table X for ICD–9–CM codes. Rates are based on the civilian population as of July 1. Starting with *Health, United States, 2003*, rates for 2000 and beyond are based on the 2000 census. Rates for 1990–1999 use population estimates based on the 1990 census adjusted for net underenumeration using the 1990 National Population Adjustment Matrix from the U.S. Census Bureau. Rates for 1990–1999 are not strictly comparable with rates for 2000 and beyond because population estimates for 1990–1999 have not been revised to reflect the 2000 census. See Appendix I, National Hospital Discharge Survey: Population Census and Population Estimates. Data for additional years are available. See Appendix III.

SOURCE: Centers for Disease Control and Prevention, National Center for Health Statistics, National Hospital Discharge Survey.

Table 101 (page 1 of 3). Discharges and average length of stay in nonfederal short-stay hospitals, by sex, age, and selected first-listed diagnoses: United States, 1990, 2000, and 2005

[Data are based on a sample of hospital records]

	Discharges			*Average length of stay*[1]		
Sex, age, and first-listed diagnosis	*1990*	*2000*	*2005*	*1990*	*2000*	*2005*
Both sexes	Number in thousands			Number of days		
Total[2]	30,788	31,706	34,667	6.4	4.9	4.8
Male						
All ages[2]	12,280	12,514	13,902	6.9	5.3	5.2
Under 18 years[2]	1,572	1,515	1,550	5.0	4.8	4.9
Pneumonia	124	95	108	4.6	3.3	3.1
Asthma	111	129	103	2.8	2.1	2.3
Injuries and poisoning	232	185	183	4.4	4.3	*4.9
Fracture, all sites	76	68	61	4.2	3.9	*3.8
18–44 years[2]	3,120	2,498	2,660	6.1	4.8	4.8
HIV infection	*15	32	20	*10.6	*9.4	7.5
Alcohol and drug[3]	201	224	203	8.9	4.7	4.5
Serious mental illness[4]	184	*296	344	13.8	*8.2	*8.3
Diseases of heart	163	148	166	5.4	3.5	3.8
Intervertebral disc disorders	138	81	60	4.2	2.2	2.3
Injuries and poisoning	704	408	452	5.0	4.5	4.6
Fracture, all sites	217	141	151	5.6	5.0	5.0
45–64 years[2]	3,115	3,424	4,076	6.7	5.1	5.0
HIV infection	*3	*15	15	*7.1	*	10.4
Malignant neoplasms	235	188	211	9.4	6.8	6.6
Trachea, bronchus, lung	60	26	29	7.1	6.0	7.3
Diabetes	65	114	110	7.3	6.0	5.3
Alcohol and drug[3]	77	106	141	8.5	4.5	4.7
Serious mental illness[4]	56	*120	167	13.7	*8.8	8.8
Diseases of heart	704	802	795	5.8	3.8	3.8
Ischemic heart disease	502	539	473	5.7	3.6	3.5
Acute myocardial infarction	165	178	151	7.5	4.7	4.6
Heart failure	68	102	137	6.9	5.2	4.9
Cerebrovascular diseases	91	116	118	10.0	5.2	5.9
Pneumonia	75	102	125	8.0	6.0	5.7
Injuries and poisoning	257	266	380	7.2	5.7	5.5
Fracture, all sites	74	77	93	7.2	6.4	5.6
65–74 years[2]	2,268	2,199	2,339	7.8	5.6	5.3
Malignant neoplasms	220	146	158	9.9	6.9	6.8
Large intestine and rectum	24	24	21	11.4	9.2	7.9
Trachea, bronchus, lung	50	23	24	8.7	6.8	7.6
Prostate	40	31	25	6.5	3.8	*3.3
Diabetes	34	39	44	9.1	6.2	5.6
Serious mental illness[4]	20	*28	24	17.4	*11.7	10.0
Diseases of heart	547	586	545	7.0	4.7	4.4
Ischemic heart disease	331	329	292	6.8	4.3	4.3
Acute myocardial infarction	110	104	102	8.8	5.3	6.1
Heart failure	93	113	113	7.9	5.7	4.9
Cerebrovascular diseases	108	109	109	8.3	4.5	4.6
Pneumonia	88	105	126	9.5	6.4	5.2
Hyperplasia of prostate	113	45	29	4.5	2.8	2.4
Osteoarthritis	44	86	108	8.8	4.7	3.8
Injuries and poisoning	139	149	165	7.9	5.9	6.2
Fracture, all sites	36	39	38	10.2	6.4	5.6
Fracture of neck of femur (hip)	12	*17	14	*11.8	*7.9	*7.2

See footnotes at end of table.

Table 101 (page 2 of 3). Discharges and average length of stay in nonfederal short-stay hospitals, by sex, age, and selected first-listed diagnoses: United States, 1990, 2000, and 2005

[Data are based on a sample of hospital records]

Sex, age, and first-listed diagnosis	Discharges			Average length of stay[1]		
	1990	2000	2005	1990	2000	2005
Male—Con.	Number in thousands			Number of days		
75 years and over[2]	2,203	2,878	3,276	8.8	6.2	5.8
Malignant neoplasms	189	135	156	10.0	7.6	6.9
Large intestine and rectum	25	26	24	15.0	10.6	9.4
Trachea, bronchus, lung	25	18	22	10.0	6.1	6.9
Prostate	45	20	13	6.8	*6.1	*5.2
Diabetes	21	40	36	11.0	6.6	6.7
Serious mental illness[4]	*12	18	14	*15.5	*11.2	*9.8
Diseases of heart	489	697	706	8.1	5.3	4.8
Ischemic heart disease	226	326	282	8.1	5.2	4.9
Acute myocardial infarction	106	141	123	9.9	5.9	6.6
Heart failure	147	190	217	7.8	5.8	5.0
Cerebrovascular diseases	139	186	167	9.9	5.7	5.5
Pneumonia	175	226	247	10.3	6.2	5.8
Hyperplasia of prostate	82	42	36	6.1	3.2	3.3
Osteoarthritis	30	44	86	10.3	4.5	3.8
Injuries and poisoning	144	207	221	10.9	7.7	6.1
Fracture, all sites	63	89	92	10.6	*8.3	6.8
Fracture of neck of femur (hip)	39	52	54	11.5	7.5	7.0
Female						
All ages[2]	18,508	19,192	20,766	6.1	4.6	4.5
Under 18 years[2]	1,500	1,397	1,470	4.7	4.1	4.5
Pneumonia	95	86	91	4.7	3.9	3.3
Asthma	71	85	61	3.1	2.3	2.2
Injuries and poisoning	138	111	113	3.9	*3.8	3.8
Fracture, all sites	42	32	31	5.0	2.5	3.0
18–44 years[2]	8,018	6,941	7,410	4.0	3.2	3.3
HIV infection	*	15	*13	*	*7.5	*
Delivery	3,815	3,588	3,888	2.8	2.5	2.6
Alcohol and drug[3]	85	*116	110	9.1	*5.2	*5.0
Serious mental illness[4]	200	*300	*381	14.8	*7.6	*6.7
Diseases of heart	73	95	96	5.4	3.7	4.4
Intervertebral disc disorders	84	58	51	4.7	2.3	2.2
Injuries and poisoning	366	237	282	5.5	4.2	4.4
Fracture, all sites	85	57	60	6.9	4.4	5.4
45–64 years[2]	3,129	3,534	4,273	6.8	4.8	4.9
HIV infection	*	*	*	*	*	*
Malignant neoplasms	303	195	228	8.5	5.7	6.3
Trachea, bronchus, lung	41	17	25	8.6	6.4	6.3
Breast	67	40	39	4.3	2.1	2.6
Diabetes	70	93	99	8.9	5.2	4.9
Alcohol and drug[3]	23	47	63	8.2	*4.8	4.2
Serious mental illness[4]	95	146	223	15.2	9.4	8.9
Diseases of heart	397	470	447	6.1	4.1	4.7
Ischemic heart disease	237	251	203	5.8	3.8	*4.5
Acute myocardial infarction	68	64	63	7.6	5.0	5.6
Heart failure	54	94	99	7.3	4.7	5.6
Cerebrovascular diseases	72	113	103	10.7	5.5	5.4
Pneumonia	78	116	126	8.0	5.7	5.3
Injuries and poisoning	225	248	324	6.7	5.3	5.3
Fracture, all sites	75	87	88	7.9	4.9	5.0

See footnotes at end of table.

Table 101 (page 3 of 3). Discharges and average length of stay in nonfederal short-stay hospitals, by sex, age, and selected first-listed diagnoses: United States, 1990, 2000, and 2005

[Data are based on a sample of hospital records]

Sex, age, and first-listed diagnosis	Discharges			Average length of stay[1]		
	1990	2000	2005	1990	2000	2005
Female—Con.	Number in thousands			Number of days		
65–74 years[2]	2,421	2,479	2,561	8.1	5.7	5.3
Malignant neoplasms	210	142	127	9.1	7.2	6.6
Large intestine and rectum	24	17	18	14.5	9.0	7.7
Trachea, bronchus, lung	26	25	24	10.2	*7.1	7.1
Breast	40	29	13	4.5	*	*3.3
Diabetes	59	47	49	8.0	5.6	4.8
Serious mental illness[4]	39	40	43	16.3	11.7	11.1
Diseases of heart	453	525	435	7.0	4.9	4.4
Ischemic heart disease	245	235	177	6.3	4.9	4.0
Acute myocardial infarction	75	81	53	7.8	6.6	5.3
Heart failure	95	128	112	8.8	5.4	4.9
Cerebrovascular diseases	114	124	104	8.5	4.8	4.3
Pneumonia	85	114	119	9.4	6.3	5.6
Osteoarthritis	78	101	179	9.5	4.7	3.8
Injuries and poisoning	179	185	187	9.3	6.0	6.2
Fracture, all sites	85	77	81	11.5	5.7	5.5
Fracture of neck of femur (hip)	36	32	30	*16.7	6.7	7.0
75 years and over[2]	3,440	4,840	5,052	9.5	6.2	5.6
Malignant neoplasms	185	186	161	11.7	7.1	7.3
Large intestine and rectum	39	36	32	15.1	8.4	9.3
Trachea, bronchus, lung	18	20	22	9.9	7.3	6.9
Breast	33	27	18	5.7	*3.5	*
Diabetes	39	67	62	11.9	5.4	4.8
Serious mental illness[4]	35	49	34	18.7	10.5	9.7
Diseases of heart	711	1,045	1,020	8.0	5.3	4.8
Ischemic heart disease	283	375	299	7.5	5.2	4.5
Acute myocardial infarction	110	174	151	9.6	6.7	5.6
Heart failure	240	343	363	8.4	5.6	5.2
Cerebrovascular diseases	249	292	244	10.2	5.7	5.0
Pneumonia	198	317	323	10.9	6.9	5.9
Osteoarthritis	52	105	146	10.1	4.7	4.0
Injuries and poisoning	389	472	517	10.6	6.2	5.4
Fracture, all sites	265	316	315	11.2	6.3	5.4
Fracture of neck of femur (hip)	158	189	168	12.5	7.0	6.0

* Estimates are considered unreliable. Data preceded by an asterisk have a relative standard error (RSE) of 20%–30%. Data not shown have an RSE of greater than 30%.

[1]Crude estimates.

[2]Includes discharges with first-listed diagnoses not shown in table.

[3]Includes abuse, dependence, and withdrawal. These estimates are for nonfederal short-stay hospitals only and do not include alcohol and drug discharges from other types of facilities or programs such as the Department of Veterans Affairs or day treatment programs.

[4]These estimates are for nonfederal short-stay hospitals only and do not include serious mental illness discharges from other types of facilities or programs such as the Department of Veterans Affairs or long-term hospitals.

NOTES: Excludes newborn infants. Diagnostic categories are based on the *International Classification of Diseases, Ninth Revision, Clinical Modification* (ICD–9–CM). See Appendix II, Diagnosis; Human immunodeficiency virus (HIV) disease; International Classification of Diseases, Clinical Modification; Table X for ICD–9–CM codes. Data for additional years are available. See Appendix III.

SOURCE: Centers for Disease Control and Prevention, National Center for Health Statistics, National Hospital Discharge Survey.

ble 102 (page 1 of 3). Discharges with at least one procedure in nonfederal short-stay hospitals, sex, age, and selected procedures: United States, average annual 1994–1995 and 2004–2005

a are based on a sample of hospital records]

Age and procedure (any listed)	Both sexes		Male		Female	
	1994–1995	*2004–2005*	*1994–1995*	*2004–2005*	*1994–1995*	*2004–2005*
18 years and over			Number in thousands[1]			
spital discharges with at least one procedure[2]	17,969	19,889	6,655	7,284	11,314	12,605
			Number per 10,000 population[3]			
spital discharges with at least one procedure, ge-adjusted[2,4]	935.2	902.6	789.6	723.1	1,091.3	1,093.8
spital discharges with at least one procedure, crude[2]	927.6	902.3	717.3	682.9	1,120.8	1,108.0
rdiac catheterization	53.5	56.1	68.3	70.2	39.9	43.0
ertion, replacement, removal, and revision of acemaker leads or device	9.3	9.0	9.5	9.5	9.1	8.4
giocardiography using contrast material	44.6	47.7	56.2	58.2	34.0	37.8
erations on vessels of heart	38.0	41.4	54.4	58.0	22.9	25.8
Removal of coronary artery obstruction and insertion of stent(s)	21.3	30.1	29.2	41.8	14.1	19.0
Insertion of coronary artery stent(s)[5]	. . .	27.0	. . .	37.8	. . .	16.9
Insertion of drug-eluting coronary artery stent(s)[5]	. . .	22.4	. . .	31.1	. . .	14.2
Coronary artery bypass graft	17.5	11.6	26.4	16.5	9.3	7.0
agnostic procedures on small intestine	43.9	47.5	41.7	43.7	45.9	51.2
agnostic procedures on large intestine	26.2	25.4	22.1	20.9	29.9	29.6
agnostic radiology	59.0	34.7	57.3	31.8	60.5	37.3
Computerized axial tomography	43.1	28.3	43.1	26.3	43.1	30.1
agnostic ultrasound	54.6	33.4	47.5	31.7	61.2	35.0
agnetic resonance imaging	10.1	10.6	9.8	9.7	10.5	11.3
int replacement of lower extremity	24.6	46.3	18.1	36.1	30.6	55.8
Total hip replacement	6.6	10.6	5.5	9.7	7.6	11.4
Partial hip replacement	4.9	10.3	2.6	7.9	7.0	12.6
Total knee replacement	10.6	21.9	8.0	15.6	13.1	27.8
eduction of fracture and dislocation	25.7	24.2	23.0	21.3	28.3	27.0
cision or destruction of intervertebral disc and spinal fusion	18.0	19.1	21.1	19.3	15.2	19.0
Excision or destruction of intervertebral disc	15.1	13.8	17.8	14.3	12.6	13.3
holecystectomy	23.7	18.6	15.3	12.9	31.4	23.9
Laparoscopic cholecystectomy	16.0	14.2	8.6	8.9	22.7	19.2
sis of peritoneal adhesions	16.6	15.3	6.3	6.5	26.0	23.4
18–44 years			Number in thousands[1]			
ospital discharges with at least one procedure[2]	7,311	7,326	1,698	1,457	5,613	5,869
			Number per 10,000 population[3]			
ospital discharges with at least one procedure[2]	668.9	653.2	312.1	258.1	1,022.5	1,053.2
epair of hernia	4.6	4.4	4.4	3.1	4.7	5.6
esarean section and removal of fetus[6]	. . .	. . .	. . .	. . .	144.2	218.8
orceps, vacuum, and breech delivery[6]	. . .	. . .	. . .	. . .	78.3	52.5
ther procedures inducing or assisting delivery[6,7]	. . .	. . .	. . .	. . .	398.7	400.8
ilation and curettage of uterus[6]	. . .	. . .	. . .	. . .	15.3	7.4
otal abdominal hysterectomy[6]	. . .	. . .	. . .	. . .	37.2	32.6
aginal hysterectomy[6]	. . .	. . .	. . .	. . .	17.7	16.6
ardiac catheterization	7.9	8.2	11.3	10.4	4.6	6.1
ngiocardiography using contrast material	7.3	7.7	10.4	9.7	4.1	5.6
)perations on vessels of heart	3.8	4.1	6.0	6.0	1.6	2.2
Removal of coronary artery obstruction and insertion of stent(s)	2.8	3.3	4.3	4.8	1.3	1.8
Insertion of coronary artery stent(s)[5]	. . .	3.0	. . .	4.4	. . .	1.6
Insertion of drug-eluting coronary artery stent(s)[5]	. . .	2.3	. . .	3.4	. . .	1.3
Coronary artery bypass graft	1.0	0.8	1.7	1.2	*	*
)iagnostic procedures on small intestine	13.3	13.4	13.7	11.7	12.8	15.2
)iagnostic procedures on large intestine	5.9	7.1	5.2	6.1	6.7	8.2
)iagnostic radiology	26.0	15.6	24.6	12.8	27.3	18.4
Computerized axial tomography	16.7	11.7	19.3	11.2	14.2	12.2
)iagnostic ultrasound	23.3	11.4	15.1	9.2	31.5	13.6
lagnetic resonance imaging	4.3	4.0	4.2	3.8	4.4	4.2
Reduction of fracture and dislocation	14.1	12.7	18.8	17.6	9.4	7.7
Excision or destruction of intervertebral disc and spinal fusion	15.2	12.2	18.8	13.3	11.7	11.2
Excision or destruction of intervertebral disc	13.0	9.6	15.8	10.4	10.3	8.8
Cholecystectomy	14.0	12.1	4.9	5.1	22.9	19.2
Laparoscopic cholecystectomy	10.9	10.4	3.5	4.1	18.3	16.8
Lysis of peritoneal adhesions	13.6	12.0	2.1	1.8	25.1	22.4

See footnotes at end of table.

Table 102 (page 2 of 3). Discharges with at least one procedure in nonfederal short-stay hospitals, by sex, age, and selected procedures: United States, average annual 1994–1995 and 2004–2005

[Data are based on a sample of hospital records]

Age and procedure (any listed)	Both sexes		Male		Female	
	1994–1995	2004–2005	1994–1995	2004–2005	1994–1995	2004–2005
45–64 years						
	Number in thousands[1]					
Hospital discharges with at least one procedure[2]	4,111	5,210	2,054	2,560	2,056	2,650
	Number per 10,000 population[3]					
Hospital discharges with at least one procedure[2]	800.2	726.4	826.3	732.5	775.8	720.5
Transurethral prostatectomy[8]	. . .	. . .	12.7	4.8	. . .	. . .
Repair of hernia	14.6	12.2	15.1	10.4	14.2	13.9
Total abdominal hysterectomy[6]	. . .	. . .	. . .	. . .	47.5	41.2
Vaginal hysterectomy[6]	. . .	. . .	. . .	. . .	21.2	20.0
Cardiac catheterization	85.0	73.3	115.4	99.3	56.6	48.7
Insertion, replacement, removal, and revision of pacemaker leads or device	5.6	3.7	6.2	4.8	5.0	2.6
Angiocardiography using contrast material	70.7	61.2	94.5	80.1	48.3	43.2
Operations on vessels of heart	61.5	54.5	94.7	83.8	30.3	26.7
Removal of coronary artery obstruction and insertion of stent(s)	36.1	40.1	53.7	61.2	19.7	20.0
Insertion of coronary artery stent(s)[5]	. . .	36.4	. . .	56.1	. . .	17.7
Insertion of drug-eluting coronary artery stent(s)[5]	. . .	30.5	. . .	46.8	. . .	14.9
Coronary artery bypass graft	26.7	14.8	43.0	23.0	11.4	7.0
Diagnostic procedures on small intestine	41.9	43.7	44.6	45.6	39.4	41.9
Diagnostic procedures on large intestine	22.8	20.6	22.4	19.0	23.3	22.2
Diagnostic radiology	58.0	32.3	61.6	31.5	54.6	33.1
Computerized axial tomography	41.0	25.5	44.3	26.1	37.9	24.9
Diagnostic ultrasound	50.8	30.9	53.1	34.5	48.6	27.4
Magnetic resonance imaging	12.0	10.8	12.9	11.2	11.2	10.4
Joint replacement of lower extremity	19.0	48.0	18.2	38.8	19.8	56.6
Total hip replacement	5.8	11.3	6.4	11.9	5.2	10.7
Partial hip replacement	1.2	9.1	*1.2	8.1	*1.2	9.9
Total knee replacement	9.8	24.5	8.1	16.3	11.5	32.2
Reduction of fracture and dislocation	21.1	18.2	21.1	18.9	21.1	17.6
Excision or destruction of intervertebral disc and spinal fusion	24.9	27.1	27.9	27.3	22.1	26.9
Excision or destruction of intervertebral disc	21.0	20.1	24.1	20.8	18.0	19.4
Cholecystectomy	28.0	18.4	19.3	13.7	36.1	22.9
Laparoscopic cholecystectomy	19.0	13.8	11.3	9.1	26.2	18.3
Lysis of peritoneal adhesions	15.9	15.1	7.5	7.2	23.8	22.6
65–74 years						
	Number in thousands[1]					
Hospital discharges with at least one procedure[2]	3,069	3,036	1,522	1,482	1,546	1,554
	Number per 10,000 population[3]					
Hospital discharges with at least one procedure[2]	1,653.2	1,636.7	1,842.0	1,748.0	1,501.6	1,543.1
Transurethral prostatectomy[8]	. . .	. . .	101.4	41.1	. . .	. . .
Repair of hernia	26.5	22.3	34.0	21.3	20.6	23.1
Total abdominal hysterectomy[6]	. . .	. . .	. . .	. . .	22.5	15.9
Vaginal hysterectomy[6]	. . .	. . .	. . .	. . .	21.0	14.8
Cardiac catheterization	170.4	172.3	227.7	225.5	124.4	127.5
Insertion, replacement, removal, and revision of pacemaker leads or device	26.0	21.5	30.7	26.5	22.3	17.3
Angiocardiography using contrast material	140.7	143.3	184.5	185.6	105.5	107.7
Operations on vessels of heart	129.2	137.5	190.2	202.0	80.2	83.2
Removal of coronary artery obstruction and insertion of stent(s)	66.3	95.6	91.7	140.8	45.8	57.6
Insertion of coronary artery stent(s)[5]	. . .	85.4	. . .	125.8	. . .	51.4
Insertion of drug-eluting coronary artery stent(s)[5]	. . .	71.7	. . .	104.8	. . .	43.9
Coronary artery bypass graft	65.7	42.9	103.0	62.9	35.8	26.0
Diagnostic procedures on small intestine	103.2	108.3	108.5	110.4	99.0	106.6
Diagnostic procedures on large intestine	65.4	58.8	60.3	51.2	69.5	65.1
Diagnostic radiology	123.4	68.9	138.3	74.3	111.5	64.3
Computerized axial tomography	91.8	55.6	99.9	58.7	85.3	53.0
Diagnostic ultrasound	124.2	73.9	133.6	78.9	116.7	69.7
Magnetic resonance imaging	24.5	23.7	24.6	21.4	24.4	25.6
Joint replacement of lower extremity	88.1	161.5	68.9	133.4	103.6	185.2
Total hip replacement	23.8	36.2	20.7	32.1	26.4	39.6
Partial hip replacement	8.7	19.4	*5.0	15.0	11.7	23.1
Total knee replacement	47.1	91.4	36.8	69.8	55.4	109.6
Reduction of fracture and dislocation	37.3	41.0	28.0	27.5	44.7	52.4
Excision or destruction of intervertebral disc and spinal fusion	20.5	32.8	19.7	29.0	21.1	36.1
Excision or destruction of intervertebral disc	16.2	19.0	15.2	16.9	17.0	20.8
Cholecystectomy	46.6	36.2	44.4	33.4	48.4	38.6
Laparoscopic cholecystectomy	27.5	26.0	22.1	22.9	31.8	28.6
Lysis of peritoneal adhesions	24.8	22.7	20.2	17.7	28.4	26.9

See footnotes at end of table.

ble 102 (page 3 of 3). Discharges with at least one procedure in nonfederal short-stay hospitals, · sex, age, and selected procedures: United States, average annual 1994–1995 and 2004–2005

ıta are based on a sample of hospital records]

Age and procedure (any listed)	Both sexes 1994–1995	Both sexes 2004–2005	Male 1994–1995	Male 2004–2005	Female 1994–1995	Female 2004–2005
	Number in thousands[1]					
75 years and over						
ɔspital discharges with at least one procedure[2]	3,479	4,317	1,380	1,785	2,098	2,532
	Number per 10,000 population[3]					
ɔspital discharges with at least one procedure[2]	2,401.8	2,399.7	2,631.9	2,623.5	2,271.2	2,263.6
ansurethral prostatectomy[8]	. . .	. . .	150.8	63.7	. . .	. . .
epair of hernia	35.9	28.6	53.6	34.7	25.9	24.8
tal abdominal hysterectomy[6]	. . .	. . .	. . .	. . .	13.0	8.9
aginal hysterectomy[6]	. . .	. . .	. . .	. . .	10.2	6.6
ardiac catheterization	135.8	166.6	185.3	222.7	107.7	132.5
sertion, replacement, removal, and revision of ɔacemaker leads or device	67.2	70.3	83.0	87.6	58.3	59.7
ngiocardiography using contrast material	111.3	144.5	147.1	189.3	90.9	117.2
perations on vessels of heart	96.2	122.1	151.4	177.8	64.9	88.2
Removal of coronary artery obstruction and insertion of stent(s)	51.1	89.3	72.7	125.9	38.8	67.1
Insertion of coronary artery stent(s)[5]	. . .	79.3	. . .	111.6	. . .	59.6
Insertion of drug-eluting coronary artery stent(s)[5]	. . .	64.5	. . .	89.0	. . .	49.7
Coronary artery bypass graft	47.2	33.6	82.8	52.3	27.0	22.2
iagnostic procedures on small intestine	206.2	212.9	212.0	215.9	202.9	211.0
iagnostic procedures on large intestine	140.4	123.7	135.5	115.9	143.3	128.4
iagnostic radiology	228.8	127.9	247.6	139.2	218.1	121.0
Computerized axial tomography	187.3	114.7	194.4	112.3	183.2	116.1
iagnostic ultrasound	215.3	139.2	221.2	144.8	211.9	135.7
agnetic resonance imaging	29.2	37.1	29.1	37.5	29.3	36.9
oint replacement of lower extremity	131.7	175.1	102.2	153.4	148.5	188.3
Total hip replacement	28.7	38.9	21.5	36.6	32.8	40.2
Partial hip replacement	49.6	50.6	30.6	37.2	60.3	58.7
Total knee replacement	43.1	72.3	41.3	69.0	44.2	74.3
eduction of fracture and dislocation	115.4	102.5	67.0	55.9	142.8	130.8
xcision or destruction of intervertebral disc and spinal fusion	11.6	16.2	15.0	16.2	9.6	16.2
Excision or destruction of intervertebral disc	8.1	9.1	11.7	9.7	6.0	8.7
holecystectomy	52.6	41.6	58.8	47.5	49.1	37.9
Laparoscopic cholecystectomy	28.8	27.5	28.0	31.0	29.2	25.4
ysis of peritoneal adhesions	30.4	28.3	22.0	28.3	35.2	28.3

Estimates are considered unreliable. Rates for inpatient procedures preceded by an asterisk are based on 5,000–8,999 estimated procedures; those based on fewer ıan 5,000 are not shown. Estimates that are not shown generally have a relative standard error of greater than 30%.

.. Category not applicable.

Average number of procedures per year.

Includes discharges for procedures not shown separately.

[3]Average annual rate.

[4]Estimates are age-adjusted to the year 2000 standard population using five age groups: 18–44 years, 45–54 years, 55–64 years, 65–74 years, and 75 years and over. See Appendix II, Age adjustment.

[5]The procedure code for insertion of coronary artery stents (36.06) first appears in the 1996 data. A second procedure code for the insertion of drug-eluting stents (36.07) first appears in the 2003 data.

[6]Rate for female population only.

[7]Includes artificial rupture of membranes, surgical and medical induction of labor, and episiotomy.

[8]Rate for male population only.

NOTES: Excludes newborn infants. Up to four procedures were coded for each hospital discharge. If more than one procedure with the same code (e.g., a coronary artery bypass graft) was performed during the hospital stay, it was counted only once (any listed). Procedure categories are based on the *International Classification of Diseases, Ninth Revision, Clinical Modification (ICD–9–CM)*. See Appendix II, International Classification of Diseases, Ninth Revision, Clinical Modification; Procedure; Table XI. Rates are based on the civilian population as of July 1. Starting with *Health, United States, 2003*, rates for 2000 and beyond are based on the 2000 census. Rates for 1990–1999 use population estimates based on the 1990 census adjusted for net underenumeration using the 1990 National Population Adjustment Matrix from the U.S. Census Bureau. Rates for 1990–1999 are not strictly comparable with rates for 2000 and beyond because population estimates for 1990–1999 have not been revised to reflect the 2000 census. See Appendix I, National Hospital Discharge Survey; Population Census and Population Estimates.

SOURCE: Centers for Disease Control and Prevention, National Center for Health Statistics, National Hospital Discharge Survey.

Table 103. Hospital admissions, average length of stay, outpatient visits, and outpatient surgery by type of ownership and size of hospital: United States, selected years 1975–2005

[Data are based on reporting by a census of hospitals]

Type of ownership and size of hospital	*1975*	*1980*	*1990*	*1995*	*2000*	*2003*	*2004*	*2005*
Admissions				Number in thousands				
All hospitals	36,157	38,892	33,774	33,282	34,891	36,611	36,942	37,00
Federal	1,913	2,044	1,759	1,559	1,034	973	1,000	95
Nonfederal[1]	34,243	36,848	32,015	31,723	33,946	35,637	35,942	36,05
Community[2]	33,435	36,143	31,181	30,945	33,089	34,783	35,086	35,23
Nonprofit	23,722	25,566	22,878	22,557	24,453	25,668	25,757	25,88
For profit	2,646	3,165	3,066	3,428	4,141	4,481	4,599	4,61
State-local government	7,067	7,413	5,236	4,961	4,496	4,634	4,730	4,74
6–24 beds	174	159	95	124	141	162	182	18
25–49 beds	1,431	1,254	870	944	995	1,098	1,092	1,17
50–99 beds	3,675	3,700	2,474	2,299	2,355	2,464	2,451	2,41
100–199 beds	7,017	7,162	5,833	6,288	6,735	6,817	6,663	6,67
200–299 beds	6,174	6,596	6,333	6,495	6,702	6,887	6,929	7,07
300–399 beds	4,739	5,358	5,091	4,693	5,135	5,590	5,765	6,02
400–499 beds	3,689	4,401	3,644	3,413	3,617	3,591	3,821	3,63
500 beds or more	6,537	7,513	6,840	6,690	7,410	8,174	8,184	8,05
Average length of stay[3]				Number of days				
All hospitals	11.4	9.9	9.1	7.8	6.8	6.6	6.5	6.
Federal	20.3	16.8	14.9	13.1	12.8	11.5	11.6	11.
Nonfederal[1]	10.9	9.6	8.8	7.5	6.6	6.4	6.4	6.
Community[2]	7.7	7.6	7.2	6.5	5.8	5.7	5.6	5.
Nonprofit	7.8	7.7	7.3	6.4	5.7	5.5	5.5	5.
For profit	6.6	6.5	6.4	5.8	5.4	5.3	5.4	5.
State-local government	7.6	7.3	7.7	7.4	6.7	6.6	6.5	6.
6–24 beds	5.6	5.3	5.4	5.5	4.2	4.0	4.1	4.
25–49 beds	6.0	5.8	6.1	5.7	5.1	5.0	5.1	4.9
50–99 beds	6.8	6.7	7.2	7.0	6.4	6.3	6.4	6.4
100–199 beds	7.1	7.0	7.1	6.4	5.7	5.6	5.7	5.6
200–299 beds	7.5	7.4	6.9	6.2	5.7	5.4	5.4	5.3
300–399 beds	7.8	7.6	7.0	6.1	5.5	5.4	5.3	5.4
400–499 beds	8.1	7.9	7.3	6.3	5.6	5.5	5.5	5.5
500 beds or more	9.1	8.7	8.1	7.1	6.2	6.1	6.0	6.0
Outpatient visits[4]				Number in thousands				
All hospitals	254,844	262,951	368,184	483,195	592,673	648,560	662,131	673,689
Federal	51,957	50,566	58,527	59,934	63,402	74,240	79,966	80,018
Nonfederal[1]	202,887	212,385	309,657	423,261	531,972	574,320	582,165	593,671
Community[2]	190,672	202,310	301,329	414,345	521,405	563,186	571,569	584,429
Nonprofit	131,435	142,156	221,073	303,851	393,168	424,215	430,262	441,653
For profit	7,713	9,696	20,110	31,940	43,378	44,246	44,962	46,016
State-local government	51,525	50,459	60,146	78,554	84,858	94,725	96,345	96,760
6–24 beds	915	1,155	1,471	3,644	4,555	6,512	7,243	7,970
25–49 beds	5,855	6,227	10,812	19,465	27,007	31,261	32,446	35,172
50–99 beds	16,303	17,976	27,582	38,597	49,385	52,959	53,051	53,382
100–199 beds	35,156	36,453	58,940	91,312	114,183	119,856	117,611	121,053
200–299 beds	32,772	36,073	60,561	84,080	99,248	100,095	99,826	107,332
300–399 beds	29,169	30,495	43,699	54,277	73,444	80,938	84,332	85,366
400–499 beds	22,127	25,501	33,394	44,284	52,205	57,203	56,122	56,023
500 beds or more	48,375	48,430	64,870	78,685	101,378	114,362	120,937	118,131
Outpatient surgery				Percent of total surgeries[5]				
Community hospitals[2]	- - -	16.3	50.5	58.1	62.7	63.3	63.3	63.3

- - - Data not available.

[1]The category of nonfederal hospitals comprises psychiatric, tuberculosis and other respiratory diseases hospitals, and long-term and short-term general and other special hospitals. See Appendix II, Hospital.

[2]Community hospitals are nonfederal short-term general and special hospitals whose facilities and services are available to the public. See Appendix II, Hospital.

[3]Average length of stay is calculated as the number of inpatient days divided by the number of admissions. See Appendix II, Average length of stay.

[4]Outpatient visits include visits to the emergency department, outpatient department, referred visits (pharmacy, EKG, radiology), and outpatient surgery. See Appendix II, Outpatient visit.

[5]Total surgeries is a measure of patients with at least one surgical procedure. Persons with multiple surgical procedures are counted only once. See Appendix II, Outpatient surgery.

SOURCES: American Hospital Association (AHA) Annual Survey of Hospitals. Hospital Statistics, 1976, 1981, 1991–2007 editions. Chicago, IL. (Copyrights 1976, 1981 1991–2007: Used with the permission of Health Forum LLC, an affiliate of the AHA.)

ble 104. Nursing home residents 65 years of age and over, by age, sex, and race: United States, selected ars 1973–2004

a are based on a sample of nursing home residents]

Age, sex, and race	Number of residents in hundreds					Residents per 1,000 population[1]				
	1973–1974	1985	1995	1999	2004	1973–1974	1985	1995	1999	2004
Age										
years and over, age-adjusted[2]	. . .	. . .	. . .	. . .	. . .	58.5	54.0	46.4	43.3	34.8
years and over, crude	9,615	13,183	14,229	14,695	13,172	44.7	46.2	42.8	42.9	36.3
–74 years	1,631	2,121	1,897	1,948	1,741	12.3	12.5	10.2	10.8	9.4
–84 years	3,849	509	5,096	5,176	4,689	57.7	57.7	46.1	43.0	36.1
years and over	4,136	5,973	7,235	7,571	6,742	257.3	220.3	200.9	182.5	138.7
Male										
years and over, age-adjusted[2]	. . .	. . .	. . .	. . .	. . .	42.5	38.8	33.0	30.6	24.1
years and over, crude	2,657	3,344	3,571	3,778	3,368	30.0	29.0	26.2	26.5	22.2
–74 years	651	806	795	841	754	11.3	10.8	9.6	10.3	8.9
–84 years	1,023	1,413	1,443	1,495	1,408	39.9	43.0	33.5	30.8	27.0
years and over	983	1,126	1,333	1,442	1,206	182.7	145.7	131.5	116.5	80.0
Female										
years and over, age-adjusted[2]	. . .	. . .	. . .	. . .	. . .	67.5	61.5	52.8	49.8	40.4
years and over, crude	6,958	9,839	10,658	10,917	9,804	54.9	57.9	54.3	54.6	46.4
5–74 years	980	1,315	1,103	1,107	988	13.1	13.8	10.7	11.2	9.8
5–84 years	2,826	3,677	3,654	3,681	3,280	68.9	66.4	54.3	51.2	42.3
5 years and over	3,153	4,847	5,902	6,129	5,536	294.9	250.1	228.1	210.5	165.2
White[3]										
5 years and over, age-adjusted[2]	. . .	. . .	. . .	. . .	. . .	61.2	55.5	45.8	41.9	34.0
5 years and over, crude	9,206	12,274	12,715	12,796	11,488	46.9	47.7	42.7	42.1	36.2
5–74 years	1,501	1,878	1,541	1,573	1,342	12.5	12.3	9.3	10.0	8.5
5–84 years	3,697	4,736	4,513	4,406	4,060	60.3	59.1	45.0	40.5	35.2
5 years and over	4,008	5,660	6,662	6,817	6,086	270.8	228.7	203.2	181.8	139.4
Black or African American[3]										
5 years and over, age-adjusted[2]	. . .	. . .	. . .	. . .	. . .	28.2	41.5	50.8	55.5	49.9
5 years and over, crude	377	820	1,229	1,459	1,454	22.0	35.0	45.5	51.0	47.7
5–74 years	122	225	296	303	345	11.1	15.4	18.5	18.2	20.2
5–84 years	134	306	475	587	546	26.7	45.3	57.8	66.5	55.5
5 years and over	121	290	458	569	563	105.7	141.5	168.2	182.8	160.7

. . Category not applicable.

Rates are calculated using estimates of the civilian population of the United States including institutionalized persons. Population data are from unpublished tabulations rovided by the U.S. Census Bureau. The 2004 population estimates are postcensal estimates as of July 1, 2004, based on the 2000 census. For more information bout the 2004 population estimates, see the Technical Notes in Kozak LJ, DeFrances CJ, Hall MJ. National Hospital Discharge Survey: 2004 annual summary with etailed diagnosis and procedure data. National Center for Health Statistics. Vital Health Stat 13(162). 2006. Available from: www.cdc.gov/nchs/products/pubs/pubd/series/ser.htm.

Age-adjusted to the year 2000 population standard using the following three age groups: 65–74 years, 75–84 years, and 85 years and over.

Starting with 1999 data, the instruction for the race item on the Current Resident Questionnaire was changed so that more than one race could be recorded. In revious years, only one racial category could be checked. Estimates for racial groups presented in this table are for residents for whom only one race was recorded. Estimates for residents where multiple races were checked are unreliable due to small sample sizes and are not shown.

NOTES: Residents are persons on the roster of the nursing home as of the night before the survey. Residents for whom beds are maintained even though they may be away on overnight leave or in a hospital are included. People residing in personal care or domiciliary care homes are excluded. See Appendix I, National Nursing Home Survey (NNHS). Numbers have been revised and differ from previous editions of *Health, United States*. Data for additional years are available. See Appendix III.

SOURCE: Centers for Disease Control and Prevention, National Center for Health Statistics, National Nursing Home Survey.

le 105. Persons employed in health service sites, by site and sex: United States, 2000–2006

are based on household interviews of a sample of the civilian noninstitutionalized population]

Site	2000	2001	2002	2003	2004	2005	2006
	Number of persons in thousands						
Both sexes							
mployed civilians [1]	136,891	136,933	136,485	137,736	139,252	141,730	144,427
ealth service sites [2]	12,211	12,558	13,069	13,615	13,817	14,052	14,352
fices and clinics of physicians	1,387	1,499	1,533	1,673	1,727	1,801	1,785
fices and clinics of dentists	672	701	734	771	780	792	852
ffices and clinics of chiropractors	120	111	132	142	156	163	163
ffices and clinics of optometrists	95	102	113	92	93	98	98
fices and clinics of other health practitioners [3]	143	140	149	250	274	275	292
utpatient care centers	772	830	850	873	885	901	919
ome health care services	548	582	636	741	750	795	928
ther health care services [4]	1,027	1,101	1,188	943	976	1,045	1,096
ospitals	5,202	5,256	5,330	5,652	5,700	5,719	5,712
ursing care facilities	1,593	1,568	1,715	1,877	1,858	1,848	1,807
esidential care facilities, without nursing	652	668	689	601	618	615	700
Men							
ealth service sites [2]	2,756	2,778	2,838	2,986	3,067	3,097	3,187
ffices and clinics of physicians	354	379	370	414	424	418	421
ffices and clinics of dentists	158	150	151	163	158	156	173
ffices and clinics of chiropractors	32	39	47	53	63	68	61
ffices and clinics of optometrists	26	27	29	29	24	27	29
ffices and clinics of other health practitioners [3]	38	41	42	63	69	80	80
utpatient care centers	186	185	172	200	203	201	199
ome health care services	45	51	54	56	65	81	91
ther health care services [4]	304	345	362	297	314	311	344
ospitals	1,241	1,187	1,195	1,263	1,333	1,347	1,337
ursing care facilities	195	189	223	267	251	246	263
esidential care facilities, without nursing	177	185	193	181	164	162	189
Women							
health service sites [2]	9,457	9,782	10,232	10,631	10,750	10,958	11,167
Offices and clinics of physicians	1,034	1,120	1,164	1,259	1,302	1,383	1,364
Offices and clinics of dentists	514	551	584	607	623	637	679
Offices and clinics of chiropractors	88	72	85	90	93	95	102
Offices and clinics of optometrists	69	75	84	64	69	71	69
Offices and clinics of other health practitioners [3]	106	99	106	186	204	195	213
Outpatient care centers	586	646	678	673	683	700	720
Home health care services	503	531	582	685	685	713	837
Other health care services [4]	723	756	826	646	662	734	752
Hospitals	3,961	4,069	4,135	4,390	4,366	4,372	4,376
Nursing care facilities	1,398	1,380	1,492	1,611	1,607	1,602	1,544
Residential care facilities, without nursing	475	483	496	420	454	453	511
	Percent of employed civilians						
Both sexes							
health service sites	8.9	9.2	9.6	9.9	9.9	9.9	9.9
	Percent distribution						
health service sites	100.0	100.0	100.0	100.0	100.0	100.0	100.0
Offices and clinics of physicians	11.4	11.9	11.7	12.3	12.5	12.8	12.4
Offices and clinics of dentists	5.5	5.6	5.6	5.7	5.6	5.6	5.9
Offices and clinics of chiropractors	1.0	0.9	1.0	1.0	1.1	1.2	1.1
Offices and clinics of optometrists	0.8	0.8	0.9	0.7	0.7	0.7	0.7
Offices and clinics of other health practitioners [3]	1.2	1.1	1.1	1.8	2.0	2.0	2.0
Outpatient care centers	6.3	6.6	6.5	6.4	6.4	6.4	6.4
Home health care services	4.5	4.6	4.9	5.4	5.4	5.7	6.5
Other health care services [4]	8.4	8.8	9.1	6.9	7.1	7.4	7.6
Hospitals	42.6	41.9	40.8	41.5	41.3	40.7	39.8
Nursing care facilities	13.0	12.5	13.1	13.8	13.4	13.2	12.6
Residential care facilities, without nursing	5.3	5.3	5.3	4.4	4.5	4.4	4.9

Excludes workers under the age of 16 years.
Data for health service sites for men and women may not sum to total for all health service sites for both sexes due to rounding.
ncludes health service sites such as psychologists' offices, nutritionists' offices, speech defect clinics, and other offices and clinics. Complete list of clinics under this ategory is available from: www.census.gov/hhes/www/ioindex/cens_797_847.html. Census Industry Code 808.
ncludes health service sites such as clinical laboratories, blood banks, CT-SCAN (computer tomography) centers, and other offices and clinics. Complete list of clinics nder this category is available from: www.census.gov/hhes/www/ioindex/cens_797_847.html. Census Industry Code 818.

OTES: Annual data are based on data collected each month and averaged over the year. Health service sites are based on the 2002 North American Industry lassification System. See Appendix II, Industry of employment, Table IX for codes for industries.

OURCES: U.S. Department of Labor, Bureau of Labor Statistics, Current Population Survey: Employment and Earnings, January 2007, available from: ww.bls.gov/cps/home.htm#annual (table 18), and unpublished data.

Table 106 (page 1 of 2). Active physicians and doctors of medicine in patient care, by geographic division and state: United States, selected years 1975–2005

[Data are based on reporting by physicians]

Geographic division and state	Total physicians[1]				Doctors of medicine in patient care[2]			
	1975	1985	1995[3]	2005[4,5]	1975	1985	1995	2005
	Number per 10,000 civilian population							
United States	15.3	20.7	24.2	26.9	13.5	18.0	21.3	23.8
New England	19.1	26.7	32.5	37.5	16.9	22.9	28.8	33.4
Connecticut	19.8	27.6	32.8	35.4	17.7	24.3	29.5	31.8
Maine	12.8	18.7	22.3	30.1	10.7	15.6	18.2	24.3
Massachusetts	20.8	30.2	37.5	42.8	18.3	25.4	33.2	38.4
New Hampshire	14.3	18.1	21.5	26.7	13.1	16.7	19.8	24.1
Rhode Island	17.8	23.3	30.4	35.8	16.1	20.2	26.7	32.0
Vermont	18.2	23.8	26.9	35.4	15.5	20.3	24.2	32.1
Middle Atlantic	19.5	26.1	32.4	35.0	17.0	22.2	28.0	30.0
New Jersey	16.2	23.4	29.3	32.6	14.0	19.8	24.9	27.6
New York	22.7	29.0	35.3	38.0	20.2	25.2	31.6	33.9
Pennsylvania	16.6	23.6	30.1	32.0	13.9	19.2	24.6	25.8
East North Central	13.9	19.3	23.3	26.6	12.0	16.4	19.8	22.8
Illinois	14.5	20.5	24.8	27.5	13.1	18.2	22.1	24.4
Indiana	10.6	14.7	18.4	21.9	9.6	13.2	16.6	19.8
Michigan	15.4	20.8	24.8	27.4	12.0	16.0	19.0	21.5
Ohio	14.1	19.9	23.8	27.7	12.2	16.8	20.0	23.4
Wisconsin	12.5	17.7	21.5	25.7	11.4	15.9	19.6	23.4
West North Central	13.3	18.3	21.8	25.0	11.4	15.6	18.9	21.7
Iowa	11.4	15.6	19.2	21.1	9.4	12.4	15.1	16.6
Kansas	12.8	17.3	20.8	23.6	11.2	15.1	18.0	20.4
Minnesota	14.9	20.5	23.4	27.9	13.7	18.5	21.5	25.7
Missouri	15.0	20.5	23.9	25.9	11.6	16.3	19.7	21.5
Nebraska	12.1	15.7	19.8	23.8	10.9	14.4	18.3	21.8
North Dakota	9.7	15.8	20.5	24.2	9.2	14.9	18.9	22.3
South Dakota	8.2	13.4	16.7	22.3	7.7	12.3	15.7	20.6
South Atlantic	14.0	19.7	23.4	26.7	12.6	17.6	21.0	23.8
Delaware	14.3	19.7	23.4	26.1	12.7	17.1	19.7	22.4
District of Columbia	39.6	55.3	63.6	75.6	34.6	45.6	53.6	65.8
Florida	15.2	20.2	22.9	25.3	13.4	17.8	20.3	22.4
Georgia	11.5	16.2	19.7	22.0	10.6	14.7	18.0	20.1
Maryland	18.6	30.4	34.1	39.9	16.5	24.9	29.9	34.4
North Carolina	11.7	16.9	21.1	24.8	10.6	15.0	19.4	22.8
South Carolina	10.0	14.7	18.9	23.0	9.3	13.6	17.6	21.3
Virginia	12.9	19.5	22.5	26.8	11.9	17.8	20.8	24.4
West Virginia	11.0	16.3	21.0	25.2	10.0	14.6	17.9	20.9
East South Central	10.5	15.0	19.2	22.8	9.7	14.0	17.8	21.0
Alabama	9.2	14.2	18.4	21.4	8.6	13.1	17.0	19.8
Kentucky	10.9	15.1	19.2	22.9	10.1	13.9	18.0	21.1
Mississippi	8.4	11.8	13.9	18.1	8.0	11.1	13.0	16.5
Tennessee	12.4	17.7	22.5	26.1	11.3	16.2	20.8	24.1
West South Central	11.9	16.4	19.5	21.8	10.5	14.5	17.3	19.5
Arkansas	9.1	13.8	17.3	20.4	8.5	12.8	16.0	18.9
Louisiana	11.4	17.3	21.7	24.5	10.5	16.1	20.3	23.2
Oklahoma	11.6	16.1	18.8	20.5	9.4	12.9	14.7	15.7
Texas	12.5	16.8	19.4	21.7	11.0	14.7	17.3	19.4
Mountain	14.3	17.8	20.2	22.8	12.6	15.7	17.8	20.0
Arizona	16.7	20.2	21.4	22.5	14.1	17.1	18.2	19.2
Colorado	17.3	20.7	23.7	26.8	15.0	17.7	20.6	23.6
Idaho	9.5	12.1	13.9	17.9	8.9	11.4	13.1	16.2
Montana	10.6	14.0	18.4	23.0	10.1	13.2	17.1	21.2
Nevada	11.9	16.0	16.7	19.6	10.9	14.5	14.6	17.5
New Mexico	12.2	17.0	20.2	23.9	10.1	14.7	18.0	21.5
Utah	14.1	17.2	19.2	21.2	13.0	15.5	17.6	19.1
Wyoming	9.5	12.9	15.3	19.4	8.9	12.0	13.9	17.7

See footnotes at end of table.

able 106 (page 2 of 2). Active physicians and doctors of medicine in patient care, by eographic division and state: United States, selected years 1975–2005

ata are based on reporting by physicians]

	Total physicians[1]				Doctors of medicine in patient care[2]			
Geographic division and state	*1975*	*1985*	*1995*[3]	*2005*[4,5]	*1975*	*1985*	*1995*	*2005*[5]
	Number per 10,000 civilian population							
acific	17.9	22.5	23.3	26.0	16.3	20.5	21.2	23.6
laska	8.4	13.0	15.7	24.1	7.8	12.1	14.2	21.3
California	18.8	23.7	23.7	25.7	17.3	21.5	21.7	23.3
Hawaii	16.2	21.5	24.8	31.2	14.7	19.8	22.8	28.2
Oregon	15.6	19.7	21.6	26.9	13.8	17.6	19.5	24.2
Washington	15.3	20.2	22.5	26.6	13.6	17.9	20.2	23.9

ncludes active doctors of medicine and active doctors of osteopathy. See Appendix II, Physician.
xcludes doctors of osteopathy (DOs); states with more than 3,000 active DOs are California, Florida, Michigan, New York, Ohio, Pennsylvania, and Texas. States with wer than 100 active DOs are North Dakota, South Dakota, Vermont, Wyoming, and the District of Columbia. Excludes doctors of medicine in medical teaching, ministration, research, and other nonpatient care activities.
ata for doctors of osteopathy are as of July 1996.
ata for doctors of osteopathy are as of June 2005.
tarting with 2003 data, federal and nonfederal physicians are included. Data prior to 2004 include nonfederal physicians only.

OTES: Data for doctors of medicine are as of December 31. Data for additional years are available. See Appendix III.

OURCES: American Medical Association (AMA). Physician distribution and medical licensure in the U.S., 1975; Physician characteristics and distribution in the U.S., 986 edition; 1996–1997 edition; 2004 edition; 2007 edition; Department of Physician Practice and Communication Information, Division of Survey and Data Resources, MA. (Copyrights 1976, 1986, 1997, 2004, 2007: Used with the permission of the AMA); American Osteopathic Association: 1975–1976 Yearbook and Directory of steopathic Physicians, 1985–1986 Yearbook and Directory of Osteopathic Physicians; American Association of Colleges of Osteopathic Medicine: 2002 Annual Report n Osteopathic Medical Education, 2002, 2005 Annual Report on Osteopathic Medical Education, 2005.

Table 107. Doctors of medicine, by activity and place of medical education: United States and outlying U.S. areas, selected years 1975–2005

[Data are based on reporting by physicians]

Activity and place of medical education	*1975*	*1985*	*1995*	*2000*	*2002*	*2003*	*2004*	*2005*
	Number of doctors of medicine							
Doctors of medicine	393,742	552,716	720,325	813,770	853,187	871,535	884,974	902,05
Professionally active[1]	340,280	497,140	625,443	692,368	719,431	736,211	744,143	762,43
Place of medical education:								
U.S. medical graduates	- - -	392,007	481,137	525,691	544,779	558,167	563,118	571,79
International medical graduates[2]	- - -	105,133	144,306	164,437	172,770	178,044	181,025	190,64
Activity:								
Nonfederal[3]	312,089	475,573	604,364	672,987	699,249	- - -	- - -	- -
Patient care[4]	287,837	431,527	564,074	631,431	658,123	691,873	700,287	718,47
Office-based practice	213,334	329,041	427,275	490,398	516,246	529,836	538,538	563,22
General and family practice	46,347	53,862	59,932	67,534	71,696	73,508	73,234	74,99
Cardiovascular diseases	5,046	9,054	13,739	16,300	16,989	17,301	17,252	17,51
Dermatology	3,442	5,325	6,959	7,969	8,282	8,477	8,651	8,79
Gastroenterology	1,696	4,135	7,300	8,515	9,044	9,326	9,430	9,74
Internal medicine	28,188	52,712	72,612	88,699	96,496	99,670	101,776	107,02
Pediatrics	12,687	22,392	33,890	42,215	46,097	47,996	49,356	51,85
Pulmonary diseases	1,166	3,035	4,964	6,095	6,672	6,919	7,072	7,32
General surgery	19,710	24,708	24,086	24,475	24,902	25,284	25,229	26,07
Obstetrics and gynecology	15,613	23,525	29,111	31,726	32,738	33,636	33,811	34,65
Ophthalmology	8,795	12,212	14,596	15,598	16,052	16,240	16,304	16,58
Orthopedic surgery	8,148	13,033	17,136	17,367	18,118	18,423	18,632	19,11
Otolaryngology	4,297	5,751	7,139	7,581	8,001	8,103	8,160	8,20
Plastic surgery	1,706	3,299	4,612	5,308	5,593	5,725	5,845	6,01
Urological surgery	5,025	7,081	7,991	8,460	8,615	8,804	8,793	8,95
Anesthesiology	8,970	15,285	23,770	27,624	28,661	29,254	29,984	31,88
Diagnostic radiology	1,978	7,735	12,751	14,622	15,896	16,403	16,828	17,61
Emergency medicine	- - -	- - -	11,700	14,541	16,907	17,727	18,961	20,17
Neurology	1,862	4,691	7,623	8,559	9,034	9,304	9,632	10,40
Pathology, anatomical/clinical	4,195	6,877	9,031	10,267	10,103	10,209	10,653	11,74
Psychiatry	12,173	18,521	23,334	24,955	25,350	25,656	25,998	27,63
Radiology	6,970	7,355	5,994	6,674	6,916	7,010	6,900	7,04
Other specialty	15,320	28,453	29,005	35,314	34,084	34,861	36,037	39,85
Hospital-based practice	74,503	102,486	136,799	141,033	141,877	162,037	161,749	155,24
Residents and interns[5]	53,527	72,159	93,650	95,125	96,547	100,033	102,563	95,39
Full-time hospital staff	20,976	30,327	43,149	45,908	45,330	62,004	59,186	59,85
Other professional activity[6]	24,252	44,046	40,290	41,556	41,126	44,338	43,856	43,96
Federal[3]	28,191	21,567	21,079	19,381	20,182	- - -	- - -	- -
Patient care	24,100	17,293	18,057	15,999	16,701	- - -	- - -	- -
Office-based practice	2,095	1,156	. . .	. . .	. . .	- - -	- - -	- -
Hospital-based practice	22,005	16,137	18,057	15,999	16,701	- - -	- - -	- -
Residents and interns	4,275	3,252	2,702	600	390	- - -	- - -	- -
Full-time hospital staff	17,730	12,885	15,355	15,399	16,311	- - -	- - -	- -
Other professional activity[6]	4,091	4,274	3,022	3,382	3,481	- - -	- - -	- -
Inactive	21,449	38,646	72,326	75,168	84,166	84,360	92,323	99,82
Not classified	26,145	13,950	20,579	45,136	49,067	50,447	48,011	39,30
Unknown address	5,868	2,980	1,977	1,098	523	517	497	48

- - - Data not available.
. . . Category not applicable.
[1]Excludes inactive, not classified, and address unknown. See Appendix II, Physician.
[2]International medical graduates received their medical education in schools outside the United States and Canada.
[3]Starting with 2003 data, separate estimates for federal and nonfederal doctors of medicine are not available.
[4]Specialty information based on the physician's self-designated primary area of practice. Categories include generalists and specialists. See Appendix II, Physician specialty.
[5]Starting with 1990 data, clinical fellows are included in this category. In prior years, clinical fellows were included in the other professional activity category.
[6]Includes medical teaching, administration, research, and other. Prior to 1990, this category also included clinical fellows.

NOTES: Data for doctors of medicine are as of December 31, except for 1990–1994 data, which are as of January 1. Outlying areas include Puerto Rico, the U.S. Virgin Islands, and the Pacific islands of Canton, Caroline, Guam, Mariana, Marshall, American Samoa, and Wake. Data for additional years are available. See Appendix III.

SOURCES: American Medical Association (AMA). Distribution of physicians in the United States, 1970; Physician distribution and medical licensure in the U.S., 1975; Physician characteristics and distribution in the U.S., 1981, 1986, 1989, 1990, 1992, 1993, 1994, 1995–1996, 1996–1997, 1997–1998, 1999, 2000–2001, 2001–2002, 2002–2003, 2003–2004, 2004, 2005, 2006, 2007 editions, Department of Physician Practice and Communications Information, Division of Survey and Data Resources, AMA. (Copyrights 1971, 1976, 1982, 1986, 1989, 1990, 1992, 1993, 1994, 1996, 1997, 1997, 1999, 2000, 2001, 2002, 2003, 2004, 2005, 2006, 2007: Used with the permission of the AMA.)

ble 108. Doctors of medicine in primary care, by specialty: United States and outlying S. areas, selected years 1949–2005

ta are based on reporting by physicians]

Specialty	1949[1]	1960[1]	1970	1980	1990	1995	2000	2002	2004	2005
					Number					
al doctors of medicine[2]	201,277	260,484	334,028	467,679	615,421	720,325	813,770	853,187	884,974	902,053
tive doctors of medicine[3]	191,577	247,257	310,929	435,545	559,988	646,022	737,504	768,498	792,154	801,742
General primary care specialists	113,222	125,359	134,354	170,705	213,514	241,329	274,653	286,294	296,495	300,022
General practice/family medicine	95,980	88,023	57,948	60,049	70,480	75,976	86,312	89,357	91,164	91,858
Internal medicine	12,453	26,209	39,924	58,462	76,295	88,240	101,353	106,499	111,800	112,934
Obstetrics/Gynecology	---	---	18,532	24,612	30,220	33,519	35,922	36,810	37,779	38,285
Pediatrics	4,789	11,127	17,950	27,582	36,519	43,594	51,066	53,628	55,752	56,945
Primary care subspecialists	---	---	3,161	16,642	30,911	39,659	52,294	57,929	62,322	65,420
Family medicine	---	---	---	---	---	236	483	627	768	835
Internal medicine	---	---	1,948	13,069	22,054	26,928	34,831	38,821	41,471	43,552
Obstetrics/Gynecology	---	---	344	1,693	3,477	4,133	4,319	4,228	4,280	4,315
Pediatrics	---	---	869	1,880	5,380	8,362	12,661	14,253	15,803	16,718
					Percent of active doctors of medicine					
General primary care specialist	59.1	50.7	43.2	39.2	38.1	37.4	37.2	37.3	37.4	37.4
General practice/family medicine	50.1	35.6	18.6	13.8	12.6	11.8	11.7	11.6	11.5	11.5
Internal medicine	6.5	10.6	12.8	13.4	13.6	13.7	13.7	13.9	14.1	14.1
Obstetrics/Gynecology	---	---	6.0	5.7	5.4	5.2	4.9	4.8	4.8	4.8
Pediatrics	2.5	4.5	5.8	6.3	6.5	6.7	6.9	7.0	7.0	7.1
Primary care subspecialists	---	---	1.0	3.8	5.5	6.1	7.1	7.5	7.9	8.2
Family medicine	---	---	---	---	---	0.0	0.1	0.1	0.1	0.1
Internal medicine	---	---	0.6	3.0	3.9	4.2	4.7	5.1	5.2	5.4
Obstetrics/Gynecology	---	---	0.1	0.4	0.6	0.6	0.6	0.6	0.5	0.5
Pediatrics	---	---	0.3	0.4	1.0	1.3	1.7	1.9	2.0	2.1

Percent greater than zero but less than 0.05.
- Data not available.
stimated by the Bureau of Health Professions, Health Resources Administration. Active doctors of medicine (M.D.s) include those with address unknown and primary ecialty not classified.
cludes M.D.s engaged in federal and nonfederal patient care (office-based or hospital-based) and other professional activities.
tarting with 1970 data, M.D.s who are inactive, have unknown address, or primary specialty not classified are excluded. See Appendix II, Physician.

OTES: See Appendix II, Physician specialty. Data are as of December 31 except for 1990–1994 data, which are as of January 1, and 1949 data, which are as of dyear. Outlying areas include Puerto Rico, the U.S. Virgin Islands, and the Pacific islands of Canton, Caroline, Guam, Mariana, Marshall, American Samoa, and ake. Data for additional years are available. See Appendix III.

OURCES: Health Manpower Source Book: Medical Specialists, USDHEW, 1962; American Medical Association (AMA). Distribution of physicians in the United States, 70; Physician characteristics and distribution in the U.S., 1981, 1992, 1996–1997, 1997–1998, 1999, 2000–2001, 2001–2002, 2002–2003, 2003–2004, 2004, 2005, 06, 2007 editions, Department of Division of Survey and Data Resources, AMA. (Copyrights 1971, 1982, 1992, 1996, 1997, 1997, 1999, 2000, 2001, 2002, 2003, 04, 2005, 2006, 2007: Used with the permission of the AMA.)

Table 109. Employees and wages, by selected healthcare occupations: United States, selected years 1999–200

[Data are based on a semi-annual mail survey of nonfarm establishments]

Occupation title	*1999*	*2000*	*2004*	*2005*	*1999–2005*	*1999*	*2000*	*2004*	*2005*	*1999–2005*
Healthcare practitioner and technical occupations	Number of employees[1]				AAPC[2]	Mean hourly wage[3]				AAPC
Audiologists	12,950	11,530	9,810	10,030	–4.2	$21.96	$22.92	$26.47	$27.72	4.0
Cardiovascular Technologists and Technicians	41,490	40,080	43,540	43,560	0.8	$16.00	$16.81	$19.09	$19.99	3.8
Dental Hygienists	90,050	148,460	155,810	161,140	10.2	$23.15	$24.99	$28.58	$29.15	3.9
Diagnostic Medical Sonographers	29,280	31,760	41,280	43,590	6.9	$21.04	$22.03	$25.78	$26.65	4.0
Dietetic Technicians	29,190	28,010	24,630	23,780	–3.4	$10.09	$10.98	$11.89	$12.20	3.2
Dietitians and Nutritionists	41,320	43,030	46,530	48,850	2.8	$17.96	$18.76	$21.46	$22.09	3.5
Emergency Medical Technicians and Paramedics	172,360	165,530	187,900	196,880	2.2	$11.19	$11.89	$13.30	$13.68	3.4
Licensed Practical and Licensed Vocational Nurse	688,510	679,470	702,740	710,020	0.5	$13.95	$14.65	$16.75	$17.41	3.8
Nuclear Medicine Technologists	17,880	18,030	17,520	18,280	0.4	$20.40	$21.56	$29.43	$29.10	6.1
Occupational Therapists	78,950	75,150	83,560	87,430	1.7	$24.96	$24.10	$27.19	$28.41	2.2
Opticians, Dispensing	58,860	66,580	62,350	70,090	3.0	$12.11	$12.67	$14.37	$14.80	3.4
Pharmacists	226,300	212,660	222,960	229,740	0.3	$30.31	$33.39	$40.56	$42.62	5.8
Pharmacy Technicians	196,430	190,940	255,290	266,790	5.2	$ 9.64	$10.38	$11.87	$12.19	4.0
Physical Therapists	131,050	120,410	142,940	151,280	2.4	$28.05	$27.62	$30.00	$31.42	1.9
Physician Assistants	56,750	55,490	59,470	63,350	1.9	$24.35	$29.17	$33.07	$34.17	5.8
Psychiatric Technicians	54,560	53,350	59,010	62,040	2.2	$11.30	$12.53	$13.43	$14.04	3.7
Radiation Therapists	12,340	13,100	14,470	14,120	2.3	$20.84	$25.59	$29.05	$30.59	6.6
Radiologic Technologists and Technicians	177,850	172,080	177,220	184,580	0.6	$17.07	$17.93	$21.41	$22.60	4.8
Recreational Therapists	30,190	26,940	23,050	23,260	–4.3	$14.08	$14.23	$16.48	$16.90	3.1
Registered Nurses	2,205,430	2,189,670	2,311,970	2,368,070	1.2	$21.38	$22.31	$26.06	$27.35	4.2
Respiratory Therapists	80,230	82,670	91,350	95,320	2.9	$17.72	$18.37	$21.24	$22.24	3.9
Respiratory Therapy Technicians	33,990	28,230	24,190	22,060	–7.0	$16.07	$16.46	$18.00	$18.57	2.4
Speech-Language Pathologists	85,920	82,850	89,260	94,660	1.6	$22.99	$23.31	$26.71	$27.89	3.3
Healthcare support occupations										
Dental Assistants	175,160	250,870	264,820	270,720	7.5	$11.60	$12.86	$13.97	$14.41	3.7
Home Health Aides	577,530	561,120	596,330	663,280	2.3	$ 9.04	$ 8.71	$ 9.13	$ 9.34	0.5
Massage Therapists	21,910	24,620	32,200	37,670	9.5	$13.82	$15.51	$17.63	$19.33	5.8
Medical Assistants	281,480	330,830	380,340	382,720	5.3	$10.89	$11.46	$12.21	$12.58	2.4
Medical Equipment Preparers	29,070	32,760	40,380	41,790	6.2	$10.20	$10.68	$12.14	$12.42	3.3
Medical Transcriptionists	97,260	97,330	92,740	90,380	–1.2	$11.86	$12.37	$14.01	$14.36	3.2
Nursing Aides, Orderlies, and Attendants	1,308,740	1,273,460	1,384,120	1,391,430	1.0	$ 8.59	$ 9.18	$10.39	$10.67	3.7
Occupational Therapist Aides	9,250	8,890	5,240	6,220	–6.4	$10.92	$11.21	$12.51	$13.20	3.2
Occupational Therapist Assistants	17,290	15,910	20,880	22,160	4.2	$15.97	$16.76	$18.49	$19.13	3.1
Pharmacy Aides	48,270	59,890	47,720	46,610	–0.6	$ 9.14	$ 9.10	$ 9.52	$ 9.76	1.1
Physical Therapist Aides	44,340	34,620	41,910	41,930	–0.9	$ 9.69	$10.06	$11.14	$11.01	2.2
Physical Therapist Assistants	48,600	44,120	57,420	58,670	3.2	$16.20	$16.52	$18.14	$18.98	2.7
Psychiatric Aides	51,100	57,680	54,520	56,150	1.6	$10.76	$10.79	$11.70	$11.47	1.1

[1]Estimates do not include self-employed workers and were rounded to the nearest 10.
[2]Average annual percent change. See Appendix II, Average annual rate of change (percentage change).
[3]The mean hourly wage rate for an occupation is the total wages that all workers in the occupation earn in an hour divided by the total employment of the occupation. More information is available from: www.bls.gov/oes/current/oes_tec.htm.

NOTES: This table excludes occupations such as dentists, physicians, and chiropractors, with a large percentage of workers who are self-employed and/or not employed by establishments. Data for additional years are available. See Appendix III.

SOURCE: U.S. Department of Labor. Bureau of Labor Statistics. Occupational Employment Statistics. Available from: www.bls.gov/oes.

Table 110. First-year enrollment and graduates of health professions schools, and number of schools, by selected profession: United States, selected years 1980–2005

[Data are based on reporting by health professions associations]

Profession	1980	1985	1990	1995	2000	2005
			Number			
First-year enrollment						
Dentistry	6,132	5,047	3,979	4,121	4,314	4,612
Medicine (Allopathic) [1]	16,930	16,997	16,756	17,085	16,856	17,059
Medicine (Osteopathic)	1,426	1,750	1,844	2,217	2,848	3,646
Nursing:						
Licensed practical	56,316	47,034	52,969	57,906	---	---
Registered, total	105,952	118,224	108,580	127,184	---	---
Baccalaureate	35,414	39,573	29,858	43,451	---	---
Associate degree	53,633	63,776	68,634	76,016	---	---
Diploma	16,905	14,875	10,088	7,717	---	---
Optometry [1]	1,202	1,187	1,258	1,390	1,410	1,429
Pharmacy [1,2]	8,035	6,986	8,267	8,740	8,382	10,506
Podiatry	695	811	561	630	606	519
Public Health [1,3]	---	---	4,392	5,332	5,840	7,206
Graduates						
Dentistry	5,256	5,353	4,233	3,908	4,171	---
Medicine (Allopathic) [1]	15,113	16,318	15,398	15,883	15,718	15,736
Medicine (Osteopathic)	1,059	1,474	1,529	1,843	2,279	2,756
Nursing:						
Licensed practical	41,892	36,955	35,417	44,234	---	---
Registered, total	75,523	82,075	66,088	97,052	---	---
Baccalaureate	24,994	24,975	18,571	31,254	---	---
Associate degree	36,034	45,208	42,318	58,749	---	---
Diploma	14,495	11,892	5,199	7,049	---	---
Occupational therapy	---	---	2,424	3,473	---	---
Optometry [1]	1,073	1,114	1,115	1,219	1,315	1,251
Pharmacy [1]	7,432	5,735	6,956	7,837	7,260	8,268
Podiatry	597	582	679	558	583	347
Public Health [1]	3,326	3,047	3,549	4,636	5,879	6,656
Schools						
Dentistry	60	60	58	54	55	56
Medicine (Allopathic) [1]	126	127	127	125	125	125
Medicine (Osteopathic)	14	15	15	16	19	20
Nursing: [4]						
Licensed practical	1,299	1,165	1,154	1,210	---	---
Registered, total	1,385	1,473	1,470	1,516	---	---
Baccalaureate	377	441	489	521	---	---
Associate degree	697	776	829	876	---	---
Diploma	311	256	152	119	---	---
Occupational therapy	50	61	69	98	142	---
Optometry [1]	16	17	17	17	17	17
Pharmacy [1]	72	72	74	75	81	92
Podiatry	5	7	7	7	7	7
Public Health [1]	21	23	25	27	28	37

- - - Data not available.

[1]Include data from schools in Puerto Rico.

[2]Data for 2005 first-year enrollment for pharmacy schools include Pharm.D.1 enrollments only. Prior to 2005, first-year enrollment data include both Pharm.D.1, B.S. Pharmacy, and B.Pharm. enrollments.

[3]Number of students entering Schools of Public Health for the first time. Starting with 2003–2004 data, first-year enrollment data for public health schools include Spring, Summer, and Fall enrollment. Prior to 2003–2004, the data are for Fall enrollment only and are not directly comparable to 2003–2004 data.

[4]Some nursing schools offer more than one type of program. Numbers shown for nursing are number of nursing programs.

NOTES: Data on the number of schools are reported as of the beginning of the academic year while data on first-year enrollment and number of graduates are reported as of the end of the academic year. Optometry, pharmacy, podiatry, and public health data on first-year enrollment are reported as of the beginning of the academic year. Some numbers in this table have been revised and differ from previous editions of *Health, United States*. Data for additional years are available. See Appendix III.

SOURCES: Association of American Medical Colleges: AAMC Data Book, Medical Schools and Teaching Hospitals by the Numbers, Washington, DC. 2004, 2005, 2006 (Copyright 2005, 2006, 2007: Used with the permission of the AAMC) and unpublished data. Bureau of Health Professions: United States Health Personnel FACTBOOK. Health Resources and Services Administration. Rockville, MD. 2003; National League for Nursing: unpublished data; American Dental Association: 2003–2004 Survey of Predoctoral Dental Education, vol. 1, Academic Programs, Enrollments, and Graduates, Chicago, IL. 2005 (Copyright 2006: Used with the permission of the ADA), Annual U.S. Dental Education at-a-Glance (available from: www.adea.org/adea.html), and unpublished data; American Association of Colleges of Osteopathic Medicine. Annual Report on Osteopathic Medical Education, Chevy Chase, MD, available from: www.aacom.org/data/annualreport/index.html; Association of Schools of Public Health: Annual Data Reports. Washington, DC., available from: www.asph.org/userfiles/ADR%202005.pdf; Association of Schools and Colleges of Optometry: Annual Student Data Report Academic Years 2003–2004, 2005–2006 and unpublished data; (Copyright 2006: Used with permission of the ASCO); American Association of Colleges of Pharmacy: Academic Pharmacy's Vital Statistics, Profile of Pharmacy Students, Fall 2005 (available from: www.aacp.org) and unpublished data; American Association of Colleges of Podiatric Medicine: unpublished data; American Medical Association: Health Professions Career and Education Directory, 29th edition. Chicago, IL. 2001.

Table 111 (page 1 of 2). Total enrollment of minorities in schools for selected health occupations, by race and Hispanic origin: United States, selected academic years 1980–1981 through 2004–2005

[Data are based on reporting by health professions associations]

Occupation, race, and Hispanic origin	*1980–1981*	*1990–1991*	*2004–2005*	*1980–1981*	*1990–1991*	*2004–2005*
Dentistry	Number of students			Percent distribution of students		
All races	22,842	15,951	18,315	100.0	100.0	100.0
Not Hispanic or Latino:						
White [1]	19,947	11,185	12,112	87.3	70.1	66.1
Black or African American	1,022	940	998	4.5	5.9	5.4
Hispanic or Latino [2]	780	1,254	1,059	3.4	7.9	5.8
American Indian or Alaska Native	53	53	93	0.2	0.3	0.5
Asian or Pacific Islander	1,040	2,519	4,053	4.6	15.8	22.1
Medicine (Allopathic) [3]						
All races [1]	65,189	65,163	66,821	100.0	100.0	100.0
Not Hispanic or Latino:						
White	55,434	47,893	42,302	85.0	73.5	63.3
Black or African American	3,708	4,241	4,947	5.7	6.5	7.4
Hispanic or Latino	2,761	3,538	4,509	4.2	5.4	6.7
Mexican	951	1,109	1,590	1.5	1.7	2.4
Puerto Rican	1,012	1,253	1,143	1.6	1.9	1.7
Other Hispanic or Latino [4]	683	1,176	1,776	1.0	1.8	2.7
American Indian or Alaska Native [5]	221	277	578	0.3	0.4	0.9
Asian or Pacific Islander	1,924	8,436	13,811	3.0	12.9	20.7
Medicine (Osteopathic)						
All races [1]	4,940	6,792	12,525	100.0	100.0	100.0
Not Hispanic or Latino:						
White	4,688	5,680	9,209	94.9	83.6	73.5
Black or African American	94	217	469	1.9	3.2	3.7
Hispanic or Latino	52	277	472	1.1	4.1	3.8
American Indian or Alaska Native	19	36	90	0.4	0.5	0.7
Asian or Pacific Islander	87	582	1,961	1.8	8.6	15.7
Nursing, registered [6]						
All races	230,966	221,170	- - -	- - -	100.0	- - -
Not Hispanic or Latino:						
White [1]	- - -	183,102	- - -	- - -	82.8	- - -
Black or African American	- - -	23,094	- - -	- - -	10.4	- - -
Hispanic or Latino	- - -	6,580	- - -	- - -	3.0	- - -
American Indian or Alaska Native	- - -	1,803	- - -	- - -	0.8	- - -
Asian or Pacific Islander	- - -	6,591	- - -	- - -	3.0	- - -
Optometry						
All races [1]	4,641	4,760	5,377	100.0	100.0	100.0
Not Hispanic or Latino:						
White	4,221	3,706	3,399	91.0	77.9	63.2
Black or African American	57	134	189	1.2	2.8	3.5
Hispanic or Latino	108	296	273	2.3	6.2	5.1
American Indian or Alaska Native	12	21	29	0.3	0.4	0.5
Asian or Pacific Islander	243	603	1,266	5.2	12.7	23.5
Pharmacy [7]						
All races [1]	21,628	29,797	43,908	100.0	100.0	100.0
Not Hispanic or Latino:						
White	19,153	21,717	26,226	88.6	80.5	59.7
Black or African American	945	2,103	3,784	4.4	5.7	8.6
Hispanic or Latino	459	1,118	1,691	2.1	4.2	3.9
American Indian or Alaska Native	36	85	210	0.2	0.3	0.5
Asian or Pacific Islander	1,035	3,346	9,103	4.8	9.4	20.7

See footnotes at end of table.

Table 111 (page 2 of 2). Total enrollment of minorities in schools for selected health occupations, by race and Hispanic origin: United States, selected academic years 1980–1981 through 2004–2005

[Data are based on reporting by health professions associations]

Occupation, race, and Hispanic origin	1980–1981	1990–1991	2004–2005	1980–1981	1990–1991	2004–2005
Podiatry	Number of students			Percent distribution of students		
All races[1]	2,577	2,221	1,584	100.0	100.0	100.0
Not Hispanic or Latino:						
White	2,353	1,671	957	91.3	75.2	60.4
Black or African American	110	235	228	4.3	10.6	14.4
Hispanic or Latino	39	149	122	1.5	6.7	7.7
American Indian or Alaska Native	6	7	9	0.2	0.3	0.6
Asian or Pacific Islander	69	159	176	2.7	7.2	11.1

- - - Data not available.
[1]Includes other and unknown races; may also include foreign students.
[2]Includes students from the University of Puerto Rico.
[3]Starting with 2002–2003 data, allopathic medical students had the option of reporting both their race and ethnicity alone or in combination with some other race or ethnicity, allowing multiple responses. Total enrollments only include unduplicated number of enrollments. Therefore, the data for 2003–2004 and subsequent years are not directly comparable to earlier years.
[4]Includes Cuban students.
[5]Starting with 1997–1998 data, includes American Indian, Alaska Native, and Native Hawaiian; prior to 1997, included only American Indian and Alaska Native
[6]In 1990, the National League for Nursing developed a new system for analyzing minority data. An evaluation of the former system revealed considerable underreporting. Therefore, race-specific data before 1990 are not comparable and not shown. Additional changes in the minority data question were introduced in academic years 2000–2001 and 2001–2002, resulting in a discontinuity in the trend.
[7]Prior to 1992–1993, pharmacy total enrollment data were only for students in the final three years of pharmacy education. Starting with 1992–1993 data, pharmacy data are for all students.

NOTES: Total enrollment data are collected at the beginning of the academic year. Data for chiropractic students, occupational and physical therapy students, and public health students were not available for this table. Some numbers have been revised and differ from previous editions of *Health, United States*.
Data for additional years are available. See Appendix III.

SOURCES: Bureau of Health Professions: Minorities and Women in the Health Fields, 1990 Edition; Association of American Medical Colleges: AAMC Data Book: Medical Schools and Teaching Hospitals by the Numbers. Washington, DC. 2005, 2006 (Copyrights 2006, 2007: Used with the permission of the AAMC); American Association of Colleges of Osteopathic Medicine: 2006 Annual Report on Osteopathic Medical Education. Chevy Chase, MD. 2007. Available from: http://www.aacom.org/data/annualreport/index.html (Copyright 2007: Used with the permission of the AACOM); American Dental Education Association: Dental Education At-A-Glance 2005, available from: www.adea.org/adea.html and unpublished data; Association of Schools and Colleges of Optometry: Annual Student Data Report Academic Year 2002–2004, 2005–2006, and unpublished data (Copyright 2005, 2006: Used with the permission of the ASCO); American Association of Colleges of Pharmacy: Profile of Pharmacy Students, Fall 2005, available from: http://www.aacp.org; American Association of Colleges of Podiatric Medicine: unpublished data; National League for Nursing: unpublished data.

Table 112. First-year and total enrollment of women in schools for selected health occupations: United States, selected academic years 1980–1981 through 2004–2005

[Data are based on reporting by health professions associations]

Enrollment and occupation	Both sexes 1980–1981	Both sexes 1990–1991	Both sexes 2004–2005[1]	Women 1980–1981	Women 1990–1991[2]	Women 2004–2005[1]
First-year enrollment	Number of students			Percent of students		
Dentistry	6,030	4,001	4,612	19.8	38.0	- - -
Medicine (Allopathic)[3]	17,186	16,876	17,059	28.9	38.8	49.4
Medicine (Osteopathic)	1,496	1,950	3,646	22.0	34.2	50.1
Nurses, registered	110,201	113,526	- - -	92.7	89.3	- - -
Optometry[3,4]	1,258	1,239	1,429	25.3	50.6	64.9
Pharmacy[3,5]	7,377	8,267	10,437	48.4	- - -	65.4
Podiatry	695	561	519	- - -	28.0	49.0
Public Health[3,6]	3,348	4,289	7,206	- - -	62.1	70.9
Total enrollment						
Dentistry	22,842	15,951	18,315	17.0	34.4	43.8
Medicine (Allopathic)[3]	65,189	65,163	67,466	26.5	37.3	48.7
Medicine (Osteopathic)	4,940	6,792	12,525	19.7	32.7	48.8
Nurses, registered	230,966	221,170	- - -	94.3	- - -	- - -
Optometry[3,4]	4,641	4,760	5,377	- - -	47.3	63.1
Pharmacy[3,5]	26,617	29,797	43,908	47.4	62.4	66.5
Podiatry	2,577	2,154	1,584	11.9	28.9	46.9
Public Health[3,6]	8,486	11,386	19,434	55.2	62.5	69.6

- - - Data not available.

[1]Starting with 2003–2004 data, osteopathic medicine data include the students of the Edward Via Virginia College of Osteopathic Medicine.

[2]Percentage of women podiatry students is for 1991–1992.

[3]Include data from schools in Puerto Rico.

[4]2004–2005 optometry data are for 2005–2006.

[5]First-year enrollment data for pharmacy schools are for students in the first year of the final three years of pharmacy education. Prior to 1992–1993, pharmacy total enrollment data were for students in the final three years of pharmacy education. Starting in 1992–1993, pharmacy total enrollment data are for all students.

[6]For 2003–2004 data, first-year enrollment data for public health schools include Spring, Summer, and Fall enrollment. All other years of data including 2004–2005 are for Fall enrollment only and are not directly comparable to 2003–2004 data.

NOTES: Total enrollment data are collected at the beginning of the academic year while first-year enrollment data are collected during the academic year. Data for chiropractic students and occupational, physical, and speech therapy students were not available for this table. Some numbers in this table have been revised and differ from previous editions of *Health, United States*. Data for additional years are available. See Appendix III.

SOURCES: Association of American Medical Colleges: AAMC Data Book: Medical Schools and Teaching Hospitals by the Numbers. Washington, DC. 2004, 2005, 2006 (Copyrights 2005, 2006, 2007: Used with the permission of the AAMC); American Association of Colleges of Osteopathic Medicine: 2005 Annual Report on Osteopathic Medical Education. Chevy Chase, MD. 2006, available from: www.aacom.org/data/annualreport/index.html; Bureau of Health Professions: Minorities and Women in the Health Fields, 1990 edition; American Dental Association: 2003–2004 Survey of Dental Education, vol.1, Academic Programs, Enrollments, and Graduates, Chicago, IL. 2005 (Copyright 2006: Used with the permission of the ADA) and unpublished data; Association of Schools and Colleges of Optometry: Annual Student Data Report Academic Years 2003–2004, 2005–2006 and unpublished data (Copyright 2006: Used with the permission of the ASCO); American Association of Colleges of Pharmacy: Profile of Pharmacy Students, Fall 2005, available from: www.aacp.org, and unpublished data; American Association of Colleges of Podiatric Medicine: unpublished data; National League for Nursing: Nursing Data Review. New York, NY. 1997; Nursing data book. New York, NY. 1982 and unpublished data; State-Approved Schools of Nursing-RN. New York, NY. 1973; Association of Schools of Public Health: 2005 Annual Data Report. Washington, DC. 2006, available from: http://www.asph.org/userfiles/ADR%202005.pdf.

Table 113. Hospitals, beds, and occupancy rates, by type of ownership and size of hospital: United States, selected years 1975–2005

[Data are based on reporting by a census of hospitals]

Type of ownership and size of hospital	*1975*	*1980*	*1990*	*1995*	*2000*	*2003*	*2005*
Hospitals				Number			
All hospitals	7,156	6,965	6,649	6,291	5,810	5,764	5,756
Federal	382	359	337	299	245	239	226
Nonfederal[1]	6,774	6,606	6,312	5,992	5,565	5,525	5,530
Community[2]	5,875	5,830	5,384	5,194	4,915	4,895	4,936
Nonprofit	3,339	3,322	3,191	3,092	3,003	2,984	2,958
For profit	775	730	749	752	749	790	868
State-local government	1,761	1,778	1,444	1,350	1,163	1,121	1,110
6–24 beds	299	259	226	278	288	327	370
25–49 beds	1,155	1,029	935	922	910	965	1,032
50–99 beds	1,481	1,462	1,263	1,139	1,055	1,031	1,001
100–199 beds	1,363	1,370	1,306	1,324	1,236	1,168	1,129
200–299 beds	678	715	739	718	656	624	619
300–399 beds	378	412	408	354	341	349	368
400–499 beds	230	266	222	195	182	172	173
500 beds or more	291	317	285	264	247	256	244
Beds							
All hospitals	1,465,828	1,364,516	1,213,327	1,080,601	983,628	965,256	946,997
Federal	131,946	117,328	98,255	77,079	53,067	47,456	45,837
Nonfederal[1]	1,333,882	1,247,188	1,115,072	1,003,522	930,561	917,800	901,160
Community[2]	941,844	988,387	927,360	872,736	823,560	813,307	802,311
Nonprofit	658,195	692,459	656,755	609,729	582,988	574,587	561,106
For profit	73,495	87,033	101,377	105,737	109,883	109,671	113,510
State-local government	210,154	208,895	169,228	157,270	130,689	129,049	127,695
6–24 beds	5,615	4,932	4,427	5,085	5,156	5,635	6,316
25–49 beds	41,783	37,478	35,420	34,352	33,333	33,613	33,726
50–99 beds	106,776	105,278	90,394	82,024	75,865	74,025	71,737
100–199 beds	192,438	192,892	183,867	187,381	175,778	167,451	161,593
200–299 beds	164,405	172,390	179,670	175,240	159,807	152,487	151,290
300–399 beds	127,728	139,434	138,938	121,136	117,220	119,903	126,899
400–499 beds	101,278	117,724	98,833	86,459	80,763	76,333	76,894
500 beds or more	201,821	218,259	195,811	181,059	175,638	183,860	173,856
Occupancy rate[3]				Percent			
All hospitals	76.7	77.7	69.5	65.7	66.1	68.1	69.3
Federal	80.7	80.1	72.9	72.6	68.2	64.8	66.0
Nonfederal[1]	76.3	77.4	69.2	65.1	65.9	68.3	69.5
Community[2]	75.0	75.6	66.8	62.8	63.9	66.2	67.3
Nonprofit	77.5	78.2	69.3	64.5	65.5	67.7	69.1
For profit	65.9	65.2	52.8	51.8	55.9	59.6	59.6
State-local government	70.4	71.1	65.3	63.7	63.2	65.3	66.7
6–24 beds	48.0	46.8	32.3	36.9	31.7	31.9	33.5
25–49 beds	56.7	52.8	41.3	42.6	41.3	44.6	47.1
50–99 beds	64.7	64.2	53.8	54.1	54.8	57.2	59.0
100–199 beds	71.2	71.4	61.5	58.8	60.0	62.6	63.2
200–299 beds	77.1	77.4	67.1	63.1	65.0	67.0	67.7
300–399 beds	79.7	79.7	70.0	64.8	65.7	68.5	70.1
400–499 beds	81.1	81.2	73.5	68.1	69.1	70.7	71.2
500 beds or more	80.9	82.1	77.3	71.4	72.2	74.2	75.9

[1]The category of nonfederal hospitals comprises psychiatric, tuberculosis and other respiratory diseases hospitals, and long-term and short-term general and other special hospitals. See Appendix II, Hospital.
[2]Community hospitals are nonfederal short-term general and special hospitals whose facilities and services are available to the public. See Appendix II, Hospital.
[3]Estimated percentage of staffed beds that are occupied. See Appendix II, Occupancy rate.

SOURCES: American Hospital Association (AHA) Annual Survey of Hospitals. Hospital Statistics, 1976, 1981, 1991–2007 editions. Chicago, IL. (Copyrights 1976, 1981, 1991–2007: Used with the permission of Health Forum LLC, an affiliate of the AHA.)

Table 114. Mental health organizations and beds for 24-hour hospital and residential treatment, by type of organization: United States, selected years 1986–2004

[Data are based on inventories of mental health organizations]

Type of organization	1986	1990	1994	1998	2000	2002	2004
	Number of mental health organizations						
All organizations	3,512	3,942	3,853	3,741	3,211	3,044	2,891
State and county mental hospitals	285	278	270	237	229	227	237
Private psychiatric hospitals	314	464	432	347	271	255	264
Nonfederal general hospital psychiatric services	1,351	1,577	1,539	1,595	1,325	1,231	1,230
Department of Veterans Affairs medical centers[1]	139	131	136	124	134	132	- - -
Residential treatment centers for emotionally disturbed children	437	501	472	462	476	510	458
All other organizations[2]	986	991	1,004	976	776	689	702
	Number of beds						
All organizations	267,613	325,529	293,139	269,148	214,186	211,040	212,231
State and county mental hospitals	119,033	102,307	84,063	71,266	61,833	57,314	57,034
Private psychiatric hospitals	30,201	45,952	42,742	31,731	26,402	24,996	28,422
Nonfederal general hospital psychiatric services	45,808	53,576	53,455	54,775	40,410	40,520	41,403
Department of Veterans Affairs medical centers[1]	26,874	24,779	21,346	17,173	8,989	9,581	- - -
Residential treatment centers for emotionally disturbed children	24,547	35,170	32,691	32,040	33,508	39,407	33,835
All other organizations[2]	21,150	63,745	58,842	62,163	43,044	39,222	51,536
	Beds per 100,000 civilian population[3]						
All organizations	111.7	128.5	110.9	94.0	74.8	72.2	71.2
State and county mental hospitals	49.7	40.4	31.8	24.9	21.6	19.6	19.1
Private psychiatric hospitals	12.6	18.1	16.2	11.1	9.2	8.6	9.5
Nonfederal general hospital psychiatric services	19.1	21.2	20.2	19.1	14.1	13.9	13.9
Department of Veterans Affairs medical centers[1]	11.2	9.9	8.1	6.0	3.1	3.3	- - -
Residential treatment centers for emotionally disturbed children	10.3	13.9	12.4	11.2	11.7	13.5	11.4
All other organizations[2]	8.8	25.2	22.2	21.7	15.0	13.4	17.3

- - - Data not available.

[1]Department of Veterans Affairs Medical Centers (VA general hospital psychiatric services and VA psychiatric outpatient clinics) were dropped from the survey as of 2004.

[2]Includes freestanding psychiatric outpatient clinics, partial care organizations, and multiservice mental health organizations. See Appendix I, Survey of Mental Health Organizations (SMHO).

[3]Civilian population estimates for 2000 and beyond are based on the 2000 census as of July 1; population estimates for 1992–1998 are 1990 postcensal estimates.

NOTES: Data for 1990, 1992, 1994, 1998, 2000, and 2002 are revised final estimates and differ from previous editions of *Health, United States*. Data for additional years are available. See Appendix III.

SOURCE: Substance Abuse and Mental Health Services Administration, Center for Mental Health Services (CMHS), Survey of Mental Health Organizations.

Table 115 (page 1 of 2). Community hospital beds and average annual percentage change, by geographic division and state: United States, selected years 1960–2005

[Data are based on reporting by a census of hospitals]

Geographic division and state	1960[1,2]	1970[1]	1980[1]	1990[3]	2000[3]	2005[3]	1960–1970[1,2]	1970–1980[1]	1980–1990[4]	1990–2000[3]	2000–2005[3]
	Beds per 1,000 resident population[5]						Average annual percent change				
United States	3.6	4.3	4.5	3.7	2.9	2.7	1.8	0.5	–1.9	–2.4	–1.4
New England	3.9	4.1	4.1	3.4	2.5	2.4	0.5	0.0	–1.9	–3.0	–0.8
Connecticut	3.4	3.4	3.5	2.9	2.3	2.2	0.0	0.3	–1.9	–2.3	–0.9
Maine	3.4	4.7	4.7	3.7	2.9	2.7	3.3	0.0	–2.4	–2.4	–1.4
Massachusetts	4.2	4.4	4.4	3.6	2.6	2.5	0.5	0.0	–2.0	–3.2	–0.8
New Hampshire	4.4	4.0	3.9	3.1	2.3	2.2	–0.9	–0.3	–2.3	–2.9	–0.9
Rhode Island	3.7	4.0	3.8	3.2	2.3	2.2	0.8	–0.5	–1.7	–3.2	–0.9
Vermont	4.5	4.5	4.4	3.0	2.7	2.2	0.0	–0.2	–3.8	–1.0	–4.0
Middle Atlantic	4.0	4.4	4.6	4.1	3.4	3.1	1.0	0.4	–1.1	–1.9	–1.8
New Jersey	3.1	3.6	4.2	3.7	3.0	2.5	1.5	1.6	–1.3	–2.1	–3.6
New York	4.3	4.6	4.5	4.1	3.5	3.3	0.7	–0.2	–0.9	–1.6	–1.2
Pennsylvania	4.1	4.7	4.8	4.4	3.4	3.2	1.4	0.2	–0.9	–2.5	–1.2
East North Central	3.6	4.4	4.7	3.9	2.9	2.7	2.0	0.7	–1.8	–2.9	–1.4
Illinois	4.0	4.7	5.1	4.0	3.0	2.7	1.6	0.8	–2.4	–2.8	–2.1
Indiana	3.1	4.0	4.5	3.9	3.2	2.8	2.6	1.2	–1.4	–2.0	–2.6
Michigan	3.3	4.3	4.4	3.7	2.6	2.6	2.7	0.2	–1.7	–3.5	0.0
Ohio	3.4	4.2	4.7	4.0	3.0	2.9	2.1	1.1	–1.6	–2.8	–0.7
Wisconsin	4.3	5.2	4.9	3.8	2.9	2.6	1.9	–0.6	–2.5	–2.7	–2.2
West North Central	4.3	5.7	5.8	4.9	3.9	3.6	2.9	0.2	–1.7	–2.3	–1.6
Iowa	3.9	5.6	5.7	5.1	4.0	3.6	3.7	0.2	–1.1	–2.4	–2.1
Kansas	4.2	5.4	5.8	4.8	4.0	3.7	2.5	0.7	–1.9	–1.8	–1.5
Minnesota	4.8	6.1	5.7	4.4	3.4	3.1	2.4	–0.7	–2.6	–2.5	–1.8
Missouri	3.9	5.1	5.7	4.8	3.6	3.3	2.7	1.1	–1.7	–2.8	–1.7
Nebraska	4.4	6.2	6.0	5.5	4.8	4.3	3.5	–0.3	–0.9	–1.4	–2.2
North Dakota	5.2	6.8	7.4	7.0	6.0	5.5	2.7	0.8	–0.6	–1.5	–1.7
South Dakota	4.5	5.6	5.5	6.1	5.7	5.6	2.2	–0.2	1.0	–0.7	–0.4
South Atlantic	3.3	4.0	4.5	3.7	2.9	2.7	1.9	1.2	–1.9	–2.4	–1.4
Delaware	3.7	3.7	3.6	3.0	2.3	2.3	0.0	–0.3	–1.8	–2.6	0.0
District of Columbia	5.9	7.4	7.3	7.6	5.8	6.4	2.3	–0.1	0.4	–2.7	2.0
Florida	3.1	4.4	5.1	3.9	3.2	2.9	3.6	1.5	–2.6	–2.0	–1.9
Georgia	2.8	3.8	4.6	4.0	2.9	2.8	3.1	1.9	–1.4	–3.2	–0.7
Maryland	3.3	3.1	3.6	2.8	2.1	2.0	–0.6	1.5	–2.5	–2.8	–1.0
North Carolina	3.4	3.8	4.2	3.3	2.9	2.7	1.1	1.0	–2.4	–1.3	–1.4
South Carolina	2.9	3.7	3.9	3.3	2.9	2.7	2.5	0.5	–1.7	–1.3	–1.4
Virginia	3.0	3.7	4.1	3.3	2.4	2.3	2.1	1.0	–2.1	–3.1	–0.8
West Virginia	4.1	5.4	5.5	4.7	4.4	4.0	2.8	0.2	–1.6	–0.7	–1.9
East South Central	3.0	4.4	5.1	4.7	3.8	3.6	3.9	1.5	–0.8	–2.1	–1.1
Alabama	2.8	4.3	5.1	4.6	3.7	3.4	4.4	1.7	–1.0	–2.2	–1.7
Kentucky	3.0	4.0	4.5	4.3	3.7	3.6	2.9	1.2	–0.5	–1.5	–0.5
Mississippi	2.9	4.4	5.3	5.0	4.8	4.4	4.3	1.9	–0.6	–0.4	–1.7
Tennessee	3.4	4.7	5.5	4.8	3.6	3.5	3.3	1.6	–1.4	–2.8	–0.6
West South Central	3.3	4.3	4.7	3.8	3.0	2.8	2.7	0.9	–2.1	–2.3	–1.4
Arkansas	2.9	4.2	5.0	4.6	3.7	3.4	3.8	1.8	–0.8	–2.2	–1.7
Louisiana	3.9	4.2	4.8	4.6	3.9	3.4	0.7	1.3	–0.4	–1.6	–2.7
Oklahoma	3.2	4.5	4.6	4.0	3.2	3.0	3.5	0.2	–1.4	–2.2	–1.3
Texas	3.3	4.3	4.7	3.5	2.7	2.5	2.7	0.9	–2.9	–2.6	–1.5
Mountain	3.5	4.3	3.8	3.1	2.3	2.2	2.1	–1.2	–2.0	–2.9	–0.9
Arizona	3.0	4.1	3.6	2.7	2.1	2.0	3.2	–1.3	–2.8	–2.5	–1.0
Colorado	3.8	4.6	4.2	3.2	2.2	2.1	1.9	–0.9	–2.7	–3.7	–0.9
Idaho	3.2	4.0	3.7	3.2	2.7	2.3	2.3	–0.8	–1.4	–1.7	–3.2
Montana	5.1	5.8	5.9	5.8	4.7	4.6	1.3	0.2	–0.2	–2.1	–0.4
Nevada	3.9	4.2	4.2	2.8	1.9	1.9	0.7	0.0	–4.0	–3.8	0.0
New Mexico	2.9	3.5	3.1	2.8	1.9	1.8	1.9	–1.2	–1.0	–3.8	–1.1
Utah	2.8	3.6	3.1	2.6	1.9	1.8	2.5	–1.5	–1.7	–3.1	–1.1
Wyoming	4.6	5.5	3.6	4.8	3.9	4.0	1.8	–4.1	2.9	–2.1	0.5
Pacific	3.1	3.7	3.5	2.7	2.1	1.9	1.8	–0.6	–2.6	–2.5	–2.0
Alaska	2.4	2.3	2.7	2.3	2.3	2.1	–0.4	1.6	–1.6	0.0	–1.8
California	3.0	3.8	3.6	2.7	2.1	1.9	2.4	–0.5	–2.8	–2.5	–2.0
Hawaii	3.7	3.4	3.1	2.7	2.5	2.4	–0.8	–0.9	–1.4	–0.8	–0.8
Oregon	3.5	4.0	3.5	2.8	1.9	1.8	1.3	–1.3	–2.2	–3.8	–1.1
Washington	3.3	3.5	3.1	2.5	1.9	1.7	0.6	–1.2	–2.1	–2.7	–2.2

See footnotes at end of table.

Table 115 (page 2 of 2). Community hospital beds and average annual percentage change, by geographic division and state: United States, selected years 1960–2005

[Data are based on reporting by a census of hospitals]

[1]Data exclude facilities for the mentally retarded. See Appendix II, Hospital.
[2]1960 data include hospital units of institutions such as prisons and college infirmaries.
[3]Starting with 1990 data, hospital units of institutions, facilities for the mentally retarded, and alcoholism and chemical dependency hospitals are excluded. See Appendix II, Hospital.
[4]1990 data used in this calculation (not shown in table) exclude only facilities for the mentally retarded, consistent with exclusions from 1980 data.
[5]Civilian population for 1997 and earlier years.

SOURCES: American Hospital Association (AHA): Hospitals. *JAHA* 35(15):383–430, 1961 (Copyright 1961: Used with permission of AHA); AHA Annual Survey of Hospitals for 1970 and 1980; Hospital Statistics 1991–1992, 2001–2007 editions. Chicago, IL. (Copyrights 1971, 1981, 1991, 2001–2007: Used with permission of Health Forum LLC, an affiliate of the AHA.)

Table 116 (page 1 of 2). Occupancy rates in community hospitals and average annual percent change, by geographic division and state: United States, selected years 1960–2005

[Data are based on reporting by a census of hospitals]

Geographic division and state	*1960[1,2]*	*1970[1]*	*1980[1]*	*1990[3]*	*2000[3]*	*2005[3]*	*1960–1970[1,2]*	*1970–1980[1]*	*1980–1990[4]*	*1990–2000[3]*	*2000–2005[3]*
	Occupancy rate[5]						Average annual percent change				
United States	75	77	75	67	64	67	0.3	–0.3	–1.1	–0.5	0.9
New England	75	80	80	74	70	74	0.6	0.0	–0.8	–0.6	1.1
Connecticut	78	83	80	77	75	81	0.6	–0.4	–0.4	–0.3	1.6
Maine	73	73	75	72	64	66	0.0	0.3	–0.4	–1.2	0.6
Massachusetts	76	80	82	74	71	74	0.5	0.2	–1.0	–0.4	0.8
New Hampshire	67	73	73	67	59	62	0.9	0.0	–0.9	–1.3	1.0
Rhode Island	76	83	86	79	72	78	0.9	0.4	–0.8	–0.9	1.6
Vermont	69	76	74	67	67	67	1.0	–0.3	–1.0	0.0	0.0
Middle Atlantic	78	82	83	81	74	75	0.5	0.1	–0.2	–0.9	0.3
New Jersey	78	83	83	80	69	73	0.6	0.0	–0.4	–1.5	1.1
New York	79	83	86	86	79	79	0.5	0.4	0.0	–0.8	0.0
Pennsylvania	76	82	80	73	68	70	0.8	–0.2	–0.9	–0.7	0.6
East North Central	78	80	77	65	61	64	0.3	–0.4	–1.7	–0.6	1.0
Illinois	76	79	75	66	60	66	0.4	–0.5	–1.3	–0.9	1.9
Indiana	80	80	78	61	56	58	0.0	–0.3	–2.4	–0.9	0.7
Michigan	81	81	78	66	65	67	0.0	–0.4	–1.7	–0.2	0.6
Ohio	81	82	79	65	61	64	0.1	–0.4	–1.9	–0.6	1.0
Wisconsin	74	73	74	65	60	63	–0.1	0.1	–1.3	–0.8	1.0
West North Central	72	74	71	62	60	63	0.3	–0.4	–1.3	–0.3	1.0
Iowa	73	72	69	62	58	59	–0.1	–0.4	–1.1	–0.7	0.3
Kansas	69	71	69	56	53	56	0.3	–0.3	–2.1	–0.5	1.1
Minnesota	72	74	74	67	67	69	0.3	0.0	–1.0	0.0	0.6
Missouri	76	79	75	62	58	63	0.4	–0.5	–1.9	–0.7	1.7
Nebraska	66	70	67	58	59	64	0.6	–0.4	–1.4	0.2	1.6
North Dakota	71	67	69	64	60	60	–0.6	0.3	–0.7	–0.6	0.0
South Dakota	66	66	61	62	65	65	0.0	–0.8	0.2	0.5	0.0
South Atlantic	75	78	76	67	65	70	0.4	–0.3	–1.3	–0.3	1.5
Delaware	70	79	82	77	75	92	1.2	0.4	–0.6	–0.3	4.2
District of Columbia	81	78	83	75	74	77	–0.4	0.6	–1.0	–0.1	0.8
Florida	74	76	72	62	61	66	0.3	–0.5	–1.5	–0.2	1.6
Georgia	72	77	70	66	63	68	0.7	–0.9	–0.6	–0.5	1.5
Maryland	74	79	84	79	73	77	0.7	0.6	–0.6	–0.8	1.1
North Carolina	74	79	78	73	70	71	0.7	–0.1	–0.7	–0.4	0.3
South Carolina	77	76	77	71	69	74	–0.1	0.1	–0.8	–0.3	1.4
Virginia	78	81	78	67	68	71	0.4	–0.4	–1.5	0.1	0.9
West Virginia	75	79	76	63	61	63	0.5	–0.4	–1.9	–0.3	0.6
East South Central	72	78	75	63	59	62	0.8	–0.4	–1.7	–0.7	1.0
Alabama	71	80	73	63	60	64	1.2	–0.9	–1.5	–0.5	1.3
Kentucky	73	80	77	62	62	62	0.9	–0.4	–2.1	0.0	0.0
Mississippi	63	74	71	59	59	58	1.6	–0.4	–1.8	0.0	–0.3
Tennessee	76	78	76	64	56	63	0.3	–0.3	–1.7	–1.3	2.4
West South Central	69	73	70	58	58	61	0.6	–0.4	–1.9	0.0	1.0
Arkansas	70	74	70	62	59	58	0.6	–0.6	–1.2	–0.5	–0.3
Louisiana	68	74	70	57	56	60	0.8	–0.6	–2.0	–0.2	1.4
Oklahoma	71	73	68	58	56	59	0.3	–0.7	–1.6	–0.4	1.0
Texas	68	73	70	57	59	62	0.7	–0.4	–2.0	0.3	1.0
Mountain	70	71	70	61	61	64	0.1	–0.1	–1.4	0.0	1.0
Arizona	74	73	74	62	63	68	–0.1	0.1	–1.8	0.2	1.5
Colorado	81	74	72	64	58	60	–0.9	–0.3	–1.2	–1.0	0.7
Idaho	56	66	65	56	53	53	1.7	–0.2	–1.5	–0.5	0.0
Montana	60	66	66	61	67	65	1.0	0.0	–0.8	0.9	–0.6
Nevada	71	73	69	60	71	74	0.3	–0.6	–1.4	1.7	0.8
New Mexico	65	70	66	58	58	63	0.7	–0.6	–1.3	0.0	1.7
Utah	70	74	70	59	56	58	0.6	–0.6	–1.7	–0.5	0.7
Wyoming	61	63	57	54	56	56	0.3	–1.0	–0.5	0.4	0.0
Pacific	71	71	69	64	65	70	0.0	–0.3	–0.7	0.2	1.5
Alaska	54	59	58	50	57	60	0.9	–0.2	–1.5	1.3	1.0
California	74	71	69	64	66	71	–0.4	–0.3	–0.7	0.3	1.5
Hawaii	62	76	75	85	76	78	2.1	–0.1	1.3	–1.1	0.5
Oregon	66	69	69	57	59	63	0.4	0.0	–1.9	0.3	1.3
Washington	63	70	72	63	60	63	1.1	0.3	–1.3	–0.5	1.0

See footnotes at end of table.

Table 116 (page 2 of 2). Occupancy rates in community hospitals and average annual percent change, by geographic division and state: United States, selected years 1960–2005

[Data are based on reporting by a census of hospitals]

---

[1]Data exclude facilities for the mentally retarded. See Appendix II, Hospital.
[2]1960 data include hospital units of institutions such as prisons and college infirmaries.
[3]Starting with 1990 data, hospital units of institutions, facilities for the mentally retarded, and alcoholism and chemical dependency hospitals are excluded. See Appendix II, Hospital.
[4]1990 data used in this calculation (not shown in table) exclude only facilities for the mentally retarded, consistent with exclusions from 1980 data.
[5]Estimated percent of staffed beds that are occupied. Occupancy rate is calculated as the average daily census (inpatient days divided by 365) divided by the number of hospital beds. Data include hospital and nursing home units. See Appendix II, Occupancy rate.

SOURCES: American Hospital Association (AHA): Hospitals. *JAHA* 35(15):383–430, 1961. (Copyright 1961: Used with permission of AHA); AHA Annual Survey of Hospitals, 1970 and 1980 unpublished; Hospital Statistics 1991–1992, 2001–2007 editions. Chicago, IL. (Copyrights 1971, 1981, 1991, 2001–2007: Used with permission of Health Forum LLC, an affiliate of the AHA.)

Table 117 (page 1 of 2). Nursing homes, beds, occupancy, and residents, by geographic division and state: United States, selected years 1995–2006

[Data are based on a census of certified nursing facilities]

Geographic division and state	Nursing homes				Beds			
	1995	*2000*	*2005*	*2006*	*1995*	*2000*	*2005*	*2006*
United States	16,389	16,886	15,995	15,899	1,751,302	1,795,388	1,724,582	1,716,102
New England	1,140	1,137	1,031	1,021	115,488	118,562	109,173	108,027
Connecticut	267	259	247	245	32,827	32,433	30,605	30,100
Maine	132	126	114	113	9,243	8,248	7,380	7,359
Massachusetts	550	526	456	453	54,532	56,030	50,708	50,416
New Hampshire	74	83	82	82	7,412	7,837	7,817	7,829
Rhode Island	94	99	91	87	9,612	10,271	9,214	8,889
Vermont	23	44	41	41	1,862	3,743	3,449	3,434
Middle Atlantic	1,650	1,796	1,741	1,734	244,342	267,772	261,054	261,537
New Jersey	300	361	363	363	43,967	52,195	51,233	52,126
New York	624	665	658	655	107,750	120,514	120,855	120,850
Pennsylvania	726	770	720	716	92,625	95,063	88,966	88,561
East North Central	3,171	3,301	3,114	3,090	367,879	369,657	343,158	339,079
Illinois	827	869	803	799	103,230	110,766	103,722	102,941
Indiana	556	564	511	511	59,538	56,762	55,793	56,964
Michigan	432	439	429	424	49,473	50,696	48,294	47,432
Ohio	943	1,009	971	958	106,884	105,038	96,134	93,210
Wisconsin	413	420	400	398	48,754	46,395	39,215	38,532
West North Central	2,258	2,281	2,154	2,144	200,109	193,754	182,044	180,287
Iowa	419	467	455	455	39,959	37,034	35,128	34,532
Kansas	429	392	358	352	30,016	27,067	26,254	25,908
Minnesota	432	433	404	399	43,865	42,149	36,660	35,837
Missouri	546	551	518	519	52,679	54,829	54,138	54,541
Nebraska	231	236	225	225	18,169	17,877	16,243	16,258
North Dakota	87	88	83	83	7,125	6,954	6,508	6,502
South Dakota	114	114	111	111	8,296	7,844	7,113	6,709
South Atlantic	2,215	2,418	2,356	2,345	243,069	264,147	264,166	263,950
Delaware	42	43	42	44	4,739	4,906	4,649	4,754
District of Columbia	19	20	20	20	3,206	3,078	3,036	2,988
Florida	627	732	686	682	72,656	83,365	82,519	82,319
Georgia	352	363	363	359	38,097	39,817	40,180	39,920
Maryland	218	255	237	233	28,394	31,495	29,306	29,020
North Carolina	391	410	423	421	38,322	41,376	43,623	43,768
South Carolina	166	178	176	176	16,682	18,102	18,310	18,415
Virginia	271	278	277	279	30,070	30,595	31,585	31,830
West Virginia	129	139	132	131	10,903	11,413	10,958	10,936
East South Central	1,014	1,071	1,058	1,053	99,707	106,250	108,908	108,675
Alabama	221	225	228	231	23,353	25,248	26,491	26,836
Kentucky	288	307	296	293	23,221	25,341	26,222	26,041
Mississippi	183	190	205	203	16,059	17,068	18,524	18,323
Tennessee	322	349	329	326	37,074	38,593	37,671	37,475
West South Central	2,264	2,199	2,022	2,011	224,695	224,100	216,776	216,867
Arkansas	256	255	236	237	29,952	25,715	24,419	24,684
Louisiana	337	337	304	293	37,769	39,430	38,260	37,043
Oklahoma	405	392	350	336	33,918	33,903	31,611	30,776
Texas	1,266	1,215	1,132	1,145	123,056	125,052	122,486	124,364
Mountain	800	827	779	773	70,134	75,152	73,209	73,353
Arizona	152	150	134	135	16,162	17,458	16,425	16,508
Colorado	219	225	213	211	19,912	20,240	19,899	19,982
Idaho	76	84	80	80	5,747	6,181	6,167	6,195
Montana	100	104	98	97	7,210	7,667	7,368	7,338
Nevada	42	51	47	47	3,998	5,547	5,442	5,615
New Mexico	83	80	75	72	6,969	7,289	7,030	6,939
Utah	91	93	93	92	7,101	7,651	7,827	7,724
Wyoming	37	40	39	39	3,035	3,119	3,051	3,052
Pacific	1,877	1,856	1,740	1,728	185,879	175,994	166,094	164,327
Alaska	15	15	14	15	814	821	727	725
California	1,382	1,369	1,295	1,283	140,203	131,762	126,016	124,416
Hawaii	34	45	45	46	2,513	4,006	4,074	4,127
Oregon	161	150	139	138	13,885	13,500	12,698	12,573
Washington	285	277	247	246	28,464	25,905	22,579	22,486

See footnotes at end of table.

Table 117 (page 2 of 2). Nursing homes, beds, occupancy, and residents, by geographic division and state: United States, selected years 1995–2006

[Data are based on a census of certified nursing facilities]

Geographic division and state	Residents				Occupancy rate[1]				Resident rate[2]			
	1995	2000	2005	2006	1995	2000	2005	2006	1995	2000	2005	2006
United States	1,479,550	1,480,076	1,436,442	1,433,523	84.5	82.4	83.3	83.5	404.5	349.1	281.9	270.6
New England	105,792	106,308	98,320	97,511	91.6	89.7	90.1	90.3	474.2	419.5	309.4	324.6
Connecticut	29,948	29,657	27,874	27,364	91.2	91.4	91.1	90.9	541.7	461.4	323.0	358.2
Maine	8,587	7,298	6,711	6,651	92.9	88.5	90.9	90.4	417.9	313.0	256.2	246.2
Massachusetts	49,765	49,805	44,986	45,068	91.3	88.9	88.7	89.4	477.3	426.8	316.1	328.9
New Hampshire	6,877	7,158	7,033	7,052	92.8	91.3	90.0	90.1	434.1	392.6	299.2	305.0
Rhode Island	8,823	9,041	8,564	8,265	91.8	88.0	92.9	93.0	476.9	432.6	310.8	329.0
Vermont	1,792	3,349	3,152	3,111	96.2	89.5	91.4	90.6	207.0	335.0	264.5	265.6
Middle Atlantic	228,649	242,674	237,362	238,468	93.6	90.6	90.9	91.2	384.0	354.2	280.6	286.3
New Jersey	40,397	45,837	44,864	45,667	91.9	87.8	87.6	87.6	351.6	337.0	262.5	274.2
New York	103,409	112,957	112,268	112,141	96.0	93.7	92.9	92.8	371.8	362.6	303.7	301.7
Pennsylvania	84,843	83,880	80,230	80,660	91.6	88.2	90.2	91.1	419.2	353.1	262.7	273.6
East North Central	294,319	289,404	275,433	273,438	80.0	78.3	80.3	80.6	476.1	414.3	322.8	325.1
Illinois	83,696	83,604	77,923	77,204	81.1	75.5	75.1	75.0	495.3	435.4	342.1	340.0
Indiana	44,328	42,328	40,386	39,758	74.5	74.6	72.4	69.8	548.9	462.3	371.8	357.6
Michigan	43,271	42,615	41,678	41,090	87.5	84.1	86.3	86.6	345.0	299.1	226.4	235.1
Ohio	79,026	81,946	81,039	81,275	73.9	78.0	84.3	87.2	499.5	463.5	372.7	374.6
Wisconsin	43,998	38,911	34,407	34,111	90.2	83.9	87.7	88.5	518.9	406.9	298.5	306.9
West North Central	164,660	157,224	144,385	143,361	82.3	81.1	79.3	79.5	489.6	429.8	350.0	337.2
Iowa	27,506	29,204	27,241	26,866	68.8	78.9	77.5	77.8	458.0	448.5	361.5	357.4
Kansas	25,140	22,230	20,214	19,785	83.8	82.1	77.0	76.4	528.9	429.4	350.5	332.4
Minnesota	41,163	38,813	33,537	32,738	93.8	92.1	91.5	91.4	537.4	453.4	325.6	322.1
Missouri	39,891	38,586	37,524	38,001	75.7	70.4	69.3	69.7	432.8	391.5	361.7	334.0
Nebraska	16,166	14,989	13,196	13,327	89.0	83.8	81.2	82.0	501.4	441.5	357.2	340.6
North Dakota	6,868	6,343	5,978	5,967	96.4	91.2	91.9	91.8	522.0	430.7	348.8	355.2
South Dakota	7,926	7,059	6,695	6,677	95.5	90.0	94.1	99.5	543.3	438.8	358.7	350.0
South Atlantic	217,303	227,818	233,076	233,404	89.4	86.2	88.2	88.4	335.4	291.9	246.4	224.4
Delaware	3,819	3,900	3,834	3,855	80.6	79.5	82.5	81.1	448.7	369.7	267.4	264.9
District of Columbia	2,576	2,858	2,804	2,760	80.3	92.9	92.4	92.4	297.6	318.4	289.8	256.3
Florida	61,845	69,050	72,879	72,552	85.1	82.8	88.3	88.1	228.2	208.4	182.5	156.9
Georgia	35,933	36,559	36,007	35,755	94.3	91.8	89.6	89.6	496.0	416.1	358.7	315.4
Maryland	24,716	25,629	24,983	25,273	87.0	81.4	85.2	87.1	432.7	383.1	279.7	294.6
North Carolina	35,511	36,658	38,305	38,362	92.7	88.6	87.8	87.6	401.1	347.6	300.6	281.6
South Carolina	14,568	15,739	16,473	16,635	87.3	86.9	90.0	90.3	366.0	313.1	259.1	242.1
Virginia	28,119	27,091	28,039	28,380	93.5	88.5	88.8	89.2	385.2	310.4	257.2	253.1
West Virginia	10,216	10,334	9,752	9,832	93.7	90.5	89.0	89.9	355.2	325.2	297.1	272.6
East South Central	91,563	96,348	95,773	95,987	91.8	90.7	87.9	88.3	416.6	385.5	374.8	324.0
Alabama	21,691	23,089	23,432	23,488	92.9	91.4	88.5	87.5	370.1	343.1	344.7	295.3
Kentucky	20,696	22,730	23,053	23,261	89.1	89.7	87.9	89.3	391.9	390.1	380.5	334.9
Mississippi	15,247	15,815	16,261	16,419	94.9	92.7	87.8	89.6	405.3	368.7	399.9	331.1
Tennessee	33,929	34,714	33,027	32,819	91.5	89.9	87.7	87.6	479.6	426.1	382.8	335.9
West South Central	169,047	159,160	155,783	155,800	75.2	71.0	71.9	71.8	486.1	397.6	367.9	317.5
Arkansas	20,823	19,317	17,476	17,970	69.5	75.1	71.6	72.8	508.3	415.5	360.0	327.4
Louisiana	32,493	30,735	28,316	27,800	86.0	77.9	74.0	75.0	639.3	523.8	454.7	411.2
Oklahoma	26,377	23,833	20,978	20,242	77.8	70.3	66.4	65.8	499.1	416.8	379.4	308.7
Texas	89,354	85,275	89,013	89,788	72.6	68.2	72.7	72.2	439.9	358.4	345.9	296.7
Mountain	58,738	59,379	57,927	58,042	83.8	79.0	79.1	79.1	335.9	271.2	205.8	190.0
Arizona	12,382	13,253	12,964	12,775	76.6	75.9	78.9	77.4	233.3	193.4	142.1	121.5
Colorado	17,055	17,045	16,410	16,579	85.7	84.2	82.5	83.0	420.6	353.5	275.5	270.8
Idaho	4,697	4,640	4,685	4,646	81.7	75.1	76.0	75.0	321.7	257.0	200.0	198.7
Montana	6,415	5,973	5,420	5,405	89.0	77.9	73.6	73.7	491.4	389.5	282.5	284.5
Nevada	3,645	3,657	4,399	4,664	91.2	65.9	80.8	83.1	312.0	215.3	171.2	167.5
New Mexico	6,051	6,503	6,184	6,019	86.8	89.2	88.0	86.7	332.0	279.0	224.7	192.2
Utah	5,832	5,703	5,400	5,480	82.1	74.5	69.0	70.9	323.5	262.2	197.5	187.4
Wyoming	2,661	2,605	2,465	2,474	87.7	83.5	80.8	81.1	468.2	386.8	328.0	295.7
Pacific	149,479	141,761	138,383	137,512	80.4	80.5	83.3	83.7	302.4	241.3	182.1	179.9
Alaska	634	595	622	640	77.9	72.5	85.6	88.3	348.0	225.9	159.2	154.3
California	109,805	106,460	106,408	105,458	78.3	80.8	84.4	84.8	302.9	250.1	195.8	189.9
Hawaii	2,413	3,558	3,777	3,828	96.0	88.8	92.7	92.8	178.5	202.6	136.6	142.4
Oregon	11,673	9,990	8,215	8,108	84.1	74.0	64.7	64.5	244.9	173.9	110.2	114.2
Washington	24,954	21,158	19,361	19,478	87.7	81.7	85.7	86.6	362.5	251.6	175.2	182.0

[1]Percentage of beds occupied (number of nursing home residents per 100 nursing home beds).

[2]Number of nursing home residents (all ages) per 1,000 resident population 85 years of age and over. Resident rates for 1995–1999 are based on population estimates projected from the 1990 census. Starting with 2000 data, resident rates are based on the 2000 census and postcensal population estimates. Available from: www.census.gov/popest/datasets.html.

NOTES: An error in the 2005 data file of the number of beds in Kansas was corrected. This affected the number of beds for Kansas, the West North Central division, and United States and the occupancy rates for these areas. See Appendix I, Online Survey Certification and Reporting Database (OSCAR). Annual numbers of nursing homes, beds, and residents are based on a 15-month OSCAR reporting cycle. Data for additional years are available. See Appendix III.

SOURCES: Cowles CM ed., 2005 Nursing Home Statistical Yearbook. McMinnville, OR: Cowles Research Group, 2006 and previous editions; and Cowles Research Group, unpublished data. Based on data from the Centers for Medicare & Medicaid Services' Online Survey Certification and Reporting (OSCAR) database.

Table 118. Medicare-certified providers and suppliers: United States, selected years 1980–2005

[Data are compiled from various Centers for Medicare & Medicaid Services data systems]

Providers or suppliers	*1980*	*1985*	*1990*	*1996*	*2000*	*2002*	*2004*	*2005*
	Number of providers or suppliers							
Home health agencies	2,924	5,679	5,730	10,807	7,857	6,813	7,519	8,090
Clinical Lab Improvement Act Facilities	- - -	- - -	- - -	164,054	171,018	173,807	189,340	196,296
End stage renal disease facilities	999	1,393	1,937	3,367	3,787	4,113	4,618	4,755
Outpatient physical therapy	419	854	1,195	2,758	2,867	2,836	2,971	2,962
Portable X-ray	216	308	443	656	666	644	608	553
Rural health clinics	391	428	551	3,673	3,453	3,283	3,536	3,661
Comprehensive outpatient rehabilitation facilities	- - -	72	186	531	522	524	635	634
Ambulatory surgical centers	- - -	336	1,197	2,480	2,894	3,371	4,136	4,445
Hospices	- - -	164	825	2,344	2,326	2,275	2,645	2,872

- - - Data not available.

NOTES: Provider and supplier data for 1980–1990 are as of July 1. Provider and supplier data for 1996–2005 are as of December. Providers and suppliers certified for Medicare are deemed to meet Medicaid standards. Data for additional years are available. See Appendix III.

SOURCE: Centers for Medicare & Medicaid Services (CMS). 2006 CMS Statistics. Baltimore, MD: CMS; 2006 and previous editions.

Table 119. Number of Magnetic Resonance Imaging (MRI) units and Computed Tomography (CT) scanners: Selected countries, selected years 1990–2004

[Data are based on reporting by countries]

Country	1990	1995	2000	2001	2002	2003	2004	1990	1995	2000	2001	2002	2003	2004
	Number of MRI units per million population							Number of CT scanners per million population						
Australia[1]	0.6	2.9	3.5	3.8	3.7	3.7	3.7	13.8	20.8	---	---	---	---	---
Austria	---	---	10.9	11.6	13.4	13.6	14.9	11.7	---	25.8	26.3	27.2	27.2	28.5
Belgium	2.0	3.3	6.0	7.0	6.6	6.8	---	16.1	---	21.8	23.1	28.8	29.8	---
Canada[2]	0.7	1.4	2.5	4.2	---	4.6	4.9	7.1	8.0	---	9.8	---	10.5	10.8
Czech Republic[3]	---	1.0	1.7	1.9	2.2	2.5	2.8	---	6.7	9.6	11.4	12.1	12.6	12.6
Denmark	2.5	---	5.4	---	8.6	9.1	10.2	4.3	7.3	11.4	13.2	13.8	14.5	14.6
Finland	1.8	4.3	9.9	11.0	12.5	13.0	14.0	9.8	11.7	13.5	13.7	13.3	14.0	14.2
France	0.8	2.1	2.6	2.4	2.7	2.8	3.2	6.7	9.2	9.5	9.0	9.7	8.4	7.5
Germany[4]	---	2.3	4.9	5.5	6.0	6.2	6.6	---	9.0	12.7	13.3	14.2	14.7	15.4
Greece	0.4	---	---	---	2.3	---	---	6.5	---	---	---	17.1	---	---
Hungary[5]	0.1	1.0	1.8	2.0	2.3	2.6	2.6	1.9	4.6	5.7	6.0	6.3	6.5	6.8
Iceland	3.9	7.5	10.7	14.0	17.4	17.3	17.1	11.8	18.7	21.3	17.5	20.9	20.7	17.1
Italy[6]	1.3	---	7.6	8.7	10.5	11.6	10.2	6.0	---	20.8	22.1	23.2	24.1	20.6
Japan[7]	6.1	---	---	---	35.3	---	---	55.2	---	---	---	92.6	---	---
South Korea	---	3.9	5.4	6.8	7.9	9.0	11.0	---	15.5	28.4	27.3	31.0	31.9	31.5
Mexico	---	---	0.6	1.1	1.2	1.3	1.7	---	---	1.4	2.5	2.9	3.0	3.1
New Zealand	---	---	---	---	---	3.7	---	3.6	---	8.8	10.6	11.2	11.5	12.1
Poland	---	---	---	---	0.9	1.0	---	---	---	4.4	5.2	5.8	6.3	---
Portugal[8]	0.8	---	---	---	---	3.9	---	4.6	---	---	---	---	12.8	---
Spain[9]	---	2.7	4.8	5.7	6.2	7.3	7.7	---	8.3	12.0	12.4	12.8	13.0	13.3
Sweden	1.5	6.8	---	---	---	---	---	10.5	---	---	---	---	---	---
Switzerland	---	---	12.9	12.9	14.1	14.2	14.3	---	---	18.5	17.6	18.0	18.0	17.9
Turkey	---	---	---	---	3.0	3.0	3.0	1.6	---	---	---	7.5	7.3	---
United Kingdom[10]	---	---	4.7	5.2	4.8	4.4	5.0	---	---	4.5	5.8	7.1	6.7	7.0
United States[11]	---	12.3	---	20.1	---	21.9	26.6	---	---	---	28.9	---	29.2	32.2
	Number of MRI units							Number of CT scanners						
Australia[1]	11	52	67	73	73	73	75	235	375	---	---	---	---	---
Austria	---	---	88	94	108	110	122	90	---	209	214	220	221	233
Belgium	20	33	61	72	68	71	---	160	---	223	238	298	309	---
Canada[2]	19	40	76	130	---	146	157	198	234	---	303	---	331	346
Czech Republic[3]	---	10	17	19	22	25	29	---	69	99	117	123	129	129
Denmark	13	---	29	---	46	49	55	22	38	61	71	74	78	79
Finland	9	22	51	57	65	68	73	49	60	70	71	69	73	74
France	45	123	156	141	163	169	191	379	534	563	531	579	503	449
Germany[4]	---	184	405	451	493	514	545	---	737	1,040	1,096	1,173	1,215	1,268
Greece	4	---	---	---	25	---	---	66	---	---	---	188	---	---
Hungary[5]	1	10	18	20	23	26	26	20	47	58	61	64	66	69
Iceland	1	2	3	4	5	5	5	3	5	6	5	6	6	5
Italy[6]	72	---	435	497	605	666	585	340	---	1,188	1,268	1,336	1,385	1,185
Japan[7]	756	---	---	---	4,501	---	---	6,821	---	---	---	11,803	---	---
South Korea	---	174	254	322	375	430	531	---	699	1,334	1,293	1,474	1,526	1,515
Mexico	---	---	60	110	123	138	174	---	---	138	248	296	309	324
New Zealand	---	---	---	---	---	15	---	12	---	34	41	44	46	49
Poland	---	---	---	---	36	39	---	---	---	169	199	222	242	---
Portugal[8]	8	---	---	---	---	41	---	45	---	---	---	---	134	---
Spain[9]	---	107	194	231	256	306	328	---	327	483	505	530	544	566
Sweden	13	60	---	---	---	---	---	90	---	---	---	---	---	---
Switzerland	---	---	93	93	103	104	106	---	---	133	127	131	132	132
Turkey	---	---	---	---	207	211	212	89	---	---	---	519	516	---
United Kingdom[10]	---	---	277	308	287	263	300	---	---	264	341	420	400	421
United States[11]	---	3,265	---	5,730	---	6,375	7,810	---	---	---	8,230	---	8,490	9,455

- - - Data not available.

[1]Starting with 2000 data, the number of MRI units include only those that are approved for billing to Medicare (Australia's national health program). In 1999, approved units represented approximately 60% of total units.

[2]The number of units in freestanding imaging facilities was imputed for years prior to 2003 based on data collected in the 2003 National Survey of Selected Medical Imaging Equipment, conducted by the Canadian Institute for Health Information. MRI units in Quebec are not included in 2000.

[3]Prior to 2000, the data include only equipment of Health Sector establishments.

[4]The data include equipment installed in acute care hospitals and prevention and rehabilitation homes.

[5]Equipment used in military hospitals and the health institutes of Hungarian State Railways are not included.

[6]1990 data include only equipment in public and private hospitals.

[7]Prior to 2000, the data include only equipment in hospitals.

[8]The data do not include equipment in all the private sectors.

[9]The data include equipment available in hospitals and do not include equipment in other health care facilities.

[10]The data include devices in public sector establishments only.

[11]Data are from the MRI Census and are comparable to the OECD definition. The devices in U.S. territories are not included.

SOURCES: Organisation for Economic Co-operation and Development (OECD); 2004 Computed Tomography (CT) and Magnetic Resonance Imaging (MRI) Census. Market Summary Report: IMV, Limited, Medical Information Division. 2004 Section B: Installed Base of CT Scanners: Installed Base of MRI Scanners (for U.S. data only).

Table 120. Total health expenditures as a percent of gross domestic product and per capita health expenditures in dollars, by selected countries: Selected years 1960–2004

[Data compiled by the Organisation for Economic Co-operation and Development]

Country	1960	1970	1980	1990	1995	1999	2000	2001	2002[1]	2003[1]	2004[1]
					Health expenditures as a percent of gross domestic product						
Australia	4.0	---	6.8	7.5	8.0	8.4	8.8	8.9	9.1	9.2	9.6
Austria	4.3	5.2	7.5	7.0	9.7	9.6	9.4	9.5	9.5	9.6	9.6
Belgium	---	3.9	6.3	7.2	8.2	8.5	8.6	8.7	8.9	10.1	---
Canada	5.4	7.0	7.1	9.0	9.2	9.0	8.9	9.4	9.7	9.9	9.9
Czech Republic	---	---	---	4.7	7.0	6.7	6.7	7.0	7.2	7.5	7.3
Denmark	---	---	8.9	8.3	8.1	8.5	8.3	8.6	8.8	8.9	8.9
Finland	3.8	5.6	6.3	7.8	7.4	6.9	6.7	6.9	7.2	7.4	7.5
France	3.8	5.3	7.0	8.4	9.4	9.2	9.2	9.3	10.0	10.4	10.5
Germany	---	6.2	8.7	8.5	10.1	10.3	10.3	10.4	10.6	10.8	10.6
Greece	---	6.1	6.6	7.4	9.6	9.6	9.9	10.4	10.3	10.5	10.0
Hungary	---	---	---	---	7.4	7.3	7.1	7.3	7.7	8.3	8.0
Iceland	3.0	4.7	6.2	7.9	8.4	9.3	9.2	9.3	10.0	10.5	10.2
Ireland	3.7	5.1	8.3	6.1	6.7	6.2	6.3	6.8	7.2	7.2	7.1
Italy	---	---	---	7.7	7.1	7.8	8.1	8.2	8.3	8.4	8.7
Japan	3.0	4.5	6.5	5.9	6.8	7.4	7.6	7.8	7.9	8.0	---
Korea	---	---	---	4.4	4.2	4.7	4.8	5.4	5.3	5.5	5.6
Luxembourg	---	3.1	5.2	5.4	5.6	5.8	5.8	6.4	6.8	7.7	8.0
Mexico	---	---	---	4.8	5.6	5.6	5.6	6.0	6.2	6.3	6.5
Netherlands	---	---	7.2	7.7	8.1	8.0	7.9	8.3	8.9	9.1	9.2
New Zealand	---	5.1	5.9	6.9	7.2	7.6	7.7	7.8	8.2	8.0	8.4
Norway	2.9	4.4	7.0	7.7	7.9	9.4	8.5	8.9	9.9	10.1	9.7
Poland	---	---	---	4.9	5.6	5.9	5.7	6.0	6.6	6.5	6.5
Portugal	---	2.6	5.6	6.2	8.2	8.7	9.4	9.3	9.5	9.8	10.1
Slovak Republic	---	---	---	---	---	5.8	5.5	5.5	5.6	5.9	---
Spain	1.5	3.5	5.3	6.5	7.4	7.3	7.2	7.2	7.3	7.9	8.1
Sweden	---	6.8	9.0	8.3	8.1	8.4	8.4	8.7	9.1	9.3	9.1
Switzerland	4.9	5.5	7.4	8.3	9.7	10.5	10.4	10.9	11.1	11.5	11.6
Turkey	---	---	3.3	3.6	3.4	6.4	6.6	7.5	7.4	7.6	7.7
United Kingdom	3.9	4.5	5.6	6.0	7.0	7.1	7.3	7.5	7.7	7.8	8.1
United States[2]	5.1	7.0	8.8	11.9	13.3	13.1	13.3	14.0	14.7	15.2	15.3
					Per capita health expenditures[3]						
Australia	$ 94	---	$ 691	$1,306	$1,741	$2,195	$2,398	$2,544	$2,724	$2,886	$3,120
Austria	77	193	770	1,328	2,229	2,539	2,667	2,748	2,857	2,958	3,124
Belgium	---	148	636	1,341	1,828	2,112	2,277	2,425	2,612	3,044	---
Canada	125	299	783	1,737	2,055	2,408	2,503	2,718	2,861	2,998	3,165
Czech Republic	---	---	---	561	902	931	980	1,089	1,188	1,296	1,361
Denmark	---	---	927	1,522	1,844	2,297	2,380	2,555	2,656	2,743	2,881
Finland	63	191	590	1,419	1,430	1,637	1,716	1,857	2,012	2,104	2,235
France	70	205	697	1,532	2,028	2,311	2,450	2,611	2,886	3,048	3,159
Germany	---	269	960	1,738	2,226	2,516	2,632	2,746	2,883	2,983	3,043
Greece	---	159	486	844	1,250	1,468	1,616	1,805	1,971	2,141	2,162
Hungary	---	---	---	---	685	819	856	975	1,115	1,249	1,276
Iceland	57	163	703	1,593	1,854	2,547	2,623	2,740	2,948	3,159	3,331
Ireland	43	117	519	794	1,216	1,627	1,809	2,099	2,395	2,455	2,596
Italy	---	---	---	1,387	1,534	1,898	2,083	2,184	2,275	2,314	2,467
Japan	30	149	580	1,116	1,541	1,829	1,967	2,082	2,138	2,249	---
Korea	---	---	---	361	540	712	778	938	975	1,068	1,149
Luxembourg	---	163	640	1,533	2,033	2,727	2,982	3,263	3,729	4,611	5,089
Mexico	---	---	---	306	388	469	506	548	578	608	662
Netherlands	---	---	755	1,435	1,822	2,134	2,257	2,519	2,775	2,909	3,041
New Zealand	---	211	506	995	1,246	1,522	1,605	1,705	1,850	1,902	2,083
Norway	49	141	665	1,393	1,893	2,816	3,080	3,286	3,616	3,769	3,966
Poland	---	---	---	300	423	566	590	646	734	748	805
Portugal	---	51	292	674	1,096	1,426	1,624	1,681	1,783	1,721	1,824
Slovak Republic	---	---	---	---	---	577	595	641	716	777	---
Spain	16	95	363	873	1,193	1,450	1,520	1,613	1,723	1,952	2,094
Sweden	---	312	944	1,589	1,734	2,118	2,271	2,404	2,593	2,745	2,825
Switzerland	166	351	1,031	2,029	2,573	3,019	3,179	3,364	3,650	3,847	4,077
Turkey	---	---	76	168	187	392	451	459	482	512	580
United Kingdom	84	163	480	987	1,385	1,713	1,858	2,029	2,228	2,317	2,508
United States[2]	147	352	1,072	2,752	3,670	4,335	4,588	4,933	5,324	5,711	6,102

--- Data not available.

[1]Preliminary figures.

[2]The Organisation for Economic Co-operation and Development (OECD) estimates for the United States differ from the National Health Expenditures estimates shown in Table 121 because of differences in methodology.

[3]Per capita health expenditures for each country have been adjusted to U.S. dollars using gross domestic product purchasing power parities for each year. See Appendix II, Gross domestic product; Purchasing power parities.

NOTE: These data include revisions in health expenditures and differ from previous editions of *Health, United States*.

SOURCE: The Organisation for Economic Co-operation and Development Health Data File 2006, incorporating revisions to the annual update. Available from: www.ecosante.org/oecd.htm.

Table 121. Gross domestic product, federal, and state and local government expenditures, national health expenditures, and average annual percent change: United States, selected years 1960–2005

[Data are compiled from various sources by the Centers for Medicare & Medicaid Services]

Gross domestic product, government expenditures, and national health expenditures	*1960*	*1970*	*1980*	*1990*	*1995*	*2000*	*2003*	*2004*	*2005*
					Amount in billions				
Gross domestic product (GDP)	$ 526	$1,039	$2,790	$5,803	$7,398	$9,817	$10,961	$11,713	$12,456
Federal government expenditures	$ 87	$ 201	$ 586	$1,254	$1,604	$1,864	$ 2,252	$ 2,383	$ 2,556
State and local government expenditures	40	113	329	731	978	1,270	1,515	1,606	1,704
National health expenditures	$ 28	$ 75	$ 254	$ 714	$1,017	$1,353	$ 1,733	$ 1,859	$ 1,988
Private	21	47	148	427	552	757	956	1,021	1,085
Public	7	28	106	287	465	596	778	838	903
Federal government	3	18	72	194	327	417	553	601	644
State and local government	4	10	35	93	138	179	225	237	259
					Amount per capita				
National health expenditures	$ 148	$ 356	$1,102	$2,813	$3,783	$4,790	$ 5,952	$ 6,322	$ 6,697
Private	111	222	640	1,684	2,053	2,680	3,282	3,472	3,656
Public	36	134	462	1,130	1,730	2,110	2,670	2,850	3,041
					Percent				
National health expenditures as percent of GDP	5.2	7.2	9.1	12.3	13.7	13.8	15.8	15.9	16.0
Health expenditures as a percent of total government expenditures									
Federal government	3.3	8.8	12.2	15.5	20.4	22.4	24.6	25.2	25.2
State and local government	9.8	9.2	10.6	12.7	14.1	14.1	14.8	14.8	15.2
					Percent distribution				
National health expenditures	100.0	100.0	100.0	100.0	100.0	100.0	100.0	100.0	100.0
Private	75.3	62.4	58.1	59.8	54.3	55.9	55.1	54.9	54.6
Public	24.7	37.6	41.9	40.2	45.7	44.1	44.9	45.1	45.4
					Average annual percent change from previous year shown				
Gross domestic product	. . .	7.0	10.4	7.6	5.0	5.8	3.7	6.9	6.3
Federal government expenditures	. . .	8.8	11.3	7.9	5.0	3.1	6.5	5.8	7.3
State and local government expenditures	. . .	10.9	11.3	8.3	6.0	5.4	6.1	6.0	6.1
National health expenditures	. . .	10.5	13.0	10.9	7.3	5.9	8.6	7.2	6.9
Private	. . .	8.5	12.2	11.2	5.2	6.5	8.1	6.8	6.3
Public	. . .	15.3	14.2	10.4	10.1	5.1	9.3	7.8	7.7
Federal government	. . .	20.0	15.0	10.5	11.0	5.0	9.8	8.6	7.2
State and local government	. . .	10.2	12.8	10.3	8.2	5.4	7.9	5.7	9.1
National health expenditures, per capita	. . .	9.2	12.0	9.8	6.1	4.8	7.5	6.2	5.9
Private	. . .	7.2	11.2	10.1	4.0	5.5	7.0	5.8	5.3
Public	. . .	13.9	13.2	9.4	8.9	4.1	8.2	6.7	6.7

. . . Category not applicable.

NOTES: These data include revisions in health expenditures and may differ from previous editions of *Health, United States*. The data reflect U.S. Census Bureau resident population estimates as of July 2006, excluding the armed forces overseas and the population of outlying areas. Federal and state and local government total expenditures reflect revisions from the Bureau of Economic Analysis. See Appendix II, Gross domestic product (GDP); Health expenditures, national. Percents are calculated using unrounded data. Percents and numbers may not add to totals due to rounding.

SOURCE: Centers for Medicare & Medicaid Services, Office of the Actuary, National Health Statistics Group, National Health Expenditure Accounts, National health expenditures, 2005. Available from: www.cms.hhs.gov/NationalHealthExpendData.

Table 122. Consumer Price Index and average annual percent change for all items, selected items, and medical care components: United States, selected years 1960–2006

[Data are based on reporting by samples of providers and other retail outlets]

Items and medical care components	1960	1970	1980	1990	1995	2000	2003	2004	2005	2006
					Consumer Price Index (CPI)					
All items	29.6	38.8	82.4	130.7	152.4	172.2	184.0	188.9	195.3	201.6
All items less medical care	30.2	39.2	82.8	128.8	148.6	167.3	178.1	182.7	188.7	194.7
Services	24.1	35.0	77.9	139.2	168.7	195.3	216.5	222.8	230.1	238.9
Food	30.0	39.2	86.8	132.4	148.4	167.8	180.0	186.2	190.7	195.2
Apparel	45.7	59.2	90.9	124.1	132.0	129.6	120.9	120.4	119.5	119.5
Housing	- - -	36.4	81.1	128.5	148.5	169.6	184.8	189.5	195.7	203.2
Energy	22.4	25.5	86.0	102.1	105.2	124.6	136.5	151.4	177.1	196.9
Medical care	22.3	34.0	74.9	162.8	220.5	260.8	297.1	310.1	323.2	336.2
Components of medical care										
Medical care services	19.5	32.3	74.8	162.7	224.2	266.0	306.0	321.3	336.7	350.6
Professional services	- - -	37.0	77.9	156.1	201.0	237.7	261.2	271.5	281.7	289.3
Physicians' services	21.9	34.5	76.5	160.8	208.8	244.7	267.7	278.3	287.5	291.9
Dental services	27.0	39.2	78.9	155.8	206.8	258.5	292.5	306.9	324.0	340.9
Eye glasses and eye care[1]	- - -	- - -	- - -	117.3	137.0	149.7	155.9	159.3	163.2	168.1
Services by other medical professionals[1]	- - -	- - -	- - -	120.2	143.9	161.9	177.1	181.9	186.8	192.2
Hospital and related services	- - -	- - -	69.2	178.0	257.8	317.3	394.8	417.9	439.9	468.1
Hospital services[2]	- - -	- - -	- - -	- - -	- - -	115.9	144.7	153.4	161.6	172.1
Inpatient hospital services[2,3]	- - -	- - -	- - -	- - -	- - -	113.8	140.1	148.1	156.6	167.5
Outpatient hospital services[1,3]	- - -	- - -	- - -	138.7	204.6	263.8	337.9	356.3	373.0	395.0
Hospital rooms	9.3	23.6	68.0	175.4	251.2	- - -	- - -	- - -	- - -	- - -
Other inpatient services[1]	- - -	- - -	- - -	142.7	206.8	- - -	- - -	- - -	- - -	- - -
Nursing homes and adult day care[2]	- - -	- - -	- - -	- - -	- - -	117.0	135.2	140.4	145.0	151.0
Health insurance[4]	- - -	- - -	- - -	- - -	- - -	- - -	- - -	- - -	- - -	103.1
Medical care commodities	46.9	46.5	75.4	163.4	204.5	238.1	262.8	269.3	276.0	285.9
Prescription drugs and medical supplies	54.0	47.4	72.5	181.7	235.0	285.4	326.3	337.1	349.0	363.9
Nonprescription drugs and medical supplies[1]	- - -	- - -	- - -	120.6	140.5	149.5	152.0	152.3	151.7	154.6
Internal and respiratory over-the-counter drugs	- - -	42.3	74.9	145.9	167.0	176.9	181.2	180.9	179.7	183.4
Nonprescription medical equipment and supplies	- - -	- - -	79.2	138.0	166.3	178.1	178.1	179.7	180.6	183.2
					Average annual percent change from previous year shown					
All items	. . .	2.7	7.8	4.7	3.1	2.5	2.2	2.7	3.4	3.2
All items excluding medical care	. . .	2.6	7.8	4.5	2.9	2.4	2.1	2.6	3.3	3.2
All services	. . .	3.8	8.3	6.0	3.9	3.0	3.5	2.9	3.3	3.8
Food	. . .	2.7	8.3	4.3	2.3	2.5	2.4	3.4	2.4	2.4
Apparel	. . .	2.6	4.4	3.2	1.2	–0.4	–2.3	–0.4	–0.7	0.0
Housing	. . .	- - -	8.3	4.7	2.9	2.7	2.9	2.5	3.3	3.8
Energy	. . .	1.3	12.9	1.7	0.6	3.4	3.1	10.9	17.0	11.2
Medical care	. . .	4.3	8.2	8.1	6.3	3.4	4.4	4.4	4.2	4.0
Components of medical care										
Medical care services	. . .	5.2	8.8	8.1	6.6	3.5	4.8	5.0	4.8	4.1
Professional services	. . .	- - -	7.7	7.2	5.2	3.4	3.2	3.9	3.8	2.7
Physicians' services	. . .	4.6	8.3	7.7	5.4	3.2	3.0	4.0	3.3	1.5
Dental services	. . .	3.8	7.2	7.0	5.8	4.6	4.2	4.9	5.6	5.2
Eye glasses and eye care[1]	. . .	- - -	- - -	- - -	3.2	1.8	1.4	2.2	2.4	3.0
Services by other medical professionals[1]	. . .	- - -	- - -	- - -	3.7	2.4	3.0	2.7	2.7	2.9
Hospital and related services	. . .	- - -	- - -	9.9	7.7	4.2	7.6	5.9	5.3	6.4
Hospital services[2]	. . .	- - -	- - -	- - -	- - -	- - -	7.7	6.0	5.3	6.5
Inpatient hospital services[2,3]	. . .	- - -	- - -	- - -	- - -	- - -	7.2	5.7	5.7	7.0
Outpatient hospital services[1,3]	. . .	- - -	- - -	- - -	8.1	5.2	8.6	5.4	4.7	5.9
Hospital rooms	. . .	9.8	11.2	9.9	7.4	- - -	- - -	- - -	- - -	- - -
Other inpatient services[1]	. . .	- - -	- - -	- - -	7.7	- - -	- - -	- - -	- - -	- - -
Nursing homes and adult day care[2]	. . .	- - -	- - -	- - -	- - -	- - -	4.9	3.8	3.3	4.1
Health insurance[4]	. . .	- - -	- - -	- - -	- - -	- - -	- - -	- - -	- - -	- - -
Medical care commodities	. . .	–0.1	5.0	8.0	4.6	3.1	3.3	2.5	2.5	3.6
Prescription drugs and medical supplies	. . .	–1.3	4.3	9.6	5.3	4.0	4.6	3.3	3.5	4.3
Nonprescription drugs and medical supplies[1]	. . .	- - -	- - -	- - -	3.1	1.2	0.6	0.2	–0.4	1.9
Internal and respiratory over-the-counter drugs	. . .	- - -	5.9	6.9	2.7	1.2	0.8	–0.2	–0.7	2.1
Nonprescription medical equipment and supplies	. . .	- - -	- - -	5.7	3.8	1.4	0.0	0.9	0.5	1.4

- - - Data not available. . . . Category not applicable.

[1]December 1986 = 100.

[2]December 1996 = 100.

[3]Special index based on a substantially smaller sample.

[4]December 2005 = 100.

NOTES: Consumer Price Index for all urban consumers (CPI-U) U.S. city average, detailed expenditure categories. 1982–1984 = 100, except where noted. Data are not seasonally adjusted. See Appendix I, Consumer Price Index; Appendix II, Consumer Price Index.

SOURCE: U.S. Department of Labor, Bureau of Labor Statistics, Consumer Price Index. Various releases. 2006 data available from: www.bls.gov/cpi/cpid06av.pdf.

Table 123. Growth in personal health care expenditures and percent distribution of factors affecting growth: United States, 1960–2005

[Data are compiled from various sources by the Centers for Medicare & Medicaid Services]

Period	Average annual percent increase	Factors affecting growth: All factors	Inflation[1]: Economy-wide	Inflation[1]: Medical	Population	Intensity
		Percent distribution[3]				
1960–2005	9.9	100	39	17	11	33
1960–1965	8.3	100	17	10	18	55
1965–1970	12.7	100	34	12	8	46
1970–1975	12.3	100	55	1	8	36
1975–1980	13.8	100	54	12	7	27
1980–1985	11.6	100	47	32	9	12
1980–1981	15.9	100	61	17	7	15
1981–1982	12.0	100	52	37	9	2
1982–1983	10.3	100	40	34	10	16
1983–1984	9.6	100	40	39	10	11
1984–1985	10.2	100	31	41	10	18
1985–1990	10.3	100	32	26	10	32
1985–1986	8.7	100	26	31	11	32
1986–1987	9.4	100	30	23	10	37
1987–1988	11.2	100	32	25	9	35
1988–1989	10.5	100	37	29	10	23
1989–1990	11.7	100	34	24	10	31
1990–1995	7.3	100	34	29	16	20
1990–1991	10.2	100	36	21	12	31
1991–1992	8.5	100	28	35	15	22
1992–1993	6.6	100	36	35	19	11
1993–1994	5.3	100	41	31	21	7
1994–1995	6.1	100	34	25	18	22
1995–2000	5.7	100	30	18	18	35
1995–1996	5.4	100	36	19	19	26
1996–1997	5.4	100	31	9	20	40
1997–1998	5.3	100	21	20	20	38
1998–1999	5.7	100	26	22	18	34
1999–2000	6.7	100	33	17	15	35
2000–2005	7.8	100	32	18	13	38
2000–2001	8.7	100	28	17	12	42
2001–2002	8.3	100	22	26	13	40
2002–2003	7.8	100	28	20	13	39
2003–2004	7.3	100	40	17	14	30
2004–2005	7.1	100	43	7	14	36

[1]Total inflation is economywide and medical inflation is the medical inflation above economywide inflation.
[2]Intensity is the residual percent of growth that cannot be attributed to price increases or population growth. It represents changes in use or kinds of services and supplies.
[3]Percents may not sum to 100 due to rounding.

NOTES: These data include revisions in health expenditures for 1960 forward and revisions in population for 1990 forward. The implicit price deflator for Gross domestic product (GDP) is used to measure economy-wide inflation for all years 1960–2005. See Appendix II, Health expenditures, national; Gross domestic product (GDP). All indexes used to calculate the factors affecting growth were rebased in 2003 with base year 2000. These data include revisions and differ from previous editions of *Health, United States*.

SOURCE: Centers for Medicare & Medicaid Services, Office of the Actuary, National Health Statistics Group, National Health Expenditure Accounts, National health expenditures, 2005. Available from: www.cms.hhs.gov/NationalHealthExpendData/. Unpublished data.

able 124 (page 1 of 2). National health expenditures, average annual percent change, and percent distribution, y type of expenditure: United States, selected years 1960–2005

ata are compiled from various sources by the Centers for Medicare & Medicaid Services]

Type of national health expenditure	*1960*	*1970*	*1980*	*1990*	*1995*	*2000*	*2002*	*2003*	*2004*	*2005*
	Amount in billions									
ational health expenditures	$27.5	$74.9	$253.9	$714.0	$1,016.5	$1,353.3	$1,602.8	$1,733.4	$1,858.9	$1,987.7
Health services and supplies	24.9	67.1	234.0	666.7	952.8	1,264.4	1,498.8	1,621.7	1,738.9	1,860.9
Personal health care	23.3	62.9	215.3	607.5	863.7	1,139.9	1,341.2	1,446.3	1,551.3	1,661.4
Hospital care	9.2	27.6	101.0	251.6	340.7	417.0	488.6	525.4	566.9	611.6
Professional services	8.3	20.6	67.3	216.8	316.5	426.7	503.1	543.0	581.1	621.7
Physician and clinical services	5.4	14.0	47.1	157.5	220.5	288.6	337.9	366.7	393.7	421.2
Other professional services	0.4	0.7	3.6	18.2	28.5	39.1	45.6	49.0	52.6	56.7
Dental services	2.0	4.7	13.3	31.5	44.5	62.0	73.3	76.9	81.5	86.6
Other personal health care	0.6	1.2	3.3	9.6	23.0	37.1	46.3	50.4	53.3	57.2
Nursing home and home health	0.9	4.3	21.4	65.2	104.6	125.8	139.9	148.5	157.7	169.3
Home health care[1]	0.1	0.2	2.4	12.6	30.5	30.5	34.2	38.0	42.7	47.5
Nursing home care[1]	0.8	4.0	19.0	52.6	74.1	95.3	105.7	110.5	115.0	121.9
Retail outlet sales of medical products	4.9	10.5	25.7	74.0	101.8	170.3	209.6	229.4	245.5	258.8
Prescription drugs	2.7	5.5	12.0	40.3	60.9	120.8	157.9	174.6	189.7	200.7
Other medical products	2.3	5.0	13.6	33.7	40.9	49.5	51.6	54.7	55.9	58.1
Government administration and net cost of private health insurance	1.2	2.8	12.2	39.2	58.1	81.2	105.2	122.6	135.2	143.0
Government public health activities[2]	0.4	1.4	6.4	20.0	31.0	43.4	52.4	52.8	52.5	56.6
Investment	2.6	7.8	19.9	47.3	63.7	88.8	104.0	111.7	119.9	126.8
Research[3]	0.7	2.0	5.4	12.7	18.3	25.6	32.5	35.8	38.3	40.0
Structures and equipment	1.9	5.8	14.5	34.7	45.4	63.2	71.5	75.9	81.7	86.8
	Average annual percent change from previous year shown									
National health expenditures	. . .	10.5	13.0	10.9	7.3	5.9	8.8	8.1	7.2	6.9
Health services and supplies	. . .	10.4	13.3	11.0	7.4	5.8	8.9	8.2	7.2	7.0
Personal health care	. . .	10.4	13.1	10.9	7.3	5.7	8.5	7.8	7.3	7.1
Hospital care	. . .	11.6	13.9	9.6	6.3	4.1	8.2	7.5	7.9	7.9
Professional services	. . .	9.5	12.5	12.4	7.9	6.2	8.6	7.9	7.0	7.0
Physician and clinical services	. . .	10.1	12.9	12.8	7.0	5.5	8.2	8.5	7.4	7.0
Other professional services	. . .	6.6	17.1	17.5	9.5	6.5	8.0	7.5	7.4	7.8
Dental services	. . .	9.1	11.1	9.0	7.1	6.9	8.8	4.8	6.0	6.3
Other personal health care	. . .	7.3	10.1	11.4	19.2	10.0	11.8	8.7	5.7	7.3
Nursing home and home health	. . .	17.2	17.5	11.8	9.9	3.8	5.5	6.1	6.2	7.3
Home health care[1]	. . .	14.5	26.9	18.1	19.4	0.0	5.9	11.1	12.3	11.1
Nursing home care[1]	. . .	17.4	16.8	10.7	7.1	5.2	5.3	4.5	4.1	6.0
Retail outlet sales of medical products	. . .	7.8	9.4	11.2	6.6	10.8	10.9	9.5	7.0	5.4
Prescription drugs	. . .	7.5	8.2	12.8	8.6	14.7	14.3	10.6	8.6	5.8
Other medical products	. . .	8.1	10.6	9.5	4.0	3.9	2.1	6.1	2.1	3.9
Government administration and net cost of private health insurance	. . .	8.6	16.0	12.4	8.2	6.9	13.8	16.6	10.3	5.7
Government public health activities[2]	. . .	12.8	16.5	12.0	9.2	7.0	9.9	0.8	–0.6	7.7
Investment	. . .	11.7	9.9	9.0	6.1	6.9	8.2	7.4	7.3	5.7
Research[3]	. . .	10.9	10.8	8.9	7.7	6.9	12.8	10.1	6.7	4.6
Structures and equipment	. . .	11.9	9.5	9.1	5.5	6.8	6.3	6.2	7.6	6.3

See footnotes at end of table.

Table 124 (page 2 of 2). National health expenditures, average annual percent change, and percent distribution by type of expenditure: United States, selected years 1960–2005

[Data are compiled from various sources by the Centers for Medicare & Medicaid Services]

Type of national health expenditure	*1960*	*1970*	*1980*	*1990*	*1995*	*2000*	*2002*	*2003*	*2004*	*2005*
	Percent distribution									
National health expenditures	100.0	100.0	100.0	100.0	100.0	100.0	100.0	100.0	100.0	100.0
Health services and supplies	90.6	89.6	92.1	93.4	93.7	93.4	93.5	93.6	93.5	93.6
Personal health care	84.7	84.0	84.8	85.1	85.0	84.2	83.7	83.4	83.5	83.6
Hospital care	33.3	36.8	39.8	35.2	33.5	30.8	30.5	30.3	30.5	30.8
Professional services	30.2	27.6	26.5	30.4	31.1	31.5	31.4	31.3	31.3	31.3
Physician and clinical services	19.4	18.7	18.5	22.1	21.7	21.3	21.1	21.2	21.2	21.2
Other professional services	1.4	1.0	1.4	2.5	2.8	2.9	2.8	2.8	2.8	2.9
Dental services	7.1	6.2	5.2	4.4	4.4	4.6	4.6	4.4	4.4	4.4
Other personal health care	2.2	1.7	1.3	1.3	2.3	2.7	2.9	2.9	2.9	2.9
Nursing home and home health	3.2	5.7	8.4	9.1	10.3	9.3	8.7	8.6	8.5	8.5
Home health care[1]	0.2	0.3	0.9	1.8	3.0	2.3	2.1	2.2	2.3	2.4
Nursing home care[1]	2.9	5.4	7.5	7.4	7.3	7.0	6.6	6.4	6.2	6.1
Retail outlet sales of medical products	18.0	14.0	10.1	10.4	10.0	12.6	13.1	13.2	13.2	13.0
Prescription drugs	9.7	7.3	4.7	5.6	6.0	8.9	9.9	10.1	10.2	10.1
Other medical products	8.2	6.6	5.4	4.7	4.0	3.7	3.2	3.2	3.0	2.9
Government administration and net cost of private health insurance	4.4	3.7	4.8	5.5	5.7	6.0	6.6	7.1	7.3	7.2
Government public health activities[2]	1.5	1.9	2.5	2.8	3.0	3.2	3.3	3.0	2.8	2.8
Investment	9.4	10.4	7.9	6.6	6.3	6.6	6.5	6.4	6.5	6.4
Research[3]	2.5	2.6	2.1	1.8	1.8	1.9	2.0	2.1	2.1	2.0
Structures and equipment	6.9	7.8	5.7	4.9	4.5	4.7	4.5	4.4	4.4	4.4

. . . Category not applicable.

[1]Freestanding facilities only. Additional services of this type are provided in hospital-based facilities and counted as hospital care.

[2]Includes personal care services delivered by government public health agencies.

[3]Research and development expenditures of drug companies and other manufacturers and providers of medical equipment and supplies are excluded. They are included in the expenditure class in which the product falls because these expenditures are covered by the payment received for that product. See Appendix II, Health expenditures, national.

NOTES: Percents are calculated using unrounded data. These data include revisions in health expenditures for past years and differ from previous editions of *Health, United States.*

SOURCE: Centers for Medicare & Medicaid Services, Office of the Actuary, National Health Statistics Group, National Health Expenditure Accounts, National health expenditures, 2005. Available from: www.cms.hhs.gov/NationalHealthExpendData/.

Table 125 (page 1 of 2). Personal health care expenditures, by source of funds and type of expenditure: United States, selected years 1960–2005

[Data are compiled from various sources by the Centers for Medicare & Medicaid Services]

Type of personal health care expenditures and source of funds	*1960*	*1970*	*1980*	*1990*	*1995*	*2000*	*2003*	*2004*	*2005*
	Amount								
Per capita	$ 125	$ 299	$ 935	$2,394	$3,214	$ 4,034	$ 4,966	$ 5,276	$ 5,598
	Amount in billions								
All personal health care expenditures[1]	$ 23.3	$ 62.9	$215.3	$607.5	$863.7	$1,139.9	$1,446.3	$1,551.3	$1,661.4
	Percent distribution								
All sources of funds	100.0	100.0	100.0	100.0	100.0	100.0	100.0	100.0	100.0
Out-of-pocket payments	55.2	39.6	27.2	22.4	16.9	16.9	15.5	15.2	15.0
Private health insurance	21.4	22.3	28.4	33.7	33.2	35.4	35.9	36.0	35.9
Other private funds	2.0	2.8	4.3	5.0	5.1	5.0	4.4	4.2	4.1
Government	21.4	35.3	40.0	38.9	44.8	42.7	44.2	44.6	45.0
Federal	8.7	22.9	28.9	28.4	34.2	32.5	33.7	34.2	34.2
State and local	12.7	12.4	11.1	10.4	10.6	10.2	10.4	10.4	10.7
	Amount in billions								
Hospital care expenditures[2]	$ 9.2	$ 27.6	$101.0	$251.6	$340.7	$ 417.0	$ 525.4	$ 566.9	$ 611.6
	Percent distribution								
All sources of funds	100.0	100.0	100.0	100.0	100.0	100.0	100.0	100.0	100.0
Out-of-pocket payments	20.7	9.0	5.4	4.5	3.0	3.3	3.2	3.3	3.3
Private health insurance	35.8	32.5	36.6	38.9	32.0	34.6	35.4	35.6	35.5
Other private funds	1.2	3.2	5.0	4.1	4.2	5.2	4.6	4.5	4.5
Government[3]	42.2	55.2	53.0	52.5	60.8	56.9	56.7	56.7	56.8
Medicaid[4]	. . .	9.6	9.1	10.6	16.7	17.0	17.2	17.1	17.3
Medicare	. . .	19.4	26.1	27.0	32.0	29.9	29.3	29.4	29.5
	Amount in billions								
Physician services expenditures	$ 5.4	$ 14.0	$ 47.1	$157.5	$220.5	$ 288.6	$ 366.7	$ 393.7	$ 421.2
	Percent distribution								
All sources of funds	100.0	100.0	100.0	100.0	100.0	100.0	100.0	100.0	100.0
Out-of-pocket payments	61.7	46.2	30.4	19.2	11.8	11.2	10.2	10.1	10.1
Private health insurance	29.8	30.1	35.5	42.7	48.1	47.4	48.3	48.3	48.3
Other private funds	1.4	1.6	3.9	7.2	8.0	7.7	7.1	6.7	6.4
Government[3]	7.2	22.1	30.1	30.9	32.1	33.8	34.3	34.9	35.3
Medicaid[4]	. . .	4.6	5.2	4.5	6.7	6.6	6.9	7.1	7.1
Medicare	. . .	11.8	17.0	18.6	18.8	20.2	20.1	20.7	21.2
	Amount in billions								
Nursing home expenditures[5]	$ 0.8	$ 4.0	$ 19.0	$ 52.6	$ 74.1	$ 95.3	$ 110.5	$ 115.0	$ 121.9
	Percent distribution								
All sources of funds	100.0	100.0	100.0	100.0	100.0	100.0	100.0	100.0	100.0
Out-of-pocket payments	77.3	52.0	37.2	36.1	28.1	30.1	27.6	26.6	26.5
Private health insurance	0.0	0.2	1.2	5.6	7.9	8.3	7.8	7.5	7.5
Other private funds	6.3	4.8	4.2	7.2	6.7	4.8	3.8	3.7	3.7
Government[3]	16.4	43.0	57.5	51.1	57.2	56.9	60.8	62.2	62.3
Medicaid[4]	. . .	23.3	53.8	45.8	46.0	44.1	45.0	44.8	43.9
Medicare	. . .	3.5	1.6	3.2	9.0	10.6	13.3	14.9	15.7

See footnotes at end of table.

Table 125 (page 2 of 2). Personal health care expenditures, by source of funds and type of expenditure: United States, selected years 1960–2005

[Data are compiled from various sources by the Centers for Medicare & Medicaid Services]

Type of personal health care expenditures and source of funds	*1960*	*1970*	*1980*	*1990*	*1995*	*2000*	*2003*	*2004*	*2005*
					Amount in billions				
Prescription drug expenditures	$ 2.7	$ 5.5	$ 12.0	$ 40.3	$ 60.9	$120.8	$174.6	$189.7	$200.7
					Percent distribution				
All sources of funds	100.0	100.0	100.0	100.0	100.0	100.0	100.0	100.0	100.0
Out-of-pocket payments	96.0	82.4	70.3	55.5	38.4	27.7	25.4	25.2	25.4
Private health insurance	1.3	8.8	14.8	26.4	40.1	49.4	48.2	47.4	47.4
Other private funds	0.0	0.0	0.0	0.0	0.0	0.0	0.0	0.0	0.0
Government[3]	2.7	8.8	14.9	18.1	21.5	22.9	26.4	27.3	27.2
Medicaid[4]	. . .	7.6	11.7	12.6	15.9	16.7	18.6	19.1	18.6
Medicare	. . .	0.0	0.0	0.5	1.1	1.7	1.4	1.8	2.0
					Amount in billions				
All other personal health care expenditures[6]	$ 5.3	$ 11.8	$ 36.2	$105.5	$167.5	$218.1	$269.0	$285.9	$306.1
					Percent distribution				
All sources of funds	100.0	100.0	100.0	100.0	100.0	100.0	100.0	100.0	100.0
Out-of-pocket payments	84.5	78.9	64.6	50.4	39.3	39.0	35.4	34.6	33.9
Private health insurance	1.6	3.3	15.3	24.6	24.7	25.1	23.6	23.6	23.5
Other private funds	4.2	3.6	4.3	4.7	4.3	3.8	3.3	3.2	3.2
Government[3]	9.8	14.2	15.8	20.2	31.7	32.2	37.8	38.6	39.5
Medicaid[4]	. . .	3.3	3.9	6.5	12.5	15.9	19.7	20.1	20.6
Medicare	. . .	1.1	3.8	7.1	13.1	9.7	11.5	12.1	12.6

. . . Category not applicable.

[1]Includes all expenditures for specified health services and supplies other than expenses for program administration, net cost of private health insurance, and government public health activities.

[2]Includes expenditures for hospital-based nursing home and home health agency care.

[3]Includes other government expenditures for these health care services, for example, Medicaid State Children's Health Insurance Program (SCHIP) expansions and SCHIP, care funded by the Department of Veterans Affairs, and state and locally financed subsidies to hospitals.

[4]Excludes Medicaid SCHIP expansions and SCHIP.

[5]Includes expenditures for care in freestanding nursing homes. Expenditures for care in hospital-based nursing homes are included with hospital care.

[6]Includes expenditures for dental services, other professional services, non-hospital home health care, nonprescription drugs and other medical nondurables, vision products and other medical durables, and other personal health care, not shown separately. See Appendix II, Health expenditures, national.

NOTES: Percents are calculated using unrounded data. Percents may not add to totals because of rounding. These data include revisions in health expenditure estimates and differ from previous editions of *Health, United States.*

SOURCE: Centers for Medicare & Medicaid Services, Office of the Actuary, National Health Statistics Group, National Health Expenditure Accounts, National health expenditures, 2005. Available from: www.cms.hhs.gov/NationalHealthExpendData/.

Table 126. National health expenditures for mental health services, average annual percent change and percent distribution, by type of expenditure: United States, selected years 1986–2003

[Data are compiled from various sources by the Substance Abuse and Mental Health Services Administration]

Type of expenditure	*1986*	*1990*	*1995*	*2000*	*2002*	*2003*
			Amount in millions			
Total expenditures	$33,125	$46,456	$61,763	$79,203	$93,135	$100,321
Total all service providers	29,355	40,636	52,163	57,740	65,790	69,918
General non-specialty hospitals	5,469	7,613	11,125	12,069	14,729	15,927
General hospital specialty units	3,038	5,729	7,953	6,445	6,455	6,568
General hospital non-specialty units	2,432	1,885	3,171	5,624	8,274	9,359
Specialty hospitals	8,251	11,069	11,473	11,005	11,328	11,673
All physicians	3,753	5,827	8,261	10,445	12,541	13,748
Psychiatrists	2,681	4,276	5,924	7,569	8,678	9,802
Non-psychiatric physicians	1,072	1,551	2,337	2,876	3,863	3,946
Other professionals	3,099	4,261	5,191	6,251	7,567	8,370
Freestanding nursing homes	4,754	5,496	5,261	5,310	5,964	6,234
Freestanding home health	113	221	592	612	749	823
Multi-service mental health organizations	3,916	6,148	10,260	12,048	12,913	13,143
Retail prescription drug	2,191	3,340	5,754	16,417	20,949	23,259
Insurance administration	1,579	2,480	3,847	5,046	6,395	7,145
			Amount in inflation-adjusted millions			
Total expenditures, inflation-adjusted dollars	$46,491	$56,938	$67,057	$79,203	$89,392	$ 94,284
			Deflator (2000=1.00)			
GDP implicit price deflator[1]	0.71	0.82	0.92	1.00	1.04	1.06
			Average annual percent change from previous year shown			
Total expenditures	. . .	8.8	5.9	5.1	8.4	7.7
Total all service providers	. . .	8.5	5.1	2.1	6.7	6.3
General non-specialty hospitals	. . .	8.6	7.9	1.6	10.5	8.1
General hospital specialty units	. . .	17.2	6.8	–4.1	0.1	1.8
General hospital non-specialty units	. . .	–6.2	11.0	12.1	21.3	13.1
Specialty hospitals	. . .	7.6	0.7	–0.8	1.5	3.0
All physicians	. . .	11.6	7.2	4.8	9.6	9.6
Psychiatrists	. . .	12.4	6.7	5.0	7.1	13.0
Non-psychiatric physicians	. . .	9.7	8.6	4.2	15.9	2.1
Other professionals	. . .	8.3	4.0	3.8	10.0	10.6
Freestanding nursing homes	. . .	3.7	–0.9	0.2	6.0	4.5
Freestanding home health	. . .	18.4	21.7	0.7	10.7	9.9
Multi-service mental health organizations	. . .	11.9	10.8	3.3	3.5	1.8
Retail prescription drug	. . .	11.1	11.5	23.3	13.0	11.0
Insurance administration	. . .	11.9	9.2	5.6	12.6	11.7
			Percent distribution			
Total expenditures	100.0	100.0	100.0	100.0	100.0	100.0
Total all service providers	88.6	87.5	84.5	72.9	70.6	69.7
General non-specialty hospitals	16.5	16.4	18.0	15.2	15.8	15.9
General hospital specialty units	9.2	12.3	12.9	8.1	6.9	6.5
General hospital non-specialty units	7.3	4.1	5.1	7.1	8.9	9.3
Specialty hospitals	24.9	23.8	18.6	13.9	12.2	11.6
All physicians	11.3	12.5	13.4	13.2	13.5	13.7
Psychiatrists	8.1	9.2	9.6	9.6	9.3	9.8
Non-psychiatric physicians	3.2	3.3	3.8	3.6	4.1	3.9
Other professionals	9.4	9.2	8.4	7.9	8.1	8.3
Freestanding nursing homes	14.4	11.8	8.5	6.7	6.4	6.2
Freestanding home health	0.3	0.5	1.0	0.8	0.8	0.8
Multi-service mental health organizations	11.8	13.2	16.6	15.2	13.9	13.1
Retail prescription drug	6.6	7.2	9.3	20.7	22.5	23.2
Insurance administration	4.8	5.3	6.2	6.4	6.9	7.1

- - - Data not available.
. . . Category not applicable.
[1]Gross Domestic Product implicit price deflator developed by the U.S. Department of Commerce, Bureau of Economic Analysis. Table 1.1.9 Implicit price deflator for Gross Domestic Product is available from: www.bea.gov/bea/dn/nipaweb/SelectTable.asp, accessed on September 13, 2006.

NOTES: Additional data on specialty and non-specialty providers are available in the internet version of this table. Available from: www.cdc.gov/nchs/hus.htm. Specialty providers include general hospital specialty units, specialty hospitals, psychiatrists, other professionals, multi-service mental health organizations, and specialty substance abuse centers. Non-specialty providers include general hospital non-specialty units, non-psychiatric physicians, freestanding nursing homes, and freestanding home health providers. This table includes expenditures for treatment provided in all settings and differs from the estimates shown in Table 135, which are expenditures for mental health treatment provided by mental health organizations. Data for additional years are available. See Appendix III.

SOURCE: Mark TL, Levit KL, Coffey RM, McKusick DR, Harwood H, King E, et al. National Expenditures for Mental Health Services and Substance Abuse Treatment, 1993–2003. SAMHSA Publication No. SMA 07-4227. Rockville, MD: Substance Abuse and Mental Health Services Administration, 2007 and unpublished data.

Table 127. National health expenditures for substance abuse treatment, average annual percent change and percent distribution, by type of expenditure: United States, selected years 1986–2003

[Data are compiled from various sources by the Substance Abuse and Mental Health Services Administration]

Type of expenditure	*1986*	*1990*	*1995*	*2000*	*2002*	*2003*
	Amount in millions					
Total expenditures	$ 9,302	$12,075	$15,561	$17,545	$19,867	$20,740
Total all service providers	8,777	11,378	14,590	16,473	18,558	19,335
General non-specialty hospitals	2,995	3,167	3,764	3,649	4,132	4,359
General hospital specialty units	2,240	2,089	3,320	2,739	2,859	2,890
General hospital non-specialty units	755	1,078	444	911	1,272	1,470
Specialty hospitals	1,453	1,346	1,315	736	738	676
All physicians	685	904	1,048	1,413	1,554	1,672
Psychiatrists	237	328	410	510	428	540
Non-psychiatric physicians	448	577	638	902	1,127	1,131
Other professionals	1,451	1,685	1,652	2,076	2,372	2,636
Freestanding nursing homes	106	126	179	254	292	301
Freestanding home health	2	3	16	10	3	4
Multi-service mental health organizations	325	657	1,012	1,492	1,312	1,246
Specialty substance abuse centers	1,761	3,490	5,605	6,845	8,156	8,441
Retail prescription drug	14	19	33	67	89	98
Insurance administration	512	679	937	1,005	1,220	1,307
	Amount in inflation-adjusted millions					
Total expenditures, inflation-adjusted dollars	$13,056	$14,800	$16,895	$17,545	$19,068	$19,492
	Deflator (2000=1.00)					
GDP implicit price deflator[1]	0.71	0.82	0.92	1.00	1.04	1.06
	Average annual percent change from previous year shown					
Total expenditures	. . .	6.7	5.2	2.4	6.4	4.4
Total all service providers	. . .	6.7	5.1	2.5	6.1	4.2
General non-specialty hospitals	. . .	1.4	3.5	–0.6	6.4	5.5
General hospital specialty units	. . .	–1.7	9.7	–3.8	2.2	1.1
General hospital non-specialty units	. . .	9.3	–16.3	15.4	18.2	15.5
Specialty hospitals	. . .	–1.9	–0.5	–11.0	0.1	–8.4
All physicians	. . .	7.2	3.0	6.2	4.9	7.5
Psychiatrists	. . .	8.4	4.6	4.5	–8.4	26.2
Non-psychiatric physicians	. . .	6.5	2.0	7.2	11.7	0.4
Other professionals	. . .	3.8	–17.6	26.6	6.9	11.2
Freestanding nursing homes	. . .	4.3	7.3	7.3	7.3	3.2
Freestanding home health	. . .	15.9	36.6	–9.2	–43.1	11.9
Multi-service mental health organizations	. . .	19.3	9.0	8.1	–6.2	–5.0
Specialty substance abuse centers	. . .	18.7	9.9	4.1	9.2	3.5
Retail prescription drug	. . .	9.0	11.6	15.0	15.0	11.3
Insurance administration	. . .	7.3	6.7	1.4	10.1	7.2
	Percent distribution					
Total expenditures	100.0	100.0	100.0	100.0	100.0	100.0
Total all service providers	94.4	94.2	93.8	93.9	93.4	93.2
General non-specialty hospitals	32.2	26.2	24.2	20.8	20.8	21.0
General hospital specialty units	24.1	17.3	21.3	15.6	14.4	13.9
General hospital non-specialty units	8.1	8.9	2.9	5.2	6.4	7.1
Specialty hospitals	15.6	11.1	8.5	4.2	3.7	3.3
All physicians	7.4	7.5	6.7	8.1	7.8	8.1
Psychiatrists	2.6	2.7	2.6	2.9	2.2	2.6
Non-psychiatric physicians	4.8	4.8	4.1	5.1	5.7	5.5
Other professionals	15.6	14.0	4.1	11.8	11.9	12.7
Freestanding nursing homes	1.1	1.0	1.1	1.4	1.5	1.5
Freestanding home health	0.0	0.0	0.1	0.1	0.0	0.0
Multi-service mental health organizations	3.5	5.4	6.5	8.5	6.6	6.0
Specialty substance abuse centers	18.9	28.9	36.0	39.0	41.1	40.7
Retail prescription drug	0.1	0.2	0.2	0.4	0.4	0.5
Insurance administration	5.5	5.6	6.0	5.7	6.1	6.3

- - - Data not available.
. . . Category not applicable.
[1]Gross Domestic Product implicit price deflator developed by the U.S. Department of Commerce, Bureau of Economic Analysis. Table 1.1.9 Implicit price deflator for Gross Domestic Product is available from: www.bea.gov/bea/dn/nipaweb/SelectTable.asp, accessed on September 13, 2006.

NOTES: Additional data on specialty and non-specialty providers are available in the internet version of this table. Available from: www.cdc.gov/nchs/hus.htm. Specialty providers include general hospital specialty units, specialty hospitals, psychiatrists, other professionals, multi-service mental health organizations, and specialty substance abuse centers. Non-specialty providers include general hospital non-specialty units, non-psychiatric physicians, freestanding nursing homes, and freestanding home health providers. Data for additional years are available. See Appendix III.

SOURCE: Mark TL, Levit KL, Coffey RM, McKusick DR, Harwood H, King E, et al. National Expenditures for Mental Health Services and Substance Abuse Treatment, 1993–2003. SAMHSA Publication No. SMA 07–4227. Rockville, MD: Substance Abuse and Mental Health Services Administration, 2007 and unpublished data.

Table 128 (page 1 of 3). Expenses for health care and prescribed medicine, by selected population characteristics: United States, selected years 1987–2004

[Data are based on household interviews of a sample of the noninstitutionalized population and a sample of medical providers]

Characteristic	Population in millions[2]			Total expenses[1] — Percent of persons with expense				Total expenses[1] — Mean annual expense per person with expense[3]			
	1997	2000	2004	1987	1997	2000	2004	1987	1997	2000	2004
All ages	271.3	278.4	293.5	84.5	84.1	83.5	84.7	$2,597	$2,853	$2,962	$3,879
Under 65 years:											
Total	237.1	243.6	256.5	83.2	82.5	81.8	82.9	2,022	2,163	2,333	3,028
Under 6 years	23.8	24.1	23.3	88.9	88.0	86.7	90.0	1,718	1,010	1,233	1,285
6–17 years	48.1	48.4	49.8	80.2	81.7	80.0	83.9	1,132	1,133	1,225	1,357
18–44 years	108.9	109.0	111.4	81.5	78.3	77.7	77.0	1,778	1,961	2,090	2,631
45–64 years	56.3	62.1	71.9	87.0	89.2	88.5	88.9	3,442	3,797	3,907	5,224
Sex											
Male	118.0	120.9	127.8	78.8	77.6	76.6	77.7	1,907	1,955	2,233	2,701
Female	119.1	122.7	128.7	87.5	87.4	87.0	88.0	2,120	2,347	2,420	3,316
Hispanic origin and race[4]											
Hispanic or Latino	29.4	32.0	39.9	71.0	69.5	69.0	69.3	1,613	1,801	1,590	1,903
Not Hispanic or Latino:											
White	166.2	169.2	166.3	86.9	87.2	86.6	87.7	2,029	2,321	2,441	3,406
Black or African American	31.3	32.1	32.5	72.2	72.1	71.3	75.2	2,446	1,735	2,478	2,635
Other	10.2	10.2	17.8	72.8	75.8	76.0	82.0	1,342	1,438	1,989	2,044
Insurance status[5]											
Any private insurance	174.0	181.6	180.1	86.5	86.5	85.9	87.9	1,939	2,204	2,222	3,154
Public insurance only	29.8	29.7	40.3	82.4	83.3	83.6	84.8	3,253	2,629	3,542	3,307
Uninsured all year	33.3	32.3	36.0	61.8	61.1	57.3	55.5	1,264	1,292	1,645	1,557
65 years and over:											
Total	34.2	34.8	37.0	93.7	95.2	95.5	97.1	6,415	6,999	6,735	8,906
Sex											
Male	14.6	15.0	16.0	92.0	94.5	93.4	96.6	6,565	7,866	7,223	9,020
Female	19.6	19.8	21.0	94.9	95.7	97.1	97.5	6,311	6,361	6,381	8,819
Hispanic origin and race[4]											
Hispanic or Latino	1.7	1.9	2.3	82.5	94.2	92.5	91.7	6,109	7,324	6,044	7,209
Not Hispanic or Latino:											
White	28.8	28.9	30.0	94.9	95.9	95.9	97.6	6,316	7,035	6,837	9,316
Black or African American	2.8	2.9	3.1	88.5	92.2	94.0	95.6	7,732	6,893	6,478	8,035
Other	*	*	1.7	*	*	*	97.5	*	*	*	5,291
Insurance status[6]											
Medicare only	8.8	12.0	11.2	85.9	92.1	94.8	96.0	5,053	6,448	5,783	7,651
Medicare and private insurance	21.7	19.2	20.4	95.4	97.0	96.0	98.0	6,347	6,826	6,907	9,299
Medicare and other public coverage	3.2	3.2	5.0	94.4	93.2	96.3	97.3	9,857	9,865	9,242	10,329

See footnotes at end of table.

Table 128 (page 2 of 3). Expenses for health care and prescribed medicine, by selected population characteristics: United States, selected years 1987–2004

[Data are based on household interviews of a sample of the noninstitutionalized population and a sample of medical providers]

Characteristic	Prescribed medicine expenses: Percent of persons with expense				Prescribed medicine expenses: Mean annual out-of-pocket expense per person with out-of-pocket expense[3,7]			
	1987	*1997*	*2000*	*2004*	*1987*	*1997*	*2000*	*2004*
All ages	57.3	62.1	62.3	62.7	$153	$238	$301	$437
Under 65 years:								
Total	54.0	58.7	58.5	58.5	113	168	218	304
Under 6 years	61.8	61.3	56.9	54.4	40	41	41	58
6–17 years	44.3	48.2	46.2	46.0	75	64	77	98
18–44 years	51.3	55.9	56.0	55.0	88	144	166	227
45–64 years	65.3	71.8	73.3	74.1	215	313	411	539
Sex								
Male	46.5	51.5	51.3	51.3	105	149	192	277
Female	61.4	65.8	65.6	65.7	120	182	239	325
Hispanic origin and race[4]								
Hispanic or Latino	41.6	47.7	45.0	43.6	81	112	160	182
Not Hispanic or Latino:								
White	57.7	63.1	63.8	64.6	118	182	235	333
Black or African American	44.1	50.0	47.6	50.6	100	135	180	269
Other	41.1	44.8	47.8	49.2	83	146	154	247
Insurance status[5]								
Any private insurance	56.5	61.6	61.6	62.9	116	160	188	275
Public insurance only	56.5	62.0	62.4	60.0	78	166	313	352
Uninsured all year	35.1	40.2	37.6	35.1	125	242	362	465
65 years and over:								
Total	81.6	86.0	88.3	91.9	353	568	683	1,027
Sex								
Male	78.0	82.8	83.9	90.1	328	512	512	839
Female	84.0	88.3	91.5	93.3	367	607	802	1,166
Hispanic origin and race[4]								
Hispanic or Latino	74.7	87.5	83.9	86.6	465	464	576	759
Not Hispanic or Latino:								
White	82.3	86.7	89.0	92.6	359	587	709	1,062
Black or African American	79.5	85.3	85.3	90.6	276	472	584	943
Other	*	*	*	89.9	*	*	*	883
Insurance status[6]								
Medicare only	70.6	82.1	87.7	89.7	389	657	816	1,381
Medicare and private insurance	83.4	88.1	89.0	93.3	366	577	632	940
Medicare and other public coverage	88.2	85.0	88.5	93.7	133	318	541	636

See footnotes at end of table.

Table 128 (page 3 of 3). Expenses for health care and prescribed medicine, by selected population characteristics: United States, selected years 1987–2004

[Data are based on household interviews of a sample of the noninstitutionalized population and a sample of medical providers]

* Estimates are considered unreliable. Data not shown are based on fewer than 100 sample cases. Data preceded by an asterisk have a relative standard error equal to or greater than 30%.

[1]Includes expenses for inpatient hospital and physician services, ambulatory physician and nonphysician services, prescribed medicines, home health services, dental services, and other medical equipment, supplies, and services that were purchased or rented during the year. Excludes expenses for over-the-counter medications, alternative care services, phone contacts with health providers, and premiums for health insurance.

[2]Includes persons in the civilian noninstitutionalized population for all or part of the year. Expenditures for persons in this population for only part of the year are restricted to those incurred during periods of eligibility (e.g., expenses incurred during periods of institutionalization and military service are not included in estimates).

[3]Estimates of expenses have been updated to 2004 dollars using the Consumer Price Index (all items) and differ from the previous edition of *Health, United States*. See Appendix II, Consumer Price Index (CPI).

[4]Persons of Hispanic origin may be of any race. Starting with 2002 data, MEPS respondents were allowed to report multiple races and these persons are included in the Other category. As a result, there is a slight increase in percentage of persons classified in the Other category in 2002 compared with prior years. Other includes Asian and American Indian race in addition to multiple race.

[5]Any private insurance includes individuals with insurance that provided coverage for hospital and physician care at any time during the year, other than Medicare, Medicaid, or other public coverage for hospital or physician services. Public insurance only includes individuals who were not covered by private insurance at any time during the year but were covered by Medicare, Medicaid, other public coverage for hospital or physician services, and/or CHAMPUS/CHAMPVA (TRICARE) at any point during the year. Individuals with Indian Health Service coverage only are considered uninsured. Uninsured includes persons not covered by either private or public insurance throughout the entire year or period of eligibility for the survey.

[6]Populations do not add to total because uninsured persons and persons with unknown insurance status were excluded.

[7]Includes expenses for all prescribed medications that were purchased or refilled during the survey year.

NOTES: 1987 estimates are based on National Medical Expenditure Survey (NMES) while estimates for other years are based on Medical Expenditure Panel Survey (MEPS). Because expenditures in NMES were based primarily on charges while those for MEPS were based on payments, NMES data were adjusted to be more comparable to MEPS using estimated charge to payment ratios for 1987. Overall, this resulted in about an 11% reduction from the unadjusted 1987 NMES expenditure estimates. See Zuvekas S, Cohen S. A guide to comparing health care expenditures in the 1996 MEPS to the 1987 NMES. Inquiry 2002;39(1):76–86. See Appendix I, Medical Expenditure Panel Survey (MEPS). Data for additional years are available. See Appendix III.

SOURCE: Agency for Healthcare Research and Quality, Center for Cost and Financing Studies. 1987 National Medical Expenditure Survey and 1996–2004 Medical Expenditure Panel Surveys.

Table 129 (page 1 of 3). Sources of payment for health care, by selected population characteristics: United States, selected years 1987–2004

[Data are based on household interviews of a sample of the noninstitutionalized population and a sample of medical providers]

Characteristic	All sources	Out of pocket 1987	Out of pocket 1997	Out of pocket 2000	Out of pocket 2004	Private insurance[1] 1987	Private insurance[1] 1997	Private insurance[1] 2000	Private insurance[1] 2004
	Percent distribution								
All ages	100.0	24.8	19.4	19.4	19.0	36.6	40.3	40.3	42.0
Under 65 years:									
Total	100.0	26.2	21.1	20.3	19.5	46.6	53.1	52.5	55.0
Under 6 years	100.0	18.5	14.2	10.3	10.5	39.5	49.3	51.2	57.7
6–17 years	100.0	35.7	29.0	27.7	25.6	47.3	53.2	48.8	47.6
18–44 years	100.0	27.4	21.1	19.9	19.4	46.8	52.9	51.2	53.0
45–64 years	100.0	24.0	20.1	20.2	19.3	47.8	53.6	54.5	57.3
Sex									
Male	100.0	24.5	21.3	18.1	18.8	44.6	50.3	52.2	54.8
Female	100.0	27.5	21.0	22.1	20.1	48.1	55.1	52.7	55.1
Hispanic origin and race[2]									
Hispanic or Latino	100.0	22.0	18.8	20.5	18.9	36.1	42.3	45.8	35.1
Not Hispanic or Latino:									
White	100.0	28.2	21.8	21.7	20.1	50.1	55.8	55.1	59.4
Black or African American	100.0	15.5	17.1	11.8	14.7	30.0	42.3	40.5	39.5
Other	100.0	27.2	21.2	17.0	21.5	46.7	45.2	51.2	50.0
Insurance status									
Any private insurance[3]	100.0	29.0	21.6	21.2	19.6	60.0	67.6	70.2	70.7
Public insurance only[4]	100.0	8.9	10.6	9.8	11.4	. . .	. . .	. . .	. . .
Uninsured all year[5]	100.0	40.6	41.3	40.4	48.0	. . .	. . .	. . .	. . .
65 years and over	100.0	22.0	16.3	17.5	17.8	15.8	16.5	14.9	15.8
Sex									
Male	100.0	21.7	14.2	14.2	16.0	17.6	20.1	16.8	18.1
Female	100.0	22.2	18.1	20.2	19.2	14.4	13.2	13.3	14.0
Hispanic origin and race[2]									
Hispanic or Latino	100.0	*13.5	13.6	13.9	14.3	*4.7	5.9	8.4	*12.4
Not Hispanic or Latino:									
White	100.0	23.7	17.0	18.3	18.2	16.7	17.9	15.2	16.7
Black or African American	100.0	11.2	11.4	13.6	14.0	*11.9	8.8	9.3	10.1
Other	100.0	*	*	*	22.1	*	*	*	*10.1
Insurance status									
Medicare only	100.0	29.8	19.8	22.2	24.2	. . .	. . .	. . .	. . .
Medicare and private insurance	100.0	23.4	17.3	17.0	17.4	18.9	25.7	25.3	26.5
Medicare and other public coverage	100.0	*6.2	5.2	9.1	8.5	. . .	. . .	. . .	. . .

See footnotes at end of table.

Table 129 (page 2 of 3). Sources of payment for health care, by selected population characteristics: United States, selected years 1987–2004

[Data are based on household interviews of a sample of the noninstitutionalized population and a sample of medical providers]

	Source of payment for health care							
	Public coverage[6]				*Other*[7]			
Characteristic	*1987*	*1997*	*2000*	*2004*	*1987*	*1997*	*2000*	*2004*
	Percent distribution							
All ages	34.1	34.4	35.4	35.2	4.5	5.9	5.0	3.9
Under 65 years:								
Total	21.3	18.1	21.3	20.8	6.0	7.7	6.0	4.7
Under 6 years	35.8	25.4	33.6	28.7	6.2	11.2	4.9	3.1
6–17 years	11.8	14.1	20.1	23.0	5.2	3.7	3.4	3.7
18–44 years	19.4	15.7	21.1	22.1	6.4	10.3	7.8	5.5
45–64 years	22.4	20.3	20.2	18.8	5.8	6.0	5.2	4.5
Sex								
Male	23.9	19.5	23.5	20.6	7.1	8.9	6.3	5.8
Female	19.2	17.0	19.5	20.9	5.2	6.8	5.7	3.9
Hispanic origin and race[2]								
Hispanic or Latino	35.8	28.9	27.5	39.1	6.0	10.0	6.2	6.9
Not Hispanic or Latino:								
White	15.9	15.3	18.0	16.2	5.8	7.1	5.2	4.3
Black or African American	47.2	30.7	38.8	39.9	7.3	9.9	8.8	5.9
Other	21.0	23.7	19.0	22.8	5.1	9.9	*12.8	5.8
Insurance status								
Any private insurance[3]	6.2	6.6	5.3	7.1	4.8	4.2	3.3	2.5
Public insurance only[4]	87.2	80.7	84.4	84.4	3.9	8.7	5.8	4.2
Uninsured all year[5]	28.6	7.5	*21.2	8.5	30.9	51.1	38.4	43.5
65 years and over	60.8	64.8	64.7	64.2	1.5	2.5	2.9	2.2
Sex								
Male	58.8	63.4	66.9	64.0	*1.9	2.3	2.2	1.9
Female	62.3	65.9	63.0	64.4	1.1	2.7	3.5	2.4
Hispanic origin and race[2]								
Hispanic or Latino	80.2	77.8	75.6	69.9	*1.6	*2.7	*2.2	*3.4
Not Hispanic or Latino:								
White	58.0	62.6	64.1	63.0	1.6	2.5	2.4	2.2
Black or African American	76.3	77.6	68.3	74.7	0.6	2.2	*8.9	1.2
Other	*	*	*	65.1	*	*	*	*2.8
Insurance status								
Medicare only	68.8	72.4	72.2	68.9	1.4	7.7	5.7	6.9
Medicare and private insurance	56.1	56.3	57.1	55.7	1.6	0.6	*0.6	0.4
Medicare and other public coverage	92.9	92.7	87.3	89.7	1.0	*2.1	*3.6	0.7

See footnotes at end of table.

Table 129 (page 3 of 3). Sources of payment for health care, by selected population characteristics: United States, selected years 1987–2004

[Data are based on household interviews of a sample of the noninstitutionalized population and a sample of medical providers]

. . . Category not applicable.
* Estimates are considered unreliable. Estimates based on fewer than 100 sample cases or with a relative standard error of 30% or higher are not shown.
[1]Private insurance includes any type of private insurance payments reported for people with private health insurance coverage during the year.
[2]Persons of Hispanic origin may be of any race. Starting with 2002 data, MEPS respondents were allowed to report multiple races and these persons are included in the Other category. As a result, there is a slight increase in the percent of persons classified in the Other category in 2002 compared with prior years.
[3]Includes individuals with insurance that provided coverage for hospital and physician care at any time during the year, other than Medicare, Medicaid, or other public coverage for hospital or physician services.
[4]Includes individuals who were not covered by private insurance at any time during the year but were covered by Medicare, Medicaid, other public coverage for hospital or physician services, and/or CHAMPUS/CHAMPVA (TRICARE) at any point during the year.
[5]Includes individuals not covered by either private or public insurance throughout the entire year or period of eligibility for the survey. However, some expenses for the uninsured were paid by sources that were not defined as health insurance coverage, such as the Department of Veterans Affairs, community and neighborhood clinics, the Indian Health Service, state and local health departments, state programs other than Medicaid, Workers' Compensation, and other unclassified sources (e.g., automobile, homeowners', or liability insurance). Individuals with Indian Health Service coverage only are considered uninsured.
[6]Public coverage includes payments made by Medicare, Medicaid, the Department of Veterans Affairs, other federal sources (e.g., Indian Health Service, military treatment facilities, and other care provided by the federal government), and various state and local sources (e.g., community and neighborhood clinics, state and local health departments, and state programs other than Medicaid).
[7]Other sources includes Workers' Compensation, unclassified sources (automobile, home, or liability insurance, and other miscellaneous or unknown sources), Medicaid payments reported for people who were not enrolled in the program at any time during the year, and any type of private insurance payments reported for people without private health insurance coverage during the year.

NOTES: 1987 estimates are based on the National Medical Expenditure Survey (NMES); estimates for other years are based on the Medical Expenditure Panel Survey (MEPS). Because expenditures in NMES were based primarily on charges while those for MEPS were based on payments, data for NMES were adjusted to be more comparable to MEPS using estimated charge to payment ratios for 1987. Overall, this resulted in an approximate 11% reduction from the unadjusted 1987 NMES expenditure estimates. For a detailed explanation of this adjustment, see Zuvekas S, Cohen S. A guide to comparing health care estimates in the 1996 Medical Expenditure Panel Survey to the 1987 National Medical Expenditure Survey. Inquiry 2002;39(1):76–86. See Appendix I, Medical Expenditure Panel Survey (MEPS). Data for additional years are available. See Appendix III.

SOURCE: Agency for Healthcare Research and Quality, Center for Cost and Financing Studies. 1987 National Medical Expenditure Survey and 1996–2004 Medical Expenditure Panel Survey.

Table 130. Out-of-pocket health care expenses among persons with medical expenses, by age: United States, selected years 1987–2004

[Data are based on household interviews for a sample of the noninstitutionalized population and a sample of medical providers]

Age and year	Percent of persons with expenses	Amount paid out of pocket among persons with expenses[1]						
		Total	$0	$1–124	$125–249	$250–499	$500–999	$1,000+
		Percent distribution						
All ages								
1987	84.5	100.0	10.4	29.2	16.6	17.4	13.3	13.1
2000	83.5	100.0	6.9	34.8	15.0	16.2	13.0	14.1
2001	85.4	100.0	7.1	31.7	14.7	16.6	13.8	16.2
2002	85.2	100.0	7.8	29.8	14.3	15.7	14.8	17.6
2003	85.6	100.0	7.6	28.0	14.0	15.8	15.2	19.5
2004	84.7	100.0	8.8	27.9	13.0	15.6	14.5	20.3
Under 6 years								
1987	88.9	100.0	19.2	38.7	18.9	14.7	5.3	3.2
2000	86.7	100.0	16.7	61.0	11.1	7.5	2.4	1.3
2001	88.8	100.0	18.5	57.8	12.9	7.6	2.1	1.1
2002	88.8	100.0	21.5	51.7	14.0	7.7	3.9	1.3
2003	91.3	100.0	20.6	51.7	13.3	8.5	4.2	1.6
2004	90.0	100.0	26.0	47.9	11.9	7.9	4.2	2.1
6–17 years								
1987	80.2	100.0	15.5	37.9	18.2	12.4	8.5	7.6
2000	80.0	100.0	14.7	46.5	14.5	11.2	6.5	6.6
2001	83.2	100.0	15.0	45.2	15.0	11.1	6.0	7.7
2002	83.6	100.0	16.6	43.2	14.7	12.0	6.8	6.7
2003	84.1	100.0	16.1	40.6	15.5	12.2	7.9	7.8
2004	83.9	100.0	18.7	40.9	13.0	12.0	7.7	7.7
18–44 years								
1987	81.5	100.0	10.1	32.3	17.7	18.2	11.9	9.8
2000	77.7	100.0	5.8	39.1	17.8	17.1	11.7	8.5
2001	79.3	100.0	6.0	34.8	17.5	18.8	13.3	9.7
2002	78.5	100.0	6.7	34.2	17.4	17.1	13.9	10.8
2003	79.0	100.0	6.4	31.6	17.4	18.3	14.0	12.3
2004	77.0	100.0	7.2	31.8	16.0	18.4	13.4	13.2
45–64 years								
1987	87.0	100.0	5.7	20.4	15.6	20.7	18.8	18.8
2000	88.5	100.0	2.6	22.3	15.6	19.9	18.8	20.9
2001	89.9	100.0	2.4	19.6	13.9	20.4	19.8	23.8
2002	90.0	100.0	2.3	18.8	12.8	19.1	21.3	25.8
2003	89.6	100.0	2.4	17.2	12.3	17.7	21.4	29.1
2004	88.9	100.0	2.7	17.6	12.0	18.1	21.2	28.4
65–74 years								
1987	92.8	100.0	5.3	15.4	11.6	18.5	22.1	27.1
2000	94.7	100.0	1.5	14.4	10.6	20.2	20.1	33.2
2001	95.6	100.0	1.5	14.4	9.9	18.3	21.7	34.2
2002	96.1	100.0	1.8	10.1	9.9	16.4	22.5	39.3
2003	95.3	100.0	1.7	9.0	8.2	15.6	24.5	41.0
2004	96.6	100.0	1.5	11.2	9.0	13.8	19.8	44.7
75 years or more								
1987	95.1	100.0	5.6	12.9	10.0	17.1	21.2	33.2
2000	96.5	100.0	2.6	14.2	8.4	18.2	22.0	34.6
2001	97.0	100.0	1.7	10.1	9.2	14.4	21.1	43.6
2002	96.5	100.0	2.2	9.0	7.7	14.4	20.4	46.2
2003	97.5	100.0	1.9	8.7	7.0	13.4	20.1	48.9
2004	97.7	100.0	1.8	8.4	8.1	11.9	18.5	51.2

[1] 1987 dollars were converted to 1998 dollars using the national Consumer Price Index. Starting with 1998 data, percent distributions are based on actual dollars (nonadjusted).

NOTES: Out-of-pocket expenses include expenditures for inpatient hospital and physician services, ambulatory physician and nonphysician services, prescribed medicines, home health services, dental services, and various other medical equipment, supplies, and services that were purchased or rented during the year. Out-of-pocket expenses for over-the-counter medications, alternative care services, phone contacts with health providers, and premiums for health insurance policies are not included in these estimates. 1987 estimates are based on the National Medical Expenditure Survey (NMES), while estimates for other years are based on the Medical Expenditure Panel Survey (MEPS). Because expenditures in NMES were based primarily on charges while those for MEPS were based on payments, data for the NMES were adjusted to be more comparable to MEPS using estimated charge to payment ratios for 1987. Overall, this resulted in an approximate 11% reduction from the unadjusted 1987 NMES expenditure estimates. For a detailed explanation of this adjustment, see Zuvekas S, Cohen S. A guide to comparing health care expenditures in the 1996 MEPS to the 1987 NMES. Inquiry 2002;39(1):76–86. See Appendix I, Medical Expenditure Panel Survey (MEPS). Data for additional years are available. See Appendix III.

SOURCES: Agency for Healthcare Research and Quality, Center for Cost and Financing Studies. 1987 National Medical Expenditure Survey and 1998–2004 Medical Expenditure Panel Survey.

Table 131 (page 1 of 2). Expenditures for health services and supplies and percent distribution, by type of payer: United States, selected years 1987–2005

[Data are compiled from various sources by the Centers for Medicare & Medicaid Services]

Type of payer	*1987*	*1993*	*1997*	*2000*	*2001*	*2002*	*2003*	*2004*	*2005*
	Amount in billions								
Total[1]	$477.8	$853.2	$1,054.3	$1,264.4	$1,376.2	$1,498.8	$1,621.7	$1,738.9	$1,860.9
Private	333.3	545.4	668.0	821.3	868.8	927.5	994.4	1,056.2	1,124.6
Private business	122.1	218.9	265.9	342.0	367.6	390.5	419.5	446.6	478.1
Employer contribution to private health insurance premiums	84.2	158.3	191.5	251.2	272.4	293.3	319.3	341.6	366.9
Private employer contribution to Medicare hospital insurance trust fund[2]	24.6	35.8	49.5	62.2	63.3	63.0	64.5	68.4	72.7
Workers compensation and temporary disability insurance	11.6	21.8	21.3	24.3	27.5	29.5	30.8	31.4	32.8
Industrial inplant health services	1.7	2.9	3.6	4.3	4.5	4.7	4.9	5.3	5.6
Household	188.7	290.6	353.3	425.5	448.0	482.2	515.1	548.5	582.4
Employee contribution to private health insurance premiums and individual policy premiums	43.9	89.9	112.4	133.7	147.1	167.0	182.7	196.9	207.1
Employee and self-employment contributions and voluntary premiums paid to Medicare hospital insurance trust fund[2]	29.4	43.7	63.0	82.5	82.9	84.2	86.2	91.1	96.6
Premiums paid by individuals to Medicare supplementary medical insurance trust fund	6.2	11.9	15.5	16.3	18.0	19.7	21.6	24.6	29.2
Out-of-pocket health spending	109.2	145.2	162.5	192.9	200.0	211.3	224.5	235.8	249.4
Other private revenues	22.4	36.0	48.7	53.7	53.1	54.8	59.7	61.1	64.1
Public	144.5	307.8	386.3	443.2	507.4	571.3	627.3	682.7	736.3
Federal government	74.1	176.2	220.0	235.6	277.1	317.5	354.4	389.1	416.9
Employer contributions to private health insurance premiums	4.9	11.5	11.4	14.3	15.8	17.7	19.7	21.6	23.1
Medicaid[3]	28.1	78.1	97.4	119.7	134.5	149.5	163.6	174.9	183.6
Other[4]	41.1	86.6	111.2	101.6	126.9	150.4	171.0	192.6	210.1
State and local government	70.5	131.6	166.3	207.6	230.3	253.7	273.0	293.6	319.4
Employer contributions to private health insurance premiums	16.0	35.8	43.9	56.0	63.5	73.1	82.1	91.4	97.1
Medicaid[3]	22.8	46.5	64.9	85.3	94.7	103.9	112.6	122.6	137.8
Other[5]	31.7	49.2	57.5	66.2	72.1	76.8	78.3	79.6	84.5
	Percent distribution								
Total	100.0	100.0	100.0	100.0	100.0	100.0	100.0	100.0	100.0
Private	69.7	63.9	63.4	65.0	63.1	61.9	61.3	60.7	60.4
Private business	25.6	25.7	25.2	27.1	26.7	26.1	25.9	25.7	25.7
Employer contribution to private health insurance premiums	17.6	18.6	18.2	19.9	19.8	19.6	19.7	19.6	19.7
Private employer contribution to Medicare hospital insurance trust fund[2]	5.2	4.2	4.7	4.9	4.6	4.2	4.0	3.9	3.9
Workers compensation and temporary disability insurance	2.4	2.6	2.0	1.9	2.0	2.0	1.9	1.8	1.8
Industrial inplant health services	0.4	0.3	0.3	0.3	0.3	0.3	0.3	0.3	0.3
Household	39.5	34.1	33.5	33.7	32.6	32.2	31.8	31.5	31.3
Employee contribution to private health insurance premiums and individual policy premiums	9.2	10.5	10.7	10.6	10.7	11.1	11.3	11.3	11.1
Employee and self-employment contributions and voluntary premiums paid to Medicare hospital insurance trust fund[2]	6.1	5.1	6.0	6.5	6.0	5.6	5.3	5.2	5.2
Premiums paid by individuals to Medicare supplementary medical insurance trust fund	1.3	1.4	1.5	1.3	1.3	1.3	1.3	1.4	1.6
Out-of-pocket health spending	22.9	17.0	15.4	15.3	14.5	14.1	13.8	13.6	13.4
Other private revenues	4.7	4.2	4.6	4.2	3.9	3.7	3.7	3.5	3.4

See footnotes at end of table.

Table 131 (page 2 of 2). Expenditures for health services and supplies and percent distribution, by type of payer: United States, selected years 1987–2005

[Data are compiled from various sources by the Centers for Medicare & Medicaid Services]

Type of payer	*1987*	*1993*	*1997*	*2000*	*2001*	*2002*	*2003*	*2004*	*2005*
					Percent distribution				
Public	30.3	36.1	36.6	35.0	36.9	38.1	38.7	39.3	39.6
Federal government	15.5	20.7	20.9	18.6	20.1	21.2	21.9	22.4	22.4
Employer contributions to private health insurance premiums	1.0	1.3	1.1	1.1	1.1	1.2	1.2	1.2	1.2
Medicaid[3]	5.9	9.2	9.2	9.5	9.8	10.0	10.1	10.1	9.9
Other[4]	8.6	10.1	10.5	8.0	9.2	10.0	10.5	11.1	11.3
State and local government	14.8	15.4	15.8	16.4	16.7	16.9	16.8	16.9	17.2
Employer contributions to private health insurance premiums	3.3	4.2	4.2	4.4	4.6	4.9	5.1	5.3	5.2
Medicaid[3]	4.8	5.5	6.2	6.7	6.9	6.9	6.9	7.1	7.4
Other[5]	6.6	5.8	5.5	5.2	5.2	5.1	4.8	4.6	4.5

[1]Excludes research and construction.
[2]Includes one-half of self-employment contribution to Medicare hospital insurance trust fund.
[3]Includes Medicaid buy-in premiums for Medicare.
[4]Includes expenditures for Medicare (with adjustments for contributions by employers and individuals and premiums paid to the Medicare insurance trust fund), maternal and child health, vocational rehabilitation, Substance Abuse and Mental Health Services Administration, Indian Health Service, federal workers' compensation, other miscellaneous general hospital and medical programs, public health activities, Department of Defense, Department of Veterans Affairs, and State Children's Health Insurance Program (SCHIP).
[5]Includes other public and general assistance, maternal and child health, vocational rehabilitation, public health activities, hospital subsidies, and employer contributions to Medicare hospital insurance trust fund.

NOTES: This table disaggregates health expenditures according to four classes of payers: businesses, households (individuals), federal government, and state and local governments with a small amount of revenue coming from nonpatient revenue sources such as philanthropy. Where businesses or households pay dedicated funds into government health programs (for example, Medicare) or employers and employees share in the cost of health premiums, these costs are assigned to businesses or households accordingly. This results in a lower share of expenditures being assigned to the federal government than for tabulations of expenditures by source of funds. Estimates of national health expenditure by source of funds aim to track government-sponsored health programs over time and do not delineate the role of business employers in paying for health care. Figures may not sum to totals due to rounding. These data were revised and differ from previous editions of *Health, United States*.

SOURCE: Centers for Medicare & Medicaid Services, Office of the Actuary, National Health Statistics Group. Sponsors of Health Care Costs: Businesses, Households, and Governments, 1987–2005. Available from: www.cms.hhs.gov/NationalHealthExpendData/.

Table 132 (page 1 of 2). Employers' costs per employee-hour worked for total compensation, wages and salaries, and health insurance, by selected characteristics: United States, selected years 1991–2006

[Data are based on surveys of a sample of employers]

Characteristic	1991	1994	1996	1998	2000	2002	2003	2004	2005	2006
					Amount per employee-hour worked					
State and local government	$22.31	$25.27	$25.73	$27.28	$29.05	$31.29	$32.62	$34.21	$35.50	$36.96
Total private industry	15.40	17.08	17.49	18.50	19.85	21.71	22.37	23.29	24.17	25.09
Industry:										
Goods producing	18.48	20.85	21.27	22.26	23.55	25.44	26.25	27.19	28.48	29.36
Service providing	14.31	15.82	16.28	17.31	18.72	20.66	21.30	22.33	23.11	24.05
Occupational group:[1]										
White collar	18.15	20.26	21.10	22.38	24.19	26.43	28.85	---	---	---
Blue collar	15.15	16.92	17.04	17.56	18.73	20.15	21.21	---	---	---
Service	7.82	8.38	8.61	9.37	9.72	10.95	13.68	---	---	---
Management, professional, and related	---	---	---	---	---	---	---	40.23	42.09	44.32
Sales and office	---	---	---	---	---	---	---	18.42	19.30	19.93
Service	---	---	---	---	---	---	---	11.66	12.07	12.3
Natural resources, construction, and maintenance	---	---	---	---	---	---	---	26.55	27.26	28.07
Production, transportation, and material moving	---	---	---	---	---	---	---	20.21	20.82	21.19
Census region:										
Northeast	17.56	20.03	20.57	20.38	22.67	25.00	25.70	26.29	27.09	28.75
Midwest	15.05	16.26	16.30	18.15	19.22	21.25	22.40	23.26	24.23	24.65
South	13.68	15.05	15.62	16.45	17.81	19.49	19.95	20.80	21.36	22.35
West	15.97	18.08	18.78	19.94	20.88	22.68	23.07	24.54	25.98	26.56
Union status:										
Union	19.76	23.26	23.31	23.59	25.88	29.42	30.68	31.94	33.17	34.07
Nonunion	14.54	16.04	16.61	17.80	19.07	20.79	21.36	22.28	23.09	24.03
Establishment employment size:										
1–99 employees	13.38	14.58	14.85	15.92	17.16	18.51	18.93	19.47	20.22	20.43
100 or more	17.34	19.45	20.09	21.20	22.81	25.48	26.42	27.81	28.94	30.34
100–499	14.31	15.88	16.61	17.52	19.30	21.99	22.62	23.91	24.44	25.91
500 or more	20.60	23.35	24.03	25.56	26.93	29.79	30.94	32.54	34.59	35.94
					Wages and salaries as a percent of total compensation					
State and local government	69.6	69.5	69.8	70.3	70.8	70.8	70.0	69.2	68.3	67.6
Total private industry	72.3	71.1	71.9	72.8	73.0	72.8	72.2	71.5	71.0	70.7
Industry:										
Goods producing	68.7	66.5	67.6	69.0	69.0	68.7	67.7	66.7	65.5	66.2
Service providing	73.9	73.1	73.8	74.4	74.5	74.2	73.7	72.9	72.6	72.0
Occupational group:[1]										
White collar	73.8	72.7	73.2	73.9	74.0	73.7	72.9	---	---	---
Blue collar	68.4	66.8	68.1	69.2	69.4	69.5	68.5	---	---	---
Service	76.2	75.5	75.8	77.4	77.9	76.9	72.4	---	---	---
Management, professional, and related	---	---	---	---	---	---	---	72.1	71.5	70.9
Sales and office	---	---	---	---	---	---	---	73.0	72.6	72.2
Service	---	---	---	---	---	---	---	75.8	75.7	75.3
Natural resources, construction, and maintenance	---	---	---	---	---	---	---	69.1	68.0	68.0
Production, transportation, and material moving	---	---	---	---	---	---	---	66.9	66.2	66.7
Census region:										
Northeast	72.0	70.5	70.9	72.1	72.2	71.9	71.2	70.4	70.4	70.0
Midwest	71.1	69.7	71.1	71.6	72.4	72.0	71.6	71.1	70.1	69.4
South	73.3	72.1	72.7	73.9	73.5	73.6	73.2	72.5	72.1	72.1
West	72.8	72.0	73.1	74.0	74.0	73.5	72.6	71.6	70.9	71.0
Union status:										
Union	65.9	63.5	64.0	65.2	65.2	65.7	65.0	63.6	62.6	62.3
Nonunion	74.1	72.9	73.6	74.2	74.4	74.0	73.5	72.8	72.4	72.1
Establishment employment size:										
1–99 employees	74.7	73.5	74.7	75.4	75.5	75.0	74.6	74.3	73.9	73.7
100 or more	70.5	69.3	69.9	70.8	71.0	70.9	70.2	69.1	68.5	68.4
100–499	72.1	71.6	71.6	72.3	72.8	72.2	71.4	70.7	70.2	70.0
500 or more	69.3	67.6	68.6	69.6	69.4	69.8	69.1	67.7	67.0	66.9

See footnotes at end of table.

Table 132 (page 2 of 2). Employers' costs per employee-hour worked for total compensation, wages and salaries, and health insurance, by selected characteristics: United States, selected years 1991–2006

[Data are based on surveys of a sample of employers]

Characteristic	*1991*	*1994*	*1996*	*1998*	*2000*	*2002*	*2003*	*2004*	*2005*	*2006*
	Health insurance as a percent of total compensation									
State and local government	6.9	8.2	7.7	7.5	7.8	8.6	9.2	9.8	10.2	10.6
Total private industry	6.0	6.7	5.9	5.4	5.5	5.9	6.3	6.6	6.8	6.9
Industry:										
Goods producing	6.9	8.1	7.2	6.6	6.9	7.2	7.5	7.8	8.0	8.4
Service providing	5.5	6.0	5.4	4.9	4.9	5.5	5.9	6.2	6.4	6.4
Occupational group:[1]										
White collar	5.6	6.2	5.5	5.0	5.0	5.4	6.4	---	---	---
Blue collar	7.0	8.0	7.2	6.7	6.8	7.3	8.0	---	---	---
Service	4.6	5.4	4.8	4.3	4.3	5.1	7.0	---	---	---
Management, professional, and related	---	---	---	---	---	---	---	5.4	5.5	5.6
Sales and office	---	---	---	---	---	---	---	7.3	7.5	7.5
Service	---	---	---	---	---	---	---	6.0	6.1	6.2
Natural resources, construction, and maintenance	---	---	---	---	---	---	---	6.9	7.5	7.7
Production, transportation, and material moving	---	---	---	---	---	---	---	8.5	8.9	9.0
Census region:										
Northeast	6.2	6.9	6.2	5.6	5.6	5.9	6.3	6.5	6.8	6.7
Midwest	6.3	7.3	6.3	5.7	5.8	6.4	6.6	7.0	7.3	7.6
South	5.5	6.3	5.9	5.3	5.4	5.8	6.2	6.5	6.6	6.7
West	5.8	6.1	5.2	4.9	5.0	5.6	6.0	6.3	6.3	6.4
Union status:										
Union	8.2	9.8	8.8	8.4	8.4	8.7	9.1	9.6	10.3	10.3
Nonunion	5.4	5.9	5.3	4.8	5.0	5.4	5.8	6.1	6.2	6.3
Establishment employment size:										
1–99 employees	5.1	5.7	5.0	4.6	4.8	5.2	5.5	5.8	5.9	6.0
100 or more	6.6	7.3	6.6	6.0	6.0	6.6	7.0	7.2	7.5	7.5
100–499	6.3	6.5	6.3	5.8	5.6	6.4	6.9	7.1	7.5	7.4
500 or more	6.8	7.9	6.9	6.2	6.4	6.7	7.0	7.3	7.6	7.6

- - - Data not available.

[1]Starting with 2004 data, sample establishments were classified by industry categories based on the 2000 North American Industry Classification (NAICS) system, as defined by the U.S. Office of Management and Budget. Within a sample establishment, specific job categories were selected and classified into about 800 occupational classifications according to the 2000 Standard Occupational Classification (SOC) system. Individual occupations were combined to represent one of five higher-level aggregations, such as management, professional, and related occupations. For more detailed information on NAICS and SOC, including background and definitions, see the websites: www.bls.gov/bls/naics.htm and www.bls.gov/soc/home.htm. NAICS and SOC have replaced the 1987 Standard Industrial Classification System (SIC) and the Occupational Classification System (OCS).

NOTES: Costs are calculated annually from March survey data. Total compensation includes wages and salaries and benefits. See Appendix II, Employer costs for employee compensation. Data for additional years are available. See Appendix III.

SOURCES: U.S. Department of Labor, Bureau of Labor Statistics, National Compensation Survey, Employer Costs for Employee Compensation, March release; News pub no 06–1049, June 21, 2006. Washington, DC. Data are available on the Bureau of Labor Statistics Web site at www.bls.gov/ncs/ect/home.htm.

Table 133. Hospital expenses, by type of ownership and size of hospital: United States, selected years 1980–2005

[Data are based on reporting by a census of hospitals]

Type of ownership and size of hospital	*1980*	*1990*	*1995*	*2000*	*2004*	*2005*	*1980–1990*	*1990–1995*	*1995–2000*	*2000–2005*
Total expenses	Amount in billions						Average annual percent change			
All hospitals	$ 91.9	$234.9	$320.3	$395.4	$ 533.9	$ 570.5	9.8	6.4	4.3	7.6
Federal	7.9	15.2	20.2	23.9	34.8	36.8	6.8	5.9	3.4	9.0
Nonfederal[1]	84.0	219.6	300.0	371.5	499.0	533.7	10.1	6.4	4.4	7.5
Community[2]	76.9	203.7	285.6	356.6	481.2	515.7	10.2	7.0	4.5	7.7
Nonprofit	55.8	150.7	209.6	267.1	359.4	386.0	10.4	6.8	5.0	7.6
For profit	5.8	18.8	26.7	35.0	49.0	51.8	12.5	7.3	5.6	8.2
State-local government	15.2	34.2	49.3	54.5	72.9	77.9	8.4	7.6	2.0	7.4
6–24 beds	0.2	0.5	1.1	1.5	2.9	3.5	9.6	17.1	6.4	18.5
25–49 beds	1.7	4.0	7.2	10.4	15.1	17.4	8.9	12.5	7.6	10.8
50–99 beds	5.4	12.6	17.8	22.3	30.2	31.9	8.8	7.2	4.6	7.4
100–199 beds	12.5	33.3	50.7	63.4	79.7	84.8	10.3	8.8	4.6	6.0
200–299 beds	13.4	38.7	55.8	67.1	86.1	93.4	11.2	7.6	3.8	6.8
300–399 beds	11.5	33.1	43.3	54.3	76.0	84.0	11.2	5.5	4.6	9.1
400–499 beds	10.5	25.3	33.7	41.3	57.4	60.2	9.2	5.9	4.2	7.8
500 beds or more	21.6	56.2	76.1	96.3	134.0	140.6	10.0	6.3	4.8	7.9
Expenses per inpatient day	Amount									
Community[2]	$ 245	$ 687	$ 968	$1,149	$ 1,450	$ 1,522	10.9	7.1	3.5	5.8
Nonprofit	246	692	994	1,182	1,501	1,585	10.9	7.5	3.5	6.0
For profit	257	752	947	1,057	1,362	1,413	11.3	4.7	2.2	6.0
State-local government	239	634	878	1,064	1,291	1,330	10.2	6.7	3.9	4.6
6–24 beds	203	526	678	896	1,222	1,233	10.0	5.2	5.7	6.6
25–49 beds	197	489	696	891	1,071	1,101	9.5	7.3	5.1	4.3
50–99 beds	191	493	647	745	916	952	9.9	5.6	2.9	5.0
100–199 beds	215	585	796	925	1,153	1,205	10.5	6.4	3.0	5.4
200–299 beds	239	665	943	1,122	1,436	1,528	10.8	7.2	3.5	6.4
300–399 beds	248	731	1,070	1,277	1,602	1,639	11.4	7.9	3.6	5.1
400–499 beds	215	756	1,135	1,353	1,756	1,917	13.4	8.5	3.6	7.2
500 beds or more	239	825	1,212	1,468	1,829	1,940	13.2	8.0	3.9	5.7
Expenses per inpatient stay										
Community[2]	$1,851	$4,947	$6,216	$6,649	$ 8,166	$ 8,535	10.3	4.7	1.4	5.1
Nonprofit	1,902	5,001	6,279	6,717	8,267	8,671	10.2	4.7	1.4	5.2
For profit	1,676	4,727	5,425	5,642	7,139	7,352	10.9	2.8	0.8	5.4
State-local government	1,750	4,838	6,445	7,106	8,473	8,793	10.7	5.9	2.0	4.4
6–24 beds	1,072	2,701	3,578	3,652	4,743	5,054	9.7	5.8	0.4	6.7
25–49 beds	1,138	2,967	3,797	4,381	5,202	5,374	10.1	5.1	2.9	4.2
50–99 beds	1,271	3,461	4,427	4,760	5,792	6,109	10.5	5.0	1.5	5.1
100–199 beds	1,512	4,109	5,103	5,305	6,608	6,826	10.5	4.4	0.8	5.2
200–299 beds	1,767	4,618	5,851	6,392	7,739	8,120	10.1	4.8	1.8	4.9
300–399 beds	1,881	5,096	6,512	6,988	8,496	8,816	10.5	5.0	1.4	4.8
400–499 beds	2,090	5,500	7,164	7,629	9,720	10,516	10.2	5.4	1.3	6.6
500 beds or more	2,517	6,667	8,531	9,149	10,995	11,621	10.2	5.1	1.4	4.9

[1]The category of nonfederal hospitals includes psychiatric, tuberculosis and other respiratory diseases hospitals, and long-term and short-term general and other special hospitals. See Appendix II, Hospital.

[2]Community hospitals are nonfederal short-term general and special hospitals whose facilities and services are available to the public. See Appendix II, Hospital.

NOTE: In 2005, employee payroll and benefit expenses comprised 51% of expenses in community hospitals and 59% in federal hospitals.

SOURCES: American Hospital Association (AHA) Annual Survey of Hospitals. Hospital Statistics, 1981, 1991–2007 editions. Chicago, IL. (Copyrights 1981, 1991–2007: Used with the permission of Health Forum LLC, an affiliate of the AHA.)

Table 134. Nursing home average monthly charges per resident, by selected facility characteristics: United States, 1985–2004

[Data are based on reporting by a sample of nursing homes]

Facility characteristic	*1985*	*1995*	*1997*	*1999*	*2004*
			Average monthly charge		
All facilities	$1,508	$ 3,132	$3,638	$3,531	$5,690
Ownership					
Proprietary	1,436	3,044	3,530	3,266	5,356
Nonprofit and government	1,659	3,293	3,834	4,013	6,214
Certification					
Both Medicare and Medicaid	1,797	3,314	3,791	3,679	5,654
Medicare only	1,550	4,189	4,490	3,696	7,541
Medicaid only	1,267	2,167	2,448	2,396	6,206
Neither	954	2,324	2,420	2,146	4,117
Bed size					
Fewer than 50 beds	1,133	*4,953	3,549	3,195	5,708
50–99 beds	1,394	2,688	3,207	3,071	5,446
100–199 beds	1,511	3,025	3,614	3,647	5,696
200 beds or more	1,785	3,561	4,258	3,858	6,162
Geographic region					
Northeast	1,936	3,895	4,597	4,256	7,229
Midwest	1,425	2,734	3,240	3,589	5,198
South	1,294	2,743	3,236	2,902	5,005
West	1,496	3,701	3,816	3,663	5,969

* Estimates are considered unreliable. Data preceded by an asterisk have a relative standard error of 20%–30%.

NOTES: Average monthly charge is for the month prior to interview. Charges do not reflect the amount that was paid for care. Residents are persons on the roster of the nursing home as of the night before the survey. Residents for whom beds are maintained even though they may be away on overnight leave or in a hospital are included. People residing in personal care or domiciliary care homes are excluded. See Appendix I, National Nursing Home Survey (NNHS). Numbers have been revised and differ from previous editions of *Health, United States.*

SOURCE: Centers for Disease Control and Prevention, National Center for Health Statistics, National Nursing Home Survey.

Table 135. Mental health expenditures, percent distribution, and per capita expenditures, by type of mental health organization: United States, selected years 1975–2002

[Data are based on an inventory of Mental Health Organizations]

Type of organization	*1975*	*1979*	*1983*	*1986*	*1990*	*1994*	*1998*	*2000*	*2002*
					Amount in millions				
All organizations	$6,564	$8,764	$14,432	$18,458	$28,410	$33,136	$38,512	$34,528	$34,302
State and county psychiatric hospitals	3,185	3,757	5,491	6,326	7,774	7,825	7,117	7,485	7,616
Private psychiatric hospitals	467	743	1,712	2,629	6,101	6,468	4,106	3,885	3,929
Nonfederal general hospital psychiatric services	621	723	2,176	2,878	4,662	5,344	5,589	5,853	5,179
Department of Veterans Affairs medical centers[1]	699	848	1,316	1,338	1,480	1,386	1,690	976	1,018
Residential treatment centers for emotionally disturbed children	279	436	573	978	1,969	2,360	3,557	3,781	4,496
All other organizations[2]	1,313	2,256	3,164	4,310	6,424	9,753	16,454	12,549	12,063
					Percent distribution				
All organizations	100.0	100.0	100.0	100.0	100.0	100.0	100.0	100.0	100.0
State and county psychiatric hospitals	48.5	42.9	38.0	34.3	27.4	23.6	18.5	21.7	22.2
Private psychiatric hospitals	7.1	8.5	11.9	14.2	21.5	19.5	10.7	11.3	11.5
Nonfederal general hospital psychiatric services	9.5	8.2	15.1	15.6	16.4	16.1	14.5	17.0	15.1
Department of Veterans Affairs medical centers[1]	10.6	9.7	9.1	7.2	5.2	4.2	4.4	2.8	3.0
Residential treatment centers for emotionally disturbed children	4.2	5.0	4.0	5.3	6.9	7.1	9.2	11.0	13.1
All other organizations[2]	20.0	25.7	21.9	23.3	22.6	29.4	42.7	36.4	35.2
					Amount per capita[3]				
All organizations	$ 31	$ 40	$ 62	$ 77	$ 116	$ 128	$ 143	$ 122	$ 119
State and county psychiatric hospitals	15	17	24	26	32	30	26	27	26
Private psychiatric hospitals	2	3	7	11	25	25	15	14	14
Nonfederal general hospital psychiatric services	3	3	9	12	19	21	21	21	18
Department of Veterans Affairs medical centers[1]	3	4	6	6	6	5	6	3	4
Residential treatment centers for emotionally disturbed children	1	2	2	4	8	9	13	13	16
All other organizations[2]	6	10	14	18	26	38	61	44	42

[1]Includes Department of Veterans Affairs neuropsychiatric hospitals, general hospital psychiatric services, and psychiatric outpatient clinics.
[2]Includes freestanding psychiatric outpatient clinics, partial care organizations, multiservice mental health organizations, residential treatment centers for adults, substance abuse organizations, and, in 1975 and 1979, federally-funded community mental health centers.
[3]Civilian population as of January 1 each year through 1998. The rates for 2000 and later years are based on the July 1 civilian population estimates from the Census Bureau.

NOTES: Changes in reporting procedures and definitions may affect the comparability of data prior to 1980 with those of later years. Starting with 1994 data, information on supportive residential clients (moderately staffed housing arrangements, such as supervised apartments, group homes, and halfway houses) is included in the totals and All Other Organizations category. This change affects the comparability of trend data prior to 1994 with data for 1994 and later years. See Appendix II, Mental health organization. Mental health expenditures include salaries, other operating expenditures, and capital expenditures. Excludes expenditures for mental health care provided in nonpsychiatric units of hospitals such as general medical units. This table includes expenditures for treatment provided by mental health organizations and differs from the estimates shown in Table 126, which are expenditures for mental health treatment provided in all settings. Data for additional years are available.. See Appendix III.

SOURCES: Substance Abuse and Mental Health Services Administration, Center for Mental Health Services. Manderscheid RW, Berry JT, editors. *Mental health, United States, 2004.* DHHS Pub. No. (SMA)-06-4195. Washington, DC. U.S. Government Printing Office, 2006.

Table 136 (page 1 of 2). Private health insurance coverage among persons under 65 years of age, by selected characteristics: United States, selected years 1984–2005

[Data are based on household interviews of a sample of the civilian noninstitutionalized population]

	Private health insurance[1]									
Characteristic	*1984*	*1989*	*1995*	*1997*[2]	*2000*	*2001*	*2002*	*2003*	*2004*	*2005*
	Number in millions									
Total[3]	157.5	162.7	164.2	165.8	174.0	175.3	172.4	173.6	174.5	174.7
	Percent of population									
Total[3]	76.8	75.9	71.3	70.7	71.5	71.2	69.4	68.9	68.8	68.2
Age										
Under 18 years	72.6	71.8	65.2	66.1	66.6	66.3	63.5	63.0	63.2	62.1
Under 6 years	68.1	67.9	59.5	61.3	62.7	62.9	60.2	58.2	58.1	56.6
6–17 years	74.9	74.0	68.3	68.5	68.5	67.9	65.1	65.3	65.6	64.7
18–44 years	76.5	75.5	70.9	69.4	70.5	70.1	68.7	67.7	67.3	66.6
18–24 years	67.4	64.5	60.8	59.3	60.3	60.3	60.2	58.8	58.2	58.0
25–34 years	77.4	75.9	70.1	68.1	70.1	70.0	68.0	65.6	65.5	65.1
35–44 years	83.9	82.7	77.7	76.4	77.0	76.2	74.6	75.1	74.8	73.7
45–64 years	83.3	82.5	80.1	79.0	78.7	78.6	77.3	77.3	77.1	76.9
45–54 years	83.3	83.4	80.9	80.4	80.0	79.4	77.5	77.9	77.8	77.4
55–64 years	83.3	81.6	79.0	76.9	76.7	77.4	76.9	76.5	76.1	76.2
Sex										
Male	77.3	76.1	71.6	70.9	71.6	71.2	69.0	69.0	68.7	68.0
Female	76.2	75.7	70.9	70.5	71.3	71.2	69.8	68.9	68.9	68.4
Race[4]										
White only	79.9	79.1	74.5	74.2	75.7	75.1	73.4	71.5	71.4	70.9
Black or African American only	58.1	57.7	53.0	54.7	55.9	56.5	55.1	54.9	53.9	52.9
American Indian or Alaska Native only	49.1	45.5	45.3	39.4	43.7	49.0	37.9	45.0	44.7	43.0
Asian only	69.9	71.9	68.4	68.0	72.1	72.3	70.9	71.4	71.6	72.2
Native Hawaiian or Other Pacific Islander only	- - -	- - -	- - -	- - -	*	*	*	*	*	*
2 or more races	- - -	- - -	- - -	- - -	61.4	61.5	57.1	56.3	62.0	57.6
Hispanic origin and race[4]										
Hispanic or Latino	55.7	51.5	46.4	46.4	47.8	46.1	44.4	41.9	41.7	42.4
Mexican	53.3	46.8	42.6	42.3	45.4	43.1	42.1	39.3	39.1	39.7
Puerto Rican	48.4	45.6	47.6	47.0	51.1	50.5	50.0	48.6	47.3	48.5
Cuban	72.5	70.3	63.6	71.0	63.9	66.1	62.0	55.9	57.9	58.1
Other Hispanic or Latino	61.6	61.0	51.4	49.9	50.7	49.9	46.2	45.3	45.1	45.6
Not Hispanic or Latino	78.7	78.4	74.4	74.0	75.2	75.3	73.7	73.7	73.7	73.0
White only	82.3	82.4	78.6	78.1	79.5	79.4	77.9	77.8	77.9	77.3
Black or African American only	58.3	57.8	53.4	54.9	56.0	56.7	55.2	55.5	54.6	53.1
Age and percent of poverty level[5]										
All ages:										
Below 100%	32.2	27.0	22.6	23.3	25.2	25.3	25.2	23.9	21.8	21.4
100%–less than 150%	62.2	55.1	47.8	43.6	41.7	41.7	38.4	37.5	39.0	38.1
150%–less than 200%	77.2	71.0	65.1	62.9	58.5	56.7	56.2	52.2	52.5	51.3
200% or more	91.5	90.8	88.3	86.4	85.7	85.5	83.9	84.6	84.2	83.7
Under 18 years:										
Below 100%	28.5	22.3	16.9	18.3	19.5	18.2	16.9	15.9	14.2	14.2
100%–less than 150%	66.2	59.6	48.5	43.5	39.8	40.7	35.2	33.9	35.9	35.0
150%–less than 200%	80.9	75.9	67.4	65.7	59.7	56.3	55.3	50.9	51.7	48.4
200% or more	92.3	92.5	89.5	87.8	86.7	86.8	84.5	85.1	85.2	84.2
Geographic region										
Northeast	80.5	82.0	75.4	74.2	76.3	76.4	73.9	74.7	74.0	74.0
Midwest	80.6	81.5	77.3	77.1	78.8	78.1	76.4	75.9	76.3	74.6
South	74.3	71.4	66.9	67.3	66.8	66.0	64.6	64.0	64.1	62.5
West	71.9	71.2	67.5	65.4	66.5	67.9	66.1	64.7	64.1	65.6
Location of residence										
Within MSA[6]	77.5	76.5	72.1	71.2	72.3	72.2	70.7	70.2	69.6	69.0
Outside MSA[6]	75.2	73.8	67.9	68.4	67.8	67.0	64.2	63.7	65.5	64.6

See footnotes at end of table.

Table 136 (page 2 of 2). Private health insurance coverage among persons under 65 years of age, by selected characteristics: United States, selected years 1984–2005

[Data are based on household interviews of a sample of the civilian noninstitutionalized population]

* Estimates are considered unreliable. Data not shown have a relative standard error of greater than 30%.
- - - Data not available.
[1]Includes all private health insurance coverage (both individual and insurance obtained through the workplace).
[2]Starting with 1997 data, the National Health Interview Survey (NHIS) was redesigned, and changes to the questions on health insurance coverage were made. See Appendix I, National Health Interview Survey and Appendix II, Health insurance coverage.
[3]Includes all other races not shown separately and, in 1984 and 1989, with unknown poverty level.
[4]The race groups, white, black, American Indian or Alaska Native, Asian, Native Hawaiian or Other Pacific Islander, and 2 or more races, include persons of Hispanic and non-Hispanic origin. Persons of Hispanic origin may be of any race. Starting with 1999 data, race-specific estimates are tabulated according to the 1997 Revisions to the Standards for the Classification of Federal Data on Race and Ethnicity and are not strictly comparable with estimates for earlier years. The five single-race categories plus multiple-race categories shown in the table conform to the 1997 Standards. Starting with 1999 data, race-specific estimates are for persons who reported only one racial group; the category 2 or more races includes persons who reported more than one racial group. Prior to 1999, data were tabulated according to the 1977 Standards with four racial groups and the Asian only category including Native Hawaiian or Other Pacific Islander. Estimates for single-race categories prior to 1999 included persons who reported one race or, if they reported more than one race, identified one race as best representing their race. Starting with 2003 data, race responses of other race and unspecified multiple race were treated as missing, and then race was imputed if these were the only race responses. Almost all persons with a race response of other race were of Hispanic origin. See Appendix II, Hispanic origin; Race.
[5]Percent of poverty level is based on family income and family size and composition using U.S. Census Bureau poverty thresholds. Poverty level was unknown for 10%–11% of persons under 65 years of age in 1984 and 1989. Missing family income data were imputed for 15%–16% of persons under 65 years of age in 1994–1996, 24% in 1997, and 28%–33% in 1998–2005. See Appendix II, Family income; Poverty.
[6]MSA is metropolitan statistical area.

NOTES: Standard errors are available in the spreadsheet version of this table. Available from: www.cdc.gov/nchs/hus.htm. Data for additional years are available. See Appendix III.

SOURCES: Centers for Disease Control and Prevention, National Center for Health Statistics, National Health Interview Survey, health insurance supplements (1984, 1989, 1994–1996). Starting with 1997 data, data are from the family core questionnaire.

Table 137 (page 1 of 2). Private health insurance coverage obtained through the workplace among persons under 65 years of age, by selected characteristics: United States, selected years 1984–2005

[Data are based on household interviews of a sample of the civilian noninstitutionalized population]

Characteristic	Private insurance obtained through workplace[1]									
	1984	1989	1995	1997[2]	2000	2001	2002	2003	2004	2005
	Number in millions									
Total[3]	141.8	146.3	150.7	155.6	162.5	164.2	161.3	159.3	161.0	161.7
	Percent of population									
Total[3]	69.1	68.3	65.4	66.3	66.7	66.7	65.0	63.3	63.5	63.1
Age										
Under 18 years	66.5	65.8	60.4	62.7	62.7	62.8	60.1	58.6	59.2	58.2
Under 6 years	62.1	62.3	55.1	58.2	58.8	59.1	57.0	53.9	54.4	53.2
6–17 years	68.7	67.7	63.3	64.9	64.6	64.5	61.7	60.9	61.5	60.7
18–44 years	69.6	68.4	65.3	65.5	66.1	65.9	64.3	62.2	62.1	61.7
18–24 years	58.7	55.3	53.5	54.7	54.9	55.3	54.3	52.3	51.6	51.6
25–34 years	71.2	69.5	65.0	64.5	66.1	66.0	63.9	60.3	60.6	60.6
35–44 years	77.4	76.2	72.7	72.6	72.8	72.1	70.8	70.0	70.2	69.3
45–64 years	71.8	71.6	72.2	72.6	72.5	72.5	71.4	70.0	70.2	70.3
45–54 years	74.6	74.4	74.7	75.4	75.3	74.5	72.9	71.5	72.0	72.1
55–64 years	69.0	68.3	68.4	68.3	68.1	69.5	69.1	68.0	67.6	67.9
Sex										
Male	69.8	68.7	65.9	66.6	67.0	66.7	64.7	63.3	63.6	63.1
Female	68.4	67.9	64.9	66.0	66.5	66.6	65.2	63.3	63.4	63.1
Race[4]										
White only	72.0	71.2	68.4	69.6	70.6	70.2	68.7	65.6	65.8	65.6
Black or African American only	52.4	52.8	49.3	52.5	53.1	54.2	52.4	51.5	51.0	50.2
American Indian or Alaska Native only	45.8	40.9	40.2	37.1	41.6	47.0	35.8	40.5	41.9	39.8
Asian only	59.0	61.1	59.6	61.4	65.1	65.9	62.5	62.1	64.9	63.6
Native Hawaiian or Other Pacific Islander only	- - -	- - -	- - -	- - -	*	*	*	*	*	*
2 or more races	- - -	- - -	- - -	- - -	59.7	57.9	54.5	53.1	57.9	54.6
Hispanic origin and race[4]										
Hispanic or Latino	52.0	47.3	43.4	43.9	45.0	43.8	41.9	38.9	39.0	39.9
Mexican	50.5	44.2	40.9	40.7	43.2	41.2	40.1	36.7	37.0	37.4
Puerto Rican	45.9	42.3	44.5	45.1	49.3	47.5	48.0	45.0	43.9	46.0
Cuban	57.4	56.5	54.0	58.1	53.4	56.6	52.1	51.1	50.7	53.2
Other Hispanic or Latino	57.4	54.7	46.7	46.9	47.0	47.6	43.1	41.6	41.3	42.6
Not Hispanic or Latino	70.6	70.4	68.2	69.4	70.2	70.5	68.8	67.6	67.9	67.4
White only	74.0	74.0	72.1	73.1	74.1	74.1	72.8	71.3	71.6	71.3
Black or African American only	52.6	53.0	49.8	52.8	53.3	54.4	52.6	52.0	51.7	50.4
Age and percent of poverty level[5]										
All ages:										
Below 100%	24.1	19.9	17.5	19.9	20.9	21.8	21.4	19.9	18.1	17.7
100%–less than 150%	52.4	46.4	42.1	38.8	37.1	37.0	34.3	31.8	34.6	33.5
150%–less than 200%	69.5	63.1	58.8	58.3	53.4	51.9	50.9	46.8	47.3	46.1
200% or more	85.0	83.7	82.3	81.9	81.0	80.9	79.3	78.6	78.5	78.3
Under 18 years:										
Below 100%	23.0	17.5	13.6	16.2	16.5	16.2	14.8	14.0	12.8	12.5
100%–less than 150%	58.3	52.5	43.6	39.6	36.3	37.0	32.5	30.1	33.5	31.7
150%–less than 200%	75.8	70.1	61.8	62.5	55.6	52.9	50.8	47.0	47.9	44.8
200% or more	86.9	86.6	84.4	83.9	82.5	82.9	80.8	79.9	80.1	79.5
Geographic region										
Northeast	74.0	75.0	69.8	70.9	72.1	72.9	70.5	69.4	69.6	70.2
Midwest	72.0	73.3	71.2	72.4	74.5	73.7	72.2	70.4	71.5	69.6
South	66.2	63.6	61.8	62.8	62.2	61.6	60.3	58.8	59.1	57.5
West	64.7	63.9	60.4	60.6	60.6	62.1	59.9	57.5	57.0	59.2
Location of residence										
Within MSA[6]	70.9	69.6	66.6	67.2	67.8	67.9	66.3	64.6	64.4	64.1
Outside MSA[6]	65.3	63.5	60.7	62.7	62.4	61.7	59.2	58.0	59.6	59.0

See footnotes at end of table.

Table 137 (page 2 of 2). Private health insurance coverage obtained through the workplace among persons under 65 years of age, by selected characteristics: United States, selected years 1984–2005

[Data are based on household interviews of a sample of the civilian noninstitutionalized population]

* Estimates are considered unreliable. Data not shown have a relative standard error of greater than 30%.
- - - Data not available.
[1]Private insurance originally obtained through a present or former employer or union. Starting with 1997 data, also includes private insurance obtained through workplace, self-employment, or professional association.
[2]Starting with 1997 data, the National Health Interview Survey (NHIS) was redesigned, and changes to the questions on health insurance coverage were made. See Appendix I, National Health Interview Survey and Appendix II, Health insurance coverage.
[3]Includes all other races not shown separately and, in 1984 and 1989, with unknown poverty level.
[4]The race groups, white, black, American Indian or Alaska Native, Asian, Native Hawaiian or Other Pacific Islander, and 2 or more races, include persons of Hispanic and non-Hispanic origin. Persons of Hispanic origin may be of any race. Starting with 1999 data, race-specific estimates are tabulated according to the 1997 Revisions to the Standards for the Classification of Federal Data on Race and Ethnicity and are not strictly comparable with estimates for earlier years. The five single-race categories plus multiple-race categories shown in the table conform to the 1997 Standards. Starting with 1999 data, race-specific estimates are for persons who reported only one racial group; the category 2 or more races includes persons who reported more than one racial group. Prior to 1999, data were tabulated according to the 1977 Standards with four racial groups and the Asian only category included Native Hawaiian or Other Pacific Islander. Estimates for single-race categories prior to 1999 included persons who reported one race or, if they reported more than one race, identified one race as best representing their race. Starting with 2003 data, race responses of other race and unspecified multiple race were treated as missing, and then race was imputed if these were the only race responses. Almost all persons with a race response of other race were of Hispanic origin. See Appendix II, Hispanic origin; Race.
[5]Percent of poverty level is based on family income and family size and composition using U.S. Census Bureau poverty thresholds. Poverty level was unknown for 10%–11% of persons under 65 years of age in 1984 and 1989. Missing family income data were imputed for 15%–16% of persons under 65 years of age in 1994–1996, 24% in 1997, and 28%–33% in 1998–2005. See Appendix II, Family income; Poverty.
[6]MSA is metropolitan statistical area.

NOTES: Standard errors are available in the spreadsheet version of this table. Available from: www.cdc.gov/nchs/hus.htm. Data for additional years are available. See Appendix III.

SOURCES: Centers for Disease Control and Prevention, National Center for Health Statistics, National Health Interview Survey, health insurance supplements (1984, 1989, 1994–1996). Starting with 1997 data, data are from the family core questionnaire.

Table 138 (page 1 of 2). Medicaid coverage among persons under 65 years of age, by selected characteristics: United States, selected years 1984–2005

[Data are based on household interviews of a sample of the civilian noninstitutionalized population]

Characteristic	1984	1989	1995	1997[1]	2000	2002	2003	2004(1)[2]	2004(2)[2]	2005[2]
	Number in millions									
Total[3]	14.0	15.4	26.6	22.9	23.2	29.4	30.9	31.1	31.6	33.2
	Percent of population									
Total[3]	6.8	7.2	11.5	9.7	9.5	11.8	12.3	12.3	12.5	12.9
Age										
Under 18 years	11.9	12.6	21.5	18.4	19.6	24.8	26.0	25.9	26.4	27.2
Under 6 years	15.5	15.7	29.3	24.7	24.7	30.0	32.3	31.8	32.4	34.0
6–17 years	10.1	10.9	17.4	15.2	17.2	22.3	23.0	23.1	23.4	23.9
18–44 years	5.1	5.2	7.8	6.6	5.6	7.1	7.4	7.5	7.7	8.3
18–24 years	6.4	6.8	10.4	8.8	8.1	9.9	9.6	10.3	10.4	11.3
25–34 years	5.3	5.2	8.2	6.8	5.5	6.6	7.8	7.6	7.8	8.0
35–44 years	3.5	4.0	5.9	5.2	4.3	5.9	5.6	5.7	5.8	6.6
45–64 years	3.4	4.3	5.6	4.6	4.5	5.3	5.3	5.4	5.5	5.5
45–54 years	3.2	3.8	5.1	4.0	4.2	5.1	5.0	5.4	5.5	5.2
55–64 years	3.6	4.9	6.4	5.6	4.9	5.8	5.8	5.4	5.5	5.8
Sex										
Male	5.4	5.7	9.6	8.4	8.2	10.6	10.9	10.8	11.0	11.6
Female	8.1	8.6	13.4	11.1	10.8	13.0	13.6	13.7	13.9	14.3
Race[4]										
White only	4.6	5.1	8.9	7.4	7.1	9.3	10.4	10.2	10.4	11.0
Black or African American only	20.5	19.0	28.5	22.4	21.2	23.2	23.7	24.5	24.9	24.9
American Indian or Alaska Native only	*28.2	29.7	19.0	19.6	15.1	21.1	18.5	18.0	18.4	24.2
Asian only	*8.7	*8.8	10.5	9.6	7.5	9.8	8.0	9.6	9.8	8.2
Native Hawaiian or Other Pacific Islander only	---	---	---	---	*	*	*	*	*	*
2 or more races	---	---	---	---	19.1	21.6	23.5	19.0	19.3	22.0
Hispanic origin and race[4]										
Hispanic or Latino	13.3	13.5	21.9	17.6	15.5	20.8	21.8	21.9	22.5	22.9
Mexican	12.2	12.4	21.6	17.2	14.0	20.2	21.7	21.9	22.4	23.0
Puerto Rican	31.5	27.3	33.4	31.0	29.4	29.0	31.0	28.5	29.1	31.9
Cuban	*4.8	*7.7	13.4	7.3	9.2	14.9	13.8	17.9	17.9	17.7
Other Hispanic or Latino	7.9	11.1	18.2	15.3	14.5	19.6	19.3	19.9	20.8	19.7
Not Hispanic or Latino	6.2	6.6	10.2	8.7	8.5	10.3	10.6	10.5	10.7	11.1
White only	3.7	4.2	7.1	6.1	6.1	7.7	8.0	7.8	7.9	8.5
Black or African American only	20.7	19.0	28.1	22.1	21.0	23.2	23.4	24.1	24.6	24.8
Age and percent of poverty level[5]										
All ages:										
Below 100%	33.0	37.6	48.4	40.5	38.4	42.8	43.2	44.2	45.0	45.7
100%–less than 150%	7.7	10.9	19.1	17.9	20.7	27.6	26.9	26.5	27.1	28.7
150%–less than 200%	3.2	5.1	8.3	8.3	11.5	16.1	17.1	16.6	16.9	18.1
200% or more	0.6	1.1	1.7	1.8	2.3	3.1	3.3	3.5	3.5	3.7
Under 18 years:										
Below 100%	43.2	47.9	66.0	58.0	58.5	66.4	67.5	69.2	70.7	71.2
100%–less than 150%	9.0	12.3	27.2	28.7	35.0	47.1	49.1	46.6	47.6	49.0
150%–less than 200%	4.4	6.1	13.1	13.0	21.3	29.1	33.6	31.9	32.4	35.3
200% or more	0.8	1.8	3.3	3.1	5.1	7.2	7.6	8.0	8.0	8.3

See footnotes at end of table.

Table 138 (page 2 of 2). Medicaid coverage among persons under 65 years of age, by selected characteristics: United States, selected years 1984–2005

[Data are based on household interviews of a sample of the civilian noninstitutionalized population]

Characteristic	*1984*	*1989*	*1995*	*1997*[1]	*2000*	*2002*	*2003*	*2004(1)*[2]	*2004(2)*[2]	*2005*[2]
Geographic region					Percent of population					
Northeast	8.6	6.6	11.7	11.3	10.6	12.5	12.9	12.8	13.0	13.3
Midwest	7.4	7.6	10.5	8.4	8.0	10.3	10.8	10.2	10.4	12.3
South	5.1	6.5	11.3	8.7	9.4	12.0	12.6	12.2	12.4	12.7
West	7.0	8.5	12.9	11.7	10.4	12.7	12.8	14.2	14.4	13.8
Location of residence										
Within MSA[6]	7.1	7.0	11.3	9.7	8.9	11.0	11.5	11.7	11.9	12.4
Outside MSA[6]	6.1	7.9	12.3	10.1	11.9	15.2	15.3	14.8	15.0	15.5

* Estimates are considered unreliable. Data preceded by an asterisk have a relative standard error (RSE) of 20%–30%. Data not shown have an RSE of greater than 30%.

- - - Data not available.

[1]Starting with 1997 data, the National Health Interview Survey (NHIS) was redesigned, and changes to the questions on health insurance coverage were made. See Appendix I, National Health Interview Survey and Appendix II, Health insurance coverage.

[2]Beginning in quarter 3 of the 2004 NHIS, persons under 65 years with no reported coverage were asked explicitly about Medicaid coverage. Estimates were calculated without and with the additional information from this question in the columns labeled 2004(1) and 2004(2), respectively, and estimates were calculated with the additional information in 2005.

[3]Includes all other races not shown separately and, in 1984 and 1989, with unknown poverty level.

[4]The race groups, white, black, American Indian or Alaska Native, Asian, Native Hawaiian or Other Pacific Islander, and 2 or more races, include persons of Hispanic and non-Hispanic origin. Persons of Hispanic origin may be of any race. Starting with 1999 data, race-specific estimates are tabulated according to the 1997 Revisions to the Standards for the Classification of Federal Data on Race and Ethnicity and are not strictly comparable with estimates for earlier years. The five single-race categories plus multiple-race categories shown in the table conform to the 1997 Standards. Starting with 1999 data, race-specific estimates are for persons who reported only one racial group; the category 2 or more races includes persons who reported more than one racial group. Prior to 1999, data were tabulated according to the 1977 Standards with four racial groups and the Asian only category included Native Hawaiian or Other Pacific Islander. Estimates for single-race categories prior to 1999 included persons who reported one race or, if they reported more than one race, identified one race as best representing their race. Starting with 2003 data, race responses of other race and unspecified multiple race were treated as missing, and then race was imputed if these were the only race responses. Almost all persons with a race response of other race were of Hispanic origin. See Appendix II, Hispanic origin; Race.

[5]Percent of poverty level is based on family income and family size and composition using U.S. Census Bureau poverty thresholds. Poverty level was unknown for 10%–11% of persons under 65 years of age in 1984 and 1989. Missing family income data were imputed for 15%–16% of persons under 65 years of age in 1994–1996, 24% in 1997, and 28%–33% in 1998–2005. See Appendix II, Family income; Poverty.

[6]MSA is metropolitan statistical area.

NOTES: Medicaid includes other public assistance through 1996. Starting with 1997 data, state-sponsored health plan coverage is included as Medicaid coverage. Starting with 1999 data, coverage by the State Children's Health Insurance Program (SCHIP) is included as Medicaid coverage. In 2005, 10.2% of persons under 65 years of age were covered by Medicaid, 1.3% by state-sponsored health plans, and 1.5% by SCHIP. Standard errors are available in the spreadsheet version of this table. Available from: www.cdc.gov/nchs/hus.htm. Data for additional years are available. See Appendix III.

SOURCES: Centers for Disease Control and Prevention, National Center for Health Statistics, National Health Interview Survey, health insurance supplements (1984, 1989, 1994–1996). Starting with 1997 data, data are from the family core questionnaire.

Table 139 (page 1 of 2). No health insurance coverage among persons under 65 years of age, by selected characteristics: United States, selected years 1984–2005

[Data are based on household interviews of a sample of the civilian noninstitutionalized population]

Characteristic	*1984*	*1989*	*1995*	*1997*[1]	*2000*	*2002*	*2003*	*2004(1)*[2]	*2004(2)*[2]	*2005*[2]
					Number in millions					
Total[3]	29.8	33.4	37.1	41.0	41.4	41.7	41.6	42.1	41.6	42.1
					Percent of population					
Total[3]	14.5	15.6	16.1	17.5	17.0	16.8	16.5	16.6	16.4	16.4
Age										
Under 18 years	13.9	14.7	13.4	14.0	12.6	10.9	9.8	9.7	9.2	9.3
Under 6 years	14.9	15.1	11.8	12.5	11.8	9.2	8.2	8.9	8.2	7.7
6–17 years	13.4	14.5	14.3	14.7	13.0	11.7	10.6	10.0	9.7	10.1
18–44 years	17.1	18.4	20.4	22.4	22.4	23.0	23.5	23.6	23.5	23.5
18–24 years	25.0	27.1	28.0	30.1	30.4	28.8	30.1	30.1	30.0	29.1
25–34 years	16.2	18.3	21.1	23.8	23.3	24.6	25.4	25.7	25.5	25.6
35–44 years	11.2	12.3	15.1	16.7	16.9	18.0	17.5	17.6	17.5	17.9
45–64 years	9.6	10.5	10.9	12.4	12.6	13.1	12.5	12.9	12.8	12.9
45–54 years	10.5	11.0	11.6	12.8	12.8	14.1	13.6	13.7	13.6	14.2
55–64 years	8.7	10.0	9.9	11.8	12.4	11.5	10.9	11.7	11.6	11.1
Sex										
Male	15.3	16.8	17.4	18.7	18.1	18.4	17.7	18.1	17.9	17.9
Female	13.8	14.4	14.8	16.3	15.9	15.2	15.3	15.2	14.9	15.0
Race[4]										
White only	13.6	14.5	15.5	16.4	15.4	15.5	16.0	16.3	16.1	15.9
Black or African American only	19.9	21.6	18.0	20.1	19.5	18.8	18.4	18.1	17.6	18.4
American Indian or Alaska Native only	22.5	28.4	34.3	38.1	38.4	39.1	35.0	35.0	34.6	32.2
Asian only	18.5	16.9	18.6	19.5	17.6	17.4	18.2	16.7	16.5	17.1
Native Hawaiian or Other Pacific Islander only	---	---	---	---	*	*	*	*	*	*
2 or more races	---	---	---	---	16.8	17.6	15.9	12.6	12.3	16.5
Hispanic origin and race[4]										
Hispanic or Latino	29.5	33.7	31.4	34.5	35.6	33.9	34.7	35.1	34.4	33.0
Mexican	33.8	39.9	35.6	39.4	39.9	37.1	37.8	38.1	37.6	36.0
Puerto Rican	18.3	24.7	17.6	19.0	16.4	19.2	17.7	21.0	20.4	16.3
Cuban	21.6	20.6	22.3	21.1	25.4	20.8	29.1	22.8	22.8	23.2
Other Hispanic or Latino	27.4	25.8	30.2	33.0	33.4	33.2	33.4	33.3	32.3	32.6
Not Hispanic or Latino	13.2	13.7	14.2	15.2	14.0	13.9	13.3	13.3	13.2	13.4
White only	12.0	12.2	13.0	13.8	12.5	12.5	11.9	12.1	12.0	12.0
Black or African American only	19.6	21.4	17.9	20.0	19.5	18.7	18.1	17.8	17.3	18.3
Age and percent of poverty level[5]										
All ages:										
Below 100%	33.9	35.0	29.6	33.7	34.2	30.3	31.1	31.8	31.0	30.6
100%–less than 150%	27.2	31.1	31.6	35.1	34.9	32.2	31.9	31.3	30.8	29.9
150%–less than 200%	17.3	21.7	24.0	26.3	27.0	25.2	27.6	27.4	27.2	27.3
200% or more	6.0	7.1	8.7	10.1	10.1	11.1	10.0	10.2	10.2	10.4
Under 18 years:										
Below 100%	29.0	31.4	20.0	23.2	22.0	17.0	16.8	16.5	15.0	14.3
100%–less than 150%	22.8	26.1	24.8	26.5	25.4	19.4	16.2	17.0	16.0	15.1
150%–less than 200%	12.7	15.8	18.0	19.9	17.7	14.3	14.9	14.5	14.1	15.0
200% or more	4.2	4.5	6.4	7.1	6.5	6.7	5.5	5.3	5.2	5.6

See footnotes at end of table.

Table 139 (page 2 of 2). No health insurance coverage among persons under 65 years of age, by selected characteristics: United States, selected years 1984–2005

[Data are based on household interviews of a sample of the civilian noninstitutionalized population]

Characteristic	*1984*	*1989*	*1995*	*1997*[1]	*2000*	*2002*	*2003*	*2004(1)*[2]	*2004(2)*[2]	*2005*[2]
Geographic region					Percent of population					
Northeast	10.2	10.9	13.3	13.5	12.2	12.8	11.3	11.9	11.8	11.3
Midwest	11.3	10.7	12.2	13.2	12.3	12.5	12.4	12.6	12.4	11.9
South	17.7	19.7	19.4	20.9	20.5	20.3	19.8	20.2	19.9	21.0
West	18.2	18.8	17.9	20.6	20.7	19.1	19.9	19.1	18.9	18.4
Location of residence										
Within MSA[6]	13.6	15.2	15.5	16.9	16.6	16.3	16.0	16.4	16.2	16.1
Outside MSA[6]	16.6	17.0	18.6	19.8	18.6	18.7	18.7	17.4	17.2	17.8

* Estimates are considered unreliable. Data not shown have a relative standard error of greater than 30%.

- - - Data not available.

[1]Starting with 1997 data, the National Health Interview Survey (NHIS) was redesigned, and changes to the questions on health insurance coverage were made. See Appendix I, National Health Interview Survey and Appendix II, Health insurance coverage.

[2]Beginning in quarter 3 of the 2004 NHIS, persons under 65 years with no reported coverage were asked explicitly about Medicaid coverage. Estimates were calculated without and with the additional information from this question in the columns labeled 2004(1) and 2004(2), respectively, and estimates were calculated with the additional information in 2005.

[3]Includes all other races not shown separately and, in 1984 and 1989, persons with unknown poverty level.

[4]The race groups, white, black, American Indian or Alaska Native, Asian, Native Hawaiian or Other Pacific Islander, and 2 or more races, include persons of Hispanic and non-Hispanic origin. Persons of Hispanic origin may be of any race. Starting with 1999 data, race-specific estimates are tabulated according to the 1997 Revisions to the Standards for the Classification of Federal Data on Race and Ethnicity and are not strictly comparable with estimates for earlier years. The five single-race categories plus multiple-race categories shown in the table conform to the 1997 Standards. Starting with 1999 data, race-specific estimates are for persons who reported only one racial group; the category 2 or more races includes persons who reported more than one racial group. Prior to 1999, data were tabulated according to the 1977 Standards with four racial groups and the Asian only category included Native Hawaiian or Other Pacific Islander. Estimates for single-race categories prior to 1999 included persons who reported one race or, if they reported more than one race, identified one race as best representing their race. Starting with 2003 data, race responses of other race and unspecified multiple race were treated as missing, and then race was imputed if these were the only race responses. Almost all persons with a race response of other race were of Hispanic origin. See Appendix II, Hispanic origin; Race.

[5]Percent of poverty level is based on family income and family size and composition using U.S. Census Bureau poverty thresholds. Poverty level was unknown for 10%–11% of persons under 65 years of age in 1984 and 1989. Missing family income data were imputed for 15%–16% of persons under 65 years of age in 1994–1996, 24% in 1997, and 28%–33% in 1998–2005. See Appendix II, Family income; Poverty.

[6]MSA is metropolitan statistical area.

NOTES: Persons not covered by private insurance, Medicaid, State Children's Health Insurance Program (SCHIP), public assistance (through 1996), state-sponsored or other government-sponsored health plans (starting in 1997), Medicare, or military plans are considered to have no health insurance coverage. Persons with only Indian Health Service coverage are considered to have no health insurance coverage. See Appendix II, Health insurance coverage. Standard errors are available in the spreadsheet version of this table. Available from: www.cdc.gov/nchs/hus.htm. Data for additional years are available. See Appendix III.

SOURCES: Centers for Disease Control and Prevention, National Center for Health Statistics, National Health Interview Survey, health insurance supplements (1984, 1989, 1994–1996). Starting with 1997 data, data are from the family core questionnaire.

Table 140 (page 1 of 2). Health insurance coverage for persons 65 years of age and over, by type of coverage and selected characteristics: United States, selected years 1992–2005

[Data are based on household interviews of a sample of the civilian noninstitutionalized population]

Characteristic	*Medicare risk Health Maintenance Organization*[1]					*Medicaid*[2]				
	1992	*1995*	*2000*	*2004*	*2005*	*1992*	*1995*	*2000*	*2004*	*2005*
Age	Number in millions									
65 years and over	1.1	2.6	5.9	4.5	4.6	2.7	2.8	2.7	3.2	3.2
	Percent of population									
65 years and over	3.9	8.9	19.3	14.3	14.5	9.4	9.6	9.0	10	10.1
65–74 years	4.2	9.5	20.6	13.9	13.9	7.9	8.8	8.5	9.3	9.9
75–84 years	3.7	8.3	18.5	15.1	15.3	10.6	9.6	8.9	10.3	9.9
85 years and over	*	7.3	16.3	13.6	13.9	16.6	13.6	11.2	12.5	11.9
Sex										
Male	4.6	9.2	19.3	12.9	13.5	6.3	6.2	6.3	6.8	7.2
Female	3.4	8.6	19.3	15.4	15.2	11.6	12.0	10.9	12.5	12.3
Race and Hispanic origin										
White, not Hispanic or Latino	3.6	8.4	18.4	13.0	13.2	5.6	5.4	5.1	6.0	6.1
Black, not Hispanic or Latino	*	7.9	20.7	15.9	17.1	28.5	30.3	23.6	24.7	23.6
Hispanic	*	15.5	27.5	28.0	27.2	39.0	40.5	28.7	27.2	29.2
Percent of poverty level[3]										
Below 100%	3.6	7.7	18.4	13.2	---	22.3	17.2	15.9	17.0	---
100%-less than 200%	3.7	9.5	23.4	17.7	---	6.7	6.3	8.4	11.0	---
200% or more	4.2	10.1	18.0	13.9	---	*	*	*	*	---
Marital status										
Married	4.6	9.5	18.7	13.9	13.8	4.0	4.3	4.3	4.8	5.4
Widowed	2.3	7.7	19.4	14.6	15.0	14.9	15.0	13.6	15.0	14.9
Divorced	*	9.7	24.4	16.4	17.1	23.4	24.5	20.2	21.9	20.0
Never married	*	*	15.8	*	13.9	19.2	19.0	17.0	20.7	21.3

Characteristic	*Employer-sponsored plan*[4]					*Medigap*[5]				
	1992	*1995*	*2000*	*2004*	*2005*	*1992*	*1995*	*2000*	*2004*	*2005*
Age	Number in millions									
65 years and over	12.5	11.3	10.7	11.5	11.6	9.9	9.5	7.6	7.8	8.2
	Percent of population									
65 years and over	42.8	38.6	35.2	36.6	36.4	33.9	32.5	25.0	24.8	25.7
65–74 years	46.9	41.1	36.6	38.4	38.1	31.4	29.9	21.7	22.1	23.2
75–84 years	38.2	37.1	35.0	36.1	35.5	37.5	35.2	27.8	26.5	27.3
85 years and over	31.6	30.2	29.4	31.0	31.8	38.3	37.6	31.1	30.4	30.8
Sex										
Male	46.3	42.1	37.7	39.4	39.4	30.6	30.0	23.4	23.4	23.8
Female	40.4	36.0	33.4	34.5	34.2	36.2	34.4	26.2	25.8	27.1
Race and Hispanic origin										
White, not Hispanic or Latino	45.9	41.3	38.6	39.6	39.5	37.2	36.2	28.3	28.2	29.1
Black, not Hispanic or Latino	25.9	26.7	22.0	28.0	27.9	13.6	10.2	7.5	8.5	9.5
Hispanic	20.7	16.9	15.8	19.5	18.6	15.8	10.1	11.3	9.2	11.1
Percent of poverty level[3]										
Below 100%	29.0	32.1	28.1	31.5	---	30.8	29.8	22.6	21.4	---
100%-less than 200%	37.5	32.0	27.0	27.0	---	39.3	39.1	28.4	28.6	---
200% or more	58.4	52.8	49.0	49.0	---	32.8	32.2	26.2	27.1	---
Marital status										
Married	49.9	44.6	41.0	42.1	41.7	33.0	32.6	25.6	26.0	27.0
Widowed	34.1	30.3	28.7	30.6	30.4	37.5	35.2	26.7	25.2	26.2
Divorced	27.3	26.6	22.4	24.6	25.1	27.9	24.1	16.9	18.4	19.8
Never married	38.0	35.1	28.5	30.9	29.1	29.1	26.2	21.9	18.6	15.4

See footnotes at end of table.

Table 140 (page 2 of 2). Health insurance coverage for persons 65 years of age and over, by type of coverage and selected characteristics: United States, selected years 1992–2005

[Data are based on household interviews of a sample of the civilian noninstitutionalized population]

Characteristic	Medicare fee-for-service only or Other[6]				
	1992	*1995*	*2000*	*2004*	*2005*
Age	Number in millions				
65 years and over	2.9	3.1	3.5	4.5	4.3
	Percent of population				
65 years and over	9.9	10.5	11.5	14.3	13.3
65–74 years	9.7	10.7	12.6	16.3	14.9
75–84 years	10.1	9.9	9.9	12.1	11.9
85 years and over	10.8	11.3	12.1	12.5	11.6
Sex					
Male	12.2	12.6	13.3	17.4	16.2
Female	8.3	8.9	10.2	11.9	11.2
Race and Hispanic origin					
White, not Hispanic or Latino	7.7	8.7	9.6	13.2	12.2
Black, not Hispanic or Latino	26.7	25.0	26.1	22.9	21.9
Hispanic	18.3	17.1	16.7	16.2	13.9
Percent of poverty level[3]					
Below 100%	14.3	13.3	15.1	17.0	---
100%-less than 200%	12.9	13.1	12.7	15.8	---
200% or more	4.0	4.5	6.3	9.8	---
Marital status					
Married	8.5	9.0	10.5	13.1	12.1
Widowed	11.2	11.9	11.6	14.6	13.5
Divorced	15.7	15.1	16.1	18.7	17.9
Never married	*	13.1	16.8	17.9	20.4

* Sample cell size is 50 or fewer.
- - - Data not available.
[1]Enrollee has Medicare risk Health Maintenance Organization (HMO) regardless of other insurance. See Appendix II, Managed care.
[2]Enrolled in Medicaid and not enrolled in a Medicare risk HMO. See Appendix II, Managed care.
[3]Percent of poverty level is based on family income and family size and composition using U.S. Census Bureau poverty thresholds. See Appendix II, Family income; Poverty.
[4]Private insurance plans purchased through employers (own, current, or former employer, family business, union, or former employer or union of spouse) and not enrolled in a Medicare risk HMO or Medicaid.
[5]Supplemental insurance purchased privately or through organizations such as AARP or professional organizations, and not enrolled in a Medicare risk HMO, Medicaid, or employer-sponsored plan.
[6]Medicare fee-for-service only or other public plans (except Medicaid).

NOTES: Insurance categories are mutually exclusive. See Appendix I, Medicare Current Beneficiary Survey (MCBS). Data for additional years are available. See Appendix III.

SOURCES: Centers for Medicare & Medicaid Services, Medicare Current Beneficiary Survey. Data compiled by the National Center for Health Statistics, Trends in Health and Aging. Available from: www.cdc.gov/nchs/agingact.htm.

Table 141 (page 1 of 2). Medicare enrollees and expenditures and percent distribution, by Medicare program and type of service: United States and other areas, selected years 1970–2006

[Data are compiled from various sources by the Centers for Medicare & Medicaid Services]

Medicare program and type of service	*1970*	*1980*	*1990*	*1995*	*2000*	*2001*	*2002*	*2003*	*2004*	*2005*	*2006*[1]
Enrollees					Number in millions						
Total Medicare[2]	20.4	28.4	34.3	37.6	39.7	40.1	40.5	41.2	41.9	42.6	43.2
Hospital insurance	20.1	28.0	33.7	37.2	39.3	39.7	40.1	40.7	41.4	42.2	42.9
Supplementary medical insurance[3]	19.5	27.3	32.6	35.6	37.3	37.7	38.0	38.6	- - -	- - -	- - -
Part B	19.5	27.3	32.6	35.6	37.3	37.7	38.0	38.6	39.1	39.7	40.3
Part D[4]	- - -	- - -	- - -	- - -	- - -	- - -	- - -	- - -	1.2	1.8	27.9
Expenditures					Amount in billions						
Total Medicare	$ 7.5	$ 36.8	$ 111.0	$184.2	$221.7	$244.8	$265.8	280.8	308.9	336.4	408.3
Total hospital insurance (HI)	5.3	25.6	67.0	117.6	131.0	143.4	152.7	154.6	170.6	182.9	191.9
HI payments to managed care organizations[5]	- - -	0.0	2.7	6.7	21.4	20.8	19.2	19.5	20.8	24.9	32.9
HI payments for fee-for-service utilization	5.1	25.0	63.4	109.5	105.1	117.0	129.3	134.5	146.5	154.7	155.7
Inpatient hospital	4.8	24.1	56.9	82.3	87.1	96.0	104.2	108.7	116.4	121.7	121.0
Skilled nursing facility	0.2	0.4	2.5	9.1	11.1	13.1	15.2	14.7	17.1	18.5	19.9
Home health agency	0.1	0.5	3.7	16.2	4.0	4.1	5.0	4.8	5.4	5.9	6.0
Hospice	- - -	- - -	0.3	1.9	2.9	3.7	4.9	6.2	7.6	8.6	8.9
Home health agency transfer[6]	- - -	- - -	- - -	- - -	1.7	3.1	1.2	–2.2	0.0	0.0	0.0
Administrative expenses[7]	0.2	0.5	0.9	1.4	2.8	2.5	3.0	2.8	3.3	3.3	3.3
Total supplementary medical insurance (SMI)[3]	2.2	11.2	44.0	66.6	90.7	101.4	113.2	126.1	138.3	153.4	216.4
Total Part B	2.2	11.2	44.0	66.6	90.7	101.4	113.2	126.1	137.9	152.4	169.0
Part B payments to managed care organizations[5]	0.0	0.2	2.8	6.6	18.4	17.6	17.5	17.3	18.7	22.1	31.5
Part B payments for fee-for-service											
Part B payments for fee-for-service utilization[8]	1.9	10.4	39.6	58.4	72.2	85.1	94.5	104.3	116.2	126.9	134.1
Physician/supplies[9]	1.8	8.2	29.6	- - -	- - -	- - -	- - -	- - -	- - -	- - -	- - -
Outpatient hospital[10]	0.1	1.9	8.5	- - -	- - -	- - -	- - -	- - -	- - -	- - -	- - -
Independent laboratory[11]	0.0	0.1	1.5	- - -	- - -	- - -	- - -	- - -	- - -	- - -	- - -
Physician fee schedule	- - -	- - -	- - -	31.7	37.0	42.0	44.8	48.3	54.1	57.7	58.4
Durable medical equipment	- - -	- - -	- - -	3.7	4.7	5.4	6.5	7.5	7.8	7.9	8.4
Laboratory[12]	- - -	- - -	- - -	4.3	4.0	4.4	5.0	5.5	6.0	6.5	7.1
Other[13]	- - -	- - -	- - -	9.9	13.6	16.0	19.6	22.6	25.0	27.5	29.3
Hospital[14]	- - -	- - -	- - -	8.7	8.4	12.8	13.6	15.3	17.4	20.2	23.8
Home health agency	0.0	0.2	0.1	0.2	4.5	4.5	5.0	5.1	5.9	7.1	7.2
Home health agency transfer[6]	- - -	- - -	- - -	- - -	–1.7	–3.1	–1.2	2.2	0.0	0.0	0.0
Administrative expenses[7]	0.2	0.6	1.5	1.6	1.8	1.8	2.3	2.4	2.8	3.2	3.1
Part D Transitional Assistance and Start-up Costs[15]	- - -	- - -	- - -	- - -	- - -	- - -	- - -	- - -	0.2	0.7	0.0
Total Part D[4]	- - -	- - -	- - -	- - -	- - -	- - -	- - -	- - -	0.4	1.0	47.4
					Percent distribution of expenditures						
Total hospital insurance (HI)	100.0	100.0	100.0	100.0	100.0	100.0	100.0	100.0	100.0	100.0	100.0
HI payments to managed care organizations[5]	- - -	0.0	4.0	5.7	16.3	14.5	12.6	12.6	12.2	13.6	17.1
HI payments for fee-for-service utilization	97.0	97.9	94.6	93.1	80.2	81.6	84.7	87.0	85.9	84.6	81.1
Inpatient hospital	91.4	94.3	85.0	70.0	66.5	67.0	68.3	70.3	68.2	66.6	63.1
Skilled nursing facility	4.7	1.5	3.7	7.8	8.5	9.1	10.0	9.5	10.0	10.1	10.4
Home health agency	1.0	2.1	5.5	13.8	3.1	2.9	3.3	3.1	3.2	3.2	3.1
Hospice	- - -	- - -	0.5	1.6	2.2	2.6	3.2	4.0	4.4	4.7	4.6
Home health agency transfer[6]	- - -	- - -	- - -	- - -	1.3	2.2	0.8	–1.4	0.0	0.0	0.0
Administrative expenses[7]	3.0	2.1	1.4	1.2	2.1	1.7	2.0	1.8	2.0	1.8	1.7

See footnotes at end of table.

Table 141 (page 2 of 2). Medicare enrollees and expenditures and percent distribution, by Medicare program and type of service: United States and other areas, selected years 1970–2006

[Data are compiled from various sources by the Centers for Medicare & Medicaid Services]

Medicare program and type of service	*1970*	*1980*	*1990*	*1995*	*2000*	*2001*	*2002*	*2003*	*2004*	*2005*	*2006*[1]
	Percent distribution of expenditures										
Total supplementary medical insurance (SMI)[3]	100.0	100.0	100.0	100.0	100.0	100.0	100.0	100.0	100.0	100.0	100.0
Total Part B	100.0	100.0	100.0	100.0	100.0	100.0	100.0	100.0	99.7	99.3	78.1
Part B payments to managed care organizations[4]	1.2	1.8	6.4	9.9	20.2	17.3	15.5	13.7	13.6	14.5	18.6
Part B payments for fee-for-service utilization[8]	88.1	92.8	90.1	87.6	79.6	84.0	83.5	82.7	84.0	82.7	79.3
Physician/supplies[9]	80.9	72.8	67.3	---	---	---	---	---	---	---	---
Outpatient hospital[10]	5.2	16.9	19.3	---	---	---	---	---	---	---	---
Independent laboratory[11]	0.5	1.0	3.4	---	---	---	---	---	---	---	---
Physician fee schedule	---	---	---	47.5	40.8	41.5	39.6	38.3	39.2	37.9	34.6
Durable medical equipment	---	---	---	5.5	5.2	5.4	5.8	6.0	5.6	5.3	5.0
Laboratory[10]	---	---	---	6.4	4.4	4.3	4.4	4.3	4.4	4.3	4.2
Other[11]	---	---	---	14.8	15.0	15.8	17.3	17.9	18.1	18.0	17.3
Hospital[12]	---	---	---	13.0	9.3	12.6	12.0	12.1	12.6	13.5	14.1
Home health agency	1.5	2.1	0.2	0.3	4.9	4.5	4.5	4.0	4.3	4.3	4.3
Home health agency transfer[6]	---	---	---	0.0	–1.9	–3.1	–1.0	1.7	0.0	0.0	0.0
Administrative expenses[7]	10.7	5.4	3.5	2.4	2.0	1.8	2.0	1.9	2.0	1.8	1.8
Part D Transitional Assistance and Start-up Costs[15]	---	---	---	---	---	---	---	---	0.2	0.4	0.0
Total Part D[4]	---	---	---	---	---	---	---	---	0.3	0.7	21.9

- - - Data not available.
0.0 Quantity greater than 0 but less than 0.05.
[1]Preliminary figures.
[2]Average number enrolled in the hospital insurance (HI) and/or supplementary medical insurance (SMI) programs for the period. See Appendix II, Medicare.
[3]Starting with 2004 data, the SMI trust fund consists of two separate accounts: Part B (which pays for a portion of the costs of physicians' services, outpatient hospital services, and other related medical and health services for voluntarily enrolled aged and disabled individuals) and Part D (Medicare Prescription Drug Account which pays private plans to provide prescription drug coverage).
[4]The Medicare Modernization Act, enacted on December 8, 2003, established within SMI two Part D accounts related to prescription drug benefits: the Medicare Prescription Drug Account and the Transitional Assistance Account. The Medicare Prescription Drug Account is used in conjunction with the broad, voluntary prescription drug benefits that began in 2006. The Transitional Assistance Account was used to provide transitional assistance benefits, beginning in 2004 and extending through 2005, for certain low-income beneficiaries prior to the start of the new prescription drug benefit.
[5]Medicare-approved managed care organizations.
[6]Starting with 1999 data, reflects annual home health HI to SMI transfer amounts.
[7]Includes research, costs of experiments and demonstration projects, fraud and abuse promotion, and peer review activity (changed to Quality Improvement Organization in 2002).
[8]Type-of-service reporting categories for fee-for-service reimbursement differ before and after 1991.
[9]Includes payment for physicians, practitioners, durable medical equipment, and all suppliers other than independent laboratory through 1990. Starting with 1991 data, physician services subject to the physician fee schedule are shown. Payments for laboratory services paid under the laboratory fee schedule and performed in a physician office are included under Laboratory beginning in 1991. Payments for durable medical equipment are shown separately beginning in 1991. The remaining services from the Physician category are included in Other.
[10]Includes payments for hospital outpatient department services, skilled nursing facility outpatient services, Part B services received as an inpatient in a hospital or skilled nursing facility setting, and other types of outpatient facilities. Starting with 1991 data, payments for hospital outpatient department services, except for laboratory services, are listed under Hospital. Hospital outpatient laboratory services are included in the Laboratory line.
[11]Starting with 1991 data, those independent laboratory services that were paid under the laboratory fee schedule (most of the independent lab category) are included in the Laboratory line; the remaining services are included in the Physician fee schedule and Other lines.
[12]Payments for laboratory services paid under the laboratory fee schedule performed in a physician office, independent lab, or in a hospital outpatient department.
[13]Includes payments for physician-administered drugs; freestanding ambulatory surgical center facility services; ambulance services; supplies; freestanding end-stage renal disease (ESRD) dialysis facility services; rural health clinics; outpatient rehabilitation facilities; psychiatric hospitals; and federally qualified health centers.
[14]Includes the hospital facility costs for Medicare Part B services that are predominantly in the outpatient department, with the exception of hospital outpatient laboratory services, which are included on the Laboratory line. Physician reimbursement is included on the Physician fee schedule line.
[15]Part D Administrative and Transitional Start-Up Costs were funded through the SMI Part B account.

NOTES: Percents are calculated using unrounded data. Totals do not necessarily equal the sum of rounded components. Estimates include service disbursements as of February 2006 for Medicare enrollees residing in the United States, Puerto Rico, Virgin Islands, Guam, other outlying areas, foreign countries, and unknown residence. Some numbers in this table have been revised and differ from previous editions of *Health, United States*.

SOURCE: Centers for Medicare & Medicaid Services, Office of the Actuary, Medicare and Medicaid Cost Estimates Group, Medicare Administrative Data.

Table 142. Medicare enrollees and program payments among fee-for-service Medicare beneficiaries, by sex and age: United States and other areas, selected years 1994–2004

[Data are compiled from administrative data by the Centers for Medicare & Medicaid Services]

Sex and age	*1994*	*1995*	*1997*	*1998*	*1999*	*2000*	*2001*	*2002*	*2003*	*2004*
	Fee-for-service enrollees in thousands									
Total	34,076	34,062	33,009	32,349	32,179	32,740	33,860	34,977	35,815	36,345
Sex										
Male	14,533	14,563	14,149	13,902	13,872	14,195	14,746	15,314	15,736	16,040
Female	19,543	19,499	18,860	18,477	18,307	18,545	19,113	19,664	20,079	20,305
Age										
Under 65 years	4,031	4,239	4,498	4,617	4,742	4,907	5,172	5,448	5,732	6,036
65–74 years	16,713	16,373	15,099	14,433	14,072	14,230	14,689	15,107	15,390	15,528
75–84 years	9,845	9,911	9,847	9,722	9,748	9,919	10,211	10,533	10,701	10,755
85 years and over	3,486	3,540	3,565	3,577	3,618	3,684	3,787	3,889	3,991	4,026
	Fee-for-service program payments in billions									
Total	$ 146.6	$ 159.0	$ 175.4	$ 168.2	$ 166.7	$ 174.3	$ 197.5	$ 215.4	$ 232.8	$ 255.3
Sex										
Male	63.9	68.8	75.4	72.9	73.2	76.2	86.3	94.3	102.2	111.8
Female	82.6	90.2	100.1	95.3	93.5	98.0	111.2	121.1	130.6	143.5
Age										
Under 65 years	18.8	21.0	25.8	23.7	24.3	25.8	29.7	33.2	37.3	42.3
65–74 years	55.1	58.1	59.7	57.3	56.0	57.5	64.6	70.0	75.2	81.6
75–84 years	50.7	55.3	61.7	59.7	59.5	62.7	70.9	77.1	82.5	89.9
85 years and over	21.8	24.6	28.2	27.3	26.9	28.3	32.3	35.1	37.8	41.5
	Percent distribution of fee-for-service program payments									
Total	100.0	100.0	100.0	100.0	100.0	100.0	100.0	100.0	100.0	100.0
Sex										
Male	43.6	43.2	43.0	43.3	43.9	43.7	43.7	43.8	43.9	43.8
Female	56.4	56.8	57.0	56.7	56.1	56.3	56.3	56.2	56.1	56.2
Age										
Under 65 years	12.9	13.2	14.7	14.1	14.6	14.8	15.0	15.4	16.0	16.6
65–74 years	37.6	36.5	34.0	34.1	33.6	33.0	32.7	32.5	32.3	32.0
75–84 years	34.6	34.8	35.2	35.5	35.7	36.0	35.9	35.8	35.4	35.2
85 years and over	14.9	15.5	16.1	16.3	16.1	16.2	16.4	16.3	16.2	16.3
	Average fee-for-service payment per enrollee									
Total	$ 4,301	$ 4,667	$ 5,314	$ 5,198	$ 5,180	$ 5,323	$ 5,833	$ 6,159	$ 6,501	$ 7,025
Sex										
Male	4,397	4,721	5,326	5,243	5,275	5,370	5,853	6,157	6,496	6,972
Female	4,229	4,627	5,306	5,165	5,108	5,286	5,818	6,159	6,505	7,067
Age										
Under 65 years	4,673	4,960	5,735	5,143	5,117	5,252	5,746	6,102	6,499	7,001
65–74 years	3,300	3,548	3,953	3,973	3,982	4,040	4,400	4,635	4,887	5,257
75–84 years	5,152	5,576	6,267	6,145	6,106	6,320	6,939	7,317	7,713	8,358
85 years and over	6,267	6,950	7,919	7,641	7,428	7,684	8,529	9,019	9,474	10,318

NOTES: Table includes data for Medicare enrollees residing in Puerto Rico, U.S. Virgin Islands, Guam, other outlying areas, foreign countries, and unknown residence. Prior to 2004, number of fee-for-service enrollees, fee-for-service program payments, and fee-for-service billing reimbursement are based on a 5% annual Denominator File derived from the Centers for Medicare & Medicaid Services' (CMS') Enrollment Database and the fee-for-service claims for a 5% sample of beneficiaries as recorded in CMS' National Claims History File. Starting with 2004 data, the 100% Denominator File was used. See Appendix II, Medicare. Data for additional years are available. See Appendix III.

SOURCE: Centers for Medicare & Medicaid Services, Office of Research, Development, and Information. Health Care Financing Review: Medicare and Medicaid Statistical Supplements for publication years 1996 to 2006. Available from: www.cms.hhs.gov/MedicareMedicaidStatSupp/LT/list.asp.

Table 143 (page 1 of 2). Medicare beneficiaries by race, ethnicity, and selected characteristics: United States, 1992, 2003, and 2004

[Data are based on household interviews of a sample of current Medicare beneficiaries and Medicare administrative records]

				Not Hispanic or Latino								
	All			*White*			*Black or African American*			*Hispanic or Latino*		
Characteristic	*1992*	*2003*	*2004*	*1992*	*2003*	*2004*	*1992*	*2003*	*2004*	*1992*	*2003*	*2004*
	Number of beneficiaries in millions											
All Medicare beneficiaries	36.8	42.3	42.9	30.9	33.0	33.5	3.3	4.0	4.1	1.9	3.3	3.2
	Percent distribution of beneficiaries											
All Medicare beneficiaries	100.0	100.0	100.0	84.2	78.4	78.2	8.9	9.6	9.6	5.2	7.9	7.5
Medical care use	Percent of beneficiaries with at least one service											
All Medicare beneficiaries:												
Long-term care facility stay	7.7	8.8	8.5	8.0	9.3	9.2	6.2	9.4	8.5	4.2	4.5	5.2
Community-only residents:												
Inpatient hospital	17.9	19.4	17.0	18.1	19.5	16.9	18.4	22.5	18.8	16.6	16.7	15.8
Outpatient hospital	57.9	72.9	75.4	57.8	73.5	76.4	61.1	72.0	75.1	53.1	68.5	70.2
Physician/supplier[1]	92.4	96.0	96.8	93.0	96.5	97.2	89.1	92.8	95.1	87.9	94.5	95.2
Dental	40.4	43.7	46.2	43.1	47.6	49.5	23.5	24.5	27.6	29.1	32.4	38.0
Prescription medicine	85.2	92.3	93.4	85.5	92.7	93.7	83.1	90.6	90.7	84.6	90.1	91.8
Expenditures	Expenditures per beneficiary											
All Medicare beneficiaries:												
Total health care[2]	$6,716	$12,512	$13,358	$6,816	$12,495	$13,064	$7,043	$14,682	$18,111	$5,784	$10,410	$12,052
Long-term care facility[3]	1,581	2,239	2,371	1,674	2,329	2,466	1,255	2,818	2,983	*758	1,171	1,429
Community-only residents:												
Total personal health care	5,054	9,921	9,689	4,988	9,801	9,537	5,530	11,329	11,419	4,938	9,117	9,593
Inpatient hospital	2,098	2,989	2,425	2,058	2,869	2,383	2,493	3,920	3,298	1,999	2,806	1,889
Outpatient hospital	504	1,112	1,122	478	1,047	1,046	668	1,591	1,777	511	1,082	1,126
Physician/supplier[1]	1,524	3,184	2,971	1,525	3,182	3,002	1,398	3,239	3,043	1,587	3,179	2,806
Dental	142	294	327	153	328	353	70	128	141	97	174	261
Prescription medicine	468	1,667	1,894	481	1,709	1,907	417	1,606	1,929	389	1,337	1,769
Long-term care facility residents only:												
Long-term care facility[4]	23,054	33,306	35,933	23,177	32,345	35,139	21,272	38,916	42,632	*25,026	*38,910	*36,287
Sex	Percent distribution of beneficiaries											
Both sexes	100.0	100.0	100.0	100.0	100.0	100.0	100.0	100.0	100.0	100.0	100.0	100.0
Male	42.9	44.0	44.1	42.7	44.3	44.2	42.0	42.9	41.8	46.7	44.7	45.8
Female	57.1	56.0	55.9	57.3	55.7	55.8	58.0	57.1	58.2	53.3	55.3	54.2
Eligibility criteria and age												
All Medicare beneficiaries[5]	100.0	100.0	100.0	100.0	100.0	100.0	100.0	100.0	100.0	100.0	100.0	100.0
Disabled	10.2	14.4	15.2	8.6	12.1	12.7	19.1	28.1	29.9	16.5	19.2	20.2
Under 45 years	3.5	3.7	3.8	2.9	3.0	3.1	7.6	7.9	8.1	6.9	5.1	4.8
45–64 years	6.5	10.7	11.4	5.8	9.0	9.6	11.5	20.2	21.8	9.6	14.1	15.4
Aged	89.8	85.6	84.8	91.4	88.0	87.2	81.0	71.9	70.2	83.5	80.8	79.9
65–74 years	51.5	44.3	43.8	52.0	44.3	43.8	48.0	40.7	40.2	49.4	45.7	45.0
75–84 years	28.8	30.2	29.8	29.5	31.9	31.5	24.0	22.4	21.3	27.1	26.5	26.3
85 years and over	9.7	11.1	11.2	9.9	11.8	11.9	9.0	8.8	8.7	6.9	8.7	8.6
Living arrangement												
All living arrangements	100.0	100.0	100.0	100.0	100.0	100.0	100.0	100.0	100.0	100.0	100.0	100.0
Alone	27.0	28.9	29.0	27.5	29.3	29.8	27.7	32.9	32.2	20.2	22.1	21.4
With spouse	51.2	49.4	48.4	53.3	52.0	50.7	33.3	27.7	27.8	50.4	49.3	47.2
With children	9.1	9.8	10.5	7.7	8.1	8.5	16.8	17.5	18.8	16.6	15.7	17.8
With others	7.6	7.4	7.7	6.2	5.8	6.2	18.1	16.5	17.1	10.8	10.4	11.5
Long-term care facility	5.1	4.6	4.4	5.3	4.7	4.8	4.0	5.4	4.1	*2.0	2.5	2.1

See footnotes at end of table.

Table 143 (page 2 of 2). Medicare beneficiaries by race, ethnicity, and selected characteristics: United States, 1992, 2003, and 2004

[Data are based on household interviews of a sample of current Medicare beneficiaries and Medicare administrative records]

				Not Hispanic or Latino								
	All			*White*			*Black or African American*			*Hispanic or Latino*		
Characteristic	*1992*	*2003*	*2004*	*1992*	*2003*	*2004*	*1992*	*2003*	*2004*	*1992*	*2003*	*2004*
Age and limitation of activity[6]	Percent distribution of beneficiaries											
Disabled	100.0	100.0	100.0	100.0	100.0	100.0	100.0	100.0	100.0	100.0	100.0	100.0
None	22.7	28.4	29.9	21.8	26.1	29.9	26.2	35.3	32.1	21.2	27.2	24.8
IADL only	39.0	36.8	35.1	38.9	38.1	34.5	35.8	34.4	37.1	46.1	37.8	38.7
1 or 2 ADL	21.2	19.6	21.4	21.5	20.4	21.4	21.2	19.5	20.6	*20.9	*15.8	*20.7
3–5 ADL	17.2	15.2	13.5	17.9	15.4	14.1	*16.8	*10.9	*10.2	*11.9	*19.3	*15.8
65–74 years	100.0	100.0	100.0	100.0	100.0	100.0	100.0	100.0	100.0	100.0	100.0	100.0
None	67.0	70.8	71.6	68.7	72.3	73.4	55.1	62.9	61.7	59.2	63.4	65.2
IADL only	17.8	15.9	15.8	17.0	15.6	15.3	22.9	18.9	17.2	*20.9	18.4	18.9
1 or 2 ADL	10.4	8.8	8.7	9.6	8.5	7.9	14.4	11.9	13.0	*15.7	*8.8	*10.5
3–5 ADL	4.8	4.4	3.9	4.6	3.6	3.3	*7.6	*6.3	*8.2	*4.2	*9.5	*5.4
75–84 years	100.0	100.0	100.0	100.0	100.0	100.0	100.0	100.0	100.0	100.0	100.0	100.0
None	46.6	54.2	55.2	47.5	55.3	55.9	42.0	44.3	51.4	44.3	52.6	53.3
IADL only	23.9	21.8	21.5	23.6	21.7	21.7	26.7	23.4	*17.8	*27.8	21.7	21.3
1 or 2 ADL	16.5	13.6	13.6	16.8	13.7	13.8	15.3	*14.0	*13.6	*14.9	*13.4	*11.9
3–5 ADL	13.0	10.4	9.7	12.2	9.5	8.6	*15.9	18.3	17.2	*13.0	*12.3	*13.5
85 years and over	100.0	100.0	100.0	100.0	100.0	100.0	100.0	100.0	100.0	100.0	100.0	100.0
None	19.9	25.9	27.6	20.2	27.0	28.5	*19.6	*22.7	*29.7	*19.7	*16.1	*15.2
IADL only	20.9	25.1	24.3	20.2	25.6	24.5	*22.1	*20.8	*24.1	*24.7	*23.2	*23.8
1 or 2 ADL	23.5	21.8	19.5	23.5	21.8	19.1	*24.3	*23.1	*15.0	*23.7	*22.8	*24.5
3–5 ADL	35.8	27.2	28.6	36.1	25.6	27.9	*34.0	33.4	*31.1	*31.8	*37.9	*36.5

* Estimates are considered unreliable. Estimates based on 50 persons or fewer or with a relative standard error of 30% or higher are not shown.

[1]Physician/supplier services include medical and osteopathic doctor and health practitioner visits; diagnostic laboratory and radiology services; medical and surgical services; and durable medical equipment and nondurable medical supplies.

[2]Total health care expenditures by Medicare beneficiaries, including expenses paid by Medicare and all other sources of payment for the following services: inpatient hospital, outpatient hospital, physician/supplier, dental, prescription medicine, home health, and hospice and long-term care facility care. Does not include health insurance premiums.

[3]Expenditures for long-term care in facilities for all beneficiaries include facility room and board expenses for beneficiaries who resided in a facility for the full year, for beneficiaries who resided in a facility for part of the year and in the community for part of the year, and expenditures for short-term facility stays for full-year or part-year community residents. See Appendix II, Long-term care facility.

[4]Expenditures for facility-based long-term care for facility-based beneficiaries include facility room and board expenses for beneficiaries who resided in a facility for the full year and for beneficiaries who resided in a facility for part of the year and in the community for part of the year. It does not include expenditures for short-term facility stays for full-year community residents. See Appendix II, Long-term care facility.

[5]Medicare beneficiaries with end-stage renal disease (ESRD) are included within the subgroups Aged and Disabled.

[6]Includes data for both community and long-term care facility residents. See Appendix II for definitions of Activities of Daily Living (ADL) and Instrumental Activities of Daily Living (IADL).

NOTES: Percents and percent distributions are calculated using unrounded numbers. Data for additional years are available. See Appendix III.

SOURCE: Centers for Medicare & Medicaid Services, Medicare Current Beneficiary Survey, Health and Health Care of the Medicare Population. Available from: www.cms.hhs.gov/mcbs. and unpublished data.

Table 144. Medicaid recipients and medical vendor payments, by basis of eligibility, and race and ethnicity: United States, selected fiscal years 1972–2004

[Data are compiled by the Centers for Medicare & Medicaid Services from the Medicaid Data System]

Basis of eligibility and race and ethnicity	*1972*	*1980*	*1990*	*1995*	*2000*	*2001*	*2002*	*2003*	*2004*
Recipients					Number in millions				
All recipients	17.6	21.6	25.3	36.3	42.8	46.0	49.3	52.0	55.6
					Percent of recipients				
Basis of eligibility:[1]									
Aged (65 years and over)	18.8	15.9	12.7	11.4	8.7	8.3	7.9	7.8	7.8
Blind and disabled	9.8	13.5	14.7	16.1	16.1	15.4	15.0	14.8	14.6
Adults in families with dependent children[2]	17.8	22.6	23.8	21.0	20.5	21.1	22.6	22.2	22.2
Children under age 21[3]	44.5	43.2	44.4	47.3	46.1	45.7	47.1	47.8	47.8
Other Title XIX[4]	9.0	6.9	3.9	1.7	8.6	9.5	7.4	7.5	7.6
Race and ethnicity:[5]									
White	- - -	- - -	42.8	45.5	- - -	40.2	40.9	41.2	41.1
Black or African American	- - -	- - -	25.1	24.7	- - -	23.1	22.8	22.4	22.1
American Indian or Alaska Native	- - -	- - -	1.0	0.8	- - -	1.3	1.3	1.4	1.3
Asian or Pacific Islander	- - -	- - -	2.0	2.2	- - -	3.0	3.4	3.3	3.3
Hispanic or Latino	- - -	- - -	15.2	17.2	- - -	17.9	19.0	19.3	19.4
Multiple race or unknown	- - -	- - -	14.0	9.6	- - -	14.6	12.6	12.5	12.7
Vendor payments[6]					Amount in billions				
All payments	$ 6.3	$ 23.3	$ 64.9	$120.1	$ 168.3	$ 186.3	$ 213.5	$ 233.2	$ 257.7
					Percent distribution				
Total	100.0	100.0	100.0	100.0	100.0	100.0	100.0	100.0	100.0
Basis of eligibility:[1]									
Aged (65 years and over)	30.6	37.5	33.2	30.4	26.4	25.9	24.4	23.7	23.1
Blind and disabled	22.2	32.7	37.6	41.1	43.2	43.1	43.3	43.7	43.3
Adults in families with dependent children[2]	15.3	13.9	13.2	11.2	10.6	10.7	10.9	11.4	11.8
Children under age 21[3]	18.1	13.4	14.0	15.0	15.9	16.3	16.8	17.1	17.2
Other Title XIX[4]	13.9	2.6	1.6	1.2	3.9	3.9	4.6	4.1	4.7
Race and ethnicity:[5]									
White	- - -	- - -	53.4	54.3	- - -	54.4	54.1	53.8	53.4
Black or African American	- - -	- - -	18.3	19.2	- - -	19.8	19.6	19.7	19.8
American Indian or Alaska Native	- - -	- - -	0.6	0.5	- - -	1.1	1.1	1.2	1.2
Asian or Pacific Islander	- - -	- - -	1.0	1.2	- - -	2.5	2.8	2.4	2.5
Hispanic or Latino	- - -	- - -	5.3	7.3	- - -	9.4	9.7	10.6	10.7
Multiple race or unknown	- - -	- - -	21.3	17.6	- - -	12.9	12.6	12.2	12.3
Vendor payments per recipient[6]					Amount				
All recipients	$ 358	$1,079	$2,568	$3,311	$ 3,936	$ 4,053	$ 4,328	$ 4,487	$ 4,639
Basis of eligibility:[1]									
Aged (65 years and over)	580	2,540	6,717	8,868	11,929	12,725	13,370	13,677	13,687
Blind and disabled	807	2,618	6,564	8,435	10,559	11,318	12,470	13,303	13,714
Adults in families with dependent children[2]	307	662	1,429	1,777	2,030	2,059	2,095	2,296	2,475
Children under age 21[3]	145	335	811	1,047	1,358	1,448	1,545	1,606	1,664
Other Title XIX[4]	555	398	1,062	2,380	1,778	1,680	2,692	2,458	2,867
Race and ethnicity:[5]									
White	- - -	- - -	3,207	3,953	- - -	5,489	5,721	5,869	6,026
Black or African American	- - -	- - -	1,878	2,568	- - -	3,480	3,733	3,944	4,158
American Indian or Alaska Native	- - -	- - -	1,706	2,142	- - -	3,452	3,774	4,001	4,320
Asian or Pacific Islander	- - -	- - -	1,257	1,713	- - -	3,283	3,562	3,328	3,513
Hispanic or Latino	- - -	- - -	903	1,400	- - -	2,126	2,215	2,463	2,563
Multiple race or unknown	- - -	- - -	3,909	6,099	- - -	3,576	4,338	4,395	4,493

- - - Data not available.

[1]In 1980 and 1985, recipients are included in more than one category. In 1990–1996, 0.2%–2.5% of recipients have unknown basis of eligibility. Starting with 1997 data, unknowns are included in Other Title XIX.

[2]Includes adults in the Aid to Families with Dependent Children (AFDC) program. Starting with 1997 data, includes adults in the Temporary Assistance for Needy Families (TANF) program. Starting with 2001 data, includes women in the Breast and Cervical Cancer Prevention and Treatment Program.

[3]Includes children in the AFDC program. Starting with 1997 data, includes children (including those in the foster care system) in the TANF program.

[4]Includes some participants in the Supplemental Security Income program and other people deemed medically needy in participating states. Starting with 1997 data, excludes foster care children and includes unknown eligibility.

[5]Race and ethnicity are as determined on initial Medicaid application. Categories are mutually exclusive. Starting with 2001 data, the Hispanic category included Hispanic persons, regardless of race. Persons indicating more than one race were included in the unknown category.

[6]Vendor payments exclude disproportionate share hospital (DSH) payments ($14.3 billion in FY2004) and DSH mental health facility payments ($2.9 billion in FY2004).

NOTES: 1972 data are for fiscal year ending June 30. All other years are for fiscal year ending September 30. Starting with 1999 data, a new Medicaid data system was introduced. Prior to 1999, recipient counts exclude those individuals who only received coverage under prepaid health care and for whom no direct vendor payments were made during the year, and vendor payments exclude payments to health maintenance organizations and other prepaid health plans ($19 billion in 1998). See Appendix II, Medical vendor payments. See Appendix I, Medicaid Data System. Data for additional years are available. See Appendix III.

SOURCE: Centers for Medicare & Medicaid Services, Office of Information Services, Enterprise Databases Group, Division of Information Distribution, Medicaid Data System. Before 1999, data are from Medicaid Statistical Report HCFA–2082. Starting with 1999, data are from Medicaid Statistical Information System, MSIS. MSIS data available from: msis.cms.hhs.gov (accessed May 22, 2007).

Table 145 (page 1 of 2). Medicaid recipients and medical vendor payments, by type of service: United States, selected fiscal years 1972–2004

[Data are compiled by the Centers for Medicare & Medicaid Services from the Medicaid Data System]

Type of service	*1972*	*1980*	*1990*	*1995*	*2000*	*2001*	*2002*	*2003*	*2004*
Recipients					Number in millions				
All recipients	17.6	21.6	25.3	36.3	42.8	46.0	49.3	52.0	55.6
					Percent of recipients				
Inpatient hospital	16.1	17.0	18.2	15.3	11.5	10.6	10.2	10.0	9.8
Mental health facility	0.2	0.3	0.4	0.2	0.2	0.2	0.2	0.2	0.2
Mentally retarded intermediate care facility	- - -	0.6	0.6	0.4	0.3	0.3	0.2	0.2	0.2
Nursing facility	- - -	- - -	- - -	4.6	4.0	3.7	3.6	3.3	3.1
Skilled	3.1	2.8	2.4	- - -	- - -	- - -	- - -	- - -	- - -
Intermediate care	- - -	3.7	3.4	- - -	- - -	- - -	- - -	- - -	- - -
Physician	69.8	63.7	67.6	65.6	44.7	43.5	44.7	44.0	43.1
Dental	13.6	21.5	18.0	17.6	13.8	15.3	16.0	16.4	16.2
Other practitioner	9.1	15.0	15.3	15.2	11.1	11.1	11.3	11.1	10.7
Outpatient hospital	29.6	44.9	49.0	46.1	30.9	29.8	30.1	29.8	28.7
Clinic	2.8	7.1	11.1	14.7	17.9	18.4	19.2	19.6	20.0
Laboratory and radiological	20.0	14.9	35.5	36.0	26.6	26.8	28.5	28.3	28.9
Home health	0.6	1.8	2.8	4.5	2.3	2.2	2.2	2.3	2.1
Prescribed drugs	63.3	63.4	68.5	65.4	48.0	47.6	49.4	50.2	50.3
Family planning	. . .	5.2	6.9	6.9	- - -	- - -	- - -	- - -	- - -
Early and periodic screening	. . .	. . .	11.7	18.2	- - -	- - -	- - -	- - -	- - -
Rural health clinic	. . .	. . .	0.9	3.4	- - -	- - -	- - -	- - -	- - -
Capitated care	- - -	- - -	- - -	- - -	49.7	50.5	51.7	53.1	54.2
Primary care case management	- - -	- - -	- - -	- - -	13.0	13.9	14.6	14.5	15.4
Personal support	- - -	- - -	- - -	- - -	10.6	10.8	11.5	11.6	11.3
Other care[1]	14.4	11.9	20.3	31.5	21.4	21.5	22.6	23.1	22.9
Vendor payments[2]					Amount in billions				
All payments	$ 6.3	$ 23.3	$ 64.9	$120.1	$168.3	$186.3	$213.5	$233.2	$257.7
					Percent distribution				
Total	100.0	100.0	100.0	100.0	100.0	100.0	100.0	100.0	100.0
Inpatient hospital	40.6	27.5	25.7	21.9	14.4	13.9	13.6	13.5	13.5
Mental health facility	1.8	3.3	2.6	2.1	1.1	1.1	1.0	0.9	0.9
Mentally retarded intermediate care facility	- - -	8.5	11.3	8.6	5.6	5.2	5.0	4.7	4.3
Nursing facility	- - -	- - -	- - -	24.2	20.5	20.0	18.4	17.3	16.3
Skilled	23.3	15.8	12.4	- - -	- - -	- - -	- - -	- - -	- - -
Intermediate care	- - -	18.0	14.9	- - -	- - -	- - -	- - -	- - -	- - -
Physician	12.6	8.0	6.2	6.1	4.0	4.0	3.9	3.9	4.0
Dental	2.7	2.0	0.9	0.8	0.8	1.0	1.1	1.1	1.1
Other practitioner	0.9	0.8	0.6	0.8	0.4	0.4	0.4	0.4	0.4
Outpatient hospital	5.8	4.7	5.1	5.5	4.2	4.0	4.0	4.0	4.0
Clinic	0.7	1.4	2.6	3.6	3.7	3.0	3.1	3.1	3.2
Laboratory and radiological	1.3	0.5	1.1	1.0	0.8	0.9	1.0	1.0	1.0
Home health	0.4	1.4	5.2	7.8	1.9	1.9	1.8	1.9	1.8
Prescribed drugs	8.1	5.7	6.8	8.1	11.9	12.7	13.3	14.5	15.3
Family planning	. . .	0.3	0.4	0.4	- - -	- - -	- - -	- - -	- - -
Early and periodic screening	. . .	. . .	0.3	1.0	- - -	- - -	- - -	- - -	- - -
Rural health clinic	. . .	. . .	0.1	0.2	- - -	- - -	- - -	- - -	- - -
Capitated care	- - -	- - -	- - -	- - -	14.5	15.7	15.8	16.0	16.5
Primary care case management	- - -	- - -	- - -	- - -	0.1	0.1	0.1	0.1	0.2
Personal support	- - -	- - -	- - -	- - -	6.9	7.0	7.2	7.4	7.2
Other care[1]	1.8	1.9	3.7	7.7	8.8	9.2	10.3	10.2	10.3

See footnotes at end of table.

Table 145 (page 2 of 2). Medicaid recipients and medical vendor payments, by type of service: United States, selected fiscal years 1972–2004

[Data are compiled by the Centers for Medicare & Medicaid Services from the Medicaid Data System]

Type of service	*1972*	*1980*	*1990*	*1995*	*2000*	*2001*	*2002*	*2003*	*2004*
Vendor payments per recipient[2]					Amount				
Total payment per recipient	$ 358	$ 1,079	$ 2,568	$ 3,311	$ 3,936	$ 4,053	$ 4,328	$ 4,487	$ 4,639
Inpatient hospital	903	1,742	3,630	4,735	4,919	5,313	5,771	6,047	6,424
Mental health facility	2,825	11,742	18,548	29,847	17,800	21,482	21,377	20,503	19,928
Mentally retarded intermediate care facility	- - -	16,438	50,048	68,613	79,330	83,227	91,588	95,287	97,497
Nursing facility	- - -	- - -	- - -	17,424	20,220	21,894	22,326	23,882	24,475
Skilled	2,665	6,081	13,356	- - -	- - -	- - -	- - -	- - -	- - -
Intermediate care	- - -	5,326	11,236	- - -	- - -	- - -	- - -	- - -	- - -
Physician	65	136	235	309	356	371	378	403	426
Dental	71	99	130	160	238	270	293	305	318
Other practitioner	37	61	96	178	139	149	151	154	160
Outpatient hospital	70	113	269	397	533	546	571	596	639
Clinic	82	209	602	804	805	662	706	720	750
Laboratory and radiological	23	38	80	90	113	131	154	161	168
Home health	229	847	4,733	5,740	3,135	3,478	3,689	3,720	3,978
Prescribed drugs	46	96	256	413	975	1,083	1,165	1,293	1,411
Family planning	. . .	72	151	206	- - -	- - -	- - -	- - -	- - -
Early and periodic screening	. . .	. . .	67	177	- - -	- - -	- - -	- - -	- - -
Rural health clinic	. . .	. . .	154	174	- - -	- - -	- - -	- - -	- - -
Capitated care	- - -	- - -	- - -	- - -	1,148	1,257	1,318	1,357	1,415
Primary care case management	- - -	- - -	- - -	- - -	30	29	28	28	58
Personal support	- - -	- - -	- - -	- - -	2,543	2,639	2,704	2,864	2,946
Other care[1]	44	172	465	807	1,600	1,734	1,963	1,975	2,086

- - - Data not available.
. . . Category not applicable.
[1]Unknown services are included with Other care (0.1% of recipients and 0.5% of payments in 2004).
[2]Vendor payments exclude disproportionate share hospital (DSH) payments ($14.3 billion in FY2004) and DSH mental health facility payments ($2.9 billion in FY2004).

NOTES: 1972 data are for fiscal year ending June 30. All other years are for fiscal year ending September 30. Starting with 1999 data, a new Medicaid data system was introduced. Prior to 1999, recipient counts exclude those individuals who only received coverage under prepaid health care and for whom no direct vendor payments were made during the year, and vendor payments exclude payments to health maintenance organizations and other prepaid health plans ($19 billion in 1998). See Appendix II, Medical vendor payments. See Appendix I, Medicaid Data System. Data for additional years are available. See Appendix III.

SOURCE: Centers for Medicare & Medicaid Services, Office of Information Services, Enterprise Databases Group, Division of Information Distribution, Medicaid Data System. Before 1999, data are from Medicaid Statistical Report HCFA–2082. Starting with 1999, data are from Medicaid Statistical Information System, MSIS and unpublished data. MSIS data available from: msis.cms.hhs.gov (accessed May 22, 2007).

Table 146. Department of Veterans Affairs health care expenditures and use, and persons treated, by selected characteristics: United States, selected fiscal years 1970–2005

[Data are compiled from patient records, enrollment information, and budgetary data by the Department of Veterans Affairs]

Type of expenditure and use	1970	1980	1990	1995	2000	2002	2003	2004	2005
Health care expenditures	Amount in millions								
All expenditures[1]	$1,689	$ 5,981	$11,500	$16,126	$19,327	$23,003	$25,647	$28,346	$30,836
	Percent distribution								
All services	100.0	100.0	100.0	100.0	100.0	100.0	100.0	100.0	100.0
Inpatient hospital	71.3	64.3	57.5	49.0	37.3	33.6	32.2	31.1	32.0
Outpatient care	14.0	19.1	25.3	30.2	45.7	48.8	49.5	49.5	50.5
Nursing home care	5.5	7.1	9.5	10.0	8.2	8.0	8.1	7.9	7.6
All other[2]	9.1	9.6	7.7	10.8	8.8	9.6	10.2	11.5	10.0
Health care use	Number in thousands								
Inpatient hospital stays[3]	787	1,248	1,029	879	579	590	588	599	600
Outpatient visits	7,312	17,971	22,602	27,527	38,370	46,058	49,760	53,745	59,570
Nursing home stays[4]	47	57	75	79	91	87	93	93	101
Inpatients[5]									
Total	- - -	- - -	598	527	417	436	443	457	587
	Percent distribution								
Total	- - -	- - -	100.0	100.0	100.0	100.0	100.0	100.0	100.0
Veterans with service-connected disability	- - -	- - -	38.9	39.3	34.4	35.2	36.2	36.5	33.6
Veterans without service-connected disability	- - -	- - -	60.3	59.9	64.7	63.9	62.9	62.6	65.8
Low income	- - -	- - -	54.8	56.2	41.7	40.9	40.8	40.9	43.7
Veterans receiving aid and attendance or housebound benefits or who are catastrophically disabled[6]	- - -	- - -	- - -	- - -	16.0	13.6	13.5	12.9	3.7
Veterans receiving medical care subject to copayments[7]	- - -	- - -	2.8	2.8	5.2	7.7	8.0	8.7	18.4
Other and unknown[8]	- - -	- - -	2.7	0.9	1.8	1.7	0.6	0.0	0.0
Nonveterans	- - -	- - -	0.8	0.8	0.9	0.9	0.8	0.9	0.6
Outpatients[5]	Number in thousands								
Total	- - -	- - -	2,564	2,790	3,657	4,456	4,715	4,894	4,603
	Percent distribution								
Total	- - -	- - -	100.0	100.0	100.0	100.0	100.0	100.0	100.0
Veterans with service-connected disability	- - -	- - -	38.3	37.5	30.7	29.5	30.3	30.8	31.7
Veterans without service-connected disability	- - -	- - -	49.8	50.5	60.8	63.9	63.4	63.1	62.6
Low income	- - -	- - -	41.1	42.2	37.6	34.1	32.7	32.8	34.4
Veterans receiving aid and attendance or housebound benefits or who are catastrophically disabled[6]	- - -	- - -	- - -	- - -	3.8	3.3	3.4	3.4	2.5
Veterans receiving medical care subject to copayments[7]	- - -	- - -	3.6	4.2	15.4	23.6	26.1	26.9	25.7
Other and unknown[8]	- - -	- - -	5.1	4.1	4.0	2.9	1.1	0.0	0.0
Nonveterans	- - -	- - -	11.8	12.0	8.5	6.6	6.3	6.1	5.7

- - - Data not available.

[1]Health care expenditures exclude construction, medical administration, and miscellaneous operating expenses at Department of Veterans Affairs headquarters.

[2]Includes miscellaneous benefits and services, contract hospitals, education and training, subsidies to state veterans hospitals, nursing homes and residential rehabilitation treatment programs (formerly domiciliaries), and the Civilian Health and Medical Program of the Department of Veterans Affairs.

[3]One-day dialysis patients were included in 1980. Interfacility transfers were included starting with 1990 data.

[4]Includes Department of Veterans Affairs nursing home and residential rehabilitation treatment programs (formerly domiciliary) stays, and community nursing home care stays.

[5]Individuals. The inpatient and outpatient totals are not additive because most inpatients are also treated as outpatients.

[6]Includes veterans who are receiving aid and attendance or housebound benefit and veterans who have been determined by the Department of Veterans Affairs to be catastrophically disabled.

[7]Includes financial means-tested veterans who receive medical care subject to copayments according to income level.

[8]Includes expenditures for services for veterans who were prisoner of war, exposed to Agent Orange, and other. Prior to fiscal year 1994, veterans who reported exposure to Agent Orange were classified as exempt. Beginning in fiscal year 1994, those veterans reporting Agent Orange exposure but not treated for it were means tested and placed in the low income or other group depending on income.

NOTES: Estimates may not add to totals due to rounding. In 1970, the fiscal year (FY) ended June 30; 1980 and in subsequent years, the FY ended September 30. The veteran population was estimated at 25.2 million at the end of FY 2003, with 38% age 65 or over, compared with 11% in FY 1980. Seventeen percent had served during World War II, 14% during the Korean conflict, 33% during the Vietnam era, 15% during the Persian Gulf War, and 25% during peacetime. These percentages add to more than 100 due to veterans serving during more than one war. Starting with FY 1995 data, categories for health care expenditures and health care use were revised. In FY 1999, a new data reporting system was introduced. Data for additional years are available. See Appendix III.

SOURCES: Department of Veterans Affairs (VA), Office of the Assistant Deputy Under Secretary for Health, National Patient Care Database, National Enrollment Database, budgetary data, and unpublished data. Veteran population estimates were provided by the VA's Office of the Actuary.

Table 147 (page 1 of 2). State mental health agency per capita expenditures for mental health services and average annual percent change, by geographic region and state: United States, selected fiscal years 1981–2004

[Data are based on reporting by state mental health agencies]

Geographic region and state[1]	1981	1985	1990	1993	1997	2001	2003	2004	1981–1990	1990–2001	2001–2004
	Amount per capita								Average annual percent change		
United States	$ 27	$35	$ 48	$ 54	$ 64	$ 81	$ 92	$ 98	6.6	4.9	6.6
New England:											
Connecticut	32	44	73	82	99	129	151	152	9.6	5.3	5.6
Maine	25	36	67	70	88	107	128	131	11.6	4.3	7.0
Massachusetts	32	46	84	83	90	107	106	104	11.3	2.2	–0.9
New Hampshire	35	42	63	78	99	112	117	117	6.7	5.4	1.5
Rhode Island	36	35	50	61	63	88	89	93	3.7	5.3	1.9
Vermont	32	44	54	74	92	130	152	166	6.0	8.3	8.5
Mideast:											
Delaware	44	46	55	56	73	93	81	85	2.5	4.9	–3.0
District of Columbia[2]	- - -	28	268	315	337	398	414	410	- - -	3.7	1.0
Maryland	33	40	61	64	76	127	147	150	7.1	6.9	5.7
New Jersey	26	36	57	68	69	90	126	133	9.1	4.2	13.9
New York	67	90	118	131	113	176	192	200	6.5	3.7	4.4
Pennsylvania	41	52	57	68	68	152	195	186	3.7	9.3	7.0
Great Lakes:											
Illinois	18	24	34	36	51	64	66	69	7.3	5.9	2.5
Indiana	19	27	47	39	40	65	72	81	10.6	3.0	7.6
Michigan	33	49	74	75	87	90	98	91	9.4	1.8	0.4
Ohio	25	30	41	47	52	61	62	64	5.7	3.7	1.6
Wisconsin	22	28	37	35	44	72	91	95	5.9	6.2	9.7
Plains:											
Iowa	8	11	17	13	29	73	74	76	8.7	14.2	1.4
Kansas	18	27	35	48	59	60	75	83	7.7	5.0	11.4
Minnesota[3]	17	32	54	69	87	105	119	121	8.8	6.2	4.8
Missouri	24	28	35	41	56	60	67	69	4.3	5.0	4.8
Nebraska	17	21	29	34	39	51	58	58	6.1	5.3	4.4
North Dakota	39	36	40	43	48	79	81	73	0.3	6.4	–2.6
South Dakota	17	22	25	47	54	61	66	69	4.4	8.4	4.2
Southeast:											
Alabama	20	28	38	43	47	57	61	59	7.4	3.8	1.2
Arkansas	17	24	26	30	30	28	30	33	4.8	0.7	5.6
Florida	20	26	37	31	44	35	38	36	7.1	–0.5	0.9
Georgia	25	23	51	49	47	46	50	51	8.2	–0.9	3.5
Kentucky	15	19	23	25	35	49	51	50	4.9	7.1	0.7
Louisiana	19	26	28	39	43	45	51	53	4.4	4.4	5.6
Mississippi	14	24	34	41	56	87	93	96	10.4	8.9	3.3
North Carolina	24	38	46	50	62	76	50	50	7.5	4.7	–13.0
South Carolina	31	33	51	56	64	74	67	67	5.7	3.4	–3.3
Tennessee	18	23	29	37	23	69	87	88	5.4	8.2	8.4
Virginia	23	32	45	40	49	65	69	70	7.7	3.4	2.5
West Virginia	20	22	24	22	23	26	49	60	2.0	0.7	32.1
Southwest:											
Arizona	10	12	27	60	68	89	126	136	11.7	11.5	15.2
New Mexico	24	25	23	24	31	33	29	28	–0.5	3.3	–5.3
Oklahoma	22	31	36	38	41	39	39	40	5.6	0.7	0.8
Texas	13	17	23	31	39	38	39	37	6.5	4.7	–0.9
Rocky Mountains:											
Colorado	24	28	34	41	57	64	66	69	3.9	5.9	2.5
Idaho	13	15	20	26	29	46	34	40	4.9	7.9	–4.6
Montana	25	29	28	34	93	124	123	126	1.3	14.5	0.5
Utah	13	17	21	25	28	33	71	74	5.5	4.2	30.9
Wyoming	23	31	35	42	43	61	103	102	4.8	5.2	18.7

See footnotes at end of table.

Table 147 (page 2 of 2). State mental health agency per capita expenditures for mental health services and average annual percent change, by geographic region and state: United States, selected fiscal years 1981–2004

[Data are based on reporting by state mental health agencies]

Geographic region and state[1]	*1981*	*1985*	*1990*	*1993*	*1997*	*2001*	*2003*	*2004*	*1981–1990*	*1990–2001*	*2001–2004*
	Amount per capita								Average annual percent change		
Far West:											
Alaska	$38	$45	$72	$86	$79	$ 81	$ 85	$288	7.4	1.1	88.6
California	28	34	42	50	58	92	109	114	4.6	7.4	11.3
Hawaii	19	23	38	71	85	175	125	148	8.0	14.9	–8.0
Nevada	22	26	33	32	45	57	63	54	4.6	5.1	–2.7
Oregon	21	25	41	60	68	97	56	61	7.7	8.1	–20.7
Washington	18	30	43	66	79	88	91	94	10.2	6.7	3.4

- - - Data not available.
[1]Data are shown for Bureau of Economic Analysis (BEA) regions that are constructed to show economically interdependent states. These BEA geographic divisions differ from U.S. Census Bureau geographic divisions shown in some *Health, United States* tables. See Appendix II, Geographic region and division.
[2]Transfer of St. Elizabeths Hospital from the National Institute of Mental Health to the District of Columbia Office of Mental Health took place over the years 1985–1993.
[3]Minnesota data for 1981 are not comparable with subsequent data. Average annual percent change is for 1983–1990.

NOTES: Expenditures are for mental illness, excluding mental retardation and substance abuse. Starting in 1990, data for Puerto Rico and starting in 1993, data for Guam are included in the U.S. total. States may vary in type of funds included in mental health expenditures. Medicaid revenues for community programs and children's mental health expenditures are not included by some states. Funds for mental health services in jails or prisons are included by some states. State data omissions and inclusions are likely to be consistent across years. Data for additional years are available. See Appendix III.

SOURCES: National Association of State Mental Health Program Directors Research Institute, Inc. Lutterman T, Hollen V, Shaw R. Funding sources and expenditures of state mental health agencies: fiscal year 2004. August 2006. Available from: www.nri-inc.org.

Table 148 (page 1 of 2). Medicare enrollees, enrollees in managed care, payment per enrollee, and short-stay hospital utilization by geographic region and state: United States, 1994 and 2004

[Data are compiled by the Centers for Medicare & Medicaid Services]

Geographic division and state[1]	Enrollment in thousands[2]	Percent of enrollees in managed care[3]		Payment per fee-for-service enrollee		Short-stay hospital utilization: Discharges per 1,000 enrollees[4]		Short-stay hospital utilization: Average length of stay in days[4]	
	2004	1994	2004	1994	2004	1994	2004	1994	2004
United States[5]	40,784	7.9	13.0	$4,375	$7,148	345	364	7.5	5.8
New England:									
Connecticut	523	2.6	5.5	4,426	7,904	287	327	8.1	6.0
Maine	231	0.1	0.2	3,464	5,719	322	303	7.6	5.4
Massachusetts	965	6.1	16.7	5,147	7,927	350	365	7.6	5.6
New Hampshire	186	0.2	1.0	3,414	6,138	281	275	7.6	5.9
Rhode Island	172	7.0	33.3	4,148	7,131	312	352	8.1	6.0
Vermont	94	0.1	0.2	3,182	5,809	283	245	7.6	5.3
Mideast:									
Delaware	123	0.2	0.7	4,712	8,008	326	357	8.1	6.5
District of Columbia	73	3.9	6.6	5,655	8,820	376	405	10.1	6.9
Maryland	683	1.4	3.9	4,997	8,247	362	403	7.5	5.3
New Jersey	1,220	2.6	7.6	4,531	8,264	354	383	10.2	6.8
New York	2,759	6.2	18.0	4,855	7,995	334	366	11.2	7.4
Pennsylvania	2,117	3.3	24.2	5,212	7,263	379	406	8.0	5.8
Great Lakes:									
Illinois	1,673	5.5	5.1	4,324	7,220	374	421	7.3	5.5
Indiana	889	2.6	2.2	3,945	6,550	345	345	6.9	5.5
Michigan	1,462	0.7	1.5	4,307	7,477	328	375	7.6	5.6
Ohio	1,738	2.4	12.9	3,982	7,189	350	392	7.1	5.4
Wisconsin	814	2.0	5.8	3,246	5,895	310	319	6.8	5.1
Plains:									
Iowa	485	3.1	4.2	3,080	5,436	322	319	6.6	5.2
Kansas	398	3.3	3.4	3,847	6,541	348	350	6.5	5.2
Minnesota	686	19.6	14.3	3,394	6,070	334	349	5.7	4.7
Missouri	897	3.4	12.4	4,191	6,717	349	399	7.3	5.5
Nebraska	259	2.2	4.0	2,926	6,157	281	286	6.3	5.4
North Dakota	103	0.6	1.0	3,218	5,456	327	285	6.3	5.2
South Dakota	123	0.1	0.3	2,952	5,214	356	297	6.1	5.0
Southeast:									
Alabama	734	0.8	7.4	4,454	6,915	413	438	7.0	5.4
Arkansas	461	0.2	0.4	3,719	6,236	366	386	7.0	5.7
Florida	2,997	13.8	18.5	5,027	8,243	326	369	7.1	5.8
Georgia	1,000	0.4	1.9	4,402	6,767	378	360	6.9	5.7
Kentucky	661	2.3	2.9	3,862	6,479	396	400	7.2	5.5
Louisiana	628	0.4	11.1	5,468	8,393	399	448	7.2	6.0
Mississippi	446	0.1	0.4	4,189	7,389	423	425	7.4	6.2
North Carolina	1,240	0.5	4.5	3,465	6,726	314	366	8.0	5.7
South Carolina	627	0.1	0.3	3,777	6,573	319	367	8.3	6.2
Tennessee	894	0.3	7.7	4,441	6,891	375	397	7.1	5.6
Virginia	967	1.5	2.0	3,748	6,031	348	348	7.3	5.8
West Virginia	350	8.3	6.6	3,798	6,408	420	422	7.1	5.5
Southwest:									
Arizona	763	24.8	27.1	4,442	6,333	292	317	5.9	5.0
New Mexico	258	13.6	16.1	3,110	5,464	301	267	6.0	5.2
Oklahoma	530	2.5	7.8	4,098	7,241	355	419	7.0	5.4
Texas	2,458	4.1	7.1	4,703	7,915	333	382	7.2	5.7
Rocky Mountains:									
Colorado	507	17.2	26.9	3,935	6,466	302	306	6.0	5.0
Idaho	185	2.5	10.1	3,045	5,255	274	243	5.2	4.8
Montana	145	0.4	0.4	3,114	5,335	306	281	5.9	4.7
Utah	228	9.4	3.3	3,443	5,862	238	263	5.4	4.6
Wyoming	70	3.3	1.7	3,537	5,825	315	283	5.6	5.3

See footnotes at end of table.

Table 148 (page 2 of 2). Medicare enrollees, enrollees in managed care, payment per enrollee, and short-stay hospital utilization by geographic region and state: United States, 1994 and 2004

[Data are compiled by the Centers for Medicare & Medicaid Services]

Geographic division and state[1]	Enrollment in thousands[2]	Percent of enrollees in managed care[3]		Payment per fee-for-service enrollee		Short-stay hospital utilization: Discharges per 1,000 enrollees[4]		Short-stay hospital utilization: Average length of stay in days[4]	
	2004	1994	2004	1994	2004	1994	2004	1994	2004
Far West:									
Alaska	50	0.6	0.4	3,687	6,737	269	264	6.3	6.2
California	4,122	30.0	32.2	5,219	7,447	366	316	6.1	6.0
Hawaii	178	29.8	33.4	3,069	5,139	301	234	9.1	6.8
Nevada	287	19.0	28.8	4,306	7,089	291	302	7.0	6.1
Oregon	527	27.7	32.5	3,285	5,985	305	282	5.2	4.8
Washington	797	12.5	16.0	3,401	5,884	269	257	5.3	4.8

0.0 less than 0.05.
[1]Data are shown for Bureau of Economic Analysis (BEA) regions that are constructed to show economically interdependent states. These BEA geographic regions differ from U.S. Census Bureau geographic divisions shown in some *Health, United States* tables. See Appendix II, Geographic region and division.
[2]Total persons enrolled in hospital insurance, supplementary medical insurance, or both, as of July 1. Includes fee-for-service and managed care enrollees.
[3]Includes enrollees in Medicare-approved managed care organizations. See Appendix II, Managed care.
[4]Data are for fee-for-service enrollees only.
[5]Includes residents of any of the 50 states and the District of Columbia. Excludes Puerto Rico, Guam, Virgin Islands, residence unknown, foreign countries, and other outlying areas not shown separately.

NOTES: Prior to 2004, enrollment and percent of enrollees in managed care are based on a 5% annual Denominator File derived from the Centers for Medicare & Medicaid Services' (CMS') Enrollment Database. Starting with 2004 data, the 100% Denominator File was used. Payments per fee-for-service enrollee are based on fee-for-service billing reimbursement for a 5% sample of Medicare beneficiaries as recorded in CMS' National Claims History File. Short-stay hospital utilization is based on the Medicare Provider Analysis and Review (MEDPAR) stay records for a 20% sample of Medicare beneficiaries. Figures may not sum to totals due to rounding. Data for additional years are available. See Appendix III.

SOURCE: Centers for Medicare & Medicaid Services, Office of Research, Development, and Information. Health Care Financing Review: Medicare and Medicaid Statistical Supplements for publication years 1996 to 2006. Available from: www.cms.hhs.gov/MedicareMedicaidStatSupp/LT/list.asp.

Table 149 (page 1 of 2). Medicaid recipients, recipients in managed care, payments per recipient, and recipients per 100 persons below the poverty level, by geographic region and state: United States, selected fiscal years 1989–2004

[Data are compiled by the Centers for Medicare & Medicaid Services from the Medicaid Data System]

Geographic region and state[2]	*Recipients in thousands*		*Percent of recipients in managed care*		*Payments per recipient*[1]			*Recipients per 100 persons below the poverty level*	
	1996	*2004*	*1996*	*2004*	*1990*	*1996*	*2004*	*1989–1990*	*2003–2004*
United States	36,118	55,553	40	61	$2,568	$3,369	$4,639	75	147
New England:									
Connecticut	329	501	61	75	4,829	6,179	7,377	167	158
Maine	167	294	1	60	3,248	4,321	8,050	88	202
Massachusetts	715	1,074	70	61	4,622	5,285	7,240	103	170
New Hampshire	100	119	16	0	5,423	5,496	6,898	53	161
Rhode Island	130	208	63	69	3,778	5,280	7,374	163	169
Vermont	102	149	–	66	2,530	2,954	4,998	108	304
Mideast:									
Delaware	82	157	78	74	3,004	3,773	5,086	68	229
District of Columbia	143	158	55	64	2,629	4,955	8,052	86	171
Maryland	399	750	64	68	3,300	5,138	6,123	74	144
New Jersey	714	960	43	68	4,054	5,217	6,900	83	133
New York	3,281	4,712	23	58	5,099	6,811	7,910	95	165
Pennsylvania	1,168	1,835	53	79	2,449	3,993	5,481	88	134
Great Lakes:									
Illinois	1,454	2,032	13	9	2,271	3,689	5,314	69	123
Indiana	594	946	31	63	3,859	4,130	4,589	45	139
Michigan	1,172	1,799	73	89	2,094	2,867	4,278	85	139
Ohio	1,478	1,896	32	31	2,566	3,729	5,999	98	145
Wisconsin	434	896	32	47	3,179	4,384	4,812	95	143
Plains:									
Iowa	308	383	41	92	2,589	3,534	5,760	80	129
Kansas	251	365	32	57	2,524	3,425	5,095	71	115
Minnesota	455	698	33	64	3,709	5,342	6,555	70	187
Missouri	636	1,140	35	44	2,002	3,171	4,286	63	172
Nebraska	191	244	27	72	2,595	3,548	5,509	61	150
North Dakota	61	78	55	63	3,955	4,889	6,096	58	127
South Dakota	77	128	65	98	3,368	4,114	4,537	51	128
Southeast:									
Alabama	546	808	11	55	1,731	2,675	4,772	43	111
Arkansas	363	708	39	65	2,267	3,375	3,332	55	159
Florida	1,638	2,952	64	66	2,273	2,851	4,347	55	136
Georgia	1,185	1,929	32	96	3,190	2,604	3,600	64	171
Kentucky	641	861	53	92	2,089	3,014	4,560	81	130
Louisiana	778	1,108	6	79	2,247	3,154	3,645	58	141
Mississippi	510	726	7	12	1,354	2,633	4,564	67	145
North Carolina	1,130	1,513	37	71	2,531	3,255	4,884	66	116
South Carolina	503	857	1	8	2,343	3,026	4,686	52	152
Tennessee	1,409	2,205	100	100	1,896	2,049	3,149	67	223
Virginia	623	732	68	66	2,596	2,849	4,883	53	101
West Virginia	395	377	30	52	1,443	2,855	5,361	80	133
Southwest:									
Arizona	528	1,070	86	89	- - -	- - -	3,633	- - -	132
New Mexico	318	474	45	65	2,120	2,757	4,802	39	142
Oklahoma	358	654	19	68	2,516	2,852	3,572	56	157
Texas	2,572	3,604	4	43	1,928	2,672	3,667	47	94
Rocky Mountains:									
Colorado	271	503	80	98	2,705	3,815	4,765	45	109
Idaho	119	206	37	79	2,973	3,402	4,796	36	146
Montana	101	113	59	67	2,793	3,478	5,191	47	83
Utah	152	307	82	89	2,279	2,775	4,416	72	130
Wyoming	51	68	1	0	2,036	3,571	5,362	59	137

See footnotes at end of table.

Table 149 (page 2 of 2). Medicaid recipients, recipients in managed care, payments per recipient, and recipients per 100 persons below the poverty level, by geographic region and state: United States, selected fiscal years 1989–2004

[Data are compiled by the Centers for Medicare & Medicaid Services from the Medicaid Data System]

Geographic region and state[1]	Recipients in thousands		Percent of recipients in managed care		Payments per recipient[1]			Recipients per 100 persons below the poverty level	
	1996	2004	1996	2004	1990	1996	2004	1989–1990	2003–2004
Far West:									
Alaska	69	118	–	0	3,562	4,027	7,665	70	194
California	5,107	10,015	23	50	1,795	2,178	2,740	88	207
Hawaii	41	218	80	78	2,252	6,574	3,946	73	192
Nevada	109	237	41	53	3,161	3,361	3,399	37	91
Oregon	450	559	91	81	2,283	2,915	3,851	74	133
Washington	621	1,109	100	77	2,128	2,242	4,445	98	149

– Quantity zero.
- - - Data not available.
[1]Vendor payments exclude disproportionate share hospital (DSH) payments ($14.3 billion in FY2004) and DSH mental health facility payments ($2.9 billion in FY2004).
[2]Data are shown for Bureau of Economic Analysis (BEA) regions that are constructed to show economically interdependent states. These BEA geographic regions differ from U.S. Census Bureau geographic divisions shown in some *Health, United States* tables. See Appendix II, Geographic region and division.

NOTES: Starting with 1999 data, a new Medicaid data system was introduced. Prior to 1999, recipient counts exclude individuals who only received coverage under prepaid health care and for whom no direct vendor payments were made during the year, and vendor payments exclude payments to health maintenance organizations and other prepaid health plans ($19 billion in 1998). Data for additional years are available. See Appendix III.

SOURCES: Centers for Medicare & Medicaid Services, Office of Information Services, Enterprise Databases Group, Division of Information Distribution, Medicaid Data System. Before 1999, data are from Medicaid Statistical Report HCFA–2082. Starting with 1999, data are from Medicaid Statistical Information System, MSIS. MSIS data available from: msis.cms.hhs.gov (accessed May 22, 2007). Poverty populations are available from: Department of Commerce, U.S. Census Bureau, Housing and Household Economic Statistics Division. Available from: pubdb3.census.gov/macro/032005/pov/new46_100125_01.htm. Managed care enrollment available from 2004 Medicaid Managed Care Enrollment report. Available from: www.cms.hhs.gov/MedicaidDataSourcesGenInfo/Downloads/mmcer04.pdf.

Table 150 (page 1 of 2). Persons enrolled in health maintenance organizations (HMOs) by geographic region and state: United States, selected years 1980–2006

[Data are based on a census of health maintenance organizations]

Geographic region and state[1]	*2006*[2]	*1980*	*1985*	*1990*	*1995*	*1998*	*2000*	*2005*	*2006*[2]
	Number in thousands	Percent of population							
United States[3]	72,707	4.0	7.9	13.4	19.4	28.6	30.0	23.4	24.5
New England:									
Connecticut	1,098	2.4	7.1	19.9	21.2	42.9	44.6	36.1	31.3
Maine	358	0.4	0.3	2.6	7.0	19.1	22.3	25.9	27.1
Massachusetts	2,668	2.9	13.7	26.5	39.0	54.2	53.0	37.4	41.7
New Hampshire	126	1.2	5.6	9.6	18.5	33.8	33.7	21.9	9.6
Rhode Island	283	3.7	9.1	20.6	19.6	29.8	38.1	25.9	26.3
Vermont	97	–	–	6.4	12.5	–	4.6	16.1	15.6
Mideast:									
Delaware	190	–	3.9	17.5	18.4	48.1	22.0	10.1	22.5
District of Columbia[4]	- - -	- - -	- - -	- - -	- - -	33.0	35.2	42.2	- - -
Maryland[5]	1,598	2.0	4.8	14.2	29.5	43.6	43.9	28.0	28.5
New Jersey	2,190	2.0	5.6	12.3	14.7	31.3	30.9	25.0	25.1
New York	6,268	5.5	8.0	15.1	26.6	37.8	35.8	24.0	32.6
Pennsylvania	3,346	1.2	5.0	12.5	21.5	37.1	33.9	29.8	26.9
Great Lakes:									
Illinois	2,214	1.9	7.1	12.6	17.2	20.8	21.0	15.7	17.3
Indiana	1,408	0.5	3.6	6.1	8.3	14.0	12.4	22.5	22.4
Michigan	2,746	2.4	9.9	15.2	20.5	25.3	27.1	26.3	27.1
Ohio	2,039	2.2	6.7	13.3	16.3	23.4	25.1	16.4	17.8
Wisconsin	1,375	8.5	17.8	21.7	24.0	30.8	30.2	26.8	24.8
Plains:									
Iowa	177	0.2	4.8	10.1	4.5	4.9	7.4	10.9	6.0
Kansas	264	–	3.3	7.9	4.7	14.4	17.9	16.6	9.6
Minnesota	710	9.9	22.2	16.4	26.5	32.4	29.9	25.4	13.8
Missouri	1,441	2.3	6.0	8.2	18.5	33.7	35.2	24.6	24.8
Nebraska	166	1.1	1.8	5.1	8.6	16.9	11.2	5.3	9.5
North Dakota	2	0.4	2.5	1.7	1.2	2.2	2.5	0.4	0.3
South Dakota	65	–	–	3.3	2.8	5.1	6.7	7.9	8.4
Southeast:									
Alabama	146	0.3	0.9	5.3	7.3	10.8	7.2	2.8	3.2
Arkansas	101	–	0.1	2.2	3.8	10.7	10.4	6.4	3.6
Florida	4,284	1.5	5.6	10.6	18.8	31.5	31.4	26.1	24.1
Georgia	1,952	0.1	2.9	4.8	7.6	15.5	17.4	16.4	21.5
Kentucky	310	0.9	1.6	5.7	16.1	35.1	31.5	10.2	7.4
Louisiana	460	0.6	0.9	5.4	7.2	16.6	17.0	10.7	10.2
Mississippi	12	–	–	–	0.7	3.6	1.1	0.1	0.4
North Carolina	742	0.6	1.6	4.8	8.3	17.1	17.8	10.5	8.5
South Carolina	321	0.2	1.0	1.9	5.5	9.9	9.9	7.1	7.5
Tennessee	1,701	–	1.8	3.7	12.2	24.1	33.0	14.4	28.5
Virginia[5]	1,084	–	1.1	6.1	7.7	16.9	18.5	22.2	14.3
West Virginia[5]	264	0.7	1.7	3.9	5.8	10.7	10.3	8.1	14.5
Southwest:									
Arizona	1,757	6.0	10.3	16.2	25.8	30.3	30.9	16.4	29.6
New Mexico	516	1.4	2.0	12.7	15.1	32.3	37.7	24.3	26.8
Oklahoma	248	–	2.1	5.5	7.6	13.8	14.7	7.1	7.0
Texas	2,960	0.6	3.4	6.9	12.0	17.8	18.5	11.8	12.9
Rocky Mountains:									
Colorado	1,298	6.9	10.8	20.0	23.3	36.4	39.5	25.6	27.8
Idaho	40	1.2	–	1.8	1.4	5.7	7.9	2.9	2.8
Montana	32	–	–	1.0	2.4	3.9	7.0	8.1	3.4
Utah	684	0.6	8.8	13.9	25.1	35.6	35.3	21.3	27.7
Wyoming	12	–	–	–	–	0.7	1.4	2.1	2.3
Far West:									
Alaska	–	–	–	–	–	–	–	–	–
California	17,930	16.8	22.5	30.7	36.0	47.1	53.5	49.1	49.6
Hawaii	582	15.3	18.1	21.6	21.0	32.8	30.0	37.4	45.7
Nevada	627	–	5.8	8.5	15.9	26.8	23.5	25.2	26.0
Oregon	1,071	12.0	14.0	24.7	40.0	45.3	41.1	16.2	29.4
Washington	1,102	9.4	8.7	14.6	18.7	26.3	15.2	18.1	17.5

See footnotes at end of table.

Table 150 (page 2 of 2). Persons enrolled in health maintenance organizations (HMOs) by geographic region and state: United States, selected years 1980–2006

[Data are based on a census of health maintenance organizations]

– Quantity less than 1,000 for number of persons and 0.02 for percent.
- - - Data not available.
[1]Data are shown for Bureau of Economic Analysis (BEA) regions that are constructed to show economically interdependent states. These BEA geographic regions differ from the U.S. Census Bureau geographic regions and divisions shown in some *Health, United States* tables. See Appendix II, Geographic region and division.
[2]Starting with 2006 data, all managed health plans offering Medicaid products, whether licensed as HMOs or not, are included in these data. Starting with 2006 data, enrollment data for Medicare HMOs are limited to Medicare Advantage HMO plans. Previously, some other types of Medicare plans were included in the enrollment data for certain plans.
[3]HMOs in Guam are included starting in 1994; HMOs in Puerto Rico are included starting in 1998.
[4]Data for the District of Columbia (DC) not included for 1980–1996 because data not adjusted for high proportion of enrollees of DC-based HMOs living in Maryland and Virginia.
[5]Includes partial enrollment for five plans serving the District of Columbia.

NOTES: Data are for midyear prior to 1990 and in 2006 and as of January 1 in all other years. Data for 1980–1990 are for pure HMO enrollment. Starting with 1994 data, pure and open-ended enrollment are included. In 1990, open-ended enrollment accounted for 3% of HMO enrollment compared with 12.5% in 2006. In 2005, 3,366 thousand enrollees in Cigna's Flexcare product were added to open-ended enrollment. Without this addition, total HMO enrollment would have continued slowly decreasing. See Appendix II, Health maintenance organization (HMO). Data for additional years are available. See Appendix III.

SOURCE: HealthLeaders-InterStudy National Health Maintenance Organization Census. HealthLeaders-InterStudy. The Competitive Edge: Part II: Managed Care Industry Report. Nashville, TN: HealthLeaders-InterStudy, 2007 and previous editions. InterStudy. The InterStudy Edge, Managed care: A decade in review 1980–1990. Excelsior, MN: InterStudy, 1991. (Copyrights 1991, 1995–2007: Used with the permission of HealthLeaders-InterStudy.)

Table 151. Persons without health insurance coverage by state: United States, average annual 1995–1997 through 2003–2005

[Data are based on household interviews of a sample of the civilian noninstitutionalized population]

Geographic region and state[1]	*1995–1997*	*1998–2000*	*2001–2003*	*2003–2005*
	Percent of population			
United States	15.7	14.4	15.1	15.7
New England:				
Connecticut	10.6	9.5	10.4	11.0
Maine	13.5	11.5	10.7	10.4
Massachusetts	12.0	9.2	9.6	10.7
New Hampshire	10.4	8.6	9.9	10.4
Rhode Island	11.0	6.9	9.3	11.0
Vermont	11.3	10.3	9.9	10.7
Mideast:				
Delaware	14.1	11.2	10.1	12.7
District of Columbia	16.1	14.5	13.3	13.5
Maryland	13.4	11.9	13.2	14.1
New Jersey	15.8	12.9	13.7	14.5
New York	16.6	15.3	15.5	13.9
Pennsylvania	9.8	8.3	10.7	11.2
Great Lakes:				
Illinois	11.6	13.3	14.0	14.2
Indiana	11.5	11.3	12.9	14.2
Michigan	10.1	10.6	11.0	11.3
Ohio	11.6	10.2	11.7	12.0
Wisconsin	7.9	9.3	9.5	10.3
Plains:				
Iowa	11.6	8.2	9.5	9.8
Kansas	11.8	11.0	10.9	10.9
Minnesota	9.1	8.2	8.2	8.7
Missouri	13.5	9.0	10.9	11.9
Nebraska	10.4	9.5	10.3	11.4
North Dakota	11.1	12.1	10.5	11.2
South Dakota	10.2	12.0	11.0	12.1
Southeast:				
Alabama	14.0	14.2	13.3	14.3
Arkansas	21.3	15.3	16.6	17.2
Florida	18.9	17.2	17.6	19.6
Georgia	17.8	15.2	16.4	17.5
Kentucky	15.0	13.1	13.3	13.6
Louisiana	18.8	19.5	19.4	18.7
Mississippi	19.4	15.7	17.0	17.3
North Carolina	15.3	13.7	16.1	16.2
South Carolina	16.2	13.8	13.1	15.6
Tennessee	14.5	10.8	11.8	13.7
Virginia	12.9	12.9	12.5	13.6
West Virginia	15.8	15.2	14.8	16.9
Southwest:				
Arizona	23.0	19.5	17.3	18.1
New Mexico	23.5	22.6	21.3	21.1
Oklahoma	18.0	17.7	18.7	19.5
Texas	24.4	22.2	24.6	24.6
Rocky Mountains:				
Colorado	15.5	14.1	16.3	16.9
Idaho	16.1	16.5	17.5	16.5
Montana	15.3	18.3	16.1	18.7
Utah	12.4	13.2	13.6	14.5
Wyoming	15.0	15.1	16.5	15.2
Far West:				
Alaska	14.7	18.1	17.8	17.8
California	20.7	19.2	18.7	18.8
Hawaii	8.3	9.8	9.9	9.5
Nevada	17.3	17.5	18.3	18.4
Oregon	13.7	13.7	14.8	16.7
Washington	12.4	12.8	14.3	14.1

[1]Data are shown for Bureau of Economic Analysis (BEA) regions that are constructed to show economically interdependent states. These BEA geographic regions differ from U.S. Census Bureau geographic divisions shown in some *Health, United States* tables. See Appendix II, Geographic region and division.

NOTES: Starting with 1997 data, people with no coverage other than access to the Indian Health Service are no longer considered covered by health insurance. The effect of this change on the estimate of number uninsured is negligible. Starting with 1999 data, estimates reflect the results of follow-up verification questions which decreased the percent uninsured by 1.2 percentage points. See Appendix I, Current Population Survey.

SOURCES: U.S. Census Bureau, Current Population Survey, DeNavas-Walt C, Proctor BD, Lee CH. Income, Poverty, and Health Insurance Coverage in the United States: 2005. Current population reports, series P–60 no 231. Washington, DC: U.S. Government Printing Office, 2006. This report and reports from earlier years available from: www.census.gov/hhes/www/hlthins/reports.html.

Appendixes

Appendix Contents

Appendix I—Data Sources **433**

Government Sources **434**

Abortion Surveillance 434
AIDS Surveillance 435
Annual Survey and Census of Jails 436
Area Resource File 436
Census of Fatal Occupational Injuries (CFOI) 437
Consumer Price Index (CPI) 438
Current Population Survey (CPS) 439
Department of Veterans Affairs National Patient Care Database and National Enrollment Database 440
Employee Benefits Survey—See National Compensation Survey.
Medicaid Data System 441
Medical Expenditure Panel Survey (MEPS) 442
Medicare Administrative Data 443
Medicare Current Beneficiary Survey (MCBS) 444
Monitoring the Future Study (MTF) 445
National Ambulatory Medical Care Survey (NAMCS) 446
National Compensation Survey 447
National Health Expenditure Accounts 449
National Health and Nutrition Examination Survey (NHANES) 450
National Health Interview Survey (NHIS) 453
National Hospital Ambulatory Medical Care Survey (NHAMCS) 454
National Hospital Discharge Survey (NHDS) 455
National Immunization Survey (NIS) 457
National Medical Expenditure Survey (NMES)—See Medical Expenditure Panel Survey.
National Notifiable Disease Surveillance System (NNDSS) 458
National Nursing Home Survey (NNHS) 459
National Prisoner Statistics (NPS) 461
National Survey on Drug Use & Health (NSDUH) 461
National Survey of Family Growth (NSFG) 463
National Vital Statistics System (NVSS) 464
  Birth File 465
  Mortality File 465
  Multiple Cause-of-Death File 466
  Linked Birth/Infant Death Data Set 467
  Compressed Mortality File 468
Occupational Employment Statistics (OES) 468
Online Survey Certification and Reporting Database (OSCAR) 469
Organ Procurement and Transplantation Network (OPTN) 470
Population Census and Population Estimates 471
  Decennial Census 471
  Race Data on the 1990 Census 471
  Race Data on the 2000 Census 471
  Modified Decennial Census Files 471
  Bridged-Race Population Estimates for Census 2000 472
  Postcensal Population Estimates 472
  Intercensal Population Estimates 473
  Special Population Estimates 473
Sexually Transmitted Disease (STD) Surveillance 474
Surveillance, Epidemiology, and End Results Program (SEER) 474
Survey of Mental Health Organizations (SMHO) 475
Survey of Occupational Injuries and Illnesses (SOII) 476
Youth Risk Behavior Survey (YRBS) 477

Private and Global Sources **478**

Alan Guttmacher Institute Abortion Provider Survey 478
American Association of Colleges of Osteopathic Medicine 479
American Association of Colleges of Pharmacy 479
American Association of Colleges of Podiatric Medicine 480
American Dental Association 480
American Hospital Association Annual Survey of Hospitals 480
American Medical Association Physician Masterfile 480
American Osteopathic Association 480
Association of American Medical Colleges 481
Association of Schools and Colleges of Optometry 481
Association of Schools of Public Health 481
Computed Tomography (CT) and Magnetic Resonance Imaging (MRI) Census 481
European Health for All Database 481
HealthLeaders-InterStudy National Health Maintenance Organization Census 482
National League for Nursing 482
Organisation for Economic Co-operation and Development Health Data 482
United Nations Demographic Yearbook 483
World Health Organization Statistical Information System (WHOSIS) 483

Appendix II—Definitions and Methods **484**

Acquired immunodeficiency syndrome (AIDS) 484
Active physician—See Physician.
Activities of daily living (ADL) 484
Addition—See Admission.
Admission 485
Age 485
Age adjustment 486
AIDS—See Acquired immunodeficiency syndrome.
Alcohol consumption 487
Any-listed diagnosis—See Diagnosis.
Average annual rate of change (percentage change) 488
Average length of stay 488
Bed, health facility 488
Binge drinking 489
Birth cohort 489
Birth rate—See Rate: Birth and related rates.
Birthweight 489
Blood pressure, elevated 489
Body mass index (BMI) 490
Cause of death 490
Cause-of-death ranking 490
Cholesterol, serum 491
Chronic condition—See Condition.
Cigarette smoking 493
Civilian noninstitutionalized population; Civilian population—See Population.
Community hospital—See Hospital.
Comparability ratio 494
Compensation—See Employer costs for employee compensation.
Computed tomography scanner 495
Condition 495
Consumer Price Index (CPI) 496
Contraception 496
Crude birth rate; Crude death rate—See Rate: Birth and related rates; Rate: Death and related rates.
Days of care 496
Death rate—See Rate: Death and related rates.
Dental caries 496
Dental visit 496
Diagnosis 497
Diagnostic and other nonsurgical procedure—See Procedure.
Discharge 497
Domiciliary care home—See Long-term care facility; Nursing home.
Drug abuse—See Illicit drug use.
Drug 497

Education 498
Emergency department 500
Emergency department or emergency room visit 500
Employer costs for employee compensation 500
Ethnicity—See Hispanic origin.
Exercise—See Physical activity, leisure-time.
Expenditures—See Health expenditures, national; Appendix I, National Health Accounts.
External cause of injury 500
Family income 500
Federal hospital—See Hospital.
Fee-for-service health insurance 501
Fertility rate—See Rate: Birth and related rates.
Foreign-born population 501
General hospital—See Hospital.
General hospital providing separate psychiatric services—See Mental health organization.
Geographic region and division 502
Gestation 502
Gross domestic product (GDP) 502
Health care contact 502
Health expenditures, national 503
Health insurance coverage 504
Health maintenance organization (HMO) 505
Health services and supplies expenditures—See Health expenditures, national.
Health status, respondent-assessed 506
Hispanic origin 506
HIV—See Human immunodeficiency virus (HIV) disease.
Home visit 507
Hospital 508
Hospital-based physician—See Physician.
Hospital day—See Days of care.
Hospital utilization 508
Human immunodeficiency virus (HIV) disease 509
Hypertension—See Blood pressure, elevated.
ICD; ICD codes—See Cause of death; *International Classification of Diseases* (ICD).
Illicit drug use 509
Incidence 510
Income—See Family income.
Individual practice association (IPA)—See Health maintenance organization (HMO).
Industry of employment 510
Infant death 510
Injury 510
Injury-related visit 511
Inpatient 511

Inpatient care—See Hospital utilization; Mental health service type.
Inpatient day—See Days of care.
Instrumental activities of daily living (IADL) 511
Insurance—See Health insurance coverage.
Intermediate care facility—See Nursing home.
International Classification of Diseases (ICD) 511
International Classification of Diseases, Ninth Revision, Clinical Modification (ICD–9–CM) 511
Late fetal death rate—See Rate: Death and related rates.
Leading causes of death—See Cause-of-death ranking.
Length of stay—See Average length of stay.
Life expectancy 513
Limitation of activity 513
Long-term care facility 513
Low birthweight—See Birthweight.
Magnetic resonance imaging (MRI) unit 513
Mammography 513
Managed care 514
Marital status 515
Maternal age—See Age.
Maternal death 516
Maternal education—See Education.
Maternal mortality rate—See Rate: Death and related rates.
Medicaid 516
Medical specialty—See Physician specialty.
Medical vendor payments 517
Medicare 517
Mental health organization 517
Mental health service type 518
Metropolitan statistical area (MSA) 518
Micropolitan statistical area 519
Multiservice mental health organization—See Mental health organization.
National Drug Code (NDC) Directory therapeutic class 519
Neonatal mortality rate—See Rate: Death and related rates.
Nonprofit hospital—See Hospital.
North American Industry Classification System (NAICS)—See Industry of employment.
Notifiable disease 520
Nursing home 520
Nursing home expenditures—See Health expenditures, national.
Obesity—See Body mass index (BMI).
Occupancy rate 522
Office-based physician—See Physician.
Office visit 522
Operation—See Procedure.
Outpatient department 522
Outpatient surgery 523
Outpatient visit 523
Overweight—See Body mass index (BMI).
Pap smear 523
Partial care organization—See Mental health organization.
Partial care treatment—See Mental health service type.
Patient—See Inpatient; Office visit; Outpatient visit.
Percent change/percentage change—See Average annual rate of change.
Perinatal mortality rate; ratio—See Rate: Death and related rates.
Personal care home with or without nursing—See Nursing home.
Personal health care expenditures—See Health expenditures, national.
Physical activity, leisure-time 524
Physician 524
Physician specialty 524
Population 525
Postneonatal mortality rate—See Rate: Death and related rates.
Poverty 526
Preferred provider organization (PPO) 526
Prenatal care 526
Prevalence 526
Primary care specialty—See Physician specialty.
Private expenditures—See Health expenditures, national.
Procedure 526
Proprietary hospital—See Hospital.
Psychiatric hospital—See Hospital; Mental health organization.
Public expenditures—See Health expenditures, national.
Purchasing power parities 527
Race 527
Rate 532
Region—See Geographic region and division.
Registered hospital—See Hospital.
Registration area 534
Relative standard error 534
Relative survival rate 534
Reporting area 534
Resident, health facility 534
Resident population—See Population.
Residential treatment care—See Mental health service type.

Residential treatment center for emotionally disturbed children—See Mental health organization.
Rural—See Urbanization.
Self-assessment of health—See Health status, respondent-assessed.
Serious psychological distress 534
Short-stay hospital—See Hospital.
Skilled nursing facility—See Nursing home.
Smoker—See Cigarette smoking.
Specialty hospital—See Hospital.
State Children's Health Insurance Program (SCHIP) 535
State mental health agency 535
Substance use 535
Suicidal ideation 536
Surgery—See Outpatient surgery; Procedure.
Surgical specialty—See Physician specialty.
Tobacco use—See Cigarette smoking.
Uninsured 536
Urbanization 536
Usual source of care 536
Wages and salaries—See Employer costs for employee compensation.
Years of potential life lost (YPLL). 537

Appendix II: Tables

I. United States standard population and age groups used to age adjust data. 485
II. United States standard population and proportion distribution by age, for age adjusting death rates prior to 2003 487
III. Numbers of live births and mother's age groups used to adjust maternal mortality rates to live births in the United States in 1970 488
IV. Revision of the *International Classification of Diseases (ICD)* by year of conference by which adopted and years in use in the United States. 491
V. Cause-of-death codes, by applicable revision of *International Classification of Diseases (ICD)* 492
VI. Comparability of selected causes of death between the Ninth and Tenth Revisions of the *International Classification of Diseases (ICD)*. 495
VII. Codes for first-listed external causes of injury from the *International Classification of Diseases, Ninth Revision, Clinical Modification*. 511
VIII. Percentage of persons under 65 years of age with Medicaid or who are uninsured, by selected demographic characteristics using Method 1 and Method 2 estimation procedures: United States, 2004 512
IX. Codes for industries, by the 2002 North American Industry Classification System (NAICS). 513
X. Codes for diagnostic categories from the *International Classification of Diseases, Ninth Revision, Clinical Modification*. 514
XI. Codes for procedure categories from the *International Classification of Diseases, Ninth Revision, Clinical Modification*. 520
XII. National Drug Code (NDC) therapeutic class analgesic drug recodes 521
XIII. Current cigarette smoking among persons 18 years of age and over, by race and Hispanic origin under the 1997 and 1977 Standards for federal data on race and ethnicity: United States, average annual 1993–1995 529
XIV. Private health care coverage among persons under 65 years of age, by race and Hispanic origin under the 1997 and 1977 Standards for federal data on race and ethnicity: United States, average annual 1993–1995 530

Appendix II: Figures

I. Census Bureau: Four Geographic Regions and 9 Divisions of the United States 502
II. Bureau of Economic Analysis: Eight Geographic Regions of the United States 503

Appendix III: Additional data years available . . . 538

Index to Trend Tables 541

Appendix I

Data Sources

Health, United States consolidates the most current data on the health of the population of the United States, the availability and use of health resources, and health care expenditures. Information was obtained from data files and published reports of many federal government and private and global agencies and organizations. In each case, the sponsoring agency or organization collected data using its own methods and procedures. Therefore, data in this report vary considerably with respect to source, method of collection, definitions, and reference period.

Although a detailed description and comprehensive evaluation of each data source are beyond the scope of this Appendix, users should be aware of the general strengths and weaknesses of the different data collection systems. For example, population-based surveys obtain socioeconomic data, data on family characteristics, and information on the impact of an illness, such as days lost from work or limitation of activity. These data are limited by the amount of information a respondent remembers or is willing to report. A respondent may not know detailed medical information, such as precise diagnoses or the types of operations performed, and therefore cannot report it. In contrast, record-based surveys, which collect data from physician and hospital records, usually have good diagnostic information but little or no information about the socioeconomic characteristics of individuals or the impact of illnesses on individuals.

The populations covered by different data collection systems may not be the same, and understanding the differences is critical to interpreting the data. Data on vital statistics and national expenditures cover the entire population. Most data on morbidity and utilization of health resources cover only the civilian noninstitutionalized population. Such statistics may not include data for military personnel, who are usually young; for institutionalized people including the prison population, who may be any age; or for nursing home residents, who are usually old.

All data collection systems are subject to error, and records may be incomplete or contain inaccurate information. Respondents may not remember essential information, a question may not mean the same thing to different respondents, and some institutions or individuals may not respond at all. It is not always possible to measure the magnitude of these errors or their effect on the data. Where possible, table notes describe the universe and method of data collection to assist users in evaluating data quality.

Some information is collected in more than one survey, and estimates of the same statistic may vary among surveys because of different survey methodologies, sampling frames, questionnaires, definitions, and tabulation categories. For example, cigarette use is measured by the National Health Interview Survey, the National Survey on Drug Use & Health, the Monitoring the Future Survey, and the Youth Risk Behavior Survey. These surveys use slightly different questions of persons of differing ages and interview in different settings (at school compared with at home), so estimates will differ.

Overall estimates generally have relatively small sampling errors, but estimates for certain population subgroups may be based on a small sample size and have relatively large sampling errors. Numbers of births and deaths from the vital statistics system represent complete counts (except for births in those states where data are based on a 50% sample for certain years). Therefore, they are not subject to sampling error. However, when the figures are used for analytical purposes, such as the comparison of rates over a period, the number of events that actually occurred may be considered as one of a large series of possible results that could have arisen under the same circumstances. When the number of events is small and the probability of such an event is rare, estimates may be unstable and considerable caution must be observed in interpreting the statistics. Estimates that are unreliable because of large sampling errors or small numbers of events are noted with asterisks in selected tables. The criteria used to designate unreliable estimates are indicated in notes to the applicable tables.

Government data sources are listed alphabetically by data set name; private and global sources are listed separately. To the extent possible, government data systems are described using a standard format. The overview is a brief, general statement about the purpose or objectives of the data system. The selected content section lists major data elements that are collected or estimated using interpolation or modeling. The data years section gives the years that the survey or data system has existed or been fielded. The coverage section describes the population that the data system represents; for example, residents of the United States, the noninstitutionalized population, persons in specific population groups, or other entities that comprise the survey. The methodology section presents a short description of methods used to collect data. Sample size and response rates are given for surveys. Issues affecting interpretation section describes major changes in the data collection methodology or other factors that must be considered when analyzing trends—for example, a major survey redesign that may introduce a discontinuity in the trend. For more information about the methodology, data files, and history of a data source, consult the references and websites at the end of each summary.

Government Sources

Abortion Surveillance

Centers for Disease Control and Prevention National Center for Chronic Disease Prevention and Health Promotion

Overview: The abortion surveillance program documents the number and characteristics of women obtaining legal induced abortions, monitors unintended pregnancy, and assists efforts to identify and reduce preventable causes of morbidity and mortality associated with abortions.

Selected Content: Content includes age, race/ethnicity, marital status, previous live births, period of gestation, and previous induced abortions of women obtaining legal induced abortions.

Data Years: Between 1973 and 1997, the number of abortions is based on reporting from 52 reporting areas: 50 states, the District of Columbia, and New York City. In 1998 and 1999, the Centers for Disease Control and Prevention (CDC) compiled abortion data from 48 reporting areas. Alaska, California, New Hampshire, and Oklahoma did not report, and data for these areas were not estimated. In 2000–2004, CDC compiled data from 49 reporting areas. Alaska, California, and New Hampshire did not report abortion data to CDC in 2000, 2001, and 2002. In 2003, California, New Hampshire, and West Virginia did not report.

Coverage: The system includes women of all ages, including adolescents, who obtain legal induced abortions.

Methodology: Starting with 2000 data, the number and characteristics of women who obtain legal induced abortions are provided for 49 reporting areas by central health agencies, such as state health departments and the health departments of New York City and the District of Columbia, and by hospitals and other medical facilities. In general, the procedures are reported by the state in which the procedure is performed (i.e., state of occurrence). Although the total number of legal induced abortions is available for those 49 reporting areas, not all areas collect information on the characteristics of women who obtain abortions. The number of areas reporting each characteristic and the number of areas with complete data for each characteristic vary from year to year. For example, in 2003, the number of areas reporting different women's characteristics ranged from 29 areas reporting Hispanic ethnicity, 35 areas reporting race, and 38 areas reporting marital status, to 48 areas reporting age. Data from reporting areas with more than 15% unknown for a given characteristic are excluded from the analysis of that characteristic.

Issues Affecting Interpretation: Between 1989 and 1997, the total number of abortions reported to CDC was about 10% less than the total estimated independently by the Alan Guttmacher Institute (AGI), a not-for-profit organization for reproductive health research, policy analysis, and public education. Between 1998 and 2003, the total number of abortions reported to CDC was about 34% less than the total estimated by AGI. The four reporting areas (the largest of which was California) that did not report abortions to CDC in 1998 accounted for 18% of all abortions tallied by AGI's 1995–1996 survey. See Appendix I, Alan Guttmacher Institute Abortion Provider Survey.

Reference:

Abortion Surveillance—United States, 2003. Centers for Disease Control and Prevention, CDC MMWR Surveillance Summaries, November 24, 2006. MMWR 2006;55(SS11):1–32. Available from: www.cdc.gov/mmwr/preview/mmwrhtml/ss5511a1.htm.

For More Information: See the NCCDPHP surveillance and research website: www.cdc.gov/reproductivehealth/Data_Stats/index.htm.

AIDS Surveillance

Centers for Disease Control and Prevention National Center for HIV, STD, and TB Prevention

Overview: Acquired immunodeficiency syndrome (AIDS) surveillance data are used to detect and monitor cases of human immunodeficiency virus (HIV) disease and AIDS in the United States, identify epidemiologic trends, identify unusual cases requiring follow-up, and inform public health efforts to prevent and control the disease.

Selected Content: Data collected on cases diagnosed with AIDS include age, sex, race/ethnicity, mode of exposure, and geographic region.

Data Years: Reports on AIDS cases are available from the beginning of the epidemic that began in 1981.

Coverage: All 50 states, the District of Columbia (D.C.), U.S. dependencies and possessions, and independent nations in free association with the United States report AIDS cases to CDC using a uniform surveillance case definition and case report form.

Methodology: AIDS surveillance is conducted by health departments in each state or territory and D.C. Although surveillance activities range from passive to active, most areas employ multifaceted active surveillance programs, which include four major reporting sources of AIDS information: hospitals and hospital-based physicians, physicians in nonhospital practice, public and private clinics, and medical record systems (death certificates, tumor registries, hospital discharge abstracts, and communicable disease reports). Using a standard confidential case report form, the health departments collect information that is then transmitted electronically without personal identifiers to CDC.

Adjustments of the estimated data on HIV infection (not AIDS) and on AIDS to account for reporting delays are calculated by a maximum likelihood statistical procedure that takes into account the differences in reporting delays among exposure, geographic, racial/ethnic, age, sex, and vital status categories and is based on the assumption that reporting delays in these categories have not changed over time. AIDS surveillance data are provisional and are updated annually.

Issues Affecting Interpretation: Although completeness of reporting of AIDS cases to state and local health departments differs by geographic region and patient population, studies conducted by state and local health departments indicate that the reporting of AIDS cases in most areas of the United States is more than 85% complete. To assess trends in AIDS cases, deaths, and prevalence, it is preferable to use case data adjusted for reporting delays and presented by year of diagnosis instead of straight counts of cases presented by year of report.

The definition of AIDS was modified in 1985 and 1987. The case definition for adults and adolescents was modified again in 1993. The revisions incorporated a broader range of AIDS-indicator diseases and conditions and used HIV diagnostic tests to improve the sensitivity and specificity of the definition. Laboratory and diagnostic criteria for the 1987 pediatric case definition were updated in 1994. Effective January 2000, the surveillance case definition for HIV infection was revised to reflect advances in laboratory HIV virologic tests. The definition incorporates the reporting criteria for HIV infection and AIDS into a single case definition for adults and children.

Decreases in AIDS incidence and in the number of AIDS deaths, first noted in 1996, have been ascribed to the effect of new treatments, which prevent or delay the onset of AIDS and premature death among HIV-infected persons and result in an increase in the number of persons living with HIV and AIDS. A growing number of states require confidential reporting of persons with HIV infection and participate in CDC's integrated HIV/AIDS surveillance system that compiles information on the population of persons newly diagnosed and living with HIV infection.

Reference:

Centers for Disease Control and Prevention, HIV/AIDS Surveillance Report, published annually. Available from: www.cdc.gov/hiv/topics/surveillance/resources/reports/index.htm.

For More Information: See the NCHSTP website: www.cdc.gov/nchstp/od/nchstp.html.

Annual Survey and Census of Jails

Bureau of Justice Statistics

Overview: The number of jail inmates is determined by a periodic census of jails and a survey of jails in the intervening years. The Census of Jails is taken every 5 to 6 years. In years between the census, the Annual Survey of Jails is conducted. The census and survey provide estimates of the characteristics of U.S. jails and the inmates they house.

Selected Content: Data are supplied on facility characteristics, staffing, inmate deaths, jail programs, admissions and releases, number of inmates held, and inmate characteristics. Inmate characteristics collected include number of adult and juvenile inmates, conviction status, sex, and race and ethnicity.

Data Years: The first census of jails was conducted in 1970; the annual survey has been conducted every year since 1982, except for years in which the Census of Jails is conducted. Data are requested for activities as of June 30 of the reference year.

Coverage: Data are collected on local jails, multijurisdiction (regional) jails, and privately contracted jails in all 50 states and the District of Columbia.

Methodology: Local jails are locally operated correctional facilities that confine persons before or after adjudication. Inmates sentenced to jails usually have a sentence of a year or less. The census is based on a facility list maintained by the U.S. Census Bureau. For the Annual Survey of Jails, there have been minor changes in the sample selection over time. For more recent surveys, all multijurisdictional jails (jails operated jointly by two or more jurisdictions) were included in the sample. Other jurisdictions were included automatically in the sample if their jails held juvenile inmates and had an average daily population of 250 or more inmates, or housed only adults and had an average daily population of 500 or more, based on the most recent census. The remaining jurisdictions were stratified into two groups: jurisdictions with jails holding at least one juvenile at last census, and jurisdictions with jails holding adults only. Using stratified probability sampling, jurisdictions were then selected from 10 strata based on the average daily population in the 1999 census. All surveys prior to the 1994 survey were based on all jails in jurisdictions with 100 or more jail inmates and a stratified random sample of jurisdictions with an average daily population of fewer than 100 inmates.

Sample Size and Response Rate: Data were obtained by mailed and Web-based survey questionnaires. After follow-up phone calls, the response rates for most years approach 100% for critical items such as rated capacity, average daily population, and number of inmates confined.

Reference:

Pastore AL, Maguire K, editors. Sourcebook of Criminal Justice Statistics [Online]. Available from: www.albany.edu/sourcebook/app4.html.

For More Information: See the Bureau of Justice Statistics website: www.ojp.usdoj.gov/bjs/correct.htm.

Area Resource File

Health Resources and Services Administration

Overview: The Area Resource File (ARF) is a data set comprised of data collected from more than 50 sources and contains more than 6,000 variables related to health care access at the county level.

Selected Content: The ARF includes information on geographic codes and classifications; health professions supply and demographics; health facility numbers and types; hospital utilization; population characteristics and economic data; land use and housing density; and health professions training resources.

Data Years: The ARF is released annually and has been maintained since the mid-1970s. The 2005 file primarily contains data from 1980 to 2004 but some fields have information dating back to 1950. Historical versions of the file can be purchased.

Coverage: The ARF includes one record for each county and independent city in the United States and one for each county equivalent in the U.S. territories Guam, Puerto Rico, and the Virgin Islands. The criteria for data to be included on the ARF are: 1) that the data be available for all or nearly all counties in the United States 2) that the data be accurate, 3) that the data be current or part of a useful time-series, and 4) that the data be potentially useful for the analysis of health occupation supply and requirements.

Expansion and maintenance of the ARF is performed on a continuing basis. The file is routinely expanded to incorporate additional variables deemed to be useful to health researchers and other users.

Methodology: The ARF integrates data from numerous data sources including: the American Hospital Association, the American Medical Association, the U.S. Census Bureau, the Centers for Medicare & Medicaid Services, Bureau of Labor Statistics, HealthLeaders-InterStudy, and the Veteran's Administration.

For More Information: See the Area Resource File website: www.arfsys.com/.

Census of Fatal Occupational Injuries (CFOI)

Bureau of Labor Statistics

Overview: The Census of Fatal Occupational Injuries (CFOI) compiles comprehensive and timely information on fatal work injuries occurring in the 50 states and the District of Columbia (D.C.) to monitor workplace safety and to inform private and public health efforts to improve workplace safety.

Selected Content: Information is collected about each workplace fatality, including occupation and other worker characteristics, equipment involved, and circumstances of the event.

Data Years: Data have been collected annually since 1992.

Coverage: The data cover all 50 states and D.C.

Methodology: CFOI is administered by the Bureau of Labor Statistics (BLS) in conjunction with participating state agencies to compile counts that are as complete as possible to identify, verify, and profile fatal work injuries. Key information about each workplace fatality (occupation and other worker characteristics, equipment or machinery involved, and circumstances of the event) is obtained by cross-referencing source records. For a fatality to be included in the census, the decedent must have been employed (that is, working for pay, compensation, or profit) at the time of the event, engaged in a legal work activity, or present at the site of the incident as a requirement of his or her job. These criteria are generally broader than those used by federal and state agencies administering specific laws and regulations. Fatalities that occur during a person's commute to or from work are excluded from the census counts.

Data for the CFOI are compiled from various federal, state, and local administrative sources including death certificates, workers' compensation reports and claims, reports to various regulatory agencies, medical examiner reports, police reports, and news reports. Diverse sources are used because studies have shown that no single source captures all job-related fatalities. Source documents are matched so that each fatality is counted only once. To ensure that a fatality occurred while the decedent was at work, information is verified from two or more independent source documents or from a source document and a follow-up questionnaire.

Issues Affecting Interpretation: The number of occupational fatalities and fatality rates are periodically revised. States have up to 1 year to update their initial published state counts. States may identify additional fatal work injuries after data collection has closed for a reference year. Fatalities initially excluded from the published count because of insufficient information to determine work relationship may subsequently be verified as work related and were included. Increases in the published counts based on additional information have averaged less than 100 fatalities per year, or less than 1.5% of the total.

Beginning with 2003 data, CFOI began using the 2002 North American Industry Classification System (NAICS) to classify industries. Prior to 2003, the program used the Standard Industrial Classification (SIC) system and the U.S. Census Bureau occupational classification system. Although some titles in SIC and NAICS are similar, there is limited comparability between the two systems because the industry groupings are defined differently. See Appendix II, Industry of employment.

Reference:

Bureau of Labor Statistics. National Census of Fatal Occupational Injuries in 2005. Washington, DC: U.S. Department of Labor, August 2006.

For More Information: See the CFOI website: www.bls.gov/iif/oshcfoi1.htm.

Consumer Price Index (CPI)

Bureau of Labor Statistics

Overview: The Consumer Price Index (CPI) is designed to produce a monthly measure of the average change in the prices paid by urban consumers for a fixed market basket of goods and services.

Selected Content: Price indexes are available for the United States, the four census regions, size of city, cross-classifications of regions and size-classes, and 26 local areas. Indexes are available for major groups of consumer expenditures (food and beverages, housing, apparel, transportation, medical care, recreation, education and communications, and other goods and services), for items within each group, and for special categories, such as services. Monthly indexes are available for the United States, the four census regions, and some local areas. More detailed item indexes are available for the United States than for regions and local areas. Indexes are available for two population groups: a CPI for All Urban Consumers (CPI-U), which covers approximately 87% of the total population, and a CPI for Urban Wage Earners and Clerical Workers (CPI-W), which covers 32% of the population.

Data Years: The index has been constructed annually since 1978.

Coverage: The all-urban index (CPI-U) introduced in 1978 covers residents of metropolitan areas as well as residents of urban parts of nonmetropolitan areas (about 87% of the U.S. population in 2000).

Methodology: In calculating the index, price changes for the various items in each location were averaged together with weights that represent their importance in the spending of all urban consumers. Local data were then combined to obtain a U.S. city average.

The index measures price changes from a designated reference date, 1982–1984, which equals 100. An increase of 22%, for example, is shown as 122. Change can also be expressed in dollars as follows: the price of a base period market basket of goods and services bought by all urban consumers has risen from $100 in 1982–1984 to $202 in 2006.

The current revision of the CPI, completed in 2000, reflects spending patterns based on the Survey of Consumer Expenditures from 1993 to 1995, the 1990 Census of Population, and the ongoing Point-of-Purchase Survey. Using an improved sample design, prices for the goods and services required to calculate the index are collected in urban areas throughout the country and from retail and service establishments. Data on rents are collected from tenants of rented housing and residents of owner-occupied housing units. Food, fuels, and other goods and services are priced monthly in urban locations. Price information is obtained through visits or calls by trained BLS field representatives using computer-assisted telephone interviews.

Issues Affecting Interpretation: A 1987 revision changed the treatment of health insurance in the cost-weight definitions for medical care items. This change has no effect on the overall index result but provides a clearer picture of the role of health insurance in the CPI. As part of the revision, three new indexes have been created by separating previously combined items, for example, eye care is separated from other professional services, and inpatient and outpatient treatment is separated from other hospital and medical care services.

Effective January 1997, the hospital index was restructured by combining the three categories—room, inpatient services, and outpatient services—into one category: hospital services. In addition, new procedures for hospital data collection identify a payor, diagnosis, and the payor's reimbursement arrangement from selected hospital bills.

References:

Bureau of Labor Statistics. Handbook of Methods. BLS Bulletin 2490. Washington: U.S. Department of Labor. April 1997; Revising the Consumer Price Index, Monthly Labor Review, Dec 1996.

Ford IK, Ginsburg DH. Medical care in the consumer price index, in Medical care output and productivity studies in income and wealth, vol 62, Cutler DM, Berndt ER, eds., Chicago, IL: University of Chicago Press, pp. 203–19, 2001.

For More Information: See the BLS/CPI website: www.bls.gov/cpi/home.htm.

Current Population Survey (CPS)

Bureau of Labor Statistics and U.S. Census Bureau

Overview: The Current Population Survey (CPS) provides current estimates and trends in employment, unemployment, and other characteristics of the general labor force, the population as a whole, and various population subgroups.

Selected Content: The CPS interview is divided into three basic parts: (1) household and demographic information, (2) labor force information, and (3) supplement information in months that include supplements. Comprehensive work experience information is gathered on the employment status, occupation, and industry of persons interviewed.

Estimates of poverty and health insurance coverage presented in *Health, United States* from the CPS are derived from the Annual Social and Economic Supplement (ASEC), formerly called the Annual Demographic Supplement (ADS), or commonly called the March Supplement. The ASEC collects data on family characteristics, household composition, marital status, migration, income from all sources, information on weeks worked, time spent looking for work or on layoff from a job, occupation and industry classification of the job held longest during the year, health insurance coverage, and receipt of noncash benefits such as food stamps, school lunch program, employer-provided group health insurance plan, employer-provided pension plan, personal health insurance, Medicaid, Medicare, CHAMPUS or military health care, and energy assistance.

Data Years: The basic CPS has been conducted since 1945, although some data were collected prior to that time. The U.S. Census Bureau has collected data in the ASEC or ADS since 1947.

Coverage: The CPS sample is located in 754 sample areas, with coverage in every state and the District of Columbia. The adult universe (i.e., population of marriageable age) is composed of persons 15 years of age and over in the civilian noninstitutionalized population for CPS labor force data. The sample for the March CPS supplement is expanded to include members of the Armed Forces who are living in a household that includes at least one civilian adult, as well as additional Hispanic households that are not included in the monthly labor force estimates.

Methodology: The basic CPS sample is selected from multiple frames using multiple stages of selection. Each unit is selected with a known probability to represent similar units in the universe. The sample design is state-based, with the sample in each state being independent of the others.

One person generally responds for all eligible members of a household. For those who are employed, employment information is collected on the job held in the reference week. The reference week is defined as the 7-day period, Sunday through Saturday, which includes the 12th of the month. In the CPS, a person with two or more jobs is classified according to the job at which he or she worked the greatest number of hours. In general, the BLS publishes labor force data only for persons age 16 years and over, because those under 16 years are substantially limited in their labor market activities by compulsory schooling and child labor laws. No upper age limit is used, and full-time students are treated the same as nonstudents.

The additional Hispanic sample is from the previous November's basic CPS sample. If a person is identified as being of Hispanic origin from the November interview and is still residing at the same address in March, that housing unit is eligible for the March survey. This amounts to a near doubling of the Hispanic sample because there is no overlap of housing units between the basic CPS samples in November and March.

For all CPS data files, a single weight is prepared and used to compute the monthly labor force status estimates. An additional weight is prepared for the earnings universe that roughly corresponds to wage and salary workers in the two outgoing rotations. The final weight is the product of (1) the basic weight, (2) adjustments for special weighting, (3) noninterview adjustment, (4) first-stage ratio adjustment factor, and (5) second-stage ratio adjustment factor. This final weight should be used when producing estimates from the basic CPS data. Differences in the questionnaire, sample, and data uses for the March CPS supplement result in the need for additional adjustment procedures to produce what is called the March supplement weight.

Sample Size and Response Rate: Beginning with 2001, the State Children's Health Insurance Program (SCHIP) sample expansion was introduced. This included an increase in the basic CPS sample to 60,000 households per month. Prior to 2001, estimates were based on 50,000 households per month. The expansion also included an additional 12,000 households that were allocated differentially across states, based on prior information of the number of uninsured children in each state, to produce statistically reliable current state data on the number of low-income children who do not have health insurance coverage. In an average month, the nonresponse rate for the basic CPS is about 7%–8%.

Issues Affecting Interpretation: Over the years, the number of income questions has expanded, questions on work experience and other characteristics have been added, and the month of interview was moved to March. In 2002, an ASEC sample increase was implemented requiring more time for data collection. Thus, additional ASEC interviews are now taking place in February and April. However, even with this sample increase, most of the data collection still occurs in March.

In 1994 major changes were introduced, which included a complete redesign of the questionnaire including new health insurance questions and the introduction of computer-assisted interviewing for the entire survey. In addition, there were revisions to some of the labor force concepts and definitions. Prior to the redesign, CPS data were primarily collected using a paper-and-pencil form. Beginning in 1994, population controls were based on the 1990 census and adjusted for the estimated population undercount. Starting with *Health, United States, 2003*, poverty estimates for data years 2000 and beyond were recalculated based on the expanded SCHIP sample, and census 2000-based population controls were implemented. Starting with 2002 health insurance data, 1997 race standards were implemented that allowed respondents to report more than one race.

Reference:

U.S. Census Bureau. Technical Paper 63RV. Current Population Survey: Design and methodology. TP63RV, March 2002. Available from: www.census.gov/prod/2002pubs/tp63rv.pdf.

For More Information: See the CPS website: www.bls.census.gov/cps/cpsmain.htm.

Department of Veterans Affairs National Patient Care Database and National Enrollment Database

Department of Veterans Affairs (VA)

Overview: The Department of Veterans Affairs (VA) compiles and analyzes multiple data sets on the health and health care of its clients and other veterans to monitor access and quality of care and to conduct program and policy evaluations.

Selected Content: The VA maintains the National Patient Care Database (NPCD) and the National Enrollment Database (NED).

The NPCD is a nationwide system that contains a statistical record for each episode of care provided under VA auspices in VA and non-VA hospitals, nursing homes, VA residential rehabilitation treatment programs (formerly called domiciliaries), and VA outpatient clinics. Three major extracts from the NPCD are the patient treatment file (PTF), the patient census file (PCF), and the outpatient clinic file (OPC).

The PTF collects data at the time of the patient's discharge on each episode of inpatient care provided to patients at VA hospitals, VA nursing homes, VA residential rehabilitation treatment programs, community nursing homes, and other non-VA facilities. The PTF record contains the scrambled social security number (SSN), dates of inpatient treatment, date of birth, state and county of residence, type of disposition, place of disposition after discharge, and ICD–9–CM diagnostic and procedure or operative codes for each episode of care.

The PCF collects data on each patient remaining in a VA medical facility at midnight at the end of each quarter of the fiscal year. The census record includes information similar to that reported in the PTF record.

The outpatient clinic file (OPC) collects data on each instance of medical treatment provided to a veteran in an outpatient setting. The OPC record includes the age, scrambled social security number, state and county of residence, VA eligibility code, clinic(s) visited, purpose of visit, and date of visit for each episode of care.

The VA also maintains the National Enrollment Database (NED) as the official repository of enrollment information for each veteran enrolled in the VA health care system.

Coverage: U.S. veterans who receive services within the VA medical system are included. Data are available for some nonveterans who receive care at VA facilities.

Methodology: The NPCD is the source data for the Veterans Health Administration (VHA) Medical SAS Datasets. NPCD is the VHA's centralized relational database (a data warehouse) that receives encounter data from VHA clinical information systems. It is updated daily. Data are collected locally at each VA medical center and are transmitted electronically to the VA Austin Automation Center for use in providing nationwide statistics, reports, and comparisons.

In all of the medical data sets each patient has a unique identifier, which is a formula-based encryption of the individual's SSN. The identifier is consistent for a given patient across data sets and fiscal years. An extract containing selected information from the NPCD, the NED, and the cost distribution system is produced by the Austin Automation Center.

Issues Affecting Interpretation: The databases include users of the VA health care system. VA eligibility is a hierarchy based on service-connected disabilities, income, age, and availability of services. Therefore, different VA programs may serve populations with different sociodemographic characteristics than other health care systems.

For More Information: See the VHA Information Systems website: www.virec.research.va.gov/Support/Training-NewUsersToolkit/IntroToVAData.htm.

Employee Benefits Survey—See National Compensation Survey

Medicaid Data System

Centers for Medicare & Medicaid Services

Overview: The Centers for Medicare & Medicaid Services (CMS) works with its state partners to collect data on persons served by the Medicaid program to monitor and evaluate access and quality of care, trends in program eligibility, characteristics of enrollees, changes in payment policy, and other program-related issues.

Selected Content: Data collected include medical vendor payments for Medicaid recipients by type of service and information on the characteristics of Medicaid recipients, including race/ethnicity, age, and basis of eligibility.

Data Years: Selected state data are available starting in 1992 and data for the 50 states and the District of Columbia are available starting in 1999.

Coverage: The data include individuals enrolled in the Medicaid program or receiving Medicaid benefits.

Methodology: The primary data sources for Medicaid statistical data are the Medicaid Statistical Information System (MSIS) and the CMS-64 reports.

MSIS is the basic source of state-reported eligibility and claims data on the Medicaid population, and their characteristics, utilization, and payments. Beginning in FY 1999, as a result of legislation enacted from the Balanced Budget Act of 1997, states are required to submit individual eligibility and claims data tapes to CMS quarterly through MSIS. Prior to FY 1999, states were required to submit an annual HCFA-2082 report, designed to collect aggregated statistical data on eligibles, recipients, services, and expenditures during a federal fiscal year (October 1 through September 30). The data reported for each year represented people on the Medicaid rolls, recipients of Medicaid services, and payments for claims adjudicated during the year. The data reflected bills adjudicated or processed during the year, rather than services used during the year. States summarized and reported the data processed through their own Medicaid claims processing and payment operations, unless they opted to participate in MSIS, in which case the HCFA-2082 report was produced by the Health Care Financing Administration (the predecessor to CMS).

The CMS-64 is a product of the financial budget and grant system. The CMS-64 is a statement of expenditures for the Medicaid program that states submit to CMS 30 days after each quarter. The report is an accounting statement of actual expenditures made by the states for which they are entitled to receive federal reimbursement under Title XIX for that quarter. The amount claimed on the CMS-64 is a summary of expenditures derived from source documents such as invoices, cost reports, and eligibility records.

The CMS-64 shows the disposition of Medicaid grant funds for the quarter being reported and previous years, the recoupments made or refunds received, and income earned on grant funds. The data on the CMS-64 are used to reconcile the monetary advance made on the basis of states' funding estimates filed prior to the beginning of the quarter on the CMS-37. As such, the CMS-64 is the primary source for making adjustments for any identified overpayments and underpayments to the states. Also incorporated into this process are disallowance actions forwarded from other federal financial adjustments. Finally, the CMS-64 provides information that forms the basis for a series of Medicaid financial reports and budget analyses. Also included are third party liability (TPL) collections tables. TPL refers to the legal obligation of certain health care sources to pay the medical claims of Medicaid recipients before Medicaid pays these claims. Medicaid pays only after the TPL sources have met their legal obligation to pay.

Issues Affecting Interpretation: Health, United States Medicaid tables are based on MSIS data. Users of Medicaid data may note apparent inconsistencies in Medicaid data that are primarily due to the difference in information captured in MSIS compared to CMS-64 reports. The most substantive difference is due to payments made to disproportionate share hospitals. Payments to disproportionate share hospitals do not appear in MSIS because states directly reimburse these hospitals and there is no fee-for-service billing. Other less significant differences between MSIS and CMS-64 occur because adjudicated claims data are used in MSIS versus actual payments reflected in the CMS-64. Differences also may occur because of internal state practices for capturing and reporting these data through two separate systems. Finally, national totals for the CMS-64 are different because they include other jurisdictions, such as the Northern Mariana Islands and American Samoa.

For More Information: See the CMS website: www.cms.hhs.gov/medicaiddatasourcesgeninfo/01_overview.asp? or the Research Data Assistance Center (ResDAC): www.resdac.umn.edu/medicaid/data_available.asp. Also see Appendix II, Medicaid.

Medical Expenditure Panel Survey (MEPS)

Agency for Healthcare Research and Quality

Overview: The Medical Expenditure Panel Survey (MEPS) produces nationally representative estimates of health care use, expenditures, sources of payment, insurance coverage, and quality of care for the U.S. civilian noninstitutionalized population.

Selected Content: MEPS data in *Health, United States* include total health care expenses and prescribed medicine expenses, presented by sociodemographic characteristics, type of health insurance, and sources of payment.

Data Years: The 1977 National Medical Care Expenditure Survey and the 1987 National Medical Expenditure Survey (NMES) are earlier versions of this survey. Since 1996, MEPS has been conducted on an annual basis.

Coverage: U.S. civilian noninstitutionalized population is the primary population represented. The 1987 and 1996 surveys also had an institutionalized population component.

Methodology: MEPS is a national probability survey conducted on an annual basis since 1996. The panel design of the survey features several rounds of interviewing covering two full calendar years. The MEPS consists of three components: the Household Component (HC), the Medical Provider Component (MPC), and the Insurance Component (IC).

The HC is a nationally representative survey of the civilian noninstitutionalized population drawn from a subsample of households that participated in the prior year's National Health Interview Survey conducted by the National Center for Health Statistics. Missing expenditure data are imputed using data collected in the MPC whenever possible.

The MPC collects data from hospitals, physicians, home health care providers, and pharmacies that were reported in the HC as providing care to MEPS sample persons. Data are collected in MPC to improve the accuracy of expenditure estimates derived solely from the HC. The MPC is particularly useful in obtaining expenditure information for persons enrolled in managed care plans and Medicaid recipients. Sample sizes for the MPC vary from year to year depending on the HC sample size and the MPC sampling rates for providers.

The IC consists of two subcomponent samples: a household sample and list sample. The household sample collects detailed information from employers on the health insurance held by and offered to respondents to the MEPS-HC. The list sample collects data on the types and costs of workplace health insurance from a total of about 40,000 business establishments and governments each year.

The MEPS updates the 1987 NMES. The NMES consists of two components: the Household Survey (HS) and the Medical Provider Survey (MPS). The NMES-HS Component was designed to provide nationally representative estimates of health insurance status, health insurance coverage, and health care use for the U.S. civilian noninstitutionalized population for the calendar year 1987. Data from the NMES-MPS component were used in conjunction with HS data to produce estimates of health care expenditures. The NMES-HS consisted of four rounds of household interviews. Income was collected in a special supplement administered early in 1988. Events under the scope of the NMES-MPS included medical services provided by or under the direction of a physician, all hospital events, and home health care. The sample of events included in the NMES-MPS was all events for persons covered by Medicaid and for a 25% sample of NMES-HS respondents. Missing expenditure data were imputed.

Sample Size and Response Rate: For MEPS first core household interview, 17,500 households were selected. The sample sizes for the MEPS-HC are approximately 10,000 families in 1996 and 1998–2000, 13,500 families in 1997 and 2001, and 13,000–15,000 families annually beginning in 2002. The full-year household core response rate has generally been about 66%. The 12-month joint core questionnaire/health questionnaire/access supplement response rate for the household component of the NMES was 80%.

Issues Affecting Interpretation: The 1987 estimates are based on the NMES, and 1996 and later years estimates are based on the MEPS. Because expenditures in NMES were based primarily on charges, whereas those for MEPS were based on payments, data for NMES were adjusted to be more comparable to MEPS using estimated charge-to-payment ratios for 1987. For a detailed explanation of this adjustment, see Zuvekas and Cohen, 2002.

References:

Hahn B, Lefkowitz D. Annual expenses and sources of payment for health care services (AHRQ pub no 93–0007). National Medical Expenditure Survey Research Findings 14, Agency for Healthcare Research and Quality pub no 93–0007. Rockville, MD: Public Health Service, November 1992.

Cohen SB. Sample design of the 1997 Medical Expenditure Panel Survey Household Component. MEPS Methodology Report No 11. AHRQ pub no. 01–0001. Rockville MD: Agency for Healthcare Research and Quality. 2000.

Zuvekas S, Cohen S. A guide to comparing health care estimates in the 1996 Medical Expenditure Panel Survey to the 1987 National Medical Expenditure Survey. Inquiry 2002;39(1):76–86.

For More Information: See the MEPS website: www.meps.ahrq.gov.

Medicare Administrative Data

Centers for Medicare & Medicaid Services

Overview: The Centers for Medicare & Medicaid Services (CMS) collects and synthesizes Medicare enrollment, spending, and claims data to monitor and evaluate access to and quality of care, trends in utilization, changes in payment policy, and other program-related issues.

Selected Content: Data include claims information for services furnished to Medicare beneficiaries and Medicare enrollment data. Claims data include type of service, procedures, diagnoses, dates of service, charge amounts, and payment amounts. Enrollment data include date of birth, sex, race or ethnicity, and reason for entitlement.

Data Years: Some data files are available as far back as 1987, but CMS no longer provides technical support for files with data prior to 1991.

Coverage: Enrollment data are for all persons enrolled in the Medicare program. Claims data include data for Medicare beneficiaries who filed claims.

Methodology: The claims and utilization data files contain extensive utilization information at various levels of summarization for a variety of providers and services. There are many types and levels of these files, including the National Claims History (NCH) files, the Standard Analytic Files (SAF), Medicare Provider and Analysis Review (MedPAR) files, Medicare enrollment files, and various other files.

The National Claims History 100% Nearline File contains all institutional and noninstitutional claims and provides records of every Medicare claim submitted, including adjustment claims. The Standard Analytical Files (SAFs) contain final action claims data in which all adjustments have been resolved. These files contain information collected by Medicare to pay for health care services provided to a Medicare beneficiary. SAFs are available for each institutional (inpatient, outpatient, skilled nursing facility, hospice, or home health agency) and noninstitutional (physician and durable medical equipment providers) claim type. The record unit of SAFs is the claim (some episodes of care may have more than one claim). SAF files include the Inpatient SAF, the Skilled Nursing Facility SAF, the Outpatient SAF, the Home Health Agency SAF, the Hospice SAF, the Clinical Laboratory SAF, the Durable Medical Equipment SAF 5%, the physician supplier SAF (5%), and the Durable Medical Equipment SAF.

Medicare Provider and Analysis Review (MedPAR) files contain inpatient hospital and skilled nursing facility (SNF) final action stay records. Each MedPAR record represents a stay in an inpatient hospital or SNF. An inpatient stay record summarizes all services rendered to a beneficiary from the time of admission to a facility through discharge. Each MedPAR record may represent one claim or multiple claims, depending on the length of a beneficiary's stay and the amount of inpatient services used throughout the stay.

The Denominator File contains demographic and enrollment information about each beneficiary enrolled in Medicare during a calendar year. The information in the Denominator File is frozen in March of the following calendar year. Some of the information contained in this file includes the beneficiary unique identifier, state and county codes, ZIP code, date of birth, date of death, sex, race, age, monthly entitlement indicators (for Medicare Part A, Medicare Part B, or Part A and Part B), reasons for entitlement, state buy-in indicators, and monthly managed care indicators (yes/no). The Denominator File is used to determine beneficiary demographic characteristics, entitlement, and beneficiary participation in Medicare Managed Care Organizations.

The Vital Status File contains demographic information about each beneficiary ever entitled to Medicare. Some of the information contained in this file includes the beneficiary unique identifier, state and county codes, ZIP code, date of birth, date of death, sex, race, and age. Often the Vital Status File is used to obtain recent death information for a cohort of Medicare beneficiaries.

The Group Health Plan (GHP) Master File contains data on beneficiaries who are currently enrolled or have ever been enrolled in a Managed Care Organization (MCO) under contract with CMS. Each record represents one beneficiary, and each beneficiary has one record. Some of the information contained in this file includes the Beneficiary Unique Identifier number, date of birth, date of death, state and county, and managed care enrollment information such as dates of membership and MCO contract number. The GHP Master File is used to identify the exact MCO in which beneficiaries were enrolled.

Issues Affecting Interpretation: Because Medicare managed care programs may not file claims, files based only on claims data will exclude care for persons enrolled in Medicare managed care programs. In addition, to maintain a manageable file size, some files are based on a sample of enrollees, rather than on all Medicare enrollees. Coding changes and interpretation of Medicare coverage rules have also changed over the life of the Medicare program.

For More Information: See the CMS Research Data Assistance Center (ResDAC) website: www.resdac.umn.edu/medicare/index.asp or the CMS website: www.cms.hhs.gov/medicare/. Also see Appendix II, Medicare.

Medicare Current Beneficiary Survey (MCBS)

Centers for Medicare & Medicaid Services

Overview: The Medicare Current Beneficiary Survey (MCBS) produces nationally representative estimates of health status, health care use and expenditures, health insurance coverage, and socioeconomic and demographic characteristics of Medicare beneficiaries. It is used to estimate expenditures and sources of payment for all services used by Medicare beneficiaries, including co-payments, deductibles, and noncovered services; to ascertain all types of health insurance coverage and relate coverage to sources of payment; and to trace processes over time, such as changes in health status and the effects of program changes.

Selected Content: The survey collects data on utilization of health services, health and functional status, health care expenditures, and health insurance and beneficiary information (such as income, living arrangement, family assistance, and quality of life).

Data Years: The first round of interviewing was conducted from September through December 1991, and the survey has been continuously in the field since then. The data are designed to support both cross-sectional and longitudinal analyses.

Coverage: The MCBS is a continuous survey of a nationally representative sample of aged, institutionalized, and disabled Medicare beneficiaries.

Methodology: The overlapping panel design of the survey allows each sample person to be interviewed three times a year for 4 years, whether he or she resides in the community or a facility or moves between the two settings, using the version of the questionnaire appropriate to the setting. Sample persons in the community are interviewed using computer-assisted personal interviewing (CAPI) survey instruments. Because long-term care facility residents often are in poor health, information about institutionalized residents is collected from proxy respondents such as nurses and other primary caregivers affiliated with the facility. The sample is selected from the Medicare enrollment files, with oversampling among disabled persons under age 65 years and among persons 80 years of age and over.

MCBS has two components: the Cost and Use file and the Access to Care file. Medicare claims are linked to survey-reported events to produce the Cost and Use file that provides complete expenditure and source of payment data on all health care services, including those not covered by Medicare. The Access to Care file contains information on beneficiaries' access to health care, satisfaction with care, and usual source of care. The sample for this file represents the always enrolled population—those who participated in the Medicare program for the entire year. In contrast, the Cost and Use file represents the ever enrolled population, including both those who entered Medicare and those who died during the year.

Sample Size and Response Rate: Each fall, about one-third of the sample is retired and roughly 6,000 new sample persons are included in the survey—the exact number chosen is based on projections of target samples of 12,000 persons with 3 years of cost and use information distributed appropriately across the sample cells. In the community, response rates for initial interviews range in the mid- to high 80s; once respondents have completed the first interview, their participation in subsequent rounds is 95% or more. In recent rounds, data have been collected from approximately 15,000–19,000 beneficiaries, with the peaks occurring in fall rounds because of the annual and HMO samples. Roughly 90% of the sample is made up of persons who live in the community, with the remaining persons living in long-term care facilities. Response rates for facility interviews approach 100%.

Issues Affecting Interpretation: Because only Medicare enrollees are included in the survey, the survey excludes a small proportion of persons age 65 years and over who are not enrolled in Medicare, which should be noted when using the MCBS to make estimates of the entire population age 65 years and over in the United States.

References:

Adler GS. A profile of the Medicare Current Beneficiary Survey. Health Care Financ Rev 1994;15(4):153–63.

Lo A, Chu A, Apodaca R. Redesign of the Medicare Current Beneficiary Survey sample, Rockville, MD: Westat, Inc., 2003. Available from: www.cms.hhs.gov/apps/mcbs/PublBIB/Mbibl8.pdf.

For More Information: See the MCBS website: www.cms.hhs.gov/MCBS.

Monitoring the Future Study (MTF)

National Institute on Drug Abuse

Overview: Monitoring the Future (MTF) is an ongoing study of the behaviors, attitudes, and values of American secondary school students, college students, and young adults.

Selected Content: Data collected include lifetime, annual, and 30-day prevalence of use of specific illegal drugs and substances, inhalants, tobacco, and alcohol. Data are also collected on usage levels, frequency of use, perceived risks associated with use, opinions about whether use is approved or disapproved by others, and opinions about availability of the substances.

Data Years: MTF has been conducted annually since 1975, initially with high school seniors; ongoing panel studies of representative samples from each graduating class have been conducted by mail since 1976; annual surveys of 8th and 10th graders were initiated in 1991.

Coverage: MTF surveys a sample of high school seniors, 10th graders, and 8th graders selected to be representative of all seniors, 10th graders, and 8th graders in public and private high schools in the continental United States.

Methodology: The survey design is a multistage random sample with stage one being selection of particular geographic areas, stage two selection of one or more schools in each area, and stage three selection of students within each school. Data are collected using self-administered questionnaires conducted in the classroom by representatives of the Institute for Social Research. Dropouts and students who are absent on the day of the survey are excluded. Recognizing that the dropout population is at higher risk for drug use, this survey was expanded in 1991 to include similar nationally representative samples of 8th and 10th graders, which have lower dropout rates than seniors and include future high-risk 12th grade dropouts. For more information on MTF adjustments for absentees and dropouts, see: Johnston, LD, O'Malley, PM, Bachman, JG, Schulenberg, JE. (2006). Monitoring the Future national survey results on drug use, 1975–2005: Volume I, Secondary school students (NIH Publication No. 06–5883). Bethesda, MD: National Institute on Drug Abuse. Appendix A. Available from: www.monitoringthefuture.org/.

Sample Size and Response Rates: In 2006, 48,460, 8th, 10th, and 12th graders in 410 schools were surveyed. The annual senior samples comprised 14,814 seniors in 136 public and private high schools nationwide. The 10th-grade samples involved 16,620 students in 123 schools, and the 8th-grade samples had 17,026 students in 151 schools. Response rates were 83%, 88%, and 91% for 12th, 10th, and 8th graders and have been relatively constant across time. Absentees constitute virtually all of the nonresponding students.

Issues Affecting Interpretation: Estimates of substance use for youth based on the National Survey on Drug Use & Health (NSDUH) are not directly comparable with estimates based on the MTF and the Youth Risk Behavior Surveillance System (YRBSS). In addition to the fact that the MTF excludes dropouts and absentees, rates are not directly comparable across these surveys because of differences in populations covered, sample design, questionnaires, interview setting, and statistical approaches to make the survey estimates generalizable to the entire population. The NSDUH survey collects data in homes, whereas the MTF and YRBSS collect data in school classrooms. The NSDUH estimates are tabulated by age, whereas the MTF and YRBSS estimates are tabulated by grade, representing different ages as well as different populations.

References:

Johnston LD, O'Malley PM, Bachman JG, Schulenberg JE. Monitoring the future national results on adolescent drug use: Overview of key findings, 2006. NIH Pub no 07–6202. Bethesda, MD: National Institute on Drug Abuse. 2007. Available from: www.monitoringthefuture.org/pubs/monographs/overview2006.pdf.

Johnston LD, O'Malley PM, Bachman JG. Monitoring the future national survey results on drug use, 1975–2002. Vol I: Secondary school students. NIH pub no 03–5375. Bethesda, MD: National Institute on Drug Abuse. 2003. Available from: monitoringthefuture.org/pubs/monographs/vol1_2002.pdf.

Cowan CD. Coverage, sample design, and weighting in three federal surveys. Journal of Drug Issues 2001;31(3):595–614.

For More Information: See the NIDA website: www.nida.nih.gov/Infofax/HSYouthtrends.html and the Monitoring the Future website: www.monitoringthefuture.org/.

National Ambulatory Medical Care Survey (NAMCS)

Centers for Disease Control and Prevention National Center for Health Statistics

Overview: The National Ambulatory Medical Care Survey (NAMCS) is a national survey designed to provide information about the provision and use of medical care services in office-based physician practices in the United States.

Selected Content: Data are collected from medical records on type of providers seen; reason for visit; diagnoses; drugs ordered, provided, or continued; and selected procedures and tests ordered or performed during the visit. Patient data include age, sex, race, and expected source of payment. Data are also collected on selected characteristics of physician practices.

Data Years: The NAMCS, which began in 1973, was conducted annually until 1981, once in 1985, and resumed an annual schedule in 1989.

Coverage: The scope of the survey covers patient encounters in the offices of nonfederally employed physicians classified by the American Medical Association or American Osteopathic Association as office-based, patient care physicians. Patient encounters with physicians engaged in prepaid practices—health maintenance organizations (HMOs), independent practice organizations (IPAs), and other prepaid practices—are included in NAMCS. Excluded are visits to hospital-based physicians, visits to specialists in anesthesiology, pathology, and radiology, and visits to physicians who are principally engaged in teaching, research, or administration. Telephone contacts and nonoffice visits are also excluded.

Methodology: A multistage probability design is employed. The first-stage sample consisted of 84 primary sampling units (PSUs) in 1985, and beginning in 1989, 112 PSUs, which were selected from about 1,900 such units into which the United States had been divided. In each sample PSU, a sample of practicing nonfederal office-based physicians is selected from master files maintained by the American Medical Association and the American Osteopathic Association. The final stage involves systematic random samples of office visits during randomly assigned 7-day reporting periods. In 1985, the survey excluded Alaska and Hawaii. Starting in 1989, the survey included all 50 states and the District of Columbia.

The U.S. Census Bureau acts as the data collection agent for the NAMCS. Screening interviews are conducted by Census field representatives to obtain information about physicians' office-based practices and to ensure that the practice is within the scope of the survey. Field representatives visit eligible physicians prior to their participation in the survey to provide them with survey materials and instruct them on how to sample patient visits and complete patient record forms. Participants are asked to complete forms for a systematic random sample of approximately 30 office visits occurring during a randomly assigned 1-week period, but increasingly patient record forms are abstracted by field representatives.

Sample data are weighted to produce national estimates. The estimation procedure used in the NAMCS has three basic components: inflation by the reciprocal of the probability of selection, adjustment for nonresponse, and ratio adjustment to fixed totals.

Sample Size and Response Rate: In 2003, a sample of 3,000 physicians was selected; 2,007 were in scope and 1,407 participated for a response rate of 67%. Data were provided for 25,288 visits. In 2004, a sample of 3,000 physicians was selected; 1,961 were in scope and 1,372 participated for a response rate of 70%. Data were provided for 25,286 visits. In 2005, a sample of 3,000 physicians was selected; 1,936 were in scope and 1,281 participated for a response rate of 66%. Data were provided for 25,665 visits.

Issues Affecting Interpretation: The NAMCS patient record form is modified approximately every 2–4 years to reflect changes in physician practice characteristics, patterns of care, and technological innovations. Examples of recent changes include increasing the number of drugs recorded on the patient record form, and adding checkboxes for specific tests or procedures performed. Sample sizes vary by survey year. For some years it is suggested that analysts combine two or more years of data if they wish to examine relatively rare populations or events. Starting with *Health, United States, 2005,* data for survey years 2001–2002 were revised to be consistent with the weighting scheme introduced in the 2003 NAMCS data. For more information on the new weighting scheme, see National Ambulatory Medical Care Survey: 2003 summary, Advance data from vital and health statistics (2005).

Reference:

Hing E, Cherry D, Woodwell, DA. National Ambulatory Medical Care Survey, 2003 summary. Advance data from vital and health statistics 2005; no 365. Hyattsville, MD: National Center for Health Statistics. Available from: www.cdc.gov/nchs/data/ad/ad365.pdf.

For More Information: See the Ambulatory Health Care Data website: www.cdc.gov/nchs/about/major/ahcd/ahcd1.htm.

National Compensation Survey

Bureau of Labor Statistics

Overview: The National Compensation Survey (NCS) provides comprehensive measures of occupational earnings, compensation cost trends, benefit incidence, and detailed plan provisions.

Selected Content: Detailed occupational earnings are collected for metropolitan and nonmetropolitan areas and broad geographic regions, and on a national basis. The Employment Cost Index (ECI) and Employer Costs for Employee Compensation (ECEC) are compensation measures derived from the NCS. ECI measures changes in labor costs. Average hourly employer cost for employee compensation is presented in the ECEC. National benefits data are presented for three broad occupational groupings: professional, technical, and related; clerical and sales; and blue-collar and service employees. Data are also available by goods- and service-producing occupations, union affiliation, and full- and part-time status.

Data Years: The NCS replaces three existing BLS surveys: Employment Cost Index (ECI), Occupational Compensation Survey Program (OCSP), and Employee Benefits Survey (EBS). The ECI and EBS were fully integrated into the NCS in 1999. Prior to 1999, the EBS was collected for small private establishments (those employing fewer than 100 workers) and from state and local governments (regardless of employment size). In odd-numbered years, data were collected for medium and large private establishments (those employing 100 workers or more). The ECI was created in the mid-1970s. The EBS was added to an existing data collection effort, the National Pay Survey, in the late 1970s. The Employer Cost for Employee Compensation product was developed in 1987.

Coverage: The NCS provides information for the Nation, for 81 metropolitan areas and 73 nonmetropolitan counties representing the United States, and for the nine census divisions (although not all areas have information for all occupations). It includes both full- and part-time workers who are paid a wage or salary. It excludes agriculture, fishing and forestry industries, private household workers, and the federal government. The NCS only includes establishments with at least 50 workers.

Methodology: Conducted quarterly by the Bureau of Labor Statistics' Office of Compensation and Working Conditions, the sample for the NCS is selected using a three-stage design. The first stage involves the selection of areas. The NCS sample consists of 154 metropolitan and nonmetropolitan areas that represent the Nation's 326 metropolitan statistical areas and the remaining portions of the 50 states. In the second stage, establishments are systematically selected with probability of selection proportionate to their relative employment size within the industry. Use of this technique means that the larger an establishment's employment, the greater its chance of selection. The third stage of sampling is a probability sample of occupations within a sampled establishment. This step is performed by the BLS field economist during an interview with the respondent establishment in which selection of an occupation is based on probability of selection proportionate to employment in the establishment and each occupation is classified under its corresponding major occupational group.

Data collection is conducted by the BLS field economists. Data are gathered from each establishment on the primary business activity of the establishment, types of occupations, number of employees, wages and salaries and benefits, hours of work, and duties and responsibilities. Wage data obtained by occupation and work level allows NCS to publish occupational wage statistics for localities, census divisions, and the Nation.

Sample: The NCS sample consists of 154 metropolitan and nonmetropolitan areas that represent the Nation's 326 metropolitan statistical areas and the remaining portions of the 50 states.

Issues Affecting Interpretation: Because the NCS merges separate surveys, trend analyses prior to 2000 should be interpreted with care. The industrial coverage, establishment size coverage, and geographic coverage for the EBS survey changed since 1990. All surveys conducted from 1979–1989 excluded part-time employees and establishments in Alaska and Hawaii. The surveys conducted from 1979–1986 covered only medium and large private establishments and excluded most of the service industries. Establishments that employed at least 50, 100, or 250 workers, depending on the industry, were included. The survey conducted in 1987 consisted of state and local governments with 50 or more employees. The surveys carried out in 1988 and 1989 included all private-sector establishments that employed 100 or more employees.

The Employer Costs for Employee Compensation (ECEC) switched to new industry and occupation classification systems with the release of the March 2004 data. The 2002 North American Industry Classification System (NAICS) is now used to classify industries and the 2000 Standard Occupational Classification (SOC) system is used to classify occupations. ECEC data by the present classification systems—the 1987 Standard Industrial Classification System (SIC) and the 1990 Occupational Classification System (OCS)—will no longer be produced. The ECEC was the first National Compensation Survey product to make this transition. For more information about this transition, see the National Compensation Survey website: www.bls.gov/ncs/ect/sp/ecsm0001.htm.

References:

U.S. Department of Labor, Bureau of Labor Statistics, Employer Costs for Employee Compensation Summary 2006, March release, available June, 2006. Available from: www.bls.gov/ncs/ect/.

The National Compensation Survey: Compensation Statistics for the 21st Century. Available from: www.bls.gov/opub/cwc/archive/winter2000art1.pdf.

For More Information: See the National Compensation Survey website: www.bls.gov/ncs.

National Health Expenditure Accounts

Centers for Medicare & Medicaid Services

Overview: National Health Expenditure Accounts provide estimates of how much money is spent on different types of health care-related services and programs in the United States.

Selected Content: National Health Expenditures measure spending for health care in the United States by type of service delivered (such as hospital care, physician services, nursing home care) and source of funding for those services (such as private health insurance, Medicare, Medicaid, and out-of-pocket spending).

Data Years: Expenditure estimates are available starting from 1960 in data files or in published articles.

Methodology: The American Hospital Association (AHA) data on hospital finances are the primary source for estimates relating to hospital care. The salaries of physicians and dentists on the staffs of hospitals, hospital outpatient clinics, hospital-based home health agencies, and nursing home care provided in the hospital setting are considered to be components of hospital care. Expenditures for home health care and for services of health professionals (for example, doctors, chiropractors, private duty nurses, therapists, and podiatrists) are estimated primarily using a combination of data from the U.S. Census Bureau Services Annual Survey and the quinquennial Census of Service Industries.

The estimates of retail spending for prescription drugs are based on household and industry data on prescription drug transactions. Expenditures for other medical nondurables and for vision products and other medical durables purchased in retail outlets are based on estimates of personal consumption expenditures prepared by the U.S. Department of Commerce's Bureau of Economic Analysis, U.S. Bureau of Labor Statistics/Consumer Expenditure Survey; the 1987 National Medical Expenditure Survey and the Medical Expenditure Panel Surveys conducted by the Agency for Healthcare Research and Quality; and spending by Medicare and Medicaid. Those durable and nondurable products provided to inpatients in hospitals or nursing homes, and those provided by licensed professionals or through home health agencies are excluded here, but they are included with the expenditure estimates of the provider service category.

Nursing home expenditures cover care rendered in establishments providing inpatient nursing and health-related personal care through active treatment programs for medical and health-related conditions. These establishments cover skilled nursing and intermediate care facilities, including those for the mentally retarded. Spending estimates are primarily based on data from the U.S. Census Bureau's Services Annual Survey and the quinquennial Census of Service Industries.

Expenditures for construction include those spent on the erection or renovation of hospitals, nursing homes, medical clinics, and medical research facilities, but not for private office buildings providing office space for private practitioners. Expenditures for noncommercial research (the cost of commercial research by drug companies is assumed to be imbedded in the price charged for the product; to include this item again would result in double counting) are developed from information gathered by the National Institutes of Health and the National Science Foundation.

Source of funding estimates likewise come from a multiplicity of sources. Data on the federal health programs are taken from administrative records maintained by the servicing agencies. Among the sources used to estimate state and local government spending for health are the U.S. Census Bureau's Government Finances and the National Academy of Social Insurance reports on state-operated workers' compensation programs. Federal and state and local expenditures for education and training of medical personnel are excluded from these measures where they are separable. For the private financing of health care, data on the financial experience of health insurance organizations come from special Centers for Medicare & Medicaid Services analyses of private health insurers and from the Bureau of Labor Statistics' survey on the cost of employer-sponsored health insurance and on consumer expenditures. Information on out-of-pocket spending from the U.S. Bureau of the Census Services Annual Survey; U.S. Bureau of Labor Statistics Consumer Expenditure Survey; the 1987 National Medical Expenditure Survey and the Medical Expenditure Panel Surveys conducted by the Agency for Healthcare Research and Quality; and from private surveys conducted by the American Hospital Association, American Medical Association, American Dental Association, and IMS Health, an organization that collects data from the pharmaceutical industry, is used to develop estimates of direct spending by customers.

Reference:

Catlin A, Cowan C, Heffler S, Washington B, and the National Health Accounts Team. National health spending in 2005: The slowdown continues. Health Aff 2007;26(1):142–153.

For More Information: See the Centers for Medicare & Medicaid Services National Health Expenditure Accounts website: www.cms.hhs.gov/NationalHealthExpendData/02_NationalHealthAccountsHistorical.asp#TopOfPage.

National Health and Nutrition Examination Survey (NHANES)

Centers for Disease Control and Prevention National Center for Health Statistics

Overview: The National Health and Nutrition Examination Survey (NHANES) program includes a series of cross-sectional nationally representative health examination surveys conducted in mobile examination units or clinics (MEC). In the first series of surveys, the National Health Examination Survey (NHES), data were collected on the prevalence of certain chronic diseases, the distributions of various physical and psychological measures, and measures of growth and development. In 1971, a nutrition surveillance component was added and the survey name changed to the National Health and Nutrition Examination Survey (NHANES). See Data Years section for more information on the survey name and years conducted.

Selected Content: The NHANES have collected data on chronic disease prevalence and conditions (including undiagnosed conditions) and risk factors such as obesity and smoking, serum cholesterol levels, hypertension, diet and nutritional status, immunization status, infectious disease prevalence, health insurance, and measures of environmental exposures. Other topics addressed include hearing, vision, mental health, anemia, diabetes, cardiovascular disease, osteoporosis, oral health, mental health, pharmaceuticals used, and physical fitness.

NHES I data were collected on the prevalence of certain chronic diseases as well as the distributions of various physical and psychological measures, including blood pressure and serum cholesterol levels. NHES II and NHES III focused on factors related to growth and development in children and youth.

For NHANES I, data were collected on indicators of the nutritional and health status of the American people through dietary intake data, biochemical tests, physical measurements, and clinical assessments for evidence of nutritional deficiency. Detailed examinations were given by dentists, ophthalmologists, and dermatologists, with an assessment of need for treatment. In addition, data were obtained for a subsample of adults on overall health care needs and behavior, and more detailed examination data were collected on cardiovascular, respiratory, arthritic, and hearing conditions. For NHANES II, the nutrition component was expanded and the medical area focused on diabetes, kidney and liver functions, allergy, and speech pathology. The third National Health and Nutrition Examination Survey (NHANES III) also included data on antibodies, spirometry, and bone health.

Beginning in 1999 with continuous data collection for NHANES, new topics include cardiorespiratory fitness, physical functioning, lower extremity disease, full body scan (DXA) for body fat as well as bone density, and tuberculosis infection.

Data Years: Data have been collected from surveys conducted during 1960–1962 (NHES I), 1963–1965 (NHES II), 1966–1970 (NHES III), 1971–1974 (NHANES I), 1976–1980 (NHANES II), 1982–1984 (HHANES), and 1988–1994 (NHANES III). Beginning in 1999, the survey has been conducted continuously.

Coverage: With the exception of the Hispanic Health and Nutrition Examination Survey (see Methodology, below), the NHES and NHANES provide estimates of the health status of the civilian noninstitutionalized population of the United States. NHES II and NHES III examined probability samples of the Nation's noninstitutionalized children ages 6–11 years and 12–17 years, respectively.

The NHANES I target population was the civilian noninstitutionalized population 1–74 years of age residing in the coterminous United States, except for people residing on any of the reservation lands set aside for the use of American Indians.

The NHANES II target population was the civilian noninstitutionalized population 6 months–74 years of age residing in the United States, including Alaska and Hawaii.

The Hispanic Health and Nutrition Examination Survey (HHANES) studied three geographically and ethnically distinct populations: Mexican Americans living in Texas, New Mexico, Arizona, Colorado, and California; Cuban Americans living in Dade County, Florida; and Puerto Ricans living in parts of New York, New Jersey, and Connecticut.

The NHANES III target population was the civilian noninstitutionalized population 2 months of age and over. The sample design provided for oversampling among children 2 months–5 years of age, persons 60 years of age and over, black persons, and persons of Mexican origin.

Beginning in 1999, NHANES oversampled low-income persons, adolescents 12–19 years of age, persons 60 years of age and over, African Americans, and persons of Mexican origin. The sample is not designed to give a nationally representative sample for the total population of Hispanics residing in the United States.

Methodology: The NHANES includes clinical examinations, selected medical and laboratory tests, and self-reported data. The NHANES and previous surveys interviewed persons in their homes and conducted medical examinations, including laboratory analysis of blood, urine, and other tissue samples. Medical examinations and laboratory tests follow very specific protocols and are as standard as possible to ensure comparability across sites and providers. From 1999–2002, as a substitute for the MEC examinations, a small number of survey participants received an abbreviated health examination in their homes if they were unable to come to the MEC.

For the first program or cycle of the NHES I, a highly stratified multistage probability sample was selected to represent the 111 million civilian noninstitutionalized adults 18–79 years of age in the United States at that time. The sample areas consisted of 42 primary sampling units (PSUs) from the 1,900 geographic units. NHES II and NHES III were also multistage stratified probability samples of clusters of households in land-based segments. NHES II and III used the same 40 PSUs.

For NHANES I the sample areas consisted of 65 PSUs. A subsample of persons 25–74 years of age was selected to receive the more detailed health examination. Groups at high risk of malnutrition were oversampled.

NHANES II used a multistage probability design that involved selection of PSUs, segments (clusters of households) within PSUs, households, eligible persons, and finally, sample persons. The sample design provided for oversampling among persons 6 months–5 years of age, 60–74 years of age, and those living in poverty areas.

HHANES was similar in content and design to NHANES I and II. The major difference between HHANES and the previous national surveys is that HHANES used a probability sample of three special subgroups of the population living in selected areas of the United States rather than a national probability sample. The three HHANES universes included approximately 84%, 57%, and 59% of the respective 1980 Mexican-, Cuban-, and Puerto Rican-origin populations in the continental United States.

The survey for the NHANES III was conducted from 1988 to 1994 and consisted of two phases of equal length and sample size. Phase 1 and Phase 2 comprised random samples of the civilian U.S. population living in households. About 40,000 persons 2 months of age and over were selected and asked to complete an extensive interview and an examination. Participants were selected from households in 81 counties across the United States. Children age 2 months–5 years and persons 60 years of age and over were oversampled to provide precise descriptive information on the health status of selected population groups of the United States.

Beginning in 1999, NHANES became a continuous, annual survey, which also allows increased flexibility in survey content. Since April 1999, NHANES collects data every year from a representative sample of the civilian U.S. population, newborns and older, by in-home personal interviews and physical examinations in the MEC. The sample design is a complex, multistage, clustered design using unequal probabilities of selection. The first-stage sample frame for continuous NHANES during 1999–2001 was the list of PSUs selected for the design of the National Health Interview Survey (NHIS). Typically, an NHANES PSU is a county. For 2002, an independent sample of PSUs (based on current census data) was selected. This independent design is used for the period 2002–2006. For 1999, because of delay in the start of data collection, 12 distinct PSUs were in the annual sample. For each year in 2000–2004, 15 PSUs were selected. The within-PSU design involves forming secondary sampling units that are nested within census tracts, selecting dwelling units within secondary units, and then selecting sample persons within dwelling units. The final sample person selection involves differential probabilities of selection according to demographic variables sex (male or female), race/ethnicity (Mexican American, black, all others), and age. Because of the differential probabilities of selection, dwelling units are screened for potential sample persons. Sample weights are available and should be used in estimation of descriptive statistics. The complex design features should be used in estimating standard errors for the descriptive estimates.

The estimation procedure used to produce national statistics for all NHANES involved inflation by the reciprocal of the probability of selection, adjustment for nonresponse, and poststratified ratio adjustment to population totals. Sampling errors also were estimated to measure the reliability of the statistics.

Sample Size and Response Rates: NHES I sampled 7,710 adults. The examination response rate was 87%. NHES II sampled 7,417 children and reported a response rate of 96% for the questionnaire sample and 73% for the examination sample. NHES III sampled 7,514 youth and reported a response rate of 90%.

A sample of 28,043 persons was selected for NHANES I. Household interviews were completed for more than 96% of the persons selected, and about 75% (20,749) were examined. A sample of 27,801 persons was selected for NHANES II; 73% (20,322 persons) were examined.

In the HHANES 9,894 persons in the Southwest were selected (75% or 7,462 were examined); in Dade County 2,244 persons were selected (60% or 1,357 were examined); and in the Northeast 3,786 persons were selected (75% or 2,834 were examined). Over the 6-year survey period of NHANES III, 39,695 persons were selected, the household interview response rate was 86%, and the medical examination response rate was 78%.

In the sample selection for NHANES 1999–2000, there were 22,839 dwelling units screened. Of these, 6,005 households had at least one eligible sample person identified for interviewing. A total of 12,160 eligible sample persons were identified. The overall response rate in NHANES 1999–2000 for those interviewed was 82% (9,965 of 12,160), and the response rate for those examined was 76% (9,282 of 12,160). For NHANES 2001–2002 there were 13,156 persons selected in the sample, of which 84% (11,039) were interviewed and 80% (10,480) of the 13,156 selected completed the health examination component of the survey. For NHANES 2003–2004 6,410 households had at least one eligible sample person identified for interviewing. A total of 12,761 eligible sample persons were identified, of which 79% (10,115) were interviewed and 76% (9,653) completed the health examination component of the survey.

Issues Affecting Interpretation: Data elements, lab tests performed, and the technological sophistication of medical examination and laboratory equipment have changed over time. Therefore, trend analyses should carefully examine how specific data elements were collected across the different NHANES and NHES surveys.

References:

Gordon T, Miller HW. Cycle I of the Health Examination Survey: Sample and response, United States, 1960–1962. National Center for Health Statistics. Vital Health Stat 11(1). 1974. Available from: www.cdc.gov/nchs/data/series/sr_11/sr11_001.pdf.

Plan, operation, and response results of a program of children's examinations. National Center for Health Statistics. Vital Health Stat 1(5). 1967. Available from: www.cdc.gov/nchs/data/series/sr_01/sr01_005.pdf.

Schaible WL. Quality control in a National Health Examination Survey. National Center for Health Statistics. Vital Health Stat 2(44). 1972. Available from: www.cdc.gov/nchs/data/series/sr_02/sr02_044.pdf.

Miller HW. Plan and operation of the Health and Nutrition Examination Survey, United States, 1971–73. National Center for Health Statistics. Vital Health Stat 1(10a) and 1(10b). 1977 and 1978. Available from: www.cdc.gov/nchs/data/series/sr_01/sr01_010a.pdf and www.cdc.gov/nchs/data/series/sr_01/sr01_010b.pdf.

Engel A, Murphy RS, Maurer K, Collins E. Plan and operation of the NHANES I Augmentation Survey of Adults 25–74 years, United States, 1974–1975. National Center for Health Statistics. Vital Health Stat 1(14). 1978. Available from: www.cdc.gov/nchs/data/series/sr_01/sr01_014.pdf.

McDowell A, Engel A, Massey JT, Maurer K. Plan and operation of the second National Health and Nutrition

Examination Survey, 1976–1980. National Center for Health Statistics. Vital Health Stat 1(15), 1981. Available from: www.cdc.gov/nchs/data/series/sr_01/sr01_015.pdf.

Maurer K. Plan and operation of the Hispanic Health and Nutrition Examination Survey, 1982–1984. National Center for Health Statistics. Vital Health Stat 1(19). 1985. Available from: www.cdc.gov/nchs/data/series/sr_01/sr01_019.pdf.

Ezzati TM, Massey JT, Waksberg J, et al. Sample design: Third National Health and Nutrition Examination Survey. National Center for Health Statistics. Vital Health Stat 2(113). 1992.

Plan and operation of the Third National Health and Nutrition Examination Survey, 1988–1994. National Center for Health Statistics. Vital Health Stat 1(32). 1994. Available from: www.cdc.gov/nchs/data/series/sr_01/sr01_032.pdf.

For More Information: See the NHANES website: www.cdc.gov/nchs/about/major/nhanes/nhanes.htm.

National Health Interview Survey (NHIS)

Centers for Disease Control and Prevention

National Center for Health Statistics

Overview: The National Health Interview Survey (NHIS) monitors the health of the U.S. population through the collection and analysis of data on a broad range of health topics. A major strength of this survey lies in the ability to analyze health measures by many demographic and socioeconomic characteristics.

Selected Content: The NHIS obtains information during household interviews on illnesses, injuries, activity limitation, chronic conditions, health insurance coverage, utilization of health care, and other health topics. Demographic data include age, sex, education, race/ethnicity (reported by respondent or proxy), place of birth, income, and place of residence. Other data collected include risk factors such as lack of exercise, smoking, alcohol consumption, and use of prevention services such as vaccinations, mammography, and pap smears. Special modules and supplements focus on different issues each year and have included topics such as HIV/AIDS, aging, cancer screening, prevention, alternative and complementary medicine, and many other topics.

Data Years: The NHIS has been conducted annually since 1957 with a major redesign every 10–15 years.

Coverage: The NHIS covers the civilian noninstitutionalized population of the United States. Excluded are patients in long-term care facilities, persons on active duty with the Armed Forces (although their dependents are included), and U.S. nationals living in foreign countries.

Methodology: The NHIS is a cross-sectional household interview survey. Sampling and interviewing are continuous throughout each year. The sampling plan follows a multistage area probability design that permits the representative sampling of households. The sampling plan was last redesigned in 1995 and will be redesigned in the 2006 survey. Information for only the current sampling plan covering the design years of 1995–2005 is presented. The first stage consists of a sample of 358 primary sampling units (PSUs) drawn from approximately 1,900 geographically defined PSUs that cover the 50 states and the District of Columbia. A PSU consists of a county, a small group of contiguous counties, or a metropolitan statistical area.

Within a PSU, two types of second-stage units are used: area segments and permit area segments. Area segments are defined geographically and contain an expected 8 or 12 addresses. Permit area segments cover geographical areas containing housing units built after the 1990 census. The permit area segments are defined using updated lists of building permits issued in the PSU since 1990 and contain an expected four addresses. Within each segment all occupied households at the sample addresses are targeted for interview.

The total NHIS sample of PSUs is subdivided into four separate panels, or subdesigns, such that each panel is a representative sample of the U.S. population. This design feature has a number of advantages, including flexibility for the total sample size. The households selected for interview each week in the NHIS are a probability sample representative of the target population.

The NHIS that was fielded from 1982–1996 consisted of two parts: (1) a set of basic health and demographic items (known as the Core questionnaire), and (2) one or more sets of questions on current health topics (known as Supplements). The Core questionnaire remained the same over that time period whereas the current health topics changed depending on data needs.

The NHIS questionnaire revision first implemented in 1997 has three parts or modules: a Basic module, a Periodic module, and a Topical module. The Basic module corresponds to the core questionnaire before revision. It remains largely unchanged from year to year and allows for trend analysis and for data from more than 1 year to be pooled to increase sample size for analytic purposes. The Basic module contains three components: the Family Core, the Sample Adult Core, and the Sample Child Core. The Family Core component collects information on everyone in the family and allows the NHIS to serve as a sampling frame for additional integrated surveys as needed. Information collected on the Family Core for all family members includes household composition and sociodemographic characteristics, tracking information, information for matches to administrative data bases, health insurance coverage, and basic indicators of health status and utilization of health care services.

From each family in the NHIS, one sample adult and, for families with children under 18 years of age, one sample child are randomly selected to participate in the Sample Adult Core and the Sample Child Core questionnaires. Because some health issues are different for children and adults, these two questionnaires differ in some items but both collect basic information on health status, use of health care services, health conditions, and health behaviors.

Sample Size and Response Rates: Since 1997, the sample numbered about 100,000 persons with about 30–36,000 persons participating in the sample adult and about 12–14,000 persons in the sample child questionnaire. In 2005, the total household response rate was 87%. Response rates for special health topics (supplements) have generally been lower. For example, the response rate was 80% for the 1994 Year 2000 Supplement, which included questions about cigarette smoking and use of such preventive services as mammography. Since 1997 the final response rate for the sample adult supplement was 70%–80% and 78%–84% for the sample child supplement.

Issues Affecting Interpretation: In 1997, the questionnaire was redesigned and some basic concepts were changed and other concepts were measured in different ways. For some questions there was a change in the reference period. Also in 1997, the collection methodology changed from paper and pencil questionnaires to computer-assisted personal interviewing (CAPI). Because of the major redesigns of the questionnaire in 1997, most trend tables in *Health, United States* begin with 1997 data. Starting with *Health, United States, 2005* estimates for 2000 and later years use weights derived from the 2000 census.

References:

Massey JT, Moore TF, Parsons VL, Tadros W. Design and estimation for the National Health Interview Survey, 1985–1994. National Center for Health Statistics. Vital Health Stat 2(110). 1989. Available from: www.cdc.gov/nchs/data/series/sr_02/sr02_110.pdf.

National Center for Health Statistics. National Health Interview Survey: Research for the 1995–2004 redesign. National Center for Health Statistics. Vital Health Stat 2(126). 1999. Available from: www.cdc.gov/nchs/data/series/sr_02/sr02_126.pdf.

Botman SL, Moore TF, Moriarity CL, Parsons VL. Design and estimation for the National Health Interview Survey, 1995–2004. National Center for Health Statistics. Vital Health Stat 2(130), 2000. Available from: www.cdc.gov/nchs/data/series/sr_02/sr02_130.pdf.

For More Information: See the NHIS website: www.cdc.gov/nchs/nhis.htm.

National Hospital Ambulatory Medical Care Survey (NHAMCS)

Centers for Disease Control and Prevention National Center for Health Statistics

Overview: The National Hospital Ambulatory Medical Care Survey (NHAMCS) collects data on the utilization and provision of medical care services provided in hospital emergency and outpatient departments.

Selected Content: Data are collected from medical records on type of providers seen; reason for visit; diagnoses; drugs ordered, provided, or continued; and selected procedures and tests performed during the visit. Patient data include age, sex, race, and expected source of payment. Data are also collected on selected characteristics of hospitals included in the survey.

Data Years: Annual data collection began in 1992.

Coverage: The survey is a representative sample of visits to emergency departments (EDs) and outpatient departments (OPDs) of nonfederal, short-stay, or general hospitals. Telephone contacts are excluded.

Methodology: A four-stage probability sample design is used in NHAMCS, involving samples of primary sampling units (PSUs), hospitals within PSUs, clinics within OPDs, and patient visits within clinics. Emergency departments are treated as their own stratum and all service areas within EDs are included. In the rare event that a sample hospital has more than five emergency service areas, a sample of five areas is selected. The first stage sample of the NHAMCS consists of 112 PSUs selected from 1,900 such units comprising the United States. Within PSUs, 600 general and short-stay hospitals were sampled and assigned to 1 of 16 panels. In any given year, 13 panels are included. Each panel is assigned to a 4-week reporting period during the calendar year.

In the NHAMCS outpatient department survey, a clinic is defined as an administrative unit of the OPD in which ambulatory medical care is provided under the supervision of a physician. Clinics where only ancillary services, such as radiology, laboratory services, physical rehabilitation, renal dialysis, and pharmacy, are provided, or other settings in which physician services are not typically provided, are considered out of scope. If a hospital OPD has five or fewer in-scope clinics, all are included in the sample. For hospital OPDs with more than five clinics, a systematic sample of clinics proportional to size is included in the survey.

The U.S. Census Bureau acts as the data collection agent for the NHAMCS. Census field representatives contact sample hospitals to determine whether they have a 24-hour ED or an OPD that offers physician services. Visits to eligible EDs and OPDs are systematically sampled over the 4-week reporting period such that about 100 ED encounters and about 200 OPD encounters are selected. Hospital staff are asked to complete patient record forms (PRFs) for each sampled visit, but census field representatives typically abstract data for more than one-half of these visits.

Sample data are weighted to produce national estimates. The estimation procedure used in the NHAMCS has three basic components: inflation by the reciprocal of the probability of selection, adjustment for nonresponse, and ratio adjustment to fixed totals.

Sample Size and Response Rates: In any given year, the hospital sample consists of approximately 500 hospitals, of which 80% have EDs and about one-half have eligible OPDs. Typically, about 1,000 clinics are selected from participating hospital OPDs. In 2002, the number of PRFs completed for EDs was 37,337 and for OPDs 35,586. In 2003, the number of PRFs completed for EDs was 40,253 and for OPDs 34,492. In 2004, the number of PRFs completed for EDs was 36,589 and for OPDs 31,783. In 2005, the number of PRFs completed for EDs was 33,605 and for OPDs 29,975. In 2002, the hospital response rate for NHAMCS was 92% for EDs and 75% for OPDs. In 2003, the hospital response rate was 85% for EDs and 73% for OPDs. In 2004, the hospital response rate was 89% for EDs and 75% for OPDs. In 2005, the hospital response rate was 89% for EDs and 80% for OPDs.

Issues Affecting Interpretation: The NHAMCS PRF is modified approximately every 2 to 4 years to reflect changes in physician practice characteristics, patterns of care, and technological innovations. Examples of recent changes are the number of drugs recorded on the PRF form, and checkboxes of specific tests or procedures performed. For analyses that present visit rates per population, the civilian noninstitutionalized population is used as the denominator. However, visits to hospital EDs can also include persons who reside in institutional settings.

Reference:

McCaig LF, McLemore T. Plan and operation of the National Hospital Ambulatory Medical Care Survey. National Center for Health Statistics. Vital Health Stat 1(34). 1994. Available from: www.cdc.gov/nchs/data/series/sr_01/sr01_034acc.pdf.

For More Information: See the National Health Care Survey (NHCS) website: www.cdc.gov/nchs/nhcs.htm or the Ambulatory Health Care website: www.cdc.gov/nchs/about/major/ahcd/ahcd1.htm.

National Hospital Discharge Survey (NHDS)

Centers for Disease Control and Prevention

National Center for Health Statistics

Overview: The National Hospital Discharge Survey (NHDS) collects and produces national estimates on characteristics of inpatient stays in nonfederal short-stay hospitals in the United States.

Selected Content: Patient information collected includes demographics, length of stay, diagnoses, and procedures.

Hospital characteristics collected include region, ownership, and bedsize.

Data Years: The NHDS has been conducted annually since 1965.

Coverage: The survey design covers the 50 states and the District of Columbia. Included in the survey are hospitals with an average length of stay of less than 30 days for all inpatients, general hospitals, and children's general hospitals. Excluded are federal, military, and Department of Veterans Affairs hospitals, as well as hospital units of institutions (such as prison hospitals), and hospitals with fewer than six beds staffed for patient use. All discharged patients from in-scope hospitals are included in the survey; however, data for newborns are not included in *Health, United States.*

Methodology: The design implemented in 1965 continued through 1987, and a redesign with a new sample of hospitals fielded in 1988 is currently in place. The sample for the 1965 NHDS was selected in 1964 from a frame of short-stay hospitals listed in the National Master Facility Inventory. A two-stage stratified sample design was used, with hospitals stratified according to bedsize and geographic region. Sample hospitals were selected with probabilities ranging from certainty for the largest hospitals to 1 in 40 for the smallest hospitals. Within each participating hospital, a systematic random sample was selected from a daily listing sheet of discharges. Within-hospital sampling rates for discharges varied inversely with the probability of hospital selection, so the overall probability of selecting a discharge was approximately the same across the sample.

Data collection was conducted by means of manual abstraction of patient information from sampled medical records. Sample selection and transcription of information from inpatient medical records to NHDS survey forms were performed by hospital staff, representatives of NCHS, or both. In 1985, a second data collection procedure was introduced. The procedure involved the purchase of computer data tapes from commercial abstracting services that contained automated discharge data for some hospitals participating in the NHDS. This procedure was used in approximately 17% of the sample hospitals for 1985–1987. Discharges on these computer files were subjected to the NHDS sampling specifications as well as the computer edits and estimation procedures. Two data collection methods, manual and automated, continue to be used in the NHDS.

A redesign of the NHDS was implemented for the 1988 survey. Under the redesign hospitals were selected using a modified three-stage stratified design. Units selected at the first stage consisted of either hospitals or geographic areas. The geographic areas were Primary Sample Units (PSUs) used for the 1985–1994 National Health Interview Survey, which are geographic areas such as counties or townships. Hospitals within PSUs were then selected at the second stage. Strata at this stage were defined by geographic region, PSU size, abstracting service status, and hospital specialty-size groups. Within these strata, hospitals were selected with probabilities proportional to their annual number of discharges. At the third stage, a sample of discharges was selected by a systematic random sampling technique. The sampling rate was determined by the hospital's sampling stratum and the type of data collection system (manual or automated) used. Discharge records from hospitals submitting data via commercial abstracting services and selected state data systems (approximately 44% of sample hospitals) were arrayed by primary diagnoses, patient sex and age group, and date of discharge, before sampling.

The NHDS hospital sample is updated every 3 years by continuing the sampling process among hospitals that become eligible for the survey during the intervening years and by deleting hospitals that were no longer eligible. This process was conducted in 1991, 1994, 1997, 2000, and 2003.

The basic unit of estimation for NHDS is a sampled discharge. The basic estimation procedure involves inflation by the reciprocal of the probability of selection. There are adjustments for nonresponding hospitals and discharges; a postratio adjustment to fixed totals is employed.

Sample Size and Response Rate: In 2005, 501 hospitals were selected: 473 were within scope, 444 participated (94%), and data were collected from medical records for approximately 375,000 discharges.

Issues Affecting Interpretation: In 1988, the NHDS was redesigned. Caution is required in comparing trend data from before and after the redesign. There are also annual modifications to the ICD–9–CM affecting diagnoses and procedure categories. See Appendix II, ICD–9–CM; Tables X and XI.

Hospital utilization rates per 1,000 population were computed using estimates of the civilian population of the United States as of July 1 of each year. Rates for 1990 through 1999 use postcensal estimates of the civilian population based on the

1990 census adjusted for net underenumeration using the 1990 National Population Adjustment Matrix from the U.S. Census Bureau. The estimates for 2000 and beyond that appear in *Health, United States, 2003* and later editions were calculated using estimates of the civilian population based on census 2000, and therefore are not strictly comparable with postcensal rates calculated for the 1990s. See Appendix I, Population Census and Population Estimates.

References:

DeFrances CJ, Hall MJ. 2005 National Hospital Discharge Survey. Advance data from vital and health statistics 2007; no 385. Hyattsville, MD. National Center for Health Statistics.

Dennison C, Pokras R. Design and operation of the National Hospital Discharge Survey: 1988 redesign. National Center for Health Statistics. Vital Health Stat 1(39). 2000. Available from: www.cdc.gov/nchs/data/series/sr_01/sr01_039.pdf.

Haupt BJ, Kozak LJ. Estimates from two survey designs: National Hospital Discharge Survey. National Center for Health Statistics. Vital Health Stat 13(111). 1992. Available from: www.cdc.gov/nchs/data/series/sr_13/sr13_111.pdf.

For More Information: See the National Health Care Survey website: www.cdc.gov/nchs.nhcs.htm or the National Hospital Discharge Survey website: www.cdc.gov/nchs/about/major/hdasd/nhds.htm.

National Immunization Survey (NIS)

Centers for Disease Control and Prevention National Center for Health Statistics and National Immunization Program

Overview: The National Immunization Survey (NIS) is a continuing nationwide telephone sample survey to monitor vaccination coverage rates among children 19–35 months of age.

Selected Content: Data collected include vaccination status and timing for Diphtheria, Tetanus toxoids, and Pertussis vaccine (DTP/DT/DTaP); Polio vaccine; Measles, Mumps, and Rubella vaccine (MMR); Haemophilius influenzae type b vaccine (Hib); Hepatitis B vaccine (Hep B); Varicella vaccine; Pneumococcal conjugate vaccine (PCV); and Combined series (4:3:1:3) by race/ethnicity, poverty level, location of residence, geographic division, state, and selected urban areas.

Data Years: Annual data collection was initiated beginning with the data year 1994. Data collection for Varicella began in July 1996; data collection for PCV began in July 2001.

Coverage: Children 19–35 months of age in the civilian noninstitutionalized population are represented in this survey. Estimates of vaccine-specific coverage are available for the Nation, states, and 28 urban areas. In 2005, about 82% of the age-eligible children were up-to-date for the 4:3:1:3 series.

Methodology: The NIS is a nationwide telephone sample survey of households with age-eligible children. The NIS uses a two-phase sample design. First, a random-digit dialing (RDD) sample of telephone numbers is drawn. When households with age-eligible children are contacted, the interviewer collects information on the vaccinations received by all age-eligible children and obtains permission to contact the children's immunization providers. In the second phase, immunization providers are sent vaccination history questionnaires by mail. Providers' responses are compared with information obtained from households to provide a more accurate estimate of vaccination coverage levels. Final estimates are adjusted for households without telephones and nonresponse.

Sample Size and Response Rates: In 2005, vaccination data were collected for 27,627 children age 19–35 months. In 2005, the overall interview response rate was 65%. Vaccination information from providers was obtained for 64% of all children who were eligible for provider follow-up in 2005.

Issues Affecting Interpretation: For data years 1998, 2002, 2004, and 2005 slight modifications to the estimation procedure were implemented to obtain vaccination coverage rates from the provider data. Published estimates of vaccination coverage based on the NIS data for years prior to 1998 (e.g., estimates published in MMWR articles) may differ slightly from estimates published in *Health, United States* and on the NIS website for the same NIS data. All released public-use data files include the sampling weight for the revised estimation procedure.

References:

Centers for Disease Control and Prevention (CDC). National, state, and urban area vaccination levels among children aged 19–35 months—United States, 2005. MMWR 2006;55(36);988–21. Available from: www.cdc.gov/mmwr/preview/mmwrhtml/mm5536a2.htm.

Centers for Disease Control and Prevention (CDC), National Center for Health Statistics. National Immunization Survey: A User's Guide for the 2005 Public-Use Data File. Hyattsville, MD; 2006. Available from: www.cdc.gov/nis/pdfs/nispuf05_dug.pdf.

Smith PJ, Hoaglin DC, Battaglia M, Michael P, Khare M, Barker LE. Statistical methodology of the National Immunization Survey, 1994–2002.

National Center for Health Statistics. Vital Health Stat Series no 2 (138). 2005. Available from: www.cdc.gov/nchs/data/series/sr_02/sr02_138.pdf.

For More Information: See the NIS website: www.cdc.gov/nis.

National Medical Expenditure Survey (NMES)—See Medical Expenditure Panel Survey

National Notifiable Disease Surveillance System (NNDSS)

Centers for Disease Control and Prevention

Overview: This system provides weekly provisional information on the occurrence of diseases defined as notifiable by the Council of State and Territorial Epidemiologists.

Selected Content: Data include incidence of reportable diseases using uniform case definitions.

Data Years: The first annual summary of The Notifiable Diseases in 1912 included reports of 10 diseases from 19 states, the District of Columbia, and Hawaii. By 1928, all states, the District of Columbia, Hawaii, and Puerto Rico were participating in national reporting of 29 specified diseases. At their annual meeting in 1950, the State and Territorial Health Officers authorized a conference of state and territorial epidemiologists whose purpose was to determine which diseases should be reported to Public Health Service. In 1961, CDC assumed responsibility for the collection and publication of data concerning nationally notifiable diseases.

Coverage: Notifiable disease reports are received from health departments in the 50 states, five territories, New York City, and the District of Columbia. Policies for reporting notifiable disease cases can vary by disease or reporting jurisdiction, depending on case status classification (i.e., confirmed, probable, or suspect).

Methodology: CDC, in partnership with the Council of State and Territorial Epidemiologists (CSTE), operates the National Notifiable Diseases Surveillance System (NNDSS). Notifiable disease surveillance is conducted by public health practitioners at local, state, and national levels to support disease prevention and control activities. The system also provides annual summaries of the data. CSTE and CDC annually review the status of national infectious disease surveillance and recommend additions or deletions to the list of nationally notifiable diseases based on the need to respond to emerging priorities. For example, Q fever and tularemia became nationally notifiable in 2000. However, reporting nationally notifiable diseases to CDC is voluntary. Reporting is currently mandated by law or regulation only at the local and state level. Therefore, the list of diseases that are considered notifiable varies slightly by state. For example, reporting of cyclosporiasis to CDC is not done by some states in which this disease is not notifiable to local or state authorities.

State epidemiologists report cases of notifiable diseases to CDC, which tabulates and publishes these data in the *Morbidity and Mortality Weekly Report* (MMWR) and the *Summary of Notifiable Diseases, United States* (titled *Annual Summary* before 1985).

Issues Affecting Interpretation: These data must be interprete[d] in light of reporting practices. Some diseases that cause severe clinical illness (for example, plague and rabies) are most likely reported accurately if diagnosed by a clinician. However, persons who have diseases that are clinically mild and infrequently associated with serious consequences (for example, salmonellosis) might not seek medical care from a health care provider. Even if these less severe diseases are diagnosed, they are less likely to be reported.

The degree of completeness of data reporting also is influenced by the diagnostic facilities available, the control measures in effect, public awareness of a specific disease, and the interests, resources, and priorities of state and local officials responsible for disease control and public health surveillance. Finally, factors such as changes in case definitions for public health surveillance, introduction of new diagnostic tests, or discovery of new disease entities can cause changes in disease reporting that are independent of the true incidence of disease.

Reference:

Centers for Disease Control and Prevention. Summary of notifiable diseases—United States, 2005. MMWR 2007; 54 (53). Available from: www.cdc.gov/mmwr/summary.html.

For More Information: See the NNDSS website: www.cdc.gov/epo/dphsi/nndsshis.htm.

National Nursing Home Survey (NNHS)

Centers for Disease Control and Prevention National Center for Health Statistics

Overview: The National Nursing Home Survey (NNHS) provides information on characteristics of nursing homes and their residents and staff.

Selected Content: The NNHS provides information on nursing homes from two perspectives—that of the provider of services and that of the recipient. Data about the facilities include characteristics such as bed size, ownership, affiliation, Medicare/Medicaid certification, specialty units, services offered, number and characteristics of staff, expenses, and charges. Data about the current residents and discharges include demographic characteristics, health status, level of assistance needed with activities of daily living, vision and hearing impairment, continence, services received, sources of payment, and discharge disposition (for discharges). The redesigned NNHS conducted in 2004 included new facility data items on Joint Commission on Accreditation of Healthcare Organization accreditation, electronic information systems, cultural competency, immunization polices and practices, end-of-life practices, special service programs, and new patient-level data items on hospitalizations and emergency department admissions, pain assessment and pain relief, medications, family and caregiver services, end-of-life care and advance directives, pressure ulcers, behavior or mood symptoms, falls, and out-of-pocket charges. In addition to these facility and resident data items, data on nurse staffing and a supplemental survey on nursing assistants working in nursing homes were also collected.

Data Years: NCHS conducted seven NNHS: the first survey August 1973–April 1974; the second May–December 1977; the third August 1985–January 1986; the fourth July–December 1995; the fifth July–December 1997; the sixth July–December 1999, and the seventh and most recent NNHS; which has undergone a major redesign, was conducted August–January 2004.

Coverage: The initial NNHS, conducted in 1973–1974, included the universe of nursing homes that provided some level of nursing care and excluded homes providing only personal or domiciliary care. The 1977 NNHS encompassed all types of nursing homes, including personal care and domiciliary care homes. The 1985 NNHS was designed to be similar to the 1973–1974 survey in that it excluded personal or domiciliary care homes. However in 1985, an unknown number of residential care facilities were present in the sampling frame. These facilities were identified in the 1986 inventory survey and can be removed from the estimate of facilities and beds for 1985. The 1995, 1997, 1999, and 2004 NNHS also included only nursing homes that provided some level of nursing care and excluded homes providing only personal or domiciliary care, similar to the 1985 and 1973–1974 surveys.

Data were collected from nursing homes in all 50 states and the District of Columbia (D.C.) in the 1995, 1997, 1999 and 2004 surveys, but in 1973–1974, 1977, and 1985, data were only collected in the 48 contiguous states and D.C. Data on current residents were collected in all surveys; data on discharges were collected in 1977, 1985, 1997, and 1999. Expense data were collected in 1977, 1985, and 1995. Data on characteristics of staff were collected in 1973–1974, 1977, 1985, and 2004.

Methodology: The survey uses a stratified two-stage probability design. The first stage is the selection of facilities, and the second stage is the selection of residents and discharges. Prior to the 2004 NNHS up to six current residents and/or six discharges were selected. The 2004 survey was designed to select only 12 current residents from each facility to participate in the survey. Information on the facility is collected through a personal interview with the administrator or staff designated by the administrator. Resident data were provided by staff familiar with the care provided to the resident. Staff relied on the medical record and personal knowledge of the resident. In addition to employee data that were collected during the interview with the administrator, in several years staffing data were collected via a self-administered questionnaire. Discharge data, when collected, were based on information recorded in the medical record.

Current residents are those on the facility's roster as of the night before the survey. Included are all residents for whom beds are maintained even though they may be away on an overnight leave or in the hospital. People residing in personal care or domiciliary care homes are excluded. Discharges are those who are formally discharged from care by the facility during a designated reference period randomly selected for each facility before data collection. Both live and deceased discharges are included. Residents were counted more than once if they were discharged more than once during the reference period. Resident rates are calculated using estimates of the civilian population of the United States including institutionalized persons. Population data are from unpublished tabulations provided by the U.S. Census Bureau. The 2004 population estimates are postcensal estimates as of July 1, 2004, based on the 2000 census. For more information about the 2004 population estimates, see the Technical Notes in Kozak LJ, DeFrances CJ, Hall MJ. National Hospital Discharge Survey: 2004 annual summary with detailed diagnosis and procedure data. National Center for Health Statistics. Vital Health Stat 13(162). 2006. Available from: www.cdc.gov/nchs/data/series/sr_13/sr13_162acc.pdf.

Statistics for the NNHS are derived by a multistage estimation procedure that has three major components: (a) inflation by the reciprocals of the probabilities of sample selection; (b) adjustment for nonresponse; and (c) ratio adjustment to fixed totals. The surveys are adjusted for four types of nonresponse: (1) when an eligible nursing facility did not respond; (2) when the facility failed to complete the sampling lists; (3) when the facility did not complete the facility questionnaire but did complete the questionnaire for residents in the facility; and (4) when the facility did not provide information to complete the questionnaire for the sample resident or discharge.

Sample Size and Response Rates: In 1973–1974 the sample of 2,118 homes was selected from the 1971 National Master Facility Inventory (NMFI) and from those that opened for business in 1972. For the 1977 NNHS the sample of 1,698 facilities was selected from nursing homes in the sampling frame, which consisted of all homes listed in the 1973 NMFI and those opening for business between 1973 and December 1976. The sample for the 1985 survey consisted of the 1,220 facilities selected from the 1982 NMFI, data for homes identified in the 1982 Complement Survey of the NMFI, data on hospital-based nursing homes obtained from the Health Care Financing Administration (now known as the Centers for Medicare & Medicaid Services), and data on nursing homes open for business between 1982 and June 1, 1984. The 1995 sample of 1,500 homes was selected from a sampling frame consisting of nursing homes from the 1991 National Health Provider Inventory (NHPI) and updated lists from the Agency Reporting System (ARS). The ARS was an ongoing system designed to periodically update the NHPI and consisted primarily of lists or directories of facilities from state agencies, federal agencies, and national voluntary organizations. For the 1997 survey, data were obtained from about 1,488 nursing homes from a sampling frame consisting of nursing homes listed on the 1991 NHPI that was updated with a current listing of nursing facilities supplied by the Health Care Finance Administration and other national organizations. The facility frame for the 1999 NNHS consisted of all nursing homes identified in the 1997 NNHS and updated with current nursing facilities listed by the Centers for Medicare & Medicaid Services and other national organizations. The 1999 sample consisted of 1,496 nursing homes. In 1995, 1997, and 1999, facility-level response rates were over 93%. For the 2004 redesigned and expanded NNHS, 1,500 nursing homes were selected and a facility response rate of 81% was achieved.

Issues Affecting Interpretation: Samples of discharges and residents contain different populations with different characteristics. The resident sample is more likely to contain long-term nursing home residents and, conversely, to underestimate short nursing home stays. Because short-term residents are less likely to be on the nursing home rolls on a given night, they are less likely to be sampled. Estimates of discharges underestimate long nursing home stays. In addition, analysts should ensure that the underlying populations are similar across survey years—for example, whether the survey includes personal or domiciliary care homes.

References:

Meiners MR. Selected operating and financial characteristics of nursing homes, United States, 1973–1974 National Nursing Home Survey. National Center for Health Statistics. Vital Health Stat Series no 13 (22). 1975. Available from: www.cdc.gov/nchs/data/series/sr_13/sr13_022.pdf.

Van Nostrand JF, Zappolo A, Hing E, et al. The National Nursing Home Survey: 1977 summary for the United States. National Center for Health Statistics. Vital Health

Stat Series no 13 (43). 1979. Available from: www.cdc.gov/nchs/data/series/sr_13/sr13_043.pdf.

Hing E, Sekscenski E, Strahan G. The National Nursing Home Survey: 1985 summary for the United States. National Center for Health Statistics. Vital Health Stat Series no 13 (97). 1989. Available from: www.cdc.gov/nchs/data/series/sr_13/sr13_097.pdf.

Strahan G. An overview of nursing homes and their current residents: Data from the 1995 National Nursing Home Survey. Advance data from vital and health statistics; no 280. Hyattsville, MD: National Center for Health Statistics. 1997. Available from: www.cdc.gov/nchs/data/ad/ad280.pdf.

The National Nursing Home Survey: 1997 summary. National Center for Health Statistics. Vital Health Stat Series no 13 (147). 2000. Available from: www.cdc.gov/nchs/data/series/sr_13/sr13_147.pdf.

The National Nursing Home Survey: 1999 summary. National Center for Health Statistics. Vital Health Stat Series no 13 (152). 2002. Available from: www.cdc.gov/nchs/data/series/sr_13/sr13_152.pdf.

For More Information: See the National Health Care Survey website: www.cdc.gov/nchs/nhcs.htm and the NNHS website: www.cdc.gov/nchs/nnhs.htm.

National Prisoner Statistics (NPS)

Bureau of Justice Statistics

Overview: National Prisoner Statistics (NPS) produces semiannual national- and state-level data on the numbers of prisoners in state and federal prison facilities. The NPS provides information on prisoners incarcerated in state and federal correctional institutions, including their characteristics, movements, and locations.

Data Years: Since 1926, the federal government has published data annually on the prisoner count in each state and the federal prison system.

Coverage: Data are collected from all 50 states. The prisoner count in the District of Columbia was included until 2001, when the District ceased operating a prison system.

Methodology: NPS obtains prisoner information from a census of prisons in the United States, conducted by the U.S. Census Bureau. The census is based on a facility list maintained by the Census Bureau. Prisons are mailed the NPS forms that may be returned by mail or facsimile. Starting with 2003 data, respondents were provided with an internet reporting option. NPS distinguishes between prisoners in custody from those under jurisdiction. To have custody of a prisoner, a state must hold that person in one of its facilities. To have jurisdiction, a state has legal authority over the prisoner. Prisoners under a state's jurisdiction may be in the custody of a local jail, another state's prison, or other correctional facility such as a privately-operated institution. NPS collects data on both prisoners in custody and under jurisdiction, though some states are unable to provide both custody and jurisdiction counts. NPS counts include all inmates in state-operated facilities in Alaska, Connecticut, Delaware, Hawaii, Rhode Island, and Vermont, which have combined jail-prison systems.

Sample Size and Response Rate: Data were obtained by mailed and web-based survey questionnaires. After follow-up phone calls, the response rates for most years approach 100%.

For More Information: See the Bureau of Justice Statistics website: www.ojp.usdoj.gov/bjs/correct.htm.

National Survey on Drug Use & Health (NSDUH)

Substance Abuse and Mental Health Services Administration

Overview: The National Survey on Drug Use & Health (NSDUH), formerly called the National Household Survey on Drug Abuse (NHSDA), collects data on substance abuse and dependence, mental health problems, and receipt of substance abuse and mental health treatment.

Selected Content: NSDUH reports on the prevalence, patterns, and consequences of drug and alcohol use and abuse in the general U.S. civilian noninstitutionalized population age 12 and over. Data are collected on the use of illicit drugs, the nonmedical use of licit drugs, and use of alcohol and tobacco products. The survey is conducted annually and is designed to produce drug and alcohol use incidence and prevalence estimates. Data are also collected periodically on special topics of interest such as criminal behavior, treatment, mental health, and attitudes about drugs.

Data Years: The NHSDA survey has been conducted since 1971. In 1999 the NHSDA underwent a major redesign affecting the method of data collection, sample design, sample size, and oversampling. In 2002 the survey underwent a name change to NSDUH as well as additional improvements and modifications to the survey.

Coverage: The survey is representative of persons 12 years of age and over in the civilian noninstitutionalized population in the United States. This includes civilians living on military bases and persons living in noninstitutionalized group quarters, such as college dormitories, rooming houses, and shelters. Persons excluded from the survey include homeless people who do not use shelters, active military personnel, and residents of institutional group quarters, such as jails and hospitals.

Methodology: The data collection method is in-person interviews conducted with a sample of individuals at their place of residence. Prior to 1999, the NSDUH used a paper-and-pencil interviewing (PAPI) methodology. Since 1999, the interview has been carried out with computer assisted interviewing (CAI) methodology. The survey uses a combination of computer-assisted personal-interviewing (CAPI), conducted by the interviewer for some basic demographic information, and audio computer-assisted self-interviewing (ACASI) for most of the questions. ACASI provides a highly private and confidential means of responding to questions to increase the level of honest reporting of illicit drug use and other sensitive behavior. The 2005 National Survey on Drug Use and Health (NSDUH) is the first survey in a coordinated 5-year sample design providing estimates for all 50 States plus the District of Columbia for the years 2005–2009. For the 50-State design, 8 States were designated as large sample States (California, Florida, Illinois, Michigan, New York, Ohio, Pennsylvania, and Texas) with samples large enough to support direct State estimates. States were first stratified into a total of 900 State sampling (SS) regions (48 regions in each large sample State and 12 regions in each small sample State). These regions were contiguous geographic areas designed to yield the same number of interviews on average. Unlike the 1999–2001 NHSDAs and the 2002–2004 NSDUHs in which the first-stage sampling units were clusters of census blocks called area segments, the first stage of selection for the 2005–2009 NSDUHs was census tracts. This stage was included to contain sample segments within a single census tract to the extent possible. A total of 48 census tracts per SS region were selected with probability proportional to size. Within sampled census tracts, adjacent census blocks were combined to form the second-stage sampling units or area segments. One segment was selected within each sampled census tract with probability proportional to population size to support the 5-year sample and any supplemental studies that the Substance Abuse and Mental Health Services Administration (SAMHSA) may choose to field. Of these segments, 24 were designated for the coordinated 5-year sample and 24 were designated as "reserve" segments. Eight sample segments per SS region were fielded during the 2005 survey year. These sampled segments were allocated equally into four separate samples, one for each 3-month period (calendar quarter) during the year, so that the survey was essentially continuous in the field.

The design also oversampled youths and young adults, so that each state's sample was approximately equally distributed among three major age groups: 12–17 years, 18–25 years, and 26 years or over.

Sample Size and Response Rate: Nationally, of the 146,912 eligible households sampled, 134,055 addresses were successfully screened for the 2005 survey, and in these screened households, a total of 83,805 sample persons were selected from which 68,308 completed interviews were obtained. The survey was conducted from January to December 2005. Weighted response rates for household screening and for interviewing were 91% and 76%, respectively.

Issues Affecting Interpretation: Several improvements to the survey were implemented in 2002. In addition to the name change, respondents were offered a $30 incentive payment for participation in the survey starting in 2002, and quality control procedures for data collection were enhanced in 2001 and 2002. Because of these improvements and modifications, estimates from the NSDUH completed in 2002 and later should not be compared with estimates from the 2001 or earlier versions of the survey. The data collected in 2002 represent a new baseline for tracking trends in substance use and other measures. Estimates of substance use for youth based on the NSDUH are not directly comparable with estimates based on Monitoring the Future (MTF) and Youth Risk Behavior Surveillance System (YRBSS). In addition to the fact that the MTF excludes dropouts and absentees, rates are not directly comparable across these surveys because of differences in populations covered, sample design, questionnaires, interview setting, and statistical approaches to make the survey estimates generalizable to the entire population. The NSDUH survey collects data in homes, whereas the MTF and YRBSS collect data in school classrooms. The NSDUH estimates are tabulated by age, whereas the MTF and YRBSS estimates are tabulated by grade, representing different ages as well as different populations.

References:

Substance Abuse and Mental Health Services Administration. (2006). Results from the 2005 National Survey on Drug Use and Health: National Findings (Office of Applied Studies, NSDUH Series H-30, DHHS Publication No. SMA 06–4194). Rockville, MD. 2006.

Wright D, Sathe N. (2005). State Estimates of Substance Use from the 2002–2003 National Surveys on Drug Use and Health (DHHS Publication No. SMA 05–3989, NSDUH Series H-26). Substance Abuse and Mental Health Services Administration. Rockville, MD: Office of Applied Studies. 2004.

Cowan CD. Coverage, Sample Design, and Weighting in Three Federal Surveys. Journal of Drug Issues 2001; 31(3):595–614.

For More Information: See the NSDUH website: nsduhweb.rti.org/ or the SAMHSA Office of Applied Studies website: oas.samhsa.gov/.

National Survey of Family Growth (NSFG)

Centers for Disease Control and Prevention National Center for Health Statistics

Overview: The National Survey of Family Growth (NSFG) provides national data on factors affecting birth and pregnancy rates, adoption, and maternal and infant health.

Selected Content: Data elements include sexual activity, marriage, divorce and remarriage, unmarried cohabitation, contraception and sterilization, infertility, breastfeeding, pregnancy loss, low birthweight, and use of medical care for family planning and infertility.

Data Years: Six cycles of the survey have been completed: 1973, 1976, 1982, 1988, 1995, and 2002.

Coverage: The 1973–1995 cycles of the National Survey of Family Growth (NSFG) were based on samples of women ages 15–44 years in the civilian noninstitutionalized population of the United States. The first and second cycles (1973 and 1976) excluded most women who had never been married. The third, fourth, and fifth cycles (1982, 1988, and 1995) included all women ages 15–44 years in the civilian noninstitutional population of the United States. The sixth cycle (2002) included men and women 15–44 years of age in the household population of the United States.

Methodology: Interviews are conducted in person by professional female interviewers using a standardized questionnaire. In all cycles black women were sampled at higher rates than white women so that detailed statistics for black women could be produced. In cycles 5 and 6 (1995 and 2002) Hispanic persons were also oversampled.

In order to make national estimates from the sample for the millions of women age 15–44 years in the United States, data for the interviewed sample women were (a) inflated by the reciprocal of the probability of selection at each stage of sampling (for example, if there was a 1 in 5,000 chance that a woman would be selected for the sample, her sampling weight was 5,000); (b) adjusted for nonresponse; and (c) poststratified, or forced to agree with benchmark population values based on data from the U.S. Census Bureau.

Sample Size and Response Rates: For cycle 1, from 101 PSUs, 10,879 women 15–44 years of age were selected, 9,797 of these were interviewed. In cycle 2, from 79 PSUs, 10,202 eligible women were identified; of these, 8,611 were interviewed. In cycle 3 household screener interviews were completed in 29,511 households (95%). Of the 9,964 eligible women identified, 7,969 were interviewed. In cycle 4, 10,566 eligible women age 15–44 years were sampled. Interviews were completed with 8,450 women. The response rate for the 1990 telephone reinterview was 68% of those responding to the 1988 survey and still eligible for the 1990 survey. In cycle 5, of the 13,795 eligible women in the sample, 10,847 were interviewed. In cycle 6, from 120 PSUs, 7,643 (about 80%) interviews were completed with eligible women and 4,928 (78%) interviews were completed with men.

References:

French DK. National Survey of Family Growth, Cycle I: Sample design, estimation procedures, and variance estimation. National Center for Health Statistics. Vital Health Stat Series no 2 (76). 1978. Available from: www.cdc.gov/nchs/data/series/sr_02/sr02_076.pdf.

Grady WR. National Survey of Family Growth, Cycle II: Sample design, estimation procedures, and variance estimation. National Center for Health Statistics. Vital Health Stat Series no 2 (87). 198l. Available from: www.cdc.gov/nchs/data/series/sr_02/sr02_087.pdf.

Bachrach CA, Horn MC, Mosher WD, Shimizu I. National Survey of Family Growth, Cycle III: Sample design, weighting, and variance estimation. National Center for Health Statistics. Vital Health Stat Series no 2 (98). 1985. Available from: www.cdc.gov/nchs/data/series/sr_02/sr02_098.pdf.

Judkins DR, Mosher WD, Botman SL. National Survey of Family Growth: Design, estimation, and inference. National Center for Health Statistics. Vital Health Stat Series no 2 (109). 1991. Available from: www.cdc.gov/nchs/data/series/sr_02/sr02_109.pdf.

Goksel H, Judkins DR, Mosher WD. Nonresponse adjustments for a telephone follow-up to a National In-Person Survey. Journal of Official Statistics 1992;8(4):417–32.

Kelly JE, Mosher WD, Duffer AP, Kinsey SH. Plan and operation of the 1995 National Survey of Family Growth. Vital Health Stat 1(36). 1997. Available from: www.cdc.gov/nchs/data/series/sr_01/sr01_036.pdf.

Potter FJ, Iannacchione VG, Mosher WD, Mason RE, Kavee JD. Sampling weights, imputation, and variance estimation in the 1995 National Survey of Family Growth. Vital Health Stat Series no 2 (124). 1998. Available from: www.cdc.gov/nchs/data/series/sr_02/sr02_124.pdf.

Groves R, Mosher W, Benson G, et al. Plan and operation of Cycle 6 of the National Survey of Family Growth. National Center for Health Statistics. Vital Health Stat Series no 1 (42). 2005. Available from: www.cdc.gov/nchs/data/series/sr_01/sr01_042.pdf.

For More Information: See the NSFG website: www.cdc.gov/nchs/nsfg.htm.

National Vital Statistics System (NVSS)

Centers for Disease Control and Prevention
National Center for Health Statistics

Overview: The National Vital Statistics System (NVSS) collects and publishes official national statistics on births, deaths, fetal deaths, and prior to 1996, marriages and divorces occurring in the United States based on U.S. Standard Certificates. Fetal deaths are classified and tabulated separately from other deaths. Detailed descriptions of the five Vital Statistics files (birth file, mortality file, multiple cause-of-death file, linked birth/infant death data set, and compressed mortality file) are presented separately below.

Data Years: The death registration area for 1900 consisted of 10 states, the District of Columbia, and a number of cities located in nonregistration states; it covered 40% of the continental U.S. population. The birth registration area was established in 1915 with 10 states and the District of Columbia. The birth and death registration areas continued to expand until 1933, when they included all 48 states and the District of Columbia. Alaska and Hawaii were added to both registration areas in 1959 and 1960, the years in which they gained statehood.

Coverage: The NVSS collects and presents U.S. resident data for the aggregate of 50 states, New York City, and the District of Columbia, as well as for each individual state and the District of Columbia. Vital events occurring in the United States to non-U.S. residents and vital events occurring abroad to U.S. residents are excluded.

Methodology: NCHS's Division of Vital Statistics obtains information on births and deaths from the registration offices of each of the 50 states, New York City, the District of Columbia, Puerto Rico, the U.S. Virgin Islands, Guam, American Samoa, and Northern Mariana Islands. Until 1972 microfilm copies of all death certificates and a 50% sample of birth certificates were received from all registration areas and processed by NCHS. In 1972 some states began sending their data to NCHS through the Cooperative Health Statistics System (CHSS). States that participated in the CHSS program processed 100% of their death and birth records and sent the entire data file to NCHS on computer tapes. Currently, data are sent to NCHS through the Vital Statistics Cooperative Program (VSCP), following the same procedures as CHSS. The number of participating states grew from 6 in 1972 to 46 in 1984. Starting in 1985 all 50 states and the District of Columbia participated in VSCP.

U.S. Standard Certificates—U.S. Standard Live Birth and Death Certificates and Fetal Death Reports are revised periodically, allowing evaluation and addition, modification, and deletion of items. Beginning with 1989 revised standard certificates replaced the 1978 versions. The 1989 revision of the birth certificate included items to identify the Hispanic parentage of newborns and to expand information about maternal and infant health characteristics. The 1989 revision of the death certificate included items on educational attainment and Hispanic origin of decedents, as well as changes to improve the medical certification of cause of death. Standard certificates recommended by NCHS are modified in each registration area to serve the area's needs. However, most certificates conform closely in content and arrangement to the standard certificate, and all certificates contain a minimum data set specified by NCHS. Following 1989, the next revisions of vital records went into effect in some states beginning in 2003, but full implementation in all states will be phased in over several years.

Birth File

Overview: Vital statistics natality data are a fundamental source of demographic, geographic, and medical and health information on all births occurring in the United States. This is one of the few sources of comparable health-related data for small geographic areas over an extended time period. The data are used to present the characteristics of babies and their mothers, track trends such as birth rates for teenagers, and compare natality trends with other countries.

Selected Content: The natality file includes characteristics about the baby such as sex, birthweight, weeks of gestation; demographic information about the parents such as age, race, Hispanic origin, parity, educational attainment, marital status, and state of residence; medical and health information such as prenatal care based on hospital records; and behavioral risk factors for the birth such as mother's tobacco use during pregnancy.

Data Years: The birth registration area began in 1915 with 10 states and the District of Columbia.

Methodology: In the United States, state laws require birth certificates to be completed for all births. The registration of births is the responsibility of the professional attendant at birth, generally a physician or midwife. The birth certificate must be filed with the local registrar of the district in which the birth occurs. Each birth must be reported promptly—the reporting requirements vary from state to state, ranging from 24 hours after the birth to as much as 10 days.

Federal law mandates national collection and publication of birth and other vital statistics data. The National Vital Statistics System is the result of cooperation between NCHS and the states to provide access to statistical information from birth certificates. Standard forms for the collection of the data and model procedures for the uniform registration of the events are developed and recommended for state use through cooperative activities of the states and NCHS. NCHS shares the costs incurred by the states in providing vital statistics data for national use.

Issues Affecting Interpretation: In 2003, two states, Pennsylvania and Washington, implemented the 2003 revision of the U.S. Standard Certificate of Live Birth, and in 2004, seven more states, Florida, Idaho, Kentucky, New Hampshire, New York state (excluding New York City), South Carolina, and Tennessee also implemented the 2003 revision. Data on mother's educational attainment, tobacco use during pregnancy, and prenatal care based on the 2003 revision are not comparable with data based on the 1989 revision of the U.S. Standard Certificate of Live Birth, and are currently excluded from *Health, United States* statistics. Prior to 2003, the number of states reporting information on maternal education, Hispanic origin, marital status, and tobacco use during pregnancy increased over the years. Interpretation of trend data should take into consideration expansion of reporting areas and immigration. For methodological and reporting area changes for the following birth certificate items, see Appendix II: Age (maternal age); Cigarette smoking; Education (maternal education); Hispanic origin; Marital status; Prenatal care; Race.

Reference:

National Center for Health Statistics, Vital Statistics of the United States 2000, Vol. I Natality, Technical Appendix. Available from: www.cdc.gov/nchs/data/techap00.pdf.

For More Information: See the Birth Data website: www.cdc.gov/nchs/births.htm.

Mortality File

Overview: Vital statistics mortality data are a fundamental source of demographic, geographic, and cause-of-death information. This is one of the few sources of comparable health-related data for small geographic areas over an extended time period. The data are used to present the characteristics of those dying in the United States, to determine life expectancy, and to compare mortality trends with other countries.

Selected Content: The mortality file includes demographic information on age, sex, race, Hispanic origin, state of residence, and educational attainment, and medical information on cause of death.

Data Years: The death registration area began in 1900 with 10 states and the District of Columbia.

Methodology: By law, the registration of deaths is the responsibility of the funeral director. The funeral director obtains demographic data for the death certificate from an informant. The physician in attendance at the death is required to certify the cause of death. Where death is from other than natural causes, a coroner or medical examiner may be required to examine the body and certify the cause of death. Data for the entire United States refer to events occurring within the United States; data for geographic areas are by place of residence. For methodological and reporting area changes for the following death certificate items, see Appendix II: Education; Hispanic origin; Race.

Issues Affecting Interpretation: International Classification of Diseases (ICD), by which cause of death is coded and classified, is revised approximately every 10 to 15 years. Revisions of the ICD may cause discontinuities in trend data by cause of death. Comparing death rates by cause of death across ICD revisions should be conducted with caution and with reference to the comparability ratio. (See Appendix II, Comparability ratio.) The death certificate has been revised periodically. A revised U.S. Standard Certificate of Death was recommended for state use beginning on January 1, 1989. Among the changes were the addition of a new item on educational attainment and Hispanic origin of decedent and changes to improve the medical certification of cause of death. The U.S. Standard Certificate of Death was revised in 2003; states are adopting this new certificate on a rolling basis. The educational attainment item was changed on the 2003 certificate. Consequently, educational attainment data collected using the 2003 certificate are not compatible with data collected using the 1989 revision. Starting with 2003 data, California, Idaho, Montana, and New York have adopted the 2003 certificate. In addition to these four states, starting with 2004 data, Connecticut, Georgia, Michigan, New Hampshire, New Jersey, Oklahoma, Rhode Island, South Dakota, Washington, and Wyoming have adopted the 2003 certificate. Because of different education profiles of the excluded states compared with the remaining reporting areas, mortality data by educational attainment in 2003 and subsequent years are not directly comparable to earlier years. For more information, see Appendix II: Education.

References:

Grove RD, Hetzel AM. Vital statistics rates in the United States, 1940–1960. Washington, DC: Government Printing Office. 1968.

Hoyert DL, Heron M, Murphy SL, Kung HC. Deaths: Final data for 2003. National vital statistics reports. Vol 54 no 13. Hyattsville, MD: National Center for Health Statistics. 2006.

National Center for Health Statistics, Vital Statistics of the United States, Vol II Mortality part A, Technical Appendix. Available from: www.cdc.gov/nchs/datawh/statab/pubd/ta.htm.

For More Information: See the Mortality Data website: www.cdc.gov/nchs/about/major/dvs/mortdata.htm.

Multiple Cause-of-Death File

Overview: Multiple cause-of-death data reflect all medical information reported on death certificates and complement traditional underlying cause-of-death data. Multiple cause data give information on diseases that are a factor in death whether or not they are the underlying cause of death; on associations among diseases; and on injuries leading to death.

Selected Content: In addition to the same demographic variables listed for the mortality file, the multiple cause-of-death file includes record axis and entity axis cause-of-death data (see Methodology section).

Data Years: Multiple cause-of-death data files are available for every data year since 1968.

Methodology: NCHS is responsible for compiling and publishing annual national statistics on causes of death. In carrying out this responsibility, NCHS adheres to the World Health Organization Nomenclature Regulations. These Regulations require that (1) cause of death be coded in accordance with the applicable revision of the *International Classification of Diseases* (ICD) (see Appendix II, Table IV and ICD); and (2) underlying cause of death be selected in accordance with international rules. Traditionally, national mortality statistics have been based on a count of deaths, with one underlying cause assigned for each death.

Starting with data year 1968, electronic files exist with multiple cause-of-death information. These files contain codes for all diagnostic terms and related codable information recorded on the death certificate. These codes make up the entity axis and are the input for a software program called TRANSAX. The TRANSAX program eliminates redundant entity axis codes and combines other entity axis codes to create the best set of ICD codes for a record. The output of the TRANSAX program is the record axis. Record axis data are generally used for research and analysis of multiple or nonunderlying cause of death. Because the function of the TRANSAX program is not to select a single underlying cause of death, record axis data may or may not include the underlying cause. Tabulations of underlying and nonunderlying cause of death in Table 48 (selected occupational diseases) are compiled by searching both underlying cause of death and record axis data.

Reference:

Multiple Causes of Death in the United States. Monthly vital statistics report; vol 32 no 10, supp 2. Hyattsville, MD: National Center for Health Statistics. February 17, 1984. Available from: www.cdc.gov/nchs/data/mvsr/supp/mv32_10s2.pdf.

For More Information: See the Mortality Multiple Cause-of-Death Data File website: www.cdc.gov/nchs/products/elec_prods/subject/mortmcd.htm.

Linked Birth/Infant Death Data Set

Overview: National linked files of live births and infant deaths are used for research on infant mortality.

Selected Content: The linked birth/infant death data set includes all variables on the natality file, including racial and ethnic information, as well as variables on the mortality file, including cause of death and age at death.

Data Years: National linked files of live births and infant deaths were first produced for the 1983 birth cohort. Birth cohort linked file data are available for 1983–1991 and period linked file data starting with 1995. National linked files do not exist for 1992–1994.

Methodology: Infant mortality rates are based on infant deaths (numerator) and live births (denominator). To create the linked data files, death certificates are linked with corresponding birth certificates for infants who die in the United States before their first birthday. About 97–99% of files can be linked. The linkage makes available extensive information about the pregnancy, maternal risk factors, infant characteristics, and health items at birth that can be used in analyses of infant mortality.

Starting with data year 1995, more timely linked file data are produced in a period data format preceding the release of the corresponding birth cohort format. Other changes to the data set starting with 1995 data include addition of record weights to correct for the 1.0%–1.4% in 2000–2004 (2.1%–2.5% in 1995–1999) of records that could not be linked and for the addition of an imputation for not stated birthweight. The 1995–2004 weighted mortality rates range from less than 1% to 4.1% higher than unweighted rates for the same period. The 1995–2004 weighted mortality rates with imputed birthweights are less than 1%–6.7% higher than unweighted rates with imputed birthweight for the same period.

Issues Affecting Interpretation: Period linked file data starting with 1995 are not strictly comparable with birth cohort data for 1983–1991. While birth cohort linked files have methodological advantages, their production incurs substantial delays in data availability, because it is necessary to wait until the close of a second data year to include all infant deaths to the birth cohort. In 2003, two states, Pennsylvania and Washington, implemented the 2003 revision of the U.S. Standard Certificate of Live Birth, and in 2004, seven more states, Florida, Idaho, Kentucky, New Hampshire, New York state (excluding New York City), South Carolina, and Tennessee also implemented the 2003 revision. Data on mother's educational attainment, tobacco use during pregnancy, and prenatal care based on the 2003 revision are not comparable with data based on the 1989 revision of the U.S. Standard Certificate of Live Birth, and are currently excluded from *Health, United States* statistics.

Reference:

Mathews TJ, MacDorman MF. Infant mortality statistics from the 2004 period linked birth/infant death data set. National vital statistics report; vol 55 no 14. Hyattsville, MD: National Center for Health Statistics. 2007. Available from: www.cdc.gov/nchs/data/nvsr/nvsr55/nvsr55_14.pdf.

For More Information: See the NCHS Linked Birth and Infant Death Data website: www.cdc.gov/nchs/linked.htm.

Compressed Mortality File

Overview: The Compressed Mortality File (CMF) is a county-level national mortality and population database.

Selected Content: The CMF contains mortality data derived from the detailed mortality files of the National Vital Statistics System and estimates of U.S. national, state, and county resident populations from the U.S. Census Bureau. Number of deaths, crude death rates, and age-adjusted death rates can be obtained by place of residence (total U.S., state, and county), age group, race (white, black, and other), sex, year of death, and underlying cause of death.

Data Years: The CMF spans the years 1968–2004. On CDC WONDER, data are available starting with 1979.

Methodology: In *Health, United States*, the CMF is used to compute death rates by urbanization level of decedent's county of residence. Counties are categorized according to level of urbanization based on the 2006 NCHS Urban-Rural Classification Scheme for Counties. This scheme assigns counties and county equivalents to one of six urbanization levels, four metropolitan and two nonmetropolitan.

For More Information: See the Compressed Mortality File website: www.cdc.gov/nchs/products/elec_prods/subject/mcompres.htm; or the CDC Wonder website: wonder.cdc.gov/mortSQL.html. See Appendix II, Urbanization.

Occupational Employment Statistics (OES)

Bureau of Labor Statistics

Overview: The Occupational Employment Statistics (OES) program conducts a semi-annual survey designed to produce estimates of employment and wages for specific occupations.

Selected Content: The OES survey produces estimates of occupational employment and wages for most sector, 3-, 4-, and 5-digit industrial groups in these industrial sectors: Forestry and logging; Mining; Utilities; Construction; Manufacturing; Wholesale trade; Retail trade; Transportation and warehousing; Information; Finance and insurance; Real estate and rental and leasing; Professional, scientific, and technical services; Management of companies and enterprises; Administrative and support and waste management and remediation services; Educational services; Health care and social assistance; Arts, entertainment, and recreation; Accommodation and food services; Other services (except public administration); and Government.

Data Years: Prior to 1996, the OES program collected only occupational employment data for selected industries in each year of the 3-year survey cycle, and produced only industry-specific estimates of occupational employment. The 1996 survey round was the first year that the OES program began collecting occupational employment and wage data in every state. In addition, the program's 3-year survey cycle was modified to collect data from all covered industries each year. 1997 is the earliest year available for which the OES program produced estimates of cross-industry as well as industry-specific occupational employment and wages.

Coverage: The OES survey covers all full-time and part-time wage and salary workers in nonfarm industries. Surveys collect data for the payroll period including the 12th day of May or November, depending upon the industry surveyed. The survey does not cover the self-employed, owners and partners in unincorporated firms, household workers, or unpaid family workers.

The OES survey produces estimates of occupational employment and wages for most sector, 3-, 4-, and 5-digit industrial groups in these industrial sectors: Forestry and logging; Mining; Utilities; Construction; Manufacturing; Wholesale trade; Retail trade; Transportation and warehousing; Information; Finance and insurance; Real estate and rental and leasing; Professional, scientific, and technical services; Management of companies and enterprises; Administrative and support and waste management and remediation services; Educational services; Health care and social assistance; Arts, entertainment, and recreation; Accommodation and food services; Other services (except public administration); and Government.

Methodology: The OES survey is a federal-state cooperative program between the Bureau of Labor Statistics (BLS) and State Workforce Agencies (SWAs). The OES program surveys approximately 200,000 establishments per panel (every six months), taking 3 years to fully collect the sample of 1.2 million establishments. Mail surveys collect data for the payroll period including the 12th day of May or November, depending upon the industry surveyed. The estimates for occupations in nonfarm establishments are based on OES data collected for the reference months of May and November. BLS provides the procedures and technical support, draws the sample, and produces the survey materials, while the SWAs collect the data. SWAs from all 50 states, plus the District of Columbia, Puerto Rico, Guam, and the Virgin Islands participate in the survey. Occupational employment and wage rate estimates at the national level are produced by BLS using data from the 50 states and the District of Columbia. Employers who respond to states' requests to participate in the OES survey make these estimates possible. The nationwide response rate for the May 2005 survey was 78% for establishments, covering 73% of employment. The survey included establishments sampled in the May 2005, November 2004, May 2004, November 2003, May 2003, and November 2002 semiannual panels.

Issues Affecting Interpretation: The OES survey began using the North American Industrial Classification System (NAICS) in 2002. Data prior to 2002 are based on the Standard Industrial Classification (SIC) system. In 1999, the OES survey began using the new Office of Management and Budget (OMB) Standard Occupational Classification (SOC) system. The new SOC system, which will be used by all federal statistical agencies for reporting occupational data, consists of 821 detailed occupations, grouped into 449 broad occupations, 96 minor groups, and 23 major groups. The OES program provides occupational employment and wage estimates at the major group and detailed occupation level. Due to the OES survey's transition to the new SOC system 1999 and 2000 OES estimates are not directly comparable with previous years' OES estimates, which were based on a classification system having seven major occupational groups and 770 detailed occupations. Approximately one-half of the detailed occupations were unchanged under the new SOC system, with the other half being new SOC occupations or occupations that are slightly different from similar occupations in the old OES classification system. Guam, Puerto Rico, and the Virgin Islands were surveyed, but their data were not included in the May 2005 survey.

Reference:

Bureau of Labor Statistics. Occupational Employment and Wages, May 2005. Washington, DC: Department of Labor. May 2006.

For More Information: See the Occupational Statistics website: www.bls.gov/OES/#overview.

Online Survey Certification and Reporting Database (OSCAR)

Centers for Medicare & Medicaid Services

Overview: The Online Survey Certification and Reporting (OSCAR) is an administrative database containing detailed information on all Medicare- and Medicaid-certified institutional health care providers, including all currently and previously certified Medicare and Medicaid nursing homes in the United States and territories. (Data for the territories are not shown in *Health, United States.)* The purpose of the nursing home survey certification process is to ensure that nursing facilities meet the current Centers for Medicare & Medicaid Services (CMS) care requirements and thus can be reimbursed for services furnished to Medicare and Medicaid beneficiaries.

Selected Content: OSCAR contains information on facility and patient characteristics and health deficiencies issued by the government during state surveys.

Data Years: OSCAR has been maintained by CMS, formerly the Health Care Financing Administration (HCFA), since 1992. OSCAR is an updated version of the Medicare and Medicaid Automated Certification System that had been in existence since 1972.

Coverage: All nursing homes in the United States that receive Medicare or Medicaid payments are included. Nursing homes that are intermediate care facilities for the mentally retarded and Department of Veterans Affairs nursing homes are excluded.

Methodology: Information on the number of beds and other facility characteristics comes from HCFA form 671, and information on residents and resident characteristics is collected on HCFA form 672. A nursing home representative fills out the forms, and they are submitted to CMS. The information provided on HCFA forms 671 and 672 can be audited at any time.

All certified nursing homes are inspected by representatives of the state survey agency (generally the department of health) at least once every 15 months. Therefore, a complete census must be based on a 15-month reporting cycle rather than a 12-month cycle. Some nursing homes are inspected twice or more often during any given reporting cycle. To avoid overcounting, the data must be edited and duplicates removed. Data editing and compilation were performed by

Cowles Research Group and published in the group's *Nursing Home Statistical Yearbook* series.

References:

Cowles CM. 1995; 1996; 1997 Nursing Home Statistical Yearbook. Anacortes, WA: Cowles Research Group (CRG). 1995; 1997; 1998.

Cowles CM, ed. 1998; 1999; 2000; 2001; 2002. Nursing home statistical yearbook. Washington, DC: American Association of Homes and Services for the Aging (AAHSA). 1999; 2000; 2001; 2002; 2003.

Cowles CM. ed. 2003; 2004; 2005. Nursing Home Statistical Yearbook. McMinnville, OR: Cowles Research Group (CRG). 2004; 2005; 2006.

For More Information: See the CRG website: www.longtermcareinfo.com/crg or the CMS website: www.cms.hhs.gov/NonIdentifiableDataFiles/.

Organ Procurement and Transplantation Network (OPTN)

The United Network for Organ Sharing (UNOS) under contract with the Health Resources and Services Administration

Overview: The OPTN is a unique public-private partnership that links all of the professionals involved in the donation and transplantation system. The primary goals of the OPTN are to: 1) increase the effectiveness and efficiency of organ sharing and equity in the national system of organ allocation; and 2) to increase the supply of donated organs available for transplantation.

Selected Content: UNet^{SM}, the transplant information database, contains transplant information that pertains to transplant candidates on the waiting list, donor/recipient matching, deceased and living donors, histocompatibility, and transplant recipients. The Patient Waiting List contains information used by the computer system to match potential organ recipients with available organ donors. Renal candidate waiting list data elements include name, gender, race, age, ABO blood group, number of previous transplants, peak and current panel reactive antibody (PRA) levels, acceptable donor characteristics, and patient human leukocyte antigens (HLAs). Kidney data collected on the Transplant Recipient Registration Form include transplant date, patient status (at time of transplant), primary renal diagnosis, pre-transplant serology, organ preservation description, and surgical information. Additional data collected as part of the Transplant Recipient Follow-Up Form include patient status (at time of follow-up), information about organ rejection, immunosuppressive medication, graft status, cause of graft loss, patient status, and cause of death.

Data Years: This system contains data regarding every organ donation and transplant event occurring in the U.S. since 1987.

Coverage: The database covers 100% of transplants occurring in the United States.

Methodology: The outcomes for all wait-listed registrants are summarized by the fraction who receive a transplant, die without a transplant, are removed from the waiting list for various reasons, are still surviving after removal from the list, and are still on the waiting list at various time points after wait-listing. The FT is a simple fraction of all wait-listed registrants who received a transplant, regardless of the program where the transplant was performed. The FT summarizes the time to transplantation at any program among all registrants in that transplant program. The Annual Report shows percentiles of waiting time based on rates of deceased donor transplantation among all registrants during the time from listing until removal from the list. For such calculations, time while inactive is excluded, and registrants are censored at removal from the list for any reason, including death, poor health, recovery of native organ function, or receiving a living donor organ transplant. This measure of waiting time reflects that which would result for a hypothetical population with transplant rates identical to those observed, if all registrants remained active on the waiting list until transplant.

Sample Size and Response Rates: All transplants are included with a 100% response rate.

Issues Affecting Interpretation: Transplant centers may have difficulties following transplant patients over time for a variety of reasons. For example, patients may move away or transfer their care to other medical professionals, or centers may just have a difficult time allocating staff to report on all patients. There are two different ways in which patients may become lost to follow-up (LTFU): (1) the transplant center reports them as being lost, or (2) the center just does not complete follow-up forms for a patient. About 13% of recipients transplanted with kidneys, livers, hearts, or lungs since 1997 were LTFU by the end of the third year after transplant; about three-quarters of these had been coded as LTFU by the transplant center, and the other quarter had no records completed for at least the last 1.5 years before the three-year anniversary.

LTFU varies both by the time since the transplant occurred and by organ. Not only does the number of patients being lost increase over time but also that the variation among transplant centers grows wider. Centers performing fewer than 10 transplants are not included here as their follow-up percentage is often quite uneven, depending on the small set of patients included. Almost all centers were able to follow at least 89% of their patients in the first year following a transplant, but after the fifth year half of the transplant programs had lost more than 14% of patients to follow-up and 5% of centers had lost over half of their patients; furthermore, a quarter of the facilities had lost more than 25% of their patients to follow-up by the fifth year, although it should be noted that this analysis only includes transplants from the first half of the period (1997–1999) due to the lack of sufficient follow-up time for later transplants.

References:

www.optn.org/data/annualReport.asp.

For More Information: See www.optn.org or www.unos.org.

Population Census and Population Estimates

U.S. Census Bureau Decennial Census

The census of population (decennial census) has been held in the United States every 10 years since 1790. The decennial census has enumerated the resident population as of April 1 of the census year ever since 1930. Data on sex, race, age, and marital status are collected from 100% of the enumerated population. More detailed information such as income, education, housing, occupation, and industry are collected from a representative sample of the population.

Race Data on the 1990 Census

The question on race on the 1990 census was based on the Office of Management and Budget's (OMB) 1977 Statistical Policy Directive 15, Race and Ethnicity Standards for Federal Statistics and Administrative Reporting. This document specified rules for the collection, tabulation, and reporting of race and ethnicity data within the federal statistical system. The 1977 standards required federal agencies to report race-specific tabulations using four single-race categories: American Indian or Alaska Native, Asian or Pacific Islander, black, and white. Under the 1977 standards, race and ethnicity were considered to be two separate and distinct concepts. Thus, persons of Hispanic origin may be of any race.

Race Data on the 2000 Census

The question on race on the 2000 census was based on OMBs 1997 Revisions to the Standards for the Classification of Federal Data on Race and Ethnicity (see Appendix II, Race and Revisions to the Standards for the Classification of Federal Data on Race and Ethnicity. Fed Regist 1997 October 30;62:58781–90). The 1997 Standards incorporated two major changes in the collection, tabulation, and presentation of race data. First, the 1997 standards increased from four to five the minimum set of categories to be used by federal agencies for identification of race: American Indian or Alaska Native, Asian, black or African American, Native Hawaiian or Other Pacific Islander, and white. Second, the 1997 standards included the requirement that federal data collection programs allow respondents to select one or more race categories when responding to a query on their racial identity. This provision means that there are potentially 31 race groups, depending on whether an individual selects one, two, three, four, or all five of the race categories. The 1997 standards continue to call for use, when possible, of a separate question on Hispanic or Latino ethnicity and specify that the ethnicity question should appear before the question on race. Thus, under the 1997 standards, as under the 1977 standards, Hispanics may be of any race.

Modified Decennial Census Files

For several decades the U.S. Census Bureau has produced modified decennial census files. These modified files incorporate adjustments to the 100% April 1 count data for 1) errors in the census data discovered subsequent to publication, 2) misreported age data, and 3) nonspecified race.

For the 1990 census, the U.S. Census Bureau modified the age, race, and sex data on the census and produced the Modified Age Race Sex (MARS) file. The differences between the population counts on the original census file and the

MARS file are primarily due to modification of the race data. Of the 248.7 million persons enumerated in 1990, 9.8 million persons did not specify their race (over 95% were of Hispanic origin). For the 1990 MARS file, these persons were assigned the race reported by a nearby person with an identical response to the Hispanic origin question.

For the 2000 census, the U.S. Census Bureau modified the race data on the census and produced the Modified Race Data Summary File. For this file, persons who reported the category, Some other race, as part of their race response were assigned to one of the 31 race groups, which are the single- and multiple-race combinations of the five race categories specified in the 1997 race and ethnicity standards. Persons who did not specify their race were assigned to one of the 31 race groups using imputation. Of the 18.5 million persons who reported the category, Some other race, as part of their race response, or who did not specify their race, 16.8 million (90.4%) were of Hispanic origin.

Bridged-Race Population Estimates for Census 2000

Race data on the 2000 census are not comparable with race data on other data systems that are continuing to collect data using the 1977 standards on race and ethnicity during the transition to full implementation of the 1997 standards. For example, most of the states in the Vital Statistics Cooperative Program will revise their birth and death certificates to conform to the 1997 standards after 2000. Thus, population estimates for 2000 and beyond with race categories comparable to the 1977 categories are needed so that race-specific birth and death rates can be calculated. To meet this need, NCHS, in collaboration with the U.S. Census Bureau, developed methodology to bridge the 31 race groups in census 2000 to the four single-race categories specified under the 1977 standards.

The bridging methodology was developed using information from the 1997–2000 National Health Interview Survey (NHIS). The NHIS provides a unique opportunity to investigate multiple-race groups because since 1982, the NHIS has allowed respondents to choose more than one race but has also asked respondents reporting multiple races to choose a primary race. The bridging methodology developed by NCHS involved the application of regression models relating person-level and county-level covariates to the selection of a particular primary race by the multiple-race respondents. Bridging proportions derived from these models were applied by the U.S. Census Bureau to the Census 2000 Modified Race Data Summary File. This application resulted in bridged counts of the April 1, 2000, resident single-race populations for four racial groups, American Indian or Alaska Native, Asian or Pacific Islander, black, and white. As bridged-race population estimates continue to be needed for the calculation of vital rates, the Census Bureau annually produces postcensal bridged-race estimates of the July 1 resident single-race populations.

For More Information about bridged-race population estimates, see Ingram DD, Parker JD, Schenker N, et al. United States Census 2000 population with bridged race categories. National Center for Health Statistics. Vital Health Stat 2(135). 2003; and the NCHS website for U.S. Census Populations with Bridged Race Categories: www.cdc.gov/nchs/about/major/dvs/popbridge/popbridge.htm.

Postcensal Population Estimates

Postcensal population estimates are estimates made for the years following a census, before the next census has been taken. National postcensal population estimates are derived annually by updating the resident population enumerated in the decennial census using a components of population change approach. Each annual series includes estimates for the current data year and revised estimates for the earlier years in the decade. The following formula is used to derive the estimates for a given year from those for the previous year, starting with the decennial census enumerated resident population as the base:

(1) resident population,
(2) + births to U.S. resident women,
(3) – deaths to U.S. residents,
(4) + net international migration,
(5) + net movement of U.S. Armed Forces and U.S. civilian citizens.

Estimates for the earlier years in a given series are revised to reflect changes in the components of change data sets (for example, births to U.S. resident women from a preliminary natality file are replaced with counts from a final natality file). To help users keep track of which postcensal estimate is being used, each annual series is referred to as a vintage and the last year in the series is used to name the series. For example, the Vintage 2001 postcensal series has estimates for July 1, 2000, and July 1, 2001, and the Vintage 2002 postcensal series has revised estimates for July 1,

2000, and July 1, 2001, as well as estimates for July 1, 2002. The estimates for July 1, 2000, and for July 1, 2001, from the Vintage 2001 and Vintage 2002 postcensal series differ.

State postcensal estimates are based on similar data and on a variety of other data series, including school statistics from state departments of education and parochial school systems. The postcensal estimates are consistent with official decennial census figures and do not reflect estimated decennial census underenumeration.

The Census Bureau has annually produced a postcensal series of estimates of the July 1 resident population of the United States based on census 2000 by applying the components of change methodology to the Modified Race Data Summary File. These series of postcensal estimates have race data for 31 race groups, in accordance with the 1997 race and ethnicity standards. So that the race data for 2000-based postcensal estimates will be comparable with race data on vital records, the Census Bureau has applied the NHIS bridging methodology to each 31-race group postcensal series of population estimates to obtain bridged-race postcensal estimates (estimates for the four single-race categories: American Indian or Alaska Native, Asian or Pacific Islander, black, and white). Bridged-race postcensal population estimates are available from: www.cdc.gov/nchs/about/major/dvs/popbridge/popbridge.htm.

Vital rates for 2000 were calculated using the bridged-race April 1, 2000 census counts, and vital rates for 2001 and beyond were calculated using bridged-race estimates of the July 1, population from the corresponding postcensal vintage.

Intercensal Population Estimates

The further from the census year on which the postcensal estimates are based, the less accurate are the postcensal estimates. With the completion of the decennial census at the end of the decade, intercensal estimates for the preceding decade were prepared to replace the less accurate postcensal estimates. Intercensal population estimates take into account the census of population at the beginning and end of the decade. Thus intercensal estimates are more accurate than postcensal estimates as they correct for the error of closure or difference between the estimated population at the end of the decade and the census count for that date. The error of closure at the national level was quite small for the 1960s (379,000). However, for the 1970s it amounted to almost 5 million; for the 1980s, 1.5 million; for the 1990s, about 6 million. The error of closure differentially affects age, race, sex, and Hispanic origin subgroup populations as well as the rates based on these populations. Vital rates that were calculated using postcensal population estimates are routinely revised when intercensal estimates become available because the intercensal estimates correct for the error of closure.

Intercensal estimates for the 1990s with race data comparable to the 1977 standards have been derived so that vital rates for the 1990s could be revised to reflect census 2000. Calculation of the intercensal population estimates for the 1990s was complicated by the incomparability of the race data on the 1990 and 2000 censuses. The Census Bureau, in collaboration with National Cancer Institute and NCHS, derived race-specific intercensal population estimates for the 1990s using the 1990 MARS file as the beginning population base and the bridged-race population estimates for April 1, 2000, as the ending population base. Bridged-race intercensal population estimates are available from: www.cdc.gov/nchs/about/major/dvs/popbridge/popbridge.htm.

Special Population Estimates

Special population estimates are prepared for the education reporting area for mortality statistics because educational attainment of decedent is not reported by all 50 states. The Housing and Household Economics Statistics Division of the U.S. Census Bureau currently produces unpublished estimates of populations by age, race, sex, and educational attainment for NCHS. These population estimates are based on the Current Population Survey, adjusted to resident population controls. The control totals are based on July 1 estimates for the relevant year. 1994–1996 data are 1990-based population estimates for 45 reporting states and the District of Columbia (D.C.); 1997–2000 data use 1990-based postcensal population estimates for 46 reporting states and D.C.; 2001–2002 data use 2000-based postcensal population estimates for 47 reporting states and D.C.; 2003 data use 2000-based postcensal population estimates for 46 reporting states and D.C.: 2004 data use 2000-based postcensal population estimates for 36 reporting states and D.C. See Appendix II, Education.

For More Information: See the U.S. Census Bureau website: www.census.gov/.

Sexually Transmitted Disease (STD) Surveillance

Centers for Disease Control and Prevention National Center of HIV, STD, and TB Prevention

Overview: Surveillance information on incidence and prevalence of sexually transmitted diseases (STDs) is used to inform public and private health efforts to control these diseases.

Selected Content: Case reporting data are available for nationally notifiable chanchroid, chlamydia, gonorrhea, and syphilis; surveillance of other STDs, such as genital herpes simplex virus (HSV), genital warts or other human papillomavirus infections, and trichomoniasis are based on estimates of office visits in physicians' office practices provided by the National Disease and Therapeutic Index (NDTI).

Data Years: STD national surveillance data have been collected since 1941.

Coverage: Case reports of STDs are reported to CDC by STD surveillance systems operated by state and local STD control programs and health departments in 50 states, the District of Columbia, selected cities, 3,139 U.S. counties, and outlying areas comprised of U.S. dependencies, possessions, and independent nations in free association with the United States. Data from outlying areas are not included in *Health, United States.*

Methodology: Information is obtained from the following sources of data: (1) case reports from STD project areas; (2) prevalence data from the Regional Infertility Prevention Program, the National Job Training Program (formerly the Job Corps), the Jail STD Prevalence Monitoring Projects, the adolescent Women Reproductive Health Monitoring Project, the Men Who Have Sex With Men (MSM) Prevalence Monitoring Project, and the Indian Health Service; (3) sentinel surveillance of gonococcal antimicrobial resistance from the Gonococcal Isolate Surveillance Project (GISP); and (4) national sample surveys implemented by federal and private organizations. STD data are submitted to CDC on a variety of hard-copy summary reporting forms (monthly, quarterly, and annually) and in electronic summary or individual case-specific (line-listed) formats via the National Electronic Telecommunications System for Surveillance (NETSS).

Issues Affecting Interpretation: Because of incomplete diagnosis and reporting, the number of STD cases reported to CDC undercounts the actual number of cases occurring among the U.S. population.

Reference:

Centers for Disease Control and Prevention. Sexually Transmitted Disease Surveillance, 2005. Atlanta, GA: Department of Health and Human Services. 2006.

For More Information: See the STD Surveillance Report website: www.cdc.gov/std/stats/ or the STD Prevention website: www.cdc.gov/std/default.htm.

Surveillance, Epidemiology, and End Results Program (SEER)

National Cancer Institute

Overview: The Surveillance, Epidemiology, and End Results (SEER) program tracks incidence of persons diagnosed with cancer during the year as well as follow-up information on all previously diagnosed patients until death.

Selected Content: SEER registries routinely collect data on patient demographics, primary tumor site, morphology, stage at diagnosis, first course of treatment, and follow-up for vital status.

Data Years: Case ascertainment for SEER began on January 1, 1973, and has continued for more than 30 years.

Coverage: SEER cancer registries were initiated in 1973 in Connecticut, Iowa, New Mexico, Utah, Hawaii, Detroit, and San Francisco-Oakland. Registries were added as follows: in 1974–1975, Atlanta and Seattle-Puget Sound; in 1978, 10 predominantly black rural counties in Georgia; in 1980, American Indians in Arizona; New Orleans, Louisiana (1974–1977, rejoined 2001); New Jersey (1979–1989, rejoined 2001); and Puerto Rico (1973–1989); in 1992, Alaska Native populations in Alaska and Hispanics in Los Angeles County and San Jose-Monterey; in 2001, Kentucky, Greater California, New Jersey, and Louisiana. The SEER Program currently collects and publishes cancer incidence and survival data from 17 population-based cancer registries covering approximately 26% of the U.S. population.

To ensure continuity in reporting areas for trend data, the following combination of SEER registries are commonly used.

for statistical analyses and are used for analysis of cancer survival rates in *Health, United States*: the SEER 9 registries of Atlanta, Connecticut, Detroit, Hawaii, Iowa, New Mexico, San Francisco-Oakland, Seattle-Puget Sound, and Utah. Analysis of cancer incidence covers residents in the following SEER 13 registries: the SEER 9 registries plus Los Angeles, San Jose-Monterey, Rural Georgia, and the Alaska Native Tumor Registry.

Methodology: A cancer registry (or tumor registry) collects and stores data on cancers diagnosed in a specific hospital or medical facility (hospital-based registry) or in a defined geographic area (population-based registry). A population-based registry is generally composed of a number of hospital-based registries. In SEER registry areas, trained coders abstract medical records using the International Classification of Diseases for Oncology, Third Edition (ICD–O–3), which provides a coding system for onset and stage of specific cancers. The third edition, implemented in 2001, is the first complete review and revision of the text and guidelines since its original publication in 1988.

Population estimates used to calculate incidence rates are obtained from the U.S. Census Bureau. NCI uses estimation procedures as needed to obtain estimates for years and races not included in data provided by the U.S. Census Bureau. Life tables used to determine normal life expectancy when calculating relative survival rates were obtained from NCHS and in-house calculations. Separate life tables are used for each race-sex-specific group included in the SEER Program.

Issues Affecting Interpretation: Because of the addition of registries over time, analysis of long-term incidence and survival trends is limited to those registries that have been in SEER for similar lengths of time. Analysis of Hispanic and American Indian and Alaska Native data is limited to shorter trends. Starting with *Health, United States, 2006*, the NAACCR Hispanic Identification Algorithm was used on a combination of variables to classify cases as Hispanic for analytic purposes. Starting with *Health, United States, 2007*, Hispanic incidence data exclude data for Alaska. Earlier editions of *Health, United States,* also excluded Hispanic data for Hawaii and Seattle. Starting with *Health, United States, 2007*, incidence estimates for the American Indian or Alaska Native population are limited to Contract Health Service Delivery Area (CHSDA) counties within SEER reporting areas. This change is believed to produce estimates that more accurately reflect the incidence rates for this population group. More information on CHSDA is available from: www.ihs.gov/NonMedicalPrograms/dqwg/dqwg-section1-home.asp.

For more information on SEER estimates by race and ethnicity, see seer.cancer.gov/seerstat/variables/seer/yr1973_2004/race_ethnicity/. Rates presented in this report may differ somewhat from previous reports due to revised population estimates and the addition and deletion of small numbers of incidence cases.

Reference:

Ries LAG, Melbert D, Krapcho M, Mariotto A, Miller BA, Feuer EJ, et al. (eds). SEER Cancer Statistics Review, 1975–2004. Bethesda, MD: National Cancer Institute; 2007; based on November 2006 SEER data submission. Available from: seer.cancer.gov/csr/1975_2004/.

For More Information: See the SEER website: www.seer.cancer.gov.

Survey of Mental Health Organizations (SMHO)

Substance Abuse and Mental Health Services Administration (SAMHSA)

Overview: The Survey of Mental Health Organizations and General Hospital Mental Health Services (SMHO/GHMHS) collects data on the number and characteristics of specialty mental health organizations in the United States.

Selected Content: The inventory collects basic information such as types of mental health organizations, ownership, number of additions and residents, and number of beds. The sample survey is a more detailed questionnaire that covers types of services provided, revenues and expenditures, staffing, and many items addressed to managed behavioral health care.

Data Years: The Inventory of Mental Health Organizations (IMHO/GHMHS) was conducted biannually from 1986 until 1994. The SMHO replaced the IMHO/GHMHS in 1998. The SMHO and the inventory used as its sampling frame have been conducted biannually starting in 1998.

Coverage: Organizations included are state and county mental hospitals, private psychiatric hospitals, nonfederal general hospitals with separate psychiatric services, Department of Veterans Affairs medical centers, residential treatment centers for emotionally disturbed children, freestanding outpatient psychiatric clinics, partial care organizations, freestanding day-night organizations, and multiservice mental health organizations not elsewhere classified.

Methodology: The IMHO was an inventory of all mental health organizations. Its core questionnaire included versions designed for specialty mental health organizations and another for non-federal general hospitals with separate psychiatric services. The data system was based on questionnaires mailed every other year to mental health organizations in the United States. In 1998, the IMHO was replaced by the SMHO. The SMHO is made up of two parts. A complete inventory is done by postcard gathering a limited amount of information. The inventory is used as a sampling frame for the SMHO, which contains most of the information from the IMHO core questionnaire as well as new items about managed behavioral health care.

Sample Size and Response Rate: In Phase I, all organizations were inventoried by postcard (about 10,000). A complete enumeration was needed to define the sampling frame for the sample survey. In Phase II, general hospitals without separate mental health units, community residential organizations, and managed behavioral health care organizations are dropped from the sampling frame. From this number, approximately 1,600–2,200 organizations are drawn for the sample survey and sent a questionnaire with a response rate of approximately 90%.

Issues Affecting Interpretation: Revisions to definitions of providers include phasing out Community Mental Health Centers as a category after 1981–1982; increasing the number of multiservice mental health organizations from 1981–1986; increasing the number of psychiatric outpatient clinics in 1981–1982, but decreasing the number in 1983–1984, 1986, 1990, and 1992; and increasing the number of partial care services in 1983–1984. These changes should be noted when interyear comparisons for the affected organizations and service types are made. The increase in the number of general hospitals with separate psychiatric services was partially due to a more concerted effort to identify these organizations. Forms had been sent only to those hospitals previously identified as having a separate psychiatric service. Beginning in 1980–1981, a screener form was sent to general hospitals not previously identified as providing a separate psychiatric service to determine whether they had such a service.

Reference:

Center for Mental Health Services. Mental Health, United States, 2004. Manderscheid RW, Berry JT, eds. DHHS pub no (SMA) 06–4195. Rockville, MD: Substance Abuse and Mental Health Services Administration. 2006. Available from: mentalhealth.samhsa.gov/publications/allpubs/SMA06–4195/.

For More Information: See the Center for Mental Health Services website: www.samhsa.gov/centers/cmhs/cmhs.html.

Survey of Occupational Injuries and Illnesses (SOII)

Bureau of Labor Statistics

Overview: The Survey of Occupational Injuries and Illnesses (SOII) is a federal/state program that collects statistics used to identify problems with workplace safety and develop programs to improve workplace safety.

Selected Content: Data include the number of injuries and illnesses by industry. The case and demographic data provide additional details on workers injured, the nature of the disabling condition, and the event and source producing that condition for those cases that involve one or more days away from work.

Data Years: The Bureau of Labor Statistics (BLS) has conducted an annual survey since 1971.

Coverage: The data represent persons employed in private industry establishments in the United States. The survey excludes the self-employed, farms with fewer than 11 employees, private households, federal government agencies, and state and local government agencies.

Methodology: Survey estimates of occupational injuries and illnesses are based on a scientifically selected probability sample of establishments, rather than a census of all establishments. An independent sample is selected for each state and the District of Columbia that represents industries in that jurisdiction. BLS includes all the state samples in the national sample.

Establishments included in the survey are instructed in a mailed questionnaire to provide summary totals of all entries for the previous calendar year to its Log and Summary of Occupational Injuries and Illnesses (OSHA No. 200 form). An occupational injury is any injury such as a cut, fracture, sprain, or amputation that results from a work-related event or from a single instantaneous exposure in the work environment. An occupational illness is any abnormal condition or disorder other than one resulting from an occupational injury, caused by exposure to factors associated with employment. It includes acute and chronic illnesses or diseases that may be caused by inhalation, absorption, ingestion, or direct contact. Prior to 2002, injury and illness cases involved days away from work, days of restricted work activity, or both (lost workday cases). Starting in 2002, injury and illness cases may involve days away from work, job transfer, or restricted work activity. Restriction may involve shortened hours, a temporary job change, or temporary restrictions on certain duties (for example, no heavy lifting) of a worker's regular job.

Sample Size and Response Rates: Employer reports were collected from about 182,400 private industry establishments in 2005. The survey response rate was 100% in 2005.

Issues Affecting Interpretation: The number of injuries and illnesses reported in any given year can be influenced by the level of economic activity, working conditions and work practices, worker experience and training, and number of hours worked. Long-term latent illnesses caused by exposure to carcinogens are believed to be understated in the survey's illness measures. In contrast, new illnesses such as contact dermatitis and carpal tunnel syndrome are easier to relate directly to workplace activity.

Effective January 1, 2002, the Occupational Safety and Health Administration (OSHA) revised its requirement for recording occupational injuries and illnesses. Because of the revised recordkeeping rule, the estimates from the 2002 survey and beyond are not comparable with those from previous years. See www.osha-slc.gov/recordkeeping/index.html for details about the revised recordkeeping requirements.

Data for the mining industry and for railroad activities are provided by the Department of Labor's Mine Safety and Health Administration and the Department of Transportation's Federal Railroad Administration. Neither of these agencies adopted the revised OSHA recordkeeping requirements for 2002. Therefore, estimates for these industries for 2002 and beyond are not comparable with estimates for other industries but are comparable with estimates for prior years. Excluded from the survey are self-employed individuals; farmers with fewer than 11 employees; private households; federal government agencies; and employees in state and local government agencies.

Beginning with the 2003 data year, SOII began using the 2002 North American Industry Classification System (NAICS) to classify industries. Prior to 2003, the program used the Standard Industrial Classification (SIC) system and the Bureau of the Census occupational classification system. Although some titles in SIC and NAICS are similar, there is limited compatibility because industry groupings are defined differently between the two systems. See Appendix II, Industry of employment.

Reference:

Bureau of Labor Statistics. Workplace Injuries and Illnesses in 2005. Washington, DC: Department of Labor. October 2006.

For More Information: See the BLS occupational safety and health website: www.bls.gov/iif/home.htm.

Youth Risk Behavior Survey (YRBS)

Centers for Disease Control and Prevention National Center for Chronic Disease Prevention and Health Promotion

Overview: The national Youth Risk Behavior Survey (YRBS) monitors health risk behaviors among students in grades 9–12 that contribute to morbidity and mortality in both adolescence and adulthood.

Selected Content: Data are collected on tobacco use, dietary behaviors, physical activity, alcohol and other drug use, sexual behaviors that contribute to unintended pregnancy and sexually transmitted diseases including HIV infection, and behaviors that contribute to unintentional injuries and violence.

Data Years: The national YRBS of high school students was conducted in 1990, 1991, 1993, 1995, 1997, 1999, 2001, 2003, and 2005.

Coverage: Data are representative of high school students in public and private schools in the United States.

Methodology: The national YRBS school-based surveys employ a three-stage cluster sample design to produce a nationally representative sample of students in grades 9–12 attending public and private high schools. The first-stage sampling frame contains primary sampling units (PSUs) consisting of large counties or groups of smaller, adjacent counties. The PSUs are then stratified based on degree of urbanization and relative percentage of black and Hispanic students in the PSU. The PSUs are selected from these strata with probability proportional to school enrollment size. At the second sampling stage, schools are selected with probability proportional to school enrollment size. To enable separate analysis of data for black and Hispanic students, schools with substantial numbers of black and Hispanic students are sampled at higher rates than all other schools. The third stage of sampling consists of randomly selecting one or two intact classes of a required subject from grades 9–12 at each chosen school. All students in the selected classes are eligible to participate in the survey. A weighting factor is applied to each student record to adjust for nonresponse and for the varying probabilities of selection, including those resulting from the oversampling of black and Hispanic students.

Sample Size and Response Rate: The sample size for the 2005 YRBS was 13,953 students in 159 schools. The school response rate was 78% and the student response rate was 86%, for an overall response rate of 67%.

Issues Affecting Interpretation: National YRBS data are subject to at least two limitations. First, these data apply only to adolescents who attend regular high school. These students may not be representative of all persons in this age group because those who have dropped out of high school or attend an alternative high school are not surveyed. Second, the extent of underreporting or overreporting cannot be determined, although the survey questions demonstrate good test-retest reliability.

Estimates of substance use for youth based on the YRBS differ from the National Survey on Drug Use & Health (NSDUH) and Monitoring the Future (MTF). Rates are not directly comparable across these surveys because of differences in populations covered, sample design, questionnaires, interview setting, and statistical approaches to make the survey estimates generalizable to the entire population. The NSDUH survey collects data in homes, whereas the MTF and YRBS collect data in school classrooms. The NSDUH estimates are tabulated by age, whereas the MTF and YRBS estimates are tabulated by grade, representing different ages as well as different populations.

References:

Brener ND, Kann L, Kinchen S, et al. Methodology of the Youth Risk Behavior Surveillance System. MMWR 2004;53(RR-12):1–13.

Eaton DK, Kann L, Kinchen S, et al. Youth Risk Behavior Surveillance—United States, 2005. In: *Surveillance Summaries June 9, 2006. MMWR 2006;55(SS-5):1–108.*

Cowan CD. Coverage, Sample Design, and Weighting in Three Federal Surveys. Journal of Drug Issues 2004;1(3):595–614.

For More Information: See the Division of Adolescent and School Health website: www.cdc.gov/HealthyYouth/index.htm.

Private and Global Sources

Alan Guttmacher Institute Abortion Provider Survey

The Alan Guttmacher Institute (AGI), a not-for-profit organization focused on reproductive health research, policy analysis, and public education, conducts periodic surveys of abortion providers to provide nationally representative statistics on abortion incidence.

Number of induced abortions; number, types, and locations of providers; and types of procedures performed, are presented by state and region. *Health, United States* presents the total for each data year. Thirteen provider surveys have been conducted for selected data years 1973 to midyear 2001. Data were collected from clinics, physicians, and hospitals identified as potential providers of abortion services. Mailed questionnaires were sent to all potential providers, with two additional mailings and telephone follow-up for nonresponse. No surveys were conducted in 1983, 1986, 1989, 1990, 1993, 1994, 1997, or 1998. For 1999–2000, a version of the survey questionnaire was created for each of the three major categories of providers, modeled on the survey questionnaire used for AGI's data collection in 1997. All surveys asked the number of induced abortions performed at the provider's location. State health statistics agencies were contacted, requesting all available data reported by providers to each state health agency on the number of abortions performed in the survey year. For states that provided data to AGI, the health agency figures were used for providers who did not respond to the survey. Estimates of the number of abortions performed by some providers were ascertained from knowledgeable sources in the community.

Of the 2,442 potential providers surveyed for 1999–2000, 1,931 performed abortions between January 1999 and June 2001. Of abortions reported for data year 2000, 77% were reported by providers, 10% came from health department data, 11% were estimated by knowledgeable sources, and 2% were projections or other estimates.

To estimate the number of abortions performed in 2001, 2002, and 2003, AGI first estimated the change in the number of abortions between 2000 and 2001, beginning with the number of abortions occurring in each state, as reported by the CDC, in each of those two years. The three states without reporting systems were excluded. AGI also eliminated the states with very incomplete or inconsistent reporting (Arizona, Maryland, Nevada, and the District of Columbia). AGI summed the number of abortions that took place in the 44 remaining states for each year. The percentage change between 2000 and 2001 was then applied to AGI's more complete nationwide count of 1,312,990 abortions in 2000 to arrive at the national estimate for 2001. The same procedure was used to estimate the change in the number of abortions between 2001 and 2002 and between 2002 and 2003, except that the data for both years were collected directly from state health departments because the CDC abortion surveillance report for the latest year was not yet available. The states without reporting systems were not included, and as before, AGI excluded states with incomplete or inconsistent reporting.

The number of abortions estimated by AGI through the mid-to-late 1980s was about 20% higher than the number reported to CDC. Between 1989 and 1997 the AGI estimates were about 12% higher than those reported by CDC. Beginning in 1998, health departments of four states did not report abortion data to CDC. The four reporting areas (the largest of which is California) that did not report abortions to CDC in 1998 accounted for 18% of all abortions tallied by AGI's 1995–1996 survey. In the first five years following FDA approval of Mifepristone (medical abortion) in September of 2000, approximately 575,000 U.S. women have used Mifepristone.

References:

Finer LB, Henshaw SK. Abortion incidence and services in the United States in 2000. Perspect Sex Reprod Health 2003;35(1):6–15.

Finer LB, Henshaw SK. Estimates of U.S. Abortion Incidence, 2001–2003. The Alan Guttmacher Institute. August 2006. Available from: www.guttmacher.org/pubs/2006/08/03/ab_incidence.pdf.

For More Information: See the AGI website: www.guttmacher.org or write to The Alan Guttmacher Institute, 120 Wall Street, New York, NY 10005.

American Association of Colleges of Osteopathic Medicine

The American Association of Colleges of Osteopathic Medicine (AACOM), founded in 1898, compiles data on various aspects of osteopathic medical education for distribution to the profession, the government, and the public. Questionnaires are sent annually to schools of osteopathic medicine requesting information on characteristics of applicants, students, and graduates, faculty, curriculum, contract and grant activity, revenues and expenditures, and clinical facilities. The response rate is 100%.

For more information: See 2006 Annual Statistical Report on Osteopathic Medical Education, 2007. American Association of Colleges of Osteopathic Medicine: 5550 Friendship Boulevard, Suite 310, Chevy Chase, Maryland 20815; or see the AACOM website: www.aacom.org.

American Association of Colleges of Pharmacy

The American Association of Colleges of Pharmacy (AACP) compiles data on the Colleges of Pharmacy, including information on student enrollment and types of degrees conferred. Data are collected through an annual survey; the response rate is 100%.

For More Information: See Fall 2005 Profile of Pharmacy Students. The American Association of Colleges of Pharmacy, 1426 Prince Street, Alexandria, VA; or the AACP website: www.aacp.org.

American Association of Colleges of Podiatric Medicine

The American Association of Colleges of Podiatric Medicine (AACPM) compiles data on the Colleges of Podiatric Medicine, including information on the schools and enrollment. Data are collected annually through written questionnaires. The response rate is 100%.

For More Information: Write to The American Association of Colleges of Podiatric Medicine, 15850 Crabbs Branch Way, Suite 320, Rockville, MD 20855; or see the AACPM website: www.aacpm.org.

American Dental Association

The Division of Educational Measurement of the American Dental Association (ADA) conducts annual surveys of predoctoral dental educational institutions. The questionnaire, mailed to all dental schools, collects information on student characteristics, financial management, and curricula.

For More Information: See the American Dental Association, *2003–2004 Survey of Dental Education, vol.1, Academic Programs, Enrollments, and Graduates*, Chicago. 2005 or the ADA website: www.ada.org.

American Hospital Association Annual Survey of Hospitals

Data from the American Hospital Association (AHA) annual survey are based on questionnaires sent to all AHA-registered and nonregistered hospitals in the United States and its associated areas. U.S. government hospitals located outside the United States are excluded. Overall, the average response rate over the past 5 years has been approximately 83%. For nonreporting hospitals and for the survey questionnaires of reporting hospitals on which some information was missing, estimates are made for all data except those on beds, bassinets, and facilities. Data for beds and bassinets of nonreporting hospitals are based on the most recent information available from those hospitals. Data for facilities and services are based only on reporting hospitals.

Estimates of other types of missing data are based on data reported the previous year, if available. When unavailable, estimates are based on data furnished by reporting hospitals similar in size, control, major service provided, length of stay, and geographic and demographic characteristics.

For More Information: Write to the AHA Annual Survey of Hospitals, Health Forum, LLC, an American Hospital Association Company, One North Franklin Street, Chicago, IL 60606; or see the AHA website: www.aha.org/aha_app/index.jsp.

American Medical Association Physician Masterfile

A masterfile of physicians has been maintained by the American Medical Association (AMA) since 1906. The Physician Masterfile contains data on all physicians in the United States, both members and nonmembers of the AMA, and on those graduates of American medical schools temporarily practicing overseas. The file also includes information on international medical graduates (IMGs), who are graduates of foreign medical schools who reside in the United States and who meet education standards for primary recognition as physicians.

A file is initiated on each individual upon entry into medical school or, in the case of IMGs, upon entry into the United States. Between 1965 and 1985, a mail questionnaire survey was conducted every 4 years to update the file information on professional activities, self-designated area of specialization, and present employment status. Since 1985, approximately one-third of all physicians are surveyed each year.

For More Information: See Division of Survey and Data Resources, American Medical Association, Physician Characteristics and Distribution in the U.S., 2007 ed. Chicago, IL. 2007; or the AMA website: www.ama-assn.org/.

American Osteopathic Association

The American Osteopathic Association (AOA) was established to promote the public health, to encourage scientific research, and to maintain and improve high standards of medical education in osteopathic colleges. The Department of Educational Affairs sets the standards for and accredits osteopathic medical colleges and hospitals, postdoctoral training and board certification programs. The AOA publishes both professional and public information materials. Professional publications include information on osteopathic education, accreditation of hospitals and other health care delivery facilities, and physician licensing. Public information materials include introductory materials on osteopathic medicine, brochures on osteopathic physicians and osteopathic medicine, and patient education materials. The AOA compiles the number of osteopathic physicals (D.O.s), the number of active D.O.s by gender, age, specialty, and by 50 states and the District of Columbia, and the number of osteopathic medical students by selected characteristics. These statistics are available annually from www.osteopathic.org/pdf/ost_factsheet.pdf.

For More Information: See the AOA website: www.osteopathic.org.

Association of American Medical Colleges

The Association of American Medical Colleges (AAMC) collects information on student enrollment in medical schools through the annual Liaison Committee on Medical Education questionnaire, the fall enrollment questionnaire, and the American Medical College Application Service (AMCAS) data system. Other data sources are the institutional profile system, the premedical students questionnaire, the minority student opportunities in medicine questionnaire, the faculty roster system, data from the Medical College Admission Test, and one-time surveys developed for special projects.

For More Information: See the Association of American Medical Colleges, Statistical Information Related to Medical Schools and Teaching Hospitals, Washington, DC. 2006; or the AAMC website: www.aamc.org.

Association of Schools and Colleges of Optometry

The Association of Schools and Colleges of Optometry (ASCO) compiles data on various aspects of optometric education including data on schools and enrollment. Questionnaires are sent annually to all schools and colleges of optometry. The response rate is 100%.

For More Information: Write to the Annual Survey of Optometric Educational Institutions, Association of Schools and Colleges of Optometry, 6110 Executive Blvd., Suite 510, Rockville, MD 20852; or see the ASCO website: www.opted.org.

Association of Schools of Public Health

The Association of Schools of Public Health (ASPH) compiles data on schools of public health in the United States and Puerto Rico. Questionnaires are sent annually to all member schools. The response rate is 100%.

Unlike health professional schools that emphasize specific clinical occupations, schools of public health offer study in specialty areas such as biostatistics, epidemiology, environmental health, occupational health, health administration, health planning, nutrition, maternal and child health, social and behavioral sciences, and other population-based sciences.

For More Information: Write to the Association of Schools of Public Health, 1101 15th Street, NW, Suite 910, Washington, DC 20005; or see the ASPH website: www.asph.org.

Computed Tomography (CT) and Magnetic Resonance Imaging (MRI) Census

CT/MRI Census is a biennial telephone survey used to query all hospital and non-hospital sites in the United States performing CT and MRI procedures. The Census details the types of procedures being performed, procedure volumes, staffing and productivity, installed equipment, planned equipment purchases and annual budgets for consumables including contrast media.

Candidate sites for MRI/CT procedures are identified in the American Hospital Association's AHA guide-The AHA Guide to the Health Care Field. U.S. territories are not included.

For More Information: See 2004 Computed Tomography (CT) and Magnetic Resonance Imaging (MRI) Census. Market Summary Report: IMV, Limited, Medical Information Division. 2004 Section B: Installed Base of CT Scanners: Installed Base of MRI Scanners; or the website: imvlimited.com/.

European Health for All Database

World Health Organization Regional Office for Europe

The WHO Regional Office for Europe (WHO/Europe) provides country-specific and topic-specific health information via the

Internet for people who influence health policy in the WHO European Region and the media.

WHO/Europe collects statistics on health and makes them widely available through:

- European Health for all Database (www.euro.who.int/hfadb) (HFA-DB), which contains data on about 600 health indicators collected from national counterparts in 52 European countries, and data from other WHO technical programs and some international organizations.
- Highlights on Health (www.euro.who.int/InformationSources/Evidence/20011015_1) from countries in the WHO European Region that give an overview of the health situation in each country in comparison with other countries. Highlights complement the public health reports produced by a number of member states in the region.
- Health Status Overview for Countries of Central and Eastern Europe (www.euro.who.int/Document/E76888.pdf) that are candidates for accession to the European Union (Bulgaria, the Czech Republic, Estonia, Hungary, Latvia, Lithuania, Poland, Romania, Slovakia, and Slovenia).

WHO/Europe helps countries strengthen their national health information systems, particularly by supporting:

- development of National Health Indicator Databases (www.euro.who.int/eprise/main/WHO/Progs/HIS/products/20020514_2)
- exchange of experience on national public health reports between countries; a database of public health reports is maintained and available for consultation and networking
- implementation of International Classifications (www.who.int/whosis/en/) and definitions in countries
- Regional Networks (www.euro.who.int/main/WHO/Home/TopPage) of health information professionals.

For More Information: See the European health for all database: data.euro.who.int/hfadb/.

HealthLeaders-InterStudy National Health Maintenance Organization Census

From 1976 to 1980, the Office of Health Maintenance Organizations conducted a census of health maintenance organizations (HMOs). Since 1981, InterStudy (now HealthLeaders-InterStudy) has conducted the census. A questionnaire is sent to all HMOs in the United States asking for updated enrollment, profit status, and federal qualification status. New HMOs are also asked to provide information on model type. When necessary, information is obtained, supplemented, or clarified by telephone. For nonresponding HMOs state-supplied information or the most current available data are used.

In 1985, a large increase in the number of HMOs and enrollment was partly attributable to a change in the categories of HMOs included in the census: Medicaid-only and Medicare-only HMOs were added. Component HMOs, which have their own discrete management, could be listed separately, whereas previously the oldest HMO reported for all of its component or expansion sites, even when the components had different operational dates or were different model types.

For More Information: See Waller RL, et al. The HealthLeaders-InterStudy Competitive Edge, September 2005, Part II: Managed Care Industry Report. Nashville, TN. Available from: www.healthleaders.com.

National League for Nursing

The division of research of the National League for Nursing (NLN) conducts The Annual Survey of Schools of Nursing in October of each year. Questionnaires are sent to all graduate nursing programs (master's and doctoral), baccalaureate programs designed exclusively for registered nurses, basic registered nursing programs (baccalaureate, associate degree, and diploma), and licensed practical nursing programs. Data on enrollments, first-time admissions, and graduates are completed for all nursing education programs. Response rates of approximately 80% are achieved for other areas of inquiry.

For More Information: See the NLN website: www.nln.org.

Organisation for Economic Co-operation and Development Health Data

The Organisation for Economic Co-operation and Development (OECD) provides annual data on statistical indicators on health and health systems collected from 30 member countries, with some time series going back to 1960. The international comparability of health expenditure estimates depends on the quality of national health accounts in OECD member countries. In recent years, an increasing number of countries have adopted the standards for health accounting defined by OECD, greatly increasing the comparability of national health expenditure data reporting. Additional limitations in international comparisons include differing boundaries between health care and other social care, particularly for the disabled and elderly, and underestimation of private expenditures on health.

The OECD was established in 1961 with a mandate to promote policies to achieve the highest sustainable economic growth and a rising standard of living among member countries. The Organisation now comprises 30 member countries: Australia, Austria, Belgium, Canada, Czech Republic, Denmark, Finland, France, Germany, Greece, Hungary, Iceland, Ireland, Italy, Japan, Korea, Luxembourg, Mexico, the Netherlands, New Zealand, Norway, Poland, Portugal, Slovak Republic, Spain, Sweden, Switzerland, Turkey, the United Kingdom, and the United States.

As part of its mission, the OECD has developed a number of activities in relation to health and health care systems. The main aim of OECD work on health policy is to conduct cross-national studies of the performance of OECD health systems and to facilitate exchanges between member countries of their experiences of financing, delivering, and managing health services. To support this work, each year the OECD compiles cross-country data in OECD Health Data, one of the most comprehensive sources of comparable health-related statistics. OECD Health Data is an essential tool to carry out comparative analyses and draw lessons from international comparisons of diverse health care systems. This international database now incorporates the first results arising from the implementation of the OECD manual, A System of Health Accounts (2000), which provide a standard framework for producing a set of comprehensive, consistent, and internationally comparable data on health spending. The OECD collaborates with other international organizations such as the WHO.

For More Information: See the OECD website: www.oecd.org/health.

United Nations Demographic Yearbook

The Statistical Office of the United Nations prepares the *Demographic Yearbook*, a comprehensive collection of international demographic statistics.

Questionnaires are sent annually and monthly to more than 220 national statistical services and other appropriate government offices. Data from these questionnaires are supplemented, to the extent possible, by data taken from official national publications and by correspondence with the national statistical services. To ensure comparability, rates, ratios, and percents have been calculated in the statistical office of the United Nations.

Lack of international comparability among estimates arises from differences in concepts, definitions, and time of data collection. The comparability of population data is affected by several factors, including (a) definitions of the total population, (b) definitions used to classify the population into its urban and rural components, (c) difficulties relating to age reporting, (d) extent of over- or underenumeration, and (e) quality of population estimates. The completeness and accuracy of vital statistics data also vary from one country to another. Differences in statistical definitions of vital events may also influence comparability.

International demographic trend data are available on a CD-ROM entitled United Nations, 2000. Demographic Yearbook—Historical Supplement 1948–1997. CD-ROM Special Issue. United Nations publication sales number E/F.99.XIII.12.

For More Information: See the United Nations, Statistics Division website: unstats.un.org/unsd/demographic/products/dyb/dyb2.htm.

World Health Organization Statistical Information System (WHOSIS)

World Health Organization

WHO Statistical Information System (WHOSIS) is a guide to health and health-related epidemiological and statistical information from the World Health Organization. Statistics are listed by country or region and by topic. WHOSIS contains the following databases: Core Health Indicators for 192 countries; World Health Statistics 2007; Statistics from WHO Regional Offices; Statistics by country or region; Burden of Disease statistics; and Family of International Classifications.

For More Information: See the World Health Organization, *World Health Statistics Annual 2007*: www3.who.int/statistics/; or the WHO website: www.who.int/en/.

Appendix II

Definitions and Methods

Appendix II is an alphabetical listing of terms used in *Health, United States*. It includes cross-references to related terms and synonyms. It also describes the methods used for calculating age-adjusted rates, average annual rates of change, relative standard errors, birth rates, death rates, and years of potential life lost. Appendix II includes standard populations used for age adjustment (Tables I, II, and III); *International Classification of Diseases* (ICD) codes for cause of death from the Sixth through Tenth Revisions and the years when the Revisions were in effect (Tables IV and V); comparability ratios between ICD–9 and ICD–10 for selected causes (Table VI); ICD–9–CM codes for external cause of injury, diagnostic, and procedure categories (Tables VII, X, and XI); an analysis of the effects of adding probe questions for Medicare and Medicaid coverage on health insurance rates in the National Health Interview Survey (Table VIII); classification of generic analgesic drugs (Table XII); and industry codes from the North American Industry Classification System (NAICS) (Table IX). Standards for presenting federal data on race and ethnicity are described, and sample tabulations of National Health Interview Survey (NHIS) data comparing the 1977 and 1997 Standards for the Classification of Federal Data on Race and Ethnicity are presented in Tables XIII and XIV.

Acquired immunodeficiency syndrome (AIDS)—Human immunodeficiency virus (HIV) is the pathogen that causes AIDS and HIV disease is the term that encompasses all the condition's stages, from infection to the deterioration of the immune system and the onset of opportunistic diseases. However, AIDS is still the name that most people use to refer to the immune deficiency caused by HIV. An AIDS diagnosis (indicating that the person has reached the late stages of the disease) is given to people with HIV who have counts below 200 CD4+ cells/mm3 (also known as T cells or T4 cells, which are the main target of HIV) or when they become diagnosed with at least one of a set of opportunistic diseases. All 50 states and the District of Columbia report AIDS cases to CDC using a uniform surveillance case definition and case report form. The case reporting definitions were expanded in 1985 (MMWR 1985; 34:373–5); 1987 (MMWR 1987; 36 (No. SS-1):1S–15S); 1993 for adults and adolescents (MMWR 1992; 41(no. RR-17):1–19); and 1994 for pediatric cases (MMWR 1994; 43(no. RR-12):1–19). The revisions incorporated a broader range of AIDS-indicator diseases and conditions and used HIV diagnostic tests to improve the sensitivity and specificity of the definition. The 1993 expansion of the case definition caused a temporary distortion of AIDS incidence trends. In 1995, new treatments (protease inhibitors) for HIV and AIDS were approved. These therapies have prevented or delayed the onset of AIDS and premature death among many HIV-infected persons, which should be considered when interpreting trend data. AIDS surveillance data are published annually by CDC in the HIV/AIDS Surveillance Report. Available from: www.cdc.gov/hiv/topics/surveillance/resources/reports/index.htm. See related Human immunodeficiency virus (HIV) disease.

Active physician—See Physician.

Activities of daily living (ADL)—Activities of daily living are activities related to personal care and include bathing or showering, dressing, getting in or out of bed or a chair, using the toilet, and eating. In the National Health Interview Survey, respondents were asked whether they or family members 3 years of age and over need the help of another person with personal care because of a physical, mental, or emotional problem. Persons are considered to have an ADL limitation if any condition(s) causing the respondent to need help with the specific activities was chronic.

In the Medicare Current Beneficiary Survey, if a sample person had any difficulty performing an activity by him or herself and without special equipment, or did not perform the activity at all because of health problems, the person was categorized as having a limitation in that activity. The limitation may have been temporary or chronic at the time of the interview. Sampled people who were administered a community interview answered health status and functioning questions themselves, if able to do so. A proxy such as a nurse answered questions about the sample person's health status and functioning for those in a long-term care facility. Beginning in 1997, interview questions for people residing in long-term care facilities were changed slightly from those administered to people living in the community to differentiate residents who were independent from those who received supervision or assistance with transferring, locomotion on unit, dressing, eating, toilet use, and bathing. See related Condition; Instrumental activities of daily living (IADL); Limitation of activity.

Table I. United States standard population and age groups used to age adjust data

Data system and age	Number
DVS mortality data	
Total	274,633,642
Under 1 year	3,794,901
1–4 years	15,191,619
5–14 years	39,976,619
15–24 years	38,076,743
25–34 years	37,233,437
35–44 years	44,659,185
45–54 years	37,030,152
55–64 years	23,961,506
65–74 years	18,135,514
75–84 years	12,314,793
85 years and over	4,259,173
NHIS, NAMCS, NHAMCS, NNHS, and NHDS	
All ages	274,633,642
18 years and over	203,852,188
25 years and over	177,593,760
40 years and over	118,180,367
65 years and over	34,709,480
Under 18 years	70,781,454
2–17 years	63,227,991
18–44 years	108,151,050
18–24 years	26,258,428
25–34 years	37,233,437
35–44 years	44,659,185
45–64 years	60,991,658
45–54 years	37,030,152
55–64 years	23,961,506
65–74 years	18,135,514
75 years and over	16,573,966
18–49 years	127,956,843
40–64 years:	
40–49 years	42,285,022
50–64 years	41,185,865
NHES and NHANES	
20 years and over	195,850,985
20–74 years	179,277,019
20–34 years	55,490,662
35–44 years	44,659,185
45–54 years	37,030,152
55–64 years	23,961,506
65–74 years	18,135,514
or	
60 years and over	45,363,782
65 years and over	34,709,480

See footnotes at end of table.

Table I. United States standard population and age groups used to age adjust data—Con.

Data system and age	Number
NHANES (Table 71 only)	
20–39 years	77,670,618
40–59 years	72,816,615
60–74 years	28,789,786
NHANES (Table 93 only)	
Under 18 years	70,781,454
18–44 years	108,151,050
45–64 years	60,991,658
65 years and over	34,709,480

SOURCE: National Institutes of Health, National Cancer Institute, Surveillance, Epidemiology, and End Results (SEER). Standard population—single ages. Available from: seer.cancer.gov/stdpopulations/stdpop.singleages.html.

Addition—See Admission.

Admission—The American Hospital Association defines admissions as persons, excluding newborns, accepted for inpatient services during the survey reporting period. See related Days of care; Discharge; Inpatient.

An admission (also sometimes referred to as an addition) to a mental health organization is defined by the Substance Abuse and Mental Health Services Administration's Center for Mental Health Services as a new admission, a re-admission, a return from long-term leave, or a transfer from another service of the same organization or another organization. See related Mental health organization; Mental health service type.

Age—Age is reported as age at last birthday, that is, age in completed years, often calculated by subtracting date of birth from the reference date, with the reference date being the date of the examination, interview, or other contact with an individual.

Mother's (maternal) age is reported on the birth certificate by all states. Birth statistics are presented for mothers age 10–49 years through 1996 and 10–54 years starting in 1997, based on mother's date of birth or age as reported on the birth certificate. The age of mother is edited for upper and lower limits. When the age of the mother is computed to be under 10 years or 55 years or over (50 years or over in 1964–1996), it is considered not stated and imputed according to the age of the mother from the previous birth record of the same race and total birth order (total of fetal deaths and live births). Before 1963, not stated ages were distributed in proportion to the known ages for each racial group. Beginning in 1997, the birth rate for the maternal age group 45–49 years includes data for mothers age 50–54 years in the numerator and is based on the population of women 45–49 years in the denominator.

Age adjustment—Age adjustment is used to compare risks of two or more populations at one point in time or one population at two or more points in time. Age-adjusted rates are computed by the direct method by applying age-specific rates in a population of interest to a standardized age distribution, to eliminate differences in observed rates that result from age differences in population composition. Age-adjusted rates should be viewed as relative indexes rather than actual measures of risk.

Age-adjusted rates are calculated by the direct method as follows:

$$\sum_{i=1}^{n} r_i \times (p_i / P)$$

where r_i = rate in age group i in the population of interest

p_i = standard population in age group i

$$P = \sum_{i=1}^{n} p_i$$

n = total number of age groups over the age range of the age-adjusted rate

Age adjustment by the direct method requires use of a standard age distribution. The standard for age adjusting death rates and estimates from surveys in *Health, United States* is the projected year 2000 U.S. resident population. Starting with *Health, United States, 2000*, the year 2000 U.S. standard population replaced the 1970 civilian non-institutionalized population for age adjusting estimates from most NCHS surveys and starting with *Health, United States, 2001* it was used uniformly and replaced the 1940 U.S. population for age adjusting mortality statistics and the 1980 U.S. resident population, which previously had been used for age adjusting estimates from the NHANES surveys.

Changing the standard population has implications for racial and ethnic differentials in mortality. For example, the mortality ratio for the black to white populations is reduced from 1.6 using the 1940 standard to 1.4 using the 2000 standard, reflecting the greater weight that the 2000 standard gives to the older population where race differentials in mortality are smaller.

Age-adjusted estimates from any data source presented in *Health, United States* may differ from age-adjusted estimates based on the same data presented in other reports if different age groups are used in the adjustment procedure.

For more information on implementing the 2000 population standard for age adjusting death rates, see Anderson RN, Rosenberg HM. Age standardization of death rates: Implementation of the year 2000 standard. National vital statistics reports; vol 47 no 3. Hyattsville, MD: National Center for Health Statistics. 1998. For more information on the derivation of age adjustment weights for use with NCHS survey data, see Klein RJ, Schoenborn CA. Age adjustment using the 2000 projected U.S. population. Healthy People Statistical Notes no. 20. Hyattsville, MD: National Center for Health Statistics. 2001. Both reports are available from the NCHS home page: www.cdc.gov/nchs. The year 2000 U.S. standard population is available from the National Cancer Institute, Surveillance, Epidemiology, and End Results, seer.cancer.gov/stdpopulations/stdpop.singleages.html.

Mortality data—Death rates are age adjusted to the year 2000 U.S. standard population (Table I). Prior to 2003 data, age-adjusted rates were calculated using standard million proportions based on rounded population numbers (Table II). Starting with 2003 data, unrounded population numbers are used to age adjust. Adjustment is based on 11 age groups with two exceptions. First, age-adjusted death rates for black males and black females in 1950 are based on nine age groups, with under 1 year and 1–4 years of age combined as one group and 75–84 years and 85 years of age and over combined as one group. Second, age-adjusted death rates by educational attainment for the age group 25–64 years are based on four 10-year age groups (25–34 years, 35–44 years, 45–54 years, and 55–64 years).

Age-adjusted rates for years of potential life lost before age 75 years also use the year 2000 standard population and are based on eight age groups (under 1 year, 1–14 years, 15–24 years, and 10-year age groups through 65–74 years).

Table II. United States standard population and proportion distribution by age, for age adjusting death rates prior to 2003

Age	*Population*	*Proportion distribution (weights)*	*Standard million*
Total	274,634,000	1.000000	1,000,000
Under 1 year	3,795,000	0.013818	13,818
1–4 years	15,192,000	0.055317	55,317
5–14 years	39,977,000	0.145565	145,565
15–24 years	38,077,000	0.138646	138,646
25–34 years	37,233,000	0.135573	135,573
35–44 years	44,659,000	0.162613	162,613
45–54 years	37,030,000	0.134834	134,834
55–64 years	23,961,000	0.087247	87,247
65–74 years	18,136,000	0.066037	66,037
75–84 years	12,315,000	*0.044842	44,842
85 years and over	4,259,000	0.015508	15,508

* Figure is rounded up instead of down to force total to 1.0.

SOURCE: Anderson RN, Rosenberg HM. Age standardization of death rates: Implementation of the year 2000 standard. National vital statistics reports; vol 47 no 3. Hyattsville, MD: National Center for Health Statistics. 1998.

Maternal mortality rates for pregnancy, childbirth, and the puerperium are calculated as the number of deaths per 100,000 live births. These rates are age adjusted to the 1970 distribution of live births by mother's age in the United States as shown in Table III. See related Rate: Death and related rates; Years of potential life lost.

National Health and Nutrition Examination Survey—Estimates based on the National Health Examination Survey and the National Health and Nutrition Examination Survey are age adjusted to the year 2000 U.S. standard population generally using five age groups: 20–34 years, 35–44 years, 45–54 years, 55–64 years, and 65–74 years or 65 years and over (see Table I). Prior to *Health, United States, 2001*, these estimates were age adjusted to the 1980 U.S. resident population.

National Health Care Surveys—Estimates based on the National Hospital Discharge Survey, the National Ambulatory Medical Care Survey, the National Hospital Ambulatory Medical Care Survey, and the National Nursing Home Survey are age adjusted to the year 2000 U.S. standard population (Table I). Information on the age groups used in the age adjustment procedure is contained in the footnotes to the relevant tables.

National Health Interview Survey—Estimates based on the National Health Interview Survey are age adjusted to the year 2000 U.S. standard population (Table I). Prior to the 2000 edition of *Health, United States*, National Health Interview Survey estimates were age adjusted to the 1970 civilian noninstitutionalized population. Information on the age groups used in the age adjustment procedure is contained in the footnotes to the relevant tables.

AIDS—See Acquired immunodeficiency syndrome.

Alcohol consumption—Alcohol consumption is measured differently in various data systems. See related Binge drinking.

Monitoring the Future Study—This school-based survey of secondary school students collects information on alcohol use using self-completed questionnaires. Information on consumption of alcoholic beverages, defined as beer, wine, wine coolers, and liquor, is based on the following question: "On how many occasions (if any) have you had alcohol to drink—more than just a few sips—in the last 30 days?" Students responding affirmatively are then asked "How many times have you had five or more drinks in a row in the last 2 weeks?" For this question, a "drink" means a 12-ounce can (or bottle) of beer, a 4-ounce glass of wine, a 12-ounce bottle or can of wine cooler, or a mixed drink or a shot of liquor.

Table III. Number of live births and mother's age group used to adjust maternal mortality rates to live births in the United States in 1970

Mother's age	*Number*
All ages	3,731,386
Under 20 years	656,460
20–24 years	1,418,874
25–29 years	994,904
30–34 years	427,806
35 years and over	233,342

SOURCE: Summary report final natality statistics, 1970. Monthly vital statistics report; vol 22 no 12, supp. Hyattsville, MD: National Center for Health Statistics. 1974.

National Health Interview Survey (NHIS)—Starting with the 1997 NHIS, information on alcohol consumption is collected in the sample adult questionnaire. Adult respondents are asked two screening questions about their lifetime alcohol consumption: "In any one year, have you had at least 12 drinks of any type of alcoholic beverage? In your entire life, have you had at least 12 drinks of any type of alcoholic beverage?" Persons who report at least 12 drinks in a lifetime are then asked a series of questions about alcohol consumption in the past year: "In the past year, how often did you drink any type of alcoholic beverage? In the past year, on those days that you drank alcoholic beverages, on the average, how many drinks did you have?"

National Survey on Drug Use and Health (NSDUH)—Starting in 1999, NSDUH information about the frequency of the consumption of alcoholic beverages in the past 30 days has been obtained for all persons surveyed who are 12 years of age and over. An extensive list of examples of the kinds of beverages covered was given to respondents prior to the question administration. A drink is defined as a can or bottle of beer, a glass of wine or a wine cooler, a shot of liquor, or a mixed drink with liquor in it. Those times when the respondent had only a sip or two from a drink are not considered consumption. Alcohol use is based on the following questions: "During the past 30 days, on how many days did you drink one or more drinks of an alcoholic beverage?" "On the days that you drank during the past 30 days, how many drinks did you usually have?" and "During the past 30 days, on how many days did you have five or more drinks on the same occasion?"

Youth Risk Behavior Survey (YRBS) Starting in 1991, the YRBS has collected information on alcohol use among high school students. Questions on alcohol use have the following introduction: "The next five questions ask about drinking alcohol. This includes drinking beer, wine, wine coolers, and liquor such as rum, gin, vodka, or whiskey. For these questions, drinking alcohol does not include drinking a few sips of wine for religious purposes." Alcohol use is based on the questions that follow, including: "During the past 30 days, on how many days did you have at least one drink of alcohol?"

Any-listed diagnosis—See Diagnosis.

Average annual rate of change (percentage change)—In *Health, United States* average annual rates of change or growth rates are calculated as follows:

$$[(P_n / P_o)^{1/N}-1] \times 100$$

where P_n = later time period

P_o = earlier time period

N = number of years in interval.

This geometric rate of change assumes that a variable increases or decreases at the same rate during each year between the two time periods.

Average length of stay—In the National Health Interview Survey, average length of stay in a hospital per discharged inpatient is computed by dividing the total number of hospital days for a specified group by the total number of discharges for that group. Similarly, in the National Hospital Discharge Survey, average length of stay is computed by dividing the total number of hospital days of care, counting the date of admission but not the date of discharge, by the number of patients discharged. The American Hospital Association computes average length of stay by dividing the number of inpatient days by the number of admissions. See related Days of care; Discharge; Inpatient.

Bed, health facility—The American Hospital Association defines the bed count as the number of beds, cribs, and pediatric bassinets that are set up and staffed for use by inpatients on the last day of the reporting period. In the Center for Medicare & Medicaid Service's Online Survey Certification and Reporting (OSCAR) database, all beds in certified facilities are counted on the day of certification inspection. The World Health Organization defines a hospital bed as one regularly maintained and staffed for the accommodation and full-time care of a succession of inpatients and situated in a part of the hospital where continuous medical care for inpatients is provided. The Center for Mental Health Services within the Substance Abuse and Mental Health Services Administration counts the number of beds set up and staffed for use in inpatient and residential treatment services on the last day of the survey reporting period. See related Hospital; Mental health organization; Mental health service type; Occupancy rate.

Binge drinking—Binge drinking and binge alcohol use are measured in three different data systems. See related Alcohol consumption.

Monitoring the Future Survey—This school-based survey of secondary school students collects information on alcohol use using self-completed questionnaires. Information on binge drinking is obtained for high school seniors (starting in 1975) and 8th and 10th graders (starting in 1991) based on the following question for the prior 2-week period: "How many times have you had five or more drinks in a row?" among students who first responded affirmatively to the question: "On how many occasions (if any) have you had alcohol to drink—more than just a few sips—in the last 30 days?" Alcoholic beverages are defined as beer, wine, wine coolers, and liquor.

National Health Interview Survey—Information about binge alcohol use is defined as "In the past year, on how many days did you have five or more drinks of any alcoholic beverage?"

National Survey on Drug Use and Health (NSDUH)—Information about binge alcohol use, defined as "Five or more drinks on the same occasion (i.e., at the same time or within a couple of hours of each other) at least once in the past 30 days." Heavy alcohol use is defined as "Five or more drinks on the same occasion (binge drinking) on at least 5 different days in the past 30 days."

Birth cohort—A birth cohort consists of all persons born within a given period of time, such as a calendar year.

Birth rate—See Rate: Birth and related rates.

Birthweight—Birthweight is the first weight of the newborn obtained after birth. Low birthweight is defined as less than 2,500 grams or 5 pounds 8 ounces. Very low birthweight is defined as less than 1,500 grams or 3 pounds 4 ounces. Before 1979, low birthweight was defined as 2,500 grams or less and very low birthweight as 1,500 grams or less.

Blood pressure, elevated—In *Health, United States*, elevated blood pressure or hypertension is defined as having an average systolic blood pressure reading of at least 140 mmHg or diastolic pressure of at least 90 mmHg, which is consistent with the Seventh Report of the Joint National Committee on Prevention, Detection, Evaluation, and Treatment of High Blood Pressure (available from: www.nhlbi.nih.gov/guidelines/hypertension/jnc7full.pdf). People are also considered to have hypertension if they report that they are taking a prescription medicine for high blood pressure, even if their blood pressure readings are within normal range.

Blood pressure is measured by averaging the blood pressure readings taken. Blood pressure readings of 0 mmHg are assumed to be in error and are not included in the estimates. The methods to measure the blood pressure of NHANES participants have changed over the different NHANES survey years. Changes include:

- Number of BP measures taken (from 1 to 4)
- Equipment maintenance procedures
- Training of persons taking readings (physician, nurse, interviewer)
- Proportion zero end digits for systolic and diastolic readings
- Published diastolic definition
- Location where the measurements were taken (Mobile Examination Component (MEC) or home)

Blood pressure is measured in 1999 and subsequent years in the MEC of the NHANES. Participants who are 50 years and older or less than 1 year of age who are unable to travel to the MEC are offered an abbreviated examination in their homes. Blood pressure measurements are taken by one of the MEC examiners. For people age 20 and over, three consecutive blood pressure readings are obtained, using the same arm. If a blood pressure measurement was interrupted or the measurer was unable to get one or more of the readings, a fourth attempt may be made. Both systolic and diastolic measurements are recorded to the nearest even number.

In NHANES III, three sets of blood pressure measurements were taken in the examination center on examinees age 5 years and over. Blood pressure measurements were also taken by trained interviewers during the household interview, on sample persons age 17 years and over. Systolic and diastolic average blood pressure were computed as the arithmetic mean of six or fewer measurements obtained at the household interview (maximum of three) and the MEC examination (maximum of three). If the examinee did not have blood pressure measurements taken in the examination center, this variable was calculated from measurements taken at the household interview. Both systolic and diastolic measurements were recorded to the nearest even number.

See Burt VL, Cutler JA, Higgings M, Horan MJ, Labarthe D, Whelton P, et al. Trends in the prevalence, awareness, treatment, and control of hypertension in the adult US population. Hypertension 1995;26(1):60–9 for more information on changes in high blood pressure measurement in the NHANES up to 1991.

Body mass index (BMI)—BMI is a measure that adjusts bodyweight for height. It is calculated as weight in kilograms divided by height in meters squared. Overweight for children and adolescents is defined as BMI at or above the sex- and age-specific 95th percentile BMI cut points from the 2000 CDC Growth Charts (www.cdc.gov/growthcharts/). Healthy weight for adults is defined as a BMI of 18.5 to less than 25; overweight, as greater than or equal to a BMI of 25; and obesity, as greater than or equal to a BMI of 30. BMI cut points are defined in the Report of the Dietary Guidelines Advisory Committee on the Dietary Guidelines for Americans, 2000. U.S. Department of Agriculture, Agricultural Research Service, Dietary Guidelines Advisory Committee, p. 23. Available from: www.health.gov/dietaryguidelines/dgac/; NHLBI Obesity Education Initiative Expert Panel on the Identification, Evaluation, and Treatment of Overweight and Obesity in Adults. Clinical guidelines on the identification, evaluation, and treatment of overweight and obesity in adults—The evidence report. Obes Res 1998. 6:51S–209S. Available from: www.nhlbi.nih.gov/guidelines/obesity/ob_gdlns.htm and in U.S. Department of Health and Human Services. Tracking Healthy People 2010. Washington, DC: U.S. Government Printing Office, November 2000. Objectives 19.1, 19.2, and 19.3. Available from: www.healthypeople.gov/document/html/volume2/19nutrition.htm.

Cause of death—For the purpose of national mortality statistics, every death is attributed to one underlying condition, based on information reported on the death certificate and using the international rules for selecting the underlying cause of death from the conditions stated on the death certificate. The underlying cause is defined by the World Health Organization (WHO) as the disease or injury that initiated the train of events leading directly to death, or the circumstances of the accident or violence that produced the fatal injury. Generally more medical information is reported on death certificates than is directly reflected in the underlying cause of death. The conditions that are not selected as underlying cause of death constitute the nonunderlying causes of death, also known as multiple cause of death.

Cause of death is coded according to the appropriate revision of the *International Classification of Diseases* (ICD) (see Table IV). Effective with deaths occurring in 1999, the United States began using the Tenth Revision of the ICD (ICD–10); during the period 1979–1998, causes of death were coded and classified according to the Ninth Revision (ICD–9). Table V lists ICD codes for the Sixth through Tenth Revisions for causes of death shown in *Health, United States.*

Each of these revisions has produced discontinuities in cause-of-death trends. These discontinuities are measured using comparability ratios that are essential to the interpretation of mortality trends. For further discussion, see the Mortality Technical Appendix on the NCHS website, Available from: www.cdc.gov/nchs/deaths.htm. See related Comparability ratio; *International Classification of Diseases* (ICD); Appendix I, National Vital Statistics System, Multiple Cause-of-Death File.

Cause-of-death ranking—Selected causes of death of public health and medical importance comprise tabulation lists and are ranked according to the number of deaths assigned to these causes. The top-ranking causes determine the leading causes of death. Certain causes on the tabulation lists are not ranked if, for example, the category title represents a group title (such as Major cardiovascular diseases and Symptoms, signs, and abnormal clinical and laboratory findings, not elsewhere classified); or the category title begins with the words Other and All other. In addition, when one of the titles that represents a subtotal (such as malignant neoplasms) is ranked, its component parts are not ranked.

Table IV. Revision of the *International Classification of Diseases* (ICD) by year of conference by which adopted and years in use in the United States

Revision of the International Classification of Diseases	*Year of conference by which adopted*	*Years in use in United States*
First	1900	1900–1909
Second	1909	1910–1920
Third	1920	1921–1929
Fourth	1929	1930–1938
Fifth	1938	1939–1948
Sixth	1948	1949–1957
Seventh	1955	1958–1967
Eighth	1965	1968–1978
Ninth	1975	1979–1998
Tenth	1990	1999–present

SOURCE: National Center for Health Statistics. Available from: www.cdc.gov/nchs/about/major/dvs/icd9des.htm.

The tabulation lists used for ranking in the *Tenth Revision of the International Classification of Diseases* (ICD) include the List of 113 Selected Causes of Death, which replaces the ICD–9 List of 72 Selected Causes, HIV infection and Alzheimer's disease; and the ICD–10 List of 130 Selected Causes of Infant Death, which replaces the ICD–9 List of 60 Selected Causes of Infant Death and HIV infection. Causes that are tied receive the same rank; the next cause is assigned the rank it would have received had the lower-ranked causes not been tied, that is, a rank is skipped. See related *International Classification of Diseases* (ICD).

Cholesterol, serum—Serum cholesterol is a measure of the total blood cholesterol. Elevated total blood cholesterol—a combination of high-density lipoproteins (HDL), low-density lipoproteins (LDL), and very-low density lipoproteins (VLDL)—is a risk factor for cardiovascular disease. According to the National Cholesterol Education Program, high serum cholesterol is defined as greater than or equal to 240 mg/dL (6.20 mmol/L). Borderline high serum cholesterol is defined as greater than or equal to 200 mg/dL and less than 240 mg/dL. Assessments of the components of total cholesterol or lower thresholds for high total cholesterol may be used for individuals with other risk factors for cardiovascular disease. (For more information on high cholesterol guidelines, see the Third Report of the Expert Panel on Detection, Evaluation, and Treatment of High Blood Cholesterol in Adults (Adult Treatment Panel III) Full Report. Available from: www.nhlbi.nih.gov/guidelines/cholesterol/atp3_rpt.htm.) In *Health, United States*, the conservative threshold of 240 mg/dL is used to define high total serum cholesterol. Individuals who take medication to lower their serum cholesterol levels and whose measured total serum cholesterol levels are below the cut-offs for high and borderline high cholesterol, are not defined as having high or borderline cholesterol, respectively.

Venous blood serum samples that are collected from National Health and Nutrition Examination Survey (NHANES) participants at mobile examination centers are frozen and shipped on dry ice to the laboratory conducting the lipid analyses. Serum total cholesterol was measured on all examined adults regardless of whether they had fasted and data were analyzed regardless of fasting status. Cholesterol measurements are standardized according to the criteria of the CDC and later the CDC-National Heart, Lung, and Blood Institute Cholesterol Standardization Program to ensure comparable and accurate measurements (for more information, see Myers GL, Cooper GR, Winn CL, Smith SJ. The CDC-National, Heart, Lung, and Blood Institute Lipid Standardization Program. Clin Lab Med 1989;9(1):105–35). A detailed summary of the procedures used for measurement of total cholesterol in the earlier NHANES survey years has been published (see Johnson CL, Rifkind BM, Sempos CT, Carroll MD, Bachorik PS, Briefel RR, et al. Declining serum total cholesterol levels among U.S. adults: The National Health and Nutrition Examination Surveys. JAMA 1993;269(23):3002–8.) A description of the laboratory procedures for the total cholesterol measurement for different NHANES survey years is published by NCHS. Available from: www.cdc.gov/nchs/nhanes.htm.

Chronic condition—See Condition.

Table V. Cause-of-death codes, by applicable revision of *International Classification of Diseases* (ICD)

Cause of death (Tenth Revision titles)	*Sixth and Seventh Revisions*	*Eighth Revision*	*Ninth Revision*	*Tenth Revision*
Communicable diseases	...	...	001–139, 460–466, 480–487, 771.3	A00–B99, J00–J22
Chronic and noncommunicable diseases	...	...	140–459, 470–478, 490–799	C00–I99, J30–R99
Meningococcal Infection	...	...	036	A39
Septicemia	...	...	038	A40–A41
Human immunodeficiency virus (HIV) disease[2]	...	...	*042–*044	B20–B24
Malignant neoplasms	140–205	140–209	140–208	C00–C97
Colon, rectum, and anus	153–154	153–154	153, 154	C18–C21
Trachea, bronchus, and lung	162–163	162	162	C33–C34
Breast	170	174	174–175	C50
Prostate	177	185	185	C61
In situ neoplasms and benign neoplasms	...	...	210–239	D00–D48
Diabetes mellitus	260	250	250	E10–E14
Anemias	...	...	280–285	D50–D64
Meningitis	...	...	320–322	G00, G03
Alzheimer's disease	...	...	331	G30
Diseases of heart	6th: 410–443 7th: 400–402, 410–443	390–398, 402, 404, 410–429	390–398, 402, 404, 410–429	I00–I09, I11, I13, I20–I51
Ischemic heart disease	...	...	410–414, 429.2	I20–I25
Cerebrovascular diseases	330–334	430–438	430–434, 436–438	I60–I69
Atherosclerosis	...	...	440	I70
Influenza and pneumonia	480–483, 490–493	470–474, 480–486	480–487	J10–J18
Chronic lower respiratory diseases	241, 501, 502, 527.1	490–493, 519.3	490–494, 496	J40–J47
Chronic liver disease and cirrhosis	581	571	571	K70, K73–K74
Nephritis, nephrotic syndrome, and nephrosis	...	...	580–589	N00–N07, N17–N19, N25–N27
Pregnancy, childbirth, and the puerperium	640–689	630–678	630–676	A34, O00–O95, O98–O99
Congenital malformations, deformations, and chromosomal abnormalities	...	...	740–759	Q00–Q99
Certain conditions originating in the perinatal period	...	...	760–779	P00–P96
Newborn affected by maternal complications of pregnancy	...	...	761	P01
Newborn affected by complications of placenta, cord, and membranes	...	...	762	P02
Disorders related to short gestation and low birthweight, not elsewhere classified	...	...	765	P07
Birth trauma	...	...	767	P10–P15
Intrauterine hypoxia and birth asphyxia	...	...	768	P20–P21
Respiratory distress of newborn	...	...	769	P22
Sudden infant death syndrome	...	...	798.0	R95
Injuries[1]	...	...	E800–E869, E880–E929, E950–E999	*U01–*U03, V01–Y36, Y85–Y87, Y89

See footnotes at end of table.

Table V. Cause-of-death codes, by applicable revision of *International Classification of Diseases* (ICD)—Con

Cause of death (Tenth Revision titles)	*Sixth and Seventh Revisions*	*Eighth Revision*	*Ninth Revision*	*Tenth Revision*
Unintentional injuries[3]	E800–E936, E960–E965	E800–E929, E940–E946	E800–E869, E880–E929	V01–X59, Y85–Y86
Motor vehicle-related injuries[3]	E810–E835	E810–E823	E810–E825	V02–V04, V09.0, V09.2, V12–V14, V19.0–V19.2, V19.4–V19.6, V20–V79, V80.3–V80.5, V81.0–V81.1, V82.0–V82.1, V83–V86, V87.0–V87.8, V88.0–V88.8, V89.0, V89.2
Suicide[1]	E963, E970–E979	E950–E959	E950–E959	*U03, X60–X84, Y87.0
Homicide[1]	E964, E980–E983	E960–E969	E960–E969	*U01–*U02, X85–Y09, Y87.1
Injury by firearms	. . .	E922, E955, E965, E970, E985	E922, E955.0–E955.4, E965.0–E965.4, E970, E985.0–E985.4	W32–W34, X72–X74, X93–X95, Y22–Y24, Y35.0

. . . Cause-of-death code numbers are not provided for causes not shown in *Health, United States.*

[1]Starting with 2001 data, NCHS introduced categories *U01–*U03 for classifying and coding deaths due to acts of terrorism. The * indicates codes are not part of the Tenth Revision.

[2]Categories for coding human immunodeficiency virus infection were introduced in 1987. The asterisk (*) indicates codes are not part of the Ninth Revision.

[3]In the public health community, the term "unintentional injuries" is preferred to "accidents" and "motor vehicle-related injuries" to "motor vehicle accidents."

SOURCE: Advance report of final mortality statistics, 1976. Monthly vital statistics report; vol 24 no 11, supp. Hyattsville, MD: National Center for Health Statistics. 1976. Available from: www.cdc.gov/nchs/data/mvsr/supp/mv24_11sacc.pdf. Hoyert DL, Kochanek KD, Murphy SL. Deaths: Final Data for 1997. National vital statistics reports; vol 47 no. 19. Hyattsville, MD: National Center for Health Statistics. 1999. Available from: www.cdc.gov/nchs/data/nvsr/nvsr47/nvs47_19.pdf. Hoyert DL, Heron MP, Murphy SL, Kung H. Deaths: Final Data for 2003. National vital statistics reports; vol 54 no 13. Hyattsville, MD: National Center for Health Statistics. 2006. Available from: www.cdc.gov/nchs/data/nvsr/nvsr54/nvsr54_13.pdf.

Cigarette smoking—Cigarette smoking and related tobacco use are measured in several different data systems.

Birth File—Information on cigarette smoking by the mother during pregnancy is based on Yes/No responses to the birth certificate item "Other risk factors for this pregnancy: Tobacco use during pregnancy" and the average number of cigarettes per day with no specificity on timing during pregnancy. This information became available for the first time in 1989 with revision of the U.S. Standard Certificate of Live Birth. In 1989, 43 states and the District of Columbia (D.C.) collected data on tobacco use. The following states did not require the reporting of tobacco use in the standard format on the birth certificate: California, Indiana, Louisiana, Nebraska, New York, Oklahoma, and South Dakota. In 1990, information on tobacco use became available from Louisiana and Nebraska, increasing the number of reporting states to 45 and the District of Columbia. In 1991–1993, with the addition of Oklahoma to the reporting area, information on tobacco use was available for 46 states and D.C.; in 1994–1998, 46 states, D.C., and New York City reported tobacco use; in 1999, information on tobacco use became available from Indiana and New York, increasing the number of reporting states to 48 and D.C.; starting in 2000, with the addition of South Dakota, the reporting area includes 49 states and D.C. During 1989–2004, California did not require the reporting of tobacco use. The area reporting tobacco use comprised 87% of U.S. births in 1999–2002. Starting in 2003, some states began implementation of the 2003 revision of the U.S. Standard Certificate of Live Birth. The 2003 revision asked for the number of cigarettes smoked at different intervals before and during pregnancy. Tobacco use during pregnancy data from the 2003 revision of the birth certificate are not comparable with data from the 1989 revision. Therefore, data on tobacco use during pregnancy were excluded for states that implemented the 2003 revision of the U.S. Standard Certificate of Live Birth: these reporting areas included Pennsylvania and Washington starting in 2003, and Florida, Idaho, Kentucky, New Hampshire, New York state (excluding New York City), South Carolina, and Tennessee starting in 2004. The reporting area for mother's tobacco use decreased to 47 states and D.C. in 2003, and 40 states, D.C., and New York City in 2004.

Monitoring the Future Survey—Information on current cigarette smoking is obtained for high school seniors (starting in 1975) and 8th and 10th graders (starting in 1991) based on the following question: "How frequently have you smoked cigarettes during the past 30 days?"

National Health Interview Survey (NHIS)—Information about cigarette smoking is obtained for adults 18 years of age and over. Starting in 1993, current smokers are identified by asking the following two questions: "Have you smoked at least 100 cigarettes in your entire life?" and "Do you now smoke cigarettes every day, some days, or not at all?" Persons who smoked 100 cigarettes and who now smoke every day or some days are defined as current smokers. Before 1992, current smokers were identified based on positive responses to the following two questions: "Have you smoked 100 cigarettes in your entire life?" and "Do you smoke now?" (traditional definition). In 1992, the definition of current smoker in the NHIS was modified to specifically include persons who smoked on some days (revised definition). In 1992, cigarette smoking data were collected for a half-sample with half the respondents (one-quarter sample) using the traditional smoking questions and the other half of respondents (one-quarter sample) using the revised smoking question ("Do you smoke every day, some days, or not at all?"). An unpublished analysis of the 1992 traditional smoking measure revealed that the crude percentage of current smokers 18 years of age and over remained the same as for 1991. The estimates for 1992 combine data collected using the traditional and the revised questions.

In 1993–1995, estimates of cigarette smoking prevalence were based on a half-sample. Smoking data were not collected in 1996. Starting in 1997, smoking data were collected in the sample adult questionnaire. For further information on survey methodology and sample sizes pertaining to the NHIS cigarette smoking data for data years 1965–1992 and other sources of cigarette smoking data available from the National Center for Health Statistics, see National Center for Health Statistics. Bibliographies and Data Sources, Smoking Data Guide, no 1, DHHS pub no (PHS) 91–1308–1, Public Health Service. Washington, DC: U.S. Government Printing Office. 1991.

The National Health Interview Survey tobacco information website, available from: www.cdc.gov/nchs/about/major/nhis/tobacco/nhis_tobhoma.htm.

National Survey on Drug Use & Health (NSDUH)—Information on current cigarette smoking is obtained for all persons surveyed who are 12 years of age and over based on the following question: "During the past 30 days, have you smoked part or all of a cigarette?"

Youth Risk Behavior Survey—Information on current cigarette smoking is obtained from high school students (starting in 1991) based on the following question: "During the past 30 days, on how many days did you smoke cigarettes?"

Civilian noninstitutionalized population; Civilian population—See Population.

Community hospital—See Hospital.

Comparability ratio—About every 10–20 years the *International Classification of Diseases* (ICD) is revised to stay abreast of advances in medical science and changes in medical terminology. Each of these revisions produces breaks in the continuity of cause-of-death statistics. Discontinuities across revisions are due to changes in classification and rules for selecting underlying cause of death. Classification and rule changes affect cause-of-death trend data by shifting deaths away from some cause-of-death categories and into others. Comparability ratios measure the effect of changes in classification and coding rules. For causes shown in Table VI, comparability ratios range between 0.6974 and 1.1404. Influenza and pneumonia had the lowest comparability ratio (0.6974), indicating that influenza and pneumonia is about 30% less likely to be selected as the underlying cause of death in ICD–10 than in ICD–9. Pregnancy, childbirth, and the puerperium had the highest comparability ratio (1.1404), indicating that pregnancy is more than 14% more likely to be selected as the underlying cause using ICD–10 coding.

For selected causes of death, the ICD–9 codes used to calculate death rates for 1980 through 1998 differ from the ICD–9 codes most nearly comparable with the corresponding ICD–10 cause-of-death category, which also affects the ability to compare death rates across ICD revisions. Examples of these causes are ischemic heart disease; cerebrovascular diseases; trachea, bronchus and lung cancer; unintentional injuries; and homicide. To address this source of discontinuity, mortality trends for 1980–1998 were recalculated, using ICD–9 codes that are more comparable with codes for corresponding ICD–10 categories. Table V shows the ICD–9 codes used for these causes. This modification may lessen the discontinuity between the Ninth and Tenth Revisions, but the effect on the discontinuity between the Eighth and Ninth Revisions is not measured.

Comparability ratios shown in Table VI are based on a comparability study in which the same deaths were coded by both the Ninth and Tenth Revisions. The comparability ratio was calculated by dividing the number of deaths classified by ICD–10 by the number of deaths classified by ICD–9. The resulting ratios represent the net effect of the Tenth Revision on cause-of-death statistics and can be used to adjust mortality statistics for causes of death classified by the Ninth Revision to be comparable with cause-specific mortality statistics classified by the Tenth Revision.

The application of comparability ratios to mortality statistics helps make the analysis of change between 1998 and 1999 more accurate and complete. The 1998 comparability-modified death rate is calculated by multiplying the comparability ratio by the 1998 death rate. Comparability-modified rates should be used to estimate mortality change between 1998 and 1999.

Caution should be taken when applying the comparability ratios presented in Table VI to age-, race-, and sex-specific mortality data. Demographic subgroups may sometimes differ with regard to their cause-of-death distribution, and this would result in demographic variation in cause-specific comparability ratios.

For more information, see Anderson RN, Miniño AM, Hoyert DL, Rosenberg HM. Comparability of cause of death between ICD–9 and ICD–10: Preliminary estimates; Kochanek KD, Smith BL, Anderson RN. Deaths: Preliminary data for 1999. National vital statistics reports; vol 49 no 2 and vol 49 no 3. Hyattsville, MD: National Center for Health Statistics. 2001; and Final ratios for 113 selected causes of death. Available from: ftp://ftp.cdc.gov/pub/Health_Statistics/NCHS/Datasets/Comparability/icd9_icd10/. See related Cause of death; *International Classification of Diseases* (ICD); Tables IV, V, and VI.

Table VI. Comparability of selected causes of death between the Ninth and Tenth Revisions of the *International Classification of Diseases* (ICD)

Cause of death[1]	*Final comparability ratio*[2]
Human immunodeficiency virus (HIV) disease	1.0821
Malignant neoplasms	1.0093
Colon, rectum, and anus	0.9988
Trachea, bronchus, and lung	0.9844
Breast	1.0073
Prostate	1.0144
Diabetes mellitus	1.0193
Diseases of heart	0.9852
Ischemic heart diseases	1.0006
Cerebrovascular diseases	1.0502
Influenza and pneumonia	0.6974
Chronic lower respiratory diseases	1.0411
Chronic liver disease and cirrhosis	1.0321
Pregnancy, childbirth, and the puerperium	1.1404
Unintentional injuries	1.0251
Motor vehicle-related injuries	0.9527
Suicide	1.0022
Homicide	1.0020
Injury by firearms	1.0012
Chronic and noncommunicable diseases	1.0100
Injuries	1.0159
Communicable diseases	0.8582
HIV disease	1.0821
Other communicable diseases	0.7997

[1]See Table V for ICD–9 and ICD–10 cause-of-death codes.
[2]Ratio of number of deaths classified by ICD–10 to number of deaths classified by ICD–9.

SOURCE: National Center for Health Statistics. Final comparability ratios for 113 selected causes of death. Available from: ftp://ftp.cdc.gov/pub/Health_Statistics/NCHS/Datasets/Comparability/icd9_icd10/Comparability_Ratio_tables.xls.

Compensation—See Employer costs for employee compensation.

Computed tomography scanner—A CT or CAT scanner is an x-ray machine which combines many x-ray images with the aid of a computer to generate cross-sectional views and, if needed, three-dimensional images of the internal organs and structures of the body.

Condition—A health condition is a departure from a state of physical or mental well-being. In the National Health Interview Survey, each condition reported as a cause of an individual's activity limitation has been classified as chronic, not chronic, or unknown if chronic, based on the nature and duration of the condition. Conditions that are not cured once acquired (such as heart disease, diabetes, and birth defects in the original response categories, and amputee and old age in the ad hoc categories) are considered chronic, whereas conditions related to pregnancy are always considered not chronic. In addition, other conditions must have been present 3 months or longer to be considered chronic. An exception is made for children less than 1 year of age who have had a condition since birth, as these conditions are always considered chronic.

Consumer Price Index (CPI)—The CPI is prepared by the U.S. Bureau of Labor Statistics. It is a monthly measure of the average change in the prices paid by urban consumers for a fixed market basket of goods and services. The medical care component of CPI shows trends in medical care prices based on specific indicators of hospital, medical, dental, and drug prices. A revision of the definition of CPI has been in use since January 1988. See related Gross domestic product (GDP); Health expenditures, national; Appendix I, Consumer Price Index.

Contraception—The National Survey of Family Growth collects information on contraceptive use as reported by women 15–44 years of age, during heterosexual vaginal intercourse. For current contraceptive use, women were asked about contraceptive use during the month of interview. Women were classified by whether they reported using each of 19 methods of contraception at any time in the month of interview. Contraceptive methods listed as other methods include the following: for 2002, the female condom, foam, cervical cap, Today Sponge®, suppository or insert, jelly or cream, or other method; for 1995, the female condom or vaginal pouch, foam, cervical cap, Today Sponge®, suppository or insert, jelly or cream, or other method; for 1988, foam, douche, Today Sponge®, suppository or insert, jelly or cream, or other method; and for 1982, foam, douche, suppository or insert, or other method.

Crude birth rate; Crude death rate—See Rate: Birth and related rates; Rate: Death and related rates.

Days of care—Days of care is defined similarly in different data systems. See related Admission; Average length of stay; Discharge; Hospital; Hospital utilization; Inpatient.

American Hospital Association—Days, hospital days, or inpatient days are the number of adult and pediatric days of care rendered during the entire reporting period. Days of care for newborns are excluded.

National Health Interview Survey (NHIS)—Hospital days during the year refer to the total number of hospital days occurring in the 12-month period before the interview week. A hospital day is a night spent in the hospital for persons admitted as inpatients. Starting in 1997, hospitalization data from NHIS are for all inpatient stays, whereas estimates for prior years published in previous editions of *Health, United States* excluded hospitalizations for deliveries and newborns.

National Hospital Discharge Survey—Days of care refers to the total number of patient days accumulated by inpatients at the time of discharge from nonfederal short-stay hospitals during a reporting period. All days from and including the date of admission but not including the date of discharge are counted.

Death rate—See Rate: Death and related rates.

Dental caries—Dental caries is evidence of dental decay on any surface of a tooth. Untreated dental caries was determined by an oral examination conducted by a trained dentist as part of the National Health and Nutrition Examination Survey. In *Health, United States*, untreated dental caries refers to coronal caries, that is, caries on the crown or enamel surface of the tooth. Treated dental caries and root caries are not included. Study participants 2 years of age and over were eligible for the examination, as long as they did not meet other exclusion criteria. Both permanent and primary (or baby) teeth were evaluated, depending on the age of the participant. For children 2–5 years of age, only caries in primary teeth were included. For children 6–11 years of age, caries in both primary and permanent teeth were included. For children 12 years of age and over, and for adults, only caries in permanent teeth were included.

Dental visit—Starting in 1997, National Health Interview Survey respondents were asked "About how long has it been since you last saw or talked to a dentist? Include all types of dentists, such as orthodontists, oral surgeons, and all other dental specialists as well as hygienists." Starting in 2001, the question was modified slightly to ask respondents how long it had been since they last saw a dentist. Questions about dental visits were not asked for children under 2 years of age for years 1997–1999 and under 1 year of age for 2000 and beyond. Starting with 1997 data, estimates are presented for ɜople with a dental visit in the past year. Prior to 1997, ɜntal visit estimates were based on a 2-week recall period.

iagnosis—Diagnosis is the act or process of identifying or etermining the nature and cause of a disease or injury ırough evaluation of patient history, examination, and review ıf laboratory data. Diagnoses in the National Hospital)ischarge Survey, the National Ambulatory Medical Care ;urvey, the National Hospital Ambulatory Medical Care ;urvey, and the National Nursing Home Survey are ıbstracted from medical records and coded to the *International Classification of Diseases, Ninth Revision, Clinical Modification* (ICD–9–CM). For a given medical care encounter, the first-listed diagnosis can be used to categorize the visit, or if more than one diagnosis is recorded on the medical record, the visit can be categorized based on all diagnoses recorded. Analyzing first-listed diagnoses avoids double-counting events such as visits or hospitalizations; the first-listed diagnosis is often, but not always, considered the most important or dominant condition among all comorbid conditions. For example, a hospital discharge would be considered a first-listed stroke discharge if the ICD–9–CM diagnosis code for stroke was recorded in the first diagnosis field on the hospital record. An any-listed stroke discharge would classify all diagnoses of stroke recorded regardless of the order in which they are listed on the hospital facesheet. Any-listed diagnoses double count events such as visits or hospitalizations with more than one recorded diagnosis but provide information on the burden a specific diagnosis presents to the health care system. See related External cause of injury; Injury; Injury-related visit.

Diagnostic and other nonsurgical procedure—See Procedure.

Discharge—The National Health Interview Survey defines a hospital discharge as the completion of any continuous period of stay of one night or more in a hospital as an inpatient. According to the National Hospital Discharge Survey, a discharge is a completed inpatient hospitalization. A hospitalization may be completed by death or by releasing the patient to the customary place of residence, a nursing home, another hospital, or other locations. See related Admission; Average length of stay; Days of care; Inpatient.

Domiciliary care home—See Long-term care facility; Nursing home.

Drug abuse—See Illicit drug use.

Drug—Drugs are pharmaceutical agents—by any route of administration—for prevention, diagnosis, or treatment of medical conditions or diseases. Data on specific drug use are collected in three NCHS surveys.

National Ambulatory Medical Care Survey (NAMCS) and *National Hospital Ambulatory Medical Care Survey (NHAMCS)*—Data collection in the NAMCS and NHAMCS outpatient and emergency department components is from the medical record of an inperson physician office, or hospital outpatient or emergency department visit, rather than from the patient. Generic or brand name drugs are abstracted from the medical record, including prescription and over-the-counter drugs, immunizations, allergy shots, and anesthetics that were prescribed, ordered, supplied, administered, or continued during the visit. Prior to 1995, up to five drugs per visit could be reported on the patient record form; in data years 1995 and beyond, up to six drugs could be reported. Starting with data year 2003, up to eight drugs could be reported, as well as a count of the total number of drugs prescribed, ordered, supplied, administered, or continued during the visit.

For more information on drugs collected by the NAMCS and NHAMCS, see the NAMCS drug database, available from: www.cdc.gov/nchs/about/major/ahcd/ambulatory.htm, or ftp://ftp.cdc.gov/pub/Health_Statistics/NCHS/Dataset_Documentation/NAMCS/doc01.pdf.
For more information on how drugs are classified into therapeutic use categories, See National Drug Code (NDC) Directory therapeutic class. See related Appendix I, National Ambulatory Medical Care Survey and National Hospital Ambulatory Medical Care Survey.

National Health and Nutrition Examination Survey (NHANES)—Drug information from NHANES III and 1999–2004 NHANES was collected during an inperson interview conducted in the participant's home. Participants were asked whether they had taken a medication in the past month for which they needed a prescription. Those who answered "yes" were asked to produce the prescription medication containers for the interviewer. For each medication reported, the interviewer entered the product's complete name from the container. If no container was available, the interviewer asked the participant to verbally report the name of the medication.

In addition, participants were asked how long they had been taking the medication and the main reason for use.

All reported medication names were converted to their standard generic ingredient name. For multi-ingredient products, the ingredients were listed in alphabetical order and counted as one drug (e.g., Tylenol #3 was listed as Acetaminophen; Codeine). No trade or proprietary names are provided on the data file.

Drug data from NHANES provide a snapshot of all prescribed drugs reported by a sample of the civilian noninstitutionalized population for a 1-month period. Drugs taken on an irregular basis such as every other day, once per week, or for a 10 day period, etc. were captured in the 1-month recall period. Data shown in *Health, United States* for the percentage of the population reporting three or more prescription drugs during the past month include a range of drug utilization patterns—for example, persons who took three or more drugs on a daily basis during the past month or persons who took a different drug three separate times—as long as at least three different drugs were taken during the past month.

For more information on prescription drug data collection and coding in the NHANES 1999–2002, see: www.cdc.gov/nchs/data/nhanes/frequency/rxq_rxdoc.pdf. For more information on NHANES III prescription drug data collection and coding, see: www.cdc.gov/nchs/data/nhanes/nhanes3/PUPREMED-acc.pdf. See related Appendix I, National Health and Nutrition Examination Survey.

Education—Several approaches to defining educational categories are used in this report. In survey data, educational categories are based on information about educational credentials, such as diplomas and degrees. In vital statistics, educational attainment is based on years of school completed.

Birth File—Information on educational attainment of mother is based on number of years of school completed, as reported by the mother on the birth certificate. Between 1970 and 1992, the reporting area for maternal education expanded.

Mother's education was reported on the birth certificate by 38 states in 1970. Data were not available from Alabama, Arkansas, California, Connecticut, Delaware, the District of Columbia (D.C.), Georgia, Idaho, Maryland, New Mexico, Pennsylvania, Texas, and Washington. In 1975, these data became available from Connecticut, Delaware, Georgia, Maryland, and D.C., increasing the number of states reporting mother's education to 42 and D.C. Between 1980 and 1988, only three states, California, Texas, and Washington, did not report mother's education. In 1988, mother's education was also missing from New York state outside New York City. In 1989–1991, mother's education was missing only from Washington and New York state outside New York City. During 1992–2002, mother's education was reported by all 50 states and D.C. Starting in 2003, some states began implementation of the 2003 revision of the U.S. Standard Certificate of Live Birth. The education item on the 2003 revision asks for the highest degree or level of school completed whereas the education item on the 1989 revision asks for highest grade completed. Data from the 1989 and 2003 certificate items on educational attainment are too dissimilar to be reliably combined. Therefore, data on maternal education were excluded for states that implemented the 2003 revision of the U.S. Standard Certificate of Live Birth: these reporting areas included Pennsylvania and Washington starting in 2003, and Florida, Idaho, Kentucky, New Hampshire, New York state (outside New York City), South Carolina, and Tennessee starting in 2004. The reporting area for education decreased to 48 states and D.C. in 2003, and 41 states, D.C., and New York City in 2004.

Mortality File—Information on educational attainment of decedent became available for the first time in 1989 because of a revision of the U.S. Standard Certificate of Death. Decedent's educational attainment is reported on the death certificate by the funeral director based on information provided by an informant such as next of kin. Mortality data by educational attainment for 1989 were based on data from 20 states and by 1994–1996, increased to 45 states and the District of Columbia (D.C.). In 1994–1996, either the following states did not report educational attainment on the death certificate or the information was more than 20% incomplete: Georgia, Kentucky, Oklahoma, Rhode Island, and South Dakota. In 1997–2000, information on decedent's education was available from Oklahoma, increasing the reporting area to 46 states and D.C. With the addition of Kentucky, the reporting area increased to 47 states and D.C. in 2001 and 2002. The U.S. Standard Certificate of Death was revised in 2003; states are adopting this new certificate on a rolling basis. Starting with 2003 data, California, Idaho, Montana, and New York implemented the 2003 revision. In addition to these four states, starting with 2004 data, Connecticut, Georgia, Michigan, New Hampshire, New Jersey, Oklahoma, Rhode Island, South Dakota, Washington, and Wyoming have adopted the 2003 certificate. Educational attainment data from the revised death certificate are not comparable with educational attainment data collected using the 1989 revision of the U.S. Standard Certificate of Death. Therefore, deaths in states adopting the revised death certificate are excluded from educational attainment mortality data beginning with 2003. Because of different education profiles of the excluded states compared with the remaining states and D.C., 2003 and subsequent data are not directly comparable to earlier years. For more information on the revised educational attainment item, see the technical notes of Hoyert DL, Heron M, Murphy SL, Kung HC. Deaths: Final data for 2003. National vital statistics reports; vol 54 no 13. Hyattsville, MD: National Center for Health Statistics. 2006. Available from: www.cdc.gov/nchs/data/nvsr/nvsr54/nvsr54_13.pdf.

Calculation of unbiased death rates by educational attainment based on the National Vital Statistics System requires that the reporting of education on the death certificate be complete and consistent with the reporting of education on the Current Population Survey (CPS), the source of population estimates for denominators for death rates. Death records that are missing information about decedent's education are not included in the calculation of rates. Therefore, the levels of death rates by educational attainment shown in this report are underestimated by approximately the percentage with not stated education, which ranges from 2%–9%.

The validity of information about the decedent's education was evaluated by comparing self-reported education obtained in the CPS with education on the death certificate for decedents in the National Longitudinal Mortality Survey (NLMS). (Sorlie PD, Johnson NJ. Validity of education information on the death certificate. Epidemiology 1996;7(4):437–9.) Another analysis compared self-reported education collected in the first National Health and Nutrition Examination Survey (NHANES I) with education on the death certificate for decedents in the NHANES I Epidemiologic Followup Study. (Makuc DM, Feldman JJ, Mussolino ME. Validity of education and age as reported on death certificates. American Statistical Association. 1996 Proceedings of the Social Statistics Section 102–6.) Results of both studies indicated that there is a tendency for some people who did not graduate from high school to be reported as high school graduates on the death certificate. This tendency results in overstating the death rate for high school graduates and understating the death rate for the group with less than 12 years of education. The bias was greater among older than younger decedents and somewhat greater among black than white decedents.

In addition, educational gradients in death rates based on the National Vital Statistics System were compared with those based on the NLMS, a prospective study of persons in the CPS. Results of these comparisons indicate that educational gradients in death rates based on the National Vital Statistics System were reasonably similar to those based on NLMS for white persons 25–64 years of age and black persons 25–44 years of age. The number of deaths for persons of Hispanic origin in NLMS was too small to permit comparison for this ethnic group. For further information on measurement of education, see Kominski R, Siegel PM. Measuring education in the Current Population Survey. Monthly Labor Review September 1993; 34–8.

National Health Interview Survey (NHIS)—Starting in 1997, the NHIS questionnaire was changed to ask "What is the highest level of school ___ has completed or the highest degree received?" Responses were used to categorize adults according to educational credentials (e.g., no high school diploma or general educational development (GED) high school equivalency diploma; high school diploma or GED; some college, no bachelor's degree; bachelor's degree or higher).

Prior to 1997, the education variable in NHIS was measured by asking, "What is the highest grade or year of regular school ___ has ever attended?" and "Did ___ finish the grade/year?" Responses were used to categorize adults according to years of education completed (e.g., less than 12 years, 12 years, 13–15 years, and 16 or more years).

Data from the 1996 and 1997 NHIS were used to compare distributions of educational attainment for adults

25 years of age and over using categories based on educational credentials (1997) with categories based on years of education completed (1996). A larger percentage of persons reported some college than 13–15 years of education and a correspondingly smaller percentage reported high school diploma or GED than 12 years of education. In 1997, 19% of adults reported no high school diploma, 31% a high school diploma or GED, 26% some college, and 24% a bachelor's degree or higher. In 1996, 18% of adults reported less than 12 years of education, 37% reported 12 years of education, 20% 13–15 years, and 25% 16 or more years of education.

Emergency department—According to the National Hospital Ambulatory Medical Care Survey, an emergency department is a hospital facility that provides unscheduled outpatient services to patients whose conditions require immediate care and is staffed 24 hours a day. Off-site emergency departments open less than 24 hours are included if staffed by the hospital's emergency department. See related Emergency department or emergency room visit; Outpatient department.

Emergency department or emergency room visit—Starting with the 1997 National Health Interview Survey, respondents to the sample adult and sample child questionnaires (generally the parent) were asked about the number of visits to hospital emergency rooms during the past 12 months, including visits that resulted in hospitalization. In the National Hospital Ambulatory Medical Care Survey, an emergency department visit is a direct personal exchange between a patient and a physician or other health care providers working under the physician's supervision, for the purpose of seeking care and receiving personal health services. See related Emergency department; Injury-related visit.

Employer costs for employee compensation—This is a measure of the average cost per employee hour worked to employers for wages and salaries and benefits. Wages and salaries are defined as the hourly straight-time wage rate or, for workers not paid on an hourly basis, straight-time earnings divided by the corresponding hours. Straight-time wage and salary rates are total earnings before payroll deductions, excluding premium pay for overtime and for work on weekends and holidays, shift differentials, nonproduction bonuses, and lump-sum payments provided in lieu of wage increases. Production bonuses, incentive earnings, commission payments, and cost-of-living adjustments are included in straight-time wage and salary rates. Benefits covered are paid leave—paid vacations, holidays, sick leave, and other leave; supplemental pay—premium pay for overtime and work on weekends and holidays, shift differentials, nonproduction bonuses, and lump-sum payments provided in lieu of wage increases; insurance benefits—life, health, and sickness and accident insurance; retirement and savings benefits—pension and other retirement plans and savings and thrift plans; legally required benefits—Social Security, railroad retirement and supplemental retirement, railroad unemployment insurance, federal and state unemployment insurance, workers' compensation, and other benefits required by law, such as state temporary disability insurance; and other benefits—severance pay and supplemental unemployment plans. See related Appendix I, National Compensation Survey.

Ethnicity—See Hispanic origin.

Exercise—See Physical activity, leisure-time.

Expenditures—See Health expenditures, national; Appendix I, National Health Expenditure Accounts.

External cause of injury—The ICD–9 External Cause Matrix is a two-dimensional array describing both the mechanism or external cause of the injury (e.g., fall, motor vehicle traffic) and the manner or intent of the injury (e.g., self inflicted or assault). Although this matrix was originally developed for mortality, it has been adapted for use with the ICD–9–CM. For more information, see the NCHS website: www.cdc.gov/nchs/about/otheract/injury/tools.htm.

Family income—For purposes of the National Health Interview Survey and the National Health and Nutrition Examination Survey, all people within a household related to each other by blood, marriage, or adoption constitute a family. Each member of a family is classified according to the total income of the family. Unrelated individuals are classified according to their own income.

National Health Interview Survey (NHIS)—In the NHIS (prior to 1997), family income was the total income received by members of a family (or by an unrelated individual) in the 12 months before the interview. Starting in 1997, the NHIS collected family income data for the calendar year prior to the interview (e.g., 2005 family income data were based on calendar year 2004 information). Family income includes wages, salaries, rents from property, interest, dividends, profits and fees from their own businesses, pensions, and help from relatives. Family income data are used in the computation of poverty level. Starting with *Health, United States, 2004* a new methodology for imputing family income data for NHIS data was implemented for data years 1997 and beyond. Multiple imputations were performed for survey years 1997 and beyond with five sets of imputed values created to allow for the assessment of variability caused by imputation. Family income was missing for 24%–29% of persons in 1997–1998 and 31%–34% in 1999–2005. A detailed description of the multiple imputation procedure, as well as data files for 1997 and beyond, are available from: www.cdc.gov/nchs/nhis.htm, via the Imputed Income Files link under that year. For data years 1990–1996, about 16%–18% of persons had missing data for family income. In those years, missing values were imputed for family income using a sequential hot deck within matrix cells imputation approach. A detailed description of the imputation procedure, as well as data files with imputed annual family income for 1990–1996, is available from NCHS on CD-ROM, NHIS Imputed Annual Family Income 1990–1996, series 10, no. 9A.

National Health and Nutrition Examination Survey (NHANES)—In the NHANES 1999 and onward, family income is asked in a series of questions about possible sources of income, including wages, salaries, interest and dividends, federal programs, child support, rents, royalties, and other possible sources of income. After the information about sources of income was obtained in the family interview income section of the questionnaire, the respondent was asked to report total combined family income for themselves and the other members of their family, in dollars. If the respondent did not provide an answer or did not know the total combined family income, they were asked if the total family income was less than $20,000 or $20,000 or more. If the respondent answered, a follow-up question asked the respondent to select an income range from a list on a printed hand card. The midpoint of the income range was then used as the total family income value. Family income values were used to calculate the poverty income ratio. NHANES III did not ask the detailed components of income questions but asked respondents to identify their income based on a set of ranges provided on a flashcard, whereas NHANES II did include questions on components of income. Family income was not imputed for individuals or families with no reported income information in any of the NHANES survey years. See related Poverty.

Federal hospital—See Hospital.

Fee-for-service health insurance—This is private (commercial) health insurance that reimburses health care providers on the basis of a fee for each health service provided to the insured person. It is also known as indemnity health insurance. Medicare Parts A and B are sometimes referred to as Medicare fee-for-service. See related Health insurance coverage; Medicare.

Fertility rate—See Rate: Birth and related rates.

Foreign-born population—The U.S. Census Bureau uses the term foreign born to refer to anyone who is not a U. S. citizen at birth. This includes naturalized U.S. citizens, lawful permanent residents (immigrants), temporary migrants (such as foreign students), humanitarian migrants (such as refugees), and persons illegally present in the United States. Prior to 1994, the foreign-born population data were enumerated from the decennial census, which was the sole source for the foreign-born population data. In order to obtain more timely data, starting with 1994, the basic and monthly Current Population Survey (CPS) began including questions on nativity of respondent and parental nativity, citizenship status, and year of entry into the United States. Whereas the universe for the decennial census is the entire resident population of the United States., the universe for the CPS is the civilian noninstitutionalized population plus Armed Forces living off post or with their families on post. Therefore, foreign-born persons in institutional settings such as nursing homes or prisons are not included in the CPS count. Estimates of the foreign-born population data starting with data year 1994 are not directly comparable to the foreign-born population data estimated from the decennial census (1970, 1980, and 1990 data in this report) because of these differences in the population denominators. See related Population; Appendix I, Current Population Survey, Population Census and Population Estimates.

General hospital—See Hospital.

Figure I. Census Bureau: Four Geographic Regions and 9 Divisions of the United States

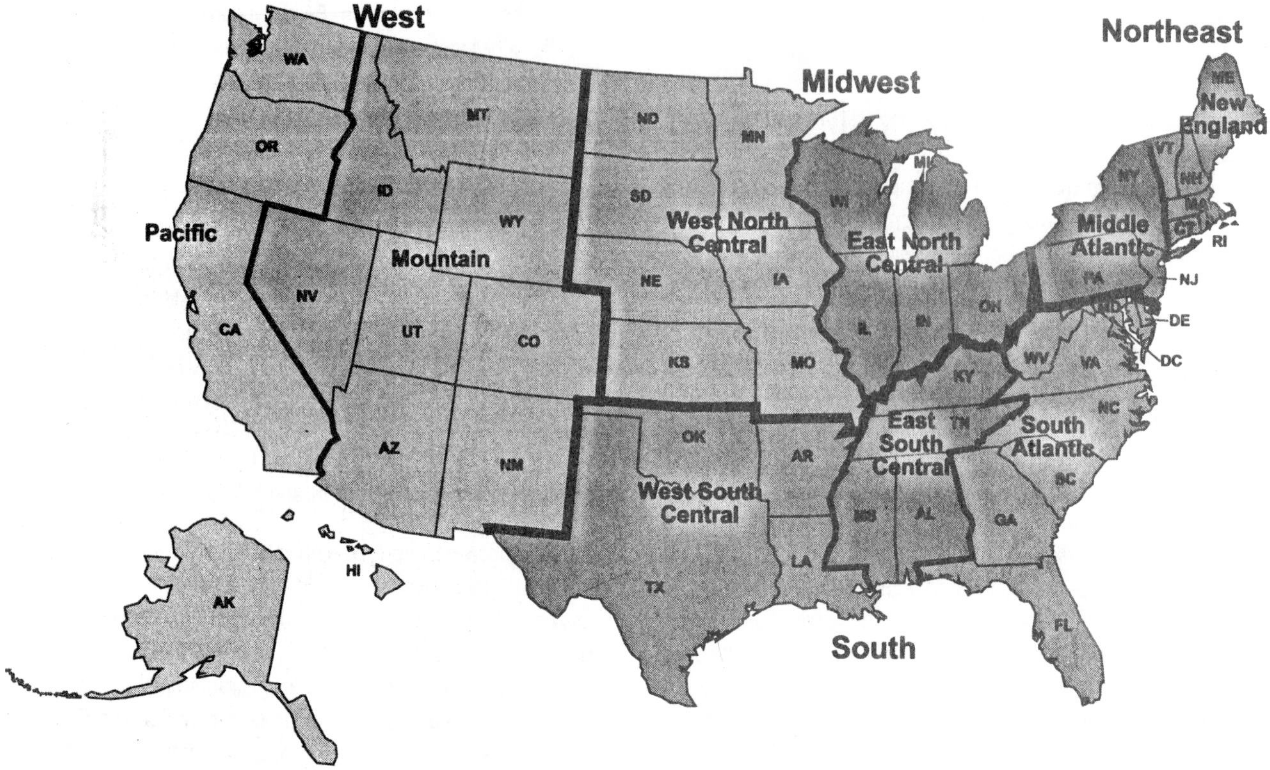

General hospital providing separate psychiatric services—See Mental health organization.

Geographic region and division—The U.S. Census Bureau groups the 50 states and the District of Columbia for statistical purposes into four geographic regions—Northeast, Midwest, South, and West—and nine divisions, based on geographic proximity. See Figure I.

The Department of Commerce's Bureau of Economic Analysis (BEA) groups states into eight regions based on their homogeneity with respect to income characteristics, industrial composition of the employed labor force, and such noneconomic factors as demographic, social, and cultural characteristics. See Figure II.

Three U.S. Census Bureau divisions—West North Central, East North Central, and New England—and three BEA regions—Plains, Great Lakes, and New England—are composed of the same states. The states composing the remaining Census Bureau divisions differ from those composing the corresponding BEA regions.

Gestation—For the National Vital Statistics System and the Centers for Disease Control and Prevention's Abortion Surveillance, the period of gestation is defined as beginning with the first day of the last normal menstrual period and ending with the day of birth or day of termination of pregnancy.

Gross domestic product (GDP)—GDP is the market value of the goods and services produced by labor and property located in the United States. As long as the labor and property are located in the United States, the suppliers (i.e., the workers and, for property, the owners) may be U.S. residents or residents of other countries. See related Consumer Price Index (CPI); Health expenditures, national.

Health care contact—Starting in 1997, the National Health Interview Survey collects information on health care contacts with doctors and other health care professionals using the

Figure II. Bureau of Economic Analysis: Eight Geographic Regions of the United States

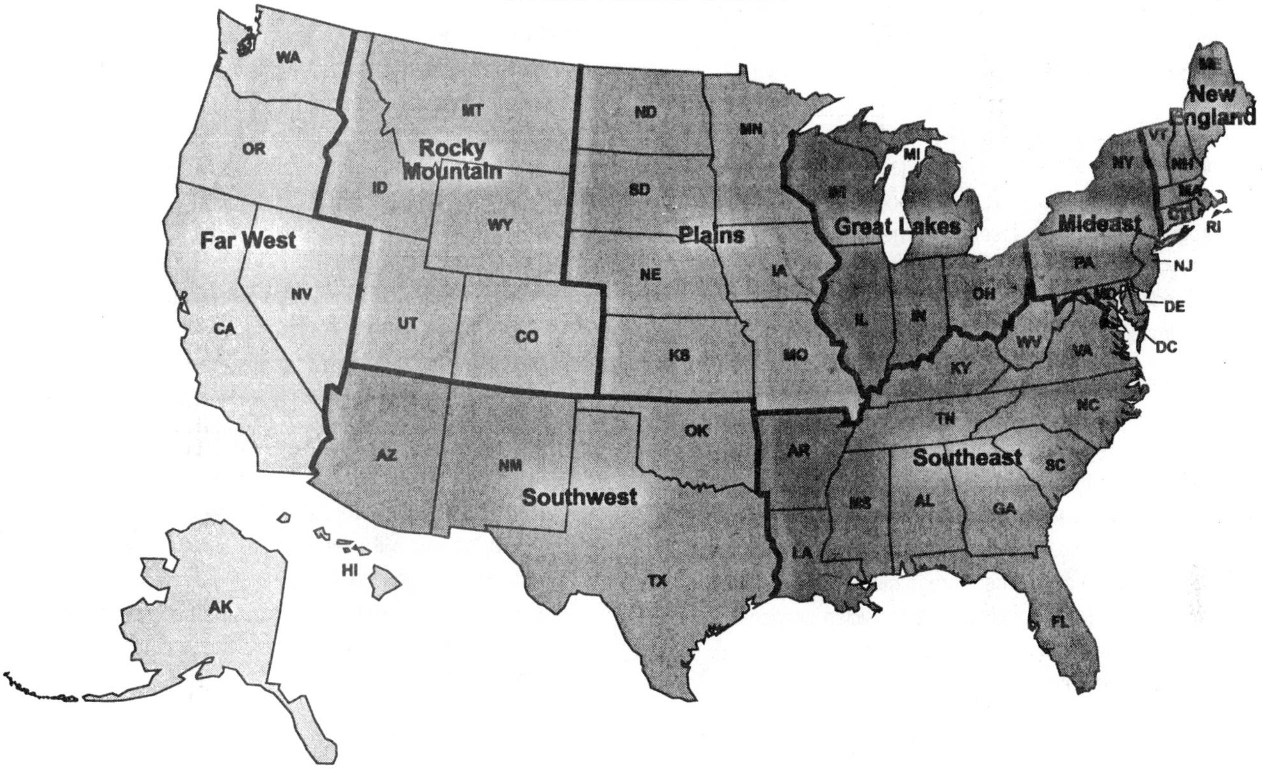

following questions: "During the past 12 months, how many times have you gone to a hospital emergency room about your own health?", "During the past 12 months, did you receive care at home from a nurse or other health care professional? What was the total number of home visits received?", and "During the past 12 months, how many times have you seen a doctor or other health care professional about your own health at a doctor's office, a clinic, or some other place? Do not include times you were hospitalized overnight, visits to hospital emergency rooms, home visits, or telephone calls." Starting with 2000 data, this question was amended to exclude dental visits also. For each question respondents were shown a flashcard with response categories of 0, 1, 2–3, 4–9, 10–12, or 13 or more visits in 1997–1999. Starting with 2000 data, response categories were expanded to 0, 1, 2–3, 4–5, 6–7, 8–9, 10–12, 13–15, or 16 or more. Analyses of the percentage of persons with health care visits were tabulated as follows: For tabulation of the 1997–1999 data, responses of 2–3 were recoded to 2, and responses of 4–9 were recoded to 6. Starting with 2000 data, tabulation of responses of 2–3 were recoded to 2, and other responses were recoded to the midpoint of the range. A summary measure of health care visits was constructed by adding recoded responses for these questions and categorizing the sum as none, 1–3, 4–9, or 10 or more health care visits in the past 12 months.

Analyses of the percentage of children without a health care visit are based upon the following question: "During the past 12 months, how many times has ____ seen a doctor or other health care professional about (his/her) health at a doctor's office, a clinic, or some other place? Do not include times ____ was hospitalized overnight, visits to hospital emergency rooms, home visits, or telephone calls." See related Emergency department or emergency room visit; Home visit.

Health expenditures, national—National Health Expenditures are estimated by the Centers for Medicare & Medicaid Services (CMS) and measure spending for health care in the United States by type of service delivered (e.g., hospital care, physician services, nursing home care) and source of funding for those services (e.g., private health insurance, Medicare, Medicaid, out-of-pocket spending). CMS produces both historical and projected estimates of health expenditures by category. See related Consumer price index (CPI); Gross domestic product (GDP).

Health services and supplies expenditures—These are outlays for goods and services relating directly to patient care plus expenses for administering health insurance programs and government public health activities. This category is equivalent to total national health expenditures minus expenditures for research and construction.

National health expenditures—This measure estimates the amount spent for all health services and supplies and health-related research and construction activities consumed in the United States during the calendar year. Detailed estimates are available by source of expenditures (e.g., out-of-pocket payments, private health insurance, and government programs) and by type of expenditures (e.g., hospital care, physician services, and drugs) and are in current dollars for the year of report. Data are compiled from a variety of sources.

Nursing home expenditures—These cover care rendered in establishments primarily engaged in providing inpatient nursing and rehabilitative services and continuous personal care services to persons requiring nursing care (skilled nursing and intermediate care facilities, including those for the mentally retarded) and continuing care retirement communities with on-site nursing care facilities. The costs of long-term care provided by hospitals are excluded.

Personal health care expenditures—These are outlays for goods and services relating directly to patient care. The expenditures in this category are total national health expenditures minus expenditures for research and construction, health insurance program administration, and government public health activities.

Private expenditures—These are outlays for services provided or paid for by nongovernmental sources—consumers, insurance companies, private industry, and philanthropic and other nonpatient care sources.

Public expenditures—These are outlays for services provided or paid for by federal, state, and local government agencies or expenditures required by governmental mandate (such as worker's compensation insurance payments).

Health insurance coverage—Health insurance is broadly defined to include both public and private payors who cover medical expenditures incurred by a defined population in a variety of settings.

National Health Interview Survey (NHIS)—For point-in-time health insurance estimates, NHIS respondents were asked about their coverage in the previous month in 1993–1996 and at the time of the interview in other years. Questions on health insurance coverage were expanded starting in 1993 compared with previous years. In 1997, the entire questionnaire was redesigned and data were collected using a computer-assisted personal interview (CAPI).

Respondents were considered to be covered by private health insurance if they indicated private health insurance or, prior to 1997, if they were covered by a single-service hospital plan. Private health insurance includes managed care such as health maintenance organizations (HMOs).

Until 1996, persons were defined as having Medicaid or other public assistance coverage if they indicated that they had either Medicaid or other public assistance or if they reported receiving Aid to Families with Dependent Children (AFDC) or Supplemental Security Income (SSI). After welfare reform in late 1996, Medicaid was delinked from AFDC and SSI. Starting in 1997, persons were considered to be covered by Medicaid if they reported Medicaid or a state-sponsored health program. Starting in 1998, persons were considered covered by Medicaid if they reported coverage by the State Children's Health Insurance Program (SCHIP). Medicare or military health plan coverage was also determined in the interview, and starting in 1997 other government-sponsored program coverage was determined as well.

If respondents did not report coverage under one of the above types of plans and they had unknown coverage under either private health insurance or Medicaid, they were considered to have unknown coverage.

The remaining respondents without any indicated coverage were considered uninsured. The uninsured are persons who did not have coverage under private health insurance, Medicare, Medicaid, public assistance, a state-sponsored health plan, other government-sponsored programs, or a military health plan. Persons with only Indian Health Service coverage were considered uninsured. Estimates of the percentage of persons who were uninsured based on the NHIS may differ slightly from those based on the March Current Population Survey (CPS) because of differences in survey questions, recall period, and other aspects of survey methodology.

In the NHIS less than 2% of people age 65 years and over reported no current health insurance coverage, but the small sample size precludes the presentation of separate estimates for this population. Therefore, the term uninsured refers only to the population under age 65.

Two additional questions were added to the health insurance section of the NHIS beginning with the third quarter of 2004 (Table VIII). One question was asked of persons 65 years and over who had not indicated that they had Medicare: "People covered by Medicare have a card which looks like this. [Are/Is] [person] covered by Medicare?" The other question was asked of persons under age 65 who had not indicated any type of coverage: "There is a program called Medicaid that pays for health care for persons in need. In this state it is also called [state name]. [Are/Is] [person] covered by Medicaid?"

Respondents who originally classified themselves as uninsured, but whose classification was changed to Medicare or Medicaid on the basis of a yes response to either question, subsequently received appropriate follow-up questions concerning periods of noncoverage for insured respondents. Of the 892 people (unweighted) who were eligible to receive the Medicare probe question in the third and fourth quarter of 2004, 55.4% indicated that they were covered by Medicare. Of the 9,146 people (unweighted) who were eligible to receive the Medicaid probe question in the third and fourth quarter of 2004, 3.0% indicated that they were covered by Medicaid. Estimates for this report are calculated using the responses to the two additional probe questions. For a complete discussion of the implications of the addition of these two probe questions on the estimates for insurance coverage, see Cohen RA and Martinez ME. Impact of Medicare and Medicaid probe questions on health insurance estimates from the National Health Interview Survey, 2004. Health E-Stat, 2005, available from: www.cdc.gov/nchs/products/pubs/pubd/hestats/impact04/impact04.htm.

Survey respondents may be covered by health insurance at the time of the interview, but may have experienced one or more lapses in coverage during the 12 months prior to the interview. Starting with *Health United States, 2006*, NHIS estimates are presented for the following three exhaustive categories: people with health insurance continuously for the full 12 months prior to the interview, those who had a period of up to 12 months prior to the interview without coverage, and those who were uninsured for more than 12 months prior to interview. This stub variable has been added to selected tables. Two additional NHIS questions were used to determine the appropriate category for the survey respondents: all persons without known comprehensive health insurance plan were asked, "About how long has it been since person last had health care coverage?" and all persons with known health insurance coverage were asked, "In the past 12 months, was there any time when person did NOT have ANY health insurance coverage?"

See related Fee-for-service health insurance; Health maintenance organization (HMO); Managed care; Medicaid; Medicare; State Children's Health Insurance Program (SCHIP); Uninsured.

Health maintenance organization (HMO)—An HMO is a health care system that assumes or shares both the financial risks and the delivery risks associated with providing comprehensive medical services to a voluntarily enrolled population in a particular geographic area, usually in return for a fixed, prepaid fee. Pure HMO enrollees use only the prepaid capitated health services of the HMO panel of medical care providers. Open-ended HMO enrollees use the prepaid HMO health services but, in addition, may receive medical care from providers who are not part of the HMO panel. There is usually a substantial deductible, copayment, or coinsurance associated with use of nonpanel providers.

HMO model types are these:

Group model HMO—A group model HMO is an HMO that contracts with a single multispecialty medical group to provide care to the HMO's membership. The group practice may work exclusively with the HMO, or it may provide services to non-HMO patients as well. The HMO pays the medical group a negotiated per capita rate, which the group distributes among its physicians, usually on a salaried basis.

Staff model HMO —A staff model HMO is a closed-panel HMO (where patients can receive services only through a limited number of providers) in which physicians are HMO employees. The providers see members in the HMO's own facilities.

Network model HMO—A network model HMO is an HMO that contracts with multiple physician groups to provide services to HMO members and may include single or multispecialty groups.

Individual practice association (IPA)—An individual practice association is a healthcare provider organization composed of a group of independent practicing physicians who maintain their own offices and band together for the purpose of contracting their services to HMOs, preferred provider organizations (PPOs), and insurance companies. An IPA may contract with and provide services to both HMO and non-HMO plan participants.

Mixed model HMO—A mixed model HMO combines features of more than one HMO model.

See related Managed care; Preferred provider organization (PPO).

Health services and supplies expenditures—See Health expenditures, national.

Health status, respondent-assessed—Health status was measured in the National Health Interview Survey by asking the family respondent about his or her health or the health of a family member: "Would you say _____'s health is excellent, very good, good, fair, or poor?"

Hispanic origin—Hispanic or Latino origin includes persons of Mexican, Puerto Rican, Cuban, Central and South American, and other or unknown Latin American or Spanish origins. Persons of Hispanic origin may be of any race.

Birth File—The reporting area for an Hispanic-origin item on the birth certificate expanded between 1980 and 1993. Trend data on births of Hispanic and non-Hispanic parentage in this report are affected by expansion of the reporting area and by immigration. These two factors affect numbers of events, composition of the Hispanic population, and maternal and infant health characteristics.

In 1980 and 1981, information on births of Hispanic parentage was reported on the birth certificate by the following 22 states: Arizona, Arkansas, California, Colorado, Florida, Georgia, Hawaii, Illinois, Indiana, Kansas, Maine, Mississippi, Nebraska, Nevada, New Jersey, New Mexico, New York, North Dakota, Ohio, Texas, Utah, and Wyoming. In 1982 Tennessee, and in 1983 the District of Columbia, began reporting this information. Between 1983 and 1987, information on births of Hispanic parentage was available for 23 states and the District of Columbia (D.C.). In 1988, this information became available for Alabama, Connecticut, Kentucky, Massachusetts, Montana, North Carolina, and Washington, increasing the number of states reporting information on births of Hispanic parentage to 30 states and D.C. In 1989, this information became available from an additional 17 states, increasing the number of Hispanic-reporting states to 47 and D.C. In 1989, only Louisiana, New Hampshire, and Oklahoma did not report Hispanic parentage on the birth certificate. With the inclusion of Oklahoma in 1989 and Louisiana in 1990 as Hispanic-reporting states, 99% of birth records included information on mother's origin. Hispanic origin of the mother was reported on the birth certificates of 49 states and D.C. in 1991 and 1992; only New Hampshire did not provide this information. Starting in 1993, Hispanic origin of mother was reported by all 50 states and D.C.

Mortality File—The reporting area for an Hispanic-origin item on the death certificate expanded between 1985 and 1997. In 1985, mortality data by Hispanic origin of decedent were based on deaths to residents of the following 17 states and the District of Columbia (D.C.) whose data on the death certificate were at least 90% complete on a place-of-occurrence basis and of comparable format: Arizona, Arkansas, California, Colorado, Georgia, Hawaii, Illinois, Indiana, Kansas, Mississippi, Nebraska, New York, North Dakota, Ohio, Texas, Utah, and Wyoming. In 1986 New Jersey began reporting Hispanic origin of decedent, increasing the number of reporting states to 18 and D.C. in 1986 and 1987. In 1988, Alabama, Kentucky, Maine, Montana, North Carolina, Oregon, Rhode Island, and Washington were added to the reporting area, increasing the number of states to 26 and D.C. In 1989, an additional 18 states were added, increasing the Hispanic reporting area to 44 states and D.C.; only Connecticut, Louisiana, Maryland, New Hampshire, Oklahoma, and Virginia were not included in the reporting area. Starting with 1990 data in this book, the criterion was changed to include states whose data were at least 80% complete. In 1990, Maryland, Virginia, and Connecticut, in 1991 Louisiana, and in 1993 New Hampshire were added, increasing the reporting area for Hispanic origin of decedent to 47 states and D.C. in 1990, 48 states and D.C. in 1991 and 1992, and 49 states and D.C. in 1993–1996. Only Oklahoma did not provide this information in 1993–1996. Starting in 1997, Hispanic origin of decedent was reported by all 50 states and D.C. Based on data from the U.S. Census Bureau, the 1990 reporting area encompassed 99.6% of the U.S. Hispanic population. In 1990, more than 96% of death records included information on Hispanic origin of decedent.

Starting with 2003 data, some states reported multiple-race data. The multiple-race data for these states were bridged to the single-race categories of the 1977 Office of Management and Budget standards for comparability with other states. In 2003, California, Hawaii, Idaho, Maine, Montana, New York, and Wisconsin reported multiple-race data. In 2004, fifteen states reported multiple-race data. In addition to the seven listed above, Michigan, Minnesota, New Hampshire, New Jersey, Oklahoma, South Dakota, Washington, and Wyoming reported multiple-race data.

National Health Interview Survey (NHIS) and *National Health and Nutrition Examination Survey (NHANES)*—Questions on Hispanic origin are self-reported in the NHANES III and subsequent years and all years of the NHIS and precede questions on race. The NHANES sample was designed to provide estimates specifically for persons of Mexican origin and not for all Hispanic-origin persons in the United States. Persons of Hispanic origin other than Mexicans were entered into the sample with different selection probabilities that are not nationally representative of the total U.S. Hispanic population.

Surveillance, Epidemiology, and End Results (SEER) Program—Data are available from the National Institutes of Health, National Cancer Institute. SEER Hispanic data used in *Health, United States* tables exclude data from Alaska. The North American Association of Central Cancer Registries, Inc. (NAACCR) Hispanic Identification Algorithm was used on a combination of variables to classify incidence cases as Hispanic for analytic purposes. See the report, NAACCR Guideline for Enhancing Hispanic-Latino Identification. Available from: seer.cancer.gov/seerstat/variables/seer/yr1973_2004/race_ethnicity/.

Youth Risk Behavior Survey (YRBS)—Prior to 1999, a single question was asked about race and Hispanic origin with the option of selecting one of the following categories: white (not Hispanic), black (not Hispanic), Hispanic or Latino, Asian or Other Pacific Islander, American Indian or Alaska Native, or other. Between 1999 and 2003, respondents were asked a single question about race and Hispanic origin with the option of choosing one or more of the following categories: White, Black or African American, Hispanic or Latino, Asian, Native Hawaiian or Other Pacific Islander, or American Indian or Alaska Native. In 2005, respondents were asked a question about Hispanic origin (Are you Hispanic or Latino?) and a second separate question about race that included the option of selecting one or more of the following categories: American Indian or Alaska Native, Asian, Black or African American, Native Hawaiian or Other Pacific Islander, or White. Because of the differences between questions, the data about race and Hispanic ethnicity for the years prior to 1999 are not strictly comparable with estimates for the later years. However, analyses of data collected between 1991 and 2003 have indicated that the data are comparable across years and can be used to study trends. See related Race.

See Brender ND, Kann L, McManus, T. A comparison of two survey questions on race and ethnicity among high school students. Public opinion quarterly 2003;67(2):227–36.

HIV—See Human immunodeficiency virus (HIV) disease.

Home visit—Starting in 1997, the National Health Interview Survey has been collecting information on home visits received during the past 12 months. Respondents are asked "During the past 12 months, did you receive care at home from a nurse or other health care professional? What was the total number of home visits received?" These data are combined with data on visits to doctors' offices, clinics, and emergency departments to provide a summary measure of health care visits. See related Emergency department or emergency room visit; Health care contact.

Hospital—According to the American Hospital Association, hospitals are licensed institutions with at least six beds whose primary function is to provide diagnostic and therapeutic patient services for medical conditions by an organized physician staff and that have continuous nursing services under the supervision of registered nurses. The World Health Organization considers an establishment to be a hospital if it is permanently staffed by at least one physician, can offer inpatient accommodation, and can provide active medical and nursing care. Hospitals may be classified by type of service, ownership, size in terms of number of beds, and length of stay. In the National Hospital Ambulatory Medical Care Survey, hospitals include all those with an average length of stay for all patients of less than 30 days (short-stay) or hospitals whose specialty is general (medical or surgical) or children's general. Federal hospitals and hospital units of institutions and hospitals with fewer than six beds staffed for patient use are excluded. See related Average length of stay; Bed, health facility; Days of care; Emergency department; Inpatient; Outpatient department.

Community hospital—Community hospitals based on the American Hospital Association definition include all nonfederal short-term general and special hospitals whose facilities and services are available to the public. Special hospitals include obstetrics and gynecology; eye, ear, nose, and throat; rehabilitation; orthopedic; and other specialty services. Short-term general and special childrens hospitals are also considered to be community hospitals. A hospital may include a nursing-home-type unit and still be classified as short-term, provided that the majority of its patients are admitted to units where the average length of stay is less than 30 days. Hospital units of institutions such as prisons and college infirmaries that are not open to the public and are contained within a nonhospital facility are not included in the category of community hospitals. Traditionally the definition included all nonfederal short-stay hospitals except facilities for the mentally retarded. In a revised definition, the following additional sites were excluded: hospital units of institutions, and alcoholism and chemical dependency facilities.

Federal hospital—Federal hospitals are operated by the federal government.

For-profit hospital—For-profit hospitals are operated for profit by individuals, partnerships, or corporations.

General hospital—General hospitals provide diagnostic, treatment, and surgical services for patients with a variety of medical conditions. According to the World Health Organization, these hospitals provide medical and nursing care for more than one category of medical discipline (e.g., general medicine, specialized medicine, general surgery, specialized surgery, and obstetrics). Excluded are hospitals, usually in rural areas, that provide a more limited range of care.

Nonprofit hospital—Nonprofit hospitals are controlled by nonprofit organizations, including religious organizations, fraternal societies, and others.

Psychiatric hospital—Psychiatric hospitals are ones whose major type of service is psychiatric care. See related Mental health organization.

Registered hospital—Registered hospitals are registered with the American Hospital Association. About 98% of hospitals are registered.

Short-stay hospital—Short-stay hospitals in the National Hospital Discharge Survey are those in which the average length of stay is less than 30 days. The National Health Interview Survey defines short-stay hospitals as any hospital or hospital department in which the type of service provided is general; maternity; eye, ear, nose, and throat; children's; or osteopathic.

Specialty hospital—Specialty hospitals such as psychiatric, tuberculosis, chronic disease, rehabilitation, maternity, and alcoholic or narcotic, provide a particular type of service to the majority of their patients.

Hospital-based physician—See Physician.

Hospital day—See Days of care.

Hospital utilization—Estimates of hospital utilization (such as hospital discharge rate, days of care rate, average length of stay, and percentage of the population with a hospitalization) presented in *Health, United States* are based on data from ree different sources—the National Health Interview Survey HIS), the National Hospital Discharge Survey (NHDS), and e American Hospital Association. NHIS data are based on usehold interviews of the civilian noninstitutionalized pulation and thus exclude hospitalizations for stitutionalized persons and those who died while spitalized. NHDS data are based on hospital discharge cords of all persons who have an inpatient stay in a nfederal short-stay hospital. NHDS includes hospital scharge records for all persons discharged alive or eceased and institutionalized persons. NHDS tables shown *Health, United States* exclude data for newborn infants. stimates for average length of stay between the NHDS and e AHA presented in *Health, United States* differ because of ifferent methods for counting days of care. See related verage length of stay; Days of care; Discharge; Appendix I, ational Health Interview Survey, National Hospital Discharge urvey.

uman immunodeficiency virus (HIV) disease—HIV isease is a serious disease caused by a cytopathic etrovirus that is the cause of Acquired Immunodeficiency yndrome (AIDS). It is also called AIDS-related virus, human -cell leukemia virus type III, human T-cell lymphotrophic virus ype III, and lymphadenopathy-associated virus. Mortality and orbidity coding for HIV disease are similar and have volved over time.

Mortality coding—Starting with 1999 data, and the introduction of the Tenth Revision of the *International Classification of Diseases* (ICD–10), the title for this cause of death was changed to HIV disease from HIV infection and the ICD codes changed to B20–B24. Starting with 1987 data, NCHS introduced category numbers *042–*044 for classifying and coding HIV infection as a cause of death in ICD–9. The asterisk before the category numbers indicates that these codes were not part of the original ICD–9. HIV infection was formerly referred to as human T-cell lymphotropic virus-III/lymphadenopathy-associated virus (HTLV-III/LAV) infection. Before 1987, deaths involving HIV infection were classified to Deficiency of cell-mediated immunity (ICD–9 279.1) contained in the title All other diseases; to Pneumocystosis (ICD–9 136.3) contained in the title All other infectious and parasitic diseases; to Malignant neoplasms, including neoplasms of lymphatic and hematopoietic tissues; and to a number of other causes. Therefore, before 1987, death statistics for HIV infection are not strictly comparable with data for 1987 and later years and are not shown in this report.

Morbidity coding—The National Hospital Discharge Survey codes diagnosis data using the *International Classification of Diseases, Ninth Revision, Clinical Modification* (ICD–9–CM). During 1984 and 1985 only data for AIDS (ICD–9–CM 279.19) were included. In 1986–1994, discharges with the following diagnoses were included: Acquired immunodeficiency syndrome (AIDS), Human immunodeficiency virus (HIV) infection and associated conditions, and Positive serological or viral culture findings for HIV (ICD–9–CM 042–044, 279.19, and 795.8). Beginning in 1995, discharges with the following diagnoses were included: Human immunodeficiency virus (HIV) disease and Asymptomatic human immunodeficiency virus (HIV) infection status (ICD–9–CM 042 and V08).

See related Acquired immunodeficiency syndrome (AIDS); Cause of death; *International Classification of Diseases* (ICD); *International Classification of Diseases, Ninth Revision, Clinical Modification* (ICD–9–CM).

Hypertension—See Blood pressure, elevated.

ICD; ICD codes—See Cause of death; *International Classification of Diseases (ICD).*

Illicit drug use—Illicit drug use refers to use and misuse of illegal and controlled drugs.

Monitoring the Future Study—In this school-based survey of secondary school students, information on marijuana use is collected using self-completed questionnaires. The information is based on the following questions: "On how many occasions (if any) have you used marijuana in the last 30 days?" and "On how many occasions (if any) have you used hashish in the last 30 days?" Questions on cocaine use include the following: "On how many occasions (if any) have you taken crack (cocaine in chunk or rock form) during the last 30 days?" and "On how many occasions (if any) have you taken cocaine in any other form during the last 30 days?"

National Survey on Drug Use & Health (NSDUH)—Information on illicit drug use is collected for survey participants 12 years of age and over. Information on any illicit drug use, including marijuana or hashish, cocaine, heroin, hallucinogens, and nonmedical use of prescription drugs is based on the following question: "During the past 30 days, on how many days did you use (specific illicit drug)?" See related Substance use.

Incidence—Incidence is the number of cases of disease having their onset during a prescribed period of time. It is often expressed as a rate (e.g., the incidence of measles per 1,000 children 5–15 years of age during a specified year). Incidence is a measure of morbidity or other events that occur within a specified period of time. Measuring incidence may be complicated because the population at risk for the disease may change during the period of interest, for example, due to births, deaths, or migration. In addition, determining that a case is new—that is, that its onset occurred during the prescribed period of time—may be difficult. Because of these difficulties in measuring incidence, many health statistics are measured using prevalence. See related Prevalence.

Income—See Family income.

Individual practice association (IPA)—See Health maintenance organization (HMO).

Industry of employment—Starting with 2003 data, industries are classified according to the 2002 North American Industry Classification System (NAICS) for the presentation of health data in *Health, United States*. The NAICS classification system groups establishments into industries based on their production or supply function—establishments using similar raw material inputs, capital equipment, and labor are classified in the same industry. This approach creates homogeneous categories well suited for economic analysis. NAICS uses a six-digit hierarchical coding system to classify all economic activity into 20 industry sectors. The first two digits of the six-digit code designate the highest level of aggregation, with 20 such two-digit industry sectors (Table IX). Five sectors are primarily goods-producing sectors, and 15 are entirely services-providing sectors. NAICS allows for the classification of 1,170 industries.

NAICS replaces the Standard Industrial Classification (SIC) system, originally designed in the 1930s and revised and updated periodically to reflect changes in the U.S. economy. The last SIC revision was in 1987. The SIC system focused on the manufacturing sector of the economy and provided significantly less detail for the now dominant service sector, including newly developed industries in information services, health care delivery, and high-tech manufacturing. Although some titles in SIC and NAICS are similar, there is little comparability between the two systems because industry groupings are defined differently. Estimates of deaths, injuries, and illnesses classified by NAICS industry should not be compared with earlier estimates that used the SIC.

Starting with *Health United States, 2005*, health data by industry from the Bureau of Labor Statistics' Census of Fatal Occupational Injuries (CFOI) and Survey of Occupational Injuries and Illnesses (SOII) data systems are classified using the NAICS system and replace trends in occupational health data based on the SIC system in previous editions of *Health, United States*.

Infant death—An infant death is the death of a live-born child before his or her first birthday. Age at death may be further classified according to neonatal and postneonatal. Neonatal deaths are those that occur before the 28th day of life; postneonatal deaths are those that occur between 28 and 365 days of age. See related Rate: Death and related rates.

Injury—The International Classification of External Causes of Injuries (ICECI) Coordination and Maintenance Group defines injury as a (suspected) bodily lesion resulting from acute overexposure to energy (this can be mechanical, thermal, electrical, chemical, or radiant) interacting with the body in amounts or rates that exceed the threshold of physiological tolerance. In some cases an injury results from an insufficiency of any of the vital elements. Acute poisonings and toxic effects, including overdoses of substances and wrong substances given or taken in error are included, as are adverse effects and complications of therapeutic, surgical, and medical care. Psychological harm is excluded. Injuries can be intentional or unintentional (i.e., accidental). External causes of nonfatal injuries in NCHS data systems are coded to the *International Classification of Diseases, Ninth Revision, Clinical Modification* Supplementary Classification of External Causes of Injury and Poisoning, often referred to as E codes. See Table VII for a list of external causes of injury categories and E codes used in *Health, United States*. See related Diagnosis; Injury-related visit. See ICECI Coordination and Maintenance Group (2004). International Classification of External Causes of Injuries (ICECI), version 1.2. Consumer Safety Institute, Amsterdam and AIHW National Injury Surveillance Unit, Adelaide. Available from: www.iceci.org.

able VII. Codes for first-listed external causes of injury om the *International Classification of Diseases, Ninth evision, Clinical Modification*

External cause of injury category	*E-Code numbers*
nintentional	E800–E869, E880–E929
Motor vehicle traffic	E810–E819
Falls	E880–E886, E888
Struck by or against objects or persons	E916–E917
Caused by cutting and piercing instruments or objects	E920
ntentional (suicide and homicide) . . .	E950–E969

njury-related visit—In the National Hospital Ambulatory ledical Care Survey an emergency department visit was onsidered injury-related if, on the patient record form (PRF), he checkbox for injury was indicated. In addition, injury visits vere identified if the physician's diagnosis was injury-related ICD–9–CM code of 800–999), an external cause-of-injury ode was present (ICD–9–CM E800–E999), or the patient's eason for visit code was injury-related. See related Emergency department or emergency room visit; External cause of injury; Injury.

Inpatient—An inpatient is a person who is formally admitted to the inpatient service of a hospital for observation, care, diagnosis, or treatment. See related Admission; Average length of stay; Days of care; Discharge; Hospital.

Inpatient care—See Hospital utilization; Mental health service type.

Inpatient day—See Days of care.

Instrumental activities of daily living (IADL)—Instrumental activities of daily living are activities related to independent living and include preparing meals, managing money, shopping for groceries or personal items, performing light or heavy housework, and using a telephone. In the National Health Interview Survey (NHIS) respondents are asked whether they or family members 18 years of age and over need the help of another person for handling routine IADL needs because of a physical, mental, or emotional problem. Persons are considered to have an IADL limitation in the NHIS if any causal condition is chronic.

In the Medicare Current Beneficiary Survey, if a sample person had any difficulty performing an activity by him- or herself and without special equipment, or did not perform the activity at all because of health problems, the person was categorized as having a limitation in that activity. The limitation may have been temporary or chronic at the time of the interview. Sample persons in the community answered health status and functioning questions themselves, if able to do so. For sample persons in a long-term care facility, a proxy such as a nurse answered questions about the sample person's health status and functioning. See related Activities of daily living (ADL); Limitation of activity.

Insurance—See Health insurance coverage.

Intermediate care facility—See Nursing home.

International Classification of Diseases (ICD)—The ICD is used to code and classify cause-of-death data. The ICD is developed collaboratively by the World Health Organization (WHO) and 10 international centers, one of which is housed at NCHS. The purpose of the ICD is to promote international comparability in the collection, classification, processing, and presentation of health statistics. Since 1900, the ICD has been modified about once every 10 years, except for the 20-year interval between ICD–9 and ICD–10 (see Table IV). The purpose of the revisions is to stay abreast with advances in medical science. New revisions usually introduce major disruptions in time series of mortality statistics (see Tables V and VI). For more information, see the NCHS website. Available from: www.cdc.gov/nchs/about/major/dvs/icd10des.htm. See related Cause of death; Comparability ratio; *International Classification of Diseases, Ninth Revision, Clinical Modification* (ICD–9–CM).

***International Classification of Diseases, Ninth Revision, Clinical Modification* (ICD–9–CM)**—The ICD–9–CM is based on and is compatible with the World Health Organization's *International Classification of Diseases, Ninth Revision* (ICD–9). The United States currently uses ICD–9–CM to code morbidity diagnoses and inpatient procedures. ICD–9–CM consists of three volumes. Volumes 1 and 2 contain the diagnosis tabular list and index. Volume 3 contains the procedure classification (tabular and index combined).

ICD–9–CM is divided into 17 chapters and two supplemental classifications. The chapters are arranged primarily by body system. In addition, there are chapters for Infectious and parasitic diseases; Neoplasms; Endocrine, nutritional, and metabolic diseases; Mental disorders; Complications of

Table VIII. Percentage of persons under 65 years of age with Medicaid or who are uninsured, by selected demographic characteristics using Method 1 and Method 2 estimation procedures: United States, 2004

Characteristic	*Medicaid*[1]		*Uninsured*[2]	
	Method 2[3]	*Method 1*[3]	*Method 2*[3]	*Method 1*[3]
	Percent (standard error)			
Age				
Under 65 years	12.0 (0.24)	11.8 (0.24)	16.4 (0.23)	16.6 (0.23)
Under 18 years	25.4 (0.49)	24.9 (0.49)	9.2 (0.30)	9.7 (0.29)
18–64 years	6.6 (0.17)	6.5 (0.17)	19.3 (0.26)	19.4 (0.26)
Percent of poverty level[4]				
Below 100%	47.5 (1.03)	46.6 (1.03)	29.6 (0.89)	30.5 (0.92)
100%–less than 200%	22.0 (0.59)	21.5 (0.60)	28.9 (0.66)	29.4 (0.66)
200% or more	2.9 (0.13)	2.8 (0.13)	9.4 (0.23)	9.5 (0.23)
Age and percent of poverty level[4]				
Under 18 years				
Below 100%	71.9 (1.35)	70.2 (1.35)	14.5 (1.15)	16.2 (1.22)
100%–less than 200%	39.2 (1.13)	38.4 (1.14)	15.0 (0.81)	15.8 (0.82)
200% or more	6.2 (0.33)	6.1 (0.33)	4.9 (0.30)	4.9 (0.30)
18–64 years				
Below 100%	31.2 (1.02)	30.8 (1.02)	39.7 (1.09)	40.1 (1.09)
100%–less than 200%	12.0 (0.48)	11.8 (0.48)	37.0 (0.72)	37.2 (0.72)
200% or more	1.7 (0.11)	1.7 (0.10)	11.0 (0.26)	11.1 (0.26)
Hispanic origin and race[5]				
Hispanic or Latino	22.2 (0.55)	21.5 (0.55)	34.4 (0.64)	35.1 (0.65)
Mexican	22.0 (0.63)	21.5 (0.63)	37.6 (0.82)	38.1 (0.83)
Not Hispanic or Latino	10.2 (0.25)	10.1 (0.25)	13.2 (0.23)	13.3 (0.23)
White only	7.4 (0.26)	7.4 (0.26)	12.0 (0.25)	12.1 (0.25)
Black or African American only	23.9 (0.80)	23.5 (0.79)	17.3 (0.58)	17.8 (0.58)

[1]The category Medicaid includes persons who do not have private coverage, but who have Medicaid or other state-sponsored health plans, including the State Children's Health Insurance Program (SCHIP).

[2]The category Uninsured includes persons who have not indicated that they are covered at the time of interview under private health insurance, Medicare, Medicaid, SCHIP, a state-sponsored health plan, other government programs, or military health plan (includes VA, TRICARE, and CHAMP-VA). This category includes persons who are only covered by Indian Health Service (IHS) or only have a plan that pays for one type of service, such as accidents or dental care.

[3]Starting with the third quarter of 2004, two additional questions were added to the NHIS insurance section to reduce potential errors in reporting of Medicare and Medicaid status. Persons 65 years of age and over not reporting Medicare coverage were asked explicitly about Medicare coverage, and persons under 65 years of age with no reported coverage were asked explicitly about Medicaid coverage. Estimates calculated without using the additional information from these questions are noted as Method 1. Estimates calculated using the additional information from these questions are noted as Method 2.

[4]Percent of poverty level is based on family income and family size and composition using the U.S. Census Bureau's poverty thresholds. The percentage of respondents with unknown poverty level was 28.2% in 2004. See the NHIS Survey Description Document for 2004. Available from: www.cdc.gov/nchs/nhis.htm.

[5]Persons of Hispanic origin may be of any race or combination of races. Similarly, the category Not Hispanic or Latino refers to all persons who are not of Hispanic or Latino origin, regardless of race.

SOURCE: Family Core component of the 2004 National Health Interview Survey. Data are based on household interviews of a sample of the civilian noninstitutionalized population. Available from: www.cdc.gov/nchs/products/pubs/pubd/hestats/impact.htm.

pregnancy, childbirth, and puerperium; Certain conditions originating in the perinatal period; Congenital anomalies; and Symptoms, signs, and ill-defined conditions. The two supplemental classifications are for factors influencing health status and contact with health services (V codes), and external causes of injury and poisoning (E codes).

In *Health, United States*, morbidity data are classified using ICD–9–CM. Diagnostic categories and codes for ICD–9–CM are shown in Table X; ICD–9–CM procedure categories and codes are shown in Table XI. For additional information about ICD–9–CM, see the NCHS website. Available from: www.cdc.gov/nchs/icd9.htm. See related *International Classification of Diseases (ICD)*.

Table IX. Codes for industries, by the 2002 North American Industry Classification System (NAICS)

Private industry	*Code numbers*
Agriculture, forestry, fishing and hunting	11
Mining	21
Utilities	22
Construction	23
Manufacturing	31–33
Wholesale trade	42
Retail trade	44–45
Transportation and warehousing	48–49
Information	51
Finance and insurance	52
Real estate and rental and leasing	53
Professional, scientific, and technical services	54
Management of companies and enterprises	55
Administrative and support and waste management services	56
Education services	61
Health and social assistance	62
Arts, entertainment, and recreation	71
Accommodation and food services	72
Other services, except public administration	81

SOURCE: Bureau of Labor Statistics. Available from: www.bls.gov/bls/naics_aggregation.htm.

Late fetal death rate—See Rate: Death and related rates.

Leading causes of death—See Cause-of-death ranking.

Length of stay—See Average length of stay.

Life expectancy—Life expectancy is the average number of years of life remaining to a person at a particular age and is based on a given set of age-specific death rates, generally the mortality conditions existing in the period mentioned. Life expectancy may be determined by race, sex, or other characteristics using age-specific death rates for the population with that characteristic. See related Rate: Death and related rates.

Limitation of activity—Limitation of activity may be defined different ways, depending on the conceptual framework. In the National Health Interview Survey, limitation of activity refers to a long-term reduction in a person's capacity to perform the usual kind or amount of activities associated with his or her age group as a result of a chronic condition. Limitation of activity is assessed by asking persons a series of questions about limitations in their or household members' ability to perform activities usual for their age group because of a physical, mental, or emotional problem. Persons are asked about limitations in activities of daily living, instrumental activities of daily living, play, school, work, difficulty walking or remembering, and any other activity limitations. For reported limitations, the causal health conditions are determined, and persons are considered limited if one or more of these conditions is chronic. Children under 18 years of age who receive special education or early intervention services are considered to have a limitation of activity. See related Activities of daily living; Condition; Instrumental activities of daily living.

Long-term care facility—A long-term care facility is a residence that provides a specific level of personal or medical care or supervision to residents. In the Medicare Current Beneficiary Survey, a residence is considered a long-term care facility if it has three or more long-term care beds and provides personal care services to residents, continuous supervision of residents, or long-term care services throughout the facility or in a separately identifiable unit. Types of long-term care facilities include licensed nursing homes, skilled nursing homes, intermediate care facilities, retirement homes (that provide services), domiciliary or personal care facilities, distinct long-term care units in a hospital complex, mental health facilities and centers, assisted and foster care homes, and institutions for the mentally retarded and developmentally disabled. See related Nursing home.

Low birthweight—See Birthweight.

Magnetic resonance imaging (MRI) unit—MRI is an imaging technique designed to visualize internal structures of the body using magnetic and electromagnetic fields which induce a resonance effect of hydrogen atoms. The electromagnetic emission created by these atoms is registered and processed by a dedicated computer to produce the images of the body structures.

Mammography—A mammogram is an x-ray image of the breast used to detect irregularities in breast tissue. In the National Health Interview Survey, questions concerning use of mammography were asked on an intermittent schedule, and question content differed across years. In 1987 and 1990, women were asked to report when they had their last mammogram. In 1991, women were asked whether they had a mammogram in the past 2 years. In 1993 and 1994, women were asked whether they had a mammogram within

Table X. Codes for diagnostic categories from the *International Classification of Diseases, Ninth Revision, Clinical Modification*

Diagnostic category	*Code numbers*
Females with delivery	V27
Human immunodeficiency virus (HIV) (1984–1985)	279.19
(1986–1994)	042–044, 279.19, 795.8
(Starting in 1995)	042, V08
Malignant neoplasms	140–208
Large intestine and rectum	153–154, 197.5
Trachea, bronchus, and lung	162, 176.4, 197.0, 197.3
Breast	174–175, 198.81
Prostate	185
Diabetes	250
Alcohol and drug	291–292, 303–305
Serious mental illness	295–298
Diseases of heart	391–392.0, 393–398, 402, 404, 410–416, 420–429
Ischemic heart disease	410–414
Acute myocardial infarction	410
Heart failure	428
Cerebrovascular disease	430–438
Pneumonia	480–486
Asthma	493
Hyperplasia of prostate	600
Osteoarthritis	715, 721
Intervertebral disc disorders	722
Injuries and poisoning	800–999
Fracture, all sites	800–829
Fracture of neck of femur (hip)	820

the past year, between 1 and 2 years ago, or over 2 years ago. In 1998, women were asked whether they had a mammogram a year ago or less, more than 1 year but not more than 2 years, or more than 2 years ago. In 1999, women were asked when they had their most recent mammogram in days, weeks, months, or years. In 1999, 10% of women in the sample responded 2 years ago, and in this analysis these women were coded as within the past 2 years although a response of 2 years ago may include women whose last mammogram was more than 2 but less than 3 years ago. Thus, estimates for 1999 are overestimated to some degree in comparison with estimates in previous years. In 2000 and 2003, women were asked when they had their most recent mammogram (give month and year). Women who did not respond were given a follow-up question that used the 1999 wording, and women who did not answer the question with the 1999 wording were asked a second follow-up question that used the 1998 wording. In 2000 and 2003, 2% of women in the sample answered 2 years ago using the 1999 wording, and they were coded as within the past 2 years. Thus, estimates for 2000 and 2003 may be slightly overestimated in comparison with estimates for years prior to 1999. In 2005, women were asked the same series of mammography questions as in the 2000 and 2003 surveys but the skip pattern was modified so that more women were asked the follow-up question using the 1998 wording. Because additional information was available for women who replied their last mammogram was 2 years ago, these women were not uniformly coded as having had a mammogram within the past 2 years. Thus, estimates for 2005 are more precise compared with estimates for 1999, 2000, and 2003 and are slightly lower than they would have been without this additional information.

Managed care—Managed care is a term originally used to refer to the prepaid health care sector (health maintenance organizations or HMOs) where care is provided under a fixed budget and costs are therein capable of being managed. Increasingly, the term is being used to include preferred provider organizations (PPOs) and even forms of indemnity insurance coverage (or fee-for-service insurance) that incorporate preadmission certification and other utilization controls.

Medicare managed care, begun in 1985, has included a combination of risk-based and cost-based plans. Risk-based plans receive a fixed pre-payment per beneficiary per month to cover the cost of all services that a beneficiary would receive. The Centers for Medicare & Medicaid Services (CMS) sets the per-member-per-month rate to reimburse risk-based plans based on the fee-for-service equivalent cost adjusted for certain demographic factors. Cost-based plans are offered by a Health Maintenance Organization (HMO) or a Competitive Medical Plan (CMP) and receive payment on a fee-for-service basis, similar to the traditional Medicare plan. While the payment system under cost-based plans is similar to the traditional Medicare plan, the cost-based plans generally cover more preventative services than the traditional Medicare plan. For current definitions of the various Medicare managed care plans, refer to the Medicare Managed Care Manual, (100–16) Chapter 1, Section 30—Types of MA Plans. Available from: www.resdac.umn.edu/Tools/TBs/TN-009.asp. Medicare enrollees have the choice to enroll in a managed care program (if available) or receive services on a fee-for-service basis.

The two major Medicaid managed care categories are risk-based plans and primary care case management (PCCM) arrangements. In risk-based plans, managed care organizations (MCO) are paid a fixed monthly fee per enrollee. The MCOs assume some or all of the financial risk for providing care. PCCM providers are usually physicians, physician group practices, or entities employing or having other arrangements with such physicians, but sometimes also including nurse practitioners, nurse midwives, or physician assistants. These PCCM providers, sometimes called gatekeepers, contract directly with the state to locate, coordinate, and monitor covered primary care (and sometimes additional services). PCCM providers are paid a per-patient case management fee and usually do not assume financial risk for the provision of services. Some states allow Medicaid enrollees to voluntarily enroll in managed care plans; other states require that certain categories of Medicaid beneficiaries join managed care plans. Within both risked-based plans and PCCM arrangements there are plans that provide specialized services to certain categories of Medicaid beneficiaries. For more information on state Medicaid managed care plans, see www.cms.hhs.gov/home/medicaid.asp.

See related Health maintenance organization (HMO); Medicare; Medicaid; Preferred provider organization (PPO).

Marital status—Marital status is classified through self-reporting into the categories married and unmarried. The term married encompasses all married people including those separated from their spouses. Unmarried includes those who are single (never married), divorced, or widowed. Prior to 1978, the Center for Disease Control and Prevention's Abortion Surveillance Program classified separated people as unmarried.

Birth File—In 1970, 39 states and the District of Columbia (D.C.) and in 1975, 38 states and D.C. included a direct question about mother's marital status on the birth certificate. Since 1980, national estimates of births to unmarried women have been based on two methods for determining marital status, a direct question in the birth registration process and inferential procedures. In 1980–1996, marital status was reported on the birth certificates of 41–45 states and D.C.; with the addition of California in 1997, 46 states and D.C.; and in 1998–2001, 48 states and D.C. In 1997, all but four states (Connecticut, Michigan, Nevada, and New York), and in 1998, all but two states (Michigan and New York) included a direct question about mother's marital status on their birth certificates. In 1998–2004, marital status was imputed as married on those 0.03–0.05% of birth records with missing information in the 48 states and D.C. where this information was obtained by a direct question.

For states lacking a direct question, marital status was inferred. Before 1980, the incidence of births to unmarried women in states with no direct question on marital status was assumed to be the same as the incidence in reporting states in the same geographic division. Starting in 1980, for states without a direct question, marital status was inferred by comparing the parents' and child's surnames. Inferential procedures in current use depend on the presence of a paternity acknowledgment or missing information on the father. Changes in reporting procedures by some states in 1995 and 1997 had little effect on national totals, but they did affect trends for age groups and some state trends. Details of the changes in reporting procedures are described in Ventura SJ, Bachrach CA. Nonmarital childbearing in the United States, 1940–1999. National vital statistics reports; vol 48 no 16. Hyattsville, MD: National Center for Health Statistics. 2000. Available from: www.cdc.gov/nchs/births.htm.

Maternal age—See Age.

Maternal death—Maternal death is defined by the World Health Organization as the death of a woman while pregnant or within 42 days of termination of pregnancy, irrespective of the duration and site of the pregnancy, from any cause related to or aggravated by the pregnancy or its management, but not from accidental or incidental causes. A maternal death is one for which the certifying physician has designated a maternal condition as the underlying cause of death. Maternal conditions are those assigned to pregnancy, childbirth, and the puerperium, ICD–10 codes A34, O00–O95, O98–O99 (Table V). Changes have been made in the classification and coding of maternal deaths between ICD–9 and ICD–10, effective with mortality data for 1999. ICD–10 changes pertain to indirect maternal causes and timing of death relative to pregnancy. If only indirect maternal causes of death (i.e., a previously existing disease or a disease that developed during pregnancy that was not due to direct obstetric causes but was aggravated by physiologic effects of pregnancy) are reported in Part I of the death certificate and pregnancy is reported in either Part I or Part II, ICD–10 classifies this as a maternal death. ICD–9 only classified the death as maternal if pregnancy was reported in Part I. Some state death certificates include a separate question regarding pregnancy status. A positive response to the question is interpreted as "pregnant" being reported in Part II of the cause-of-death section of the death certificate. If the medical certifier did not specify when death occurred relative to the pregnancy, it is assumed that the pregnancy terminated 42 days or less prior to death.

In 2003, 21 states had a separate question related to pregnancy status of female decedents around the time of their death, and two states had a prompt encouraging certifiers to report recent pregnancies on the death certificate; however, there were at least six different questions used. The 2003 revision of the U.S. Standard Certificate of Death introduced a standard question format with categories designed to utilize additional codes available in ICD–10 for deaths associated with pregnancy, childbirth, and the puerperium. As states revise their certificates, most states are expected to introduce the standard item or replace pre-existing questions with the standard item, so that there will be wider adoption of a pregnancy status item across the country and greater standardization of the particular item used. See related Rate: Death and related rates.

Maternal education—See Education.

Maternal mortality rate—See Rate: Death and related rates.

Medicaid—Medicaid was authorized by Title XIX of the Social Security Act in 1965 as a jointly funded cooperative venture between the federal and state governments to assist states in the provision of adequate medical care to eligible needy persons. Within broad federal guidelines, each of the states establishes its own eligibility standards; determines the type, amount, duration, and scope of services; sets the rate of payment for services; and administers its own program.

Medicaid is the largest program providing medical and health-related services to America's poorest people. However, Medicaid does not provide medical assistance to all poor persons. Under the broadest provisions of the federal statute, Medicaid does not provide health care services even for very poor childless adults under age 65 years unless they are disabled. Except as noted, all states must provide Medicaid coverage to the following:

- Individuals who meet the requirements for the Aid to Families with Dependent Children (AFDC) program that were in effect in their state on July 16, 1996, or, at state option, more liberal criteria (with some exceptions).
- Children under age 6 whose family income is at or below 133% of the federal poverty level.
- Pregnant women whose family income is below 133% of the federal poverty level (services to these women are limited to those related to pregnancy, complications of pregnancy, delivery, and postpartum care).
- Supplemental Security Income (SSI) recipients in most states (some states use more restrictive Medicaid eligibility requirements that predate SSI).
- Recipients of adoption or foster care assistance under Title IV of the Social Security Act.
- Special protected groups (typically individuals who lose their cash assistance because of earnings from work or from increased Social Security benefits but who may keep Medicaid for a period of time).
- Children age 6–18 years in families with incomes at or below the federal poverty level.
- Certain Medicare beneficiaries (low income is only one

test for Medicaid eligibility for those within these groups; their resources also are tested against threshold levels, as determined by each state within federal guidelines).

States also have the option of providing Medicaid coverage for other groups.

Medicaid operates as a vendor payment program. States may pay health care providers directly on a fee-for-service basis, or states may pay for Medicaid services through various prepayment arrangements, such as health maintenance organizations (HMOs) or other forms of managed care. Within federally imposed upper limits and specific restrictions, each state for the most part has broad discretion in determining the payment methodology and payment rate for services. Thus, the Medicaid program varies considerably from state to state, as well as within each state over time. For more information see www.cms.hhs.gov/MedicaidEligibility/. See related Health expenditures, national; Health insurance coverage; Health maintenance organization (HMO); Managed care; Appendix I, Medicaid Data System.

Medical specialty—See Physician specialty.

Medical vendor payments—Under the Medicaid program, medical vendor payments are payments (expenditures) to medical vendors from the state through a fiscal agent or to a health insurance plan. Adjustments are made for Indian Health Service payments to Medicaid, cost settlements, third party recoupments, refunds, voided checks, and other financial settlements that cannot be related to specific provided claims. Excluded are payments made for medical care under the emergency assistance provisions, payments made from state medical assistance funds that are not federally matchable, disproportionate share hospital payments, cost sharing or enrollment fees collected from recipients or a third party, and administration and training costs.

Medicare—This is a nationwide health insurance program providing health insurance protection to people 65 years of age and over, people entitled to Social Security disability payments for 2 years or more (with limited exceptions for people with specific diagnoses), and people with end-stage renal disease, regardless of income. The program was enacted July 30, 1965, as Title XVIII, Health Insurance for the Aged of the Social Security Act, and became effective on July 1, 1966. From its inception, it has included two separate but coordinated programs: hospital insurance (Part A) and supplementary medical insurance (Part B). In 1999, additional choices were allowed for delivering Medicare Part A and Part B benefits. Medicare Advantage, previously Medicare+Choice, (Part C) is an expanded set of options for the delivery of health care under Medicare, created in the Balanced Budget Act passed by Congress in 1997. The term Medicare Advantage refers to options other than original Medicare. While all Medicare beneficiaries can receive their benefits through the original fee-for-service (FFS) program, most beneficiaries enrolled in both Part A and Part B can choose to participate in a Medicare Advantage plan instead. Organizations that seek to contract as Medicare Advantage plans must meet specific organizational, financial, and other requirements. Most Medicare Advantage plans are coordinated care plans, which include health maintenance organizations (HMOs), provider-sponsored organizations (PSOs), preferred provider organizations (PPOs), and other certified coordinated care plans and entities that meet the standards set forth in the law. The Medicare Advantage program also includes Medical savings account (MSA) plans, which provide benefits after a single high deductible is met, and private, unrestricted FFS plans, which allow beneficiaries to select certain private providers. These programs are available in only a limited number of states. For those providers who agree to accept the plan's payment terms and conditions, this option does not place the providers at risk, nor does it vary payment rates based on utilization. Only the coordinated care plans are considered managed care plans. Except for MSA plans, all Medicare Advantage plans are required to provide at least the current Medicare benefit package, excluding hospice services. Plans may offer additional covered services and are required to do so (or return excess payments) if plan costs are lower than the Medicare payments received by the plan.

The Medicare Prescription Drug, Improvement, and Modernization Act (MMA) was passed on December 8, 2003. The MMA established a voluntary drug benefit for Medicare beneficiaries and created a new Medicare Part D. People eligible for Medicare could begin to enroll in Part D beginning in January of 2006. For more information see www.medicare.gov/publications/pubs/pdf/10050.pdf.

See related Fee-for-service health insurance; Health insurance coverage; Health maintenance organization (HMO); Managed care; Appendix I, Medicare Administrative Data.

Mental health organization—The Center for Mental Health Services of the Substance Abuse and Mental Health Services

Administration defines a mental health organization as an administratively distinct public or private agency or institution whose primary concern is provision of direct mental health services to the mentally ill or emotionally disturbed. Excluded are private office-based practices of psychiatrists, psychologists, and other mental health providers; psychiatric services of all types of hospitals or outpatient clinics operated by federal agencies other than the Department of Veterans Affairs (e.g., Public Health Service, Indian Health Service, Department of Defense, and Bureau of Prisons); general hospitals that have no separate psychiatric services but admit psychiatric patients to nonpsychiatric units; and psychiatric services of schools, colleges, halfway houses, community residential organizations, local and county jails, state prisons, and other human services providers. The major types of mental health organizations are described below.

Freestanding psychiatric outpatient clinic—These clinics provide only outpatient mental health services on either a regular or emergency basis. A psychiatrist generally assumes the medical responsibility for services.

Psychiatric hospital—These hospitals (public or private) primarily provide 24-hour inpatient care and treatment in a hospital setting to persons with mental illnesses. Psychiatric hospitals may be under state, county, private for profit, or private nonprofit auspices.

General hospital psychiatric service—These are organizations that provide psychiatric services with assigned staff for 24-hour inpatient or residential care and/or less than 24-hour outpatient care in a separate ward, unit, floor, or wing of the hospital.

Department of Veterans Affairs medical center—These are hospitals operated by the Department of Veterans Affairs (formerly Veterans Administration) and include Department of Veterans Affairs general hospital psychiatric services (including large neuropsychiatric units) and Department of Veterans Affairs psychiatric outpatient clinics.

Residential treatment center for emotionally disturbed children—These centers must meet all of the following criteria: (a) provide 24-hour residential services; (b) are not licensed as a psychiatric hospital and have the primary purpose of providing individually planned mental health treatment services in conjunction with residential care; (c) include a clinical program directed by a psychiatrist, psychologist, social worker, or psychiatric nurse with a graduate degree; (d) serve children and youth primarily under the age of 18; and (e) have the primary diagnosis as mental illness, classified as other than mental retardation, developmental disability, or substance-related disorders, according to DSM–II/ICDA–8 or DSM–IIIR/ICD–9–CM codes, for the majority of admissions.

Multiservice mental health organization—These organizations provide services in both 24-hour and less than 24-hour settings and are not classifiable as a psychiatric hospital, general hospital, or residential treatment center for emotionally disturbed children. (The classification of a psychiatric or general hospital or residential treatment center for emotionally disturbed children takes precedence over a multiservice classification, even if two or more services are offered.)

Partial care organization—These organizations provide a program of ambulatory mental health services or rehabilitation, habitation, or education programs.

See related Admission; Mental health service type.

Mental health service type—This term refers to the following types of mental health services:

24-hour mental health care, formerly called inpatient care, provides care in a mental health hospital setting.

Less than 24-hour care, formerly called outpatient or partial care treatment, provides mental health services on an ambulatory basis.

Residential treatment care provides overnight mental health care in conjunction with an intensive treatment program in a setting other than a hospital. Facilities may offer care to emotionally disturbed children or mentally ill adults.

See related Admission; Mental health organization.

Metropolitan statistical area (MSA)—The Office of Management and Budget (OMB) defines metropolitan areas according to published standards that are applied to U.S. Census Bureau data. In the 2000 standards, an MSA is a county or group of contiguous counties that contains at least one urbanized area of 50,000 or more population. In addition to the county or counties that contain all or part of the urbanized area, an MSA may contain other counties that are economically and socially integrated with the central county as measured by commuting. Counties that are not within an MSA are considered to be nonmetropolitan. For additional information see: www.census.gov/population/www/estimates/metrodef.html. See related Urbanization.

For National Health Interview Survey (NHIS) data before 1995, metropolitan population is based on MSAs as defined by OMB using the 1980 standards and the 1980 census. Starting with the 1995 NHIS, metropolitan population is based on MSAs as defined by OMB using the 1990 standards and the 1990 census. The 1990 standards for designating MSAs differs from the 2000 standards. For example, under the 1990 standards the metropolitan character of a county could be considered in determining whether to classify a county as metropolitan.

Micropolitan statistical area—The Office of Management and Budget (OMB) defines micropolitan areas based on published standards that are applied to U.S. Census Bureau data. A micropolitan statistical area is a nonmetropolitan county or group of contiguous nonmetropolitan counties that contains an urban cluster of 10,000 to 49,999 persons. A micropolitan statistical area may include surrounding counties if there are strong economic ties between the counties, based on commuting patterns. Nonmetropolitan counties that are not classified as part of a micropolitan statistical area are considered nonmicropolitan. For additional information about micropolitan statistical areas, see www.census.gov/population/www/estimates/metrodef.html. See related Urbanization.

Multiservice mental health organization—See Mental health organization.

National Drug Code (NDC) Directory therapeutic class—The NDC system was originally established as an essential part of an out-of-hospital drug reimbursement program under Medicare. The NDC serves as a universal product identifier for human drugs. The current edition of the NDC is limited to prescription drugs and a few selected over-the-counter (OTC) products. The directory consists of prescription and selected OTC insulin and domestic and foreign drug products that are in commercial distribution in the United States. The products have been listed in accordance with the Drug Listing Act and applicable Code of Federal Regulations for submitting drug product information to the Food and Drug Administation (FDA). NDC therapeutic class codes are used to identify each of 20 major drug classes to which the drug entry may belong, adapted from Standard Drug Classifications in the NDC Directory, 1995. The two-digit categories are general and represent all subcategories (e.g., Antimicrobial agents), and the specific four-digit categories represent the breakouts of the general category (e.g., Penicillin). The general two-digit codes include medications that do not fit into any of the subcategories (four-digit codes). Starting in 1995, the NDC four-digit classes were changed to include more classes than the previous classification in 1985. Therefore, some drugs switched from a general two-digit class into a more specific four-digit class. In addition, drugs may be approved for several different therapeutic classes. Some drugs receive approval for additional therapeutic uses after their initial approval, so the same drug can change classes because of new uses.

Numerous drug products have many uses or indications. In an effort to categorize the vast number of the broad analgesic or pain-relief individual products in the marketplace into manageable and nonoverlapping categories, all four-digit categories within the analgesic two-digit therapeutic class were recoded by staff of the FDA's Center for Drug Evaluation and Research. Thus, the codes presented in *Health, United States* do not match the published NDC codes for analgesic therapeutic categories. The NDC contains the following four-digit analgesic therapeutic categories: 1720—general analgesic, 1721—narcotic analgesic, 1722—nonnarcotic analgesic, 1724—antiarthritics, 1723—antimigraine/headache, 1726—central pain syndrome, 1727—nonsteroidal anti-inflammatory drugs (NSAID), 1728—antipyretic, and 1729—menstrual products. These categories were collapsed into broader and mutually exclusive categories of narcotic analgesics, nonnarcotic analgesics, and NSAIDs. Under the NDC system, aspirin is coded as an NSAID because of its anti-inflammatory properties, but also as an analgesic, an antiarthritic, and an antipyretic. In this report aspirin has been recoded into the nonnarcotic analgesic category. Aspirin was not included as an NSAID because of its common use for cardiac therapy and its many other indications.

Table XII shows how generic analgesic drugs were reclassified for *Health, United States*. Analgesic drugs were

Table XI. Codes for procedure categories from the *International Classification of Diseases, Ninth Revision, Clinical Modification*

Procedure category	*Code numbers*
Operations on vessels of heart	36
Removal of coronary artery obstruction and insertion of stent(s)	36.0
Insertion of coronary artery stent(s)[1]	36.06, 36.07
Insertion of drug-eluting stent(s)	36.07
Coronary artery bypass graft	36.1
Cardiac catheterization	37.21–37.23
Insertion, replacement, removal, and revision of pacemaker leads or device	37.7–37.8
Diagnostic procedures on small intestine	45.1
Diagnostic procedures on large intestine	45.2
Cholecystectomy	51.2
Laparoscopic cholecystectomy	51.23
Repair of hernia	53
Lysis of peritoneal adhesions	54.5
Transurethral prostatectomy	60.2
Total abdominal hysterectomy	68.4
Vaginal hysterectomy	68.5, 68.7
Dilation and curettage of uterus	69.0
Forceps, vacuum, and breech delivery	72
Other procedures inducing or assisting delivery	73
Cesarean section and removal of fetus	74
Reduction of fracture and dislocation	79
Excision or destruction of intervertebral disc and spinal fusion	80.5 and 81.0
Excision or destruction of intervertebral disc	80.5
Joint replacement of lower extremity	81.5
Total hip replacement	81.51
Partial hip replacement	81.52
Total knee replacement	81.54
Diagnostic radiology	87
Computerized axial tomography	87.03, 87.41, 87.71, 88.01, 88.38
Angiocardiography using contrast material	88.5
Diagnostic ultrasound	88.7
Magnetic resonance imaging	88.91–88.97

[1]The procedure code for insertion of coronary artery stents (36.06) first appears in the 1996 data. A second procedure code for the insertion of drug-eluting stents (36.07) first appears in the 2003 data.

reclassified based on the product's main ingredients or indication of use. For example, Robitussin AC contains several ingredients, one of which is codeine, a narcotic. However, its main use is not for pain but for cough suppression, and it is therefore categorized as a cough and cold product as opposed to a narcotic analgesic product.

Neonatal mortality rate—See Rate: Death and related rates.

Nonprofit hospital—See Hospital.

North American Industry Classification System (NAICS)—See Industry of employment.

Notifiable disease—A notifiable disease is one that, when diagnosed, health providers are required, usually by law, to report to state or local public health officials. Notifiable diseases are those of public interest by reason of their contagiousness, severity, or frequency.

Nursing home—In the Online Survey Certification and Reporting database, a nursing home is a facility that is certified and meets the Center for Medicare & Medicaid Services' long-term care requirements for Medicare and Medicaid eligibility.

In the National Master Facility Inventory (NMFI), which provided the sampling frame for the 1973–1974, 1977, and

Table XII. National Drug Code (NDC) therapeutic class analgesic drug recodes

Narcotic analgesics	*Nonnarcotic analgesics*	*Nonsteroidal anti-inflammatory drugs (NSAIDs)*
Alfentanil Hydrochloride	Acetaminophen	Bromfenac Sodium
Alphaprodine	Acetylsalicylic Acid	Celecoxib
Bupernorphine	Aminobenzoic Acid	Diclofenac Potassium
Butorphanol	Aspirin	Diclofenac Sodium
Codeine	Auranofin	Difunisal
Dihydrocodeine	Aurothioglucose	Etodolac
Fentanyl	Butalbital	Fenoprofen
Hydrocodone Bitartrate	Capsaicin	Flurbiprofen Sodium
Hydromorphone	Carbaspirin Calcium	Ibuprofen
Levorphanol	Choline Salicylate	Indomethacin
Meperidine	Etanercept	Ketoprofen
Meperidine HCl	Fluprednisolone	Ketorolac Tromethamine
Methadone	Gold Sodium Thiomalate	Meclofenamate
Morphine	Gold Sodium Thiosulfate	Meclofenamic Acid
Morphine Sulfate	Hyaluronic Acid	Mefenamic Acid
Nalbuphine	Leflunomide	Meloxicam
Opium	Magnesium Salicylate	Nabumetone
Oxycodone	Menthol	Naproxen
Oxycodone HCl	Methotrexate	Oxaprozin
Pentazocine	Methylprednisolone	Piroxicam
Propoxyphene	Methylsulfonylmethane	Rofecoxib
Remifentanyl	Oxyphenbutazone	Sulindac
	Phenyl Salicylate	Suprofen
	Phenylbutazone	Tolmetin
	Prednisolone	Valdecoxib
	Salicylamide	
	Salsalate	
	Sodium Hyaluronate	
	Sodium Salicylate	
	Sodium Thiosalicylate	
	Tramadol	
	Triamcinilone	
	Zomepirac	

NOTE: Drugs originally classified as National Drug Code (NDC) therapeutic category 1720 (general analgesics); 1721 (narcotic analgesics); 1722 (non-narcotic analgesics); 1724 (antiarthritics); 1727 (NSAIDs); 1728 (antipyretics); and 1729 (menstrual products) were recoded into the three mutually exclusive categories shown above. NDC codes for the analgesic categories 1723 (antimigraine) and 1725 (antigout) were not recoded.

1985 National Nursing Home Surveys, a nursing home was an establishment with three or more beds that provided nursing or personal care services to the aged, infirm, or chronically ill. The 1977 National Nursing Home Survey included personal care homes and domiciliary care homes, whereas the National Nursing Home Surveys of 1973–1974, 1985, 1995, 1997, 1999, and 2004 excluded them. The following definitions of nursing home types applied to facilities listed in the NFMI:

Nursing care home—These homes employ one or more full-time registered or licensed practical nurses and provide nursing care to at least one-half the residents.

Personal care home with nursing—These homes have fewer than one-half the residents receiving nursing care. In addition, such homes employ one or more registered or licensed practical nurses or provided administration of medications and treatments in accordance with physicians' orders, supervision of self-administered medications, or three or more personal services.

Personal care home without nursing—These homes have no residents who receive nursing care. These homes provide administration of medications and treatments in accordance with physicians' orders, supervise self-administered medications, or provide three or more personal services.

Domiciliary care home—These homes primarily provide supervisory care and one or two personal services.

The following definitions of certification levels apply to data collected in the National Nursing Home Surveys of 1973–1974, 1977, and 1985:

Skilled nursing facility—These facilities provide the most intensive nursing care available outside a hospital. Facilities certified by Medicare provide posthospital care to eligible Medicare enrollees. Facilities certified by Medicaid as skilled nursing facilities provide skilled nursing services on a daily basis to individuals eligible for Medicaid benefits.

Intermediate care facility—These facilities are certified by the Medicaid program to provide health-related services on a regular basis to Medicaid eligibles who do not require hospital or skilled nursing facility care but do require institutional care above the level of room and board.

Not certified facility—These facilities are not certified as providers of care by Medicare or Medicaid.

Beginning with the 1995 National Nursing Home Survey, nursing homes have been defined as facilities that routinely provide nursing care services and have three or more beds set up for residents. Facilities may be certified by Medicare or Medicaid or not certified but licensed by the state as a nursing home. The facilities may be freestanding or a distinct unit of a larger facility.

After October 1, 1990, long-term care facilities that met the Omnibus Budget Reconciliation Act of 1987 (OBRA 87) nursing home reform requirements that were formerly certified under the Medicaid program as skilled nursing, nursing home, or intermediate care facilities were reclassified as nursing facilities. The Medicare program continues to certify skilled nursing facilities, but not intermediate care facilities. State Medicaid programs can certify intermediate care facilities for the mentally retarded or developmentally disabled. Nursing facilities must also be certified to participate in the Medicare program to be certified for participation in Medicaid except those facilities that have obtained waivers. Thus, most nursing home care is now provided in skilled care facilities.

See related Long-term care facility; Nursing care; Resident.

Nursing home expenditures—See Health expenditures, national.

Obesity—See Body mass index (BMI).

Occupancy rate—In American Hospital Association statistics, hospital occupancy rate is calculated as the average daily census divided by the number of hospital beds, cribs, and pediatric bassinets set up and staffed on the last day of the reporting period, expressed as a percentage. Average daily census is calculated by dividing the total annual number of inpatients, excluding newborns, by 365 days to derive the number of inpatients receiving care on an average day during the annual reporting period. The occupancy rate for facilities other than hospitals is calculated as the number of residents at the facility reported on the day of the interview divided by the number of reported beds. In the Online Survey Certification and Reporting database, occupancy is determined as of the day of certification inspection as the total number of residents on that day divided by the total number of beds on that day.

Office-based physician—See Physician.

Office visit—In the National Ambulatory Medical Care Survey, a physician's ambulatory practice (office) can be in any location other than in a hospital, nursing home, other extended care facility, patient's home, industrial clinic, college clinic, or family planning clinic. Offices in health maintenance organizations and private offices in hospitals are included. An office visit is any direct personal exchange between an ambulatory patient and a physician or members of his or her staff for the purposes of seeking care and rendering health services. See related Outpatient visit.

Operation—See Procedure.

Outpatient department—According to the National Hospital Ambulatory Medical Care Survey (NHAMCS), an outpatient department (OPD) is a hospital facility where nonurgent ambulatory medical care is provided. The following types of OPDs are excluded from the NHAMCS: ambulatory surgical centers, chemotherapy, employee health services, renal dialysis, methadone maintenance, and radiology. See related Emergency department; Outpatient visit.

Outpatient surgery—According to the American Hospital Association, outpatient surgery is a surgical operation, whether major or minor, performed on patients who do not remain in the hospital overnight. Outpatient surgery may be performed in inpatient operating suites, outpatient surgery suites, or procedure rooms within an outpatient care facility. A surgical operation involving more than one surgical procedure is considered one surgical operation. See related Procedure.

Outpatient visit—The American Hospital Association defines outpatient visits as visits for receipt of medical, dental, or other services at a hospital by patients who are not lodged in the hospital. Each appearance by an outpatient to each unit of the hospital is counted individually as an outpatient visit, including all clinic visits, referred visits, observation services, outpatient surgeries, and emergency department visits. In the National Hospital Ambulatory Medical Care Survey, an outpatient department visit is a direct personal exchange between a patient and a physician or other health care provider working under the physician's supervision for the purpose of seeking care and receiving personal health services. See related Emergency department or emergency room visit; Outpatient department.

Overweight—See Body mass index (BMI).

Pap smear—A Pap smear (also known as a Papanicolaou smear or Pap test) is a microscopic examination of cells scraped from the cervix that is used to detect cancerous or precancerous conditions of the cervix or other medical conditions. In the National Health Interview Survey questions concerning Pap smear use were asked on an intermittent schedule, and the question content differed slightly across years. In 1987, women were asked to report when they had their most recent Pap smear in days, weeks, months, or years. Women who did not respond were asked a follow-up question, "Was it 3 years ago or less, between 3 and 5 years, or 5 years or more ago?" Pap smear data in the past 3 years were not available in 1990 and 1991. In 1993 and 1994, women were asked whether they had a Pap smear within the past year, between 1 and 3 years ago, or more than 3 years ago. In 1998, women were asked whether they had a Pap smear 1 year ago or less, more than 1 year but not more than 2 years, more than 2 years but not more than 3 years, more than 3 years but not more than 5 years, or more than 5 years ago. In 1999, women were asked when they had their most recent Pap smear in days, weeks, months, or years. In 1999, 4% of women in the sample responded 3 years ago. In this analysis these women were coded as within the past 3 years, although a response of 3 years ago may include women whose last Pap smear was more than 3 but less than 4 years ago. Thus, estimates for 1999 are overestimated to some degree in comparison with estimates for previous years. In 2000 and 2003, women were asked when they had their most recent Pap smear (give month and year). Women who did not respond were given a follow-up question that used the 1999 wording and women who did not answer the follow-up question were asked a second follow-up question that used the 1998 wording. In 2000 and 2003, less than 1% of women in the sample answered 3 years ago using the 1999 wording, and they were coded as within the past 3 years. Thus, estimates for 2000 and 2003 may be slightly overestimated in comparison with estimates for years prior to 1999. In 2005, women were asked the same series of questions about Pap smear use as in the 2000 and 2003 surveys but the skip pattern was modified so that more women were asked the follow-up question using the 1998 wording. Because additional information was available for women who replied their last Pap smear was 3 years ago, these women were not uniformally coded as having had a Pap smear within the past 3 years. Thus, estimates for 2005 are more precise compared with estimates for 1999, 2000, and 2003 and are slightly lower than they would have been without this additional information.

Partial care organization—See Mental health organization.

Partial care treatment—See Mental health service type.

Patient—See Inpatient; Office visit; Outpatient visit.

Percent change/percentage change—See Average annual rate of change.

Perinatal mortality rate; ratio—See Rate: Death and related rates.

Personal care home with or without nursing—See Nursing home.

Personal health care expenditures—See Health expenditures, national.

Physical activity, leisure-time—All questions related to leisure-time physical activity were phrased in terms of current behavior and lack a specific reference period. Starting with 1998 data, leisure-time physical activity is assessed in the National Health Interview Survey by asking adults a series of questions about how often they do vigorous or light/moderate physical activity of at least 10 minutes duration and for about how long these sessions generally last. Vigorous physical activity is described as causing heavy sweating or a large increase in breathing or heart rate and light/moderate as causing light sweating or a slight to moderate increase in breathing or heart rate. Adults classified as inactive did not report any sessions of light/moderate or vigorous leisure-time physical activity of at least 10 minutes duration or reported they were unable to perform leisure-time physical activity. Adults classified with some leisure-time activity reported at least one session of light/moderate or vigorous activity of at least 10 minutes duration but did not meet the requirement for regular leisure-time activity. Adults classified with regular leisure-time activity reported at least three sessions per week of vigorous leisure-time physical activity lasting at least 20 minutes in duration or at least five sessions per week of light/moderate physical activity lasting at least 30 minutes in duration.

Physician—Data on physician characteristics are obtained through physician self-report from the American Medical Association's (AMA) Physician Masterfile. The AMA tabulates data only for doctors of medicine (MDs), but some tables in *Health, United States* include data for both MDs and doctors of osteopathy (DOs).

Active (or professionally active) physician—These physicians are currently engaged in patient care or other professional activity for a minimum of 20 hours per week. Other professional activity includes administration, medical teaching, research, and other activities, such as employment with insurance carriers, pharmaceutical companies, corporations, voluntary organizations, medical societies, and the like. Physicians who are retired, semiretired, working part-time, or not practicing are classified as inactive and are excluded. Also excluded are physicians with address unknown and physicians who did not provide information on type of practice or present employment (not classified).

Hospital-based physician—These physicians are employed under contract with hospitals to provide direct patient care and include physicians in residency training (including clinical fellows) and full-time members of the hospital staff.

Office-based physician—These physicians are engaged in seeing patients in solo practice, group practice, two-physician practice, other patient care employment, or inpatient services such as those provided by pathologists and radiologists.

Data for physicians are presented by type of education (doctors of medicine and doctors of osteopathy); place of education (U.S. medical graduates and international medical graduates); activity status (professionally active and inactive); area of specialty; and geographic area. See related Physician specialty.

Physician specialty—A physician specialty is any specific branch of medicine in which a physician may concentrate. Data are based on physician self-reports of their primary area of specialty. Physician data are broadly categorized into two areas of practice: those who provide primary care, and those who provide specialty care.

Primary care generalist—These physicians practice in the general fields of family medicine, general practice, internal medicine, obstetrics and gynecology, and pediatrics. They specifically exclude primary care specialists associated with these generalist fields.

Primary care specialist—These specialists practice in the primary care subspecialties of family medicine, internal medicine, obstetrics and gynecology, and pediatrics. Family medicine subspecialties include geriatric medicine and sports medicine. Internal medicine subspecialties include adolescent medicine, critical care medicine, diabetes, endocrinology, diabetes and metabolism, hematology, hepatology, hematology/oncology, cardiac electrophysiology, infectious diseases, clinical and laboratory immunology, geriatric medicine, sports medicine, nephrology, nutrition, medical oncology, pulmonary critical care medicine, and rheumatology. Obstetrics and gynecology subspecialties include gynecological oncology, gynecology, maternal and fetal medicine, obstetrics, critical care medicine, and reproductive endocrinology. Pediatric subspecialties include adolescent medicine, pediatric critical care medicine, pediatrics/internal medicine, neonatal-perinatal medicine, pediatric allergy, pediatric cardiology, pediatric endocrinology, pediatric infectious disease, pediatric pulmonology, medical toxicology (pediatrics), pediatric emergency medicine, pediatric gastroenterology, pediatric hematology/oncology, clinical and laboratory immunology (pediatrics), pediatric nephrology, pediatric rheumatology, and sports medicine (pediatrics).

Specialty care physician—These physicians are sometimes called specialists, and include primary care specialists listed above in addition to all other physicians not included in the generalist definition. Specialty fields include allergy and immunology, aerospace medicine, anesthesiology, cardiovascular diseases, child and adolescent psychiatry, colon and rectal surgery, dermatology, diagnostic radiology, forensic pathology, gastroenterology, general surgery, medical genetics, neurology, nuclear medicine, neurological surgery, occupational medicine, ophthalmology, orthopedic surgery, otolaryngology, psychiatry, public health and general preventive medicine, physical medicine and rehabilitation, plastic surgery, anatomic and clinical pathology, pulmonary diseases, radiation oncology, thoracic surgery, urology, addiction medicine, critical care medicine, legal medicine, and clinical pharmacology.

See related Physician.

Population—The U.S. Census Bureau collects and publishes data on populations in the United States according to several different definitions. Various statistical systems then use the appropriate population for calculating rates. See related Appendix I, Population Census and Population Estimates.

Total population—This is the population of the United States, including all members of the Armed Forces living in foreign countries, Puerto Rico, Guam, and the U.S. Virgin Islands. Other Americans abroad (e.g., civilian federal employees and dependents of members of the Armed Forces or other federal employees) are not included.

Resident population—This population includes persons whose usual place of residence (i.e., the place where one usually lives and sleeps) is in one of the 50 states or the District of Columbia. It includes members of the Armed Forces stationed in the United States and their families. It excludes international military, naval, and diplomatic personnel and their families located in this country and residing in embassies or similar quarters. Also excluded are international workers and international students in this country and Americans living abroad. The resident population is the denominator for calculating birth and death rates and incidence of disease.

Civilian population—The civilian population is the resident population excluding members of the Armed Forces. However, families of members of the Armed Forces are included. This population is the denominator in rates calculated for the National Hospital Discharge Survey, and the National Nursing Home Survey.

Civilian noninstitutionalized population—This is the civilian population not residing in institutions such as correctional institutions, detention homes, and training schools for juvenile delinquents; homes for aged and dependent persons (e.g., nursing homes and convalescent homes); homes for dependent and neglected children; homes and schools for mentally or physically handicapped persons; homes for unwed mothers; psychiatric, tuberculosis, and chronic disease hospitals; and residential treatment centers. U.S. Census Bureau estimates of the civilian noninstitutionalized population are used to calculate sample weights for the National Health Interview Survey, National Health and Nutrition Examination Survey, and National Survey of Family Growth, and as denominators in rates calculated for the National Ambulatory Medical Care Survey and the National Hospital Ambulatory Medical Care Survey.

Introduction of census 2000 population estimates—Health United States, 2003 marked the transition to the use of year 2000 resident population estimates based on the 2000 census for calculation of rates. Previously, 1991–2000 rates were based on post-1990 population estimates. Birth rates and death rates for 1991–1999 were revised using intercensal population estimates based on the 2000 census. Rates for 2000 were revised using Census 2000 counts. Data systems and surveys that use civilian and civilian noninstitutionalized population estimates as denominators for computation of rates for the period 1991–1999 have not been updated with intercensal estimates based on the 2000 civilian and civilian noninstitutionalized populations. See related Appendix I, Population Census and Population Estimates.

Postneonatal mortality rate—See Rate: Death and related rates.

Poverty—Poverty statistics are based on definitions originally developed by the Social Security Administration. These include a set of money income thresholds that vary by family size and composition. Families or individuals with income below their appropriate thresholds are classified as below poverty. These thresholds are updated annually by the U.S. Census Bureau to reflect changes in the Consumer Price Index for all urban consumers (CPI-U). For example, the average poverty threshold for a family of four was $19,971 in 2005, $17,603 in 2000, and $13,359 in 1990. For more information, see Income, poverty and health insurance coverage in the United States: 2005 (P60–231). Series P–60 No 231. Washington, DC. U.S. Government Printing Office. 2005 and the Census website. Available from: www.census.gov/hhes/www/poverty.html.

National Health Interview Survey (NHIS) and *National Health and Nutrition Examination Survey (NHANES)*—Percent of poverty level, for years prior to 1997, was based on family income and family size using U.S. Census Bureau poverty thresholds. Starting with 1997 data, percent of poverty level is based on family income, family size, number of children in the family, and for families with two or fewer adults, the age of the adults in the family. Percent of poverty level in the NHANES is also based on family income and family size and composition. See related Consumer Price Index (CPI); Family income; Appendix I, Current Population Survey; National Health Interview Survey; National Health and Nutrition Examination Survey.

Preferred provider organization (PPO)—A PPO is a type of medical plan where coverage is provided to participants through a network of selected health care providers (such as hospitals and physicians). The enrollees may go outside the network, but they would pay a greater percentage of the cost of coverage than within the network. See related Health maintenance organization (HMO); Managed care.

Prenatal care—Prenatal care is medical care provided to a pregnant woman to prevent complications and decrease the incidence of maternal and prenatal mortality. Information on when pregnancy care began is recorded on the birth certificate. Between 1970 and 1980, the reporting area for prenatal care expanded. In 1970, 39 states and the District of Columbia (D.C.) reported prenatal care on the birth certificate. Data were not available from Alabama, Alaska, Arkansas, Connecticut, Delaware, Georgia, Idaho, Massachusetts, New Mexico, Pennsylvania, and Virginia. In 1975, these data were available from three additional states—Connecticut, Delaware, and Georgia—increasing the number of states reporting prenatal care to 42 and D.C. During 1980–2002, prenatal care information was available for the entire United States. Starting in 2003, some states began implementation of the 2003 revision of the U.S. Standard Certificate of Live Birth. While all states collected information on prenatal care, the prenatal care item on the 2003 certificate, Date of first prenatal visit, is not comparable with the prenatal care item on the 1989 revision, Month prenatal care began. In addition, the 2003 revision recommends that information on prenatal care be gathered from prenatal care or medical records whereas the 1989 revision did not recommend a source for these data. Therefore, data on prenatal care were excluded for states that implemented the 2003 revision of the U.S. Standard Certificate of Live Birth: these reporting areas included Pennsylvania and Washington starting in 2003, and Florida, Idaho, Kentucky, New Hampshire, New York state (excluding New York City), South Carolina, and Tennessee starting in 2004. The reporting area for prenatal care decreased to 48 states and D.C. in 2003, and 41 states, D.C., and New York City in 2004.

Prevalence—Prevalence is the number of cases of a disease, infected persons, or persons with some other attribute present during a particular interval of time. It is often expressed as a rate (e.g., the prevalence of diabetes per 1,000 persons during a year). See related Incidence.

Primary care specialty—See Physician specialty.

Private expenditures—See Health expenditures, national.

Procedure—The National Hospital Discharge Survey (NHDS) used to classify a procedure as a surgical or nonsurgical operation, diagnostic procedure, or therapeutic procedure (such as respiratory therapy); however, the distinction between types of procedures has become less meaningful because of the development of minimally invasive and noninvasive surgery. Thus, the practice of classifying the type of procedure has been discontinued. Procedures are coded according to the *International Classification of Diseases, Ninth Revision, Clinical Modification* (see Table XI). Up to four different procedures are coded in the NHDS. Procedures per hospital stay can be classified as any-listed—that is, if more than one procedure with the same code is performed it is counted only once—or all-listed where multiple occurrences of the same procedure would be counted the number of times it appears on the medical record up to the maximum of four available codes. All-listed procedures double-count the number of procedures of a given type that are performed, thus all listed procedure counts are greater than the number of hospital stays that occurred. Any-listed procedure counts approximate the number of hospital stays where a procedure was performed at any time during the stay. See related Outpatient surgery.

Proprietary hospital—See Hospital.

Psychiatric hospital—See Hospital; Mental health organization.

Public expenditures—See Health expenditures, national.

Purchasing power parities—Purchasing power parities (PPP) are calculated rates of currency conversion that equalize the purchasing power of different currencies by eliminating the differences in price levels between countries. PPP show the ratio of prices in national currencies of the same good or service in different countries. PPP can be used to make inter-country comparisons of the gross domestic product (GDP) and its component expenditures. See related Gross domestic product.

Race—In 1977, the Office of Management and Budget (OMB) issued Race and Ethnic Standards for Federal Statistics and Administrative Reporting to promote comparability of data among federal data systems. The 1977 Standards called for the federal government's data systems to classify individuals into the following four racial groups: American Indian or Alaska Native, Asian or Pacific Islander, Black, and White. Depending on the data source, the classification by race was based on self-classification or on observation by an interviewer or other person filling out the questionnaire.

In 1997, revisions were announced for classification of individuals by race within the federal government's data systems (Revisions to the Standards for the Classification of Federal Data on Race and Ethnicity. Fed Regist 1997 October 30;62:58781–90). The 1997 Standards have five racial groups: American Indian or Alaska Native, Asian, Black or African American, Native Hawaiian or Other Pacific Islander, and White. These five categories are the minimum set for data on race in federal statistics. The 1997 Standards also offer an opportunity for respondents to select more than one of the five groups, leading to many possible multiple-race categories. As with the single-race groups, data for the multiple-race groups are to be reported when estimates meet agency requirements for reliability and confidentiality. The 1997 Standards allow for observer or proxy identification of race but clearly state a preference for self-classification. The federal government considers race and Hispanic origin to be two separate and distinct concepts. Thus, Hispanics may be of any race. Federal data systems were required to comply with the 1997 Standards by 2003.

National Health Interview Survey (NHIS)—Starting with *Health, United States, 2002*, race-specific estimates based on the NHIS were tabulated using the 1997 Standards for data year 1999 and beyond and are not strictly comparable with estimates for earlier years. The 1997 Standards specify five single-race categories plus multiple-race categories. Estimates for specific race groups are shown when they meet requirements for statistical reliability and confidentiality. The race categories White only, Black or African American only, American Indian or Alaska Native only, Asian only, and Native Hawaiian or Other Pacific Islander only include persons who reported only one racial group; the category 2 or more races includes persons who reported more than one of the five racial groups in the 1997 Standards or one of the five racial groups and "some other race." Prior to data year 1999, data were tabulated according to the 1977 Standards with four racial groups, and the Asian only category included Native Hawaiian or Other Pacific Islander. Estimates for single-race categories prior to 1999 included persons who reported one race or, if they reported more than one race, identified one race as best representing their race. Differences between estimates tabulated using the two standards for data year 1999 are discussed in the footnotes for each NHIS table in the *Health, United States, 2002, 2003, and 2004 editions.*

Tables XIII and XIV illustrate NHIS data tabulated by race and Hispanic origin according to the 1997 and 1977 Standards for two health statistics (cigarette smoking and private health insurance coverage). In these illustrations, three separate tabulations using the 1997 Standards are shown: 1) Race: mutually exclusive race groups, including several multiple-race combinations; 2) Race, any mention: race groups that are not mutually exclusive because each race category includes all persons who mention that race; and 3) Hispanic origin and race: detailed race and Hispanic origin with a multiple-race total category. Where applicable, comparison tabulations by race and Hispanic origin are shown based on the 1977 Standards. Because there are more race groups with the 1997 Standards, the sample size of each race group under the 1997 Standards is slightly smaller than the sample size under the 1977 Standards. Only those few multiple-race groups with sufficient numbers of observations to meet standards of statistical reliability are shown. Tables XIII and XIV also illustrate changes in labels and group categories in the 1997 Standards. The race designation of black was changed to Black or African American, and the ethnicity designation of Hispanic was changed to Hispanic or Latino.

Data systems included in *Health, United States,* other than the NHIS, the National Survey of Drug Use & Health (NSDUH), and the National Health and Nutrition Examination Survey (NHANES), generally do not permit tabulation of estimates for the detailed race and ethnicity categories shown in Tables XIII and XIV, either because race data based on the 1997 standard categories are not yet available or because there are insufficient numbers of observations in certain subpopulation groups to meet statistical reliability or confidentiality requirements.

In an effort to improve the quality of data on ethnicity and race in the NHIS, hot-deck imputation of selected race and ethnicity variables was done for the first time in the 2000 NHIS and continued to be used for subsequent data years. Starting with 2003 data, records for persons for whom "other race" was the only race response were treated as having missing data on race, and were added to the pool of records for which selected race and ethnicity variables were imputed. Prior to the 2000 NHIS, a crude imputation method that assigned a race to persons with missing values for the variable MAINRACE (the respondent's classification of the race he or she most identified with) was used. Under these procedures, if an observed race was recorded by the interviewer, it was used to code a race value. If there was no observed race value, all persons who had a missing value for MAINRACE and were identified as Hispanic on the Hispanic origin question were coded as white. In all other cases, non-Hispanic persons were coded as "other race." Additional information on the NHIS methodology for imputing race and ethnicity is available from the survey documentation: www.cdc.gov/nchs/about/major/nhis/quest_data_related_1997_forward.htm and from the NHIS race and Hispanic origin home page at: www.cdc.gov/nchs/about/major/nhis/rhoi/rhoi.htm.

National Health and Nutrition Examination Survey (NHANES)—Starting with *Health, United States, 2003* race-specific estimates based on NHANES were tabulated using the 1997 Standards for data years 1999 and beyond. Prior to data year 1999, the 1977 Standards were used. Because of the differences between the two standards, the race-specific estimates shown in trend tables based on the NHANES for 1999–2004 are not strictly comparable with estimates for earlier years. Race in NHANES I and II was determined primarily by interviewer observation; starting with NHANES III, race was self-reported by survey participants.

The NHANES sample was designed to provide estimates specifically for persons of Mexican origin and not for all Hispanic-origin persons in the United States. Persons of Hispanic origin other than Mexicans were entered into the sample with different selection probabilities that are not nationally representative of the total U.S. Hispanic population. Estimates are shown for non-Hispanic white, non-Hispanic black, and Mexican-origin persons. Although data were collected according to the 1997 Standards, there are insufficient numbers of observations to meet statistical reliability or confidentiality requirements for reporting estimates for additional race categories.

National Survey on Drug Use & Health (NSDUH)—Race-specific estimates based on NSDUH are tabulated using the 1997 Standards. Estimates in the NSDUH trend table begin with the data year 1999. Estimates for specific race groups are shown when they meet requirements for statistical reliability and confidentiality. The race categories White only, Black or African American only, American Indian or Alaska Native only, Asian only, and Native Hawaiian or Other Pacific Islander only include persons who reported only one racial group; and the category 2 or more races includes persons who reported more than one of the five racial groups in the 1997 Standards or one of the five racial groups and "some other race."

Table XIII. Current cigarette smoking among persons 18 years of age and over, by race and Hispanic origin under the 1997 and 1977 Standards for federal data on race and ethnicity: United States, average annual 1993–1995

1997 Standards	*Sample size*	*Percent*	*Standard error*	*1977 Standards*	*Sample size*	*Percent*	*Standard error*
White only	46,228	25.2	0.26	White	46,664	25.3	0.26
Black or African American only	7,208	26.6	0.64	Black	7,334	26.5	0.63
American Indian or Alaska Native only	416	32.9	2.53	American Indian or Alaska Native	480	33.9	2.38
Asian only	1,370	15.0	1.19	Asian or Pacific Islander	1,411	15.5	1.22
2 or more races total	786	34.5	2.00				
Black or African American; white	83	*21.7	6.05				
American Indian or Alaska Native; white	461	40.0	2.58				
Race, any mention							
White, any mention	46,882	25.3	0.26				
Black or African American, any mention	7,382	26.6	0.63				
American Indian or Alaska Native, any mention	965	36.3	1.71				
Asian, any mention	1,458	15.7	1.20				
Native Hawaiian or Other Pacific Islander, any mention	53	*17.5	5.10				
Hispanic origin and race							
Not Hispanic or Latino:				Non-Hispanic:			
White only	42,421	25.8	0.27	White	42,976	25.9	0.27
Black or African American only	7,053	26.7	0.65	Black	7,203	26.7	0.64
American Indian or Alaska Native only	358	33.5	2.69	American Indian or Alaska Native	407	35.4	2.53
Asian only	1,320	14.8	1.21	Asian or Pacific Islander	1,397	15.3	1.24
2 or more races total	687	35.6	2.15				
Hispanic or Latino	5,175	17.8	0.65	Hispanic	5,175	17.8	0.65

* Relative standard error is 20%–30%.

NOTES: The 1997 Standards for the Classification of Federal Data on Race and Ethnicity specified five race groups (white, black or African American, American Indian or Alaska Native, Asian, and Native Hawaiian or Other Pacific Islander) and allow respondents to report one or more race groups. Estimates for single-race and multiple-race groups not shown above do not meet standards for statistical reliability or confidentiality (relative standard error greater than 30%). Race groups under the 1997 Standards were based on the question, What is the group or groups which represents _____ race? For persons who selected multiple groups, race groups under the 1977 Standards were based on the additional question, Which of those groups would you say best represents _____ race? Race-specific estimates in this table were calculated after excluding respondents of other and unknown race. Other published race-specific estimates are based on files in which such responses have been edited. Estimates are age adjusted to the year 2000 standard population using five age groups: 18–24 years, 25–34 years, 35–44 years, 45–64 years, and 65 years and over. See Appendix II, Age adjustment.

SOURCE: Centers for Disease Control and Prevention, National Center for Health Statistics. National Health Interview Survey.

National Vital Statistics System—Most of the states in the Vital Statistics Cooperative Program are still revising their birth and death records to conform to the 1997 standards on race and ethnicity. During the transition to full implementation of the 1997 Standards, vital statistics data will continue to be presented for the four major race groups—White, Black or African American, American Indian or Alaska Native, and Asian or Pacific Islander—in accordance with 1977 Standards.

Birth File—Information about the race and Hispanic ethnicity of the mother and father are provided by the mother at the time of birth and recorded on the birth certificate and fetal death record. Since 1980, birth rates, birth characteristics, and fetal death rates for live-born infants and fetal deaths are presented in this report according to race of mother. Before 1980, data were tabulated by race of newborn and fetus, taking into account the race of both parents. If the parents were of different races and one parent was white, the child was

Table XIV. Private health care coverage among persons under 65 years of age, by race and Hispanic origin under the 1997 and 1977 Standards for federal data on race and ethnicity: United States, average annual 1993–1995

1997 Standards	*Sample size*	*Percent*	*Standard error*	*1977 Standards*	*Sample size*	*Percent*	*Standard error*
White only	168,256	76.1	0.28	White	170,472	75.9	0.28
Black or African American only	30,048	53.5	0.63	Black	30,690	53.6	0.63
American Indian or Alaska Native only	2,003	44.2	1.97	American Indian or Alaska Native	2,316	43.5	1.85
Asian only	6,896	68.0	1.39	Asian and Pacific Islander	7,146	68.2	1.34
Native Hawaiian or Other Pacific Islander only	173	75.0	7.43				
2 or more races total	4,203	60.9	1.17				
Black or African American; white	686	59.5	3.21				
American Indian or Alaska Native; white	2,022	60.0	1.71				
Asian; white	590	71.9	3.39				
Native Hawaiian or Other Pacific Islander; white	56	59.2	10.65				
Race, any mention							
White, any mention	171,817	75.8	0.28				
Black or African American, any mention	31,147	53.6	0.62				
American Indian or Alaska Native, any mention	4,365	52.4	1.40				
Asian, any mention	7,639	68.4	1.27				
Native Hawaiian or Other Pacific Islander, any mention	283	68.7	6.23				
Hispanic origin and race							
Not Hispanic or Latino:				Non-Hispanic:			
White only	146,109	78.9	0.27	White	149,057	78.6	0.27
Black or African American only	29,250	53.9	0.64	Black	29,877	54.0	0.63
American Indian or Alaska Native only	1,620	45.2	2.15	American Indian or Alaska Native	1,859	44.6	2.05
Asian only	6,623	68.2	1.43	Asian and Pacific Islander	6,999	68.4	1.40
Native Hawaiian or Other Pacific Islander only	145	76.4	7.79				
2 or more races total	3,365	62.6	1.18				
Hispanic or Latino	31,040	48.8	0.74	Hispanic	31,040	48.8	0.74

NOTES: The 1997 Standards for the Classification of Federal Data on Race and Ethnicity specified five race groups (white, black or African American, American Indian or Alaska Native, Asian, and Native Hawaiian or Other Pacific Islander) and allow respondents to report one or more race groups. Estimates for single-race and multiple-race groups not shown above do not meet standards for statistical reliability or confidentiality (relative standard error greater than 30%). Race groups under the 1997 Standards were based on the question, "What is the group or groups which represents _____ race?" For persons who selected multiple groups, race groups under the 1977 Standards were based on the additional question, "Which of those groups would you say best represents _____ race?" Race-specific estimates in this table were calculated after excluding respondents of other and unknown race. Other published race-specific estimates are based on files in which such responses have been edited. Estimates are age adjusted to the year 2000 standard population using three age groups: Under 18 years, 18–44 years, and 45–64 years of age. See Appendix II, Age adjustment.

SOURCE: Centers for Disease Control and Prevention, National Center for Health Statistics. National Health Interview Survey.

classified according to the race of the other parent. When neither parent was white, the child was classified according to father's race, with one exception: if either parent was Hawaiian, the child was classified Hawaiian. Before 1964, if race was unknown, the birth was classified as white. Starting in 1964, unknown race was classified according to information on the birth record. Starting with 2000 data, the race and ethnicity data used for denominators (population) to calculate birth rates are collected in accordance with 1997 revised OMB standards for race and ethnicity. However, the numerators (births) will not be compatible with the denominators until all the states revise their birth certificates to reflect the new standards. In order to compute rates, it is necessary to bridge population data for multiple-race persons to single-race categories. See related Appendix I, Population Census and Population Estimates, Bridged-Race Population Estimates for Census 2000.

Starting with 2003 data, multiple-race data were reported by both Pennsylvania and Washington, which used the 2003 revision of the U.S. Standard Certificate of Live Birth, as well as California, Hawaii, Ohio (for births occurring in December only), and Utah, which used the 1989 revision of the U.S. Standard Certificate of Live Birth. In 2004, multiple race was reported on the revised birth certificates of Florida, Idaho, Kentucky, New Hampshire, New York state (excluding New York City), Pennsylvania, South Carolina, Tennessee, and Washington, as well as on the unrevised certificates of California, Hawaii, Michigan, Minnesota, Ohio, and Utah (a total of 15 states). These 15 states, which account for 43% of births in the United States in 2004, reported 3% of the mothers as multiracial. Data from the vital records of the remaining 35 states, New York City, and the District of Columbia followed the 1977 OMB standards in which a single race is reported. In order to provide uniformity and comparability of the data during the transition period, before multiple-race data are available for all reporting areas, it is necessary to bridge the responses of those who reported more than one race to a single race. See Martin JA, Hamilton BE, et al. Births: Final data for 2003. National vital statistics report; vol 54 no 2. Hyattsville, MD: National Center for Health Statistics. 2005. Although the bridging procedure imputes multiple-race of mothers to one of the four minimum races stipulated in the 1977 race and ethnicity standards, mothers of a specified Asian or Pacific Islander (API) subgroup (Chinese, Japanese, Hawaiian, or Filipino) in combination with another race (American Indian or Alaska Native, black, and/or white) or another API subgroup cannot be imputed to a single Asian or Pacific Islander subgroup. In 2003, API mothers were disproportionately represented in the six states reporting multiple-race (44%). Data are not shown for the API subgroups or reported alone or in combination with other races or other API subgroups because the bridging technique cannot be applied in this detail. These data are available in the 2003 Natality public-use data file, which can be found at www.cdc.gov/nchs/births.htm.

Mortality File—Information about the race and Hispanic ethnicity of the decedent is reported by the funeral director as provided by an informant, often the surviving next of kin, or, in the absence of an informant, on the basis of observation. Death rates by race and Hispanic origin are based on information from death certificates (numerators of the rates) and on population estimates from the Census Bureau (denominators). Race and ethnicity information from the census is by self-report. To the extent that race and Hispanic origin are inconsistent between these two data sources, death rates will be biased. Studies have shown that persons self-reported as American Indian, Asian, or Hispanic on census and survey records may sometimes be reported as white or non-Hispanic on the death certificate, resulting in an underestimation of deaths and death rates for the American Indian, Asian, and Hispanic groups. Bias also results from undercounts of some population groups in the census, particularly young black males, young white males, and elderly persons, resulting in an overestimation of death rates. The net effects of misclassification and undercoverage result in overstated death rates for the white population and black population are estimated to be 1% and 5%, respectively; understated death rates for other population groups are estimated as follows: American Indians, 21%; Asian or Pacific Islanders, 11%; and Hispanics, 2%. For more information, see Rosenberg HM, Maurer JD, Sorlie PD, et al. Quality of death rates by race and Hispanic origin: A summary of current research, 1999. National Center for Health Statistics. Vital Health Stat 2(128). 1999.

Denominators for infant and maternal mortality rates are based on number of live births rather than population estimates. Race information for the denominator is supplied from the birth certificate. Before 1980, race of child for the denominator took into account the races of both parents. Starting in 1980, race information for the denominator was based solely on race of mother. Race information for the numerator is supplied from the death certificate. For the infant mortality rate, race information for the numerator is race of the deceased child; for the maternal mortality rate, it is race of the mother.

Vital event rates for the American Indian or Alaska Native population shown in this book are based on the total U.S. resident population of American Indians and Alaska Natives, as enumerated by the U.S. Census Bureau. In contrast, the Indian Health Service calculates vital event rates for this population based on U.S. Census Bureau county data for American Indians and Alaska Natives who reside on or near reservations. Interpretation of trends for the American Indian and Alaska Native population should take into account that population estimates for these groups increased by 45% between 1980 and 1990, partly because of better enumeration techniques in the 1990 decennial census and the increased tendency for people to identify themselves as American Indian in 1990.

Interpretation of trends for the Asian population in the United States should take into account that this population more than doubled between 1980 and 1990, primarily because of immigration. Between 1990 and 2000, the increase in the Asian population was 48% for persons reporting that they were Asian alone, and 72% for persons who reported they were either Asian alone or in combination with another race.

For more information on coding race using vital statistics, see National Center for Health Statistics, Technical Appendix. Vital Statistics of the United States, Vol. I, Natality, and Vol. II, Mortality, Part A. Available from: www.cdc.gov/nchs/nvss.htm.

Youth Risk Behavior Survey (YRBS)—Prior to 1999, the 1977 Standards were used. Respondents could select only one of the following categories: white (not Hispanic), black (not Hispanic), Hispanic or Latino, Asian or Pacific Islander, American Indian or Alaska Native, or other. Beginning in 1999, the 1997 Standards were used for race-specific estimates and respondents were given the option of selecting more than one category to describe their race and ethnicity. Between 1999 and 2003, students were asked a single question about race and Hispanic origin with the option of choosing more than one of the following responses: White, Black or African American, Hispanic or Latino, Asian, Native Hawaiian or Other Pacific Islander, or American Indian or Alaska Native. In 2005, students were asked a question about Hispanic origin (Are you Hispanic or Latino?) and a second separate question about race that included the option of selecting more than one of the following categories: American Indian or Alaska Native, Asian, Black or African American, Native Hawaiian or Other Pacific Islander, or White. Because of the differences between questions, the data about race and Hispanic ethnicity for the years prior to 1999 are not strictly comparable with estimates for the later years. However, analyses of data collected between 1991 and 2003 have indicated that the data are comparable across years and can be used to study trends.

See Brender ND, Kann L, McManus, T. A comparison of two survey questions on race and ethnicity among high school students. Public opinion quarterly. 2003;67(2) 227–236.

See related Hispanic origin; Appendix I, Population Census and Population Estimates.

Rate—A rate is a measure of some event, disease, or condition in relation to a unit of population, along with some specification of time. See related Age adjustment; Population.

- *Birth and related rates*

Birth rate is calculated by dividing the number of live births in a population in a year by the midyear resident population. For census years, rates are based on unrounded census counts of the resident population, as of April 1. For the noncensus years 1981–1989, rates were based on national estimates of the resident population, as of July 1, rounded to 1,000s. Rounded population estimates for 5-year age groups were calculated by summing unrounded population estimates before rounding to 1,000s. Starting in 1991, rates were based on unrounded national population estimates. Beginning in 1997, the birth rate for the maternal age group 45–49 years includes data for mothers age 50–54 years in the numerator and is based on the population of women age 45–49 years in the denominator. Birth rates are expressed as the number of live births per 1,000 population. The rate may be restricted to births to women of specific age, race, marital status, or geographic location (specific rate), or it may be related to the entire population (crude rate).

Fertility rate is the total number of live births, regardless of age of mother, per 1,000 women of reproductive age, 15–44 years.

■ *Death and related rates*

Death rate is calculated by dividing the number of deaths in a population in a year by the midyear resident population. For census years, rates are based on unrounded census counts of the resident population, as of April 1. For the noncensus years 1981–1989, rates were based on national estimates of the resident population, as of July 1, rounded to thousands. Rounded population estimates for 10-year age groups were calculated by summing unrounded population estimates before rounding to 1,000s. Starting in 1991 rates were based on unrounded national population estimates. Rates for the Hispanic and non-Hispanic white populations in each year are based on unrounded state population estimates for states in the Hispanic reporting area. Death rates are expressed as the number of deaths per 100,000 population. The rate may be restricted to deaths in specific age, race, sex, or geographic groups or from specific causes of death (specific rate), or it may be related to the entire population (crude rate).

Birth cohort infant mortality rates are based on linked birth and infant death files. In contrast to period rates in which the births and infant deaths occur in the same period or calendar year, infant deaths constituting the numerator of a birth cohort rate may have occurred in the same year as, or in the year following, the year of birth. The birth cohort infant mortality rate is expressed as the number of infant deaths per 1,000 live births. See related Birth cohort.

Fetal death rate is the number of fetal deaths with stated or presumed gestation of 20 weeks or more divided by the sum of live births plus fetal deaths, per 1,000 live births plus fetal deaths.

Infant mortality rate based on period files is calculated by dividing the number of infant deaths during a calendar year by the number of live births reported in the same year. It is expressed as the number of infant deaths per 1,000 live births. *Neonatal mortality rate* is the number of deaths of children under 28 days of age, per 1,000 live births. *Postneonatal mortality rate* is the number of deaths of children that occur between 28 days and 365 days after birth, per 1,000 live births. See related Infant death.

Late fetal death rate is the number of fetal deaths with stated or presumed gestation of 28 weeks or more divided by the sum of live births plus late fetal deaths, per 1,000 live births plus late fetal deaths. See related Gestation.

Maternal mortality rate is defined as the number of maternal deaths per 100,000 live births. The maternal mortality rate is a measure of the likelihood that a pregnant woman will die from maternal causes. The number of live births used in the denominator is a proxy for the population of pregnant women who are at risk of a maternal death. See related Maternal death.

Perinatal relates to the period surrounding the birth event. Rates and ratios are based on events reported in a calendar year. *Perinatal mortality rate* is the sum of late fetal deaths plus infant deaths within 7 days of birth divided by the sum of live births plus late fetal deaths, per 1,000 live births plus late fetal deaths. *Perinatal mortality ratio* is the sum of late fetal deaths plus infant deaths within 7 days of birth divided by the number of live births, per 1,000 live births.

Visit rate is a basic measure of service utilization for event-based data. Examples of events include physician office visits with drugs provided or hospital discharges. In the visit rate calculation, the numerator is the number of estimated events, and the denominator is the corresponding U.S. population estimate for those who possibly could have had events during a given period of time. The interpretation is that for every person in the population there were, on average, *x* events. It does not mean that *x* percentage of the population had events, because some persons in the population had no events while others had multiple events. The only exception is when an event can occur just once for a person (e.g., if an appendectomy were performed during a hospital stay). The visit rate is best used to compare utilization across various subgroups of interest such as age or race groups or geographic regions (e.g., the rate of hospital discharges in 2002 was 43.4 per 1,000 population for children under 18 years of age and 466.6 per 1,000 population for adults 75 years and over).

Region—See Geographic region and division.

Registered hospital—See Hospital.

Registration area—The United States has separate registration areas for birth, death, marriage, and divorce statistics. In general, registration areas correspond to states and include two separate registration areas for the District of Columbia (D.C.) and New York City. The term reporting area may be used interchangeably for the term registration area. All states have adopted laws that require registration of births and deaths and reporting of fetal deaths. It is believed that more than 99% of births and deaths occurring in this country are registered.

The death registration area was established in 1900 with 10 states and D.C., and the birth registration area was established in 1915, also with 10 states and D.C. Beginning in 1933, all states were included in the birth and death registration areas. The specific states added year by year are shown in History and Organization of the Vital Statistics System. Reprinted from Vital Statistics of the United States Vol. I, 1950, chapter 1. National Center for Health Statistics, 1978. Currently, Puerto Rico, U.S. Virgin Islands, and Guam each constitutes a separate registration area, although their data are not included in statistical tabulations of U.S. resident data. See related Reporting area.

Relative standard error—The relative standard error (RSE) is a measure of an estimate's reliability. The RSE of an estimate is obtained by dividing the standard error of the estimate (SE(r)) by the estimate itself (r). This quantity is expressed as a percentage of the estimate and is calculated as follows: RSE = 100 x (SE(r)/r). Estimates with large RSEs are considered unreliable. In *Health, United States*, most statistics with large RSEs are preceded by an asterisk or are not presented.

Relative survival rate—The relative survival rate is the ratio of the observed survival rate for the patient group to the expected survival rate for persons in the general population similar to the patient group with respect to age, sex, race, and calendar year of observation. The 5-year relative survival rate is used to estimate the proportion of cancer patients potentially curable. Because over one-half of all cancers occur in persons 65 years of age and over, many of these individuals die of other causes with no evidence of recurrence of their cancer. Thus, because it is obtained by adjusting observed survival for the normal life expectancy of the general population of the same age, the relative survival rate is an estimate of the chance of surviving the effects of cancer.

Reporting area—In the National Vital Statistics System, the reporting area for such basic items on the birth and death certificates as age, race, and sex is based on data from residents of all 50 states in the United States, the District of Columbia (D.C), and New York City (NYC). The term reporting area may be used interchangeably for the term registration area. The reporting area for selected items such as Hispanic origin, educational attainment, and marital status is based on data from those states that require the item to be reported, whose data meet a minimum level of completeness (such as 80% or 90%), and are considered to be sufficiently comparable to be used for analysis. In 1993–1996, the reporting area for Hispanic origin of decedent on the death certificate included 49 states and D.C. Starting in 1997, the Hispanic reporting area includes all 50 states and D.C. See related Registration area; Appendix I, National Vital Statistics System.

Resident, health facility—In the Online Survey Certification and Reporting database, all residents in certified facilities are counted on the day of certification inspection. In the National Nursing Home Survey, a resident is a person on the roster of the nursing home as of the night before the survey. Included are all residents for whom beds are maintained even though they may be on overnight leave or in a hospital. See related Nursing home.

Resident population—See Population.

Residential treatment care—See Mental health service type.

Residential treatment center for emotionally disturbed children—See Mental health organization.

Rural—See Urbanization.

Self-assessment of health—See Health status, respondent-assessed.

Serious psychological distress—The K6 instrument is a measure of psychological distress associated with unspecified but potentially diagnosable mental illness that may result in a higher risk for disability and higher utilization of health services. The K6 was asked of adults 18 years of age and older. The K6 is designed to identify persons with serious psychological distress using as few questions as possible. The six items included in the K6 are as follows:

During the past 30 days, how often did you feel:

So sad that nothing could cheer you up?
Nervous?
Restless or fidgety?
Hopeless?
That everything was an effort?
Worthless?

Possible answers are all of the time (4 points), most of the time (3 points), some of the time (2 points), a little of the time (1 point), and none of the time (0 points).

To score the K6, the points are added together yielding a possible total of 0 to 24 points. A threshold of 13 or more is used to define serious psychological distress. Persons answering some of the time to all six questions would not reach the threshold for serious psychological distress, because to achieve a score of 13 they would need to answer most of the time to at least one item.

For more information, see Kessler RC, Barker PR, Colpe LJ, et al. Screening for serious mental illness in the general population. Arch Gen Psychiatry 2003; 60:184–189.

Short-stay hospital—See Hospital.

Skilled nursing facility—See Nursing home.

Smoker—See Cigarette smoking.

Specialty hospital—See Hospital.

State Children's Health Insurance Program (SCHIP)—Title XXI of the Social Security Act, known as the State Children's Health Insurance Program (SCHIP), is a program initiated by the Balanced Budget Act of 1997 (BBA). SCHIP provides more federal funds for states to provide health care coverage to low-income, uninsured children. SCHIP gives states broad flexibility in program design while protecting beneficiaries through federal standards. Funds from SCHIP may be used to expand Medicaid or to provide medical assistance to children during a presumptive eligibility period for Medicaid. This is one of several options from which states may select to provide health care coverage for more children, as prescribed within the BBA's Title XXI program. See related Health insurance coverage; Medicaid.

State mental health agency—Refers to the agency or department within state government, headed by the state or territorial health official, dealing with mental health issues. Generally, the state mental health agency is responsible for setting statewide mental health priorities, carrying out national and state mandates, responding to mental health hazards, and assuring access to mental health care for underserved state residents.

Substance use—refers to the use of selected substances including alcohol, tobacco products, drugs, inhalants, and other substances that can be consumed, inhaled, injected, or otherwise absorbed into the body with possible detrimental effects.

The Monitoring the Future Study (MTF)—The MTF collects information on use of selected substances using self-completed questionnaires to a school-based survey of secondary school students. MTF has tracked 12th graders' illicit drug use and attitudes towards drugs since 1975. In 1991, 8th and 10th graders were added to the study. The survey includes questions on abuse of substances including (but not limited to) marijuana, inhalants, illegal drugs, alcohol, cigarettes, and other tobacco products. A standard set of three questions is used to assess use of the substances in the past month. Past month refers to an individual's use of a substance at least once during the month preceding their response to the survey. See related Appendix I, Monitoring the Future Study.

National Survey on Drug Use & Health (NSDUH)—The NSDUH conducts in-person interviews of a sample of individuals 12 years of age and older at their place of residence. For illicit drug use, alcohol use, and tobacco use, information is collected about use in past month. For information on illicit drug use, respondents in the NSDUH are asked about use of marijuana/hashish, cocaine (including crack), inhalants, hallucinogens, heroin, and prescription-type drugs used nonmedically (pain relievers, tranquilizers, stimulants, and sedatives). A series of questions is asked about each substance: "Have you ever, even once, used [e.g., Ecstasy, also known as MDMA/substance]?" "Think specifically about the past 30 days, from [date] up to and including today. During the past 30 days, on how many days did you use [substance]?" Numerous probes and checks are included in the computer-assisted interview system.
Nonprescription medications and legitimate uses under a doctor's supervision are not included in the survey.
Summary measures, such as, any illicit drug use, are

produced. See related Alcohol consumption; Cigarette smoking; Illicit drug use; Appendix I, National Survey on Drug Use & Health.

Suicidal ideation—Suicidal ideation is having thoughts of suicide or of taking action to end one's own life. Suicidal ideation includes all thoughts of suicide, both when the thoughts include a plan to commit suicide and when they do not include a plan. Suicidal ideation is measured in the Youth Risk Behavior Survey by the question "During the past 12 months, did you ever seriously consider attempting suicide?"

Surgery—See Outpatient surgery; Procedure.

Surgical specialty—See Physician specialty.

Tobacco use—See Cigarette smoking.

Uninsured—In the Current Population Survey (CPS) persons are considered uninsured if they do not have coverage through private health insurance, Medicare, Medicaid, State Children's Health Insurance Program, military or Veterans coverage, another government program, a plan of someone outside the household, or other insurance. Persons with only Indian Health Service coverage are considered uninsured. In addition, if the respondent has missing Medicaid information but has income from certain low-income public programs, then Medicaid coverage is imputed. The questions on health insurance are administered in March and refer to the previous calendar year.

In the National Health Interview Survey (NHIS), the uninsured are persons who do not have coverage under private health insurance, Medicare, Medicaid, public assistance, a state-sponsored health plan, other government-sponsored programs, or a military health plan. Persons with only Indian Health Service coverage are considered uninsured. Estimates of the percentage of persons who are uninsured based on the NHIS (Table 139) may differ slightly from those based on the March CPS (Table 151) because of differences in survey questions, recall period, and other aspects of survey methodology. Estimates for the uninsured are shown only for the population under age 65.

Survey respondents may be covered by health insurance at the time of the interview, but may have experienced one or more lapses in coverage during the year prior to the interview. Starting in *Health United States, 2006*, NHIS estimates for people with health insurance coverage for all 12 months prior to the interview, for those who were uninsured for any period up to 12 months, and for those who were uninsured for more than 12 months were added as stub variables to selected tables. See related Health insurance coverage; Appendix I, Current Population Survey.

Urbanization—Urbanization is the degree of urban (city-like) character of a particular geographic area. Urbanization can be measured in a variety of ways. In this report, the two measures used to categorize counties by urbanization level are the Office of Management and Budget's (OMB) metropolitan statistical area (MSA) classification and the 2006 NCHS Urban-Rural Classification Scheme for Counties. For more information on the OMB classification of counties, see related Metropolitan statistical area (MSA); Micropolitan statistical area.

The 2006 NCHS Urban-Rural Classification Scheme for Counties is a six-level classification scheme developed by NCHS to categorize the 3,141 U.S. counties and county-equivalents based on their urban and rural characteristics. The classification scheme includes four metropolitan (or urban) categories and two nonmetropolitan (or rural) categories. The county classifications are based on the following information: (1) the 2003 OMB definitions of metropolitan and nonmetropolitan counties (with revisions through 2005); (2) the 2003 Rural-Urban Continuum Codes developed by the Economic Research Service of the U.S. Department of Agriculture; (3) 2004 postcensal county population estimates; and (4) county-level data on several settlement density, socioeconomic, and demographic variables from Census 2000. The six categories of the 2006 NCHS Urban-Rural Classification Scheme for Counties are large central metro (central counties of metro areas of 1 million or more population), large fringe metro (outlying counties of metro areas of 1 million or more population), medium metro (metro areas of 250,000 to 999,999 population), small metro (metro areas of 50,000 to 249,000 population), nonmetropolitan micropolitan, and nonmetropolitan noncore. For more information on this classification scheme, see www.cdc.gov/nchs/r&d/rdc_urbanrural.htm.

Usual source of care—Usual source of care was measured in the National Health Interview Survey (NHIS) in 1993 and 1994 by asking the respondent "Is there a particular person or place that ____ usually goes to when ____ is sick or needs advice about ___ health?" In the 1995 and 1996 NHIS, the respondent was asked "Is there one doctor, person, or place that ____ usually goes to when ____ is sick or needs advice about health?" Starting in 1997 the respondent was asked "Is there a place that ____ usually goes when he/she is sick or you need advice about (his/her) health?" Persons who report the emergency department as their usual source of care are defined as having no usual source of care in this report.

Wages and salaries—See Employer costs for employee compensation.

Years of potential life lost (YPLL)—YPLL is a measure of premature mortality. Starting with *Health, United States, 1996–1997*, YPLL is presented for persons under 75 years of age because the average life expectancy in the United States is over 75 years. YPLL-75 is calculated using the following eight age groups: under 1 year, 1–14 years, 15–24 years, 25–34 years, 35–44 years, 45–54 years, 55–64 years, and 65–74 years. The number of deaths for each age group is multiplied by years of life lost, calculated as the difference between age 75 years and the midpoint of the age group. For the eight age groups, the midpoints are 0.5, 7.5, 19.5, 29.5, 39.5, 49.5, 59.5, and 69.5. For example, the death of a person 15–24 years of age counts as 55.5 years of life lost. Years of potential life lost is derived by summing years of life lost over all age groups. In *Health, United States, 1995* and earlier editions, YPLL was presented for persons under 65 years of age. For more information, see Centers for Disease Control. MMWR 35(2S):suppl. 1986. Available from: www.cdc.gov/mmwr/preview/mmwrhtml/00001773.htm.

Appendix III

Additional Data Years Available

For trend tables spanning long periods, only selected data years are shown to highlight major trends. Additional years of data are available for some of the tables in electronic spreadsheets available through the Internet and on CD-ROM.

To access spreadsheet files on the Internet, go to the *Health, United States* website at www.cdc.gov/nchs/hus.htm, scroll down to "Spreadsheet Files," and click on 2007 Edition.

Downloadable spreadsheet files for trend tables, many of which include more data years than are shown in the printed report, are available in Excel. Standard errors are included in spreadsheet files for trend tables based on the National Health Interview Survey (NHIS), National Health and Nutrition Examination Survey (NHANES), and National Survey of Family Growth (NSFG).

Spreadsheet files in Excel are also available on a CD-ROM. A limited supply of CD-ROMs are available from the National Center for Health Statistics upon request, while supplies last, or CD-ROMs may be purchased from the Government Printing Office.

Table number	Table topic	Additional data years available
1	Resident population	2001–2002
2	Inmates in state or federal prisons and local jails	2001–2002
3	Poverty	1986–1989, 1991–1994, 1996–1999, 2001–2002
4	Fertility rates and birth rates	1981–1984, 1986–1989, 1991–1994, 1996–1999, 2001
5	Live births	1972–1974, 1976–1979, 1981–1984, 1986–1989, 1991–1994, 1996–1999, 2001–2002
6	Twin births	1972–1974, 1976–1979, 1981–1984, 1986–1989, 1991–1994, 1996, 1998–1999, 2001
7	Prenatal care	1981–1984, 1986–1989, 1991–1994, 1996–1999, 2001
9	Teenage childbearing	1981–1984, 1986–1989, 1991–1994, 1996–1999
10	Nonmarital childbearing	1981–1984, 1986–1989, 1991–1994, 1996–1999
11	Maternal education	1981–1984, 1986–1989, 1991–1994, 1996–1999, 2001
12	Maternal smoking	1991–1994, 1996–1999, 2001
13	Low birthweight	1981–1984, 1986–1989, 1991–1994, 1996–1998, 2001
14	Low birthweight	1991–1994, 1996–1999, 2001
16	Abortions	1981–1984, 1986–1989, 1991–1994, 1996–1998
18	Breastfeeding	1972–1974
19	Infant mortality rates	1996–1999, 2001, 1996–1998, 1997–1999, 1998–2000, 2000–2002, 2001–2003
20	Infant mortality rates	1984, 1986–1989, 1991, 1996–1999, 2001
21	Infant mortality rates	1984, 1986–1989, 1991, 1996–1999, 2001
22	Infant mortality rates	1981–1989, 1991–1994, 1996–1997
25	International mortality rates and rankings	2001, ranking 2003
26	International life expectancy	1999, 2001, ranking 2002
27	Life expectancy	1975, 1981–1989, 1991–1994
29	Age-adjusted death rates for selected causes	1981–1989, 1991–1999, 2001
30	Years of potential life lost	1991–1999 2001, crude 1999–2003
35	Death rates for all causes	1981–1989, 1991–1999, 2001–2002
36	Diseases of heart	1981–1989, 1991–1999, 2001–2002
37	Cerebrovascular diseases	1981–1989, 1991–1999, 2001–2002
38	Malignant neoplasms	1981–1989, 1991–1999, 2001–2002
39	Malignant neoplasms of trachea, bronchus, and lung	1981–1989, 1991–1999, 2001–2002
40	Malignant neoplasm of breast	1981–1989, 1991–1999, 2001–2002
41	Chronic lower respiratory diseases	1981–1989, 1991–1994, 1996–1999, 2001
42	Human immunodeficiency virus (HIV) disease	1988–1989, 1991–1994, 1996–1999, 2001

Table number	Table topic	Additional data years available
43	Maternal mortality	1981–1989, 1991–1999, 2001
44	Motor vehicle-related injuries	1981–1989, 1991–1999, 2001–2002
45	Homicide	1981–1989, 1991–1999, 2001–2002
46	Suicide	1981–1989, 1991–1999, 2001–2002
47	Firearm-related injuries	1981–1989, 1991–1994, 1996–1999, 2001
48	Occupational diseases	1981–1984, 1986–1989, 1991–1994, 1996–1999, 2001
49	Occupational injury deaths	1993–1994, 1996–1998
51	Notifiable diseases	1985, 1988–1989, 1991–1999, 2001–2002
53	Cancer incidence rates	1991–1994, 1996–1998
54	Five-year relative cancer survival rates	1978–1980, 1984–1986
55	Diabetes	1999–2002
56	Severe headache or migraine, low back pain, and neck pain	1998–2003
57	Joint pain	2003
58	Limitation of activity	1999–2002
59	Vision and hearing limitations	1998–1999, 2001–2002
60	Respondent-assessed health status	1998–1999, 2001
61	Serious psychological distress	1998–1999, 1999–2000, 2001–2002, 2003–2004
63	Cigarette smoking	1983, 1987–1988, 1991–1994, 1997–1999
64	Cigarette smoking	1983, 1987–1988, 1991–1994, 1997–1999
65	Cigarette smoking	1993–1995, 1994–1997, 2002–2004
66	Use of selected substances	2003
67	Use of selected substances	1981–1989, 1992–1994, 1996–1999, 2001–2002
68	Alcohol consumption	1998–2002
70	Hypertension (elevated blood pressure)	1999–2002
71	Serum cholesterol levels	1999–2002
73	Leisure-time physical activity	1999, 2000–2003
74	Overweight, obesity, and healthy weight	1999–2002
75	Overweight among children and adolescents	1999–2002
76	Untreated dental caries	1999–2000, 1999–2002
77	No usual source of health care	1995–1996, 1997–1998, 1999–2000
79	Reduced access to medical care	1998–2003
81	No heath care visits	1999–2000, 2003–2004
82	Health care visits	1998–2003
83	Vaccinations	1996–1999
84	Vaccination coverage among children	1996–1997
85	Influenza vaccination	1991, 1993–1994, 1997–1999
86	Pneumococcal vaccination	1991, 1993–1994, 1997–1999
87	Mammography	1993–1994
89	Emergency department visits for children	1998–2003
90	Emergency department visits for adults	1998–1999, 2001–2003
91	Injury-related visits	1997–1998, 1998–1999, 2000–2001, 2001–2002, 2002–2003, 2003–2004
92	Ambulatory care visits	1997–1999, 2001–2002, 2004
93	Ambulatory care visits	1997–1999, 2001–2004
94	Dental visits	1998–2003
96	Prescription drug use	1999–2000
97	Additions to mental health organizations	1992, 1994, 1998, 2000
98	Discharges	1998–2003
99	Discharges	1991–1994, 1996–1999, 2001
100	Rates of discharges	1995–1999, 2001–2004

Table number	Table topic	Additional data years available
101	Discharges	1995–1999, 2001–2004
102	Inpatient procedures	1991–1992, 1992–1993, 1993–1994, 2001–2002, 2002–2003, 2003–2004
104	Nursing home residents	1997
106	Active physicians and doctors of medicine	2002–2003
107	Physicians	1970, 1980, 1987, 1989–1990, 1992–1994, 1996–1999, 2001
108	Primary care doctors of medicine	1994, 1996–1999, 2001, 2003
109	Employees and wages	2001–2003
110	Health professions schools	1996, 1998–1999, 2001–2004
111	Total enrollment of minorities in schools	2000–2001, 2001–2002, 2002–2003, 2003–2004
112	Enrollment of women in schools	2000–2001, 2001–2002, 2002–2003, 2004–2005
114	Mental health organizations	1992
117	Nursing homes	1996–1999, 2001–2004
118	Medicare-certified providers and suppliers	1975, 1996, 1998, 2001, 2003
126	Expenditures for mental health services	1987–1989, 1991–1994, 1996–1999, 2001
127	Expenditures for substance abuse treatment	1987–1989, 1991–1994, 1996–1999, 2001
128	Expenditures for health care	1996, 1998–1999, 2001–2003
129	Sources of payment for health care	1996, 1998–1999, 2001–2003
130	Out-of-pocket health care expenses	1998–1999
132	Employers' costs and health insurance	1992–1993, 1995, 1997, 1999, 2001
134	Nursing home average monthly charges	1997, 1999
135	Mental health expenditures	1992
136	Private health insurance	1994, 1996, 1998–1999
137	Private health insurance	1994, 1996, 1998–1999
138	Medicaid coverage	1994, 1996, 1998–1999, 2001
139	No health insurance coverage	1994, 1996, 1998–1999, 2001
140	Health care coverage	1993–1994, 1996–1999, 2001–2003
142	Medicare	1996
143	Medicare	All: 1999–2002, 1993–2002
144	Medicaid	1975, 1985–1989, 1991–1994, 1996–1999
145	Medicaid	1975, 1985–1989, 1991–1994, 1996–1999
146	Department of Veterans Affairs	1985, 1988–1989, 1991–1994, 1996–1999, 2001
147	State mental health agency per capita expenditures	1983, 1987, 2002
148	Medicare	1995–2003
149	Medicaid	1998, 2000–2001, 2003
150	Health maintenance organizations	1994, 1996–1997, 1999, 2001–2004

Index to Trend Tables

(Numbers refer to table numbers)

A

Table

Abortion 16
Access to care (see also Burden of expenditures; Delayed medical care; Dental visits; Drugs prescribed during medical visits; Emergency department visits; Health insurance; Hospital utilization; Physician supply; Transportation; Undiagnosed medical conditions; Unmet need)
  Health care visits, all persons 82
  No recent health care visit, children 81
  No usual source of care 77, 78
  Special Feature on Access to Health Care . . . . . Figures 21–36
Accidents, see Motor vehicle-related injuries; Unintentional injuries.
Activities of Daily Living (ADL), see Limitation of activity.
ADHD (Attention deficit/hyperactivity disorder) . . . . Figure 14
Adolescents, see Child and adolescent health.
AIDS, see HIV/AIDS.
Alcohol consumption 66, 67, 68
Alzheimer's disease 31, 32
Ambulatory surgery centers, Medicare certified 118
American Indian or Alaska Native population
  Access to care 77, 78, 79, 81, 82
  AIDS cases 52
  Alcohol consumption 66, 68
  Back pain, low 56
  Birth rates 4, 6, 10
  Births, number 5
  Birthweight, low 13, 14, 15
  Cancer incidence rates 53
  Cigarette smoking 12, 65, 66
  Death rates, all causes 28, 29, 35
  Death rates, geographic division and state 28
  Death rates, selected causes 29, 36, 37, 38, 39, 40, 41, 42, 43, 44, 45, 46, 47
  Deaths, leading causes 31
  Dental visits 94
  Education of mother 11, 14, 20
  Emergency department visits 89, 90
  Headache, severe or migraine 56
  Health insurance 136, 137, 138, 139
  Health status, respondent-assessed 60
  Hearing trouble 59
  Hospital utilization, inpatient 98
  Illicit drug use 66
  Infant mortality 19, 20, 23, 24
  Joint pain 57
  Limitation of activity 58

A—Con.

Table

American Indian or Alaska Native population—Con.
  Mammography 87
  Maternal mortality 43
  Neck pain 56
  Occupational injury deaths 49
  Pap smear 88
  Physical activity 73
  Population, resident . . . . . 1, Figure 3
  Prenatal care 7, 8
  Serious psychological distress 61
  Smoking status of mother 12
  Students, health occupations 111
  Teenage childbearing 4, 9
  Twin, triplet, and higher order multiple births 5, 6
  Unmarried mothers 10
  Unmet need 79
  Vaccinations 83, 85, 86
  Vision trouble 59
  Years of potential life lost 30
Antidepressant drugs . . . . . Figure 36
Asian or Pacific Islander population
  Access to care . . . . . 77, 78, 79, 81, 82, Figure 30
  AIDS cases 52
  Alcohol consumption 66, 68
  Back pain, low 56
  Births, number 5
  Birthweight, low 13, 14, 15
  Cancer incidence rates 53
  Cigarette smoking 12, 65, 66
  Death rates, all causes 28, 29, 35
  Death rates, geographic division and state 28
  Death rates, selected causes 29, 36, 37, 38, 39, 40, 41, 42, 43, 44, 45, 46, 47
  Deaths, leading causes 31
  Dental visits 94
  Education of mother 11, 14, 20
  Emergency department visits 89, 90
  Headache, severe or migraine 56
  Health insurance . . . . . 136, 137, 138, 139, 140, Figures 29, 30
  Health status, respondent-assessed 60
  Hearing trouble 59
  Hospital utilization, inpatient 98
  Illicit drug use 66
  Infant mortality 19, 23, 24
  Joint pain 57

A—Con.

Table

Asian or Pacific Islander population—Con.
- Kidney transplant . . . . Figures 24, 25
- Limitation of activity 58
- Mammography 87
- Maternal mortality 43
- Neck pain 56
- Occupational injury deaths 49
- Pap smear 88
- Physical activity 73
- Population, resident . . . . 1, Figure 3
- Poverty . . . . 3, Figure 5
- Prenatal care 7, 8
- Serious psychological distress 61
- Smoking status of mother 12
- Students, health occupations 111
- Teenage childbearing 4, 9
- Twin, triplet, and higher order multiple births 5, 6
- Unmarried mothers 10
- Unmet need 79
- Vaccinations 83, 85, 86
- Vision trouble 59
- Years of potential life lost 30

Asian subgroups (Chinese; Filipino; Hawaiian; Japanese)
- Birth rates 6, 10
- Births, number 5
- Birthweight, low 13, 14
- Education of mother 11, 14
- Infant mortality 19
- Prenatal care 7
- Smoking status of mother 12
- Teenage childbearing 9
- Twin, triplet, and higher order multiple births 5, 6
- Unmarried mothers 10

Atherosclerosis 31

B

Back pain, low 56

Bed, health facility 117, 133, 134

Birth control, see Contraception.

Births
- Age of mother 4, 10, 12
- Birth rates 4, 6, 10
- Births, number 5, 10
- Birthweight, low 13, 14, 15
- Education of mother 11, 12, 14
- Fertility rates 4
- Geographic division and state 15
- Hospital discharges 100, 101
- Prenatal care 7, 8
- Smoking status of mother . . . . 12, 13, Figure 9

B—Con.

Table

Births—Con.
- Teenage childbearing 9
- Twin, triplet, and higher order multiple births 5, 6
- Unmarried mothers 10

Black or African American population
- Abortion 16
- Access to care . . . . 77, 78, 79, 81, 82, Figures 26, 29, 30, 35, 36
- AIDS cases 52
- Alcohol consumption 66, 67, 68
- Antidepressant drugs . . . . Figure 36
- Back pain, low 56
- Birth rates 4, 6, 10
- Births, number 5
- Birthweight, low 13, 14, 15
- Breastfeeding 18
- Cancer incidence rates 53
- Cancer survival, 5-year relative 54
- Cholesterol, serum 71
- Cigarette smoking 12, 63, 64, 65, 66, 67
- Cocaine use 67
- Colorectal scope procedures . . . . Figure 35
- Contraception 17
- Death rates, all causes 28, 33, 35
- Death rates, geographic division and state 28
- Death rates, selected causes 29, 36, 37, 38, 39, 40, 41, 42, 43, 44, 45, 46, 47
- Death rates, urbanization 33
- Deaths, leading causes 31
- Dental caries (cavities), untreated 76
- Dental visits 94, 143
- Diabetes 55
- Drugs, prescription, use in past month 96
- Education of mother 11, 14, 20
- Emergency department visits 89, 90, 92
- Expenses, health care 128
- Fetal mortality 22
- Headache, severe or migraine 56
- Health insurance . . . . 136, 137, 139, 140, Figures 29, 30
- Health status, respondent-assessed 60
- Hearing trouble 59
- Hospital utilization, inpatient 98, 143
- Hospital utilization, outpatient department 92, 143
- Hypertension 70
- Illicit drug use 66, 67
- Infant mortality 19, 20, 22, 23, 24
- Inhalants 67
- Inmates, prisons and jails 2
- Joint pain 57
- Kidney transplant . . . . Figures 24, 25
- Life expectancy . . . . 27, Figure 18

B—Con.

Table

Black or African American population—Con.
- Limitation of activity . . . 58
- Mammography . . . 87
- Marijuana use . . . 66, 67
- Maternal mortality . . . 43
- Medicaid . . . 129, 138, 140, 144
- Medicare . . . 129, 140, 143
- Neck pain . . . 56
- Nursing home utilization . . . 104
- Occupational injury deaths . . . 49
- Out-of-pocket health care expenditures . . . 128, 129
- Overweight and obesity . . . 74, 75
- Pap smear . . . 88
- Physical activity . . . 73
- Population, resident . . . 1, Figure 3
- Poverty . . . 3, Figures 5, 35
- Prenatal care . . . 7, 8
- Serious psychological distress . . . 61
- Smoking status of mother . . . 12
- Students, health occupations . . . 111
- Suicidal ideation, suicide attempts . . . 62
- Teenage childbearing . . . 4, 9
- Twin, triplet, and higher order multiple births . . . 5, 6
- Unmarried mothers . . . 10
- Unmet need . . . 79
- Vaccinations . . . 83, 85, 86
- Vision trouble . . . 59
- Years of potential life lost (YPLL) . . . 30

Blood cotinine levels . . . Figure 10

Blood pressure, elevated, see Hypertension.

Breastfeeding . . . 18

Burden of expenditures . . . Figure 31

C

Calories, see Energy and macronutrient intake.

Cancer (Malignant neoplasms)
- Breast . . . 29, 30, 40, 53, 54, 100, 101
- Deaths and death rates . . . 29, 31, 32, 38, 39, 40, Figure 20
- Hospital discharges . . . 100, 101
- Incidence rates . . . 53
- Site-specific data . . . 29, 30, 39, 40, 53, 54, 100, 101
- Survival, 5-year relative . . . 54
- Trachea, bronchus, lung . . . 29, 39, 53, 54, 100, 101
- Years of potential life lost . . . 30

Cardiac procedures, see Heart disease, procedures.

Central and South American population, see Hispanic subgroups.

C—Con.

Table

Cerebrovascular disease (stroke)
- Deaths and death rates . . . 29, 31, 32, 37, Figure 20
- Hospital discharges . . . 100, 101
- Years of potential life lost . . . 30

Cesarean section . . . 102

Chancroid, see Diseases, notifiable.

Child and adolescent health
- Abortion . . . 16
- Access to care . . . 77, 81, 82
- AIDS cases . . . 52
- Alcohol consumption . . . 66, 67, Figure 11
- Birthweight . . . 13, 14, 15
- Blood cotinine levels . . . Figure 10
- Breastfeeding . . . 18
- Cigarette smoking . . . 66, 67, Figure 9
- Cocaine use . . . 67
- Contraception . . . 17
- Death rates, all causes . . . 35
- Death rates, selected causes . . . 41, 42, 44, 45, 46, 47
- Deaths, leading causes . . . 32
- Dental caries (cavities), untreated . . . 69
- Dental visits . . . 94, Figure 34
- Drugs, during physician and hospital outpatient department visits . . . 95
- Drugs, prescription, use in past month . . . 96
- Emergency department visits . . . 89, 91, 92, Figure 11
- Expenses, health care . . . 128, 130
- Health insurance . . . 136, 137, 138, 139, Figures 29, 30
- Health status, respondent-assessed . . . 60
- Hospital utilization, inpatient . . . 98, 99, 100, 101
- Hospital utilization, outpatient department . . . 92
- Illicit drug use . . . 66, 67
- Infant mortality . . . 19, 20, 21, 22, 23, 24, 25, Figure 19
- Inhalants . . . 67
- Injury . . . 91
- Limitation of activity . . . 58, Figure 14
- Marijuana use . . . 66, 67
- Medicaid . . . 129, 138, 144
- Out-of-pocket health care expenditures . . . 128, 129, 130
- Overweight . . . 69, 75, Figure 13
- Population, resident . . . 1, Figure 3
- Poverty . . . 3, Figures 4, 5
- Residential treatment centers for emotionally disturbed children . . . 97, 114
- Restaurant meal consumption . . . Figure 12
- Suicidal ideation, suicide attempts . . . 62
- Teenage childbearing . . . 4, 9
- Vaccinations . . . 83, 84

C—Con.

Table

Chinese population, see Asian subgroups.
Chiropractors 105
Chlamydia, see Diseases, notifiable.
Cholesterol, serum . . . . . 69, 71, Figure 32
Chronic liver disease and cirrhosis . . . . . 29, 30, 31, 32, Figure 20
Chronic lower respiratory diseases
- Deaths and death rates . . . . . 29, 31, 32, 41, Figure 20
- Years of potential life lost 30

Cigarette smoking (see also Births, smoking status of mother) . . . . . 63, 64, 65, 66, 67, Figure 9
Cirrhosis, see Chronic liver disease and cirrhosis.
Citizenship, see Foreign-born population.
Cocaine use 67
Colorectal scope procedures . . . . . Figure 35
Communicable diseases (see also Diseases, notifiable) 34
Computed Tomography (CT) scanners (see also Magnetic Resonance Imaging (MRI) units) 119
Congenital anomalies 31, 32
Consumer Price Index (CPI) 122
Contraception 17
Cost, see Employers' costs.
Cuban population, see Hispanic subgroups.

D

Deaths, death rates (see also Cancer (malignant neoplasms); Cerebrovascular disease (stroke); Chronic lower respiratory diseases; Diabetes; Firearm-related injuries; Heart disease; HIV/AIDS; Homicide; Infant mortality; Life expectancy; Maternal mortality; Motor vehicle-related injuries; Occupational diseases deaths; Occupational injuries; Suicide; Years of potential life lost (YPLL))
- All causes 35
- Educational attainment 34
- Leading causes . . . . . 31, 32, Figure 20
- Selected causes 29
- State 28
- Urbanization 33

Delayed medical care
- Due to cost 79, 80
- Transportation . . . . . Figure 27

Dental caries (cavities), untreated 76
Dental visits . . . . . 94, 143, Figures 21, 34
Dentists 105, 110, 111, 112
Diabetes . . . . . 29, 30, 31, 32, 55, 69, 100, 101, Figure 26
- Deaths and death rates 29, 31, 32
- Drugs prescribed during medical visits 95
- Hospital discharges 100, 101
- Prevalence 55
- Years of potential life lost (YPLL) 30

D—Con.

Table

Diagnostic procedures, during hospitalizations 102
Diphtheria, see Diseases, notifiable; Vaccinations.
Disability
- Blind and disabled Medicaid expenditures 144
- Limitation of activity 58
- Medicare beneficiaries 143
- Veterans with service-connected disabilities 146

Diseases, notifiable 51
Doctors of medicine, see Physicians
Drug use, illicit, see Alcohol consumption; Cigarette smoking; Cocaine use; Illicit drug use; Inhalants; Marijuana use.
Drugs prescribed during medical visits 95
Drugs, prescription, use in past month 96
DTP (Diphtheria, Tetanus, Pertussis), see Vaccinations.

E

Education
- Alcohol consumption 67
- Back pain, low 56
- Births 11, 12, 14
- Breastfeeding 18
- Cigarette smoking 64, 65, 67
- Cocaine use 67
- Colorectal scope procedures . . . . . Figure 35
- Death rates 34
- Headache, severe or migraine 56
- Hearing trouble 59
- Infant mortality 20
- Inhalants 67
- Joint pain 57
- Mammography 87
- Marijuana use 67
- Neck pain 56
- Pap smear 88
- Physical activity 73
- Suicidal ideation, suicide attempts 62
- Unmet need 79
- Vision trouble 59

Elderly population, see Older population age 65 years and over.
Emergency department visits . . . . . 82, 89, 90, 91, 92, Figure 11
Employed health service personnel 105
Employers' costs for health insurance 132
End stage renal disease facilities, Medicare certified 118
Energy and macronutrient intake . . . . . 72, Figure 12
Ethnicity, see Hispanic or Latino population.
Exercise, see Physical activity.

E—Con.

Table

Expenditures, national health (see also Consumer Price Index (CPI); Hospital care expenditures; Medicaid; Medicare; Mental health, expenditures; Nursing home expenditures; Physician services expenditures; Prescription drug expenditures; Substance abuse treatment expenditures; Veterans' medical care)
- Amount per capita . . . 120, 121, 125
- Factors affecting growth . . . 123, Figure 6
- Government . . . 121, 125
- International . . . 120
- Percent of Gross Domestic Product . . . 120, 121, Figures 7, 8
- Personal health care . . . 125, Figure 6
- Source of funds . . . 121, 125, Figure 6
- Type of expenditure . . . 124, 125, 126, 127, Figure 6
- Type of payer . . . 131

Expenses, health care . . . 128, 130

F

Fertility rates, see Births.

Fetal mortality . . . 22

Filipino population, see Asian subgroups.

Firearm-related injuries, death rates . . . 47

Food intake, see Energy and macronutrient intake.

Foreign-born population . . . Figure 2

G

Geographic region
- Access to care . . . 77, 78, 79, 81, 82, Figures 22, 23
- Alcohol . . . 68
- Back pain, low . . . 56
- Death rates . . . 33
- Dental visits . . . 94
- Emergency department visits . . . 89, 90
- Headache, severe or migraine . . . 56
- Health insurance . . . 136, 137, 138, 139
- Health status, respondent-assessed . . . 60
- Hearing trouble . . . 59
- Hospital utilization . . . 98
- Joint pain . . . 57
- Limitation of activity . . . 58
- Neck pain . . . 56
- Physical activity . . . 73
- Serious psychological distress . . . 61
- Unmet need . . . 79
- Vaccinations . . . 83, 84, 85, 86
- Vision trouble . . . 59

Gonorrhea, see Diseases, notifiable.

Gross Domestic Product (GDP) . . . 120, 121

H

Table

Haemophilus influenzae, invasive, see Diseases, notifiable.

Hawaiian population, see Native Hawaiian or Other Pacific Islander population.

Headache, severe or migraine . . . 56

Health expenditures, national, see Expenditures, national health.

Health insurance (see also Access to care; Emergency department visits; Medicaid; Medicare)
- Burden of expenditures . . . Figure 31
- Employer costs . . . 132
- Employment related . . . 137, 140
- Hospital utilization, inpatient . . . 98
- Race and Hispanic origin . . . 136, 137, 138, 139, 140
- 65 years of age and over . . . 140
- Under 65 years of age . . . 136, 137, 138, 139
- Uninsured . . . 139, 151, Figures 28, 29, 30, 32, 33, 35

Health care expenses, see Expenses, health care.

Health professionals visits, see Visits to health professionals.

Health status, respondent-assessed . . . 60

Hearing trouble . . . 59

Heart disease
- Deaths and death rates . . . 29, 31, 32, 36, Figure 20
- Drugs prescribed during medical visits . . . 95
- Hospital discharges . . . 100, 101
- Ischemic heart disease . . . 29, 30
- Procedures (angiocardiography; cardiac catheterization; coronary artery bypass graft; insertion of stent; pacemaker) . . . 102
- Serious heart conditions . . . Figure 26
- Years of potential life lost . . . 30

Hepatitis, see Diseases, notifiable; Vaccinations.

Hib (Haemophilus influenzae type b), see Vaccinations.

Hispanic or Latino population
- Abortion . . . 16
- Access to care . . . 77, 78, 79, 81, 82, Figures 26, 29, 30, 35
- AIDS cases . . . 52
- Alcohol consumption . . . 66, 68
- Back pain, low . . . 56
- Birth rates . . . 4, 6, 10
- Births, number . . . 5
- Birthweight, low . . . 13, 14, 15
- Breastfeeding . . . 18
- Cancer incidence rates . . . 53
- Cigarette smoking . . . 12, 65, 66
- Colorectal scope procedures . . . Figure 35
- Contraception . . . 17
- Death rates, all causes . . . 28, 29, 35
- Death rates, geographic division and state . . . 28
- Death rates, selected causes . . . 29, 36, 37, 38, 39, 40, 41, 42, 43, 44, 45, 46, 47

H—Con.

Table

Hispanic or Latino population—Con.
- Deaths, leading causes . . . 31
- Dental caries (cavities), untreated . . . 76
- Dental visits . . . 94, 143
- Education of mother . . . 11, 14, 20
- Emergency department visits . . . 82, 89, 90
- Expenses, health care . . . 128
- Headache, severe or migraine . . . 56
- Health insurance . . . 136, 137, 139, 140, Figures 29, 30
- Health status, respondent-assessed . . . 60
- Hearing trouble . . . 59
- Hospital utilization, inpatient . . . 98
- Illicit drug use . . . 66
- Infant mortality . . . 19, 20, 23, 24
- Inmates, prisons and jails . . . 2
- Joint pain . . . 57
- Kidney transplant . . . Figures 24, 25
- Limitation of activity . . . 58, 143
- Mammography . . . 87
- Marijuana use . . . 66
- Maternal mortality . . . 43
- Medicaid . . . 129, 138, 140, 144
- Medicare . . . 129, 140, 143
- Neck pain . . . 56
- Occupational injury deaths . . . 49
- Out-of-pocket health care expenditures . . . 128, 129
- Pap smear . . . 88
- Physical activity . . . 73
- Poverty . . . 3, Figure 5
- Population, resident . . . 1, 2, Figure 3
- Prenatal care . . . 7, 8
- Serious psychological distress . . . 61
- Smoking status of mother . . . 12
- Students, health occupations . . . 111
- Suicidal ideation, suicide attempts . . . 62
- Teenage childbearing . . . 4, 9
- Twin, triplet, and higher order multiple births . . . 5, 6
- Unmarried mothers . . . 10
- Unmet need . . . 79
- Vaccinations . . . 83, 85, 86
- Vision trouble . . . 59
- Years of potential life lost . . . 30

H—Con.

Table

Hispanic subgroups (Central and South American; Cuban; Mexican; Puerto Rican) (see also Mexican; Puerto Rican)
- Birth rates . . . 6, 10
- Births, number . . . 5
- Birthweight, low and very low . . . 13, 14
- Education of mother . . . 11, 14, 20
- Health insurance . . . 136, 137, 138, 139, Figure 29
- Infant mortality . . . 19, 20
- Prenatal care . . . 7
- Smoking status of mother . . . 12
- Teenage childbearing . . . 9
- Twin, triplet, and higher order multiple births . . . 5, 6
- Unmarried mothers . . . 10
- Unmet need . . . 79

HIV/AIDS
- AIDS cases . . . 52
- Deaths and death rates . . . 29, 31, 32, 42
- Educational attainment, death rates . . . 34
- Hospital discharges . . . 100, 101
- Years of potential life lost . . . 30

Home health agencies, Medicare certified . . . 118

Homicide, death rates . . . 29, 30, 31, 32, 45

Hospices, Medicare certified . . . 118

Hospital care expenditures (see also Consumer Price Index (CPI); Medicaid; Medicare) . . . 125, 126, 127, 133

Hospital discharges . . . 100, 101

Hospital employees . . . 105

Hospital utilization (see also Access to care; Emergency department visits; Medicaid; Medicare; Veterans' medical care)
- Admissions . . . 103
- Average length of stay . . . 98, 99, 101, 103, 148
- Days of care . . . 98, 99, 100
- Diagnoses, selected . . . 100, 101
- Discharges for inpatients . . . 98, 99, 100, 101
- Outpatient department . . . 92, 103, 143
- Procedures . . . 102
- Race and Hispanic origin . . . 98, 143

Hospitals (see also Hospital employees; Mental health; Nursing homes)
- Beds . . . 113
- Geographic division and state . . . 115, 116
- Occupancy rate . . . 113, 116

Hypertension . . . 69, 70, Figures 26, 32

I

Table

Illicit drug use 66, 67
Immunizations, see Vaccinations.
Influenza, see Vaccinations.
Incidence (Cancer) 53
Income, family, see Poverty.
Infant mortality (see also Fetal mortality)
  Age at death . . . . 19, 22, 24, Figure 19
  Birth cohort data 19, 20, 21
  Birthweight 21
  Cause of death 32
  Education of mother 20
  Geographic division and state 23, 24
  International 25
  Race and Hispanic origin 19, 20, 22, 23, 24
Influenza and pneumonia 29, 30, 31, 32
Influenza vaccination, see Vaccinations.
Inhalants 67
Injuries, see Emergency department visits; Firearm-related injuries; Hospital utilization, diagnoses, selected; Motor vehicle-related injuries; Occupational injuries; Suicide; Unintentional injuries.
Inmates, prisons and jails 2
Inpatient care, see Hospital utilization; Mental health, admissions, mental health organizations; Nursing home, utilization.
Instrumental activities of daily living (IADL), see Limitation of activity.
Insurance, see Health insurance.
International health (see also Expenditures, international; Infant mortality; Life expectancy) 25, 26, 120
Intervertebral disc disorders 100, 101, 102
Ischemic heart disease, see Heart disease.

J

Jails, see Inmates, prisons and jails.
Japanese population, see Asian subgroups.
Joint pain 57

K

Kidney transplants . . . . Figures 24, 25

L

Table

Leading causes of death, see Deaths, leading causes.
Leisure-time activity, see Physical activity.
Life expectancy . . . . 26, 27, Figure 18
Limitation of activity . . . . 58, 143, Figures 14, 15, 16
Liver disease, see Chronic liver disease and cirrhosis.
Low birthweight, see Births; Infant mortality.
Low income, see Poverty.
Lyme disease, see Diseases, notifiable.

M

Magnetic Resonance Imaging (MRI) units (see also Computed Tomography (CT) scanners 119
Malignant neoplasms, see Cancer.
Mammography 87
Marijuana use 66, 67
Maternal health, see Women's health.
Maternal mortality 43
Measles (Rubella), see Diseases, notifiable; Vaccinations.
Medicaid (see also Health insurance)
  Basis of eligibility 144
  Coverage . . . . 138, 140, Figure 28
  Expenditures . . . . 125, 131, Figures 7, 8
  Geographic region and state 149
  Race and Hispanic origin 138, 144
  Recipients and payments 129, 144, 145, 149
  Type of service 145
Medical doctors, see Physicians.
Medicare (see also Health insurance)
  Age and sex of beneficiaries 140, 142
  Certified providers and suppliers 118
  Coverage 140
  Enrollment 141, 142, 143, 148
  Expenditures . . . . 125, 141, Figures 7, 8
  Geographic region and state 148
  Hospital utilization 148
  Payments 129, 142, 148
  Race and Hispanic origin 140, 143
  Type of service 140, 141
Meningococcal disease 32, 51
Men's health
  AIDS cases 52
  Alcohol consumption 66, 67, 68
  Antidepressant drugs . . . . Figure 36
  Back pain, low 56
  Cancer incidence rates 53
  Cancer survival, 5-year relative 54

M—Con.

Table

Men's health—Con.
- Cholesterol, serum . . . 71
- Cigarette smoking . . . 63, 64, 65, 66, 67, Figure 9
- Death rates, all causes . . . 29, 35
- Death rates, educational attainment . . . 34
- Death rates, selected causes . . . 29, 36, 37, 38, 39, 40, 41, 42, 44, 45, 46, 47
- Death rates, urbanization . . . 33
- Deaths, leading causes . . . 31
- Dental caries (cavities), untreated . . . 76
- Dental visits . . . 94
- Diabetes . . . 55
- Drugs prescribed during medical visits . . . 95
- Drugs, prescription, use in past month . . . 96
- Emergency department visits . . . 82, 90, 91, 92
- Energy and macronutrient intake . . . 72
- Headache, severe or migraine . . . 56
- Health status, respondent-assessed . . . 60
- Hearing trouble . . . 59
- Hospital utilization, inpatient . . . 98, 99, 100, 101
- Hospital utilization, outpatient department . . . 92
- Hypertension . . . 70
- Illicit drug use . . . 66
- Inhalants . . . 67
- Joint pain . . . 57
- Life expectancy . . . 26, 27, Figure 18
- Limitation of activity . . . 58
- Marijuana use . . . 66, 67
- Neck pain . . . 56
- Nursing home utilization . . . 104
- Occupational injury deaths . . . 49
- Overweight and obesity . . . 74, 75
- Physical activity . . . 73
- Serious psychological distress . . . 61
- Vaccinations . . . 85, 86
- Vision trouble . . . 59
- Years of potential life lost . . . 30

Mental health (see also Suicide)
- Admissions, mental health organizations . . . 97
- Beds and organizations . . . 114
- Drugs prescribed during medical visits . . . 95
- Expenditures . . . 126, 135, 141, 147, Figure 7
- Hospital discharges . . . 100, 101
- Mental illness, serious . . . 100, 101, Figure 36
- Serious psychological distress . . . 61

M—Con.

Table

Metropolitan/nonmetropolitan data
- Access to care . . . 77, 78, 79, 81, 82
- Alcohol . . . 68
- Back pain, low . . . 56
- Death rates . . . 33
- Dental visits . . . 94
- Emergency department visits . . . 89, 90
- Headache, severe or migraine . . . 56
- Health insurance . . . 136, 137, 138, 139
- Health status, respondent-assessed . . . 60
- Hearing trouble . . . 59
- Hospital utilization . . . 98
- Joint pain . . . 57
- Limitation of activity . . . 58
- Neck pain . . . 56
- Physical activity . . . 73
- Serious psychological distress . . . 61
- Unmet need . . . 79
- Vaccinations . . . 83, 84, 86
- Vision trouble . . . 59

Mexican population (see also Hispanic subgroups)
- Antidepressant drugs . . . Figure 36
- Back pain, low . . . 56
- Cholesterol, serum . . . 71
- Cigarette smoking . . . 65
- Dental caries (cavities), untreated . . . 76
- Diabetes . . . 55
- Drugs, prescription in past month . . . 96
- Headache, severe or migraine . . . 56
- Health insurance . . . 136, 137, 138, 139
- Health status, respondent-assessed . . . 60
- Hearing trouble . . . 59
- Hypertension . . . 70
- Joint pain . . . 57
- Limitation of activity . . . 58
- Medical students . . . 111
- Neck pain . . . 56
- No usual source of care . . . 78
- Overweight and obesity . . . 74, 75
- Physical activity . . . 73
- Poverty . . . 3
- Serious psychological distress . . . 61
- Vaccinations . . . 85, 86
- Vision trouble . . . 59

MMR (Measles, Mumps, Rubella), see Vaccinations.

Motor vehicle-related injuries . . . 29, 30, 44, 91

Mumps, see Diseases, notifiable; Vaccinations.

N

Table

National health expenditures, see Expenditures, national health.
Native Hawaiian or Other Pacific Islander population
- Occupational injuries 49
- Vaccinations 83

Neonatal mortality, see Infant mortality, age at death.
Nephritis, nephrotic syndrome, and nephrosis 31, 32
Neck pain 56
Nurses 110, 111, 112
Nursing homes
- Beds, occupancy 117
- Employees 105
- Expenditures 125, 134, 143
- Utilization 104, 117, 143, 146

Nutrition, see Energy and macronutrient intake.

O

Obesity . . . . . 69, 74, Figure 13
Occupational diseases deaths 48
Occupational injuries 49, 50
Occupational therapists 110
Office visit 92, 93
Older population age 65 years and over
- AIDS cases 52
- Alcohol consumption 68
- Back pain, low 56
- Bed, health facility 117
- Cholesterol, serum 71
- Cigarette smoking 63, 65
- Colorectal scope procedures . . . . . Figure 35
- Death rates, all causes 35
- Death rates, selected causes 36, 37, 38, 39, 40, 41, 42, 44, 45, 46, 47
- Deaths, leading causes 32
- Delayed medical care . . . . . Figure 27
- Dental caries (cavities), untreated 69, 76
- Dental visits . . . . . 94, 143, Figures 21, 34
- Drugs prescribed during medical visits 95
- Drugs, prescription, use in past month 96
- Emergency department visits 82, 90, 91, 92
- Expenses, health care 128, 130
- Headache, severe or migraine 56
- Hearing trouble 59
- Health insurance . . . . . 140, Figure 35
- Health status, respondent-assessed 60
- Hospital utilization, inpatient 98, 99, 100, 101, 102, 143, 148
- Hospital utilization, outpatient department 92, 143
- Hypertension 70
- Injury 91

O—Con.

Table

Older population age 65 years and over—Con.
- Joint pain 57
- Life expectancy at age 65, age 75 . . . . . 26, 27, Figure 18
- Limitation of activity . . . . . 58, Figure 16
- Mammography 87
- Medicaid 129, 140, 144
- Medicare . . . . . 129, 140, 141, 142, 143, 148, Figure 21
- Neck pain 56
- Nursing home expenditures 134, 143
- Nursing home utilization 104, 117, 134, 143
- Nursing homes 117
- Occupational injury deaths 49
- Out-of-pocket health care expenses 128, 129, 130
- Overweight and obesity . . . . . 74, Figure 13
- Pap smear 88
- Physical activity 73
- Population, resident . . . . . 1, Figure 1
- Poverty status . . . . . Figures 4, 5, 17, 27
- Restaurant meal consumption . . . . . Figure 12
- Serious psychological distress 61
- Unmet need 79
- Vaccinations 83, 85, 86
- Vision trouble . . . . . 59, Figure 21

Optometrists 110, 111, 112
Osteoarthritis 100, 101
Osteopaths, see Physicians
Out-of-pocket health care expenses . . . . . 128, 129, 130, 131, Figures 7, 8
Outpatient department, see Hospital utilization, outpatient department.
Overweight . . . . . 69, 74, 75, Figure 13

P

Pacemakers 102
Pap smear 88
Perinatal mortality, see Infant mortality, age at death.
Personal health care expenditures, see Expenditures, national health.
Pertussis (whooping cough), see Diseases, notifiable; Vaccinations.
Pharmacists 109, 110, 111, 112
Physical activity 73
Physician services expenditures (see also Consumer Price Index (CPI); Medicaid; Medicare) 125, 126, 127
Physician utilization 92, 93
Physicians
- Doctors of osteopathy 110, 111, 112
- Employees, in offices of 105
- Geographic division and state 106
- International medical school graduates 107

P—Con.

Table

Physicians—Con.
- Physician supply .... Figures 22, 23
- Primary care 93, 108
- Primary specialty 93, 107, 108
- Schools and students 110, 111, 112

Pneumococcal vaccinations, see Vaccinations.
Pneumonia (see also Influenza and pneumonia) 100, 101
Podiatrists 110, 111, 112
Poliomyelitis (Polio), see Diseases, notifiable; Vaccinations.
Population, resident .... 1, Figures 1, 3
Postneonatal mortality, see Infant mortality, age at death.
Poverty
- Access to care 77, 78, 81
- Back pain, low 56
- Blood cotinine .... Figure 10
- Chronic conditions .... Figure 17
- Colorectal scope procedures .... Figure 35
- Dental caries (cavities), untreated 76
- Dental visits .... 94, Figure 34
- Emergency department visits 89, 90
- Headache, severe or migraine 56
- Health care visits 82
- Health insurance .... 136, 137, 138, 139, 140, Figures 29, 30
- Health status, respondent-assessed 60
- Hearing trouble 59
- Hospital utilization, inpatient 98
- Joint pain 57
- Limitation of activity 58
- Mammography 87
- Medicaid 138, 140
- Neck pain 56
- Pap smear 88
- Physical activity 73
- Serious psychological distress 61
- Unmet need 79
- Vaccinations 83, 85, 86
- Vision trouble 59

Prenatal care 7, 8
Prescription drug expenditures (see also Consumer Price Index (CPI); Medicaid; Medicare) 125, 126, 127, 128
Prescription drug use, see Drugs, prescription, use in past month.
Primary care physicians, see Physicians.
Prisons, see Inmates, prisons and jails.
Private health insurance, see Health insurance.
Procedures 102
Public Health, schools of, students 110

P—Con.

Table

Puerto Rican population (see also Hispanic subgroups)
- Health insurance 136, 137, 138, 139
- Medical students 111
- Poverty 3

R

Race, see specific race groups.
Restaurant meal consumption .... Figure 12
Rocky Mountain spotted fever, see Diseases, notifiable.
Rubella (German measles), see Diseases, notifiable; Vaccinations.
Rural data, see Metropolitan/nonmetropolitan data.

S

Salmonellosis, see Diseases, notifiable.
Self-assessment of health, see Health status, respondent-assessed.
Septicemia 31, 32
Serious psychological distress, (see also Mental health) 61
Shigellosis, see Diseases, notifiable.
Smoking, see Cigarette smoking.
Socioeconomic status, see Education; Poverty.
Source of funds or payments (see also Expenditures, national health; Health insurance; Medicaid; Medicare) ...... 125, 129, 131, 134, Figures 6, 7, 8
State data
- Access to care 80
- Bed, health facility 117
- Birthweight, low 15
- Death rates 28
- Expenditures, state mental health agency 147
- Hospital beds 115
- Hospital occupancy rates 116
- Infant mortality 23, 24
- Medicaid 149
- Medicare 148
- Nursing homes, beds, occupancy, residents 117
- Physicians 106
- Prenatal care 8
- Uninsured, health 151
- Vaccinations 84

Stent, cardiac, see Heart disease, procedures.
Sterilization, see Contraception.
Stroke, see Cerebrovascular disease.
Substance abuse treatment expenditures .... 127, Figure 8
Sudden infant death syndrome, see Infant mortality, cause of death.

S—Con.

Table

Suicidal ideation, suicide attempts 62
Suicide 29, 30, 31, 32, 46
Surgery, see Hospital utilization.
Syphilis, see Diseases, notifiable.

T

Tetanus, see Diseases, notifiable; Vaccinations.
Tobacco use, see Cigarette smoking.
Transportation . . . . Figure 27
Tuberculosis, see Diseases, notifiable.
Twin, triplet, and higher order multiple births 5, 6

U

Undiagnosed medical conditions . . . . Figure 32
Uninsured, health, see Health insurance, uninsured.
Unintentional injuries . . . . 29, 30, 31, 32, Figure 20
Unmet need 80
Urban and rural data, see Metropolitan/nonmetropolitan data.
Usual source of care, see Access to care.

V

Vaccinations 83, 84, 85, 86
Varicella, see Vaccinations.
Veterans' medical care 146
Vision trouble . . . . 59, Figure 21
Visits to health professionals 82

W

Wages and salaries 132
Wages, healthcare occupations 109
Women's health
- Abortion 16
- Access to care 78, 82
- AIDS cases 52
- Alcohol consumption 66, 67, 68
- Antidepressant drugs . . . . Figure 36
- Back pain, low 56
- Birth rates, fertility rates 4, 10
- Births, number 5, 10
- Breast cancer 40, 53, 54, 100, 101
- Cancer incidence rates 53
- Cancer survival, 5-year relative 54
- Cesarean section 102
- Cholesterol, serum 71
- Cigarette smoking . . . . 12, 13, 63, 64, 65, 66, 67, Figure 9
- Contraception 17

W—Con.

Table

Women's health—Con.
- Death rates, all causes 29, 35
- Death rates, educational attainment 34
- Death rates, selected causes 29, 36, 37, 38, 39, 40, 41, 42, 43, 44, 45, 46, 47
- Death rates, urbanization 33
- Deaths, leading causes 31
- Dental caries (cavities), untreated 76
- Dental visits 94
- Diabetes 55
- Drugs prescribed during medical visits 95
- Drugs, prescription, use in past month 96
- Emergency department visits 82, 90, 91, 92
- Energy and macronutrient intake 72
- Headache, severe or migraine 56
- Health status, respondent-assessed 60
- Hearing trouble 59
- Hospital utilization, inpatient 98, 99, 100, 101
- Hospital utilization, outpatient department 92
- Hypertension 70
- Illicit drug use 66
- Inhalants 67
- Joint pain 57
- Life expectancy . . . . 26, 27, Figure 18
- Limitation of activity 58
- Mammography 87
- Marijuana use 66, 67
- Maternal mortality 43
- Neck pain 56
- Nursing home utilization 104
- Occupational injury deaths 49
- Overweight and obesity 74, 75
- Pap smear 88
- Physical activity 73
- Poverty 3
- Prenatal care 7, 8
- Serious psychological distress 61
- Teenage childbearing 4, 9
- Unmarried mothers 10
- Vaccinations 85, 86
- Vision trouble 59
- Years of potential life lost 30

Y

Years of potential life lost (YPLL) 30